P9-CKX-719

Handbuch der experimentellen Pharmakologie

Vol. 49 Heffter-Heubner New Series

Handbook of Experimental Pharmacology

Ergot Alkaloids and Related Compounds

Contributors

W. H. Aellig · B. Berde · Th. Bucher · D. Chu · B. J. Clark
E. B. van Deusen · H. Eckert · A. Fanchamps · E. Flückiger
J. Grauwiler · R. W. Griffith · D. Hauser · Ch. Hodel
J. R. Kiechel · K. H. Leist · D. M. Loew · B. Matter
W. Meier-Ruge · E. Müller-Schweinitzer · T. J. Petcher
E. del Pozo · B. P. Richardson · J. Rosenthaler · J. Rutschmann
K. Saameli · R. Salzmann · H. O. Schild · R. Schmidt
E. Schreier · P. A. Stadler · E. Stürmer · R. D. Venn · H. Wagner
H. P. Weber · H. Weidmann

Editors

B. Berde and H.O. Schild

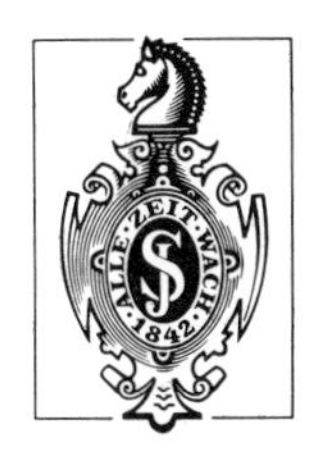

Springer-Verlag Berlin Heidelberg New York 1978

B. Berde, Forschung und Entwicklung, Pharmazeutisches Departement,
Sandoz AG, 4002 Basel, Schweiz

H.O. Schild, Emeritus Professor of Pharmacology in the University of London,
University College London, London WC1, Great Britain

With 159 Figures

ISBN 3-540-08475-4 Springer-Verlag Berlin Heidelberg New York
ISBN 0-387-08475-4 Springer-Verlag New York Heidelberg Berlin

Library of Congress Cataloging in Publication Data. Main entry under title: Ergot alkaloids and related compounds. (Handbook of experimental pharmacology: New series; v. 49) Bibliography: p. . Includes index. 1. Ergot. 2. Alkaloids. I. Aellig, W.H. II. Berde, Botond, 1919– . III. Schild, Heinz Otto. IV. Series: Handbuch der experimentellen Pharmakologie: New series; v. 49. QP905.H3 vol. 49 [RM666.E8] 615'.1'08s [615'.7] 77-14126

Type setting, printing, and binding: Universitätsdruckerei H. Stürtz, Würzburg

2122-3130/543210

Preface

> Une découverte scientifique... n'est jamais l'œuvre d'un seul homme et chacun de ceux qui y ont concouru lui ont donné bien des veilles.
>
> Louis Pasteur

Traditionally every volume of the Handbook of Experimental Pharmacology is expected to give a comprehensive account of the topic it is devoted to. This is a relatively easy task if the subject has a short history, but if the problems in question have been worked on for half a century or longer the feasibility of integral coverage becomes questionable. In such cases more attention is usually given to the literature of the last decades, whereas older findings are dealt with in a summary fashion—with due exception to findings which can be considered classic. The situation is particularly complex if the origin of the subject is a natural drug whose actions—proven or alleged—were first recorded several centuries ago and where medical use can be traced back at least one and a half centuries (STEARNS, 1808)—as is the case of ergot of rye.

As editors of the present volume of this Handbook, we did not have to face the full impact of these difficulties as two previous volumes have already been devoted to the pharmacologic actions of substances extracted from ergot of rye. The first of these, written by Arthur Cushny in 1914, was published in 1924 [A.R. CUSHNY: Mutterkorn. Handb. exper. Pharmakol. II, 2, 1297–1354 (1924)]. The second, by George Barger, appeared in 1938 [G. BARGER: The Alkaloids of Ergot. Handb. exper. Pharmakol. (Erg.-Werk) VI, 84–226 (1938)]. Nevertheless, the present volume had to bridge a gap of nearly four decades during which time tremendous developments have taken place in this field. Besides reviewing this progress, we have attempted a synopsis of the whole field in which recent work is of course treated preferentially, but without neglecting the older literature whenever this was necessary for the understanding of the present state of knowledge. Only data obtained with chemically defined compounds, namely chemical entities containing the tetracyclic ergolene- or ergoline-ring system, were considered.

A history of ergot with its colorful medieval aspects—mainly the history of ergot intoxication due to the agricultural standards of the time—has been excluded from this volume. This subject is dealt with in considerable detail in a number of treatises such as DE JUSSIEU et al., 1779; FALCK, 1855; KOBERT, 1889; HUSEMANN, 1903; BARGER, 1931; STOLL, 1943; GUGGISBERG, 1954; HOFMANN, 1964; LEDERER, 1961; BOVE, 1970; BAUER, 1973, and there is not much to be added to the story.

An important question was, of course, where the limits of "pharmacology" were to be drawn in this volume. That human pharmacology or clinical pharmacology had to be included seemed self-evident, the aim of the development of agents with therapeutic usefulness being ultimately directed for usage in man. Admittedly, it is not always easy to draw the line between clinical pharmacology and therapeutics, the latter being outside the scope of this volume. We aimed at a rather restrictive definition of clinical pharmacology, and pharmacologic findings in man were in principle incorporated in individual chapters in relation to specific groups of problems such as circulation and nervous system. Only in two instances (Chapters VII and VIII) have chapters exclusively devoted to human pharmacologic aspects been included, due to the complexity of the topics in question.

According to tradition, but also of necessity, a chapter dealing with chemical aspects (Chapter II) is included. Its aim is to give an overview of the complex chemistry of ergot alkaloids. It is deliberately entitled "chemical background," but is addressed particularly to pharmacologists, biologists, and doctors, rather than to chemists.

Pharmacokinetics and data concerning drug metabolism are dealt with in a separate chapter (Chapter XI). This aspect is of evident importance although as in most other well-studied fields of pharmacology, much more is known of what the compounds do to the living body than what the living body does to the active compounds.

We believe that the description of a group of biologically active substances is incomplete without their toxicologic characterization. The chapter in question (Chapter XII), however, makes no attempt at completeness. It should rather serve to give the reader some degree of general orientation.

The bulk of the book is devoted to traditional pharmacology. It includes an introductory section placing the therapeutically important ergot alkaloids in perspective (Chapter I) and a series of main sections dealing with fundamental receptor considerations (Chapter III) and various body systems on which ergot alkaloids exert their effects.

The Subject Index was prepared by Dr. U. BRÜCKNER. We wish to thank him for making this important contribution. Our gratitude is also expressed to Mr. E. ERFLING for compiling the Author Index.

Basel and London, May 1977

B. BERDE and H.O. SCHILD

References

Barger, G.: Ergot and Ergotism. Edinburgh: Gurney & Jackson 1931
Barger, G.: The alkaloids of ergot. Handb. exper. Pharmakol. (Erg.-Werk) **6**, 84–226 (1938)
Bauer, V.H.: Das Antonius-Feuer in Kunst und Medizin. In: Sitzungsberichte der Heidelberger Akademie der Wissenschaften. Mathematisch-Naturwissenschaftliche Klasse. Suppl. Jahrgang 1973. Berlin-Heidelberg-New York: Springer 1973
Bové, F.J.: The Story of Ergot. Basel-New York: Karger 1970
Cushny, A.R.: Mutterkorn. Handb. exper. Pharmakol. II/2, 1297–1354 (1924)
De Jussieu, A.-L., Paulet, Saillant, Tessier, H.A.: Recherches sur le feu Saint-Antoine. Histoire de la Société Royale de Médicine. Année 1776, pp. 260–302. Paris: Pierres 1779
Hofmann, A.: Die Mutterkorn-Alkaloide. Stuttgart: Enke 1964
Falck, C.Ph.: Vergiftungen durch Mutterkorn. In: Handb. der speziellen Pathologie und Therapie, Vol. II, Part 1, pp. 311–327. Erlangen: Enke 1855
Guggisberg, H.: Mutterkorn. Vom Gift zum Heilstoff. Basel-New York: Karger 1954
Husemann, T.: Ergotismus. In: Handb. der Geschichte der Medizin. Neuburger, M., Pagel, J. (eds.), Vol. II, pp. 916–926. Jena: G. Fischer 1903

Kobert, R.: Zur Geschichte des Mutterkorns. In: Historische Studien aus dem Pharmakologischen Institute der Kaiserlichen Universität Dorpat, Vol. I, pp. 1–47. Halle a.S.: von Tausch & Grosse 1889

Lederer, J.: Les mendiants de Bruegel, un document pour l'histoire des Flandres sous l'occupation espagnole. Scrinium Lovaniense Mélanges historiques Etienne van Cauwenbergh. Louvain 1961, pp. 452–465 (Univ. de Louvain, Recueil de travaux d'histoire et de philol. 4e série, fasc. 24)

Stearns, J.: Account of the pulvis parturiens, a remedy for quickening child-birth. Med. Repository N.Y. **5**, 308 (1808)

Stoll, A.: Altes und Neues über Mutterkorn. Mitteilungen der Naturforschenden Gesellschaft Bern aus dem Jahre 1942, pp. 45–80. Bern: P. Haupt 1943

Contents

CHAPTER III

Basic Pharmacological Properties. E. MÜLLER-SCHWEINITZER and H. WEIDMANN. With Contributions by R. SALZMANN, D. HAUSER, H.P. WEBER, T.J. PETCHER, and TH. BUCHER. With 42 Figures

CHAPTER VI

CHAPTER VII

Clinical Pharmacology of Ergot Alkaloids in Senile Cerebral Insufficiency. R.D. VENN. With 7 Figures

CHAPTER VIII

Some Compounds With Hallucinogenic Activity. A. FANCHAMPS. With 3 Figures

CHAPTER XI

Biopharmaceutical Aspects. Analytical Methods, Pharmacokinetics, Metabolism and Bioavailability. H. ECKERT, J.R. KIECHEL, J. ROSENTHALER, R. SCHMIDT, and E. SCHREIER. With 7 Figures

CHAPTER XII

Toxicologic Considerations. R.W. GRIFFITH, J. GRAUWILER, CH. HODEL, K.H. LEIST, and B. MATTER

List of Contributors

W.H. Aellig, Experimentelle Therapie, Medizinisch-Biologische Forschung, Sandoz A.G., 4002 Basel, Schweiz.

B. Berde, Forschung und Entwicklung Pharma, Sandoz A.G., 4002 Basel, Schweiz.

Th. Bucher. Pharmakologie, Medizinisch-Biologische Forschung, Sandoz A.G., 4002 Basel, Schweiz.

D. Chu, Pharmakologie, Medizinisch-Biologische Forschung, Sandoz A.G., 4002 Basel, Schweiz.

B.J. Clark, Pharmakologie. Medizinisch-Biologische Forschung, Sandoz A.G., 4002 Basel, Schweiz.

E.B. van Deusen, Pharmakologie, Medizinisch-Biologische Forschung, Sandoz A.G., 4002 Basel, Schweiz.

H. Eckert, Biopharmazeutik, Pharmazeutische Entwicklung, Sandoz A.G., 4002 Basel, Schweiz.

A. Fanchamps, Medizinische Beratung Pharma-Forschung, Sandoz A.G., 4002 Basel, Schweiz.

E. Flückiger, Pharmakologie, Medizinisch-Biologische Forschung, Sandoz A.G., 4002 Basel, Schweiz.

J. Grauwiler, Toxikologie, Medizinisch-Biologische Forschung, Sandoz A.G., 4002 Basel, Schweiz.

R.W. Griffith, Klinische Forschung, Medizinisch-Biologische Forschung, Sandoz A.G., 4002 Basel, Schweiz.

D. Hauser, Biochemie, Pharmazeutisch-Chemische Forschung, Sandoz A.G., 4002 Basel, Schweiz.

Ch. Hodel, Toxikologie, Medizinisch-Biologische Forschung, Sandoz A.G., 4002 Basel, Schweiz.

J.R. Kiechel, Biopharmazeutik, Pharmazeutische Entwicklung, Sandoz A.G., 4002 Basel, Schweiz.

K.H. Leist, Toxikologie, Medizinisch-Biologische Forschung, Sandoz A.G., 4002 Basel, Schweiz.

D.M. Loew, Pharmakologie, Medizinisch-Biologische Forschung, Sandoz A.G., 4002 Basel, Schweiz.

B. Matter, Toxikologie, Medizinisch-Biologische Forschung, Sandoz A.G., 4002 Basel, Schweiz.

W. Meier-Ruge, Medizinische Grundlagenforschung, Sandoz A.G., 4002 Basel, Schweiz.

E. Müller-Schweinitzer, Pharmakologie, Medizinisch-Biologische Forschung, Sandoz A.G., 4002 Basel, Schweiz.

T.J. Petcher, Physikalische Chemie, Pharmazeutisch-Chemische Forschung, Sandoz A.G., 4002 Basel, Schweiz.

E. del Pozo, Experimentelle Therapie, Medizinisch-Biologische Forschung, Sandoz A.G., 4002 Basel, Schweiz.

B.P. Richardson, Toxikologie, Medizinisch-Biologische Forschung, Sandoz A.G., 4002 Basel, Schweiz.

J. Rosenthaler, Biopharmazeutik, Pharmazeutische Entwicklung, Sandoz A.G., 4002 Basel, Schweiz.

J. Rutschmann, Pharmazeutisch-Chemische Forschung, Sandoz A.G., 4002 Basel, Schweiz.

K. Saameli, Medizinisch-Biologische Forschung, Sandoz A.G., 4002 Basel, Schweiz.

R. Salzmann, Pharmakologie, Medizinisch-Biologische Forschung, Sandoz A.G., 4002 Basel, Schweiz.

H.O. Schild, Department of Pharmacology, University College London, London WC1, Great Britain.

R. Schmidt, Experimentelle Therapie, Medizinisch-Biologische Forschung, Sandoz A.G., 4002 Basel, Schweiz.

E. Schreier, Biopharmazeutik, Pharmazeutische Entwicklung, Sandoz A.G., 4002 Basel, Schweiz.

P.A. Stadler, Pharmazeutisch-Chemische Forschung, Sandoz A.G., 4002 Basel, Schweiz.

E. Stürmer, Pharmakologie, Medizinisch-Biologische Forschung, Sandoz A.G., 4002 Basel, Schweiz.

R.D. Venn, Medical Research, Pharmaceutical Research & Development, Sandoz Inc., East Hanover, N.J. 07936, USA.

H. Wagner, Pharmakologie, Medizinisch-Biologische Forschung, Sandoz A.G., 4002 Basel, Schweiz.

H.P. Weber, Physikalische Chemie, Pharmazeutisch-Chemische Forschung, Sandoz A.G., 4002 Basel, Schweiz.

H. Weidmann, Präklinische Forschung, Medizinisch-Biologische Forschung, Sandoz A.G., 4002 Basel, Schweiz.

CHAPTER I

Introduction to the Pharmacology of Ergot Alkaloids and Related Compounds as a Basis of Their Therapeutic Application

B. BERDE and E. STÜRMER

"Truth is rarely pure and never simple"
OSCAR WILDE

This chapter, rather unorthodox for a volume of the Handbook of Experimental Pharmacology, is not intended as a summary of the wealth of information accumulated in this book. It is an attempt at a compact synopsis to help those teaching pharmacology or writing a textbook of pharmacology not to overlook the essential chemical and biological basis of the therapeutically most important compounds and those of their activities which are believed to be relevant for their therapeutic effects.

The present volume, entitled *Ergot Alkaloids and Related Compounds,* deals with *chemical entities containing the tetracyclic ergolene- or ergoline-ring system.* They can be obtained by extraction of different strains of the fungus claviceps—grown on rye or cultivated in fermentation tanks—or alternatively by partial or total synthesis. These compounds can be divided into four main structural groups: clavine alkaloids, lysergic acids, simple lysergic acid-amides, and peptide alkaloids. One example of each type of molecule is given in Figure 1.

The degree of oxidation is a criterion for further differentiation in the group of clavine alkaloids, all of which are compounds of minor biological importance.

The naturally occurring lysergic acids are divided into compounds with a double bond in the 8–9 position (8-ergolenes) and in the 9–10 position (9-ergolenes). All congeners are methylated in position 6. The two asymmetric carbon atoms in position 5 and 10 (in the case of 8-ergolenes) or 5 and 8 (in the case of

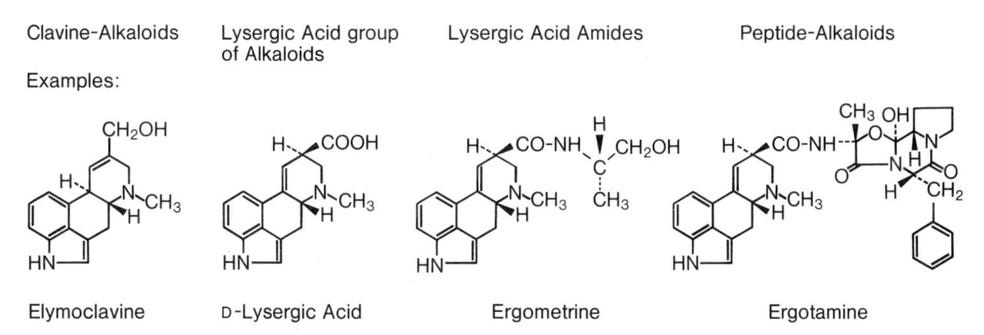

Fig. 1. One characteristic representative of each of the four main groups of ergot alkaloids

9-ergolenes) allow a further classification according to the steric position of the substituents in positions 8 or 10. (The 5-H atom always has the β-configuration.) Lysergic acid is inactive; only its derivatives are pharmacologically active.

In the group of the lysergic acid-amides the lysergic acid is in amide linkage to relatively small nonpeptide moieties.

For the group of peptide alkaloids, a relatively simple nomenclature has been adopted in this volume. The expression ergopeptine stands for the basic skeleton of a natural D-lysergic acid linked to a tricyclic peptide moiety by a peptide bond (see Fig. 2).

Only isomers that are derivatives of the natural D-lysergic acid have pharmacologic importance; derivatives of D-isolysergic acid are much less active. For convenience, the isomers of D-lysergic acid have been given endings in "-ine," while D-isolysergic acid isomers end in "-inine." Isomerization occurs during storage of the sclerotia and extraction of alkaloids and at a high rate in an alkaline milieu.

It is known that the biological activity of the ergopeptines depends largely on their configuration. This results from studies with the optical antipodes of ergotamine and dihydroergotamine and the corresponding diastereomers (natural D-lysergic acid combined with the antipode peptide moiety and antipode L-lysergic acid combined with the natural peptide moiety) which have been shown to be devoid of biological activity (STADLER and STÜRMER, 1970, 1972).

The chemical diversity of ergot alkaloids corresponds to the *diversity of the biological activities of these compounds.* It is probably correct to state that there are few chemical groups which comprise substances with such diversified actions. It has been accurately said that "ergot has been of the nature of a treasure chest to pharmacologists," (MOIR, 1932) and that it has become a "treasure-house for drugs" (STOLL, 1965). Many ergot compounds show a considerable spectrum of pharmacologic actions, and if the doses necessary to obtain a certain effect are taken into account, exhibit a high degree of specificity (selectivity). In Table 1 an attempt is made to demonstrate this, correlating ten biological activities and seven compounds. These figures are extracted from the pool of experimental data accumulated in our laboratories during the last decades. The figures should be regarded as working averages, as they were not always obtained synchronously, and they apply of course to particular species and methodologies. On the other hand, the methodologies employed in each case are uniform, and the data of Table 1 therefore provide a good idea of the range of variation encountered.

With regard to α-adrenoreceptor blocking activity on the isolated guinea pig seminal vesicle, dihydroergotoxine mesylate (Hydergine) is the most active compound, the ED_{50} being 0.7 ng/ml. The activity of dihydroergotamine and bromocriptine is lower but in the same range; that of ergotamine is 20 times weaker. At the other end of the scale are methylergometrine and methysergide, which are inactive or at least 2500 times less active than dihydroergotoxine mesylate.

The most potent antagonist of serotonin (5-HT) on the estrous rat uterus in vitro is methysergide—the ED_{50} being 0.6 ng/ml—followed by methylergometrine and LSD. Considerably less active than methysergide are dihydroergotamine (25 times), ergotamine and dihydroergotoxine mesylate (100 times), and bromocriptine (~300 times).

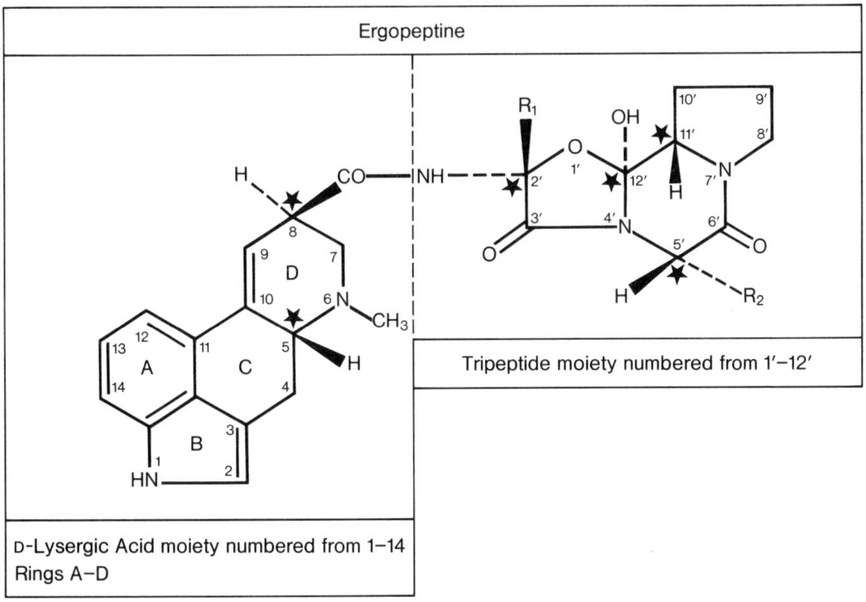

Ergopeptine

D-Lysergic Acid moiety numbered from 1–14
Rings A–D

Tripeptide moiety numbered from 1′–12′

Substitutions possible in positions: 1, 2, 6, 9, 10 (Dihydro-compounds), 10, 12, 13, 14.
✶ asymmetric centers: 6; in case of 9, 10 dihydrogenation: 7
(carbon atom 10 additionally).

2′ β R_1 / 5′ α R_2	CH_3	CH_2-CH_3	$CH(CH_3)_2$
$CH(CH_3)_2$	Ergovaline	Ergonine	Ergocornine
CH_2-$CH(CH_3)_2$	Ergosine	Ergoptine	Ergokryptine
$CH(CH_3)$-CH_2-CH_3	β-Ergosine	β-Ergoptine	β-Ergokryptine
CH_2-C_6H_5 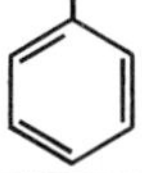	Ergotamine	Ergostine	Ergocristine

Trivial names if coined are used in this volume.
Otherwise the ergopeptine nomenclature is used. In this terms
Ergotamine is 2′β-Methyl-5′α-benzyl-ergopeptine
Ergocornine is 2′β-5′α-Diisopropyl-ergopeptine

Fig. 2. The ergopeptines consist of a D-lysergic-acid moiety linked to a tricyclic peptide moiety by a peptide bond. Ergopeptines occurring in nature have a double bond in position 9,10. Dihydro-compounds are hydrogenated in positions 9 and 10. They do not occur in nature. Six asymmetry centers marked with * are present in natural—so called genuine—ergopeptines. Dihydrogenation in position 9,10 generates an additional asymmetry center in position 10

Table 1. Activity profiles of some ergot compounds. The relative activities of seven compounds on 10 biological parameters are listed. The potency of the most active compound in each test being arbitrarily set as 1000. These figures are extracted from the pool of experimental data accumulated in our laboratories during the last decades. A ratio between the highest and the lowest activity in each test is also given. For numerical data concerning effective doses—or concentrations—see text

Parameter \ Substance	Ergotamine	Bromocriptine	Dihydroergotamine	Dihydroergotoxine mesylate[a]	Methylergometrine	Methysergide	LSD	Max./Min.
α-Adrenoceptor blockade isol. guinea pig seminal vessel	50	230	350	1000	<0.4	<0.4	1	>2500
5HT-receptor blockade isol. rat uterus	10	3	40	10	250	1000	250	330
Pressor activity spinal cat, i.v.	1000	<10	120	30	<10	30	10	>100
Uterotonic activity rabbit in situ, i.v.	500	Inhibition of Me-ergometrine	Inhibition of Me-ergometrine	Inhibition of Me-ergometrine	1000	40	670	>1000
Inhibition of fertility in rats, s.c.	50	1000	<40	70	<80	<40	<40	>25
Influence on body temperature, rabbit, i.v.	+ 3	+ 2.5	−	−	+ 14	+ 0.2	+ 1000	>5000
Emetic activity in the dog, i.v.	1000	410	85	540	210	<1	<3	>1000
Dopaminergic stereotyped behaviour in rats, i.p.	<1	630	<1	<1	310	<1	1000	>1000
Contralateral turning behaviour in rats, 6-OHDA leasioned, s.c.	<1	1000	<1	10	400	<1	730	>1000
Inhibition of NA-stimulated cAMP-synthesis in rat cerebral cortex slices in vitro	400	190	240	1000	2.5	5	60	400

[a] Hydergine.

Considering the blood pressure increasing activity on the spinal cat, ergotamine is the most active compound, eliciting clear-cut rises of blood pressure from doses of 1 μg/kg i.v. Taking its activity as 1000, that of dihydroergotamine is 120, and that of the other substances ranges between 30 and 10 or less.

If the uterotonic activity in situ—anesthetized nonpregnant rabbit in spontaneous estrous—of methylergometrine (effective submaximal doses in the range of 0.1–0.2 mg/kg i.v.) is taken as 1000, that of LSD is 670, that of ergotamine 500, and that of methysergide around 40 (and not easily reproducible), whereas bromocriptine, dihydroergotamine, and dihydroergotoxine mesylate are devoid of this activity and inhibit spontaneous uterine motility and the uterotonic effect of methylergometrine.

Bromocriptine is the only compound in this table which, due to a long-lasting inhibition of prolactin secretion, has an outstanding antifertility effect in the rat when given on day 5 after insemination ($ED_{50}=0.75$ mg/kg s.c.). Other compounds listed are either more than 10 times less effective or are ineffective in this test.

If the influence on the body temperature of the nonanesthetized rabbit is considered, the seven compounds—given i.v.—show not only quantitative but also qualitative differences: LSD is the most potent inducer of hyperthermia (3 μg/kg eliciting on the average a rise of 1° C), methylergometrine, ergotamine, bromocriptine, and methysergide being 70–5000 times less potent. Dihydroergotamine and dihydroergotoxine mesylate—in rather high doses such as 2–3 mg/kg—lower body temperature.

Emetic activity in the nonanesthetized dog is most pronounced with ergotamine ($ED_{50}=3.1$ μg/kg i.v.), dihydroergotoxine mesylate and bromocriptine being somewhat less active. Methylergometrine is 5 times and dihydroergotamine 12 times less active than ergotamine; LSD and methysergide are devoid of this activity even if administered in doses 300 to 1000 times higher than ergotamine.

In eliciting stereotyped behavior in the rat—probably due to central dopaminergic stimulation—LSD is the most active compound (2 mg/kg i.p. being an effective dose). If its activity is taken as 1000, that of bromocriptine is 630 and that of methylergometrine 310, whereas ergotamine, dihydroergotamine, dihydroergotoxine mesylate, and methysergide are for all practical purposes ineffective.

Another test for central dopaminergic action is the (apomorphine type) contralateral turning behavior of rats with 6-OH-dopamine-induced degeneration of the nigro-neostriatal dopaminergic pathway. The most potent compound in this test is bromocriptine (effective dose 1 mg/kg s.c.). If this activity is taken as 1000, those of LSD and methylergometrine are 730 and 400, respectively. Dihydroergotoxine mesylate is about 100 times less effective. Ergotamine, dihydroergotamine, and methysergide are ineffective.

Noradrenaline-stimulated cyclic AMP synthesis in the rat cerebral cortex in vitro is inhibited by some ergot compounds, the most active being dihydroergotoxine mesylate (ED_{50} 5.8 ng/ml), pA_2 value ~ 8.0). If this activity is taken as 1000, that of ergotamine is 400, of dihydroergotamine 240, of bromocriptine 190, of LSD 60, and those of methysergide and methylergometrine 5 and 2.5, respectively.

In the last column of Table 1, a ratio is given between the highest and lowest activity for each listed pharmacologic activity. These ratios range between >25 and >5000. Considering the whole pharmacologic profile of the substances, qualita-

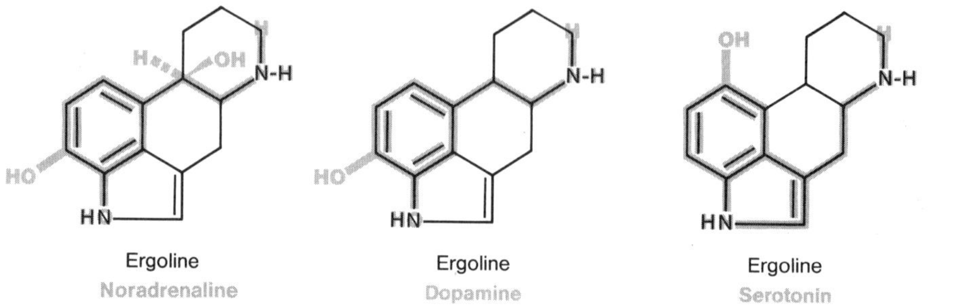

Fig. 3. Structural relationship between ergoline and three biogenic amines: noradrenaline, dopamine, and serotonin

tive rather than quantitative differences would appear to be more appropriate in distinguishing between at least some of the compounds.

There is indeed no evidence available which would suggest that these highly diversified activities could be explained by one "basic mechanism" on cellular or molecular level. The opposite seems to be more likely, and in a recent review (BRADLEY and BRIGGS, 1974) it was pointed out that "it is unlikely that a unified explanation of all the actions of these drugs can be formulated." Nevertheless, *this diversity of actions may be at least partially explained* by assuming that:

1. Ergot alkaloids interfere at more than one type of specific receptor site.
2. The population of receptor sites to which ergot alkaloids have access varies from organ to organ.
3. Affinity and efficacy (=intrinsic activity) vary from alkaloid to alkaloid as a function of their chemical configuration.

A specific relationship between ergoline—a vital part of all ergot alkaloids—and the biogenic amines noradrenaline, adrenaline, dopamine, and serotonin is evident from Figure 3. All the biogenic amines mentioned can be regarded as structural elements of ergoline. This structural relationship may contribute to the ability of different ergot alkaloids to interfere with various specific receptors. On the other hand, the structural differences between the ergot alkaloids and the biogenic amines can explain why some of the former act as partial agonists and/or antagonists on receptor sites of the biogenic amines mentioned.

An example for an ergot alkaloid eliciting partial agonism is given in Figure 4. This figure shows dose-response curves for noradrenaline, the so-called full agonist (its maximal effect is therefore set at 100%) and for ergotamine, a partial agonist, which reaches about 30% of the maximal possible stimulation in spiral strips of isolated canine femoral veins. Moreover it takes about three times longer with ergotamine than with noradrenaline for the rise in tone to develop fully and that it lasts much longer. Additionally, it is clear from Figure 4 that ergotamine is active in concentrations about 350 times lower than noradrenaline. In terms of receptor pharmacology, ergotamine is a partial agonist (30% efficacy compared with the full agonist noradrenaline) but possesses a higher affinity to the stimulating receptor sites of this vascular smooth muscle (ED_{50} for noradrenaline 7.6×10^{-7} M, while the ED_{50} for ergotamine was 2.2×10^{-9} M.)

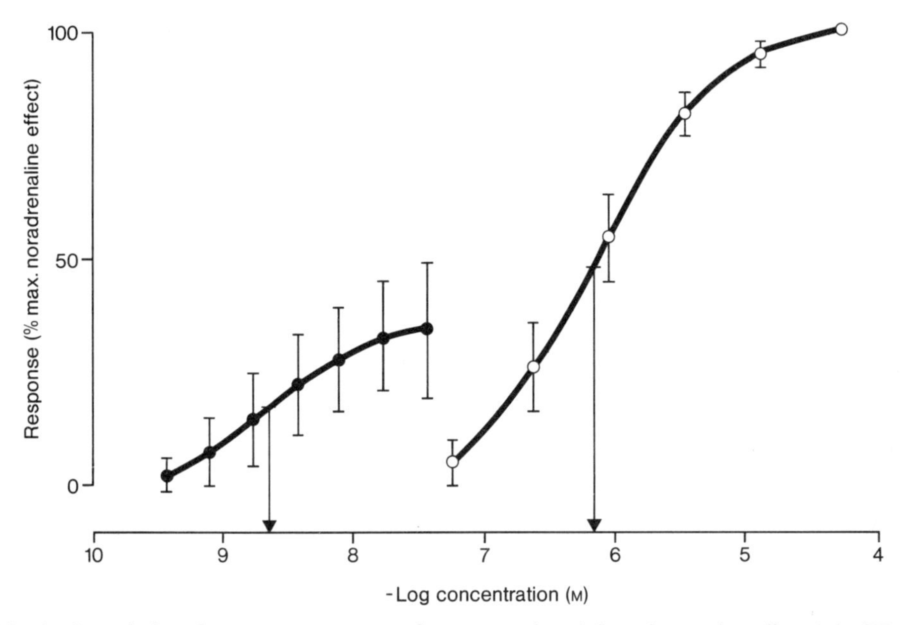

Fig. 4. Cumulative dose response curves for ergotamine (●) and noradrenaline (○). ED_{50} is represented by an arrow in each case. Organ: femoral vein of the dog. Recording: isometric. Vertical bars indicate s.d. (n=36) (MÜLLER-SCHWEINITZER and STÜRMER, 1974)

The combination of increasing concentrations of ergotamine with noradrenaline produced a series of log dose-response curves which are depicted in Figure 5. They start from progressively higher baselines but with similar maxima and show approximate parallelism in the upper reaches. In terms of receptor pharmacology, these curves correspond to curves calculated for the interaction of a full agonist and a partial agonist (so-called competitive dualist). They support the idea, that the stimulating action of ergotamine is due, at least in part, to stimulation followed by block of α-adrenoceptors. If two agonists (noradrenaline and ergotamine) act on the same receptor, they can be expected to be replaced in a similar fashion by a competitive antagonist. Indeed, it has been shown that this is the case, and that ergotamine fulfills the criteria of a partial agonist to α-adrenoceptors on this vascular smooth muscle.

It appears, therefore, that there is no reason to maintain the old concept of a "direct site of action"—as opposed to receptor sites for biogenic amines—as the mechanism of action of the agonistic (=stimulating) effect of ergot alkaloids on vascular and uterine smooth muscle.

An example of an ergot alkaloid antagonistic to serotonin (5-HT) (without partial agonistic stimulant activity) is given in Figure 6. On spiral strips from bovine basilar arteries the maxima of the log dose-response curves for 5-HT progressively decrease with increasing concentrations of methysergide: characteristic for noncompetitive antagonism.

An example in which the effect of an ergot alkaloid is probably due to stimulation (agonism) of central dopaminergic receptors is the induction of turning behav-

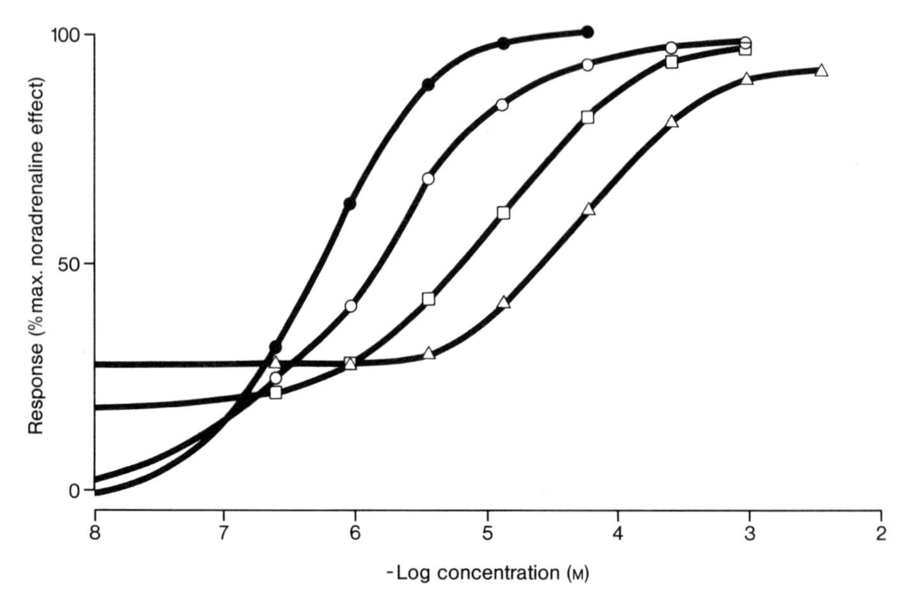

Fig. 5. Cumulative dose response curves for noradrenaline. Organ: femoral vein of the dog. Recording: isometric. (●) control curve (n=18); 15 min after ergotamine in the final concentrations of $10^{-8.76}$ (○), $10^{-7.76}$ (□) and $10^{-6.76}$M (△). n=6 for each curve (MÜLLER-SCHWEINITZER and STÜRMER, 1974)

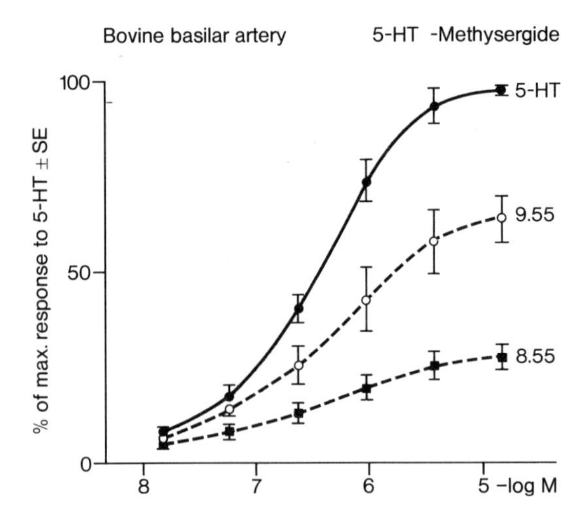

Fig. 6. Cumulative dose response curves for 5-HT without (●, n=5) and 60 min after methysergide in the final concentrations of $10^{-9.55}$M ($=2.8 \times 10^{-10}$M) (○, n=4) and $10^{-8.55}$M ($=2.8 \times 10^{-9}$M) (■, n=5) on spiral strips from bovine basilar arteries. Changes in tension were recorded isometrically (MÜLLER-SCHWEINITZER, unpublished)

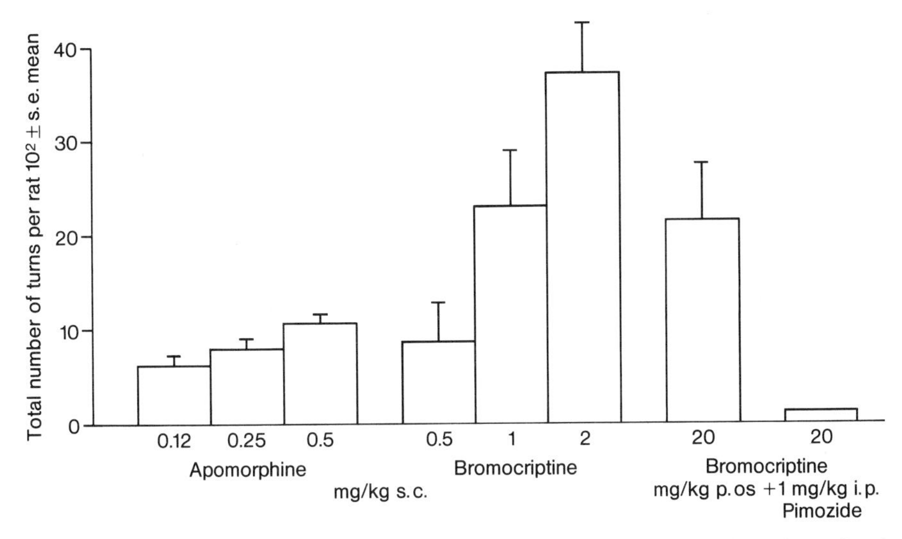

Fig. 7. The induction of turning behavior in rats lesioned unilaterally in the substantia nigra by a local injection of 6-hydroxydopamine after subcutaneous administration of bromocriptine and apomorphine. This effect of bromocriptine is blocked by pretreatment with pimozide (LOEW et al., 1976)

ior by bromocriptine in the rat with unilateral lesions in the substantia nigra produced by previous injection of 6-hydroxy-dopamine (CORRODI et al., 1973). Figure 7 shows that bromocriptine, like apomorphine, increases the number of turns in a dose-dependent way. This effect is blocked by the dopaminergic antagonist pimozide.

In many in vitro testing systems—particularly those involving vascular smooth muscle—the effective concentrations of many ergot compounds are extremely low: 10^{-8}–10^{-9} M. This corresponds to the relatively low therapeutic doses and blood levels (BERDE, 1975; MEIER and SCHREIER, 1976), e.g., steady-state plasma levels for dihydroergotamine are between 2.5 and 6.5 ng/ml after oral doses of 1 mg t.i.d. and 2.5 mg t.i.d. per os, respectively, and for methysergide 20 ng and 40 ng/ml after 1 mg t.i.d. and 2 mg t.i.d., respectively. It is widely accepted that the prophylactic effect of methysergide in migraine headache is connected with its modification of the effects of serotonin and/or metabolic handling of serotonin. On the isolated rat uterus, the serotonin antagonistic concentration of methysergide is in the range of 1 ng/ml (CERLETTI et al., 1960). The stimulating effect (irregular) of the same alkaloid on serotonin uptake in the perfused cat spleen was observed at concentrations around 100 ng/ml, and the inhibition of serotonin uptake (regular) was observed in the same system with those around 1000 ng/ml (OWEN et al., 1971). When considering the mechanism of action of methysergide, the exclusion of this last-mentioned phenomenon would not be necessary for the following reasons:

The aim of a rational therapy is the maintenance of a sufficient drug concentration at the receptor sites in order to achieve the desired pharmacologic effect during a certain time interval. Unfortunately, it is almost impossible to measure and control the drug concentrations at the receptor site or even in the tissues. The next best alternative is to measure the concentrations of the active substance in the blood, plasma, or urine of the patients. These pharmacokinetic data can be used in connection with pharmacodynamic observations for the evaluation and the planning of dosage schemes of the drug. An important condition for such a procedure is the existence of a certain correlation between drug concentration in the plasma and the time course of pharmacologic action. This correlation is not required to be simple and direct. Even a very low drug concentration in the plasma may coincide with a sufficient drug action, if for instance, the active substance has a higher binding affinity to the receptor than to the plasma proteins. Plasma is thus considered in pharmacokinetics to be the central transport compartment and not a direct correlate of the biologic activity.

The *wide field of therapeutic application* of ergot alkaloids and related compounds corresponds to their chemical and pharmacologic diversity. Migraine and other vascular headaches, uterine atonia, orthostatic circulatory disturbances, senile cerebral insufficiency, and infertility due to hyperprolactinemia are probably the most important of a great number of indications. Considering the implications of some of the diseases mentioned in terms of human suffering, medical effort, and socio-economic consequences, the therapeutic importance of the ergot alkaloids and related compounds is indeed formidable. Due to the multiple pharmacologic actions of ergot alkaloids, the relationship between their pharmacologic activity and therapeutic effectiveness is not always obvious. In some cases their clinical use stems clearly from a pharmacologic action, e.g., the use of ergometrine in obstetrics; in others the connection is less evident. Thus, although much is known about the various receptor interactions of ergotamine, it is not clear which of these is responsible for the undoubted effectiveness of this drug in migraine therapy. For this reason, we thought it appropriate in this short introductory chapter to depart from the usual sequence in which all the pharmacologic actions of certain types of compounds are described. We intend instead to describe a few prototype compounds with established therapeutic value and to concentrate on those pharmacologic qualities which are currently considered to be relevant for the therapeutic action.

The use of ergot *in obstetrics*—namely increasing uterine motor activity—is the oldest therapeutic use of this drug. Although several ergot alkaloids have a more or less pronounced effect on the uterus, the prototype compounds used today to treat uterine bleeding of various origin are *ergometrine* (=ergonovine) (DUDLEY and MOIR, 1935; BROWN and DALE, 1935; KHARASCH et al., 1936) and *methylergometrine* (STOLL and HOFMANN, 1943; KIRCHHOF et al., 1944). They influence all three parameters of uterine contractility positively, namely frequency, amplitude, and basal tone. Whereas small doses increase only frequency and/or amplitude of contractions, higher doses also elevate the basic tone, thus decreasing blood loss from the postpartum uterus. This stimulant effect holds true for many species, including man in vivo as well as in vitro, indicating a peripheral site of action.

Two types of adrenergic receptors have been postulated to be present in the uterus: one for uterine stimulation (α) and one for inhibition (β) (AHLQUIST, 1948). The nonpregnant rabbit uterus in situ—in spontaneous or induced estrus—

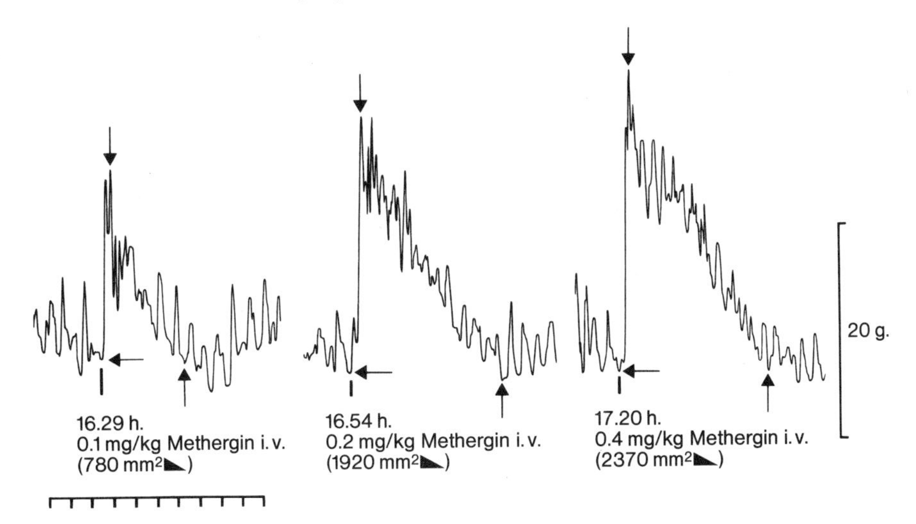

Fig. 8. Isometric recording of the uterotonic effect of methylergometrine on the estrous rabbit uterus in situ. Increased uterine activity is expressed in terms of the area of the time-response curve (BERDE and SAAMELI, 1966)

has been regarded as a particularly suitable experimental setup for the study of the uterotonic effect of many ergot alkaloids and related compounds (ROTHLIN, 1938) (Fig. 8). In this preparation, the uterine stimulating effect of methylergometrine, ergometrine, ergotamine, and some other ergot compounds—in doses between 0.1 and 0.4 mg/kg i.v.—seems to be mediated by α-adrenergic receptors; it can be blocked by α-adrenergic blocking agents such as phenoxybenzamine, phentolamine, dihydroergotamine, and dihydroergotoxine and its components (KONZETT, 1960; HOOL-ZULAUF and STÜRMER, 1976, 1977; ROTHLIN, 1947; ROTHLIN and BIRCHER, 1952) (Fig. 9). It seems that a cyclic change of the sensitivity of the uterus to uterotonic stimuli is due to changes in the number of and proportion of α- and β-adrenergic receptors brought about by the sexual hormone cycles (MILLER and MARSHALL, 1965; MILLER, 1967; BRODY and DIAMOND, 1967). It was regarded as a "rule" that on the estrous rabbit uterus, ergot compounds with a double bond in position 9,10 are oxytocics, whereas compounds dihydrogenated in this position are not oxytocic but, on the contrary, inhibit both spontaneous and induced uterine activity (ROTHLIN, 1947; ROTHLIN and BIRCHER, 1952). This is true for many compounds tested in our laboratories but not without exception, e.g., bromocriptine has no uterotonic activity (STÜRMER and FLÜCKIGER, 1974), and the dihydrogenated compound dibromo-dihydrolysergic-acid-glycinamide is a strong oxytocic (BERDE and SAAMELI, 1966) and so are some 6-Nor-6-isopropyl-9,10-dihydroergopeptines (HOOL-ZULAUF and STÜRMER, 1976, 1977). It appears, therefore, that the presence of the double bond in position 9,10 of the lysergic acid moiety is not the structural element exclusively responsible for determining α-adrenergic stimulation or inhibition.

Furthermore, there is no complete parallel between the estrous rabbit uterus

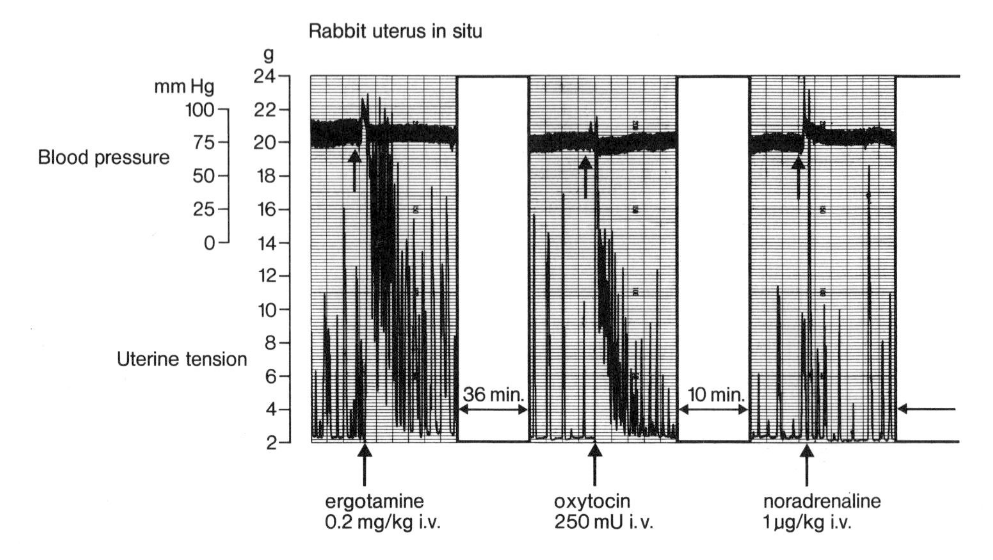

Fig. 9. Original trace of an experiment in the rabbit demonstrating the effects of ergotamine, oxytocin, and noradrenaline on blood pressure (upper tracing) and uterine tension (lower tracing) before and after phentolamine injection. It can be seen from the tracings that blockade

and the human myometrium near term with regard to their response to ergot alkaloids. It was found, for example, that some compounds hydrogenated in position 9,10, such as dihydroergotamine and dihydroergotoxine mesylate, have some uterotonic activity on the human uterus near term both in vivo and in vitro (ALTMAN et al., 1952; EMBREY and GARRETT, 1955; ROTHLIN and BERDE, 1954) and on the cat uterus in situ (BERDE and ROTHLIN, 1953). The reason for these interspecies differences is not known.

Note that the receptor involved in the uterotonic effect of some ergot compounds is different from that involved in the uterotonic effect of oxytocin. The uterine effect of the latter is not antagonized by α-adrenergic blocking agents (Fig. 9).

The prototype compound for the treatment of the *migraine attack*, as well as for cluster headache and some other vascular headaches, is *ergotamine tartrate*. The possible relevance of its various pharmacologic qualities for its therapeutic effect has recently been reviewed and discussed (FOZARD, 1975a, b). It was emphasized that only those effects elicited by very low doses can be considered as relevant. These effects are vasoconstriction (ROTHLIN, 1923; ROTHLIN and CERLETTI, 1949), sensitization of vascular smooth muscle to nervous and chemical stimuli (e.g. ROTHLIN and CERLETTI, 1949; WEIDMANN and TAESCHLER, 1966), and inhibition of circulatory baroreceptor reflexes (e.g. v. EULER and SCHMITERLÖW, 1944). Based on the extensive clinical pharmacologic studies of the behavior of the extracerebral vessels before and during the migraine attack and under the influence of ergotamine (WOLFF, 1963), however, it is now generally accepted that the therapeutic effect of ergotamine is closely related to its long lasting peripheral vasoconstrictor activity in the dilated branches of the external carotid artery

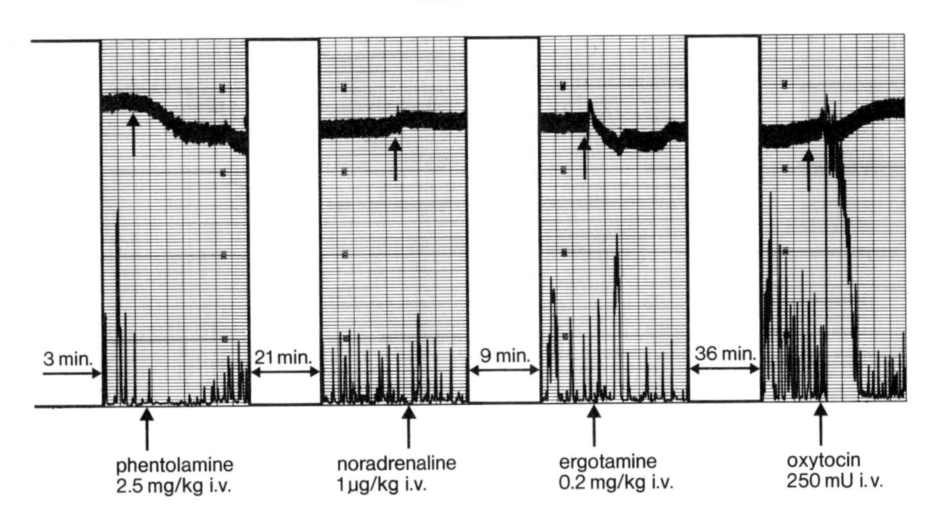

of α-adrenoceptors by phentolamine decreased mean arterial blood pressure and completely abolished the uterotonic effect of noradrenaline and ergotamine but not that of oxytocin. Time: 2.4 min between the vertical lines (HOOL-ZULAUF and STÜRMER, unpublished)

(Fig. 10). Studies employing various experimental arrangements have indeed demonstrated that (1) the preexisting vascular tone is determinant for the vasoconstrictor effect of ergotamine (AELLIG and BERDE, 1969), (2) different vascular beds in the cat show different sensitivities to ergotamine (ROTHLIN and CERLETTI, 1949), and (3) the carotid artery bed in the dog is more sensitive to this substance than some other vascular beds (CARPI and VIRNO, 1957; SAXENA and DE VLAAM-SCHLUTER, 1974).

The most effective way of administering ergotamine to abort a migraine attack is by parenteral injection. For practical reasons, however, oral administration of ergotamine is preferred, usually in combination with caffeine, in order to accelerate and enhance absorption (BERDE et al., 1970; SCHMIDT and FANCHAMPS, 1974).

Studies of isolated arteries of dogs and man (PICHLER et al., 1953; TODA and FUJITA, 1973; MÜLLER-SCHWEINITZER, 1976) have shown that they respond to serotonin (5-HT), which stimulates arterial vascular smooth muscle in concentrations about 10 times lower than noradrenaline. If the maximal effect (efficacy or intrinsic activity) of serotonin is expressed in terms of the maximal effect of noradrenaline, it varies considerably in different types of arterial smooth muscle: in the dog saphenous artery the efficacy of serotonin is 60% of noradrenaline efficacy; in the dog external carotid artery and basilar artery it is 160% and 540%, respectively. Isolated dog arteries also respond to ergotamine (MÜLLER-SCHWEINITZER, 1976), which stimulates the three above-mentioned preparations in concentrations about 100 times lower than that of noradrenaline. The efficacy of ergotamine in the three preparations, measured in terms of noradrenaline, was found to be less than that of serotonin but paralleled it, being 20%, 50%, and

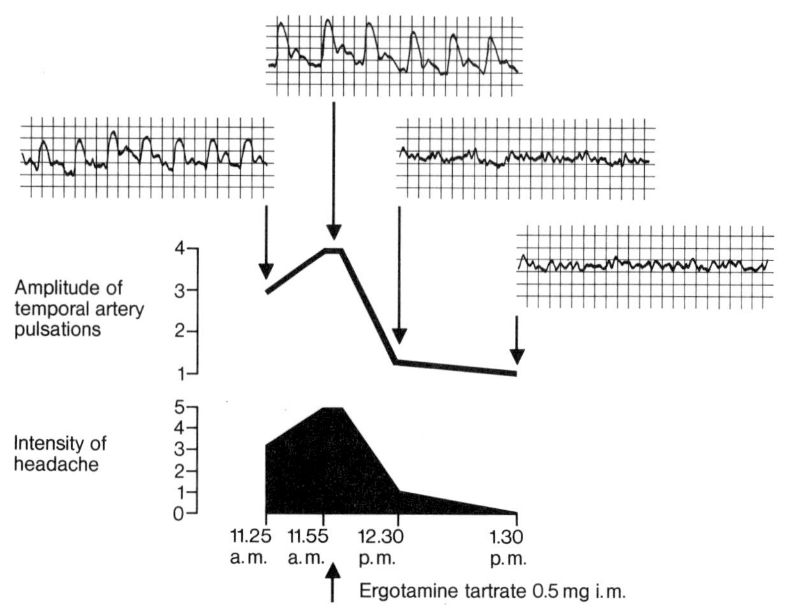

Fig. 10. Migraine attack in a woman of 22. The intensity of the pain runs parallel to the amplitude of pulsation of the temporal artery. Intramuscular injection of ergotamine tartrate exerts a tonic action on the vessels and terminates the headache. After a case of WOLFF (1955)—redrawn by permission of the author (FANCHAMPS, 1958)

210%, respectively, of noradrenaline efficacy (Fig. 11). These findings suggest that ergotamine stimulation of arterial smooth muscle may be partly mediated through serotonin receptor sites.

There is evidence that in man, a decrease in the serotonin blood level precedes the migraine attack and may be a factor in the fall of vascular tone responsible for the headache (LANCE, 1969). It is conceivable that the therapeutic effect of ergotamine is due to stimulation of serotonin receptors of cranial arteries.

Ergotamine also has a powerful effect on capacitance vessels, producing constriction (OWEN and STÜRMER, 1972; CHU et al., 1976). These effects of ergotamine on the venous site of the circulation are mediated by α-adrenoceptors, as previously mentioned. It is not known if this is of relevance to the antimigraine effect.

For the *prophylactic treatment of migraine*—and of some other vascular headaches—*methysergide* (1-Methyl-D-lysergic-acid-L-2-butanolamide-hydrogen-maleinate=Deseril=Sansert) is the prototype ergot compound.

Ever since the possible involvement of serotonin in the pathophysiology of migraine was first discussed by H.G. Wolff's research team (OSTFELD et al., 1957), a steadily increasing body of evidence has supported the view that this autacoid indeed does play a rôle in these forms of headache (see e.g. LANCE, 1969). The first successful therapeutic experiment with methysergide (SICUTERI, 1959) was based on this assumption, methysergide being given for its serotonin-antagonistic effect. It was thereafter generally maintained that the key pharmacologic quality of methysergide in this application is its outstanding serotonin-antagonistic effect; the com-

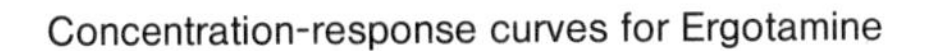

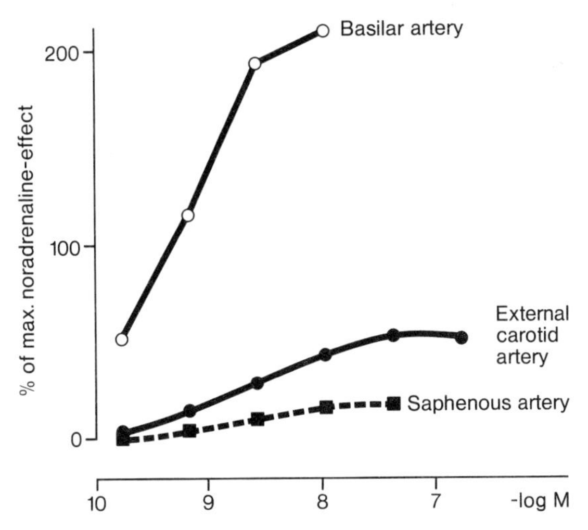

Fig. 11. Dose—response curves for ergotamine in spiral strips from canine saphenous arteries (■ ---- ■, for each point, n=6), external carotid arteries (● —— ●, for each point, n=6) and basilar arteries (○ —— ○, for each point, n=5) expressed as percentages of the maximum responses to noradrenaline (MÜLLER-SCHWEINITZER, 1976)

pound shows a high antiserotonin activity in many pharmacologic tests—not only on different types of smooth muscle, blood pressure, etc., but also on the inflammatory effect of subcutaneously injected serotonin—whereas it is practically devoid of uterotonic and vasoconstrictor activity in tests generally used for the characterization of ergot compounds (CERLETTI et al., 1960; FANCHAMPS et al., 1960; BERDE, 1972). It has recently been shown (SAXENA, 1972, 1974), however, that in the carotid artery bed of the dog, low doses of methysergide bring about a selective dose-dependent vasoconstrictor effect (Fig. 12). Although this effect of methysergide is much less pronounced than that of ergotamine, it is remarkable in itself; the threshold dose is about 20 μg/kg i.v. (that of ergotamine being about 1 μg/kg i.v.). Furthermore, it was shown that the antiserotonin effect of methysergide is present but not prominent in this particular vascular bed (SAXENA, 1972). These findings opened up new possibilities for the pharmacologic explanation of the therapeutic effect of methysergide, since it has been established (TODA and FUJITA, 1973; MÜLLER-SCHWEINITZER, 1976) that in the cerebral arteries of the dog serotonin is a potent vasoconstrictor, and the vasoconstrictor effect of ergotamine in these arteries is mediated by serotoninergic receptors. It has indeed been suggested recently that methysergide may exert its therapeutic effect as an agonist rather than an antagonist of serotonin in the carotid vascular bed (LANCE, 1974).

The pharmacologic effects of the peptide alkaloid *dihydroergotamine* (as methansulfonate = Dihydergot) differ quantitatively rather than qualitatively from those of its nonhydrogenated parent compound ergotamine. Thus, the peripheral vasoconstrictor effect of dihydroergotamine both in dogs and cats is considerably weaker than that of ergotamine (AELLIG and BERDE, 1969; OWEN and STÜRMER, 1972),

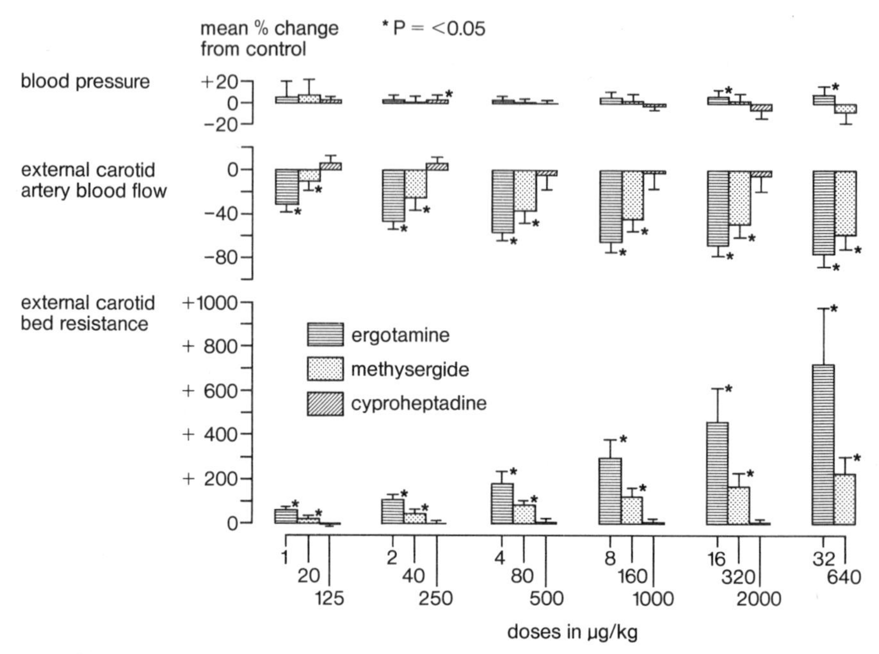

Fig. 12. Effect of the antimigraine drugs on the mean arterial blood pressure and the mean flow and resistance in the external carotid bed of the dog. Note the decrease in the carotid flow and the increase in the resistance by ergotamine and methysergide but not by cyproheptadine (SAXENA, 1972)

whereas the α-adrenergic blocking activity on smooth muscle is (several times) stronger than that of ergotamine (BRÜGGER, 1945; ROTHLIN, 1947). Dihydroergotamine is also a relatively strong antagonist of serotonin (GADDUM and HAMEED, 1954). It inhibits baroreceptor circulatory reflexes (v. EULER and HESSER, 1947) and sensitizes some smooth muscle preparations to the effect of sympathetic stimulation and noradrenaline (WEIDMANN and TAESCHLER, 1966) and, like ergotamine, inhibits the re-uptake of noradrenaline at sympathetic nerve endings (PACHA and SALZMANN, 1970) (Fig. 13).

Interestingly, dihydroergotamine is of therapeutic value both for the treatment of the *migraine attack* and for the *prophylaxis of migraine* and some other vascular headaches. For the discussion of the possible or probable relevance of different pharmacologic properties for these therapeutic applications see the above paragraphs concerning ergotamine and methysergide.

For the therapeutic use of dihydroergotamine in *orthostatic hypotension,* its constrictor effect, which is mainly confined to the capacitance vessels, is of relevance. Experiments on the autoperfused hind limb of the cat have shown that some ergot alkaloids increase the tone of capacitance vessels dose-dependently in the vascular beds of skin and skeletal muscle. Dihydroergotamine is more selective than ergotamine in that it influences resistance vessels less at the same dosage, the difference being more pronounced in skin (OWEN and STÜRMER, 1972; CHU et al., 1976) (Fig. 14). The effect of dihydroergotamine on venous tone is compar-

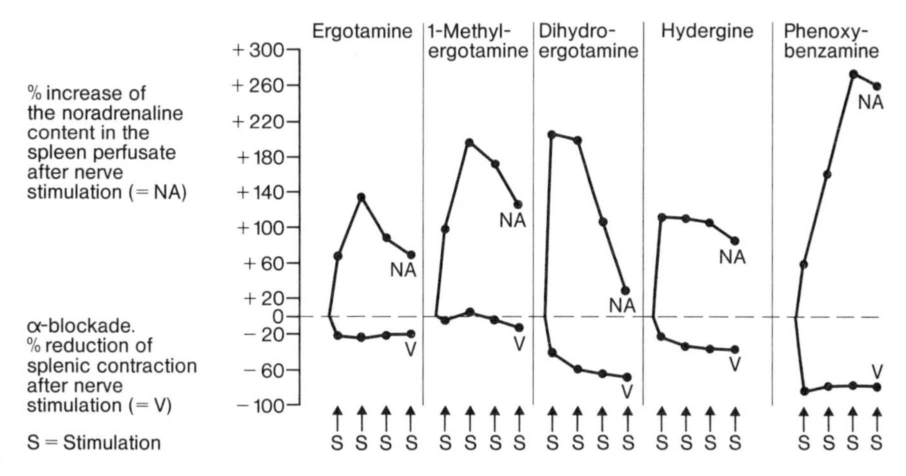

Fig. 13. The altered response of the isolated perfused spleen of the cat to postganglionic sympathetic stimulation (contraction, noradrenaline output) after administration of 1 μg/min i.a. of ergotamine, l-methylergotamine, dihydroergotamine, Hydergine, and phenoxybenzamine (PACHA and SALZMANN, 1970)

able with that of electric sympathetic stimulation, but dihydroergotamine is more selective than sympathetic stimulation in that it constricts capacitance vessels while having a negligible effect on resistance. The effect of dihydroergotamine on capacitance vessels is most probably mediated by long-lasting α-adrenoceptor stimulation, because it is abolished by α-adrenoceptor blocking drugs.

The venoconstrictor effect of dihydroergotamine was first described in man (MELLANDER and NORDENFELT, 1970) when it was shown that in resting normal subjects 10 μg/kg i.v. of dihydroergotamine mobilized about 350 ml of blood by contracting capacitance vessels in skin and skeletal muscle. In patients with orthostatic hypotension, the same doses increased cardiac output by somewhat less than half a liter in the supine position and somewhat more than half a liter in the erect position (NORDENFELT and MELLANDER, 1972).

It has been known for some time that certain ergot alkaloids may interfere with lactation and/or reproduction. It was observed, for example, that ergotoxine prevented the formation of deciduomas in the uteri of pseudo-pregnant rats, and it was suggested that this effect may be due to an influence—possibly via the hypothalamus—on the pituitary gland, resulting in inhibition of prolactin secretion (SHELESNYAK, 1954, 1958).

The prototype of an ergot compound which selectively inhibits prolactin secretion is *bromocriptine* (= CB 154 = Parlodel). This is the compound which is now clinically used to suppress normal or pathologically increased prolactin secretion in man, i.e., for *suppression of lactation* and for *treatment of certain types of hypogonadism due to hyperprolactinemia* in both males and females. It has also helped to better our understanding of how prolactin secretion is controlled and what role this hormone plays in the physiology of different species.

This substance was developed from ergotoxine with the aim of retaining the

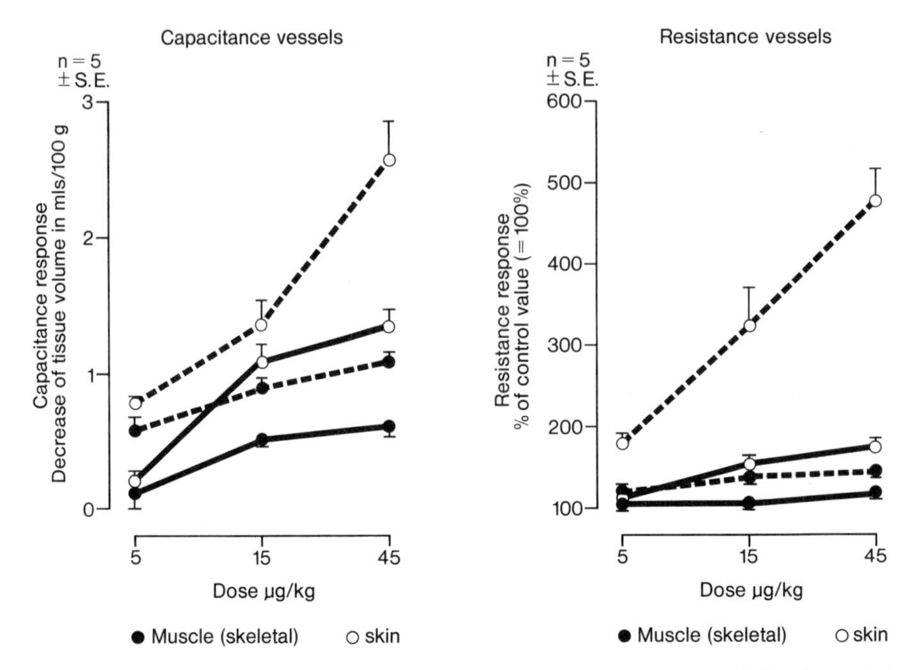

Fig. 14. Effects of ergotamine (broken lines) and dihydroergotamine (solid lines) on skeletal muscle (●) and skin (○) vasculature of the cat. The capacitance response was calculated from the rapid reduction in tissue volume on drug administration and is expressed as ml/100 g tissue. The resistance response is plotted as the post-treatment value expressed as a percentage of the pre-treatment value. The doses are expressed as µg/kg (calf muscle: µg/kg muscle i.a.; skin: µg/kg cat body weight) (CHU et al., 1976)

prolactin-inhibiting effect and eliminating the oxytocic and cardiovascular side-effects of the parent compound (FLÜCKIGER, 1972, 1975; FLÜCKIGER et al., 1976b).

As a result of many observations, the inhibition of prolactin secretion was suggested as the mode of action of bromocriptine: termination of pseudo-pregnancy in the rat (FLÜCKIGER, 1972) and prevention of implantation—an "all or nothing" type reaction—with an ED_{50} of 0.7 mg/kg s.c. in the rat (FLÜCKIGER and WAGNER, 1968), lack of effect on early pregnancy in the rabbit (FLÜCKIGER, 1972), increase in ovarian weight and number of persisting corpora lutea after daily administration of 3 mg/kg p.o. and more to adult rats (BILLETER and FLÜCKIGER, 1971), inhibition of milk secretion in several animal species at different dose levels (FLÜCKIGER and WAGNER, 1968; FLÜCKIGER, 1972; FLÜCKIGER et al., 1976a; MAYER and SCHÜTZE, 1973), suppression of the development of chemically induced mammary tumors with 6 mg/kg i.p. daily (STÄHELIN et al., 1971), etc.

With the development of highly sensitive and specific bioassays (FRANTZ et al., 1972) and radioimmunoassays (FRIESEN et al., 1972), the direct measurement of plasma prolactin levels became possible. Bromocriptine was demonstrated to decrease plasma prolactin concentration in several species, e.g., in mice (SINHA et al., 1974), in rats (MARKO and FLÜCKIGER, 1974; DÖHLER and WUTTKE, 1974), in sheep (NISWENDER, 1974), in goats (HART, 1973), in cows (KARG et al., 1972;

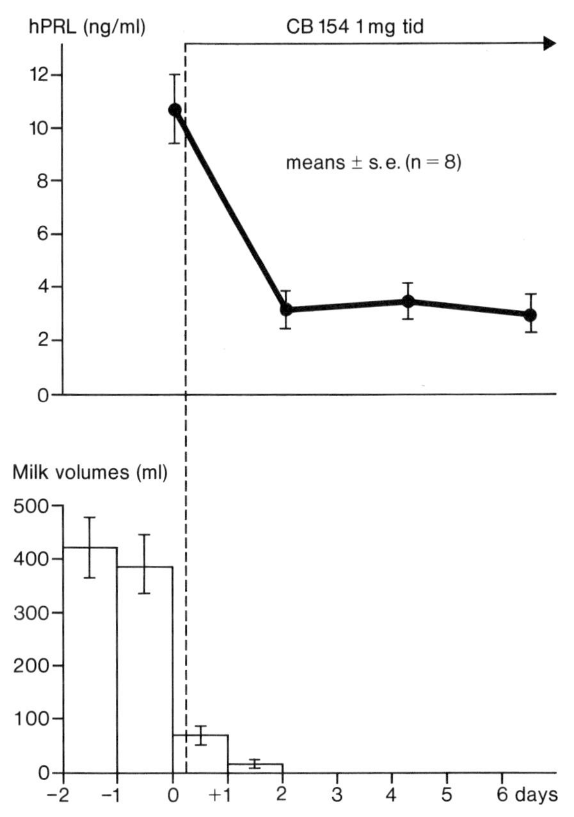

Fig. 15. Inhibition of prolactin plasma levels and milk secretion in eight lactating women exhibiting normal basal plasma prolactin concentrations (DEL POZO et al., 1975)

SCHAMS et al., 1972), and in man with a few milligrams per os (DEL POZO et al., 1972; DEL POZO et al., 1975) (Fig. 15).

The mechanism of action of bromocriptine is not fully understood. It is, however, clear that bromocriptine is not a prolactin antagonist in the sense that it would compete for peripheral prolactin-receptor sites. Its effect is the inhibition of the release of prolactin from the pituitary: it was found by in vitro studies on rat pituitary glands (PASTEELS et al., 1971; NAGASAWA et al., 1973) and pituitary cell cultures (TASHJIAN and HOYT, 1972) to inhibit prolactin secretion by a direct action on the prolactin secreting cell. In the mammal, prolactin release by the adenohypophysis is under tonic inhibition by the hypothalamus. The inhibitory effect is maintained hormonally, but the identity of the hypothalamic hormone responsible for inhibiting prolactin secretion is uncertain, some authors maintaining that it is a specific polypeptide acting on dopamine receptors, others suggesting that it may be dopamine itself. The action of bromocriptine bears some resemblance to the hypothetical hypothalamic factor which inhibits prolactin secretion. It is probable that the membrane-stabilizing effect of bromocriptine at the prolactin secreting cell itself is also due to dopamine receptor stimulation (TAKAHARA et al., 1974; MACLEOD and LEHMEYER, 1974; HILL-SAMLI and MACLEOD, 1975).

Other findings suggest an additional hypothalamic effect brought about by dopaminergic stimulation of tuberoinfundibular neurones which control both prolactin and gonadotrophin secretion (HÖKFELT and FUXE, 1972). The two sites of action, the prolactin cell of the pituitary and the hypothalamic dopaminergic stimulation, do not necessarily suggest two different mechanisms of action.

Inhibition of prolactin secretion is of course only one consequence of *stimulation of dopaminergic receptor sites* by bromocriptine. It is well established that this alkaloid also stimulates dopaminergic neurone systems in the central nervous system which are involved in nonendocrine functions (CORRODI et al., 1973; JOHNSON et al., 1973; JOHNSON et al., 1976). This long-acting central dopamine receptor stimulating activity is probably the basis of the therapeutic effect of bromocriptine in *Parkinson's disease* (e.g. CALNE et al., 1976).

The therapeutic use of bromocriptine is not restricted to prevention or inhibition of lactation, but it is also successfully used to treat certain types of infertility. With regard to the mechanism of this effect, one has to consider that inhibition of prolactin secretion increases gonadotrophin secretion and vice versa. Both are under the control of the hypothalamus; therefore, bromocriptine can be used to increase gonadotrophin secretion in cases of hypogonadism due to an imbalance in hypothalamic control, i.e., to an unduly high prolactin secretion. This was demonstrated in mice (YANAI and NAGASAWA, 1970), in rats (FLÜCKIGER et al., 1972), and in man (LUTTERBECK et al., 1971; BESSER et al., 1972; DEL POZO and FLÜCKIGER, 1973).

From animal work in the goat (HART, 1974), the cow (SMITH et al., 1974), and in the mouse (SINHA et al., 1974), there is no evidence that bromocriptine significantly alters the secretion of TSH, ACTH, or growth hormone. An apparent paradox is that bromocriptine depresses growth hormone secretion in acromegalic patients but not in normal subjects (e.g., THORNER and BESSER, 1976).

The ergoline derivative *lergotrile* (=2-chloro-6-methyl-ergoline-8β-acetonitrile mesylate) shows effects similar to those of the peptide alkaloid bromocriptine. It inhibits dose-dependent prolactin secretion as well as milk secretion in vitro and in vivo in rats (CLEMENS et al., 1975) and in humans (CLEARY et al., 1975). There is evidence to show that this compound also acts as an agonist on some dopaminergic receptor sites (CLEMENS et al., 1975; LIEBERMAN et al., 1975).

Amongst ergot compounds which have been shown to be of therapeutic value in *senile cerebral insufficiency* (=psycho-organic disease or psycho-organic defect of aging=the syndrome of mental and behavioral deterioration in aging) *dihydroergotoxine mesylate* (Hydergine=equal parts of the mesylates of dihydroergocornine, dihydroergocristine and dihydroergokryptine [dihydro-α-ergokryptine and dihydro-β-ergokryptine in the proportion 2 to 1]) is the prototype. It is therapeutically the most widely used preparation and the one for which a modern clinical pharmacologic methodology has been developed.

The mechanism of its action in the human is not fully understood, and it is not possible to say which of the measurable pharmacologic effects of dihydroergotoxine mesylate in animal experiments are relevant for the clinical activity. There is, however, some reason to believe that receptor-mediated interactions involving

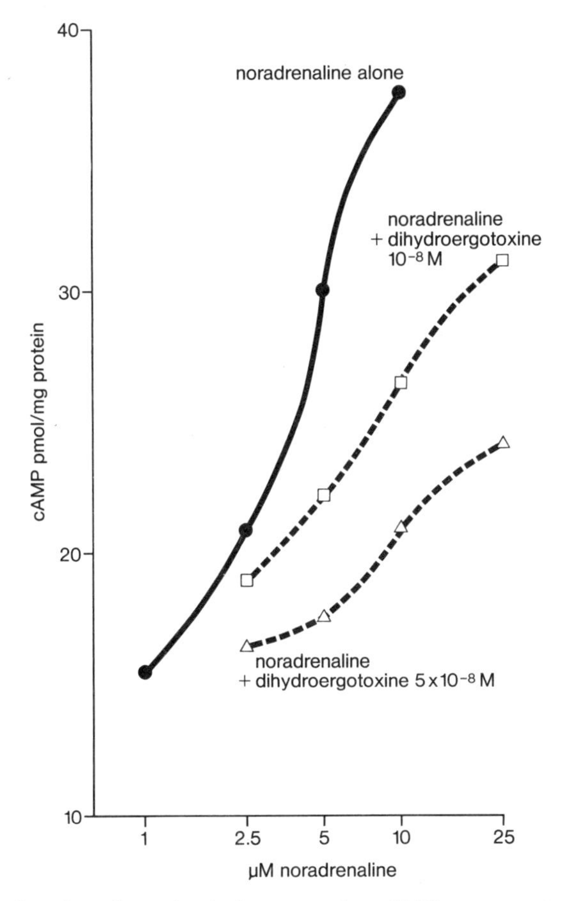

Fig. 16. Noradrenaline dose-dependently increases the cAMP content of rat cerebral cortex slices in vitro by stimulating adenyl cyclase activity. Pretreatment with dihydroergotoxine mesylate inhibits dose-dependently the effect of noradrenaline (MARKSTEIN and WAGNER, 1978)

cyclic AMP and other metabolic parameters, rather than effects on cerebral blood flow, are of primary importance (MEIER-RUGE et al., 1975). The following findings underline this aspect.

The influence of dihydroergotoxine mesylate on cyclic adenosine monophosphate (cAMP) of the brain was investigated in in vitro systems. In rat cortex slices it inhibited dose-dependently ($EC_{50} = 10^{-8}$ M) the noradrenaline-stimulated adenyl cyclase activity, resulting in a decrease of cAMP synthesis as depicted in Figure 16 (MARKSTEIN and WAGNER, 1978). In homogenates of cat cerebral cortex, dihydroergotoxine mesylate inhibits—albeit in higher concentrations (range 10^{-5} M)—the predominantly membrane-located so-called "low-K_m phosphodiesterase," resulting in a relative increase of the cAMP concentration (IWANGOFF et al., 1975).

In the more complex system of the perfused cat brain preparation some metabolic parameters were studied by means of semiquantitative histochemical methods

(EMMENEGGER and MEIER-RUGE, 1968). Changes in some enzyme activities following the reduction of the temperature of the perfusion fluid from 36° C to 29° C were shifted in the direction of the prae-hypothermic values by adding to the perfusion fluid a few μg/min dihydroergotoxine mesylate. In the same experimental setting, hypothermia-induced increase of cerebral lactic acidosis was counteracted by dihydroergotoxine mesylate (8 μg/min for 30 min) which increased the ratio of ΔAV-pyruvate to ΔAV-L-lactate (CERLETTI et al., 1973).

In the isolated perfused cat brain preparation, infusion of 8 μg/min dihydroergotoxine mesylate facilitates EEG-recovery after temporary ischemia (CERLETTI et al., 1973). In superficially anesthetized cats a marked reduction of cerebral blood flow leads to a decrease of EEG activity. This can be partially prevented by the infusion of 4 μg/kg/min dihydroergotoxine mesylate for 20 min, although the reduced cerebral blood flow is not significantly altered (GYGAX et al., 1976). In the curarized cat 0.1–0.8 mg/kg dihydroergotoxine mesylate i.v. reduced the number of reserpine-induced spike potentials in the pontogeniculo-occipital system ("PGO-spikes") in a dose-dependent way and reversed reserpine-induced electroencephalographic arousal to a high-amplitude, slow-wave pattern in cortical recordings (DEPOORTERE et al., 1975). In the rat 1 mg/kg dihydroergotoxine mesylate i.p. altered the electroencephalographically monitored sleep/wakefulness cycle by prolonging wakefulness and by shortening classical and paradoxical sleep (LOEW et al., 1976).

There is evidence that dihydroergotoxine mesylate can interfere with at least three types of receptors in the brain: In the case of inhibition of noradrenaline-stimulated adenyl-cyclase activity, adrenergic receptors in the cortex are involved (MARKSTEIN and WAGNER, 1975); in the case of inhibition of reserpine-induced potentials, a serotoninergic structure located in the pontine reticular formation is probably involved (DEPOORTERE et al., 1975). It could further be shown that i.v. administration of 2.5–10 mg/kg dihydroergotoxine mesylate reduced, in a dose-dependent manner, the antinociceptive effect of morphine in the rabbit, probably via a dopaminergic system close to the fourth ventricle (DEPOORTERE et al., 1975).

Obviously most of the above-mentioned experimental parameters cannot be investigated in man. However, EEG-studies have revealed characteristic effects of dihydroergotoxine mesylate. Electrical brain activity undergoes steady changes in frequencies and abundance during life. With age, there is a slowing of the dominant alpha frequency, an increase of the slow delta and theta activities, and a decrease in the percentage of alpha activity (ROUBICEK et al., 1972, 1973; MATEJCEK and DEVOS, 1976). In hospitalized, nonpsychotic geriatric patients, daily oral doses of 4.5 mg dihydroergotoxine mesylate brought about a shift in the dominant frequency to the fast part of the electrical spectrum and an increase in the amplitude and a better modulation of the alpha frequency (ROUBICEK et al., 1972).

Among other ergot alkaloids, *dihydroergonine* (DN 16-457) has in many respects effects similar to those of dihydroergotoxine mesylate, both in animal models (MEIER-RUGE et al., 1975) and in the human EEG (MATEJCEK and DEVOS, 1976).

Nicergoline (Sermion) was also reported to be of therapeutic value in senile cerebral insufficiency. Of its pharmacologic effects, the following may be relevant in this respect: The recovery of a normal EEG-pattern after cerebral ischemia in the cat was accelerated by 150 μg/kg nicergoline i.v. or 15 μg/kg injected into the carotid artery (SUCHOWSKY and PEGRASSI, 1974). The same is true for the postischemic recovery of cortical-evoked potentials of the cerebral hemispheres in the cat; unilateral intracarotid injection of 20–400 μg nicergoline produced a more rapid recovery on the treated side (BOISMARE and LORENZO, 1975). On the isolated dog brain in situ in the recovery phase following hypoxia, intracarotid infusion of the compound increased glucose utilization and decreased pyruvic acid formation (BENZI et al., 1972).

References

Aellig, W.H., Berde, B.: Studies of the effect of natural and synthetic polypeptide type ergot compounds on a peripheral vascular bed. Brit. J. Pharmacol. **36**, 561–570 (1969)

Ahlquist, R.P.: A study of the adrenotropic receptors. Amer. J. Physiol. **153**, 586–600 (1948)

Altman, S.G., Waltman, R., Lubin, S., Reynolds, S.R.M.: Oxytocic and toxic actions of dihydroergotamine-45. Amer. J. Obstet. Gynec. **64**, 101–109 (1952)

Benzi, G., De Bernardi, M., Manzo, L., Ferrara, A., Panceri, P., Arrigoni, E., Berté, F.: Effect of lysergide and nimergoline on glucose metabolism investigated on the dog brain isolated in situ. J. pharm. Sci. **61**, 348–352 (1972)

Berde, B.: Recent progress in the elucidation of the mechanism of action of ergot compounds used in migraine therapy. Med. J. Aust. Spec. Suppl. **2**, 15–26 (1972)

Berde, B.: Human plasma levels of anti-migraine drugs contrasted with their active concentrations in isolated organ systems. The Bergen Migraine Symposium, Bergen, 4–6 June, 1975

Berde, B., Cerletti, A., Dengler, H.J., Zoglio, M.A.: Studies of the interaction between ergot alkaloids and xanthine derivatives. In: Background to Migraine. Cochrane, A.L. (ed.), pp. 80–102. London: William Heinemann Medical Books 1970

Berde, B., Rothlin, E.: Über die Uteruswirkung hydrierter Mutterkornalkaloide an Kaninchen und Katzen vor, während und nach der Geburt. Helv. physiol. pharmacol. Acta **11**, 274–282 (1953)

Berde, B., Saameli, K.: Evaluation of substances acting on the uterus. In: Methods in Drug Evaluation. Mantegazza, P., Piccinini, F. (eds.), pp. 481–514. Amsterdam: North Holland Publ. 1966

Besser, G.M., Parke, L., Edwards, C.R.W., Forsyth, I.A., McNeilly, A.S.: Galactorrhoea: successful treatment with reduction of plasma prolactin levels by brom-ergocryptine. Brit. med. J. **3**, 669–672 (1972)

Billeter, E., Flückiger, E.: Evidence for a luteolytic function of prolactin in the intact cyclic rat using 2-Br-α-Ergokryptine (CB 154). Experientia (Basel) **27**, 464–465 (1971)

Boismare, F., Lorenzo, J.: Study of the protection afforded by nicergoline against the effects of cerebral ischemia in the cat. Arzneimittel-Forsch. **25**, 410–413 (1975)

Bradley, P.B., Briggs, I.: Ergot alkaloids and related substances. In: Neuropoisons—Their Pathophysiological Actions. Poisons of Plant Origin. Simpson, L.L., Curtis, D.R. (eds.), Vol. II, pp. 249–296. New York-London: Plenum Press 1974

Brody, T.M., Diamond, J.: Blockade of the biochemical correlates of contraction and relaxation in uterine and intestinal smooth muscle. Ann. N.Y. Acad. Sci. **139**, 772–780 (1967)

Brown, G.L., Dale, Sir Henry: The pharmacology of ergometrine. Proc. roy. Soc. B. **118**, 446–477 (1935)

Brügger, J.: Die isolierte Samenblase des Meerschweinchens als biologisches Testobjekt zur quantitativen Differenzierung der sympathikolytischen Wirkung der genuinen Mutterkornalkaloide und ihrer Dihydroderivate. Helv. physiol. pharmacol. Acta **3**, 117–134 (1945)

Calne, D.B., Kartzinel, R., Shoulson, I.: An ergot derivative in the treatment of Parkinson's disease. Postgrad. med. J. **52** (Suppl. 1), 81–82 (1976)

Carpi, A., Virno, M.: The action of ergotamine on the intracranial venous pressure and on the cerebral venous outflow of the dog. Brit. J. Pharmacol. **12**, 232–239 (1957)
Cerletti, A., Berde, B., Doepfner, W., Emmenegger, H., Konzett, H., Schalch, W.R., Taeschler, M., Weidmann, H.: Deseril® (methysergide, UML-491), a specific serotonin antagonist. Sci. Exhibit 6th Internat. Congr. Int. Medicine, Basle, 24–27 August, 1960
Cerletti, A., Emmenegger, H., Enz, A., Iwangoff, P., Meier-Ruge, W., Musil, J.: Effects of ergot DH-alkaloids on the metabolism and function of the brain. An approach based on studies with DH-ergonine. In: Central Nervous System—Studies on Metabolic Regulation and Function. Genazzani, E., Herken, H. (eds.), pp. 201–212. Berlin-Heidelberg-New York: Springer 1973
Chu, D., Owen, D.A.A., Stürmer, E.: Effects of ergotamine and dihydroergotamine on the resistance and capacitance vessels of skin and skeletal muscle in the cat. Postgrad. med. J. **52** (Suppl. 1), 32–36 (1976)
Cleary, R.E., Crabtree, R., Lemberger, L.: The effect of lergotrile on galactorrhea and gonadotropin secretion. J. clin. Endocr. **40**, 830–833 (1975)
Clemens, J.A., Smalstig, E.B., Shaar, C.J.: Inhibition of prolactin secretion by lergotrile mesylate: mechanism of action. Acta endocr. (Kbh.) **79**, 230–237 (1975)
Corrodi, H., Fuxe, K., Hökfelt, T., Lidbrink, P., Ungerstedt, U.: Effect of ergot drugs on central catecholamine neurons: evidence for a stimulation of central dopamine neurons. Letters to the Editor. J. Pharm. Pharmacol. **25**, 409–412 (1973)
Del Pozo, E., Flückiger, E.: Prolactin inhibition: experimental and clinical studies. In: Human Prolactin. Pasteels, J.L., Robyn, C. (eds.), pp. 291–301. Amsterdam: Excerpta Medica 1973
Del Pozo, E., Goldstein, M., Friesen, H., Brun Del Re, R., Eppenberger, U.: Lack of action of prolactin suppression on the regulation of the human menstrual cycle. Amer. J. Obstet. Gynec. **123**, 719–723 (1975)
Del Pozo, E., Brun del Re, R., Varga, L., Friesen, H.: The inhibition of prolactin secretion in man by CB-154 (2-Br-α-ergocryptine). J. clin. Endocr. **35**, 768–771 (1972)
Depoortere, H., Loew, D.M., Vigouret, J.M.: Neuropharmacological studies on Hydergine®. Triangle **14**, 73–79 (1975)
Döhler, K.D., Wuttke, W.: Total blockade of phasic pituitary prolactin release in rats: effect on serum LH and progesterone during the estrous cycle and pregnancy. Endocrinology **94**, 1595–1600 (1974)
Dudley, H.W., Moir, Ch.: The substance responsible for the traditional clinical effect of ergot. Brit. med. J. **I**, 520–523 (1935)
Embrey, M.P., Garrett, W.J.: A study of the effects of dihydroergotamine on the intact human uterus. J. Obstet. Gynaec. Brit. Emp. **62**, 150–154 (1955)
Emmenegger, H., Meier-Ruge, W.: The actions of Hydergine® on the brain. A histochemical, circulatory and neurophysiological study. Pharmacology **1**, 65–78 (1968)
Euler, U.S. v., Hesser, C.M.: Beobachtungen über Hemmungen der Sinusdruckreflexe durch Ergotamin, Dihydroergotamin und Hyperventilation. Schweiz. med. Wschr. **77**, 20–21 (1947)
Euler, U.S. v., Schmiterlöw, C.G.: The action of ergotamine on the chemical and mechanical reflexes from the carotid sinus region. Acta physiol. pharmacol. scand. **8**, 122–133 (1944)
Fanchamps, A.: Migraine and related types of headache—Pathogenesis and Therapy. S. Afr. Practit. **3**, 33–40 (1958)
Fanchamps, A., Doepfner, W., Weidmann, H., Cerletti, A.: Pharmakologische Charakterisierung von Deseril®, einem Serotonin-Antagonisten. Schweiz. med. Wschr. **90**, 1040–1046 (1960)
Flückiger, E.: Drugs and the control of prolactin secretion. In: Prolactin and Carcinogenesis. Proc. 4th Tenovus Workshop. Boyns, A.R., Griffiths, K. (eds.), pp. 162–180. Cardiff: Alpha Omega Alpha 1972
Flückiger, E.: Pharmacological characterization of CB 154 (bromocriptin). Triangle **14**, 153–157 (1975)
Flückiger, E., Billeter, E., Wagner, H.R.: Inhibition of lactation in rabbits by 2-Br-α-ergokryptine-mesilate (CB 154). Arzneimittel-Forsch. **26**, 51–53 (1976a)
Flückiger, E., Doepfner, W., Markó, M., Niederer, W.: Effects of ergot alkaloids on the hypothalamic-pituitary axis. Postgrad. med. J. **52** (Suppl. 1), 57–61 (1976b)

Flückiger, E., Lutterbeck, P.M., Wagner, H.R., Billeter, E.: Antagonism of 2-Br-α-ergokryptine-methanesulfonate (CB 154) to certain endocrine actions of centrally active drugs. Experientia (Basel) **28**, 924–925 (1972)

Flückiger, E., Wagner, H.R.: 2-Br-α-Ergokryptin: Beeinflussung von Fertilität und Laktation bei der Ratte. Experientia (Basel) **24**, 1130–1131 (1968)

Fozard, J.R.: The animal pharmacology of drugs in the treatment of migraine. In: Migraine and Related Headaches. Saxena, P.R. (ed.), pp. 93–118. Rotterdam: Erasmus University 1975a

Fozard, J.R.: The animal pharmacology of drugs used in the treatment of migraine. J. Pharm. Pharmacol. **27**, 297–321 (1975b)

Frantz, A.G., Kleinberg, D.L., Noel, G.L.: Studies on prolactin in man. Recent Progr. Hormone Res. **28**, 527–590 (1972)

Friesen, H., Hwang, P., Guyda, H., Tolis, G., Tyson, J., Myers, R.: A radioimmunoassay for human prolactin. In: Prolactin and Carcinogenesis. Proc. 4th Tenovus Workshop. Boyns, A.R., Griffiths, K. (eds.), pp. 64–80. Cardiff: Alpha Omega Alpha 1972

Gaddum, J.H., Hameed, K.A.: Drugs which antagonise 5-hydroxy-tryptamine. Brit. J. Pharmacol. **9**, 240–248 (1954)

Gygax, P., Meier-Ruge, W., Schulz, U., Enz, A.: Experimental studies on the action of metabolic and vasoactive substances in the oligemically disturbed brain. Arzneimittel-Forsch. **26**, 1245–1246 (1976)

Hart, I.C.: Effect of 2-bromo-α-ergocryptine on milk yield and the level of prolactin and growth hormone in the blood of the goat at milking. J. Endocr. **57**, 179–180 (1973)

Hart, I.C.: The relationship between lactation and the release of prolactin and growth hormone in the goat. J. Reprod. Fertil. **39**, 485–499 (1974)

Hill-Samli, M., MacLeod, R.M.: Thyrotropin-releasing hormone blockade of the ergocryptine and apomorphine inhibition of prolactin release in vitro. Proc. Soc. exp. Biol. (N.Y.) **149**, 511–514 (1975)

Hökfelt, T., Fuxe, K.: On the morphology and the neuroendocrine role of the hypothalamic catecholamine neurons. In: Brain-Endocrine Interaction. Knigge, K.M., Scott, D.E., Weindl, A. (eds.), pp. 181–223. Basel: Karger 1972

Hool-Zulauf, B., Stürmer, E.: Oxytocic activity of two dihydro-ergot peptide alkaloids on the rabbit uterus in situ. Naunyn-Schmiedeberg's Arch. Pharmacol. **293**, (Suppl.) R 35 (1976)

Hool-Zulauf, B., Stürmer, E.: Oxytocic activity of two dihydrogenated ergot peptide alkaloids on the rabbit uterus in situ. Arzneimittel-Forsch. **27**, 2323–2325 (1977)

Iwangoff, P., Enz, A., Chappuis, A.: Inhibition of cAMP-phosphodiesterase of different cat organs by DH-ergotoxine in the micromolar substrate range. Int. Res. Commun. System med. Sci. **3**, 403 (1975)

Johnson, A.M., Loew, D.M., Vigouret, J.M.: Stimulant properties of bromocriptine on central dopamine receptors in comparison to apomorphine, (+)-amphetamine and L-dopa. Brit. J. Pharmacol. **56**, 59–68 (1976)

Johnson, A.M., Vigouret, J.M., Loew, D.M.: Central dopaminergic actions of ergotoxine alkaloids and some derivatives. Experientia (Basel) **29**, 763 (1973)

Karg, H., Schams, D., Reinhardt, V.: Effects of 2-Br-α-ergocryptine on plasma prolactin level and milk yield in cows. Experientia (Basel) **28**, 574–576 (1972)

Kharasch, M.S., King, H., Stoll, A., Thompson, M.R.: The new ergot alkaloid. Science **83**, 206–207 (1936)

Kirchhof, A.C., Racely, C.A., Wilson, W., David, N.A.: An ergonovine-like oxytocic synthesized from lysergic acid. West. J. Surg. **52**, 197–208 (1944)

Konzett, H.: Specific antagonism of dibenamine to ergometrine. Ciba Foundation Symposium on Adrenergic Mechanisms. Wolstenholme, G.E.W., O'Connor, M. (eds.), pp. 463–465. London: Churchill 1960

Lance, J.W.: The Mechanism and Management of Headache. London: Butterworths 1969

Lance, J.W.: The pathophysiology and treatment of migraine. N.Z. med. J. **79**, 954–960 (1974)

Lieberman, A., Miyamoto, T., Battista, A.F., Goldstein, M.: Studies on the antiparkinsonian efficacy of lergotrile. Neurology (Minneap.) **25**, 459–462 (1975)

Loew, D.M., Vigouret, J.M., Jaton, A.L.: Neuropharmacological investigations with two ergot alkaloids, Hydergine and bromocriptine. Postgrad. med. J. **52** (Suppl. 1), 40–46 (1976)
Lutterbeck, P.M., Pryor, J.S., Varga, L., Wenner, R.: Treatment of non-puerperal galactorrhoea with an ergot alkaloid. Brit. med. J. **3**, 228–229 (1971)
MacLeod, R.M., Lehmeyer, J.E.: Studies on the mechanism of the dopamine-mediated inhibition of prolactin secretion. Endocrinology **94**, 1077–1085 (1974)
Markó, M., Flückiger, E.: Inhibition of spontaneous and induced ovulation in rats by non-steroidal agents. Experientia (Basel) **30**, 1174–1176 (1974)
Markstein, R., Wagner, H.: The effect of dihydroergotoxin, phentolamine and pindolol on catecholamine-stimulated adenylcyclase in rat cerebral cortex. FEBS Lett. **55**, 255–257 (1975)
Markstein, R., Wagner, H.: Effect of dihydroergotoxine on cyclic AMP generating systems in rat cerebral cortex slices. Gerontology (1978) (in press)
Matejcek, M., Devos, J.E.: Selected methods of quantitative EEG analysis and their applications in psychotropic drug research. In: Quantitative Analytic Studies in Epilepsy. Kellaway, P., Petersen, I. (eds.), pp. 183–205. New York: Raven Press 1976
Mayer, P., Schütze, E.: Effect of 2-Br-α-ergokryptine (CB 154) on lactation in the bitch. Experientia (Basel) **29**, 484–485 (1973)
Meier, J., Schreier, E.: Human plasma levels of some anti-migraine drugs. Headache **16**, 96–104 (1976)
Meier-Ruge, W., Enz, A., Gygax, P., Hunziker, O., Iwangoff, P., Reichlmeier, K.: Experimental pathology in basic research of the aging brain. In: Aging. Gershon, S., Raskin, A. (eds.), Vol. II, pp. 55–126. New York: Raven Press 1975
Mellander, S., Nordenfelt, I.: Comparative effects of dihydroergotamine and noradrenaline on resistance, exchange and capacitance functions in the peripheral circulation. Clin. Sci. **39**, 183–201 (1970)
Miller, J.W.: Adrenergic receptors in the myometrium. Ann. N.Y. Acad. Sci. **139**, 788–798 (1967)
Miller, M.D., Marshall, J.M.: Uterine response to nerve stimulation; relation to hormonal status and catecholamines. Amer. J. Physiol. **209**, 859–865 (1965)
Moir, C.: The action of ergot preparations on the puerperal uterus. Brit. med. J. **I**, 1119–1122 (1932)
Müller-Schweinitzer, E.: Responsiveness of isolated canine cerebral and peripheral arteries to ergotamine. Naunyn-Schmiedeberg's Arch. Pharmacol. **292**, 113–118 (1976)
Müller-Schweinitzer, E., Stürmer, E.: Investigations on the mode of action of ergotamine in the isolated femoral vein of the dog. Brit. J. Pharmacol. **51**, 441–446 (1974)
Nagasawa, H., Yanai, R., Flückiger, E.: Counteraction by 2-Br-α-ergocryptine of pituitary prolactin release promoted by dibutyryladenosine 3′,5′-monophosphate in rats. In: Human Prolactin. Pasteels, J.L., Robyn, C. (eds.), pp. 313–315. Amsterdam: Excerpta Medica 1973
Niswender, G.D.: Influence of 2-Br-α-ergocryptine on serum levels of prolactin and the estrous cycle in sheep. Endocrinology **94**, 612–615 (1974)
Nordenfelt, I., Mellander, S.: Central haemodynamic effects of dihydroergotamine in patients with orthostatic hypotension. Acta med. scand. **191**, 115–120 (1972)
Ostfeld, A.M., Chapman, L.F., Goodell, H., Wolff, H.G.: Studies in headache. Summary of evidence concerning a noxious agent active locally during migraine headache. Psychosom. Med. **19**, 199–208 (1957)
Owen, D.A.A., Herd, J.K., Kalberer, F., Pacha, W., Salzmann, R.: The influence of ergotamine and methysergide on the storage of biogenic amines. In: Proceedings of the International Headache Symposium, Elsinore, 16–18 May, 1971. Dalessio, D.J., Dalsgaard-Nielsen, T., Diamond, S. (eds.), pp. 153–161. Basle: Sandoz 1971
Owen, D.A.A., Stürmer, E.: The effects of ergotamine and dihydroergotamine on skin and skeletal muscle vasculature. Experientia (Basel) **28**, 743 (1972)
Pacha, W., Salzmann, R.: Inhibition of the re-uptake of neuronally liberated noradrenaline and alpha-receptor blocking action of some ergot alkaloids. Brit. J. Pharmacol. **38**, 439–440 (1970)
Pasteels, J.L., Danguy, A., Frérotte, M., Ectors, F.: Inhibition de la sécrétion de prolactine

par l'ergocornine et la 2-Br-α-ergocryptine: action directe sur l'hypophyse en culture. Ann. Endocr. (Paris) **32**, 188–192 (1971)

Pichler, E., Lazarini, W., Filippi, R.: Über schraubenförmige Struktur von Arterien. II. Mitt.: Pharmakologische Strukturanalyse von Hirnarterien. Naunyn-Schmiedeberg's Arch. exp. Path. Pharmac. **219**, 420–439 (1953)

Rothlin, E.: Recherches expérimentales sur l'ergotamine, alcaloïde spécifique de l'ergot de seigle. Arch. int. Pharmacodyn. **27**, 459–479 (1923)

Rothlin, E.: Beitrag zur differenzierenden Analyse der Mutterkornalkaloide. Schweiz. med. Wschr. **33**, 971–975 (1938)

Rothlin, E.: The pharmacology of the natural and dihydrogenated alkaloids of ergot. Bull. schweiz. Akad. med. Wiss. **2**, 249–272 (1947)

Rothlin, E., Berde, B.: Über die Wirkung hydrierter Mutterkornalkaloide auf isolierte Muskelstreifen des menschlichen Uterus nahe am Termin, am Termin und während der Geburt. Helv. physiol. pharmacol. Acta **12**, 191–205 (1954)

Rothlin, E., Bircher, R.: Allergy, the autonomic nervous system and ergot alkaloids. Progr. Allergy **3**, 434–484 (1952)

Rothlin, E., Cerletti, A.: Untersuchungen über die Kreislaufwirkung des Ergotamin. Helv. physiol. pharmacol. Acta **7**, 333–370 (1949)

Roubicek, J., Geiger, Ch., Abt, K.: An ergot alkaloid preparation (Hydergine) in geriatric therapy. J. Amer. Geriat. Soc. **20**, 222–229 (1972)

Roubicek, J., Matejcek, M., Montague, S.: The EEG in old age. Electroenceph. clin. Neurophysiol. **34**, 718 (1973)

Saxena, P.R.: The effects of antimigraine drugs on the vascular responses by 5-hydroxytryptamine and related biogenic substances on the external carotid artery bed of dogs: Possible pharmacological implications to their antimigraine action. Headache **12**, 44–54 (1972)

Saxena, P.R.: Selective vasoconstriction in carotid vascular bed by methysergide: Possible relevance to its antimigraine effect. Europ. J. Pharmacol. **27**, 99–105 (1974)

Saxena, P.R., Vlaam-Schluter, G.M. de: Role of some biogenic substances in migraine and relevant mechanism in antimigraine action of ergotamine—studies in an experimental model for migraine. Headache **13**, 142–163 (1974)

Schams, D., Reinhardt, V., Karg, H.: Effects of 2-Br-α-ergokryptine on plasma prolactin level during parturition and onset of lactation in cows. Experientia (Basel) **28**, 697–699 (1972)

Schmidt, R., Fanchamps, A.: Effect of caffeine on intestinal absorption of ergotamine in man. Europ. J. clin. Pharmacol. **7**, 213–216 (1974)

Shelesnyak, M.C.: Ergotoxine inhibition of deciduoma formation and its reversal by progesterone. Amer. J. Physiol. **179**, 301–304 (1954)

Shelesnyak, M.C.: Maintenance of gestation in ergotoxine-treated pregnant rats by exogenous prolactin. Acta endocr. (Kbh.) **27**, 99–109 (1958)

Sicuteri, F.: Prophylactic and therapeutic properties of 1-methyl-lysergic acid butanolamide in migraine. Int. Arch. Allergy **15**, 300–307 (1959)

Sinha, Y.N., Salocks, C.B., Lewis, U.J., Vanderlaan, W.P.: Influence of nursing on the release of prolactin and GH in mice with high and low incidence of mammary tumors. Endocrinology **95**, 947–954 (1974)

Sinha, Y.N., Selby, F.W., Vanderlaan, W.P.: Effects of ergot drugs on prolactin and growth hormone secretion, and on mammary nucleic acid content in C3H/Bi mice. J. nat. Cancer Inst. **52**, 189–191 (1974)

Smith, V.G., Beck, T.W., Convey, E.M., Tucker, H.A.: Bovine serum prolactin, growth hormone, cortisol and milk yield after ergocryptine. Neuroendocrinology **15**, 172–181 (1974)

Stadler, P.A., Stürmer, E.: Comparative studies on the pharmacological properties of stereoisomers of ergotamine and dihydroergotamine. Naunyn-Schmiedeberg's Arch. Pharmac. **266**, 457 (1970)

Stadler, P.A., Stürmer, E.: Synthese und biologische Aktivitäten einiger Stereoisomeren von Ergotamin und Dihydro-ergotamin. Chimia **26**, 321 (1972)

Stähelin, H., Burckhardt-Vischer, B., Flückiger, E.: Rat mammary cancer inhibition by a prolactin suppressor, 2-bromo-α-ergokryptine (CB 154). Experientia (Basel) **27**, 915–916 (1971)

Stoll, A.: Ergot—a treasure house for drugs. Pharm. J. **194**, 605–613 (1965)
Stoll, A., Hofmann, A.: Partialsynthese von Alkaloiden vom Typus des Ergobasins. 6. Mitt. über Mutterkornalkaloide. Helv. chim. Acta **26** (Fasc. 3), 944–965 (1943)
Stürmer, E., Flückiger, E.: In vivo smooth muscle stimulant activity of 2-bromo-α-ergokryptine mesylate (CB 154) as compared with that of ergotamine. Int. Res. Commun. System med. Sci. **2**, 1591 (1974)
Suchowsky, G.K., Pegrassi, L.: Action of nicergoline on electroencephalographic recovery after cat brain ischemia. Naunyn-Schmiedeberg's Arch. Pharmacol. **284**, 311–318 (1974)
Takahara, J., Arimura, A., Schally, A.V.: Suppression of prolactin release by a purified porcine PIF preparation and catecholamines infused into a rat hypophysial portal vessel. Endocrinology **95**, 462–465 (1974)
Tashjian, A.H., Hoyt, R.F.: Transient control on organ specific functions in pituitary cells in culture. In: Molecular Genetics and Development Biology. Sussman, M. (ed.), pp. 353–387. New Jersey: Englewood Cliffs 1972
Thorner, M.O., Besser, G.M.: Successful treatment of acromegaly with bromocriptine. Postgrad. med. J. **52** (Suppl. 1), 71–74 (1976)
Toda, N., Fujita, Y.: Responsiveness of isolated cerebral and peripheral arteries to serotonin, norepinephrine and transmural electrical stimulation. Circulat. Res. **33**, 98–104 (1973)
Weidmann, H., Taeschler, M.: Influence des substances antimigraineuses sur les effets des catécholamines, de la sérotonine et de la stimulation des nerfs sympathiques. Discussion du mode d'action des antimigraineux. In: Symposium International sur les Céphalées Vasculaires, St. Germain-en-Laye, 15–16 octobre, 1966, pp. 33–40
Wolff, H.G.: Pain mechanisms and headache. Triangle **2**, 53–64 (1955)
Wolff, H.G.: Headache and Other Head Pain. London-New York: Oxford U. Pr. 1963
Yanai, R., Nagasawa, H.: Effects of ergocornine and 2-Br-α-ergokryptin (CB-154) on the formation of mammary hyperplastic alveolar nodules and the pituitary prolactin levels in mice. Experientia (Basel) **26**, 649–650 (1970)

CHAPTER II

Chemical Background

J. RUTSCHMANN and P.A. STADLER

The scope of this book covers a class of natural alkaloids and their synthetic derivatives containing the tetracyclic ergoline ring system (Fig. 1), which is a partly hydrogenated indolo[4,3-fg]quinoline.

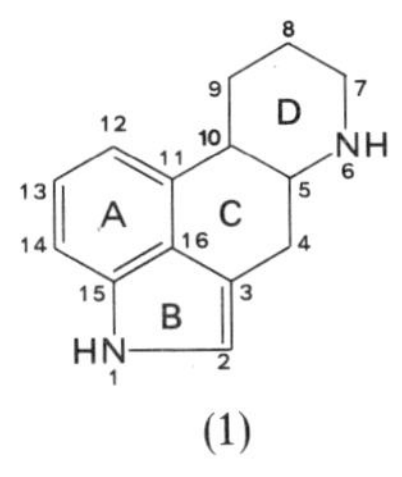

(1)

Fig. 1. Ergoline

It is the purpose of this chapter to provide in short form the chemical background to the pharmacologically oriented reader of the present volume. The more chemically inclined are referred to the detailed monographs on ergot alkaloid chemistry (HOFMANN, 1964; STOLL and HOFMANN, 1965; STADLER and STÜTZ, 1975; BERNARDI, 1969; SEMONSKY, 1970).

A. Occurrence, Biosynthesis, and Production

1. Presence of Ergot Alkaloids in the Plant Kingdom

Ergoline alkaloids have been found in scattered species of fungi belonging to different groups (phycomycetes, ascomycetes, basidiomycetes). Their main occurrence, however, is in ergot—the sclerotia of species of Claviceps—parasitic fungi living on the ears of rye and other grasses. Interestingly enough, representatives of the different classes of ergot alkaloids identical with some of the fungal metabolites have also been found in one group of flowering plants, the convolvulaceae (HOFMANN and TSCHERTER, 1960; HOFMANN, 1961).

2. Biogenesis

The problem of the biogenesis of ergot alkaloids has been solved as far as the building blocks used by the Claviceps fungus are concerned, but many questions on the mechanism of the formation of rings C and D, the formation of the amides, and especially of the cyclol moiety of the peptide alkaloids remain to be answered.

The ergolene system is assembled from a molecule of L-tryptophan (2) and an isoprenoid unit originating from mevalonic acid (3) (Fig. 2). The intermediate 4-dimethylallyl-L-tryptophan (4) is then transformed in a number of steps, including decarboxylation, oxidation, and cyclization, into agroclavine (5), which is further oxidized in the 8-methyl group to elymoclavine (6) and 6-methyl-8-ergolene-8-carboxylic acid (7). This ultimately isomerizes to d-lysergic acid (8) or its derivatives, respectively. The N-methyl group in 6 is introduced in one of the steps between (4) and (5) by L-methionine. The literature up to 1968 is covered by review articles of RAMSTAD, 1968; VOIGT, 1968a, 1968b, 1968c; GRÖGER, 1969.

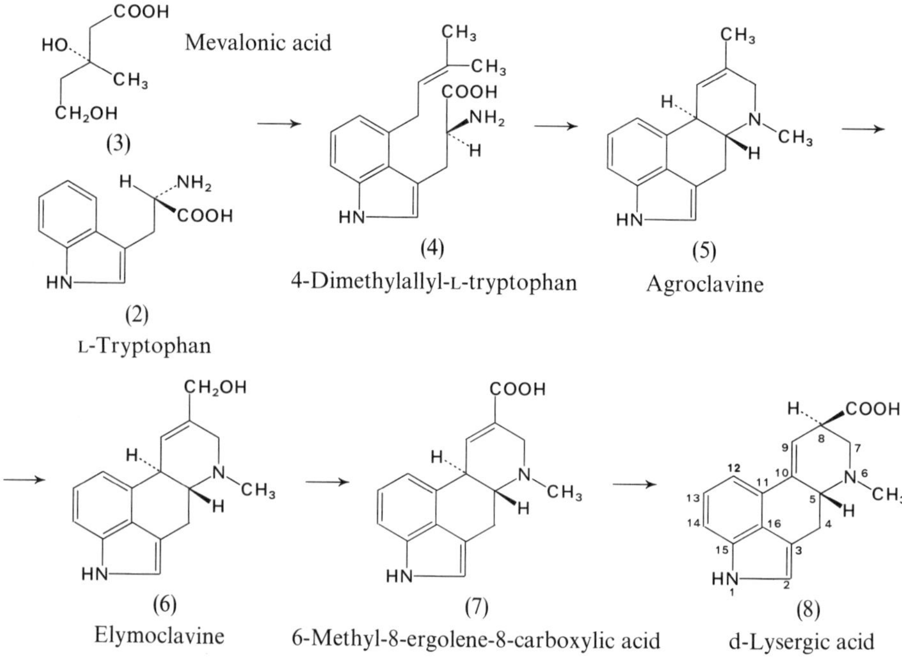

(3) Mevalonic acid

(2) L-Tryptophan

(4) 4-Dimethylallyl-L-tryptophan

(5) Agroclavine

(6) Elymoclavine

(7) 6-Methyl-8-ergolene-8-carboxylic acid

(8) d-Lysergic acid

Fig. 2. Biogenesis of lysergic acid

For the biosynthesis of the peptide alkaloids (Fig. 3) the evidence collected so far is best compatible with the hypothesis that the tricyclic cyclol moiety is built up linearly, presumably on an enzyme carrier, from L-proline and two other variable L-α-amino acids. The tripeptide (9) is then acylated with d-lysergic acid to (10) and cyclized to (11). The cyclization involves the formation of a lactam ring on the L-proline and formation of the cyclol system for which α-hydroxylation of the amino acid neighboring lysergic acid is a probable prerequisite (FLOSS et al., 1974).

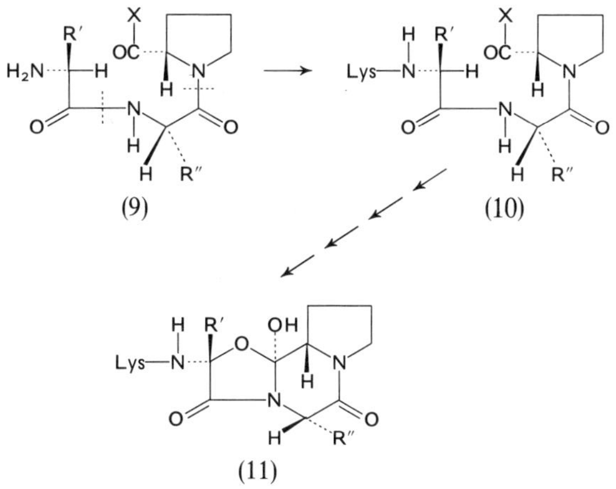

Lys = d-lysergoyl
X = supposedly a sulfur atom linked to an enzyme

Fig. 3. Biogenesis of peptide alkaloids

3. Production

The classical method for the manufacture of ergot alkaloids is isolation from the Claviceps sclerotia. A considerable part of the medicinally important peptide alkaloids are still prepared in this way, the fungal material being mainly produced by artificial infection of rye (grown in the field) with selected strains of the Claviceps fungus (STOLL, 1942).

There are, however, two alternative paths for the preparation of the compounds. The first (Fig. 4) consists in the production of lysergic acid by saprophytic cultivation of appropriate ergot strains in fermenters (KELLEHER, 1970) and subsequent chemical manipulation of the primary products. These are, depending on the strains

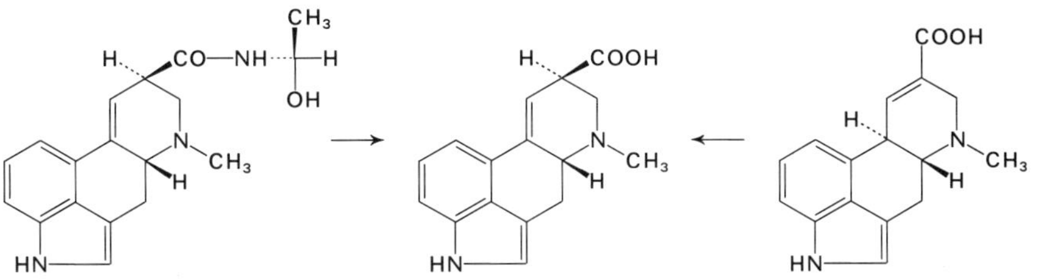

(12) d-Lysergic acid methylcarbinolamide

(8) d-Lysergic acid

(7) 6-Methyl-8-ergolene-8-carboxylic acid

Fig. 4. Technical preparation of lysergic acid

used, either lysergic acid methylcarbinolamide (12) (ARCAMONE et al., 1960), which has to be hydrolyzed, or 6-methyl-8-ergolene-8-carboxylic acid (7), (KOBEL et al., 1964), which isomerizes under mild conditions to lysergic acid (8). (This is a simplification insofar as both cases result in mixtures of lysergic and isolysergic acid.) From the key intermediates (7) and (8), all the important natural alkaloids, their analogues, and numerous derivatives can be synthetically produced.

The second route, which is gaining increasing technical importance, is the direct production of peptide alkaloids by fermentation of suitable ergot strains (KOBEL, 1974).

B. Structure and Synthesis of the Natural Alkaloids

1. General Structural Aspects

In the naturally occurring compounds, the basic ergoline system (1), (Fig. 1), is methylated at the nitrogen atom in position 6 and carries a further C-atom at position 8. Furthermore, in most cases there is a double bond in the 8-9 or 9-10 positions. The corresponding systems are called 8-ergolene and 9-ergolene. In consequence of this substitution pattern, there are in the ergolene derivatives two asymmetric centers giving rise to stereoisomerism in position 5 and 10 or 5 and 8, respectively. The relative and absolute configurations of all important alkaloids have been elucidated (STOLL and HOFMANN, 1950; STOLL et al., 1954; STADLER et al., 1963; HOFMANN et al., 1963). The 5-H-atom always has the β-configuration (LEEMANN and FABBRI, 1959; STADLER and HOFMANN, 1961). In all 8-ergolenes, general formula (13), (with one minor exception) the 10-H-atom is α, that is trans to the 5-H. In the 9-ergolenes, the asymmetric center in position 8 generally gives rise to pairs of diastereomers, an aspect of ergot chemistry which will be discussed below (STOLL et al., 1949a). Traditionally, in many important instances, the α-isomer (15) is distinguished from the β-form (14) (e.g., d-lysergic acid, ergotamine) by the prefix iso- (e.g., d-isolysergic acid) or by the ending -inine (e.g., ergotaminine).

These statements may be summarized in the following general structural formulae:

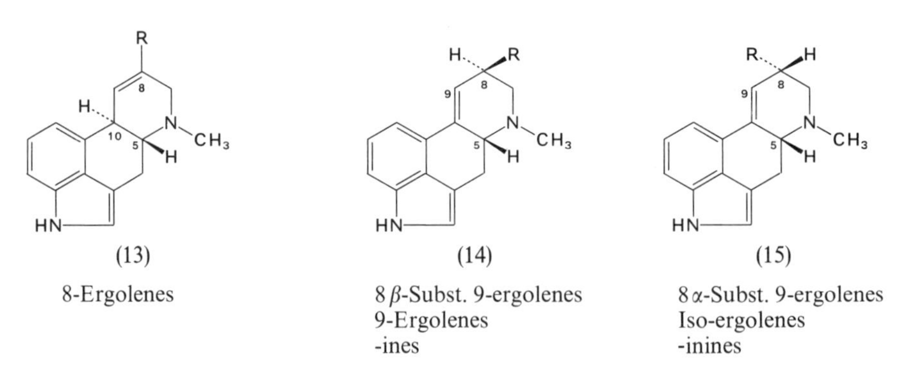

Fig. 5. General structural formulae of ergot derivatives

Although concerning mainly partially synthetic derivatives, one further feature of the stereochemistry of the lysergic acid skeleton may conveniently be mentioned here: If the double bond of the 9-ergolene alkaloids is hydrogenated, as is the case for a number of medicinally important compounds, a new asymmetric center is created at position 10 and consequently, at least in principle, two stereochemical series of derivatives arise (JACOBS and CRAIG, 1936c; STOLL and HOFMANN, 1943c; STOLL et al., 1946). Only the 5,10-trans compounds of general formula (16), (Fig. 6), however, have hitherto been of importance.

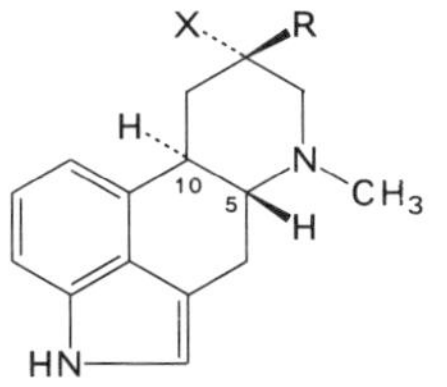

(16)

e.g.:
(16a): d-Dihydrolysergic acid
X = H, R = COOH

Fig. 6. General structural formula of dihydro ergot derivatives

For sake of simplicity, a semirational nomenclature is used for ergot peptide alkaloids, which is presented in Figure 7. The basic skeleton of the ergot peptide alkaloids, represented by formula (17), is called ergopeptine. It contains a complete lysergic acid half and a peptide part reduced to the tricyclic ring system, all hetero atoms and the four asymmetric centers in their natural configurations. Additional groups of atoms can simply be described by prefixes, supplied with the corresponding numbers of the position to which they are attached. To indicate stereochemistry of substituents the prefixes α and β are used: β means that the substituents are cis to the hydrogen atom in 5; the prefix α is used for trans-substituents.

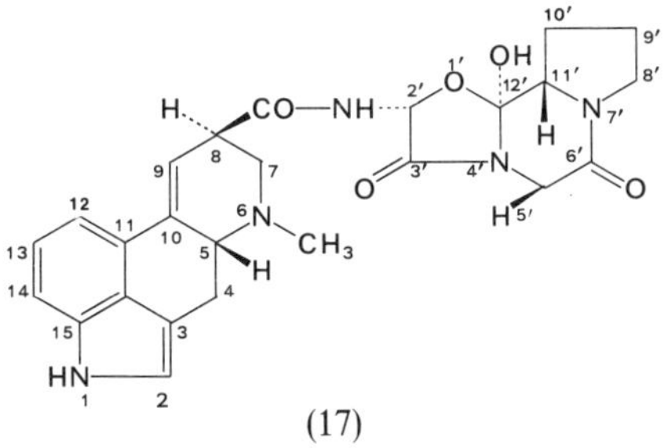

(17)

"Ergopeptine"

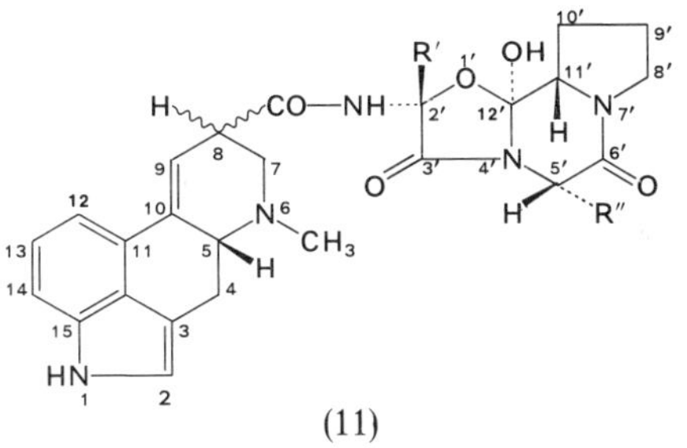

(11)

General formula of ergot peptide alkaloids
R′ = Methyl, ethyl, isopropyl
R″ = Isopropyl, sec. butyl, isobutyl, benzyl

Fig. 7. Semirational nomenclature and general formula of peptide alkaloids

2. Structure of Ergot Alkaloids

Depending on the nature of the substituent R in Figure 5, four main classes of ergot alkaloids can be distinguished:

1. The clavine alkaloids, where R is methyl or hydroxymethyl. (A number of compounds with modified or opened ring D and additional substitution are also included in this group but will not be referred to in this volume.)
2. The lysergic acids, where R is a carboxyl group.
3. The simple lysergic acid amides, having an unsubstituted or substituted carboxamide group.
4. The peptide alkaloids in which the nitrogen of the carboxamide group is part of a complex tripeptide moiety of the cyclol type, general formula (11) (Stoll et al., 1951).

The naturally found members of groups 1 and 2 belong predominantly to the 8-ergolenes (13), whereas the amides of groups 3 and 4 seem to occur exclusively as 9-ergolenes (14) and (15).

The ergot alkaloids contain a number of unique structural features and are stereochemically complicated. Their structure elucidation is a long and complicated story and cannot be presented here, but a good review is available in Hofmann (1964). In principle, it involved the hydrolysis of the compounds into the lysergic acid moiety on the one hand (Jacobs and Craig, 1934a, 1934b, 1935a) and the products resulting from the amide or peptide part on the other (Jacobs and Craig, 1935b, 1935c, 1935d, 1936b; Stoll, 1945; Stoll and Hofmann, 1950).

The structure of lysergic acid was arrived at mainly by the classical means of chemical degradation (Jacobs and Craig, 1934b, 1935a, 1936a, 1936c, 1938,

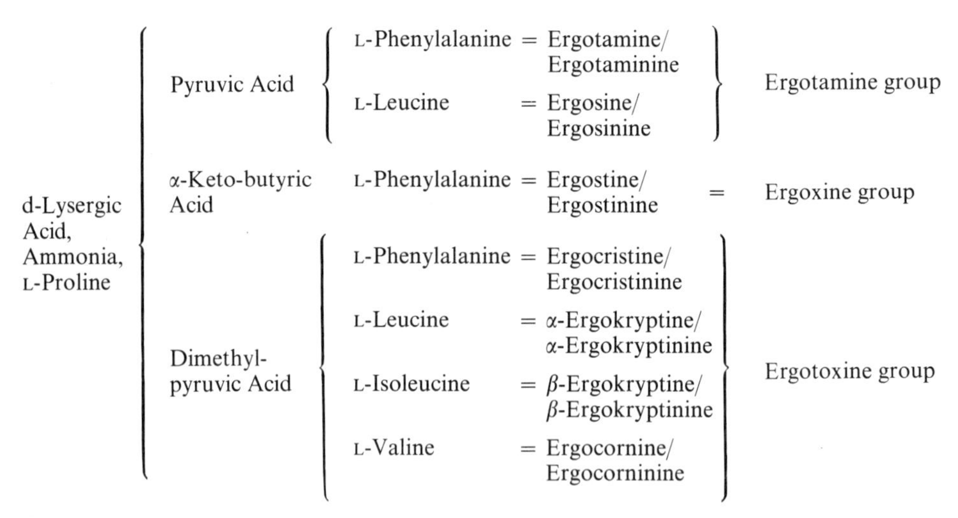

Fig. 8. The natural groups of ergot peptide alkaloids and their cleavage products resulting from hydrolysis

1939; STOLL et al., 1949a). Only for the clarification of the final details, especially the stereochemistry, were the more modern tools of physical chemistry available and used (COOKSON, 1953; STENLAKE, 1953; STOLL et al., 1954).

In Figure 8 the fission products of the natural ergot peptide alkaloids are represented. The single alkaloids form part of natural groups according to the type of keto acid they develop on hydrolysis.

One feature of the structure and chemical behavior of ergot alkaloids which complicated the chemical work all along must especially be mentioned. It is of great practical importance in the handling and application of all ergot alkaloids containing lysergic acid. This is the easy and spontaneous isomerization of the carboxy substituent at the asymmetric center in position 8, brought about by the neighborhood of the 9,10 double bond (STOLL et al., 1949a). This isomerization leads to equilibrium mixtures of derivatives of d-lysergic acid and d-isolysergic acid, the proportions of diastereomers in the equilibrium being determined by the nature of the amide substituent. The isomers show great differences in their chemical properties, such as basicity and solubility. *Only the d-lysergic acid derivatives with 8β-configuration are biologically active* and will be considered further on.

Figures 9 and 10 depict the structure and stereochemistry of the biologically important simple amide alkaloids d-lysergic acid amide (18), its isomer in 8 (18a), ergometrine (19), and the natural members of the peptide alkaloids.

The crystal structures of a number of ergopeptines have been determined (WEBER and PETCHER, Chapter III, Section E). The significance of the observed conformations in the solid state for the presumptive shape of the molecules in solution and when interacting with biological receptors will be discussed in the same chapter, where the three-dimensional structures of ergotamine and dihydroergotamine are also depicted.

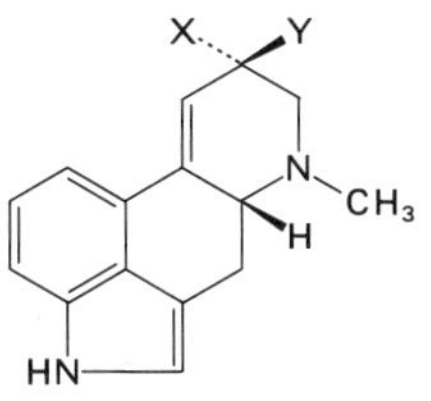

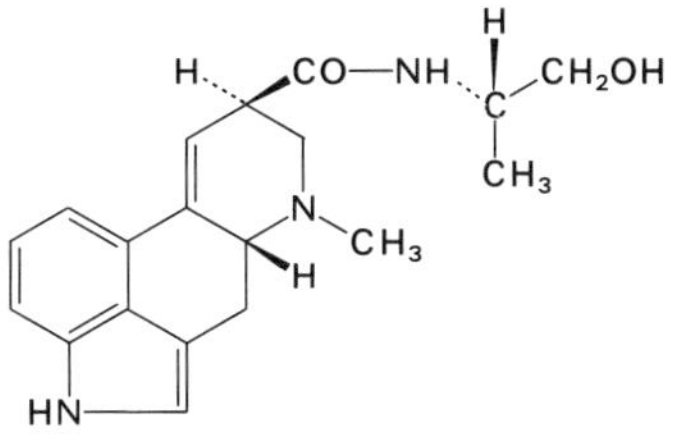

(19)

(18): d-Lysergic acid amide, ergine
X = H, Y = $CONH_2$

(18a): d-Isolysergic acid amide, isoergine
X = $CONH_2$, Y = H

Ergometrine
Ergobasine
Ergonovine
Ergotocine

Trade names:
Basergin
Ergometrin-S

Fig. 9. Structure of simple lysergic acid amides occurring in nature

Ergotamine group

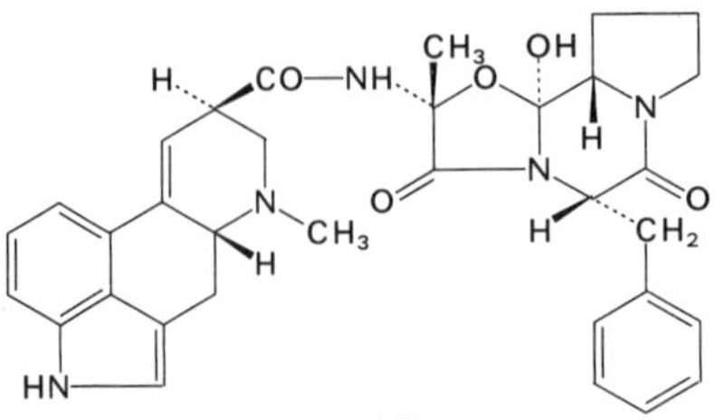

(20)
Ergotamine

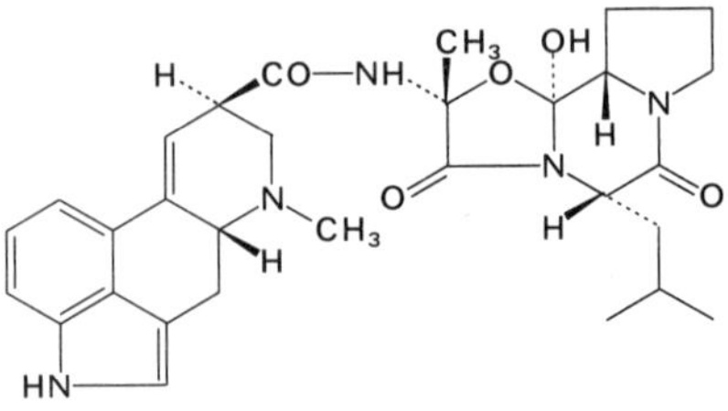

(21)
Ergosine

Ergoxine group

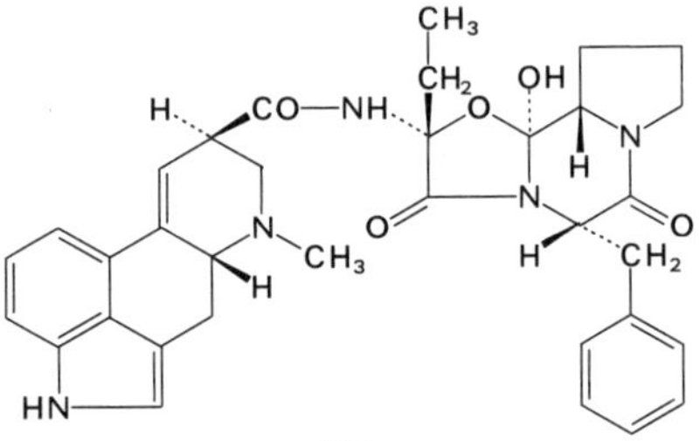

(22)
Ergostine

Ergotoxine group

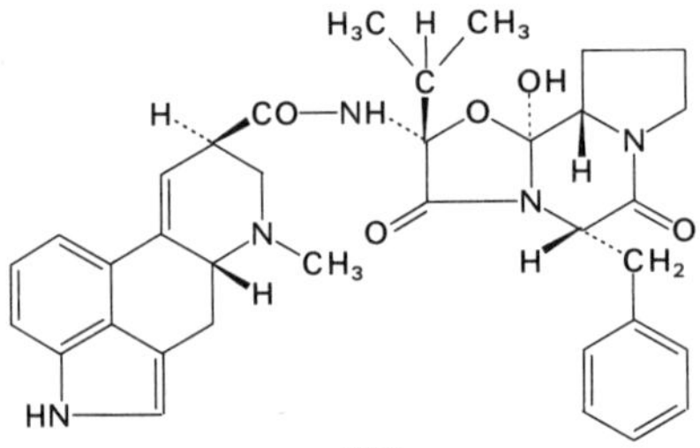

(23)
Ergocristine

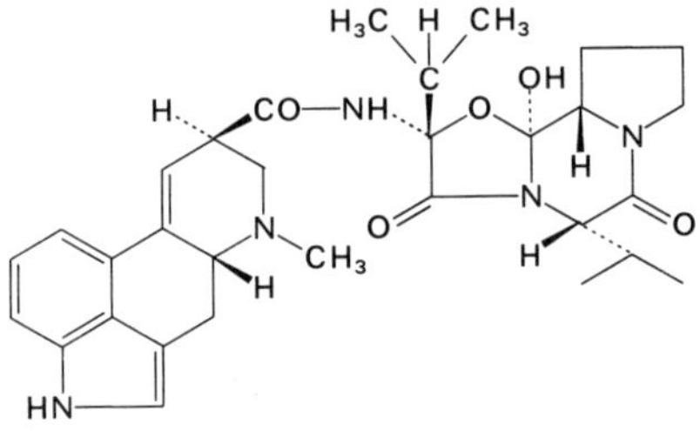

(24)
Ergocornine

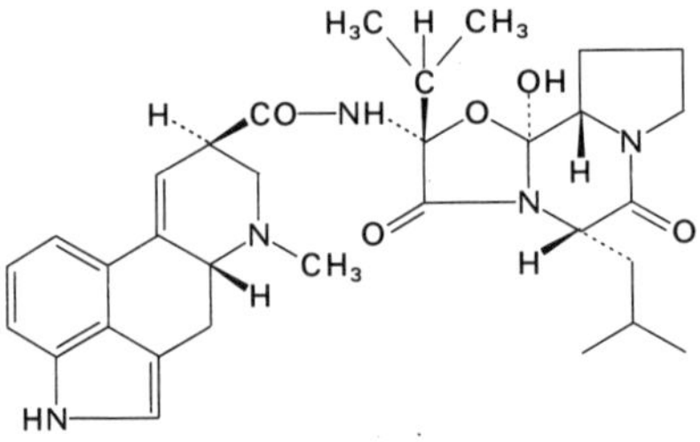

(25)
α-Ergokryptine

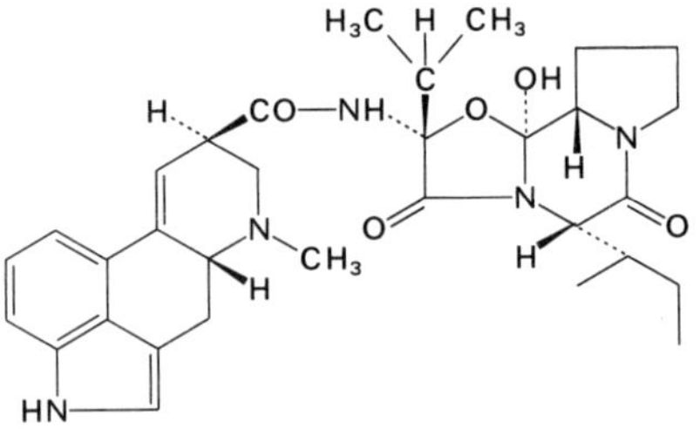

(26)
β-Ergokryptine

Fig. 10. Structure of natural ergot peptide alkaloids

From the stereoformulae of the levorotatory forms of ergot peptide alkaloids, listed above, the formulas of the corresponding dextrorotatory isoforms (e.g., ergotamine → ergotaminine) are obtainable by exchange of the substituents in position 8, i.e., substitution of the d-lysergyl moiety of the molecule by a d-isolysergyl half.
For sake of simplicity, the absolute configuration of the secondary butyl substituent at position 5′ in β-ergokryptine (26) and its derivatives (102f), (107e), (109a), (109b), (112a), and (112b) is not given; however, it has been determined in its parent substance L-isoleucine to be S (TROMMEL and BIJVOET, 1954).

3. Synthesis of Ergot Alkaloids

The total synthesis of all ergot alkaloids, and thus the formal confirmation of their structures, has been accomplished in two separate parts, the synthesis of the lysergic acid moiety on the one hand and of the peptide part on the other.

Preceded by two syntheses of d,l- and d-dihydrolysergic acid (UHLE and JACOBS, 1945; STOLL and RUTSCHMANN, 1950, 1953; STOLL et al., 1950a), d-lysergic acid was prepared by KORNFELD et al., (1954, 1956). All three synthetic sequences as well as an alternative for d-lysergic acid (JULIA et al., 1969) have, however, proved to be too complicated for practical application. As d-lysergic acid had already been transformed into its amides much earlier by procedures involving the activation of the carboxyl group by essentially classical procedures (STOLL and HOFMANN, 1937, 1938, 1943a, 1943b), the total synthesis of the simple alkaloids was solved by that of lysergic acid.

The total synthesis of the peptide part, including the novel cyclol and α-amino-α-hydroxy-acid elements and its coupling to lysergic acid, was realized later (HOFMANN et al., 1961; STADLER et al., 1963; HOFMANN et al., 1963; SCHLIENTZ et al., 1964; STADLER et al., 1969a). As this process is of technical importance for the preparation of certain natural peptide alkaloids as well as a number of artificial analogues, it is shown in Figure 11 in simple outline.

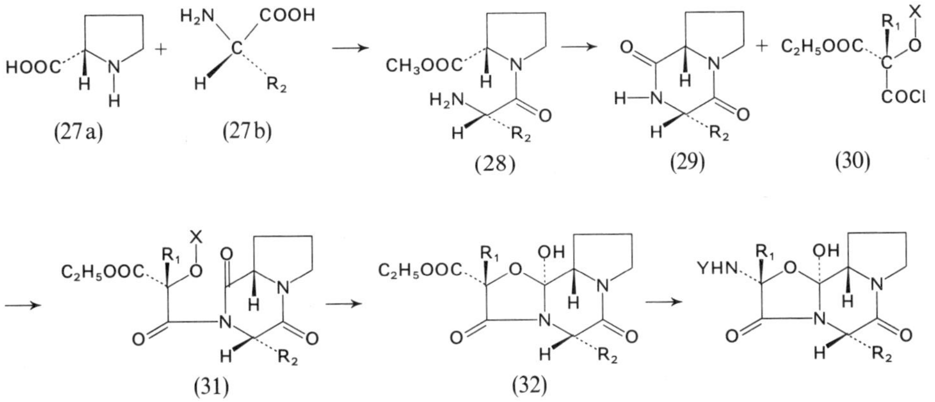

(27a) (27b) (28) (29) (30)

(31) (32)

R_1 = methyl, ethyl, isopropyl
R_2 = isopropyl, isobutyl, sec-butyl, benzyl
X = protecting group (benzyl)

(33a) Y = H · HCl
(33b) Y = Lysergoyl

Fig. 11. Total synthesis of ergot peptide alkaloids

Following established methods of peptide chemistry, L-proline (27a) was combined with a second L-amino acid (27b) to a dipeptide ester of general structure (28). Cyclization of (28) yielded the lactam (29), which was acylated with a third building block (30) containing an α-hydroxy-α-amino acid in masked form to give (31). This intermediate already contains the complete carbon skeleton of the peptide half, but it lacks the cyclol ring. This was formed spontaneously on removal of the protecting group X in (31), giving rise to (32). A modified Curtius degradation of the carbethoxy group in (32) finally led to (33a), the peptide half of ergot peptide alkaloids. Acylation of the free peptide part with d-lysergic acid chloride resulted in the corresponding ergot peptide alkaloids (33b).

C. Chemical Modifications in the Lysergic Acid Half of Ergot Alkaloids

Much work has been devoted to the chemical modification of biologically potent ergot alkaloids. Sections C and D cover this area.

1. Substitutions in Position 1

a) Alkylation

Derivatives of lysergic acid can be alkylated in liquid ammonia with alkyl halides under the influence of a strong base (TROXLER and HOFMANN, 1957a). In lysergic acid amides only does methylation proceed well to 1-methyl-lysergic acid amides of general formula (34) while dihydrolysergic acid amides are readily transformed to 1-alkyl-, 1-allyl-, or 1-benzyl-derivatives of general formula (35).

When tested on the isolated rat uterus, 1-methyl-d-lysergic acid L-2-butanolamide (34a) is a strong antagonist of serotonin. Its hydrogenmaleinate has been introduced into therapy under the trade names Deseril, Desernil, and Sansert, the generic name being Methysergide. 1-Methyl-d-lysergic acid diethylamide (34b) has gained some importance as starting material for the preparation of MBL-61 (37b). 1-Methyl-ergotamine (34c) has been in clinical investigation; the code name of its tartrate is MY-25. In the dihydro series, 1-methyl-dihydroergocristine, (35a) is an example.

b) Acylation and Mannich-Like Alkylations in Position 1

As already mentioned, the basicity of lysergic acid amides stems from the nitrogen atom in position 6 and not from the indole nitrogen in position 1, the latter being by no means basic. It may be for this reason that only special methods, i.e., the reaction of monoketene with lysergic acid amides, lead to 1-acetyl derivatives of general formula (36a), while 1-aceto-acetyl derivatives (36b) are formed from diketene. These substitution products are of limited stability, especially under basic conditions, and have found no applications (TROXLER and HOFMANN, 1957b).

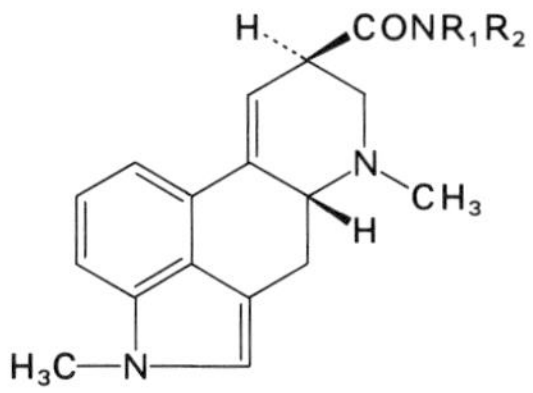

(34)

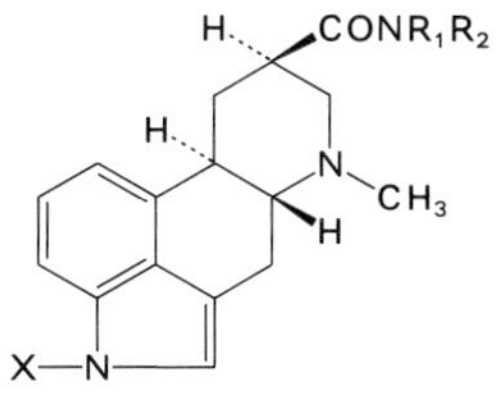

(35)

(34a): 1-Methyl-d-lysergic acid-L-2-butanolamide
R_1 = —H, R_2 = —$CH(CH_2OH)C_2H_5$
Trade names of the hydrogenmaleinate: Deseril, Desernil, Sansert
Generic: Methysergide

(34b): 1-Methyl-d-lysergic acid diethylamide
$R_1 = R_2$ = —C_2H_5

(34c): 1-Methyl-ergotamine
R_1 = —H, R_2 = -tripeptide part of ergotamine
Code name of tartrate: MY-25

(34d): 1-Methyl-lysergic acid pyrrolidide, (MPD 75)
R_1, R_2 = —$(CH_2)_4$—

(34e): 1-Methyl-lysergic acid ethylamide, (MLA 74)
$R_1 = C_2H_5$, R_2 = H

(35a): 1-Methyl-dihydroergocristine
X = CH_3, R_1 = —H, R_2 = -tripeptide part of ergocristine

(35b): 1-Methyl-dihydrolysergic acid L-2-butanolamide
R_1 = —H, R_2 = —$CH(CH_2OH)C_2H_5$
X = CH_3

Fig. 12. Ergot derivatives alkylated in position 1

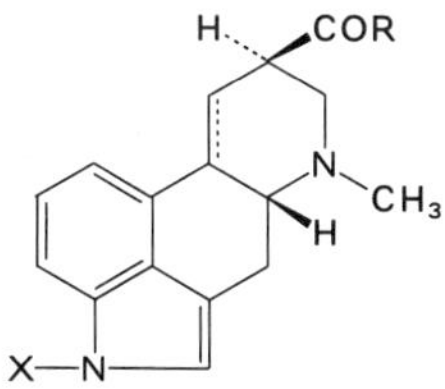

(36)

(36a): X = $COCH_3$
(36b): X = $COCH_2COCH_3$
(36c): X = CH_2OH
(36d): X = $CH_2N(CH_3)_2$
(36e): X = CH_2CH_2CN

R = OCH_3, NHR′, NR'_2

Examples

(36f): 1-Acetyl-LSD, (ALD 52)
X = $COCH_3$, R = $N(C_2H_5)_2$, Δ 9,10

(36g): 1-Acetyl-lysergic acid ethylamide, (ALA 10)
X = $COCH_3$, R = NHC_2H_5, Δ 9,10

(36h): 1-Hydroxymethyl-lysergic acid diethylamide, (OML 632)
X = CH_2OH, R = $N(C_2H_5)_2$, Δ 9,10

Fig. 13. Some further types of substitutions in position 1

Reaction of formaldehyde with lysergic acid esters or amides easily yielded the corresponding 1-hydroxymethyl derivatives of general formula (36c). It was, therefore, no surprise that a reaction of the Mannich type with formaldehyde and dimethylamine led to 1-dimethylaminomethyl lysergic acid derivatives, (36d). Michael addition of acrylonitrile gave rise to 1-cyanoethyl derivatives, formula (36e). All these compounds proved to be moderately stable against acids and bases. (TROXLER and HOFMANN, 1957b).

2. Substitutions in Position 2

From the chemical point of view, position 2 of the lysergic acid skeleton is very suitable for variation by partial synthesis. Subsequently, much synthetic work has been done in this direction, and it was found that some chemical variations in position 2 are able to induce great and sometimes selective changes in the biological potency of ergot derivatives.

a) Halogenation in Position 2

Ergot alkaloids can be halogenated by reagents capable of producing positive halogen ions; bromination of a variety of ergot substances could be achieved selectively in position 2 by application of N-bromosuccinimide in dioxane. Iodination was similarly performed by N-iodosuccinimide. Chlorination needed a somewhat more active chlorination agent. It has been shown to be effected best by application of the N-chloro-derivative of 2,6-dichloro-4-nitro-acetanilide (TROXLER and HOFMANN, 1957c).

By application of these halogenation reagents, a great number of 2-halogen derivatives of ergot substances have been prepared. Some of them that have attained pharmacologic or clinical significance are presented in Figure 14.

2-Bromo-d-lysergic acid diethylamide or 2-Bromo-LSD (37a) is known in the form of hydrogen tartrate under the code name BOL-148. A closely related compound is 1-methyl-2-bromo-lysergic acid diethylamide (37b), used as tartrate under the code name MBL-61. Both compounds are antagonists of serotonin of the same order of potency as LSD but lacking its central action (TROXLER and HOFMANN, 1957c).

2-Bromo-α-ergokryptine (38) has been discovered to be an inhibitor of prolactin secretion (FLÜCKIGER and WAGNER, 1968). Its methanesulfonate is known under the code name CB-154 and was introduced into therapy under the trade name Parlodel, with the generic name Bromocriptine.

2-Chloro-6-methyl-8β-cyanomethyl-ergoline (39), generic name Lergotrile, was synthesized in the research laboratories of Eli Lilly and Co. It proved to be an inhibitor of prolactin release (CLEMENS et al., 1974).

When dihydrolysergic acid or its derivatives are treated with excess pyridine hydrobromide perbromide, a double bromination results in position 2 and 13. Out of a series of semisynthetic compounds of this type, 2,13-dibromo-dihydrolysergic acid glycine-amide (40) has marked oxytocic activity in the rabbit uterus in situ. Its hydrogen tartrate is known under the code name RN-76 (RUTSCHMANN and SCHREIER, 1965).

(37)

(37a): 2-Bromo-LSD
$X = H$, $R_1 = R_2 = C_2H_5$
Hydrogen tartrate: BOL-148

(37b): 1-Methyl-2-bromo-LSD
$X = CH_3$, $R_1 = R_2 = C_2H_5$
Tartrate: MBL-61

(37c): 2-Bromo-ergocornine
$X = H$, $R_1 = H$, $R_2 =$ -tripeptide part of ergocornine

(38)

2-Bromo-α-ergokryptine-methansulfonate: CB-154, Parlodel, bromocriptine

(39)

(39): 2-Chloro-6-methyl-8β-cyanomethyl-ergoline, Lergotrile
$R = H$, $X = Cl$

(39a): 2-Bromo-6-methyl-8β-cyanomethyl-ergoline
$R = H$, $X = Br$

(39b): 2-Jodo-6-methyl-8β-cyanomethyl-ergoline
$R = H$, $X = J$

(39c): 1,6-Dimethyl-2-chloro-8β-cyanomethyl-ergoline
$R = CH_3$, $X = Cl$

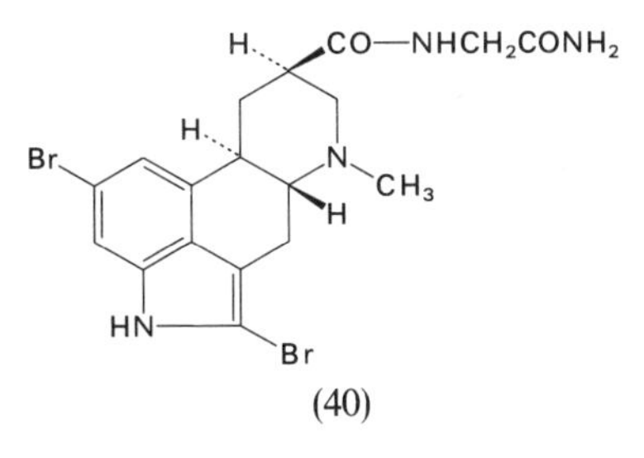

(40)

2.13-Dibromo-dihydrolysergic acid glycineamide
Hydrogen tartrate: RN-76

Fig. 14. Ergot derivatives substituted in position 2 by halogen

b) Miscellaneous Substitutions in Position 2

A series of different substitutions in positions 2 and 3, which have found only minor attention, are presented here in short.

Thus, treatment of dihydrolysergic acid or its amides with fuming nitric acid in acetic acid anhydride leads to the corresponding 2-nitro-derivatives in moderate yields (41). They could be reduced by catalytic hydrogenation to the unstable 2-amino-derivatives of general formula (42) which on acetylation give rise to the 2-acetamido-dihydrolysergic acid amides (43) (FRANCESCHI et al., 1965).

Under the influence of weak Lewis acids, e.g., of titanium tetrachloride, lysergic acid methylester reacted with 2-methoxy-1,3-dithiolane in a special Friedel-Crafts reaction to 2-dithiolanoyl-lysergic acid methylester, formula (44), $R=COOCH_3$. This compound was either hydrolyzed to the 2-formyl derivative (46) or reductively desulfurized with Raney nickel to 2-methyl-lysergic acid methylester (45) (STÜTZ and STADLER, 1972). A similar Friedel-Crafts type of reaction was performed with acetic acid anhydride and boron trifluoride (Fig. 15). It led to 2-acetyl-lysergic acid amides of the general formula (47).

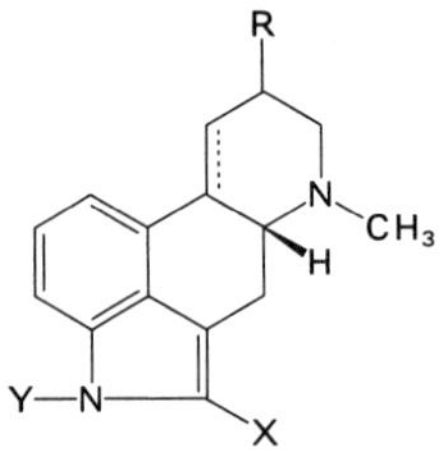

(41): $X = NO_2$
(42): $X = NH_2$
(43): $X = NHCOCH_3$

(44): X = 1,3-dithiolan-2-yl, $R = COOCH_3$
(45): $X = CH_3$, $R = COOCH_3$
(46): $X = CHO$, $R = COOCH_3$
(47): $X = COCH_3$, $R = CONR_1R_2$
(44)–(47): Δ 9,10

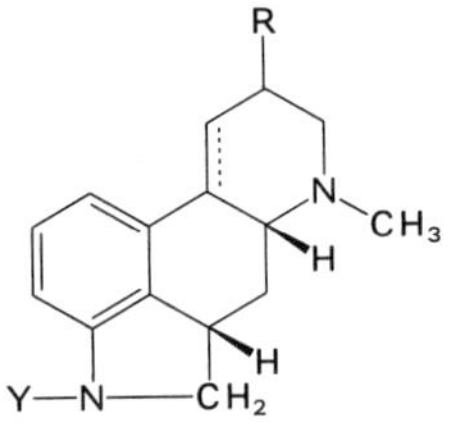

(48a): 1-Methyl-N-carbobenzoxy-2,3-9,10-tetrahydro-lysergylamine
$Y = CH_3$, $R = CH_2NHCOOCH_2C_6H_5$

(48b): 2,3-Dihydroergometrine
Y = H, R = CO · L-alaninol, Δ 9,10

(49): X = H, $R = CON(C_2H_5)_2$
(50): X = OH, $R = CON(C_2H_5)_2$

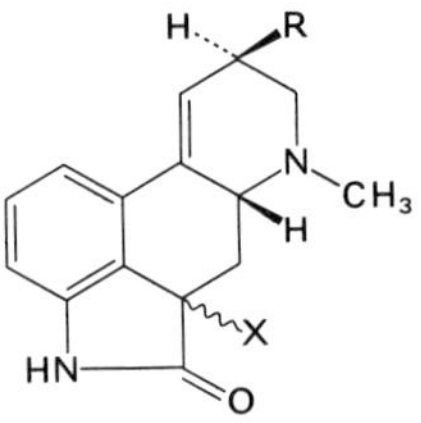

$R = COOH$, $COOCH_3$, $CONH_2$, CONH-Alkyl, $CON(Alkyl)_2$, CO-tripeptide
$Y = H$, CH_3

Fig. 15. Miscellaneous substitutions in positions 2 and 3

By reduction with zinc dust in hydrochloric acid, lysergic acid derivatives may be transformed to the corresponding 2,3-dihydro derivatives, examples being (48a) and (48b). The reaction is stereoselective in position 3; the double bond in position 9,10 is left unchanged (STADLER et al., 1964b; JOHNSON et al., 1973). Another method for the hydrogenation of the indole double bond in ergot derivatives has been described (ARCAMONE and FRANCESCHI, 1967). It is less general, as it is restricted to the preparation of 2,3-9,10-tetrahydro derivatives.

In 1956, it was observed that an enzyme system oxidizes LSD to a physiologically inactive metabolite, presumably of structure (49) (AXELROD et al., 1956). In context with this observation, work was initiated to prepare this metabolite synthetically. In a first approach, LSD was reacted with disulfur dichloride to a dimeric compound which on reduction in acidic medium gave a product identical with the metabolite (FRETER et al., 1957). Another method consisted in oxidation of LSD with hypochlorite to 2-oxo-3-hydroxy-2,3-dihydrolysergic acid diethylamide, formula (50), which could be reduced with zinc to the same metabolite (TROXLER and HOFMANN, 1959).

At last a special case of substitution in position 2 may be mentioned: When dihydrolysergic acid methylester was treated with strong acids, a dimer resulted in which a molecule of dihydrolysergic acid methylester was directly connected in position 2 by a chemical bond with position 2 of 2,3-9,10-tetrahydrolysergic acid methylester (BACH and KORNFELD, 1973).

3. Chemical Transformations in Positions 4 and 5

Until now, no chemical variations in position 4 of ergot substances have been published.

Concerning position 5, only one, but fundamental operation, namely the racemization, has been published. By means of a reaction sequence depicted in Figure 16, the *unnatural 1-form* of ergot alkaloids became accessible via the basic 1-isolysergic acid hydrazide (51) (STOLL and HOFMANN, 1937).

When ergot alkaloids of the peptide type were heated in hydrazine, the peptide part of the molecule was cleft off; however, in the lysergic acid half racemization and concomitant isomerization occurred to lead to *racemic* isolysergic acid hydrazide as the only product (STOLL and HOFMANN, 1937; STOLL et al., 1950b). By addition of di-(p-toluyl)-L-tartaric acid to racemic isolysergic acid hydrazide, a sparingly soluble salt, d-isolysergic acid hydrazide-di-(p-toluyl)-L-tartrate, was formed, which allowed the separation from the easily soluble diastereomeric salt by crystallization. Cleavage of this salt led to *d*-isolysergic acid hydrazide. Applying the antipodal di-(p-toluyl)-D-tartaric acid to racemic isolysergic acid hydrazide in the same procedure, the *unnatural l*-isolysergic acid hydrazide (51) was isolated (STOLL and HOFMANN, 1943a).

Starting from this compound the *optical antipodes* and some of the many possible *diastereomers* of ergot derivatives have been synthesized for the determination of structure-activity relations.

By transformations of (51) into the azide (52) an activated form of the carboxyl group became available, which reacted with almost any primary and secondary amine to the corresponding amide. Thus, condensation of (52) with D-alaninol consequently led to the antipode of ergometrinine (53), which was equilibrated to the antipode of ergometrine (56) in alkaline medium. Following the same procedure, all eight isomers of ergometrine, 1-lysergic acid amide (59), 1-isolysergic acid amide (60), 1-LSD (61), 1-iso-LSD (62), 1-lysergic acid 1-norephedride (63),

Ergot peptide alkaloids $\xrightarrow{\text{hydrazine}}$ *Racemic* isolysergic acid hydrazide

↓ di-(p-toluyl)-D-tartaric acid

(54): R = $CONHNH_2$ 1-Lysergic acid hydrazide	(51): R = $CONHNH_2$ 1-Isolysergic acid hydrazide
(55): R = CON_3 1-Lysergic acid azide	(52): R = CON_3 1-Isolysergic acid azide
(56): R = CO · D-alaninol, antipode of ergometrine	(53): R = CO · D-alaninol, antipode of ergometrinine
(57): R = COOH 1-Lysergic acid	(58): R = COOH 1-Isolysergic acid
(59): R = $CONH_2$ 1-Lysergic acid amide	(60): R = $CONH_2$ 1-Isolysergic acid amide
(61): R = $CO \cdot N(C_2H_5)_2$ 1-LSD	(62): R = $CO \cdot N(C_2H_5)_2$ 1-Iso-LSD
(63): R = $CO \cdot NH \cdot CHCH_3 \cdot CHOH \cdot C_6H_5$ 1-Lysergic acid 1-norephedride	(64): R = $CO \cdot NH \cdot CHCH_3 \cdot CHOH \cdot C_6H_5$ 1-Isolysergic acid 1-norephedride
(65): R = $NH \cdot CO \cdot N(C_2H_5)_2$	(66): R = $NH \cdot CO \cdot N(C_2H_5)_2$ 1-Lysenyl
(67): R = CO · peptide part in D-configuration, antipode of ergotamine	(68): R = CO · peptide part in D-configuration, antipode of ergotaminine
(69): R = CO · peptide part in L-configuration	(70): R = CO · peptide part in L-configuration

Fig. 16. Racemization in position 5, derivatives of 1-lysergic acid

and 1-isolysergic acid 1-norephedride (64) were synthesized (STOLL and HOFMANN, 1938, 1943b).

When 1-isolysergic acid azide (52) was heated in an inert solvent, it lost nitrogen. The intermediate isocyanate was converted to the antipode of Lysenyl (66) by addition of diethylamine. An analogous reaction sequence was performed with 1-lysergic acid azide (55). It gave rise to (65) (ZIKAN and SEMONSKY, 1963a).

When ergot peptide alkaloids had become available by total synthesis, these investigations were further extended: Saponification of 1-lysergic acid hydrazide (54) led to 1-lysergic acid (57), which was condensed with an antipodal peptide part of all-D-configuration to the antipodes of ergotamine (67) and ergotaminine

(68). Condensation of l-lysergic acid (57) with the natural peptide part of ergotamine led to the diastereomers (69) and (70) (STADLER and STÜRMER, 1970).

4. Replacement of the N-Methyl Group in Position 6 by Other Substituents

The total synthesis of racemic 6-nor-dihydrolysergic acid methylester (71 a) provided the first possibility for chemical variations in position 6: It was found that catalytic hydrogenation of (71a) in presence of aliphatic aldehydes led in good yield to racemic dihydrolysergic acid methylester (71 b) and its 6-alkyl-homologues. As an example, application of acetaldehyde gave (71c); hydrogenation in presence of n-hexanal led to (71 d) (STOLL and RUTSCHMANN, 1954).

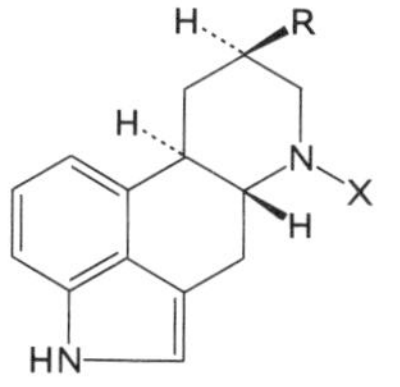

(71a): R = $COOCH_3$, X = H
(71b): R = $COOCH_3$, X = CH_3
(71c): R = $COOCH_3$, X = C_2H_5
(71d): R = $COOCH_3$, X = C_6H_{13}(n) } rac.
(71e): 6-Nor-6-isopropyl-dihydroergotamine
R = CO · tripeptide part of ergotamine,
X = isopropyl
(71f): 6-Nor-6-isopropyl-dihydroergocristine
R = CO · tripeptide part of ergocristine,
X = isopropyl

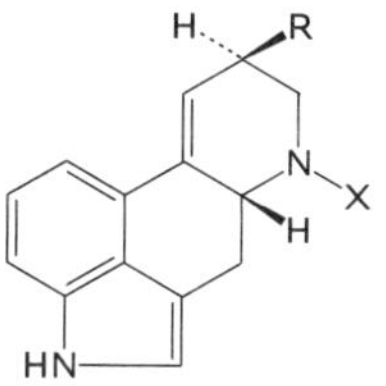

(72a): R = $COOCH_3$, X = CH_3
(72b): R = $COOCH_3$, X = CN
(72c): R = $COOCH_3$, X = H
(72d): R = $COOCH_3$, X = C_2H_5
(72e): R = COOH, X = C_2H_5
(72f): 6-Nor-6-isopropyl-ergotamine
R = CO · tripeptide part of ergotamine,
X = C_3H_7
(72g): R = CO · $N(C_2H_5)_2$, X = CN
(72h): R = CO · $N(C_2H_5)_2$, X = $CONH_2$
(72i): R = CO · $N(C_2H_5)_2$, X = H
(72k): R = CO · $N(C_4H_9)_2$, X = CN

Fig. 17. Substitutions in position 6

Direct demethylation at the nitrogen in position 6 of d-lysergic acid methylester (72a) could be realized later by new modifications of the von Braun degradation: By the action of cyanogen bromide on (72a), 6-nor-6-cyano-lysergic acid methylester (72b) was obtained, which could be reduced to 6-nor-d-lysergic acid methylester (72c) with zinc in acetic acid. It could then be selectively alkylated in position 6 by alkyl halogenides, e.g., to (72d). Saponification of (72d) finally led to (72e), the homologue of d-lysergic acid in position 6 (FEHR et al., 1970). Starting from homologues of type (72e), many new derivatives of d-lysergic acid, peptide alkaloids included, have been prepared (FEHR and STADLER, 1973a, 1973b). Here should be mentioned 6-nor-6-isopropyl-ergotamine (72f) and its dihydro-derivative (71e) (FEHR and STADLER, 1975).

A degradation of LSD has been described by a Japanese group (NAKAHARA and NIWAGUCHI, 1971). These authors saponified the intermediate 6-nor-6-cyano-LSD (72 g) by alkali to the urea (72h), which led to 6-nor-LSD (72i) on treatment with nitrous acid. Some 6-nor-6-cyano lysergic acid amides, e.g., the dibutyl amide (72k), have been prepared lately by PORTLOCK et al. (1975).

5. Reactions Involving Position 7

The only chemical transformation known at present is the preparation of an isomer of lysergic acid methylester with the double bond in position 7,8 (STÜTZ and STADLER, 1973).

6. Modifications of the Carboxylic Acid Function of d-Lysergic Acid

The synthetic versatility of the carboxyl group of d-lysergic acid has been the basis of its extended molecular manipulation.

a) Semisynthetic Lysergic- and Dihydrolysergic Acid Amides

Chronologically, the first method for new amides of lysergic acid was the azide process. It was successfully used for the first synthesis of ergometrine (19) (STOLL and HOFMANN, 1938), of ergine (18), and of a great number of secondary and tertiary amides of d-lysergic acid (STOLL and HOFMANN, 1943a, 1943b). Two of them have found medical application:

d-Lysergic acid-L-2-butanolamide (73a), the next higher homologue of the natural ergot alkaloid ergometrine (19), is a strong uterotonic agent; its hydrogen maleinate finds application in obstetrics under the trade name Methergine to reduce post-partum bleeding. Its generic names are Methylergometrine, Methylergobasine, and Methylergonovine.

d-Lysergic acid diethylamide (73b) is a powerful hallucinogenic agent. Its tartrate is known under the code name LSD-25; its trade name is Delyside; its generic name is Lysergidum.

Not being restricted to the synthesis of lysergic acid amides, the azide process was shown to be well suited also for the preparation of dihydrolysergic acid amides (STOLL et al., 1950c; STOLL and HOFMANN, 1955). An example is the synthesis of dihydrolysergic acid amide (74a), intermediates being (74d) and (74e).

During the last fifteen years, more economic processes for the technical preparation of amides of lysergic acid have been developed. They all start with d-lysergic acid, which has become easily accessible by microbiologic procedures (ARCAMONE et al., 1960; KOBEL et al., 1964). For example, one method of Eli Lilly and Co. employs the mixed anhydride of lysergic acid and sulfuric acid (GARBRECHT, 1959), while a second employs the mixed lysergic acid-trifluoroacetic anhydride (PIOCH, 1956). In a process of Spofa, N,N′-carbonyldiimidazole is used as condensation agent (CERNY and SEMONSKY, 1962). A process originating from the Sandoz Laboratories employs d-lysergic acid chloride hydrochloride for the preparation of the corresponding amides of lysergic acid (HOFMANN et al., 1961; FREY, 1965).

b) Esters of Lysergic and Dihydrolysergic Acid

Esterification of d-lysergic acid and its derivatives can be easily performed by the usual methods. Under acidic conditions, d-lysergic acid methylester (72a) can

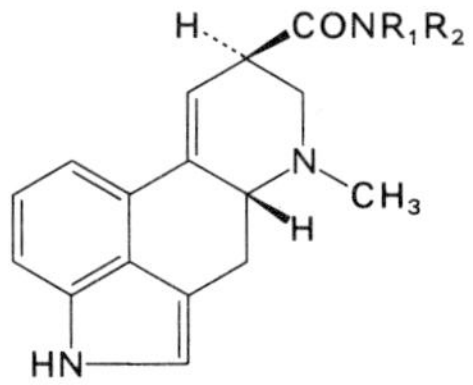

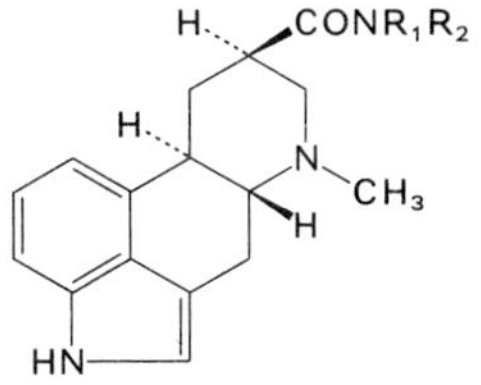

(73a): d-Lysergic acid-L-2-butanolamide
$R_1 = H$, $R_2 = CH(C_2H_5)CH_2OH$
Hydrogen maleinate:
Trade name: Methergine
Generics: Methylergobasine
Methylergometrine
Methylergonovine

(73b): d-Lysergic acid diethylamide
$R_1 = R_2 = C_2H_5$
Tartrate: LSD-25
Trade name: Delyside
Generic: Lysergidum

(73c): Lysergic acid dimethylamide, (DAM 57)
$R_1 = R_2 = CH_3$

(73d): Lysergic acid dipropylamide
$R_1 = R_2 = C_3H_7(n)$

(73e): Lysergic acid dibutylamide, (LBB 66)
$R_1 = R_2 = C_4H_9(n)$

(73f): Lysergic acid pyrrolidide, (LPD 824)
$R_1, R_2 = —(CH_2)_4—$

(73g): Lysergic acid morpholidide, (LSM 775)
$R_1, R_2 = —CH_2CH_2—O—CH_2CH_2—$

(73h): Lysergic acid ethyl amide, (LAE 32)
$R_1 = H$, $R_2 = C_2H_5$

(74a): Dihydrolysergic acid amide
$R_1 = R_2 = H$

(74b): Dihydrolysergic acid diethylamide
$R_1 = R_2 = C_2H_5$

(74c): Dihydroergometrine
$R_1 = H$, $R_2 = CH(CH_3)CH_2OH$

(74d): Dihydrolysergic acid hydrazide
$R_1 = H$, $R_2 = NH_2$

(74e): Dihydrolysergic acid azide
$R_1 = N$, $R_2 = N$

Fig. 18. Synthetic amides of d-lysergic acid and dihydrolysergic acid

be prepared in good yields, the resulting equilibrium with the 8α-epimer (75a) lying practically on the side of d-lysergic acid methylester. A great number of esters of d-lysergic acid and of its derivatives (1-methyl, dihydro, 1-methyl-dihydro e.c.) especially with diols have been described [(75c), GARBRECHT, 1969; (75d), HOFMANN and TROXLER, 1968].

c) Nitriles

d-Lysergic acid nitrile (77) is formed after treatment of d-lysergic acid amide, ergine (18) with phosphorous oxychloride or acetic acid anhydride (HOFMANN et al., 1964). An analogous reaction can be performed on dihydrolysergic acid amide (74a) with pyridine and p-toluenesulfonyl chloride which leads to dihydrolysergic acid nitrile (78) (BOSISIO et al., 1963).

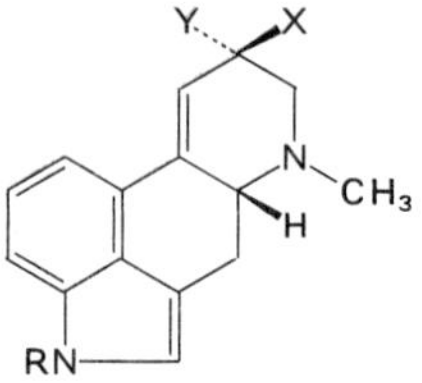

(72a): d-Lysergic acid methylester
R = H, X = $COOCH_3$, Y = H

(75a): d-Isolysergic acid methylester
R = H, X = H, Y = $COOCH_3$

(75b): 1-Methyl-d-lysergic acid methylester
R = CH_3, X = $COOCH_3$, Y = H

(75c):
R = H, X = $COOCH_2CH_2OH$, Y = H

(75d): R = H, X = $COOCH_2$–(3-pyridyl)
Y = H

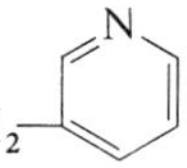

(77d): d-Lysergic acid nitrile
R = H, X = CN, Y = H

(79a): Lysergol
R = H, X = CH_2OH, Y = H

(79b): Lysergol acetate
R = H, X = CH_2OCOCH_3, Y = H

(79c): 6,8β-Dimethyl-9-ergolene
R = H, X = CH_3, Y = H

(79d): 6,8α-Dimethyl-9-ergolene
R = H, X = H, Y = CH_3

(79e): Isolysergol
R = H, X = H, Y = CH_2OH

(79f): Lysergene
R = H, X, Y = $=CH_2$

(79g): 6-Methyl-8-acetoxymethylen-9-ergolene
R = H, X, Y = $=CHOCOCH_3$

(79h): 6-Methyl-9-ergolene
R, X, Y = H

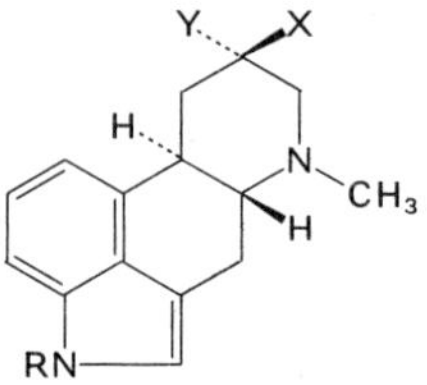

(76a): Dihydrolysergic acid methylester
R = H, X = $COOCH_3$, Y = H

(76b): 1-Methyl-dihydrolysergic acid methylester
R = CH_3, X = $COOCH_3$, Y = H

(78): Dihydrolysergic acid nitrile
R = H, X = CN, Y = H

(80): Dihydrolysergal
R = H, X = CHO, Y = H

(81a): Dihydrolysergol
R = H, X = CH_2OH, Y = H

(81b): 1-Methyl-dihydrolysergol
R = CH_3, X = CH_2OH, Y = H

Fig. 19. Ester-type derivatives of d-lysergic and dihydrolysergic acids and their reduction products

d) Lysergol and its Derivatives

Lysergol (79a) is a natural alkaloid of the clavine series (ABE et al., 1961). Moreover, it has been found in Rivea corymbosa (Convolvulaceae) (HOFMANN and TSCHERTER, 1960) and had already been obtained by reduction of d-lysergic acid methylester

(72a) with lithium aluminium hydride (STOLL et al., 1949b). The intermediate aldehyde of the dihydro series, dihydrolysergal (80), could be prepared by reduction of dihydrolysergic acid nitrile (78) with Raney nickel and sodium hypophosphite (TROXLER et al., 1968).

Besides lysergol, some of its derivatives, e.g., dihydrolysergol (81a) and 1-methyl-dihydrolysergol (81b), are important intermediates for partial synthesis on the side chain. Esters of lysergol with fatty acids, e.g., lysergol acetate (79b), are also pharmacologically active (EICH and ROCHELMEYER, 1970; BERNARDI and GOFFREDO, 1963).

e) Homolysergic Acid and its Derivatives

Upon comparison with d-lysergic acid, this amino acid (84a) shows clear differences in its chemical behavior, e.g., in its tendency to isomerize. Its synthesis proceeds from lysergol (79a) to lysergol tosylate (82a), a highly reactive intermediate suitable for further substitution reactions. Thus, (82a) reacted smoothly with sodium cyanide to homolysergic acid nitrile (83a). Homolysergic acid (84a) itself was obtained by alkaline saponification. A series of amides was prepared, e.g. homolysergic acid diethylamide (86a) (TROXLER, 1966; TROXLER and STADLER, 1968).

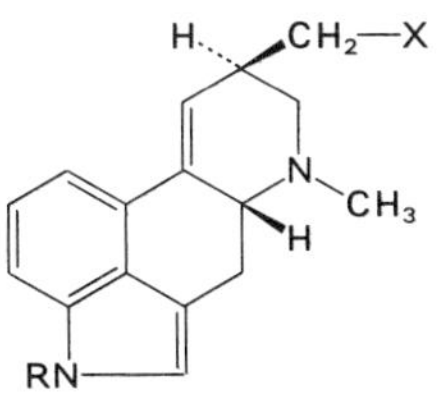

H CH2—X N CH3 H RN

(82a): Lysergol tosylate
R = H, X = O—SO_2—$C_6H_4CH_3$

(83a): Homolysergic acid nitrile
R = H, X = CN

(84a): Homolysergic acid
R = H, X = COOH

(85a): Homolysergic acid methylester
R = H, X = $COOCH_3$

(86a): Homolysergic acid diethylamide
R = H, X = CO · $N(C_2H_5)_2$

(87a): Homolysergol
R = H, X = CH_2OH

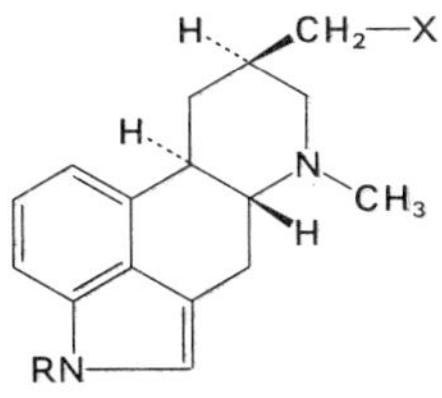

H CH2—X H N CH3 H RN

(82b): 6-Methyl-8β-chloromethyl ergoline
R = H, X = Cl

(83b): Dihydrohomolysergic acid nitrile, VUFB-6605
R = H, X = CN

(83c): 1-Methyl-dihydrohomolysergic acid nitrile
R = CH_3, X = CN

(83d): 1-Formyl-dihydrohomolysergic acid nitrile
R = CHO, X = CN

(84b): Dihydrohomolysergic acid
R = H, X = COOH

(85b): Dihydrohomolysergic acid methylester
R = H, X = $COOCH_3$

(86b): Dihydrohomolysergic acid amide, VUFB-6683, Deprenone
R = H, X = $CONH_2$

(87b): Homodihydrolysergol
R = H, X = CH_2OH

Fig. 20. Synthesis of homolysergic acid and its derivatives

Practically the same synthesis was effected somewhat later in the dihydro-series, the single steps being represented by the formulae (82b), (83b), and (84b) (SEMONSKY and KUCHARCZYK, 1968). The nitrile (83b), known under the code VUFB-6605, proved to be a strong inhibitor of prolactin secretion (REZABEK et al., 1969). Application of the azide method led to a series of amides of dihydrohomolysergic acid (SEMONSKY et al., 1971). The primary amide (86b) has been shown to reduce prolactin concentration in the anterior pituitary of rats. Its tartrate is known under the code VUFB-6683 and the generic name Deprenone (KREJCI et al., 1973).

Reduction of the methylesters (85a) and (85b) led to homolysergol (87a) and dihydrohomolysergol (87b), respectively (BERAN et al., 1969), from which some esters were prepared. They displayed antifertility effects in rats (BERAN et al., 1974).

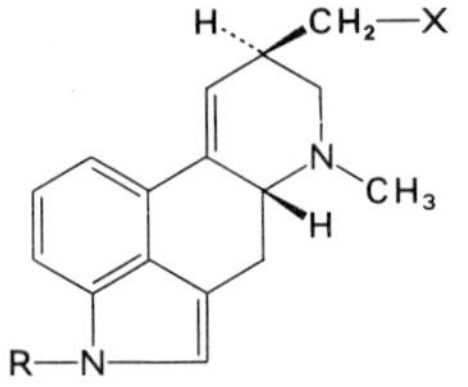

H CH₂—X N CH₃ H R—N

(88a): Lysergylamine
$R = H,\ X = NH_2$

(88b): N,N-Diethyl-lysergylamine
$R = H,\ X = N(C_2H_5)_2$

(88c): N,N-Pentamethylenlysergylamine
$R = H,\ X = C_5H_{10}N$

(88d):
$R = CH_3,\ X = N(COC_6H_5)$ (Alkyl)

(88e): 6-Methyl-8β-[4-(p-methoxyphenyl)-1-piperazinyl]methyl-9-ergolene

$R = H,\ X = N\ \ N—C_6H_4(OCH_3)$

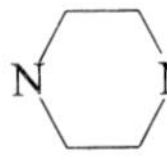

(88f): N-(6-Methyl-8β-methyl-9-ergolenyl)-azabicyclo(3,2,2)nonane

$R = H,\ X = N$

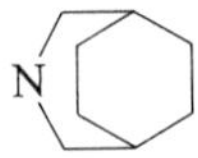

(88g): 6-Methyl-8β-azidomethyl-9-ergolene
$R = H,\ X = N_3$

(88h): 1,1-Dimethyl-3-[6-methyl-8β-(9-ergolenyl)-methyl]urea
$R = H,\ X = NHCON(CH_3)_2$

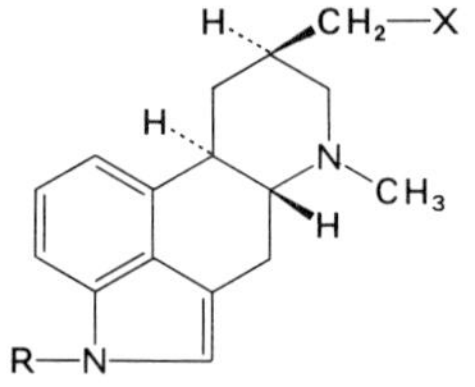

H CH₂—X H N CH₃ H R—N

(89a): Dihydrolysergylamine
$R = H,\ X = NH_2$

(89b): 1-Methyl-dihydrolysergylamine
$R = CH_3,\ X = NH_2$

(89c): N-Acetyl-dihydrolysergylamine
Acetergamina, Uterdina
$R = H,\ X = NHCOCH_3$

(89d): 1-Methyl-N-carbobenzoxy-dihydrolysergylamine, MCE, Methergoline
$R = CH_3,\ X = NHCOOCH_2C_6H_5$

(89e):
$R = H,\ X = NHC(NH)NH_2$

(89f):
$R = CH_3,\ X = NHC(NH)NH_2$

(89g): 1,6-Dimethyl-8β-[4,6-dimethyl-2-pyrimidino-aminomethyl]-ergoline

$R = CH_3,\ X = NH—$ (N, N, CH_3, CH_3)

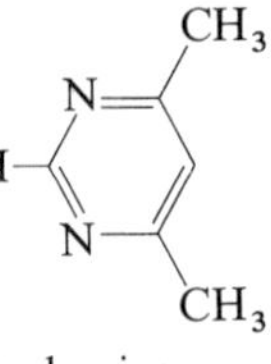

Fig. 21. Derivatives of lysergylamine and dihydrolysergylamine

f) Lysergylamine and its Derivatives

Although direct reduction of ergine (18) with lithium aluminium hydride to lysergylamine (88a) has not been successful, derivatives of lysergylamine can be easily obtained by this method. Thus, the first representative of the series, (88b), was prepared by reduction of LSD (STOLL and HOFMANN, 1952). Pentamethylen-lysergylamine (88c) was similarly obtained (RUTSCHMANN and SCHREIER, 1964) as well as a series of amides of type (88d) which showed prolonged serotonin-antagonistic activity when tested in the rat paw edema (TROXLER and HOFMANN, 1969).

6-Methyl-8β-[4-(p-methoxyphenyl)-1-piperazinyl]methylergolene (88e), code name PTR 17-402, is a stimulator of the central nervous system in mice and rats (TROXLER and HOFMANN, 1971). Another complex derivative of lysergylamine, compound (88f), produces sedative effects in mice and an inhibition of conditioned avoidance behavior in rats (STADLER and STÜTZ, 1974).

Finally, lysergylamine (88a) itself was obtained in a new synthetic way: Lysergol tosylate (82a) was transformed to 6-methyl-8β-azidomethyl-ergolene (88g) by sodium azide. Reduction of the azide with lithium aluminium hydride then led to (88a). Starting from this basic compound, many derivatives, amides, urethanes, and ureas have been prepared, e.g., treatment of lysergylamine with dimethylcarbamoyl chloride gave rise to 1,1-dimethyl-3-(6-methyl-8β-ergolenyl-methyl) urea (88h) which produced a prolonged fall in blood pressure in the hypertensive rat (FEHR et al., 1974).

g) Dihydrolysergylamine and its Derivatives

In contrast to the lysergyl series, lithium aluminium hydride reduction of dihydrolysergic acid amide (74a) leads to dihydrolysergylamine (89a) in good yields. This compound and the similarly obtained 1-methyl-dihydrolysergylamine (89b) served as starting materials for the synthesis of a great number of amides, urethanes, and ureas (BERNARDI et al., 1964a). Thus, N-acetyl-dihydrolysergylamine (89c), called Acetergamina or Uterdina, has a specific oxytocic activity comparable with that of ergometrine (FREGNAN and GLÄSSER, 1968). Treatment of 1-methyl-dihydrolysergylamine (89b) with chloroformic acid benzylester gave rise to 1-methyl-N-carbobenzoxy-dihydrolysergylamine (89d), known under the name Methergoline and the code MCE (BERNARDI et al., 1964a). It has high specific antiserotonin activity when tested on the isolated rat uterus (BERETTA et al., 1965). Another potent serotonin antagonist has been discovered in its 2,3-dihydro-derivative, formula (48a) (Fig. 15) (ARCAMONE and FRANCESCHI, 1973).

Starting from dihydrolysergylamine (89a) or its 1-methyl-analogue (89b), the corresponding guanidino-derivatives (89e) and (89f) have been prepared by reaction, e.g., with cyanamide. These compounds reacted with 1,3-diketones to the corresponding pyrimidines, e.g., to (89 g). Compounds of this type exhibit alpha-adrenergic blocking activity (ARCARI et al., 1973).

h) Thiolysergol and its Derivatives

Upon heating lysergol mesylate (90a) or lysergol tosylate (82a) with sulfur anions in polar solvents, a substitution reaction takes place. Sodium hydrogensulfide

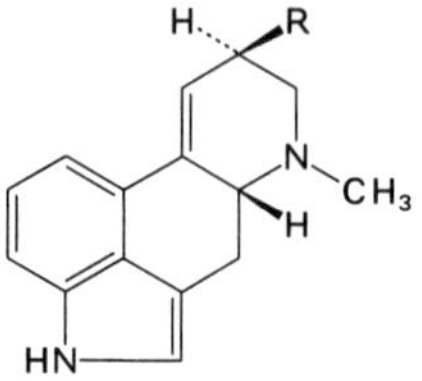

(90)

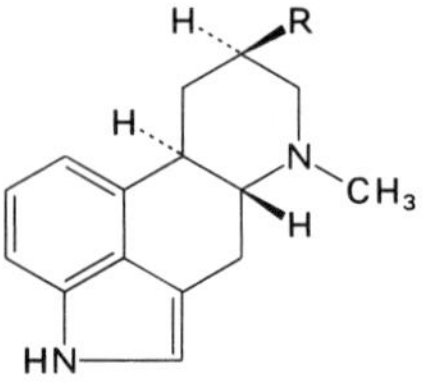

(91)

(90a): Lysergol mesylate
$R = CH_2—O—SO_2—CH_3$

(90b): Thiolysergol
$R = CH_2SH$

(90c): 6-Methyl-8β-rhodanomethyl-9-ergolene
$R = CH_2SCN$

(90d): 6-Methyl-8β-(2-pyridyl-thiomethyl)-9-ergolene

$R = CH_2—S—$(2-pyridyl)

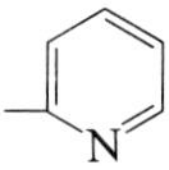

(91a): Dihydrolysergol mesylate
$R = CH_2—O—SO_2—CH_3$

(91b): 6-Methyl-8β-(2-pyridyl-thiomethyl)-ergoline

$R = CH_2—S—$(2-pyridyl)

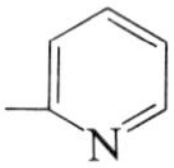

(92): 6-Methyl-8β-acetyl-ergoline
$R = COCH_3$

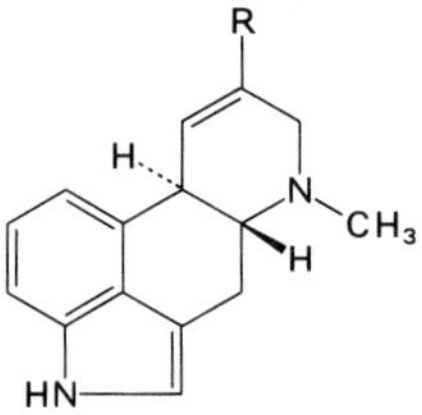

(6)

(6): Elymoclavine
$R = CH_2OH$

(6a): Elymoclavine pyridinium tosylate

$R = CH_2—N^{\oplus}$(pyridinium) $\cdot H_3C—C_6H_4—SO_3^{\ominus}$

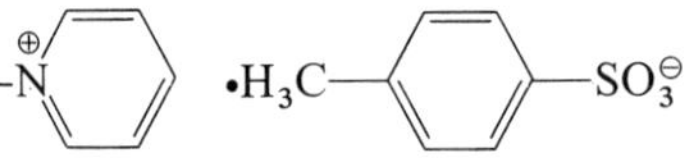

(6b): 6-Methyl-8-piperidinomethyl-8-ergolene

$R = CH_2—N$(piperidino)

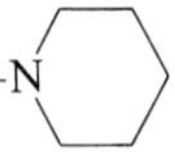

(6c): 6-Methyl-8-diethylaminomethyl-8-ergolene
$R = CH_2—N(C_2H_5)_2$

(6d): 6-Methyl-8-chloromethyl-8-ergolene
$R = CH_2Cl$

(6e): 6-Methyl-8-cyanomethyl-8-ergolene
$R = CH_2CN$

(6f): 6-Methyl-8-carboxamidomethyl-8-ergolene
$R = CH_2CONH_2$

(6g): 6-Methyl-8-pyrrolidinomethyl-8-ergolene

$R = CH_2—N$(pyrrolidino)

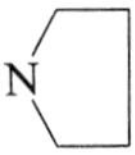

(6h): 6-Methyl-8-anilinomethyl-8-ergolene
$R = CH_2NHC_6H_5$

(6i): 6-Methyl-8-acetylanilinomethyl-8-ergolene
$R = CH_2N(COCH_3)C_6H_5$

Fig. 22. Thiolysergols, 6-methyl-8-ergolenes

yielded thiolysergol (90b), potassium rhodanide 6-methyl-8β-rhodanomethyl-9-ergolene (90c), and 2-mercapto-pyridine 6-methyl-8β-(2-pyridyl-thiomethyl)-9-ergolene (90d). Thiolysergol (90b) and especially its two derivatives mentioned above cause rotary effects in rats after nigro-striatal degeneration, suggesting central stimulation of dopaminergic pathways.

A corresponding reaction could be performed with dihydrolysergol mesylate (91a) which reacted with 2-mercapto-pyridine to 6-methyl-8β-(2-pyridyl-thiomethyl)-ergoline (91b) (STÜTZ and STADLER, 1975).

i) Ketones

Some ketones of the ergoline series have been prepared by reaction of dihydro-LSD (74b) with Grignard reagents (BERNARDI et al., 1964b). Thus, treatment of dihydro-LSD with methyl magnesium bromide led to 6-methyl-8β-acetyl-ergoline (92) (Fig. 22).

k) 6-Methyl-8-ergolenes

Up to 1975 very few 6-methyl-8-ergolenes have been reported in the literature, and the routes to these compounds have been specific. Examples are elymoclavine pyridinium tosylate (6a), its reduction product 6-methyl-8-piperidino-methyl-8-ergolene (6b) (SCHREIER, 1958), and 6-methyl-8-diethylaminomethyl-8-ergolene (6c) (TROXLER, 1968). Lately, a new access to such compounds has been found (LI et al., 1975) which starts from elymoclavine (6). Via the key intermediate 6-methyl-8-chloromethyl-8-ergolene (6d) a variety of new derivatives, listed in Figure 22, have been prepared.

7. Reactions at Position 8

a) 8-Amino-ergolenes, 8-Amino-ergolines

Isomeric 6-methyl-8-amino-ergolenes and -ergolines were produced by a modified, stereoselective Curtius degradation of the corresponding d-lysergic- and dihydrolysergic acid hydrazides. Treatment of d-lysergic acid hydrazide (93a) with nitrous acid led to the intermediate d-lysergic acid azide, which on heating in dilute acid gave rise to the degradation product 6-methyl-8β-amino-ergolene (94a). Similarly, the degradation reaction of d-isolysergic acid hydrazide (93b) led to the isomer (94b). In the dihydro series the degradation reaction was also performed, leading to the isomeric ergolines (94c) and (94d), respectively (HOFMANN, 1947).

Heating the azides in benzene containing an alcohol led (via intermediate isocyanates) directly to urethanes of type (95). By this procedure, urethane derivatives of all four amines (94a) to (94d) and their methylation products in position 1 were prepared (TROXLER, 1946; HOFMANN et al., 1967).

Similarly, ureas of type (96) were obtained by heating the azides in benzene containing a primary or secondary amine (SEMONSKY and ZIKAN, 1960; HOFMANN and TROXLER, 1962, 1965).

Some of these compounds deserve special attention. The best known is perhaps N-(6-methyl-8α-ergolenyl)-N′,N′-diethylurea (96a) (ZIKAN and SEMONSKY, 1960,

1963b, 1968). Its hydrogenmaleinate has been introduced into therapy under the trade name Lysenyl. Its methylation product in position 1 (96b) has the generic name Mesenyl (ZIKAN and SEMONSKY, 1963a). These substances have antiserotonin activity of the order of LSD when tested by the paw edema in rats, but they lack the typical central effects of LSD in man. The dihydro-derivative of Lysenyl,

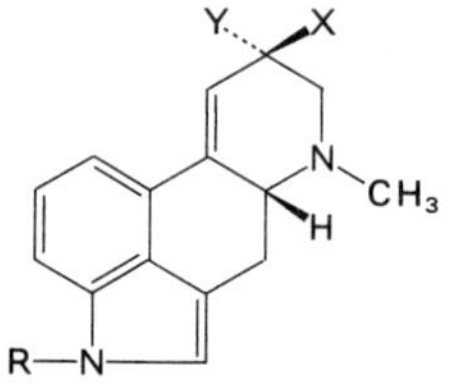

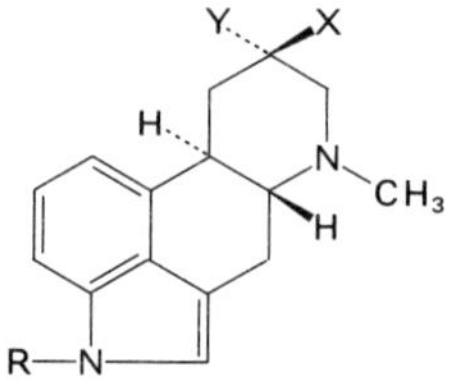

(93): d-Isolysergic acid
R = H, X = H, Y = COOH

(93a): d-Lysergic acid hydrazide
R = H, X = $CONHNH_2$, Y = H

(93b): d-Isolysergic acid hydrazide
R = H, X = H, Y = $CONHNH_2$

(93c): d-Isolysergic acid diethylamide, Iso-LSD
R = H, X = H, Y = $CON(C_2H_5)_2$

(94a): 6-Methyl-8β-amino-9-ergolene
R = H, X = NH_2, Y = H

(94b): 6-Methyl-8α-amino-9-ergolene
R = H, X = H, Y = NH_2

(95): (6-Methyl-8β-amino-9-ergolenyl)-carbamidic acid methylester
R = H, X = $NHCOOCH_3$, Y = H

(96a): N-[6-Methyl-8α-(9-ergolenyl)]-N′,N′-diethylurea, Hydrogenmaleinate: Generics: Lysuride, Lisuride, Mesorgydine; Trade name: Lysenyl
R = H, X = H, Y = $NHCON(C_2H_5)_2$

(96b): N-[1,6-Dimethyl-8α-(9-ergolenyl)]-N′,N′-diethylurea, Hydrogenmaleinate: Mesenyl
R = CH_3, X = H, Y = $NHCON(C_2H_5)_2$

(99a): 1,8-Dimethyl-LSD
R = Y = CH_3, X = $CON(C_2H_5)_2$

(99b): 8-Methyl-LSD
R = H, Y = CH_3, X = $CON(C_2H_5)_2$

(99c): 8-Methyl-ergotamine
R = H, Y = CH_3, X = tripeptide moiety of ergotamine

(94c): 6-Methyl-8β-amino-ergoline
R = H, X = NH_2, Y = H

(94d): 6-Methyl-8α-amino-ergoline
R = H, X = H, Y = NH_2

(96c): N-(6-Methyl-8α-ergolinyl)-N′,N′-diethyl-urea, Hydrogenmaleinate: VUFB-6638
R = H, X = H, Y = $NHCON(C_2H_5)_2$

(96d): Compound PAI
R = H, X = NHCO—N (pyrazolyl, with CH_3 and CH_3), Y = H

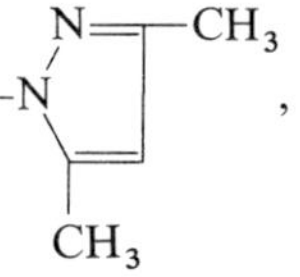

(96e): Methoquizine
R = CH_3, X = NHCO—N (pyrazolyl, with CH_3 and CH_3), Y = H

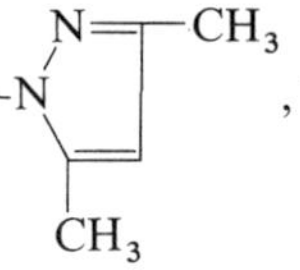

(96f): Toquizine
R = C_2H_5, X = NHCO—N (pyrazolyl, with CH_3 and CH_3), Y = H

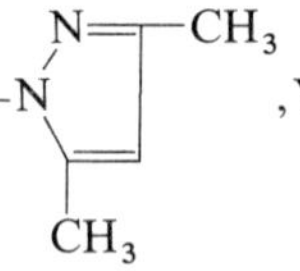

(97): 6-Methyl-8-oxo-ergoline
R = H, X + Y = O

(98): 6-Methyl-8α-(3-pyridyl-amino)-ergoline
R = H, X = H, Y = HN—(3-pyridyl)

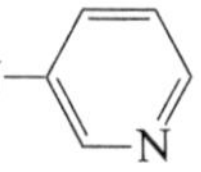

(99d): 8-Methyl-dihydroergotamine
R = H, Y = CH_3, X = tripeptide moiety of ergotamine

Fig. 23. Substitution products in position 8

N-(6-methyl-8α-ergolinyl)-N′,N′-diethylurea (96c), has antilactation and antifertility effects in rats (ZIKAN et al., 1972).

Heterocyclic ureas of this type have also been prepared, such as PAI (96d) and its derivatives in position 1, Methoquizine (96e) and Toquizine, (96f) (GARBRECHT and TSUNG-MIN LIN, 1965). PAI is an α-adrenoceptor blocking agent which reduces the blood pressure in renal hypertensive dogs (WILLARD and POWELL, 1968). Methoquizine and Toquizine are antiulcer agents (ELI LILLY and Co., 1966).

Derivatives of the epimeric 6-methyl-8-amino-ergolines (94c) and (94d) may be obtained by a completely different sequence of reactions: 6-methyl-8-ergolene-8-carboxylic acid (7) was transformed to 6-methyl-8-oxo-ergoline (97) by a Curtius degradation of its intermediate azide. Upon catalytic hydrogenation of (97) in the presence of amines, substituted 8-amino-ergolines were obtained. 6-Methyl-8α-(3-pyridylamino)-ergoline (98) proved to be an inhibitor of prolactin release (HAUTH and TSCHERTER, 1975).

b) Alkylation in Position 8

Upon methylation of LSD (73b), it was observed that besides 1-methyl-LSD (34b) two by-products were formed, which could be identified as 1,8-dimethyl-LSD, (99a) and 8-methyl-LSD (99b) (TROXLER and HOFMANN, 1957a). Later on, reaction conditions for selective alkylations in position 8 were found. Interesting compounds resulted, e.g., 8-methyl-ergotamine (99c) and its dihydro-derivative (99d).

8. Derivatives of 6-Methyl-8-ergolene-8-carboxylic Acid

a) Amides of 6-Methyl-8-ergolene-8-carboxylic Acid

Nature has provided a considerable number of clavine alkaloids carrying a double bond in position 8,9, e.g., elymoclavine (6). It seems surprising that until now no derivative of its biosynthetic oxidation product 6-methyl-8-ergolene-8-carboxylic acid (7) has been observed in nature. For the establishment of structure-activity relations it seemed therefore worthwhile to prepare a series of amides of 6-methyl-8-ergolene-8-carboxylic acid and some of its 1-methyl-derivatives. Consequently, (7) was transformed to its acid chloride hydrochloride (100a), which reacted smoothly with primary and secondary amines to the corresponding amides. Thus, (100a) and diethylamine led to 6-methyl-8-ergolene-8-carboxylic acid diethylamide (100d), the Δ-8,9-isomer of LSD. A series of other amides of this type has been prepared, e.g., (100e), Δ-8,9-ergometrine and (100f), Δ-8,9-Methergine (TROXLER, 1968).

For the synthesis of derivatives methylated in position 1, direct methylation of amides could be effected, leading from (100d) to (100g). A second, more general way of synthesis was found by the methylation of the free acid (7) to 1,6-dimethyl-8-ergolene-8-carboxylic acid (100b). Correspondingly, (100b) could be transformed into its acid chloride hydrochloride (100c), which on treatment with amines led directly to a series of amides of type (100h) (TROXLER, 1968).

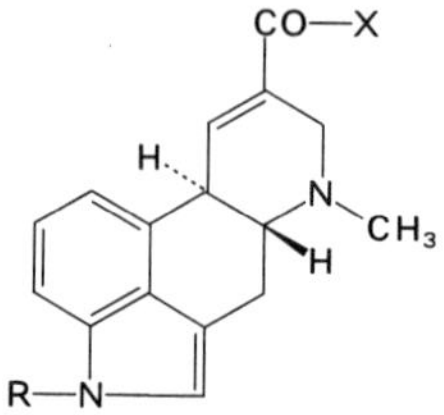

(100a): 6-Methyl-8-ergolene-8-carboxylic acid chloride · HCl
R = H, X = Cl

(100b): 1,6-Dimethyl-8-ergolene-8-carboxylic acid
$R = CH_3$, X = OH

(100c): 1,6-Dimethyl-8-ergolene-8-carboxylic acid chloride · HCl
$R = CH_3$, X = Cl

(100d): Δ-8,9-LSD
R = H, $X = N(C_2H_5)_2$

(100e): Δ-8,9-Ergometrine
R = H, X = L-alaninol

(100f): Δ-8,9-Methergine
R = H, X = L-2-aminobutanol

(100g): 1-Methyl-Δ-8,9-LSD
$R = CH_3$, $X = N(C_2H_5)_2$

(100h): Δ-8,9-Deseril
$R = CH_3$, X = L-2-aminobutanol

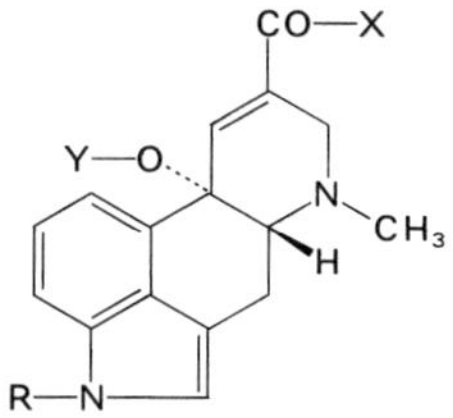

(101a): 6-Methyl-10α-methoxy-8-ergolene-8-carboxylic acid amide
R = H, $Y = CH_3$, $X = NH_2$

(101b): 1,6-Dimethyl-10α-methoxy-8-ergolene-8-carboxylic acid amide
$R = CH_3$, $Y = CH_3$, $X = NH_2$

(101c): 6-Methyl-10α-methoxy-8-ergolene-8-carboxylic acid L-2-amino-butanol-amide
R = H, $Y = CH_3$,
$X = NH \cdot CH(C_2H_5)CH_2OH$

(101d): 8,9-Didehydro-10α-methoxy-9,10-dihydroergotamine
R = H, $Y = CH_3$, X = peptide part of ergotamine

(101e): 1-Methyl-8,9-didehydro-10α-ethoxy-9,10-dihydroergokryptine
$R = CH_3$, $Y = C_2H_5$, X = peptide part of α-ergokryptine

Fig. 24. Derivatives of 6-methyl-8-ergolene-8-carboxylic- and 6-methyl-10α-alkoxy-8-ergolene-8-carboxylic acid

b) Amides of 6-Methyl-10α-alkoxy-8-ergolene-8-carboxylic Acid

Besides the direct hydroboration of d-lysergic acid to 9α-hydroxy-dihydrolysergol (CAINELLI et al., 1967), of which only some esters have been prepared, Italian chemists have developed an elegant synthesis for 10α-alkoxy-8-ergolenes: By treatment of d-lysergic acid amide, ergine, (18), first with mercury(II)chloride in methanol followed by a reduction with sodium borohydride, 6-methyl-10α-methoxy-8-ergolene-8-carboxylic acid amide (101a) is formed. The reaction proceeds as well with amides methylated in position 1 [see (101b)]. Considering the kind of amide, the reaction is a very general one, as ergot peptide alkaloids react with ease, but is restricted to lower primary alcohols for alkoxy source (BERNARDI et al., 1972).

To demonstrate the reaction further, some of the prepared derivatives are listed in Figure 24. Thus, Methergine (73a) gave rise to (101c); ergotamine (20) led to (101d), both reactions being performed in methanol. When 1-methyl-α-ergokryptine was reacted with the reagents mentioned above in ethanol, (101e) was obtained.

9. Chemical Transformations on the Double Bond in Position 9,10

a) Catalytic Hydrogenation

Early investigations (JACOBS and CRAIG, 1936a, 1936c) revealed an alicyclic double bond to occur in the lysergic acid moiety of natural ergot alkaloids which could be saturated by chemical reduction or more conveniently by catalytic hydrogenation.

Dihydroergometrine (74c) (Fig. 18) is the first known dihydro derivative of a natural ergot alkaloid prepared by catalytic hydrogenation of ergometrine (19) using a platinum catalyst (JACOBS and CRAIG, 1936a). However, (74c) has found no therapeutical application.

Up to now dihydroergosine (102a) is the only dihydro derivative of an ergot peptide alkaloid known to occur in nature. It has been found to be the main alkaloid in sclerotia of Sphacelia sorghi grown on Sorghum vulgare in Nigeria (MANTLE and WAIGHT, 1968). Like the other dihydro peptide alkaloids depicted in Figure 25, dihydroergosine may be prepared in a stereospecific manner by catalytic hydrogenation of the corresponding levorotatory, genuine alkaloid, i.e., ergosine (21) by application of a palladium catalyst (STOLL and HOFMANN, 1943c).

In the form of its methanesulfonate, dihydroergotamine (102b) increases the tone of capacitance vessels in the cat. Its code is DHE-45; its trade name Dihydergot.

The four dihydro derivatives, (102c) to (102f), of the alkaloids of the ergotoxine group may be prepared in the same manner as dihydroergosine. In the form of their methanesulfonates a mixture of these four compounds is used in therapy under the trade name Hydergine. It consists of one-third of (102c) and a second third of (102d), the rest being a mixture of (102e) and (102f) in a proportion of about 2:1, according to their naturally occuring ratio in the raw alkaloids of ergot.

In contrast to the levorotatory alkaloids of ergot, the strongly dextrorotatory genuine isoforms (e.g., ergotaminine) form two isomeric dihydro derivatives upon catalytic hydrogenation. One hydrogenation product (dihydroergotaminine-I) is the epimer in position 8 to the dihydro alkaloids depicted in Figure 25; the other one (in our example dihydroergotaminine-II) was found to be epimeric in positions 8 and 10 (STOLL et al., 1946).

b) Light-Catalyzed Addition of Water and Alcohols

Ergot alkaloids have been known for a very long time to be sensitive to light. Some years ago it was stated that lysergic acid derivatives add one molecule of water in dilute acidic medium upon illumination. The reaction leads to a mixture of two diastereomers, both carrying a hydroxy group in position 10. The main products (which have been called lumi-I-derivatives) are the 10α-hydroxy derivatives, the hydroxy group being trans to the hydrogen atom in position 5. The diastereomeric lumi-II-by-products have a cis-junction of rings C and D; they lack biological activity. A considerable number of lumi-I-derivatives of ergot compounds have been prepared by application of the method mentioned above, a

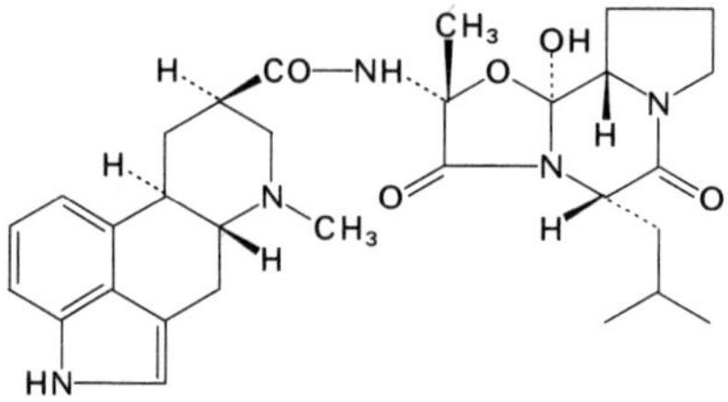

(102a)

Dihydroergosine

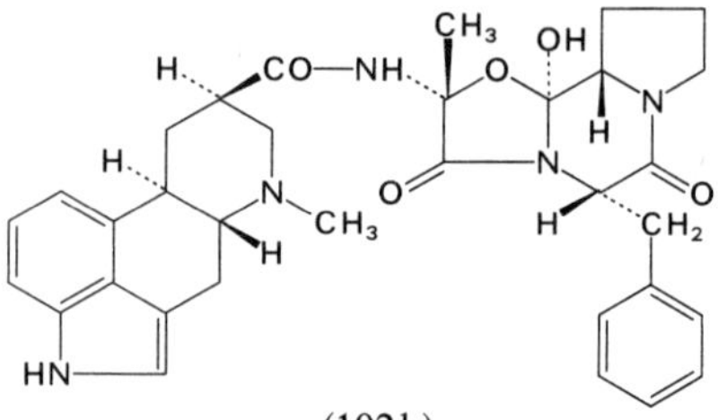

(102b)

Dihydroergotamine,
Methanesulfonate = DHE-45,
Dihydergot

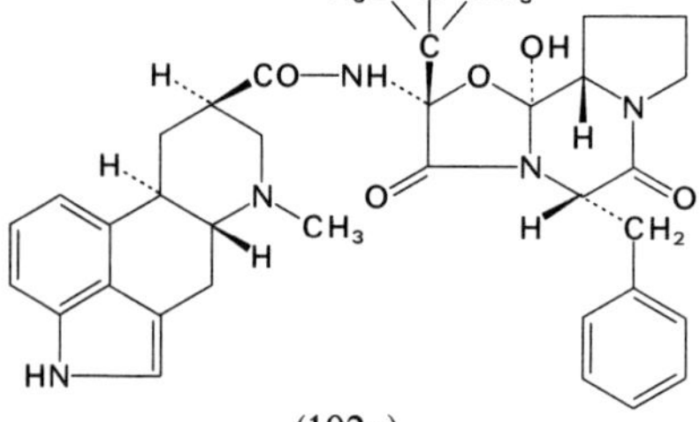

(102c)

Dihydroergocristine

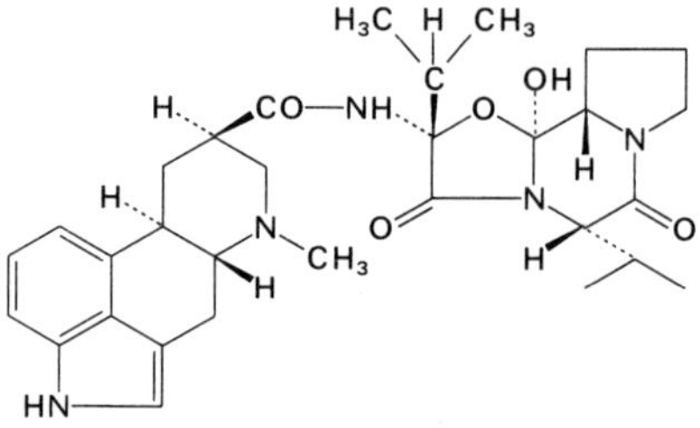

(102d)

Dihydroergocornine

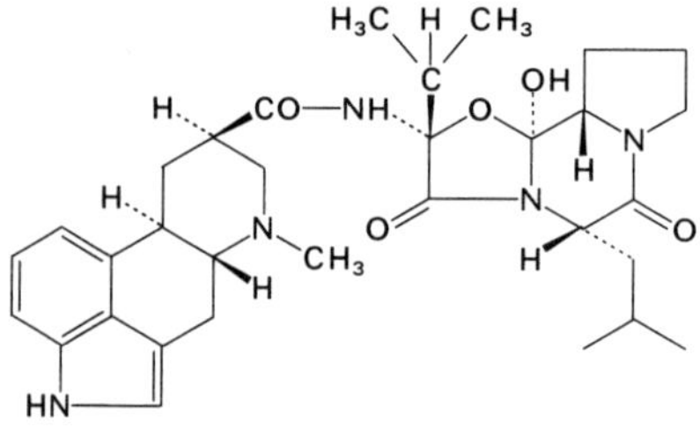

(102e)

Dihydro-α-ergokryptine

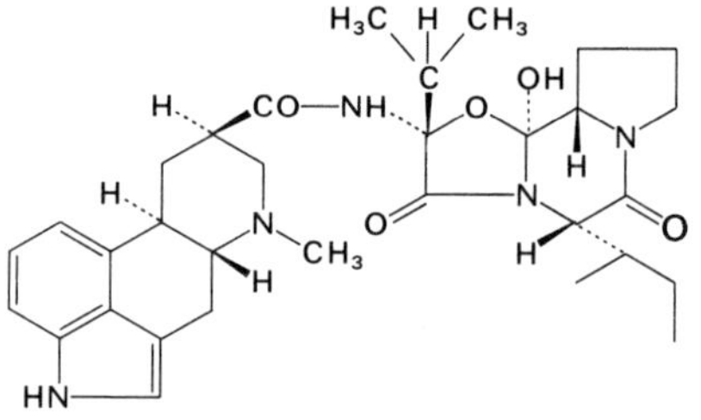

(102f)

Dihydro-β-ergokryptine

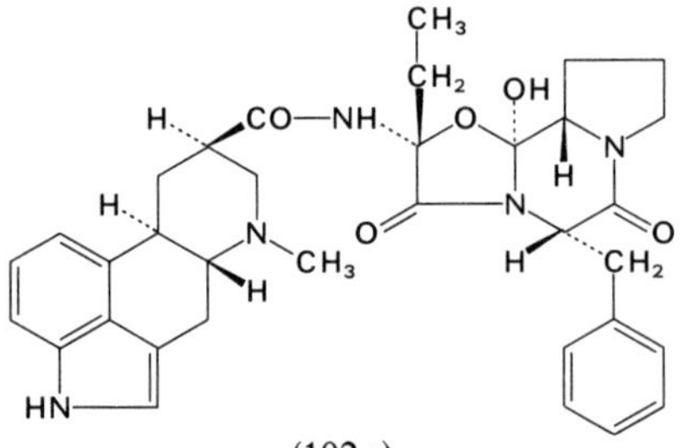

(102g)

Dihydroergostine

Fig. 25. Dihydro derivatives of ergot alkaloids

few representatives being shown in Figure 26 (STOLL and SCHLIENTZ, 1955, 1958). The reaction has been shown to be not only light-catalyzed but also pH-dependent (HELLBERG, 1957). An unequivocal chemical proof of their structure and stereochemistry has been published (BERNARDI et al., 1964c).

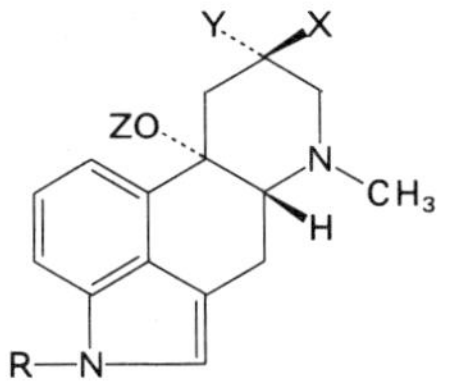

(103a): Lumi-I-lysergic acid
R = H, X = COOH, Y = H, Z = H

(103b): Lumi-I-ergometrine
R = H, X = CO-L-alaninol, Y = H, Z = H

(103c): Lumi-I-LSD
R = H, X = $CON(C_2H_5)_2$, Y = H, Z = H

(103d): Lumi-I-ergotamine
R = H, X = CO · peptide part of ergotamine, Y = H, Z = H

(104a): 10α-Methoxy-dihydrolysergic acid methylester
R = H, X = $COOCH_3$, Y = H, Z = CH_3

(104b): 1-Methyl-10α-methoxy-dihydrolysergic acid methylester
R = CH_3, X = $COOCH_3$, Y = H, Z = CH_3

(104c): 10α-Methoxy-dihydrolysergol
R = H, X = CH_2OH, Y = H, Z = CH_3

(104d): 1-Methyl-10α-methoxy-dihydrolysergol
R = CH_3, X = CH_2OH, Y = H, Z = CH_3

(104e): Nicergoline, MNE, Sermion

R = CH_3, X =
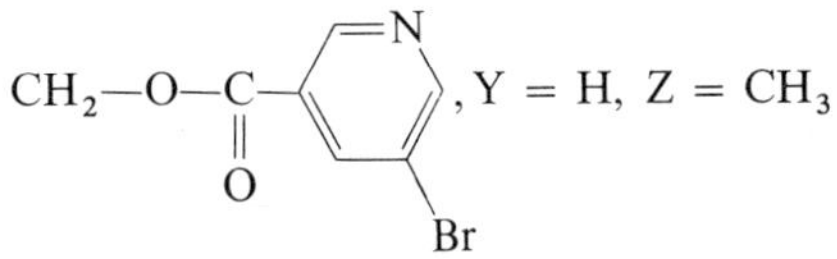

, Y = H, Z = CH_3

Fig. 26. Some lumi-I-derivatives

The hydroxy group of lumi-I-lysergic acid (103a) is not very stable. 10α-methoxy-dihydrolysergic acid methylester (104a) was obtained after acid catalyzed methanol treatment of (103a) (BERNARDI et al., 1966; BARBIERI et al., 1969). The compound could be obtained directly from d-lysergic acid (8) by illumination of its acidic methanol solution. The reaction is not limited to esters; amides of lysergic acid and even the peptide alkaloids react to 10α-methoxy-dihydro-derivatives (ARCAMONE et al., 1971).

Methylation of (104a) in the usual way (see Section 1 of this chapter) led to (104b). Reduction of these esters with lithium aluminium hydride gave rise to 10α-methoxy-dihydrolysergol (104c) and its 1-methyl derivative (104d), which were used as starting materials for the preparation of a great series of esters (BERNARDI et al., 1966, 1975; ARCARI et al., 1972). Among these esters of (104d), the 5-bromo-nicotinic acid ester (104e) proved to be an α-blocking agent. It is known under the code MNE, the generic Nicergoline, and the trade name Sermion.

10. Substitution Reactions in the Benzene Ring

There are only a few methods at our disposal to directly attack a benzene ring of an indole system. Two of them have been successfully applied to ergot derivatives leading to new substitution products:

a) Hydroxylation in Position 12

On treatment of 2,3-dihydro-derivatives of ergoline or ergolenes [general formula (48)] with potassium nitroso disulfonate, an oxidation via free radical takes place: The indoline ring system is oxidized back to the indole state, and at the same time a phenolic hydroxy group is introduced in position 12, giving rise to 12-hydroxy-ergot derivatives. Thus, 2,3-dihydroergometrine (48b) led to 12-hydroxy-ergometrine (105a), which could be hydrogenated to 12-hydroxy-dihydroergometrine (105b). Applying the same method, 12-hydroxy-LSD (105c), a metabolite of LSD, 12-hydroxy-lysergic acid L-2-butanolamide (105d) (=12-Hydroxy-methergine), and its methylation product, 12-hydroxy-1-methyl-lysergic acid L-2-butanolamide (105e), were prepared from the corresponding 2,3-dihydro-derivatives. For example, with (105d) it was shown that the phenolic hydroxy group in position 12 could be etherified by diazomethane, the reaction leading to (105f) (STADLER et al., 1964b).

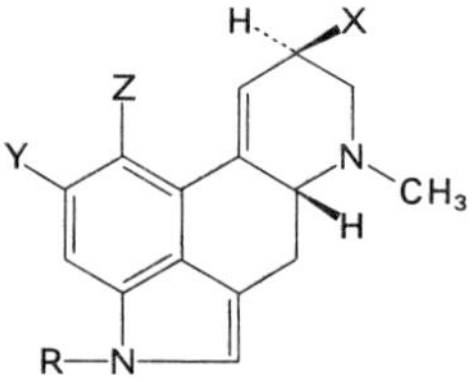

(105a): 12-Hydroxy-ergometrine
R = H, X = CO · L-alaninol
Y = H, Z = OH

(105c): 12-Hydroxy-LSD
R = H, X = $CON(C_2H_5)_2$
Y = H, Z = OH

(105d): 12-Hydroxy-methergine
R = H, X = CO · L-2-aminobutanol
Y = H, Z = OH

(105e): 12-Hydroxy-deseril
R = CH_3, X = CO · L-2-aminobutanol
Y = H, Z = OH

(105f): 12-Methoxy-methergine
R = H, X = CO · L-2-aminobutanol
Y = H, Z = OCH_3

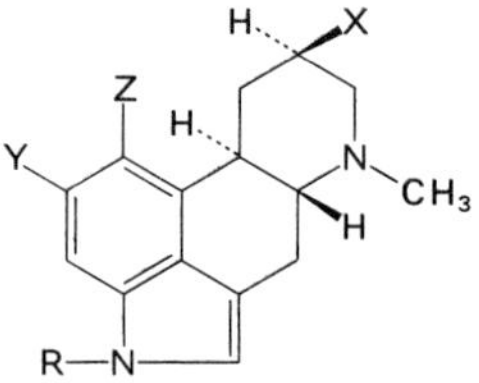

(105b): 12-Hydroxy-dihydroergometrine
R = H, X = CO · L-alaninol
Y = H, Z = OH

(106a): 13-Bromo-dihydroergotamine
R = H, X = CO · peptide part of ergotamine,
Y = Br, Z = H

(106b): 13-Bromo-dihydrolysergic acid
R = H, X = COOH, Y = Br, Z = H

(106c): 13-Bromo-MNE
R = CH_3, X = CH_2—O—CO—(5-bromo-3-pyridyl)
Y = Br
Z = H
In position 10α: OCH_3

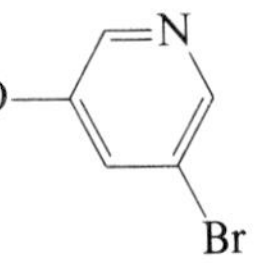

Fig. 27. Ergot derivatives substituted in the benzene ring

b) 13-Bromo-ergolines

The synthesis of 2,13-dibromoergolines from the corresponding ergolines was discussed earlier. Two laboratories have found, independently, that 13-bromo-ergolines of the general formula (106) can be prepared from 2,13-dibromo-ergolines by a selective reduction procedure. This reduction, in which only the bromo-atom in position 2 is removed, can be effected by zinc in acetic acid (FEHR and HAUTH, 1975) or by sodium borohydride in presence of cobalt salts (ARCARI et al., 1974). The first method is appropriate for sensitive compounds; it has been used, for example, for the preparation of 13-bromo-dihydroergotamine (106a). By application of the second method, a series of 13-bromo-ergolines has been synthesized: Upon reduction of free 2,13-dibromo-dihydrolysergic acid with sodium borohydride, the basic compound of the series, 13-bromo-dihydrolysergic acid (106b), has been obtained. The same method has been used to synthesize 13-bromo-MNE (106c), a compound with stronger α-adrenergic blocking activity than MNE.

D. Chemical Modifications in the Peptide Part of Ergot Alkaloids

As a consequence of their lability, only a few chemical reactions can be carried out on natural ergot peptide alkaloids. With the exception of the aci-rearrangement, all these partial syntheses concern modifications in the lysergic acid half of the molecule, which were discussed in Section C.

The total synthesis of ergot peptide alkaloids, summarized in Section B, was a genuine breakthrough in ergot chemistry. From that time on, the preparation of new analogues of ergot peptide alkaloids with modifications in the peptide part became possible.

1. The Aci-Rearrangement

In 1961 a new rearrangement of ergot peptide alkaloids was discovered: When dihydroergotamine (102b) was heated in dilute acetic acid, a reversible reaction took place, leading to an equilibrium between the starting material and a new isomer of dihydroergotamine which was called aci-dihydroergotamine (107a). The same reaction was observed with the single constituents of dihydroergotoxine mesylate (Hydergin) (102c) to (102f), leading to (107b) to (107e).

In genuine alkaloids of the peptide type, the reaction is more complex, as the well-known isomerization in position 8 of the lysergic acid moiety occurs simultaneously. For example, heating of ergotamine (20) in dilute acetic acid led to an equilibrium with ergotaminine (the isomer in C-8), which is further equilibrated together with ergotamine to the corresponding aci-forms, aci-ergotamine (107f), and aci-ergotaminine (107g). Thus, four compounds are in an equilibrium (SCHLIENTZ et al., 1961a, 1961b).

An X-ray analysis of an aci-derivative and further chemical evidence compiled later led to the conclusion that the aci-rearrangement consisted in an epimerization of the substituents in position 2′ of the peptide moiety (MCPHAIL et al., 1966; OTT et al., 1966). To give an example, in aci-dihydroergotamine (107a), the methyl group in position 2′ is in α-position, while it is β in dihydroergotamine (102b).

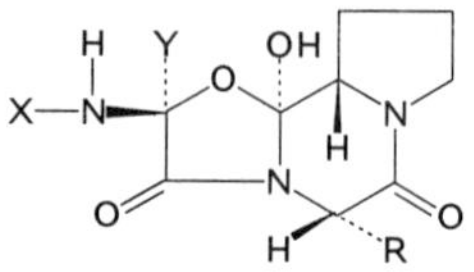

(107a): Aci-dihydroergotamine
X = dihydrolysergoyl, Y = methyl, R = benzyl

(107b): Aci-dihydroergocristine
X = dihydrolysergoyl, Y = isopropyl, R = benzyl

(107c): Aci-dihydroergocornine
X = dihydrolysergoyl, Y = R = isopropyl

(107d): Aci-dihydro-α-ergokryptine
X = dihydrolysergoyl, Y = isopropyl, R = isobutyl

(107e): Aci-dihydro-β-ergokryptine
X = dihydrolysergoyl, Y = isopropyl, R = sec. butyl

(107f): Aci-ergotamine
X = lysergoyl, Y = methyl, R = benzyl

(107g): Aci-ergotaminine
X = isolysergoyl, Y = methyl, R = benzyl

Fig. 28. Structure of important aci-isomers

2. Synthesis of Analoga of Natural Ergot Peptide Alkaloids

In Figure 10 all ergot peptide alkaloids found hitherto in nature are described and assigned to one of the three natural groups, according to their structural features.

Only one natural group, the ergotoxine group, contains four alkaloids. The ergotamine group consists of two natural alkaloids, ergotamine (20) and ergosine (21) and the ergoxine group of only one member, ergostine (22). It seems possible that some "missing links" which have been synthetically prepared for the establishment of structure-activity relationships may later be detected in nature.

a) The Ergotamine Group, Syntheses of Ergovaline and β-Ergosine

In the ergotamine group of alkaloids, the peptide part consists, besides L-proline, of L-α-hydroxy-alanine and a third variable amino acid. In ergotamine (20), this third amino acid is L-phenylalanine; in ergosine (21) it is L-leucine. In analogy to the four known members of the ergotoxine group, two new peptide alkaloids, called ergovaline (108a) and β-ergosine (109a), had to be synthesized to complete the ergotamine group.

In ergovaline (108a) the variable amino acid is, as its name already expresses, L-valine; thus, it is related to ergocornine (24). Together with its dihydro-derivative (108b), it has been synthesized in complete analogy to the synthesis of ergotamine (STADLER et al., 1964a).

The second periodic gap, β-ergosine (109a) contains L-isoleucine instead of the L-leucine of ergosine (21). It has now been synthesized in pursuit of an analogous pathway to that of ergosine (STADLER et al., 1978).

b) The Ergoxine Group, Synthesis of Ergoptine, β-Ergoptine and Ergonine

Until now, only one representative of the ergoxine group is known to occur in nature, ergostine (22). Its peptide moiety contains L-α-hydroxy-α-amino-butyric

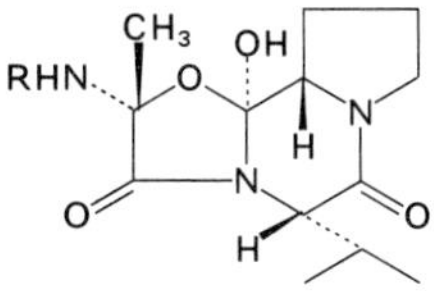

(108a): Ergovaline
R = lysergoyl

(108b): Dihydroergovaline
R = dihydrolysergoyl

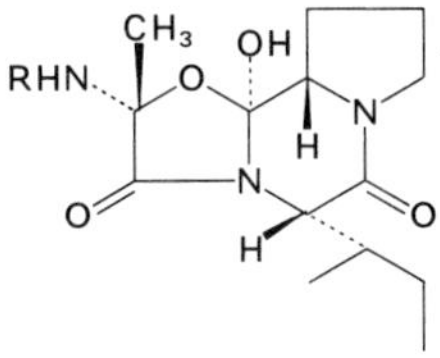

(109a): β-Ergosine
R = lysergoyl

(109b): Dihydro-β-ergosine
R = dihydrolysergoyl

Fig. 29. Synthetic peptide alkaloids of the ergotamine group

acid, L-proline, and L-phenylalanine as the variable amino acid. The ergoxine group has now also been completed by the synthesis of the following three peptide alkaloids:

Ergonine (110a) stands between ergocornine (24) and ergovaline (108a); all three compounds contain L-valine as the third amino acid. Dihydroergonine (110b), code name DN-16-457, has been recognized as a compound of high biological potency.

Ergoptine (111a), which should now correctly be called α-ergoptine, is closely related to ergosine (21) on the one hand and to α-ergokryptine (25) on the other, as all three compounds contain L-leucine as the variable amino acid.

The synthesis of ergonine and ergoptine has been reported to proceed in close analogy to that of ergostine (Stütz et al., 1970) as well as that of β-ergoptine (112a), which has been verified recently (Stadler et al., 1977). β-Ergoptine is the lower analogue of β-ergokryptine (26). The two compounds differ only in the α-hydroxy-α-amino acid, as their common characteristic building block is, besides L-proline, L-isoleucine.

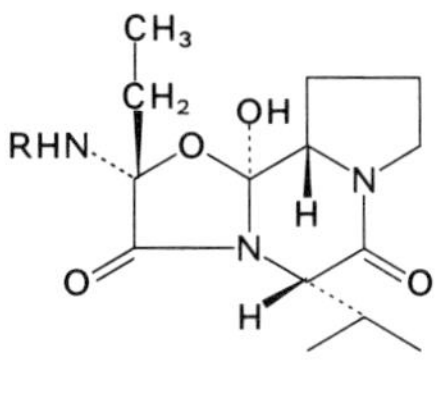

(110a): Ergonine
R = lysergoyl

(110b): Dihydroergonine
R = dihydrolysergoyl
DN-16-457

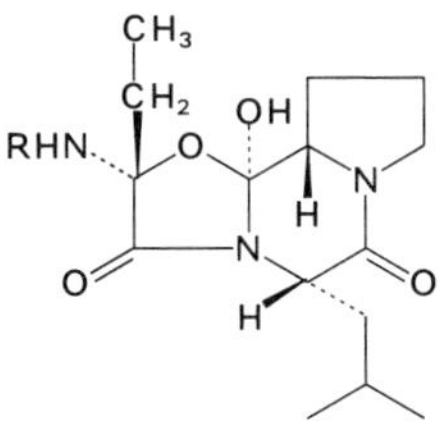

(111a): Ergoptine
R = lysergoyl

(111b): Dihydroergoptine
R = dihydrolysergoyl

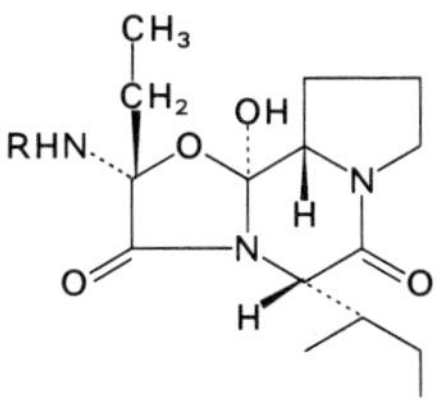

(112a): β-Ergoptine
R = lysergoyl

(112b): Dihydro-β-ergoptine
R = dihydrolysergoyl

Fig. 30. Synthetic members of the ergoxine group

3. Substitution of L-Proline by Other Amino Acids in Ergot Peptide Alkaloids

L-Proline is the only amino acid which is a constituent of all natural ergot peptide alkaloids. It therefore seemed worthwhile to synthesize some ergot peptide alkaloids in which L-proline was replaced by other amino acids.

A first attempt with D-proline, which would have led to the epimer in position 11′, failed because of the low stability of intermediates; yet syntheses with α-methyl-L-proline proved to be viable. Thus, 11′β-methyl-ergotamine (113a) and some derivatives, e.g., (113b), were prepared as well as 11′β-methyl-ergocristine (114a) (STADLER et al., 1969b, 1970a, 1970b).

By incorporation of L-pipecolinic acid instead of L-proline into the peptide part of ergotamine, a homologue of ergotamine with a six-membered ring, formula (115a), and its dihydroderivative, (115b), could be obtained. The synthesis of these products proved to be tedious, their stability insufficient, and their pharmacologic activities distinctly lower than those of ergotamine and dihydroergotamine.

In other synthetic peptide alkaloids, (115c) and its dihydro-derivative (115d), the five-membered ring of L-proline was left out. Taking sarcosine as the building block of the peptide part instead of L-proline, in addition to L-phenylalanine and α-hydroxy-L-alanine, a peptide alkaloid of the ergotamine group resulted in which the cyclol hydroxy group was etherified (HOFMANN and STADLER, 1966).

4. Synthetic Ergot Peptide Alkaloids Modified in Position 5′

In Section D, II of this chapter the procedure was discussed which allowed the synthesis of missing links in the natural groups of ergot peptide alkaloids. To summarize, it formally consists of an exchange of the variable amino acid by another one at the very beginning of the synthesis. This method has also been used to synthesize ergot peptide alkaloids with new substituents in position 5′.

Taking the natural amino acid L-norvaline as a building block instead of L-valine, a new analogue of the ergotoxine group, 2′β-isopropyl-5′α-propyl-ergopeptine (116a), has been obtained (GUTTMANN and HUGUENIN, 1971, 1972). Called ergonorcornine, its characteristic feature is a n-propyl group in 5′α. Its dihydro-derivative, (116b), is an inhibitor of prolactin release in rats; 1-methyl-dihydroergonorcornine (116d) acts as a promotor thereof.

An interesting derivative of ergotamine is 2′β-methyl-5′α-(p-methoxy-benzyl)-ergopeptine, called 5′p-methoxy-ergotamine (117a). In this synthesis the amino acid L-tyrosine was transformed into its methylether, and this compound was used as a building block for the variable amino acid (STADLER and STÜTZ, 1973). It stimulates the rabbit uterus in situ.

The simplest ergot peptide alkaloid with a complete tricyclic peptide part is represented by compound (118a). Having no substituents in position 5′, it is composed of the amino acids glycine, L-proline, and α-hydroxy-L-alanine.

In addition, it has been shown that it is possible to introduce two substituents into position 5′ of the peptide part of ergot alkaloids, starting from α-alkyl-amino acids, such as α-methyl-alanine, which lacks optical activity and is easily obtainable from acetone by a cyanhydrine synthesis. Thus, 2′β-methyl-5′-dimethyl-ergopeptine,

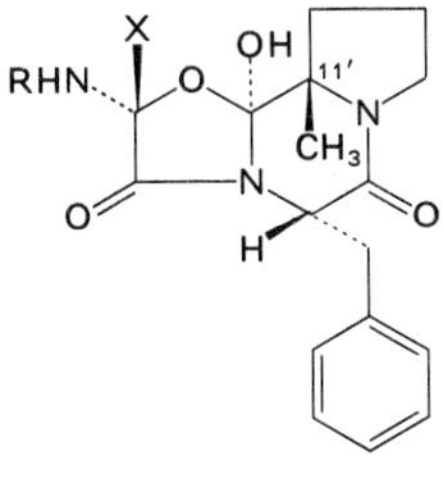

(113a): 11′β-Methyl-ergotamine,
2′β-11′β-dimethyl-5′α-benzyl-ergopeptine
R = lysergoyl, X = methyl

(113b): 11′β-Methyl-dihydroergotamine
R = dihydrolysergoyl, X = methyl

(114a): 11′β-Methyl-ergocristine, 2′β-isopropyl-5′α-benzyl-11′β-methyl-ergopeptine
R = lysergoyl, X = isopropyl

(114b): 11′β-Methyl-dihydroergocristine
R = dihydrolysergoyl
X = isopropyl

(114c): 1,11′β-Dimethyl-dihydroergocristine
R = 1-methyl-dihydrolysergoyl
X = isopropyl

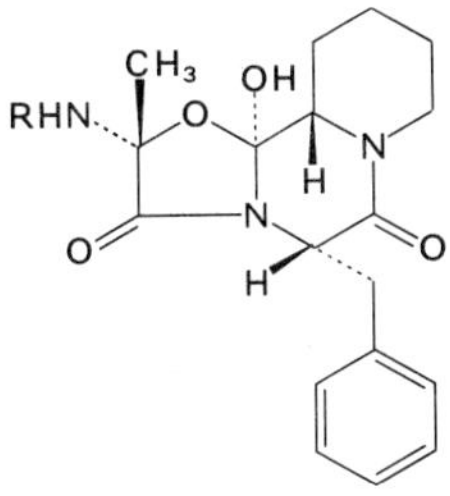

(115a): 2′β-Methyl-5′α-benzyl-11′β-homo-ergopeptine
R = lysergoyl

(115b): 2′β-Methyl-5′α-benzyl-11′β-homo-dihydroergopeptine
R = dihydrolysergoyl

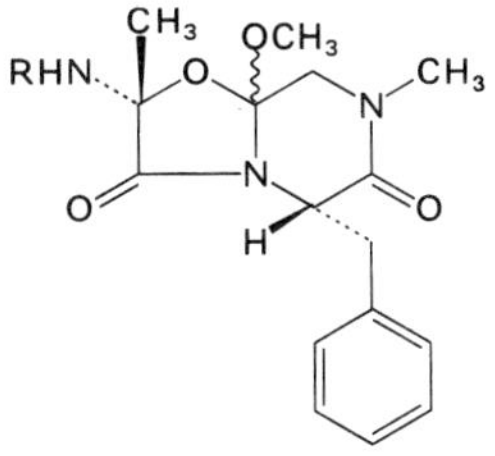

(115c): R = lysergoyl

(115d): R = dihydrolysergoyl

Fig. 31. Synthetic ergot peptide alkaloids modified in the proline building block

called 5′β-methyl-ergoalanine (119a), is known under the code MD-121 as a vasoconstrictor. Moreover, the two substituents in position 5′ can form an additional spirocyclic ring: When 1-amino-cyclohexyl-1-carboxylic acid was taken as variable amino acid for the synthesis of a new member of the ergotamine group, the corresponding peptide alkaloid with a spirocyclic structure (120a) resulted. When the two substituents X and Y differ structurally, the α-alkyl-amino acid at the basis of the synthesis contains an asymmetric center and has to be separated

(116a): 2′β-Isopropyl-5′α-n-propyl-ergopeptine, Ergonorcornine
R = lysergoyl

(116b): Dihydroergonorcornine
R = dihydrolysergoyl

(116c): 1-Methyl-ergonorcornine
R = 1-methyl-lysergoyl

(116d): 1-Methyl-dihydroergonorcornine
R = 1-methyl-dihydrolysergoyl

(117a): 2′β-Methyl-5′α-(p-methoxy-benzyl)-ergopeptine, 5′p-Methoxy-ergotamine
R = lysergoyl

(117b): 5′p-Methoxy-dihydroergotamine
R = dihydrolysergoyl

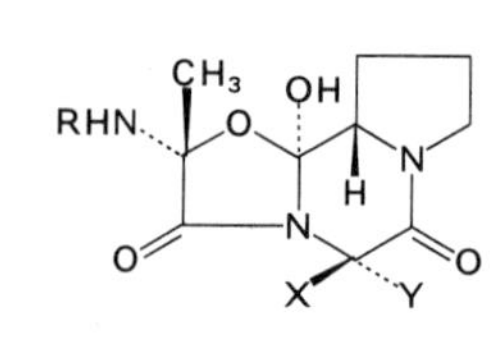

(118a): 2′β-Methyl-ergopeptine
R = lysergoyl, X = Y = H

(118b): 2′β-Methyl-dihydroergopeptine
R = dihydrolysergoyl, X = Y = H

(119a): 2′β,5′,5′-Trimethyl ergopeptine, 5′β-Methyl-ergoalanine, MD-121
R = lysergoyl, X = Y = CH_3

(119b): 5′β-Methyl-dihydroergoalanine
R = dihydrolysergoyl, X = Y = CH_3

(120a): 2′β-Methyl-5′-pentamethylen-ergopeptine
R = lysergoyl, X and Y = $-(CH_2)_5-$

(120b): 2′β-Methyl-5′-pentamethylen-dihydroergopeptine
R = dihydrolysergoyl, X and Y = $-(CH_2)_5-$

(121a): 2′β,5′β-Dimethyl-5′α-benzyl-ergopeptine, 5′β-Methyl-ergotamine
R = lysergoyl, X = methyl, Y = benzyl

(121b): 5′β-Methyl-dihydroergotamine
R = dihydrolysergoyl, X = methyl, Y = benzyl

(122a): 2′β,5′α-Dimethyl-ergopeptine, Ergoalanine
R = lysergoyl, X = H, Y = methyl

Fig. 32. Modifications in position 5′ of ergot peptide alkaloids

into its antipodes prior to its use as variable amino acid. Thus, benzylmethyl-ketone has been transformed to L-α-methyl-phenylalanine, which has then been used to synthesize 5′β-methyl-ergotamine, (121a), and its dihydro derivative, (121b) (STADLER et al., 1971).

E. Some Analytical Tools for the Determination of Ergot Alkaloids

Progress in analytical chemistry has provided, especially since about 1950, a series of very sensitive new methods which are widely used in ergot chemistry. It cannot be the aim of this chapter to give detailed information of all these analytical tools, as good reviews already exist in HOFMANN (1964), FOSTER (1955), and GYENES and BAYER (1961), but we shall briefly present the most important methods here.

1. Separation of Ergot Alkaloids

a) Column Chromatography and Crystallization

Group-wise separation of ergot alkaloids on a preparative scale is best performed by column chromatography on aluminium oxide or silicagel with chloroform or methylene chloride containing increasing amounts of methanol or ethanol as eluents (HOFMANN, 1964). Further purification may be effected by transformation of alkaloid fractions into suitable salts. Di-para-toluyl-tartaric acid has proved to be especially useful for this purpose (STOLL and HOFMANN, 1943a). Purification of raw ergot alkaloids by direct crystallization of the free bases is often tedious or even unsuccessful, as they often form isomorphic mixtures (see, e.g., "ergotoxine").

High pressure chromatography, now under rapid development, is increasingly proving to be a very valuable tool in separation and analysis of ergot alkaloids.

b) Paper Chromatography

The first success of this analytical method was the separation of ergometrine (30) and ergometrinine (31) (FOSTER et al., 1949). The method was rapidly developed, and as early as 1954 a series of different systems was known which allowed the semiquantitative separation of practically all natural ergot alkaloids on paper (STOLL and RÜEGGER, 1954; MACEK and VANECEK, 1955). Today, a battery of highly specific systems of solvents and special papers are at our disposal, and trace amounts of less than a microgram of an ergot alkaloid can be identified.

c) Thin-Layer Chromatography

Thin-layer chromatography was developed somewhat later than the paper methods. A good monograph on the technique is available (STAHL, 1962). Today, plates of aluminium oxide and silicagel are widely used, the predominant solvent system being methylene chloride and methanol. The spots are either checked by direct observation of the fluorescence of lysergic acid derivatives in ultraviolet light or made directly visible by development with the color reaction of Van Urk-Smith. The method is simpler and faster than paper chromatography; the sensitivity is about the same.

2. Assay of Ergot Alkaloids

Ergot alkaloids contain two structural subunits suitable for quantitative determination, the indole ring system and the basic nitrogen atom in 6. The latter can be used as a basis for titration methods, while color reactions and some spectroscopic methods depend on the indole ring.

a) Titration with Perchloric Acid

In galenic preparations ergot alkaloids are usually not used as free bases but in the form of salts, e.g., ergotamine tartrate and ergometrine hydrogen maleinate. For a simple and quantitative determination of the alkaloid content in such preparations, a method had to be worked out which allowed a direct titration of the alkaloids as salts. The method generally used in such cases is titration with perchloric acid: The sample of the alkaloid salt is dissolved in glacial acetic acid and titrated with perchloric acid in the same medium, free of water. As an indicator, crystal violet is used, which changes color from blue to a bluish green. Due to its extreme strength, perchloric acid expels the other, weaker acid from its salt with the ergot alkaloid (GYENES and BAYER, 1961; RENNEBERG and SZENDEY, 1958).

b) Color Reactions

The Keller reaction (KELLER, 1896) was the first characteristic color test for ergot alkaloids. A trace of an ergot alkaloid is dissolved in glacial acetic acid containing a little iron(III)chloride; the solution is carefully added to concentrated sulfuric acid in a test tube, whereupon a blue ring appears at the interface. When the solutions are homogenized, an intensely colored solution is obtained. Simple derivatives of lysergic acid, e.g., LSD or ergometrine, and the alkaloids of the ergotamine group exhibit a pure, deep blue color; the alkaloids of the ergotoxine group give green to olive-green solutions. Its limit sensitivity lies at about 30 to 50 μg.

A second color reaction was detected by VAN URK (VAN URK, 1929). He observed that ergot alkaloids give an intensive blue color reaction when treated with p-dimethylamino-benzaldehyde in the presence of a strong acid. The reaction was substantially improved by Smith (SMITH, 1930) and somewhat later developed further to a standard procedure for quantitative determination of ergot alkaloids (ALLPORT and COCKING, 1932). In this procedure the blue solution obtained from the specimen to be determined is compared with a standard VAN URK solution of ergometrine hydrogen maleinate in a colorimeter. The sensitivity of the reaction is high, in favorable circumstances about one microgram being detectable.

c) UV Spectroscopy

Ergolines contain an indole ring system, substituted in positions 3 and 4. Because of this chromophore they exhibit an intense absorption band in the ultraviolet part of the spectrum (JACOBS et al., 1936). The maximum lies at 281 nm, its extinction amounting to 7200. In 9-ergolenes, e.g., in ergotamine, the chromophore is more complex, as the additional double bond in position 9,10 lies in conjugation to the indole system, as a result of which the observed absorption band is shifted to longer wavelengths, its maximum now lying at 312–313 nm with a considerably higher (~9100) extinction.

A measurement of the absorbance at the absorption maximum allows a quantitative determination of individual alkaloids and their sum in alkaloid mixtures. It does not, however, allow one to distinguish between individual alkaloids.

Like the Van Urk-Smith color reaction, the ultraviolet absorption of the alkaloids is characteristic of the lysergoyl- and isolysergoyl-portion present in a mixture. It is therefore proportional to the total alkaloid content and not necessarily to the biological potency of the material under examination.

d) IR Spectroscopy

The IR spectra of ergot alkaloids are very useful for the identification of individual, pure alkaloids. The IR spectra of natural ergot alkaloids in Nujol have been published; they all differ distinctly one from another (Hofmann, 1964). The method has especially been used for the determination of LSD-25 (Hale and Taylor, 1967).

e) Fluorescence Spectroscopy

All ergot alkaloids carrying the additional double bond in position 9,10 show a very intense, blue fluorescence when irradiated with ultra-violet light. In ergolines, which lack the additional double bond, this fluorescence emission is shifted into the ultra-violet region of the spectrum. Based on this fluorescence, a versatile method for the determination of ergot alkaloids has been elaborated (Bowman et al., 1955). Due to its extreme sensitivity, it is especially suitable for the determination of tiny traces of ergot derivatives, e.g., of LSD-25, in biological fluids (Doepfner, 1962) or narcotic seizures (Genest and Farmilo, 1964; Dal Cortivo et al., 1966). It has been found that the fluorometric method is sensitive to one nanogram of LSD-25 (Aghajanian and Bing, 1964).

F. Subject Index

Most commonly used names of substances are italicized. The names of important synonyms are given. The stereoformulas of compounds may be found in this chapter under the indicated figure and number.

Names	Fig.	Nr.
1-Acetyl-lysergic acid derivatives, (general formula)	13	(36a)
1-Acetyl-lysergic acid ethylamide, (ALA 10)	13	(36g)
Aci-dihydroergocornine	28	(107c)
Aci-dihydroergocristine	28	(107b)
Aci-dihydro-α-ergokryptine	28	(107d)
Aci-dihydro-β-ergokryptine	28	(107e)
Aci-dihydroergotamine	28	(107a)
Aci-ergotamine	28	(107f)
Aci-ergotaminine	28	(107g)
Acylation product, (general formula)	11	(31)
Agroclavine	2	(5)
ALA 10, *1-Acetyl-lysergic acid ethylamide*	13	(36g)
ALD 52, *1-Acetyl-LSD*	13	(36f)
1-Alkyl-dihydrolysergic acid amides, (general formula)	12	(35)
2-Amino-dihydrolysergic acid derivatives, (general formula)	15	(42)
Antipode of ergometrine	16	(56)
Antipode of ergometrinine	16	(53)
Antipode of ergotamine	16	(67)
Antipode of ergotaminine	16	(68)
Antipode of Lysenyl®, l-Lysenyl®, 8β-N[1]-(l-6-Methyl-9-ergolenyl)-N[2]-diethyl-urea	16	(66)
Basergin®, *Ergometrine®*, Ergobasine, Ergonovine, Ergotocine	9	(19)
BOL-148, *2-Bromo-d-lysergic acid diethylamide,* 2-Bromo-LSD	14	(37a)
Bromocriptine, *2-Bromo-α-ergokryptine,* 2′β-Isopropyl-5′α-isobutyl-2-bromo-ergopeptine, Parlodel®, CB-154	14	(38)
13-Bromo-dihydroergotamine	27	(106a)
13-Bromo-dihydrolysergic acid	27	(106b)
2-Bromo-ergocornine	14	(37c)
2-Bromo-α-ergokryptine, 2′β-Isopropyl-5′α-isobutyl-2-bromo-ergopeptine, CB-154, Parlodel®, Bromocriptine	14	(38)
2-Bromo-LSD, *2-Bromo-d-lysergic acid diethylamide,* BOL-148	14	(37a)
2-Bromo-d-lysergic acid diethylamide, 2-Bromo-LSD, BOL-148	14	(37a)
2-Bromo-6-methyl-8β-cyanomethyl-ergoline	14	(39a)
13-Bromo-MNE	27	(106c)
CB-154, *2-Bromo-α-ergokryptine,* 2′β-Isopropyl-5′a-isobutyl-2-bromo-ergopeptine, Parlodel®, Bromocriptine	14	(38)
2-Chloro-6-methyl-8β-cyanomethyl-ergoline, Lergotrile	14	(39)
1-Cyanoethyl lysergic acid derivatives, (general formula)	13	(36e)
Cyclol ester, (general formula)	11	(32)
DAM 57, *Lysergic acid dimethylamide*	18	(73c)
Delyside®, *LSD-25, LSD, d-LSD,* d-Lysergic acid diethylamide, Lysergidum	18	(73b)
Deprenone, *VUFB-6683*, Dihydrohomolysergic acid amide	20	(86b)
Δ-8,9-Deseril, 1,6-Dimethyl-8-ergolene-8-carboxylic acid L-2-butanolamide	24	(100h)
Deseril®, *1-Methyl-lysergic acid L-2-butanolamide,* Desernil®, Sansert®, Methysergide	12	(34a)
Desernil®, *1-Methyl-lysergic acid L-2-butanolamide,* Deseril®, Sansert®, Methysergide	12	(34a)
DHE-45, *Dihydroergotamine,* Dihydergot®	25	(102b)
Diastereomer of ergotamine	16	(69)
Diastereomer of ergotaminine	16	(70)
2,13-Dibromo-dihydrolysergic acid glycine amide, RN-76	14	(40)
8,9-Didehydro-10α-methoxy-9,10-dihydroergotamine	24	(101d)

Names	Fig.	Nr.
N,N-Diethyl-lysergylamine, 6-Methyl-8β-diethylamino-methyl-9-ergolene	21	(88b)
Dihydergot®, *Dihydroergotamine*, DHE-45	25	(102b)
Dihydroergocornine	25	(102d)
Dihydroergocristine	25	(102c)
Dihydro-α-ergokryptine	25	(102e)
Dihydro-β-ergokryptine	25	(102f)
Dihydroergometrine, Dihydrolysergic acid L-alaninol-amide	18	(74c)
2,3-Dihydroergometrine	15	(48b)
Dihydroergonine, 2′β-Ethyl-5′α-isopropyl-dihydroergopeptine, DN-16-457	30	(110b)
Dihydroergonorcornine, 2′β-Isopropyl-5′-α-n-propyl-dihydroergopeptine	32	(116b)
Dihydroergopeptine, 2′β-Ethyl-5′α-isobutyl-dihydroergopeptine	30	(111b)
Dihydro-β-ergoptine, 2′β-Ethyl-5′α-sec.butyl-dihydroergopeptine	30	(112b)
Dihydroergosine	25	(102a)
Dihydro-β-ergosine, 2′β-Methyl-5′α-sec.butyl-dihydroergopeptine	29	(109b)
Dihydroergostine	25	(102g)
Dihydroergotamine, DHE-45, Dihydergot®	25	(102b)
Dihydroergotoxine mesylate, Hydergin®	25	
Dihydroergovaline, 2′β-Methyl-5′α-isopropyl-dihydroergopeptine	29	(108b)
Dihydrohomolysergic acid	20	(84b)
Dihydrohomolysergic acid amide, *VUFB-6683*, Deprenone	20	(86b)
Dihydrohomolysergic acid methylester	20	(85b)
Dihydrohomolysergic acid nitrile, VUFB-6605	20	(83b)
Dihydrohomolysergol	20	(87b)
Dihydro-LSD, *Dihydrolysergic acid diethylamide*	18	(74b)
Dihydrolysergal	19	(80)
d-Dihydrolysergic acid	6	(16a)
Dihydrolysergic acid L-alaninolamide, *Dihydroergometrine*	18	(74c)
Dihydrolysergic acid amide	18	(74a)
Dihydrolysergic acid azide	18	(74e)
Dihydrolysergic acid diethylamide, Dihydro-LSD	18	(74b)
Dihydrolysergic acid hydrazide	18	(74d)
Dihydrolysergic acid methylester	19	(76a)
Dihydrolysergic acid nitrile	19	(78)
Dihydrolysergol	19	(81a)
Dihydrolysergol mesylate	22	(91a)
Dihydrolysergylamine, 6-Methyl-8β-aminomethyl-ergoline	21	(89a)
2′β-5′α-Diisopropyl-ergopeptine, *Ergocornine*	10	(24)
4-Dimethylallyl-L-tryptophan	2	(4)
1,6-Dimethyl-8β-aminomethyl-ergoline, *1-Methyl-dihydrolysergylamine*	21	(89b)
1-Dimethylaminomethyl-lysergic acid derivatives (general formula)	13	(36d)
2′β-12′-Dimethyl-5′α-benzyl-9′,10′-bisdesmethylendihydroergopeptine	31	(115d)
2′β-12′-Dimethyl-5′α-benzyl-9′,10′-bisdesmethylen-ergopeptine	31	(115c)
2′β,5′β-Dimethyl-5′α-benzyl-dihydroergopeptine, 5′β-Methyl-dihydro-ergotamine	32	(121b)
2′β,11′β-Dimethyl-5′α-benzyl-dihydroergopeptine, *11′β-Methyl-dihydro-ergotamine*	31	(113b)
8,2′β-Dimethyl-5′α-benzyl-dihydroergopeptine, *8-Methyl-dihydroergotamine*	23	(99d)
2′β,5′β-Dimethyl-5′α-benzyl-ergopeptine, 5′β-Methyl-ergotamine	32	(121a)
2′β,11′β-Dimethyl-5′α-benzyl-ergopeptine, *11′β-Methyl-ergotamine*	31	(113a)
8,2′β-Dimethyl-5′α-benzyl-ergopeptine, *8-Methyl-ergotamine*	23	(99c)
1,6-Dimethyl-8β-carbobenzoxyaminomethyl-ergoline, *1-Methyl-N-carbo-benzoxy-dihydrolysergylamine*, MCE, Methergoline	21	(89d)
1,6-Dimethyl-8β-[4,6-dimethyl-2-pyrimidino-amino-methyl]-ergoline	21	(89g)
6,8α-Dimethyl-9-ergolene	19	(79d)
6,8β-Dimethyl-9-ergolene	19	(79c)

Names	Fig.	Nr.
1,6-Dimethyl-8-ergolene-8-carboxylic acid	24	(100b)
1,6-Dimethyl-8-ergolene-8-carboxylic acid L-2-butanolamide, *Δ-8-9-Deseril*	24	(100h)
1,6-Dimethyl-8-ergolene-8-carboxylic acid chloride.HCl	24	(100c)
1,6-Dimethyl-8-ergolene-8-carboxylic acid diethylamide, *1-Methyl-Δ-8,9-LSD*	24	(100g)
N-[1,6-Dimethyl-8α-(9-ergolenyl)]-N′N′-diethyl-urea, Mesenyl	23	(96b)
2′β,5′α-Dimethyl-ergopeptine, Ergoalanine	32	(122a)
1,6-Dimethyl-8β-guanidinomethyl-ergoline	21	(89f)
1,8-Dimethyl-LSD, 1,8α-Dimethyl-lysergic acid diethylamide	23	(99a)
1,8-Dimethyl-lysergic acid diethylamide, *1,8-Dimethyl-LSD*	23	(99a)
1,6-Dimethyl-10α-methoxy-8-ergolene-8-carboxylic acid amide	24	(101b)
1,1-Dimethyl-3-[6-methyl-8β-(9-ergolenyl)-methyl] urea	21	(88h)
Dipeptide ester, (general formula)	11	(28)
2-Dithiolanoyl-d-lysergic acid methylester	15	(44)
DN-16-457, *Dihydroergonine,* 2′β-Ethyl-5′α-isopropyl-dihydroergopeptine	30	(110b)
Elymoclavine	2	(6)
Elymoclavine pyridinium tosylate	22	(6a)
Ergine, d-Lysergic acid amide	9	(18)
Ergoalanine, *2′β,5′α-Dimethyl-ergopeptine*	32	(122a)
Ergobasine, *Ergometrine®*, Ergonovine, Ergotocine, Basergin®	9	(19)
Ergocornine, 2′β,5′α-Diisopropyl-ergopeptine	10	(24)
Ergocristine, 2′β-Isopropyl-5′α-benzyl-ergopeptine	10	(23)
α-Ergokryptine, 2′β-Isopropyl-5′α-isobutyl-ergopeptine	10	(25)
β-Ergokryptine, 2′β-Isopropyl-5′α-sec.butyl-ergopeptine	10	(26)
8-Ergolenes, (general formula)	5	(13)
9-Ergolenes, 8α-isomers, (general formula)	5	(15)
9-Ergolenes, 8β-isomers, (general formula)	5	(14)
Ergoline	1	(1)
Ergometrine, Ergobasine, Ergonovine, Ergotocine, Basergin®, Ergometrine®	9	(19)
Δ-8,9-Ergometrine, 6-Methyl-8-ergolene-8-carboxylic acid L-alaninolamide	24	(100e)
Ergonine, 2′β-Ethyl-5′α-isopropyl-ergopeptine	30	(110a)
Ergonorcornine, 2′β-Isopropyl-5′α-n-propyl-ergopeptine	32	(116a)
Ergonovine, *Ergometrine®*, Ergobasine, Ergotocine, Basergin®	9	(19)
Ergopeptine, (general formula)	7	(17a)
Ergoptine, 2′β-Ethyl-5′α-isobutyl-ergopeptine	30	(111a)
β-Ergoptine, 2′β-Ethyl-5′α-sec.butyl-ergopeptine	30	(112a)
Ergosine, 2′β-Methyl-5′α-isobutyl-ergopeptine	10	(21)
β-Ergosine, 2′β-Methyl-5′α-sec.butyl-ergopeptine	29	(109a)
Ergostine, 2′β-Ethyl-5′α-benzyl-ergopeptine	10	(22)
Ergotamine, 2′β-Methyl-5′α-benzyl-ergopeptine, Gynergene®	10	(20)
Ergotaminine, 2′β-Methyl-5′a-benzyl-ergopeptinine	10	
Ergotocine, *Ergometrine®*, Ergobasine, Ergonovine, Basergin®	9	(19)
Ergot Peptide Alkaloids (general formula)	3, 7	(11)
Ergovaline, 2′β-Methyl-5′α-isopropyl-ergopeptine	29	(108a)
2′β-Ethyl-5′α-benzyl-ergopeptine, *Ergostine*	10	(22)
2′β-Ethyl-5′α-sec.butyl-dihydroergopeptine, *Dihydro-β-ergoptine*	30	(112b)
2′β-Ethyl-5′α-sec.butyl-ergopeptine, *β-Ergoptine*	30	(112a)
2′β-Ethyl-5′α-isobutyl-dihydroergopeptine, *Dihydroergoptine*	30	(111b)
2′β-Ethyl-5′α-isobutyl-ergopeptine, *Ergoptine*	30	(111a)
2′β-Ethyl-5′α-isopropyl-dihydroergopeptine, *Dihydroergonine,* DN-16-457	30	(110b)
2′β-Ethyl-5′α-isopropyl-ergopeptine, *Ergonine*	30	(110a)
1-Formyl-dihydrohomolysergic acid nitrile	20	(83d)
2-Formyl-d-lysergic acid methylester	15	(46)

Names	Fig.	Nr.
Gynergene®, *Ergotamine,* 2′β-Methyl-5′α-benzyl-ergopeptine	10	(20)
Homolysergic acid	20	(84a)
Homolysergic acid diethylamide	20	(86a)
Homolysergic acid methylester	20	(85a)
Homolysergic acid nitrile, 6-Methyl-8β-cyanomethyl-9-ergolene	20	(83a)
Homolysergol	20	(87a)
Hydergin®, *Dihydroergotoxine mesylate*	25	
α-Hydroxy-α-amino acid, (general formula)	11	(30)
12-Hydroxy-deseril, *12-Hydroxy-1-methyl-lysergic acid L-2-butanolamide,* 12-Hydroxy-methysergide	27	(105e)
12-Hydroxy-dihydroergometrine	27	(105b)
10α-Hydroxy-dihydroergotamine, *Lumi-I-ergotamine*	26	(103d)
10α-Hydroxy-dihydrolysergic acid, *Lumi-I-lysergic acid*	26	(103a)
10α-Hydroxy-dihydrolysergic acid L-alaninolamide, *Lumi-I-ergometrine*	26	(103b)
10α-Hydroxy-dihydrolysergic acid diethylamide, *Lumi-I-LSD*	26	(103c)
12-Hydroxy-ergometrine	27	(105a)
12-Hydroxy-LSD, 12-Hydroxy-d-lysergic acid diethylamide	27	(105c)
12-Hydroxy-lysergic acid L-2-butanolamide, 12-Hydroxy-methergine, 12-Hydroxy-methylergometrine	27	(105d)
12-Hydroxy-d-lysergic acid diethylamide, *12-Hydroxy-LSD*	27	(105c)
12-Hydroxy-methergine, *12-Hydroxy-lysergic acid L-2-butanolamide,* 12-Hydroxy-methylergometrine	27	(105d)
12-Hydroxy-methylergometrine, *12-Hydroxy-lysergic acid L-2-butanolamide,* 12-Hydroxy-methergine	27	(105d)
12-Hydroxy-1-methyl-lysergic acid L-2-butanolamide, 12-Hydroxy-deseril, 12-Hydroxy-methysergide	27	(105e)
1-Hydroxymethyl lysergic acid derivatives, (general formula)	13	(36c)
1-Hydroxymethyl lysergic acid diethylamide (OML 632)	13	(36h)
12-Hydroxy-methysergide, *12-Hydroxy-1-methyl-lysergic acid-L-2-butanolamide,* 12-Hydroxy-deseril	27	(105e)
Isoergine, d-Isolysergic acid amide	9	(18a)
Iso-LSD, *d-Isolysergic acid diethylamide*	23	(93c)
l-Iso-LSD, l-Isolysergic acid diethylamide	16	(62)
d-Isolysergic acid	23	(93)
l-Isolysergic acid	16	(58)
d-Isolysergic acid amide, *Isoergine*	9	(18a)
l-Isolysergic acid amide	16	(60)
l-Isolysergic acid azide	16	(52)
d-Isolysergic acid diethylamide, Iso-LSD	23	(93c)
l-Isolysergic acid diethylamide, *l-Iso-LSD*	16	(62)
d-Isolysergic acid hydrazide	23	(93b)
l-Isolysergic acid hydrazide	16	(51)
d-Isolysergic acid methylester	19	(75a)
l-Isolysergic acid l-norephedride	16	(64)
Isolysergol, 6-Methyl-8α-hydroxymethyl-9-ergolene	19	(79e)
2′β-Isopropyl-5′α-benzyl-ergopeptine, *Ergocristine*	10	(23)
2′β-Isopropyl-5′α-benzyl-11′β-methyl-dihydroergopeptine, *11′β-Methyl-dihydroergocristine*	31	(114b)
2′β-Isopropyl-5′α-benzyl-11′β-methyl-ergopeptine, *11′β-Methyl-ergocristine*	31	(114a)
2′β-Isopropyl-5′α-isobutyl-2-bromo-ergopeptine, *2-Bromo-α-ergokryptine,* Parlodel®, Bromocriptine, CB-154	14	(38)
2′β-Isopropyl-5′α-isobutyl-ergopeptine, *α-Ergokryptine*	10	(25)
2′β-Isopropyl-5′α-isobutyl-ergopeptine, *β-Ergokryptine*	10	(26)

Names	Fig.	Nr.
2′β-Isopropyl-5′α-n-propyl-dihydroergopeptine, *Dihydroergonorcornine*	32	(116b)
2′β-Isopropyl-5′α-n-propyl-ergopeptine, *Ergonorcornine*	32	(116a)
2-Jodo-6-methyl-8β-cyanomethyl-ergoline	14	(39b)
Lactam, (general formula)	11	(29)
LAE, *Lysergic acid ethylamide*	18	(73h)
LBB 66, *Lysergic acid dibutylamide*	18	(73e)
Lergotrile, *2-Chloro-6-methyl-8β-cyanomethyl-ergoline*	14	(39)
Lisuride, *N-[6-Methyl-8α-(9-ergolenyl)]-N′,N′-diethyl-urea,* Lysuride, Mesorgydine, Lysenyl®	23	(96a)
LPD 824, *Lysergic acid pyrrolidide*	18	(73f)
l-LSD, l-Lysergic acid diethylamide	16	(61)
Δ-8,9-LSD, 6-Methyl-8-ergolene-8-carboxylic acid diethylamide	24	(100d)
LSD-25, LSD, d-LSD, d-Lysergic acid diethylamide, Lysergidum, Delyside®	18	(73b)
LSM 775, *Lysergic acid morpholidide*	18	(73g)
Lumi-I-ergometrine, 10α-Hydroxy-dihydrolysergic acid L-alaninolamide	26	(103b)
Lumi-I-ergotamine, 10α-Hydroxy-dihydroergotamine	26	(103d)
Lumi-I-LSD, 10α-Hydroxy-dihydrolysergic acid diethylamide	26	(103c)
Lumi-I-lysergic acid, 10α-Hydroxy-dihydrolysergic acid	26	(103a)
Lysenyl®, *N-[6-Methyl-8α-(9-ergolenyl)]-N′,N′-diethyl-urea,* Lysuride, Lisuride, Mesorgydine	23	(96a)
l-Lysenyl®, *Antipode of Lysenyl®,* 8β-N[1]-(l-6-Methyl-9-ergolenyl)-N[2]-diethyl-urea	16	(66)
Lysergene, 6-Methyl-8-methylen-9-ergolene	19	(79f)
d-Lysergic acid	2, 4	(8)
l-Lysergic acid	16	(57)
d-Lysergic acid amide, *Ergine*	9	(18)
l-Lysergic acid amide	16	(59)
l-Lysergic acid azide	16	(55)
d-Lysergic acid L-2-butanolamide, Methylergometrine, Methylergobasine, Methylergonovine, Methergine®	18	(73a)
Lysergic acid dibutylamide, (LBB 66)	18	(73e)
l-Lysergic acid diethylamide, *l-LSD*	16	(61)
d-Lysergic acid diethylamide, *LSD-25, LSD, d-LSD,* Lysergidum, Delyside®	18	(73b)
Lysergic acid dimethylamide, (DAM 57)	18	(73c)
Lysergic acid dipropylamide	18	(73d)
Lysergic acid ethylamide, (LAE 32)	18	(73h)
d-Lysergic acid hydrazide	23	(93a)
l-Lysergic acid hydrazide	16	(54)
d-Lysergic acid 2-hydroxy-ethylester	19	(75c)
d-Lysergic acid methylcarbinolamide	4	(12)
d-Lysergic acid methylester	17	(72a)
Lysergic acid morpholidide, (LSM 775)	18	(73g)
d-Lysergic acid nitrile	19	(77)
l-Lysergic acid 1-norephedride	16	(63)
d-Lysergic acid 3-pyridylcarbinolester	19	(75d)
Lysergic acid pyrrolidide, (LPD 824)	18	(73f)
Lysergidum, *LSD-25, LSD, d-LSD,* d-Lysergic acid diethylamide, Delyside®	18	(73b)
Lysergol, 6-Methyl-8β-hydroxymethyl-9-ergolene	19	(79a)
Lysergol acetate	19	(79b)
Lysergol mesylate	22	(90a)
Lysergol tosylate	20	(82a)
N-Lysergoyl-tripeptide, (general formula)	3	(10)
Lysergylamine, 6-Methyl-8β-aminomethyl-9-ergolene	21	(88a)

Names	Fig.	Nr.
Lysuride, *N-[6-Methyl-8α-(9-ergolenyl)]-N′,N′-diethyl-urea,* Lisuride, Mesorgydine Lysenyl®	23	(96a)
MBL-61, 1-Methyl-2-bromo-LSD	14	(37b)
MCE, *1-Methyl-N-carbobenzoxy-dihydrolysergylamine,* 1,6-Dimethyl-8β-carbobenzoxyaminomethyl-ergoline, Methergoline	21	(89d)
MD-121, *2′β,5′,5′-Trimethyl-ergopeptine,* 5′β-Methylergoalanine	32	(119a)
Mesenyl, *N-[1,6-Dimethyl-8α-(9-ergolenyl)]-N′,N′-diethyl-urea*	23	(96b)
Mesorgydine, *N-[6-Methyl-8α-(9-ergolenyl)]-N′,N′-diethyl-urea,* Lysuride, Lisuride, Lysenyl®	23	(96a)
Methergine®, *d-Lysergic acid L-2-butanolamide,* Methylergometrine, Methylergobasine, Methylergonovine	18	(73a)
Δ-8,9-Methergine, 6-Methyl-8-ergolene-8-carboxylic acid L-2-butanolamide	24	(100f)
Methergoline, *1-Methyl-N-carbobenzoxy-dihydrolysergylamine,* 1,6-Dimethyl-8β-carbobenzoxyaminomethyl-ergoline, MCE	21	(89d)
Methoquizine	23	(96e)
5′p-Methoxy-dihydroergotamine, 2′β-Methyl-5′α-(p-methoxybenzyl)-dihydro-ergopeptine	32	(117b)
10α-Methoxy-dihydrolysergic acid methylester	26	(104a)
10α-Methoxy-dihydrolysergol	26	(104c)
5′p-Methoxy-ergotamine, 2′β-Methyl-5′α-(p-methoxy-benzyl)-ergopeptine	32	(117a)
12-Methoxy-lysergic acid L-2-butanolamide, 12-Methoxy-methergine	27	(105f)
12-Methoxy-methergine, *12-Methoxy-lysergic acid L-2-butanolamide*	27	(105f)
6-Methyl-8-acetoxymethylen-9-ergolene	19	(79g)
6-Methyl-8β-acetylaminomethyl ergoline, *N-Acetyl-dihydrolysergylamine,* Acetergamina, Uterdina	21	(89c)
6-Methyl-8-acetylanilinomethyl-8-ergolene	22	(6i)
6-Methyl-8β-acetyl-ergoline	22	(92)
1-Methyl-N-alkyl-N-benzoyl-lysergylamines, (general formula)	21	(88d)
6-Methyl-8α-amino-9-ergolene	23	(94b)
6-Methyl-8β-amino-9-ergolene	23	(94a)
(6-Methyl-8β-amino-9-ergolenyl)-carbamidic acid methylester	23	(95)
6-Methyl-8α-amino-ergoline	23	(94d)
6-Methyl-8β-amino-ergoline	23	(94c)
6-Methyl-8β-aminomethyl-9-ergolene, *Lysergylamine*	21	(88a)
6-Methyl-8β-aminomethyl-ergoline, *Dihydrolysergylamine*	21	(89a)
6-Methyl-8-anilinomethyl-8-ergolene	22	(6h)
6-Methyl-8β-azidomethyl-9-ergolene	21	(88g)
2′β-Methyl-5′α-benzyl-ergopeptine, *Ergotamine,* Gynergene®	10	(20)
2′β-Methyl-5′α-benzyl-ergopeptinine, *Ergotaminine*	10	
2′β-Methyl-5′α-benzyl-11′β-homo-dihydroergopeptine	31	(115b)
2′β-Methyl-5′α-benzyl-11′β-homo-ergopeptine	31	(115a)
1-Methyl-2-bromo-LSD, *MBL-61*	14	(37b)
2′β-Methyl-5′α-sec.butyl-dihydroergopeptine, *Dihydro-β-ergosine*	29	(109b)
2′β-Methyl-5′α-isobutyl-ergopeptine, *Ergosine*	10	(21)
2′β-Methyl-5′α-sec.butyl-ergopeptine, *β-Ergosine*	29	(109a)
1-Methyl-N-carbobenzoxy-dihydrolysergylamine, 1,6-Dimethyl-8β-carbobenzoxyaminomethyl-ergoline, MCE, Methergoline	21	(89d)
1-Methyl-N-carbobenzoxy-2,3-9,10-tetrahydrolysergylamine	15	(48a)
6-Methyl-8-carboxamidomethyl-8-ergolene	22	(6f)
6-Methyl-8-chloromethyl-8-ergolene	22	(6d)
6-Methyl-8β-chloromethyl-ergoline	20	(82b)
6-Methyl-8-cyanomethyl-8-ergolene	22	(6e)
6-Methyl-8β-cyanomethyl-9-ergolene, *Homolysergic acid nitrile*	20	(83a)
1-Methyl-8,9-didehydro-10α-ethoxy-9,10-dihydroergokryptine	24	(101e)

Names	Fig.	Nr.
6-Methyl-8-diethylaminomethyl-8-ergolene	22	(6c)
6-Methyl-8β-diethylaminomethyl-9-ergolene, *N,N-Diethyl-lysergylamine*	21	(88b)
1-Methyl-dihydroergocristine, 1-Methyl-2′β-isopropyl-5′α-benzyl-dihydroergopeptine	12	(35a)
11′β-Methyl-dihydroergocristine, 2′β-Isopropyl-5′α-benzyl-11′β-methyl-dihydroergopeptine	31	(114b)
1-Methyl-dihydroergonorcornine, 1-Methyl-2′β-isopropyl-5′α-n-propyl-dihydroergopeptine	32	(116d)
2′β-Methyl-dihydroergopeptine	32	(118b)
5′β-Methyl-dihydroergotamine, *2′β,5′β-Dimethyl-5′α-benzyl-dihydroergopeptine*	32	(121b)
8-Methyl-dihydroergotamine, 8,2′β-Dimethyl-5′α-benzyl-dihydroergopeptine	23	(99d)
11′β-Methyl-dihydroergotamine, 2′β,11′β-Dimethyl-5′α-benzyl-dihydroergopeptine	31	(113b)
1-Methyl-dihydrohomolysergic acid nitrile	20	(83c)
1-Methyl-dihydrolysergic acid L-2-butanolamide	12	(35b)
1-Methyl-dihydrolysergol	19	(81b)
1-Methyl-dihydrolysergylamine, 1,6-Dimethyl-8β-aminomethyl-ergoline	21	(89b)
5′β-Methyl-ergoalanine, *2′β,5′-Trimethyl-ergopeptine,* MD-121	32	(119a)
Methylergobasine, *d-Lysergic acid L-2-butanolamide,* Methylergometrine, Methylergonovine, Methergine®	18	(73a)
11′β-Methyl-ergocristine, 2′β-Isopropyl-5′α-benzyl-11′β-methyl-ergopeptine	31	(114a)
6-Methyl-9-ergolene	19	(79h)
6-Methyl-8-ergolene-8-carboxylic acid	2, 4	(7)
6-Methyl-8-ergolene-8-carboxylic acid L-alaninolamide, *Δ-8,9-Ergometrine*	24	(100e)
6-Methyl-8-ergolene-8-carboxylic acid L-2-butanolamide, *Δ-8,9-Methergine*	24	(100f)
6-Methyl-8-ergolene-8-carboxylic acid chloride.HCl	24	(100a)
6-Methyl-8-ergolene-8-carboxylic acid diethylamide, *Δ-8,9-LSD*	24	(100d)
8α-N¹-(l-6-Methyl-9-ergolenyl)-N²-diethyl-urea	16	(65)
8β-N¹-(l-6-Methyl-9-ergolenyl)-N²-diethyl-urea, *Antipode of Lysenyl®,* l-Lysenyl®	16	(66)
N-[6-Methyl-8α-(9-ergolenyl)]-N′,N′-diethyl-urea, Lysuride, Lisuride, Mesorgydine, Lysenyl®	23	(96a)
N-(6-Methyl-8α-ergolinyl)-N′,N′-diethyl-urea, VUFB-6638	23	(96c)
Methylergometrine, *d-Lysergic acid L-2-butanolamide,* Methylergobasine, Methylergonovine, Methergine®	18	(73a)
1-Methyl-ergonorcornine, 1-Methyl-2′β-isopropyl-5′α-n-propyl-ergopeptine	32	(116c)
Methylergonovine, *d-Lysergic acid L-2-butanolamide,* Methylergometrine, Methylergobasine, Methergine®	18	(73a)
2′β-Methyl-ergopeptine	32	(118a)
1-Methyl-ergotamine, MY-25	12	(34c)
5′β-Methyl-ergotamine, *2′β,5′β-Dimethyl-5′α-benzyl-ergopeptine*	32	(121a)
8-Methyl-ergotamine, 8,2′β-Dimethyl-5′α-benzyl-ergopeptine	23	(99c)
11′β-Methyl-ergotamine, 2′β,11′β-Dimethyl-5′α-benzyl-ergopeptine	31	(113a)
6-Methyl-8β-guanidinomethyl-ergoline	21	(89e)
6-Methyl-8α-hydroxymethyl-9-ergolene, *Isolysergol*	19	(79e)
6-Methyl-8β-hydroxymethyl-9-ergolene, *Lysergol*	19	(79a)
1-Methyl-2′β-isopropyl-5′α-benzyl-dihydroergopeptine, *1-Methyl-dihydroergocristine*	12	(35a)
2′β-Methyl-5′α-isopropyl-dihydroergopeptine, *Dihydroergovaline*	29	(108b)
2′β-Methyl-5′α-isopropyl-ergopeptine, *Ergovaline*	29	(108a)
1-Methyl-2′β-isopropyl-5′α-n-propyl-dihydroergopeptine, *1-Methyl-dihydroergonorcornine*	32	(116d)
1-Methyl-2′β-isopropyl-5′α-n-propyl-ergopeptine, *1-Methyl-ergonorcornine*	32	(116c)
1-Methyl-LSD	12	(34b)
8-Methyl-LSD	23	(99b)

Names	Fig.	Nr.
1-Methyl-Δ-8,9-LSD, 1,6-Dimethyl-8-ergolene-8-carboxylic acid diethylamide	24	(100g)
1-Methyl-lysergic acid amides, (general formula)	12	(34)
1-Methyl-d-lysergic acid L-2-butanolamide, Deseril®, Desernil®, Sansert®, Methysergide	12	(34a)
1-Methyl-lysergic acid ethylamide, (MLA 74)	12	(34e)
1-Methyl-d-lysergic acid methylester	19	(75b)
2-Methyl-d-lysergic acid methylester	15	(45)
1-Methyl-lysergic acid pyrrolidide, (MPD 75)	12	(34d)
2′β-Methyl-5′α-(p-methoxybenzyl)-dihydroergopeptine, *5′p-Methoxy-dihydroergotamine*	32	(117b)
2′β-Methyl-5′α-(p-methoxybenzyl)-ergopeptine, *5′p-Methoxy-ergotamine*	32	(117a)
1-Methyl-10α-methoxy-dihydrolysergic acid methylester	26	(104b)
1-Methyl-10α-methoxy-dihydrolysergol	26	(104d)
1-Methyl-10α-methoxy-dihydrolysergol-5-bromonicotinate, *MNE,* Nicergoline, Sermion®	26	(104e)
6-Methyl-10α-methoxy-8-ergolene-8-carboxylic acid amide	24	(101a)
6-Methyl-10α-methoxy-8-ergolene-8-carboxylic acid L-2-aminobutanolamide	24	(101c)
6-Methyl-8β-[4-(p-methoxyphenyl)-1-piperazinyl] methyl-9-ergolene, PTR 17-402	21	(88e)
6-Methyl-8-methylen-9-ergolene, *Lysergene*	19	(79f)
N-(6-Methyl-8β-methyl-9-ergolenyl)-azabicyclo(3,2,2)nonane	21	(88f)
6-Methyl-8-oxo-ergoline	23	(97)
6-Methyl-8β-[N,N-pentamethylen-aminomethyl]-9-ergolene, *N,N-Pentamethylenlysergylamine*	21	(88c)
2′β-Methyl-5′-pentamethylen-dihydroergopeptine	32	(120b)
2′β-Methyl-5′-pentamethylen-ergopeptine	32	(120a)
6-Methyl-8-piperidinomethyl-8-ergolene	22	(6b)
6-Methyl-8α-(3-pyridylamino)-ergoline	23	(98)
6-Methyl-8β-(2-pyridyl-thiomethyl)-9-ergolene	22	(90d)
6-Methyl-8β-(2-pyridyl-thiomethyl)-ergoline	22	(91b)
6-Methyl-8-pyrrolidinomethyl-8-ergolene	22	(6g)
6-Methyl-8β-rhodanomethyl-9-ergolene	22	(90c)
Methysergide, *1-Methyl-lysergic acid L-2-butanolamide,* Deseril®, Desernil®, Sansert®	12	(34a)
Mevalonic acid	2	(3)
MLA 74, *1-Methyl-lysergic acid ethylamide*	12	(34e)
MNE, Nicergoline, Sermion®, 1-Methyl-10α-methoxy-dihydrolysergol-5-bromo-nicotinate	26	(104e)
MPD 75, *1-Methyl-lysergic acid pyrrolidide*	12	(34d)
My-25, *1-Methyl-ergotamine*	12	(34c)
Nicergoline, *MNE,* Sermion®, 1-Methyl-10α-methoxy-dihydrolysergol-5-bromo-nicotinate	26	(104e)
2-Nitro-dihydrolysergic acid derivatives, (general formula)	15	(41)
6-Nor-6-carboxamido-d-lysergic acid diethylamide	17	(72h)
6-Nor-6-cyano-LSD, *6-Nor-6-cyano-d-lysergic acid diethylamide*	17	(72g)
6-Nor-6-cyano-d-lysergic acid dibutylamide	17	(72k)
6-Nor-6-cyano-d-lysergic acid diethylamide, 6-Nor-6-cyano-LSD	17	(72g)
6-Nor-6-cyano-d-lysergic acid methylester	17	(72b)
6-Nor-6-ethyl-d-lysergic acid	17	(72e)
6-Nor-6-ethyl-d-lysergic acid methylester	17	(72d)
6-Nor-6-isopropyl-dihydroergocristine	17	(71f)
6-Nor-6-isopropyl-dihydroergotamine	17	(71e)
6-Nor-6-isopropyl-ergotamine	17	(72f)
6-Nor-LSD, *6-Nor-d-lysergic acid diethylamide*	17	(72i)

Names	Fig.	Nr.
6-Nor-d-lysergic acid diethylamide, 6-Nor-LSD	17	(72i)
6-Nor-d-lysergic acid methylester	17	(72c)
OML 632, *1-Hydroxymethyl lysergic acid diethylamide*	13	(36h)
2-Oxo-2,3-dihydrolysergic acid diethylamide	15	(49)
2-Oxo-3-hydroxy-2,3-dihydrolysergic acid diethylamide	15	(50)
PAI	23	(96d)
Parlodel®, *2-Bromo-α-ergokryptine*, 2′β-Isopropyl-5′α-isobutyl-2-bromo-ergopeptine, Bromocriptine, CB-154	14	(38)
N,N-Pentamethylen-lysergylamine, 6-Methyl-8β-[N,N-pentamethylen-aminomethyl]-9-ergolene	21	(88c)
Peptide half of ergot peptide alkaloids, (general formula)	11	(33a)
L-Proline	11	(27a)
PTR-17-402, *6-Methyl-8β-[4-(p-methoxyphenyl)-1-piperazinyl]methyl-9-ergolene*	21	(88e)
Racemic Dihydrolysergic acid methylester	17	(71b)
Racemic Isolysergic acid hydrazide	16	
Racemic 6-Nor-dihydrolysergic acid methylester	17	(71a)
Racemic 6-Nor-6-ethyl-dihydrolysergic acid methylester	17	(71c)
Racemic 6-Nor-6-n-hexyl-dihydrolysergic acid methylester	17	(71d)
RN-76, *2,13-Dibromo-dihydrolysergic acid glycine amide*	14	(40)
Sansert®, *1-Methyl-lysergic acid L-2-butanolamide*, Deseril®, Desernil®, Methysergide	12	(34a)
Sermion®, *MNE*, Nicergoline, 1-Methyl-10α-methoxy-dihydrolysergol-5-bromo-nicotinate	26	(104e)
Thiolysergol	22	(90b)
Toquizine	23	(96f)
2′β,5′,5′-Trimethyl-dihydroergopeptine	32	(119b)
2′β,5′,5′-Trimethyl-ergopeptine, 5′β-Methyl-ergoalanine, MD-121	32	(119a)
Tripeptide (general formula)	3	(9)
L-Tryptophan	2	(2)
Uterdina, *N-Acetyl-dihydrolysergylamine*, 6-Methyl-8β-acetylaminomethyl-ergoline, Acetergamina	21	(89c)
VUFB-6605, *Dihydrohomolysergic acid nitrile*	20	(83b)
VUFB-6638, *N-(6-Methyl-8α-ergolinyl)-N′,N′-diethyl-urea*	23	(96c)
VUFB-6683, Dihydrohomolysergic acid amide, Deprenone	20	(86b)

G. References

Abe, M., Yamatodani, S., Yamano, T., Kusumoto, M.: Isolation of lysergol, lysergene and lysergine from the saprophytic cultures of ergot fungi. J. Agric. Biol. Chem. Jpn. **25**, 594–595 (1961)

Aghajanian, G.K., Bing, O.H.L.: Persistence of lysergic acid diethylamide in the plasma of human subjects. Clin. Pharmacol. Ther. **5**, 611–614 (1964)

Allport, N.L., Cocking, T.T.: The colorimetric assay of ergot. Quart. J. Pharm. Pharmacol. **5**, 341 (1932)

Arcamone, F., Bonino, C., Chain, E.B., Ferretti, A., Pennella, P., Tonolo, A., Vero, L.: Production of lysergic acid derivatives by a strain of Claviceps paspali Stevens and Hall in submerged culture. Nature (Lond.) **187**, 238–239 (1960)
Arcamone, F., Dorigotti, L., Glaesser, A., Redaelli, S.: 10-Alkoxy-9,10-dihydro-ergoline derivatives. U.S. Patent 3′585′201 (1971)
Arcamone, F., Franceschi, G.: 1,6-Dimethyl-10α-ergoline derivatives. Belg. Pat. 702′014 (1967)
Arcamone, F., Franceschi, G.: 1,6-Dimethyl-8β-N-carbobenzoxyamino-methyl-2,3-dihydro-10α-ergoline und ein Verfahren zu seiner Herstellung. Ger. Auslegeschrift 1′695′752 (1973)
Arcari, G., Bernardi, L., Bosisio, G., Coda, S., Fregnan, G.B., Glaesser, A.H.: 10-Methoxyergoline derivatives as α-adrenergic blocking agents. Experientia (Basel) **28**, 819–820 (1972)
Arcari, G., Bernardi, L., Foglio, M., Glaesser, A., Temperilli, A.: Ergolinderivate. Ger. Offenlegungsschrift 2′259′012 (1973)
Arcari, G., Bernardi, L., Glaesser, A., Patelli, B.: Neue Bromergolinverbindungen und Verfahren zu deren Herstellung. Ger. Offenlegungsschrift 2′330′912 (1974)
Axelrod, J., Brady, R.O., Witkop, B., Evarts, E.V.: Metabolism of lysergic acid diethylamide. Nature (Lond.) **178**, 143–144 (1956)
Bach, N.J., Kornfeld, E.C.: Dimerization of ergot alkaloids. Tetr. Lett. **1973**, 3315–3316
Barbieri, W., Bernardi, L., Bosisio, G., Temperilli, A.: Ergoline derivatives—IX. Configuration and conformation of 10-methoxydihydrolysergic acid derivatives. Tetrahedron **25**, 2401–2405 (1969)
Beran, M., Rĕzábek, K., Seda, M., Semonský, M.: Some O-acyl derivatives of D-6-methyl-8-(2-hydroxyethyl)ergolene and D-6-methyl-8-(2-hydroxyethyl)ergoline(I). Coll. Czech. Chem. Commun. **39**, 1768–1772 (1974)
Beran, M., Semonský, M., Rĕzábek, K.: Ergot alkaloids. XXXV. Synthesis of D-6-methyl-8-β-hydroxyethylergolene. Coll. Czech. Chem. Commun. **34**, 2819–2823 (1969)
Beretta, C., Ferrini, R., Glaesser, A.: 1-Methyl-8β-carbobenzyloxyaminomethyl-10α-ergoline, a potent and long-lasting 5-hydroxytryptamine antagonist. Nature (Lond.) **207**, 421–422 (1965)
Bernardi, L.: Recenti sviluppi della chimica degli alcaloidi dell′ ergot. Chimica Industria **51**, 563–569 (1969)
Bernardi, L., Goffredo, O.: Nouveaux dérivés de 6-méthylergolineI et de 1,6-diméthylergolineI et procédé pour les préparer. Belg. Patent 635′411 (1963)
Bernardi, L., Camerino, B., Patelli, P., Redaelli, S.: Derivati della ergolina. Nota I. Derivati della D.6-metil-8β-aminometil-10α-ergolina. Gazz. Chim. Ital. **94**, 936–946 (1964a)
Bernardi, L., Bosisio, G., Camerino, B.: Derivati dell’ergolina Nota IV. 8-Acetilergoline. Gazz. Chim. Ital. **94**, 961–968 (1964b)
Bernardi, L., Bosisio, G., Goffredo, O., Patelli, B.: Derivati dell’ergolina. Nota VII. Lumilisergamidi. Gazz. Chim. Ital. **95**, 384–392 (1964c)
Bernardi, L., Bosisio, G., Goffredo, O.: Lumilysergol derivatives. U.S. Patent 3′228′943 (1966)
Bernardi, L., Bosisio, G., Elli, C., Patelli, B., Temperilli, A., Arcari, G., Glaesser, H.A.: Ergoline Derivatives. Note XIII. (−)-α-Adrenergic blocking drugs. Farmaco [Sci.] **30**, 789–801 (1975)
Bernardi, L., Patelli, B., Temperilli, A.: Ergolenderivate. Ger. Offenlegungsschrift 2′155′578 (1972)
Bosisio, G., Goffredo, O., Redaelli, S.: Nouveaux dérivés 6-méthylergoline et 1,6-diméthylergoline. Belg. Patent 624′729 (1963)
Bowman, R.L., Caulfield, P.A., Udenfriend, S.: Spectrophotofluorometric assay in the visible and ultraviolet. Science **122**, 32–33 (1955)
Cainelli, G., Caglioti, L., Barbieri, W.: l’Idroborazione come mezzo per ottenere prodotti farmacoligicamente attivi: Idroborazione di prodotti ergolinici. Farmaco [Sci.] **22**, 456–462 (1967)
Černý, A., Semonský, M.: Mutterkornalkaloide XIX. Über die Verwendung von N,N′-Carbonyl-diimidazol zur Synthese der D-Lysergsäure-, D-Dihydrolysergsäure(I)- und 1-Methyl-D-dihydrolysergsäure(I)amide. Coll. Czech. Chem. Commun. **27**, 1585–1592 (1962)
Clemens, J.A., Kornfeld, E.C., Bach, N.J.: D-6-Methyl-2,8-disubstituierte Ergoline. Ger. Offenlegungsschrift 2′335′750 (1974)
Cookson, R.C.: The stereochemistry of alkaloids. Chem. Ind. **1953**, 337–340

Dal Cortivo, L.A., Broich, J.R., Dihrberg, A., Newman, B.: Identification and estimation of lysergic acid diethylamide by thin layer chromatography and fluorometry. Anal. Chem. **38**, 1959–1960 (1966)

Doepfner, W.: Biochemical observations on LSD-25 and deseril. Experientia (Basel) **18**, 256–257 (1962)

Eich, E., Rochelmeyer, H.: O-Acyl-lysergole und Verfahren zu ihrer Herstellung. Belg. Patent 753′635 (1970)

Eli Lilly and Company: Metoquizine, Toquizine. J. Amer. med. Ass. **195**, 675–676 (1966)

Fehr, T., Hauth, H.: 13-Bromolysergic acid compounds. U.S. Patent 3′901′891 (1975)

Fehr, T., Stadler, P.: Verfahren zur Herstellung neuer reaktionsträger Lysergsäurederivate. Swiss Patent 535′235 (1973a)

Fehr, T., Stadler, P.: Verfahren zur Herstellung neuer reaktionsträger Lysergsäurederivate. Swiss Patent 535′236 (1973b)

Fehr, T., Stadler, P.: Verfahren zur Herstellung neuer heterocyclischer Verbindungen. Ger. Offenlegungsschrift 2′454′619 (1975)

Fehr, T., Stadler, P.A., Hofmann, A.: Demethylierung des Lysergsäuregerüstes. Helv. chim. Acta **53**, 2197–2201 (1970)

Fehr, T., Stuetz, P., Stadler, P.A., Hummel, R., Salzmann, R.: Antihypertensiv wirksame Harnstoffderivate des 8 β-Aminomethyl-6-methyl-ergolens. Europ. J. med. Chem. **9**, 597–601 (1974)

Floss, H.G., Tcheng-Lin, M., Kobel, H., Stadler, P.: On the biosynthesis of peptide ergot alkaloids. Experientia (Basel) **30**, 1369–1370 (1974)

Flückiger, E., Wagner, H.R.: 2-Br-α-Ergokryptin: Beeinflussung von Fertilität und Laktation bei der Ratte. Experientia (Basel) **24**, 1130–1131 (1968)

Foster, G.E.: Review article. The assay of ergot and its preparations. J. Pharm. Pharmacol. **7**, 1–15 (1955)

Foster, G.E., Macdonald, J., Jones, T.S.G.: The separation and identification of ergot alkaloids by paper partition chromatography. J. Pharm. Pharmacol. **1**, 802–812 (1949)

Franceschi, G., Mondelli, R., Redaelli, S., Arcamone, F.: Sulla nitrazione di derivati della 6-metil-10α-ergolina. Chimica Industria **47**, 1334–1336 (1965)

Fregnan, G.B., Glässer, A.: Structure-activity relationships of various acyl derivatives of 6-methyl-8β-aminomethyl-10α-ergoline (Dihydrolysergamine). Experientia (Basel) **24**, 150–151 (1968)

Freter, K., Axelrod, J., Witkop, B.: Studies on the chemical and enzymatic oxidation of lysergic acid diethylamide. J. Amer. chem. Soc. **79**, 3191–3193 (1957)

Frey, A.: Verfahren zur Herstellung von Halogeniden der Lysergsäure- resp. Dihydrolysergsäure-Reihe. Swiss Patent 392′529 (1965)

Garbrecht, W.L.: Synthesis of amides of lysergic acid. J. Org. Chem. **24**, 368–372 (1959)

Garbrecht, W.L.: Hydroxyesters of hexa- and octahydroindoloquinolines. U.S. Patent 3′580′916 (1969)

Garbrecht, W.L., Tsung-Min Lin: Octahydroindoloquinolines. U.S. Patent 3′183′234 (1965)

Genest, K., Farmilo, C.G.: The identification and determination of lysergic acid diethylamide in narcotic seizures. J. Pharm. Pharmacol. **16**, 250–257 (1964)

Gröger, D.: Ergolinalkaloide. In: Biogenese der Alkaloide. Mothes, K. Schütte, H.R. (eds.). Berlin: VEB Deutscher Verlag der Wissenschaften 1969

Guttmann, S., Huguenin, R.: Verfahren zur Herstellung neuer heterocyclischer Verbindungen. Swiss Patent 508′628 (1971)

Guttmann, S., Huguenin, R.: Verfahren zur Herstellung neuer Mutterkornpeptidalkaloide. Swiss Patent 517′099 (1972)

Gyenes, J., Bayer, J.: Über verschiedene Verfahren zur quantitativen Bestimmung der Mutterkornalkaloide. Pharmazie **16**, 211–217 (1961)

Hale, D., Taylor, C.: The identification of d-lysergic acid diethylamide (LSD) by IR-spectrophotometry. Instrument News **18**, 6 (1967)

Hauth, H., Tscherter, H.: Nouveaux dérivés de l'ergoline, leur préparation et leur application comme médicaments. Belg. Patent 827′930 (1975)

Hellberg, H.: On the photo-transformation of ergot alkaloids. Acta chem. scand. **11**, 219–229 (1957)

Hofmann, A.: Über den Curtius'schen Abbau der isomeren Lysergsäuren und Dihydro-lysergsäuren. Helv. chim. Acta **30**, 44–51 (1947)
Hofmann, A.: Die Wirkstoffe der mexikanischen Zauberdroge „Ololiuqui". Planta Med. **9**, 354–367 (1961)
Hofmann, A.: Die Mutterkornalkaloide. Sammlung chemischer und chemisch-technischer Beiträge. Neue Folge Nr. 60. Stuttgart: Ferdinand Enke 1964
Hofmann, A., Stadler, P.: Nouveaux dérivés de l'acide lysergique et leur préparation. French Patent 1'432'556 (1966)
Hofmann, A., Stadler, P., Troxler, F.: Verfahren zur Herstellung von neuen Urethanen. Swiss Patent 415'658 (1967)
Hofmann, A., Troxler, F.: Nouveaux composés contenant le squelette de l'acide lysergique et leur préparation. French Patent 1'298'661 (1962)
Hofmann, A., Troxler, F.: Verfahren zur Herstellung von neuen Harnstoff-Derivaten. Swiss Patent 392'533 (1965)
Hofmann, A., Troxler, F.: Verfahren zur Herstellung von neuen Lysergsäurederivaten. Swiss Patent 463'524 (1968)
Hofmann, A., Tscherter, H.: Isolierung von Lysergsäure-Alkaloiden aus der mexikanischen Zauberdroge Ololiuqui (Rivea Corymbosa (L.) Hall. f). Experientia (Basel) **16**, 414 (1960)
Hofmann, A., Frey, A.J., Ott, H.: Die Totalsynthese des Ergotamins. Experientia (Basel) **17**, 206 (1961)
Hofmann, A., Ott, H., Griot, R., Stadler, P.A., Frey, A.J.: Die Synthese und Stereochemie des Ergotamins. Helv. chim. Acta **46**, 2306–2328 (1963)
Hofmann, A., Rutschmann, J., Frey, A., Schreier, E., Troxler, F.: Nouveaux dérivés hétérocycliques et leur préparation. Belg. Patent 638'511 (1964)
Jacobs, W.A., Craig, L.C.: The degradation of ergotinine with alkali. Lysergic acid. J. biol. Chem. **104**, 547–551 (1934a)
Jacobs, W.A., Craig, L.C.: On lysergic acid. J. biol. Chem. **106**, 393–399 (1934b)
Jacobs, W.A., Craig, L.C.: Lysergic acid. J. biol. Chem. **111**, 455–465 (1935a)
Jacobs, W.A., Craig, L.C.: On an alkaloid from ergot. Science **82**, 16–17 (1935b)
Jacobs, W.A., Craig, L.C.: The ergot alkaloids V. The hydrolysis of ergotinine. J. biol. Chem. **110**, 521–530 (1935c)
Jacobs, W.A., Craig, L.C.: The hydrolysis of ergotinine and ergoclavine. J. Amer. chem. Soc. **57**, 960–961 (1935d)
Jacobs, W.A., Craig, L.C.: The structure of lysergic acid. J. biol. Chem. **113**, 767–778 (1936a)
Jacobs, W.A., Craig, L.C.: The ergot alkaloids. X. On ergotamine and ergoclavine. J. Org. Chem. **1**, 245–253 (1936b)
Jacobs, W.A., Craig, L.C.: The ergot alkaloids. XI. Isomeric dihydrolysergic acids and the structure of lysergic acid. J. biol. Chem. **115**, 227–238 (1936c)
Jacobs, W.A., Craig, L.C., Rothen, A.: The ultraviolet absorption spectra of lysergic acid and related substances. Science **83**, 166–167 (1936)
Jacobs, W.A., Craig, L.C.: The position of the carboxyl group in lysergic acid. J. Amer. chem. Soc. **60**, 1701–1702 (1938)
Jacobs, W.A., Craig, L.C.: The dimethylindole from dihydrolysergic acid. J. biol. chem. **128**, 715–719 (1939)
Johnson, F.N., Ary, I.E., Teiger, D.G.: Emetic activity of reduced lysergamides. J. med. Chem. **16**, 532–537 (1973)
Julia, M., Le Goffic, F., Igolen, J., Baillarge, M.: Une nouvelle synthèse de l'acide lysergique. Tetr. Lett. **1969**, 1569–1571
Kelleher, W.J.: Ergot alkaloid fermentations. In: Advances in Applied Microbiology. Vol. II, pp. 211–244. New York: Academic Press 1970
Keller, C.C.: Neue Studien über Secale cornutum, Ergotinin, Cornutin, Spasmotin. Schweiz. Wschr. Chem. Pharm. **34**, 65–74 (1896)
Kreijci, P., Auskova, M., Rezabek, K., Bilek, J., Semonsky, M.: The effect of the ergoline derivative VUFB-6683 on the adenohypophysial prolactin concentration in rats. Experientia (Basel) **29**, 1262–1263 (1973)
Kobel, H.: Möglichkeiten zur fermentativen Herstellung von Mutterkornpeptidalkaloiden. Chem. Rundschau **27**, 57–59 (1974)

Kobel, H., Schreier, E., Rutschmann, J.: 6-Methyl-$\Delta^{8,9}$-ergolen-8-carbonsäure, ein neues Ergolinderivat aus Kulturen eines Stammes von Claviceps paspali Stevens et Hall. Helv. chim. Acta **47**, 1052–1064 (1964)

Kornfeld, E.C., Fornefeld, E.J., Kline, G.B., Mann, M.J., Jones, R.G., Woodward, R.B.: The total synthesis of lysergic acid and ergonovine. J. Amer. chem. Soc. **76**, 5256 (1954)

Kornfeld, E.C., Fornefeld, E.J., Kline, G.B., Mann, M.J., Morrison, D.E., Jones, R.G., Woodward, R.B.: The total synthesis of lysergic acid. J. Amer. chem. Soc. **78**, 3087–3114 (1956)

Leemann, H.G., Fabbri, S.: Über die absolute Konfiguration der Lysergsäure. Helv. chim. Acta **42**, 2696–2709 (1959)

Li, G.S., Robinson, M., Floss, H.G., Cassady, J.M., Clemens, J.A.: Ergot alkaloids. Synthesis of 6-methyl-8-ergolenes as inhibitors of prolactin release. J. med. Chem. **18**, 892–895 (1975)

Macek, K., Vanecek, S.: Mutterkornalkaloide IV. Bewertung von Alkaloiden in einzelnen Sklerotien mittels Papierchromatographie. Pharmazie **10**, 422–429 (1955)

Mantle, P.G., Waight, E.S.: Dihydroergosine: a new naturally occuring alkaloid from the sclerotia of sphacelia sorghi (McRae). Nature (Lond.) **218**, 581–582 (1968)

Mcphail, A.T., Sim, G.A., Frey, A.J., Ott, H.: Fungal metabolites Part V. X-Ray determination of the structure and stereochemistry of new isomers of the ergot alkaloids of the peptide type. J. chem. Soc. (B), **1966**, 377–395

Nakahara, Y., Niwaguchi, T.: Studies on lysergic acid diethylamide and related compounds. I Synthesis of d-N^{6}-demethyllysergic acid diethylamide. Chem. Pharm. Bull. Jpn. **19**, 2337–2341 (1971)

Ott, H., Hofmann, A., Frey, A.J.: Acid-catalyzed isomerization in the peptide part of ergot alkaloids. J. Amer. chem. Soc. **88**, 1251–1256 (1966)

Pioch, R.P.: Preparation of lysergic acid amides. U.S. Patent 2'736'728 (1956)

Portlock, D.E., Schwarzel, W.C., Ghosh, A.C., Dalzell, H.C., Razdan, R.K.: Potential central nervous system antineoplastic agents. Amides of 6-cyano-6-norlysergic acid. J. med. Chem. **18**, 764–765 (1975)

Ramstad, E.: Chemistry of alkaloid formation in ergot. Lloydia **31**, 327–341 (1968)

Renneberg, K.H., Szendey, G.L.: Ergometrinhydrogenmaleinat und Ergotaminhydrogentartrat. Arch. Pharm. (Weinheim) **291/63**, 406–413 (1958)

Rězábek, K., Semonský, M., Kucharczyk, N.: Suppression of conception with D-6-methyl-8-cyanomethylergoline(I) in rats. Nature (Lond.) **221**, 666–667 (1969)

Rutschmann, J., Schreier, E.: Verfahren zur Herstellung von neuen, basisch substituierten 6-Methyl-ergolen(9)-Derivaten. Swiss Patent 375'364 (1964)

Rutschmann, J., Schreier, E.: Verfahren zur Herstellung von neuen Dibrom-Derivaten der Dihydro-lysergsäure. Swiss Patent 394'225 (1965)

Schlientz, W., Brunner, R., Thudium, F., Hofmann, A.: Eine neue Isomerisierungsreaktion der Mutterkornalkaloide vom Peptidtypus. Experientia (Basel) **17**, 108 (1961a)

Schlientz, W., Brunner, W., Hofmann, A., Berde, B., Stuermer, E.: Umlagerung von Mutterkornalkaloid-Präparaten in schwach sauren Lösungen. Pharmakologische Wirkungen der Isomerisierungsprodukte. Pharm. Acta Helv. **36**, 472–488 (1961b)

Schlientz, W., Brunner, R., Stadler, P.A., Frey, A.J., Ott, H., Hofmann, A.: Isolierung und Synthese des Ergosins, eines neuen Mutterkorn-Alkaloids. Helv. chim. Acta **47**, 1921–1933 (1964)

Schreier, E.: Zur Stereochemie der Mutterkornalkaloide vom Agroclavin- und Elymoclavin-Typus. Helv. chim. Acta **41**, 1984–1997 (1958)

Semonský, M.: Mutterkornalkaloide und ihre Analoga. Pharmazie **32**, 899–907 (1970)

Semonský, M., Kucharczyk, N.: Ergot alkaloids. XXX. Synthesis of D-6-methyl-8-ergolin-I-ylacetic and some of its derivatives. Coll. Czech. Chem. Commun. **33**, 577–582 (1968)

Semonský, M., Zikan, V.: Mutterkornalkaloide XV. Partialsynthese der Cycloalkylamide der D-Dihydrolysergsäure(I) und N-[D-6-Methylergolin(I)-yl]-N'-cycloalkylharnstoffe. Coll. Czech. Chem. Commun. **25**, 1190–1198 (1960)

Semonský, M., Kucharczyk, N., Beran, M., Rězábeck, K., Seda, M.: Ergot alkaloids. XXXVIII. Some amides of D-6-methyl-8-ergolinyl (I)acetic acid. Coll. Czech. Chem. Commun. **36**, 2200–2204 (1971)

Smith, M.I.: A quantitative colorimetric reaction for the ergot alkaloids and its application in the chemical standardization of ergot preparations. U.S. Public Health Rep. **45**, 1466–1481 (1930)
Stadler, P.A., Hofmann, A.: Chemische Bestimmung der absoluten Konfiguration der Lysergsäure. Helv. chim. Acta **45**, 2005–2011 (1961)
Stadler, P.A., Stürmer, E.: Vergleichende Untersuchungen der pharmakologischen Eigenschaften von Stereoisomeren des Ergotamin und Dihydro-Ergotamin. Naunyn-Schmiedebergs Arch. Pharmak. **266**, 457 (1970)
Stadler, P., Stütz, P.: Verfahren zur Herstellung neuer Mutterkornpeptidalkaloide. Swiss Patent 534′683 (1973)
Stadler, P., Stütz, P.: (5R,8R)-8-(3-Aza-bicyclo[3,2,2]nonan-3-ylmethyl)-6-methylergolene. U.S. Patent 3′833′585 (1974)
Stadler, P.A., Stütz, P.: The ergot alkaloids. In: The Alkaloids. Chap. 1, Vol. XV, pp. 1–44. Manske, R.H.F. (ed.). New York-San Francisco-London: Academic Press 1975
Stadler, P.A., Frey, A.J., Hofmann, A.: Herstellung der optisch aktiven Methyl-benzyloxy-malonsäure-halbester und Bestimmung ihrer absoluten Konfiguration. Helv. chim. Acta **46**, 2300–2305 (1963)
Stadler, P.A., Frey, A.J., Ott, H., Hofmann, A.: Die Synthese des Ergosins und des Valin-Analogen der Ergotamingruppe. Helv. chim. Acta **47**, 1911–1921 (1964a)
Stadler, P.A., Frey, A.J., Troxler, F., Hofmann, A.: Selektive Reduktions- und Oxydationsreaktionen an Lysergsäure-Derivaten. 2,3-Dihydro- und 12-Hydroxy-lysergsäure-amide. Helv. chim. Acta **47**, 756–769 (1964b)
Stadler, P.A., Guttmann, St., Hauth, H., Huguenin, R.L., Sandrin, Ed., Wersin, G., Willems, H., Hofmann, A.: Die Synthese der Alkaloide der Ergotoxin-Gruppe. Helv. chim. Acta **52**, 1549–1564 (1969a)
Stadler, P., Troxler, F., Hofmann, A.: Verfahren zur Herstellung neuer synthetischer Alkaloide. Swiss Patent 469′006 (1969b)
Stadler, P., Troxler, F., Hofmann, A.: Verfahren zur Herstellung neuer synthetischer Alkaloide. Swiss Patent 489′501 (1970a)
Stadler, P., Troxler, F., Hofmann, A.: Verfahren zur Herstellung neuer Mutterkornpeptidalkaloide. Swiss Patent 494′762 (1970b)
Stadler, P., Hofmann, A., Troxler, F.: Verfahren zur Herstellung heterocyclischer Verbindungen. Swiss Patent 503′031 (1971)
Stadler, P.A., Stütz, P., Stürmer, E.: Completition of the Natural Groups of Ergot Alkaloids: Syntheses and Pharmacological Profiles of β-Ergosine and β-Ergoptine. Experientia **34**, 1552–1554 (1977)
Stahl, E.: Dünnschicht-Chromatographie. Berlin-Göttingen-Heidelberg: Springer 1962
Stenlake, J.B.: The stereochemistry of lysergic acid. Chem. Ind. **1953**, 1089–1090
Stoll, A.: Altes und Neues über Mutterkorn. Mitt. Naturforsch. Ges. Bern **1942**, 45–80
Stoll, A.: Über Ergotamin. Helv. chim. Acta **28**, 1283–1308 (1945)
Stoll, A., Hofmann, A.: Racemische Lysergsäure und ihre Auflösung in die optischen Antipoden. Hoppe-Seylers Z. physiol. Chem. **250**, 7 (1937)
Stoll, A., Hofmann, A.: Partialsynthese des Ergobasins, eines natürlichen Mutterkornalkaloids sowie seines optischen Antipoden. Hoppe-Seylers Z. physiol. Chem. **251**, 155–163 (1938)
Stoll, A., Hofmann, A.: Die optisch aktiven Hydrazide der Lysergsäure und der Isolysergsäure. Helv. chim. Acta **26**, 922–928 (1943a)
Stoll, A., Hofmann, A.: Partialsynthese von Alkaloiden vom Typus des Ergobasins. Helv. chim. Acta **26**, 944–965 (1943b)
Stoll, A., Hofmann, A.: Die Dihydroderivate der natürlichen linksdrehenden Mutterkornalkaloide. Helv. chim. Acta **26**, 2070–2081 (1943c)
Stoll, A., Hofmann, A., Petrzilka, Th.: Die Dihydroderivate der rechtsdrehenden Mutterkornalkaloide. Helv. chim. Acta **29**, 635–653 (1946)
Stoll, A., Hofmann, A.: Zur Kenntnis des Polypeptidteils der Mutterkornalkaloide II (partielle alkalische Hydrolyse der Mutterkornalkaloide). Helv. chim. Acta **33**, 1705–1711 (1950)
Stoll, A., Hofmann, A.: Verfahren zur Herstellung eines Amins mit dem Ringsystem der Lysergsäure. Swiss Patent 280′366 (1952)

Stoll, A., Hofmann, A.: Amide der stereoisomeren Lysergsäuren und Dihydro-lysergsäuren. Helv. chim. Acta **38**, 421–433 (1955)

Stoll, A., Hofmann, A.: The ergot alkaloids. In: The Alkaloids. Chap. 21, Vol. VIII, pp. 725–783. Manske, R.H.F. New York: Academic Press 1965

Stoll, A., Rüegger, A.: Zur papierchromatographischen Trennung der Mutterkornalkaloide. Helv. chim. Acta **37**, 1725–1732 (1954)

Stoll, A., Rutschmann, J.: Die Synthese der rac. Dihydro-norlysergsäuren. Helv. chim. Acta **33**, 67–75 (1950)

Stoll, A., Rutschmann, J.: Über die vierte isomere Dihydrolysergsäure und eine neuartige Epimerisierungsreaktion. Helv. chim. Acta **36**, 1512–1526 (1953)

Stoll, A., Rutschmann, J.: Über die Alkylierung der rac. Dihydro-nor-lysergsäuren und Berichtigung zur 32. Mitteilung dieser Reihe. Helv. chim. Acta **37**, 814–820 (1954)

Stoll, A., Schlientz, W.: Über Belichtungsprodukte von Mutterkornalkaloiden. Helv. chim. Acta **38**, 585–594 (1955)

Stoll, A., Schlientz, W.: Verfahren zur Herstellung von neuen Derivaten der Mutterkornalkaloide. Ger. Patent 1′015′810 (1958)

Stoll, A., Hofmann, A., Troxler, F.: Über die Isomerie von Lysergsäure und Isolysergsäure. Helv. chim. Acta **32**, 506–521 (1949a)

Stoll, A., Hofmann, A., Schlientz, W.: Die stereoisomeren Lysergole und Dihydro-lysergole. Helv. chim. Acta **32**, 1947–1956 (1949b)

Stoll, A., Rutschmann, J., Schlientz, W.: Synthese der optisch aktiven Dihydro-lysergsäuren. Helv. chim. Acta **33**, 375–388 (1950a)

Stoll, A., Petrzilka, Th., Becker, B.: Beitrag zur Kenntnis des Polypeptidteils von Mutterkornalkaloiden. (Spaltung der Mutterkornalkaloide mit Hydrazin.) Helv. chim. Acta **33**, 57–67 (1950b)

Stoll, A., Hofmann, A., Jucker, E., Petrzilka, Th., Rutschmann, J., Troxler, F.: Peptide der isomeren Lysergsäuren und Dihydro-lysergsäuren. Helv. chim. Acta **33**, 108–116 (1950c)

Stoll, A., Hofmann, A., Petrzilka, Th.: Die Konstitution der Mutterkornalkaloide. Struktur des Peptidteils. III. Helv. chim. Acta **34**, 1544–1576 (1951)

Stoll, A., Petrzilka, Th., Rutschmann, J., Hofmann, A., Guenthard, Hs.H.: Über die Stereochemie der Lysergsäure und der Dihydro-lysergsäuren. Helv. chim. Acta **37**, 2039–2057 (1954)

Stütz, P., Stadler, P.A.: Synthese der 2-Methyl-lysergsäure. Eine neue Friedel-Crafts-Methode. Helv. chim. Acta **55**, 75–82 (1972)

Stütz, P., Stadler, P.A.: A novel approach to cyclic β-carbonyl-enamines, $\Delta^{7,8}$-lysergic acid derivatives via the polonovski reaction. Tetr. Lett. **1973**, 5095–5098

Stütz, P., Stadler, P.: Nouveaux dérivés de l'acide lysergique, leur préparation et leur application comme médicaments. Belg. Patent 826.605 (1975)

Stütz, P., Stadler, P.A., Hofmann, A.: Synthese von Ergonin und Ergoptin, zweier Mutterkorn-Analoga der Ergoxin-Gruppe. Helv. chim. Acta **53**, 1278–1285 (1970)

Trommel, J., Bijvoet, J.M.: Crystal structure and absolute configuration of the hydrochloride and hydrobromide of D(−)-isoleucine. Acta cryst. **7**, 703–709 (1954)

Troxler, F.: Urethane mit dem Ringsystem der Lysergsäure und Isolysergsäure. Helv. chim. Acta **30**, 163–167 (1946)

Troxler, F.: Nouveaux dérivés de l'ergolène et leur préparation. French Pat. 1′439′953 (1966)

Troxler, F.: Beiträge zur Chemie der 6-Methyl-8-ergolen-8-carbonsäure. Helv. chim. Acta **51**, 1372–1381 (1968)

Troxler, F., Hofmann, A.: Substitutionen am Ringsystem der Lysergsäure II. Alkylierung. Helv. chim. Acta **40**, 1721–1732 (1957a)

Troxler, F., Hofmann, A.: Substitutionen am Ringsystem der Lysergsäure I. Substitutionen am Indol-Stickstoff. Helv. chim. Acta **40**, 1706–1720 (1957b)

Troxler, F., Hofmann, A.: Substitutionen am Ringsystem der Lysergsäure. III. Halogenierung. Helv. chim. Acta **40**, 2160–2170 (1957c)

Troxler, F., Hofmann, A.: Oxydation von Lysergsäure-Derivaten in 2,3-Stellung. Helv. chim. Acta **42**, 793–802 (1959)

Troxler, F., Hofmann, A.: Verfahren zur Herstellung neuer Lysergsäure-Derivate. Swiss Patent 473′127 (1969)

Troxler, F., Hofmann, A.: Verfahren zur Herstellung neuer heterocyclischer Verbindungen. Swiss Patent 505'828 (1971)
Troxler, F., Stadler, P.A.: Partialsynthese von 6-Methyl-9-ergolen-8β-essigsäure und einiger ihrer Derivate. Helv. chim. Acta **51**, 1060–1067 (1968)
Troxler, F., Rutschmann, J., Schreier, E.: Verfahren zur Herstellung von neuen Lysergalen. Swiss Patent 459'243 (1968)
Uhle, F.C., Jacobs, W.A.: The ergot alkaloids. XX. The synthesis of dihydro-dl-lysergic acid. A new synthesis of 3-substituted quinolines. J. Org. Chem. **10**, 76–86 (1945)
Urk, H.W. Van: Een Niewe Gevoelige Reaktie op de Moederkoornalkaloiden Ergotamine, Ergotoxine en Ergotinine en de Toepassing voor het Onderzoek en de Colorimetrische Bepaling in Moederkoorn Preparaten. Pharm. Weekblad **66**, 473–481 (1929)
Voigt, R.: Biogenese der Mutterkornalkaloide. Teil 1: Alkaloidbildung in Sklerotien und saprophytischer Kultur. Pharmazie **23**, 285–296 (1968a)
Voigt, R.: Biogenese der Mutterkornalkaloide. Teil 2: Biosynthese des Ergolingrundkörpers. Pharmazie **23**, 353–359 (1968b)
Voigt, R.: Biogenese der Mutterkornalkaloide. Teil 3: Biogenetische Beziehungen zwischen Einzelalkaloiden und Alkaloidgruppen. Pharmazie **23**, 419–436 (1968c)
Willard, P.W., Powell, C.E.: In vivo and in vitro activity of a vasoactive drug 9-(3,5-dimethylpyrazol-1-carboxamido)-7-methyl-4,6,6a,7,8,9,10,10a-octahydroindolo[4,3-fg]quinoline maleate. J. Pharm. Sci. **57**, 1390–1394 (1968)
Zikan, V., Semonský, M.: Mutterkornalkaloide XVI. Einige N-(D-6-Methylisoergolenyl-8)-, N-(D-6-Methylergolenyl-8)- und N-(D-6-Methylergolin(I)-yl-8)-N'-substituierte Harnstoffe. Coll. Czech. Chem. Commun. **25**, 1922–1928 (1960)
Zikan, V., Semonský, M.: Mutterkornalkaloide XXVII. N-(D-1,6-Dimethyl-8-isoergolenyl)-N',N'-diäthylharnstoff, seine Stereoisomeren und das N',N'-Dimethylanalogen. Coll. Czech. Chem. Commun. **28**, 1196–1201 (1963a)
Zikan, V., Semonský, M.: Mutterkornalkaloide XXVI. Einige weitere N-(D-6-Methyl-8-isoergolenyl)- und N-(D-6-Methyl-8-ergolenyl)-N'-Substituierte Harnstoffe. Coll. Czech. Chem. Commun. **28**, 1080–1083 (1963b)
Zikan, V., Semonský, M.: Mutterkornalkaloide 31. Mitteilung: Ein Beitrag zur Herstellung von N-[D-6-Methyl-8-isoergolenyl]-N',N'-diäthylharnstoff. Pharmazie **23**, 147–148 (1968)
Zikan, V., Semonský, M., Rĕzábek, K., Auskova, M., Seda, M.: Ergot alkaloids XL. Some N-(D-6-methyl-8-isolergolin-(I)-yl)- and N-(D-6-methyl-8-isoergolin-II-yl)-N'-substituted ureas. Coll. Czech. Chem. Commun. **37**, 2600–2605 (1972)

CHAPTER III

Basic Pharmacological Properties

E. MÜLLER-SCHWEINITZER and H. WEIDMANN

With Contributions by R. SALZMANN, D. HAUSER, H.P. WEBER, T.J. PETCHER, and TH. BUCHER *

A. Introduction

This chapter intends to portray the present knowledge on site and mechanism of action of the ergot alkaloids. The presentation is based chiefly on selected work performed in defined isolated systems in which the interference with specific substrates usually called receptors has been sufficiently proven. We hope that this presentation will contribute to the understanding of the complexity of ergot pharmacology as presented in the following chapters.

For many years it was considered that the stimulant activity of ergot alkaloids in different test preparations was due to a "direct" effect on smooth muscle cells, although the antagonism against catecholamines or 5-HT (5-hydroxytryptamine), indicating an affinity to specific receptor sites, was already regarded as a characteristic property of ergot compounds.

It must be assumed now that not only the inhibitory but also the stimulant activities of several ergot alkaloids and related compounds are mediated by interference with those specific constituents of a cell which are called drug receptors. Receptors are thought to be of molecular dimensions and probably form part of the surface of the cell membrane. A characteristic property of receptors is their specificity, which implies that structurally different drug molecules interact with structurally specific receptors. A three-point alignment between drug and receptor may be the minimal requirement for pharmacologic activity of drugs. However, the effect of an interaction of an ergot alkaloid with a receptor depends not only on the type of ergot compound but probably also on the environment in which the receptor exists. Accessory receptor areas might increase the affinity of an ergot alkaloid to the receptor site or lead to the formation of a slowly reversible complex between an ergot alkaloid and a receptor. In addition to the living substrate employed, the time pattern, e.g., the extent of latency period for maximum action of the drug, is also of importance. Nevertheless, drug action throughout this chapter will be considered within the simplified framework of the classical drug-receptor interaction theory.

A brief outline of receptor theory, insofar as it is relevant to the action of ergot alkaloids, is given below.

It is generally assumed that the first event in drug action is the formation of a reversible complex between receptor R and drug D, following the laws of second order reaction kinetics, $R+D \rightleftharpoons RD$, and that this leads to a pharmacologic

* The authors wish to express their gratitude to Prof. H.O. SCHILD for his exceptionally generous encouragement and advice in preparing this chapter.

response through several intermediate stages. If the law of mass action applies to the combination between drug and receptor, the proportion y of receptors activated by the drug is

$$y=\frac{K_1 A}{K_1 A+1} \tag{1}$$

where A is concentration of drug and K_1 the affinity constant (reciprocal of dissociation constant) of the drug-receptor complex.

Competitive Drug Antagonism

When an agonist and antagonist compete for the same receptor

$$y=\frac{K_1 A}{K_1 A+1}=\frac{K_1 A x}{K_1 A x+K_2 B+1} \tag{2}$$

where y is the proportion of receptors occupied by agonist, A and B are the respective concentrations of agonist and antagonist, and K_1 and K_2 the respective affinity constants of the agonist-receptor complex and antagonist-receptor complex, and x is the dose ratio. The dose ratio is the multiple of the agonist dose required to maintain an unchanged response in the presence of an antagonist. The dose ratio is particularly relevant in competitive antagonism when the log dose-response curves of the agonist in the absence and presence of antagonist are parallel.

It must be understood that the term y does not refer to a physiologic response but to the fraction of agonist-occupied receptors. Nevertheless, it is usually assumed that in a series of parallel log dose-response curves, equal responses correspond to equal fractions y of agonist-occupied receptors. Competitive antagonists produce parallel log dose-response curves (ARUNLAKSHANA and SCHILD, 1959; SCHILD, 1969). Furthermore, in the simplest type of competitive antagonism in which one molecule of drug or antagonist occupies one receptor, the degree of displacement of the curves obtained in the presence of different concentrations of antagonist is determined. Examples of experimental curves showing competitive antagonism in an isolated preparation are shown in Figures 1 and 2.

From such curves the affinity constant of the antagonist-receptor complex may be obtained. By algebraic transformation of eq. (2)

$$K_2=\frac{x-1}{B} \tag{3}$$

and since the terms x and B are known, K_2 may be calculated. When $x=2$

$$K_2=\frac{1}{B}$$

and

$$\log K_2=-\log B=pA_2$$

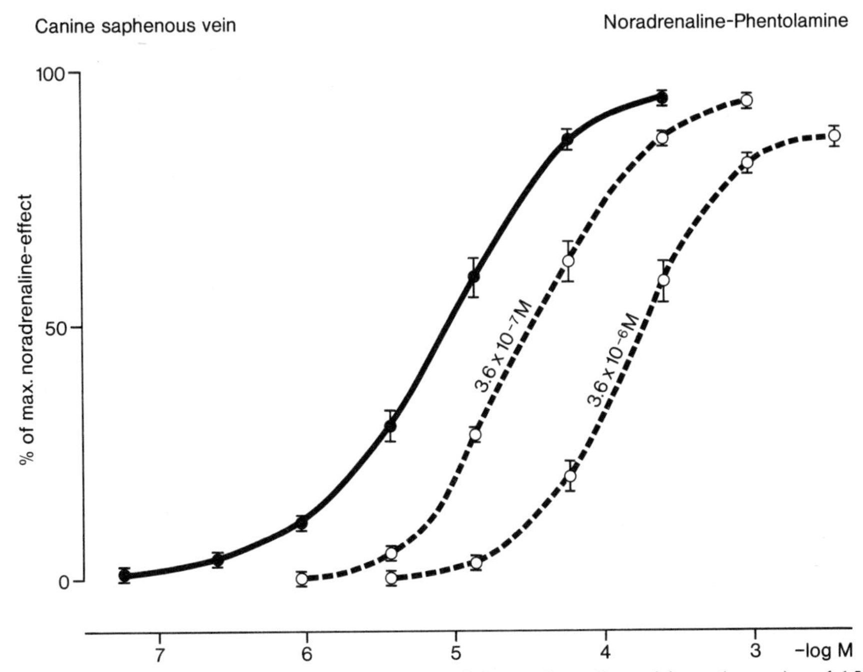

Fig. 1. Cumulative concentration-response curves for noradrenaline without (●—●) and 15 min after phentolamine (○---○) in the final concentrations of 3.6×10^{-7} and 3.6×10^{-6} M on spiral strips from canine saphenous veins. The bars represent ±SEM. [From Figure 4, MÜLLER-SCHWEINITZER, E., STÜRMER, E.: Blood Vessels **11**, 186 (1974)]

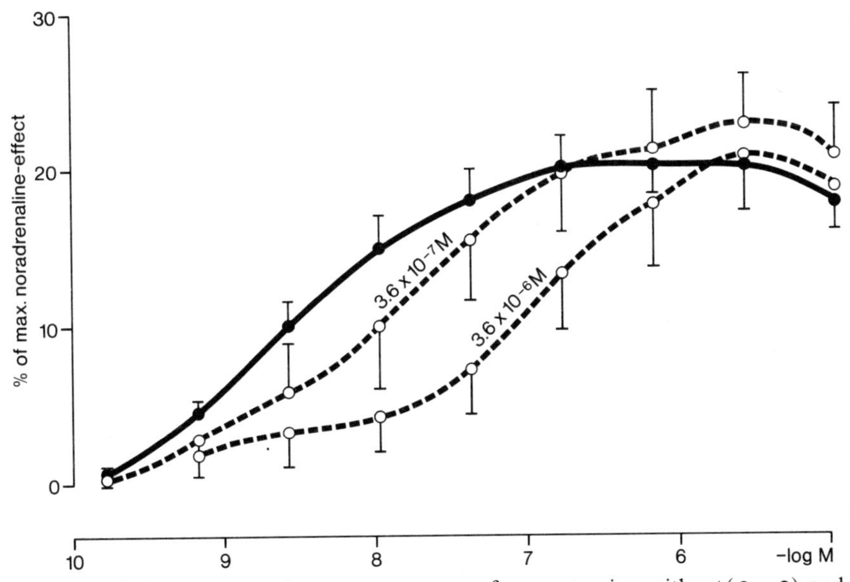

Fig. 2. Cumulative concentration-response curves for ergotamine without (●—●) and 15 min after phentolamine (○---○) in the final concentrations of 3.6×10^{-7} and 3.6×10^{-6} M on spiral strips from canine saphenous veins. The bars represent ±SEM. [From Figure 5, MÜLLER-SCHWEINITZER, E., STÜRMER, E.: Blood Vessels **11**, 187 (1974)]

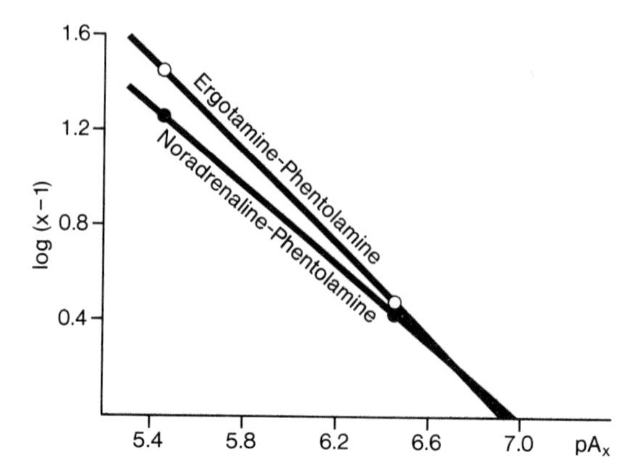

Fig. 3. Plot of the data from Figures 1 and 2 according to ARUNLAKSHANA and SCHILD (1959). The slope of the line for noradrenaline-phentolamine is $n = -0.83$, whereas the ergotamine-phentolamine line has a slope of $n = -0.97$. [From Figure 6, MÜLLER-SCHWEINITZER, E., STÜRMER, E.: Blood Vessels **11**, 187 (1974)]

wise, pA_2 can be considered as an empirical measure by which the activity of an antagonist can be expressed. It can then be defined as the decimal logarithm of the molar concentration of antagonist, which reduces the effect of a double dose of agonist to that of a single dose (SCHILD, 1947). It follows from eq. (3) that plotting log $(x-1)$ against log B (or $-\log B$ or pA_x) should give a straight line with slope unity which cuts the x-axis at a point corresponding to pA_2.

Corollaries of Competitive Antagonism

Two important corollaries of the theory of competitive antagonism have been emphasised by ARUNLAKSHANA and SCHILD (1959):

1. When two different agonists acting on the same receptor are tested with the same competitive antagonist, the affinity constant of the latter should be the same. This can be used as a test whether two agonists act on the same receptor. For example, Figure 3 shows that using this criterion ergotamine and noradrenaline probably stimulate the same receptor (α-adrenoceptor) in an isolated preparation of dog veins.

2. Identical receptors in different preparations should produce the same affinity constants with the same competitive antagonist. The method of classifying receptors is quantitative and has been shown to be applicable to receptors for acetylcholine, histamine, noradrenaline and 5-HT (ARUNLAKSHANA and SCHILD, 1959; FURCHGOTT, 1967; MÜLLER-SCHWEINITZER, 1976b).

Affinity and Intrinsic Activity (Efficacy)

The activity of a competitive antagonist at equilibrium is described by its affinity constant. In the case of agonists it was postulated by ARIENS (1954) and STEPHENSON (1956) that in addition to the affinity, a further variable, the intrinsic activity

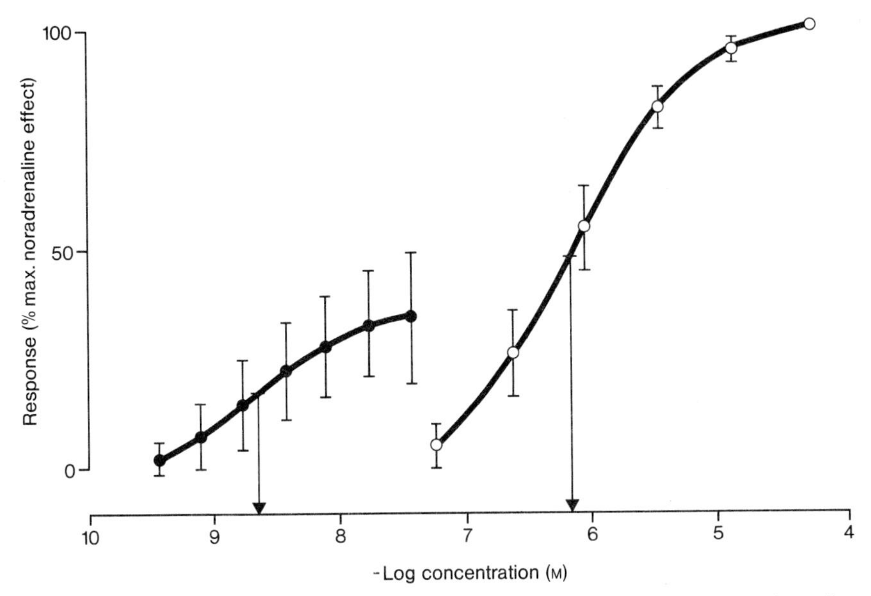

Fig. 4. Cumulative concentration-response curves for ergotamine (●) and noradrenaline (○) on spiral strips from canine femoral veins. pD_2 is represented by an arrow in each case. The bars indicate SD. [From Figure 1, MÜLLER-SCHWEINITZER, E., STÜRMER, E.: Brit. J. Pharmacol. **51**, 442 (1974)]

or efficacy, is needed to account for their effects. Efficacy can be regarded as a measure of the effectiveness with which the drug, once combined, activates the receptor.

Efficacy is an empirical constant which ranges from zero for an antagonist, upwards. Drugs with intermediate efficacy are termed partial agonists and those having the greatest efficacy of which the particular tissue is capable (a not well-defined concept) are termed full agonists. Drugs with high efficacy may be able to produce the maximal response of which the particular preparation is capable by occupying only a small fraction of receptors. The preparation is then said to contain a substantial proportion of spare receptors. Drugs with low efficacy produce flatter log dose-response curves than those with high efficacy, and their maximal responses may be reduced. Figure 4 shows the effects of a drug with low efficacy and high affinity (ergotamine) and a drug with lower affinity and high efficacy (noradrenaline).

Figure 5 shows the effect of combined administration of ergotamine, a partial agonist acting on α-adrenergic receptors, and noradrenaline, a full agonist acting on the same receptors. The partial agonist causes a rise of the base line. With increasing doses it occupies all the receptors and then acts as a typical competitive antagonist of noradrenaline.

Receptor Classification

Two main approaches to receptor classification and identification have been employed:

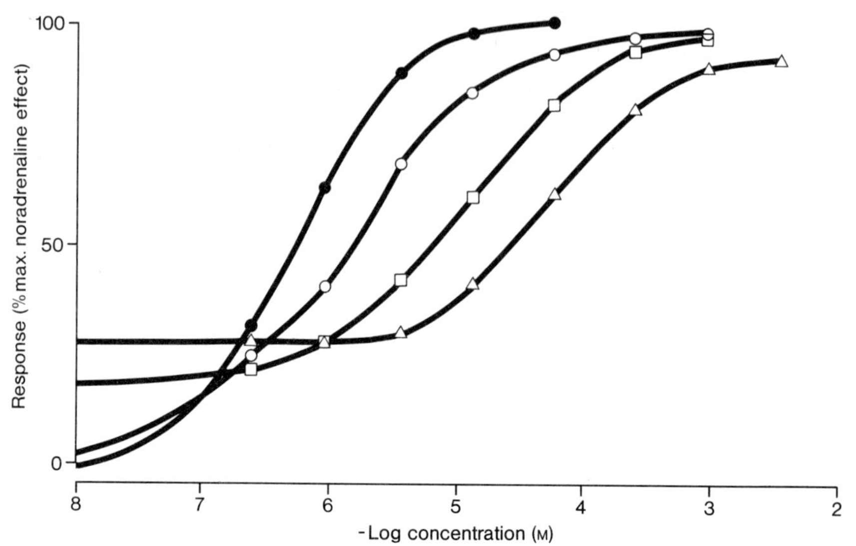

Fig. 5. Cumulative concentration-response curves for noradrenaline without (●) and 15 min after ergotamine in the final concentrations of 1.7×10^{-9} (○), 1.7×10^{-8} (□) and 1.7×10^{-7} M (△) on spiral strips from canine femoral veins. [From Figure 2, MÜLLER-SCHWEINITZER, E., STÜRMER, E.: Brit. J. Pharmacol. **51**, 443 (1974)]

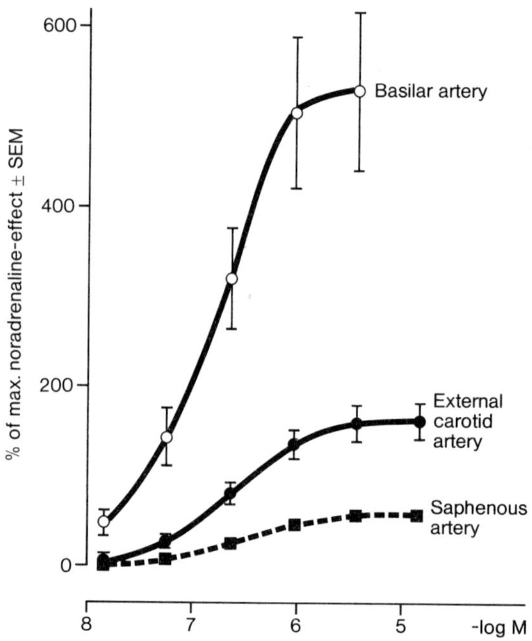

Fig. 6. Cumulative concentration-response curves for 5-HT (serotonin) on spiral strips from canine saphenous arteries (■---■), external carotid arteries (●—●) and basilar arteries (○—○) expressed as percentages of the maximum responses to noradrenaline. [From Figure 1, MÜLLER-SCHWEINITZER, E.: Naunyn Schmiedebergs Arch. Pharmacol. **292**, 114 (1976)]

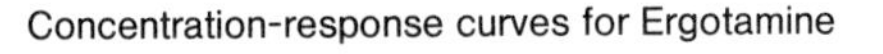

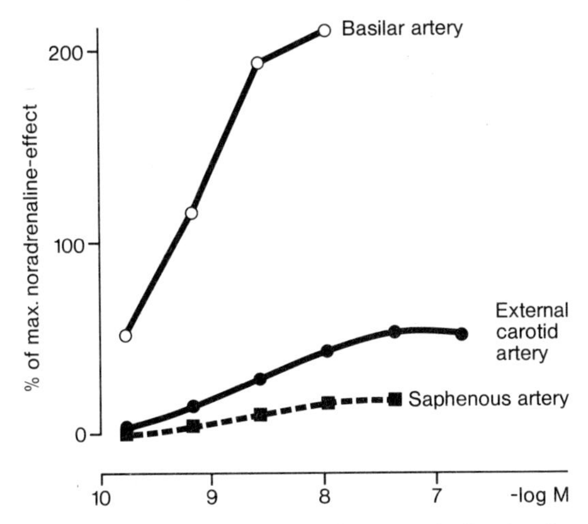

Fig. 7. Concentration-response curves for ergotamine on spiral strips from canine saphenous arteries (■---■), external carotid arteries (●—●) and basilar arteries (○—○) expressed as percentages of the maximum responses to noradrenaline. [From Figure 2, MÜLLER-SCHWEINITZER, E.: Naunyn Schmiedebergs Arch. Pharmacol. **292**, 114 (1976)]

1. Classification by antagonists. This is based on the principle, previously discussed, that similar receptors will give similar affinity constants (pA_2 values) with a competitive antagonist.

2. Classification by agonists. This is based on the idea that the potency ratios of agonists acting on the same receptor are independent of the preparation used. Although this is not strictly correct in theory (FURCHGOTT, 1972), it is a sufficient approximation to be useful in practice which has helped in the classification of beta adrenoceptor subclasses.

A variant of this approach which has been employed in the ergot field is illustrated in Figures 6, 7, and 8. They show that when ergotamine and 5-HT are tested in different arterial preparations their relative efficacies remain the same. This may indicate that the two drugs act on the same (5-HT) receptors in these preparations.

Noncompetitive Antagonism

A mass law equation for noncompetitive drug antagonism may be derived (ARIENS et al., 1956; SCHILD, 1954) based on the hypothesis that the agonist and the antagonist react with accessory sites of the same receptor or with consecutive sites of the activated effector system, so that the effect of the antagonist cannot be overcome (surmounted) by increasing the concentration of the agonist. This assumption gives rise to non-parallel log dose-response curves with decreasing slopes and maxima. Curves of this type are frequently seen: In the ergot field they tend to occur particularly when the ergot alkaloids are used as 5-HT antagonist (cf. Figs. 9, 11, and 12). True noncompetitive antagonists are probably rare, but curves

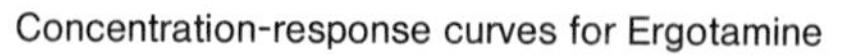

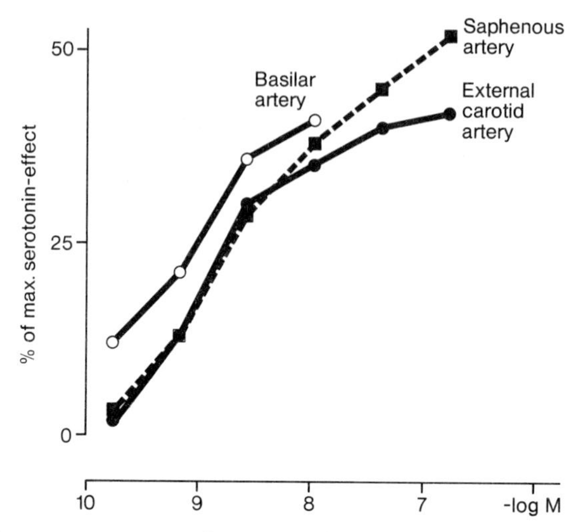

Fig. 8. Concentration-response curves for ergotamine on spiral strips from canine saphenous arteries (■---■), external carotid arteries (●—●) and basilar arteries (○—○) expressed as percentages of the maximum responses to 5-HT (serotonin). [From Figure 3, MÜLLER-SCHWEINITZER, E.: Naunyn Schmiedebergs Arch. Pharmacol. **292**, 114 (1976)]

of the noncompetitive type (pseudo-noncompetitive) are frequently seen experimentally.

As basis of drug antagonism throughout this chapter, it must be presumed that the antagonist will not react chemically with the agonist and will not interfere with the formation or metabolism of the agonist.

Besides specific action of ergot alkaloids on receptor sites, there are also interactions with other cell components such as enzymes and membranes which, however, occur only in 100 to 1000 times higher concentrations compared to those showing affinity to receptor sites. These interactions may be the consequence of the strong affinity of ergot alkaloids to several cell constituents, such as proteins and lipoproteins.

B. Actions of Ergot Alkaloids at 5-HT Receptors

I. Actions of Ergot Alkaloids at Extraneuronal 5-HT Receptors

a) General Description of "Specific Tryptamine Receptors"

Since the discovery of 5-HT as a widely occurring and potent biogenic amine, many investigations have supported the idea of the existence of tissue receptors which preferentially react to 5-HT. The first evidence for an interaction of ergot alkaloids with 5-HT receptor sites was provided when GADDUM (1953) described the marked antagonism between D-LSD (d-lysergic acid diethylamide) and 5-HT on the isolated rat uterus. Testing 5-HT and several antagonists on different isolated organs, GADDUM and HAMEED (1954) concluded that more than one receptor type for 5-HT must exist. One type was found to be present in the smooth muscle of the rat uterus and rabbit ear artery and could be specifically blocked by D-LSD. The second type was considered to be present in the post-ganglionic nerves in AUERBACH's plexus of the guinea-pig ileum and could be blocked by low concentrations of atropine, indicating the involvement of an indirect cholinergic mechanism, e.g., release of acetylcholine (ROCHA E SILVA et al., 1953; CAMBRIDGE and HOLGATE, 1955). Later studies on the isolated guinea-pig ileum (GADDUM and PICARELLI, 1957) led to the differentiation between D-receptors, which can be blocked by phenoxybenzamine, ergot derivatives or 5-benzyl-oxygramine, and M-receptors, the stimulation of which is antagonized by morphine, methadone, atropine, and cocaine but not by ergot alkaloids. Antagonism of stimulation of M-receptors may be indirect, e.g., atropine is believed to antagonize the effects of acetylcholine released from postganglionic nerve endings of AUERBACH's plexus.

Thus, although in some preparations, e.g., rabbit ear artery (APPERLEY et al., 1974, 1976; FOZARD, 1973b), guinea-pig umbilical vessels (NAIR and DYER, 1974), and cat spleen (INNES, 1962b), 5-HT and catecholamines seem to act on a common receptor, it is probably justified to accept the existence of specific receptor sites for 5-HT.

Evidence for the existence of two types of receptors for 5-HT in the nasal vessels from dogs – a constrictor receptor and a vasodilator receptor – has been provided by VARGAFTIG and LEFORT (1974). Whereas 5-HT activated both receptor types, tryptamine stimulated only the constrictor receptor, leaving the vasodilator unchallenged. GADDUM and PICARELLI (1957) referred to 5-HT receptors as tryptamine receptors, and this has tended to persist in the literature (e.g., VANE, 1960), although there is evidence that receptors for 5-HT and for tryptamine may be either different or at least differentially accessible. A tryptamine receptor different from the classical "D-type" is assumed to be involved in the mediation of the constrictor response of the external carotid vascular bed from dogs to 5-HT and ergotamine (SAXENA and DE VLAAM-SCHLUTER, 1974) and may also be involved in the action of methysergide in this vascular bed (SAXENA, 1974a, b).

A further type of tryptamine receptor mediating the phenomenon of sensitization to the vasoconstrictor activity of biogenic amines has been suggested for the vascular smooth muscle cells of several branches of the external carotid vascular bed (CARROLL and GLOVER, 1973; CARROLL et al., 1974).

b) Ergot Alkaloids as Stimulants at 5-HT Receptors

α) Common Pharmacologic Properties of Ergot Alkaloids and 5-HT

5-HT often has a dual action, e.g., stimulation and – especially at higher concentrations – self-blockade, which results in the well-known phenomenon of tachyphylaxis. Both pharmacologic properties are also characteristic of various ergot alkaloids when interacting as agonists with 5-HT receptors. D-LSD was found to be a very potent agonist in human and sheep umbilical vessels. On both preparations, however, concentration-response curves for D-LSD could be established only with single doses, since addition of increasing amounts of D-LSD to the bath without changing the fluid evoked no further contraction (DYER and GANT, 1973;

GANT and DYER, 1971). Similar observations have been made when the vasoconstrictor activity of dihydroergotamine was investigated on perfused human umbilical cords (GOKHALE et al., 1966) and when the mode of action of ergotamine was studied in canine arteries from different vascular beds (MÜLLER-SCHWEINITZER, 1976a) or in the rat stomach strip (FRANKHUIJZEN, 1975). As observed with D-LSD, the stimulating activity of ergotamine could be investigated only with a single dose-response technique. In the rat stomach strip the dose-response curve obtained with ergotamine was bell shaped, reaching its maximum at a bath concentration of 3 μM. The addition of higher ergotamine concentrations resulted in a decrease of the contraction height, indicating self-blockade.

β) Stimulation of D-Receptors by Ergot Alkaloids

As has been mentioned, ergot alkaloids specifically block D-receptors but do not antagonize effects exerted on M-receptors, thus indicating a selective affinity to those receptor sites of smooth muscles which are directly stimulated by 5-HT. When used as serotoninergic blocking agents, ergot compounds often showed considerable stimulant activity suggesting that they may act as partial agonists on 5-HT receptors. Umbilical and placental vessels are usually extremely sensitive to the vasoconstrictor activity of both 5-HT and ergot alkaloids. Human umbilical and placental vessels are stimulated by D-LSD (GANT and DYER, 1971), methylergometrine (PANIGEL, 1959, 1962), methysergide and BOL-148 (DYER and GANT, 1973), and by dihydroergotamine (GOKHALE et al., 1966; PANIGEL, 1959, 1962). Similarly, D-LSD, ergometrine, and ergotamine caused contraction of sheep umbilical vessels (DYER, 1969, 1970, 1974; DYER and GANT, 1973). Using BOL-148 and cinanserin as selective 5-HT antagonists, evidence has been provided that on both human and sheep umbilical vessels the vasoconstrictor activity of D-LSD is mediated through serotoninergic receptor sites. Moreover, since atropine failed to reduce responses to D-LSD, it was confirmed that the LSD-induced vasoconstriction was mediated solely by stimulation of D-receptors (DYER and GANT, 1973). Further evidence for this suggestion was provided by using the technique of selective receptor protection (DYER, 1974).

Methysergide, like 5-HT, caused vasoconstriction of in vitro perfused human temporal arteries. Responses to both 5-HT (0.1 μg) and methysergide (1 μg) could be abolished by perfusion of serotoninergic blocking agents such as cyproheptadine or pizotifen at a concentration of 10 ng/ml, suggesting the involvement of serotoninergic receptor sites in the vasoconstrictor response of the human temporal artery to methysergide (CARROLL and GLOVER, 1973; CARROLL et al., 1972, 1974). Injected at doses of 10 nmol to 2.5 μmol, methysergide also induced reproducible constriction of the rabbit ear artery (APPERLEY et al., 1974, 1976; CARROLL and GLOVER, 1973; CARROLL et al., 1972, 1974; FOZARD, 1973a, b, 1976a, b). As observed with the human temporal artery, this vasoconstrictor effect of methysergide could be prevented by perfusion of 1–10 ng/ml cyproheptadine or pizotifen, concentrations which also selectively antagonized responses to 5-HT but not those to noradrenaline (CARROLL and GLOVER, 1973; CARROLL et al., 1974).

While these observations suggest that methysergide constricts the rabbit ear artery via serotoninergic receptor sites, comparative studies of the antagonism by pizotifen and phentolamine against methysergide, 5-HT, and noradrenaline provided evidence that in the rabbit ear artery 5-HT and noradrenaline combine with the same receptor, which can also be activated by methysergide. APPERLEY et al. (1974, 1976) found that in the rabbit ear artery 100–300 nM pizotifen and 4–8 nM phentolamine were equipotent in antagonizing methysergide, 5-HT, and noradrenaline, thus indicating that the receptor stimulated by the three agonists may probably be identical with the α-adrenoceptor. These conclusions were confirmed by FOZARD (1976b), who found that on the isolated rabbit ear artery pA_2 values for phentolamine against noradrenaline, 5-HT, and methysergide did not differ significantly from each other.

The mode of the vasoconstrictor action of ergotamine has been investigated on canine arterial strips from different vascular beds, e.g., saphenous, external carotid, and basilar arteries. Compared with the maximum noradrenaline effect, ergotamine, like 5-HT, had different intrinsic activities in different vessels. The intrinsic activity (efficacy) of both ergotamine and 5-HT was found to be in the ascending order of saphenous < external carotid < basilar artery. Expressed as percentages of the maximum 5-HT effects, however, the intrinsic activity of ergotamine was about 50% in the three arteries (Figs. 6, 7, and 8). These results suggested that the relative efficacies of ergotamine and 5-HT in different vascular beds are the same and that in canine arterial vascular smooth muscle the stimulant activity of ergotamine might be mediated through 5-HT receptor sites. Further evidence for this was provided in experiments where 5-HT antagonists such as cyproheptadine and pizotifen and the α-adrenergic blocking drug phentolamine were used. Comparing the concentrations necessary to inhibit ergotamine effects with those required to antagonize responses to 5-HT and noradrenaline, respectively, it could be demonstrated that in canine arterial smooth muscle cells the ergotamine-induced vasoconstriction is mediated mainly through specific 5-HT receptors (MÜLLER-SCHWEINITZER, 1976a, b).

Similar conclusions were reached by FRANKHUIJZEN (1975), who investigated the mode of action of ergotamine on the isolated rat stomach preparation. Using ergotamine, 5-HT, and acetylcholine as agonists and ergotamine, methysergide, and piperoxan as antagonists, it was shown that ergotamine acts as a partial agonist on the classical D-receptors of the isolated rat stomach preparation.

It is interesting to note that ergotamine stimulated the smooth muscle cells from preparations as different as canine arteries and rat stomach strip in similar concentration ranges and with similar relative intrinsic activities compared to the maximum 5-HT effects, which implies structural similarities between the D-receptors in these different smooth muscle preparations.

An example where D-LSD effects could be blocked by 5-HT is the melanophore expansion test on the female guppy *Lebistes reticulatus*. In this test, increasing concentrations of D-LSD caused dose-dependent expansion of the melanophores, thus inducing a progressive darkening of the skin. This effect could be reversed in vivo as well as in vitro by high doses of 5-HT (BERDE and CERLETTI, 1956, 1957; CERLETTI, 1955; CERLETTI and BERDE, 1955). Although the darkening of the skin could be regarded as an agonistic action of D-LSD, the reversal by 5-HT indicates that these experimental results are a typical example of reversed antagonism, where the effect of an antagonist, D-LSD, could be inhibited by an agonist,

5-HT. Nevertheless, these results support the notion that D-LSD and 5-HT combine with the same receptor sites.

In the frog *Rana temporaria* D-LSD, like 5-HT, produces melanin dispersion, an effect which appears to be mediated indirectly through the pituitary, since responses to both D-LSD and 5-HT were absent in hypophysectomized specimens of *Rana temporaria* (KAHR and FISCHER, 1957).

Isolated hearts of various molluscs, e.g., *Venus mercenaria,* which respond to 5-HT at concentrations which are surprisingly small are also stimulated by several ergot alkaloids, e.g., ergometrine (GADDUM and PAASONEN, 1955; WELSH, 1953; WRIGHT et al., 1962), methylergometrine (CHONG and PHILLIS, 1965; WRIGHT et al., 1962), ergotoxine (CHONG and PHILLIS, 1965; WELSH, 1953, WRIGHT et al., 1962), ergotamine (CHONG and PHILLIS, 1965), dihydroergotamine and dihydroergotoxine mesylate (GADDUM and PAASONEN, 1955; WRIGHT et al., 1962), but D-LSD proved to be the most excitatory ergot alkaloid on the molluscan heart (GADDUM and PAASONEN, 1955; GREENBERG, 1960b; LIEBESWAR et al., 1975; SHAW and WOOLLEY, 1956; WELSH, 1955, 1957; WRIGHT et al., 1962). When an isolated *Venus* heart is bathed in a solution of D-LSD in sea-water at a concentration as low as 10^{-16} M, it absorbs a sufficient amount of the drug to produce a maximal increase in frequency and amplitude of heart beats within 1 to 4 h. The generally similar actions of D-LSD and 5-HT on molluscan hearts suggested that both stimulate the muscle cells through the same receptor. Evidence for this was provided by the observation that responses to both D-LSD and 5-HT could be selectively abolished by pretreatment of the heart with BOL-148 or methysergide (CHONG and PHILLIS, 1965; WELSH and MCCOY, 1957; WRIGHT et al., 1962).

The liver fluke *Fasciola hepatica* responds with increased motility to the addition of 5-HT at μM concentrations, which seems to be a peripheral effect since following removal of the central ganglia, isolated strips of the parasite exhibited a smilar response to the stimulatory action of 5-HT. When used at 5–50 nM, D-LSD temporarily reduced the spontaneous activity of the worms. At concentrations of 0.1 μM and higher, D-LSD, like 5-HT, increased the motility of the flukes, thus being more potent than 5-HT. BOL-148, having no or rather depressant effects on spontaneous motility, antagonized the stimulatory activity of both 5-HT and D-LSD, indicating that responses to D-LSD were mediated by stimulation of 5-HT receptor sites (ABRAHAMS, 1974; MANSOUR, 1956, 1957; MANSOUR et al., 1957). BEERNINK et al. (1963) performed a comparative study of a number of lysergic acid derivatives, calculating those concentrations which stimulated 50% of the preparations. It was found that all compounds tested, except for BOL-148 and L-LSD, stimulated the fluke in lower concentrations than 5-HT.

An increase in basal motility by 5-HT has also been observed in *Schistosoma mansoni.* In this preparation, dihydroergotamine was found to be more potent than methysergide in causing excitation (HILLMAN et al., 1974; TOMOSKY et al., 1974).

Experiments with isolated salivary glands from the blow fly *Calliphora erythrocephala* have shown that D-LSD, BOL-148, and lysergic acid, like 5-HT, can stimulate secretion. In this experimental model, D-LSD produced the same physiological and biochemical events that have been associated with the action of 5-HT. For example, the addition of D-LSD caused the transepithelial potential to go negative, and it also raised the intracellular concentration of cyclic 3′,5′-adenosine monophosphate (cyclic AMP) as did 5-HT. But unlike 5-HT, the D-LSD-induced secretion continued despite repeated washings, indicating that D-LSD disengaged slowly from the receptor. Thus, salivary glands which had been treated with D-LSD appeared to be insensitive to the immediate action of 5-HT antagonists. Prolonged treatment with high concentrations of the 5-HT antagonist gramine, however, caused a gradual inhibition of the D-LSD-induced secretion. Similarly, the D-LSD-induced secretion could be inhibited by prolonged exposure of the salivary glands to high concentrations of either 5-HT or tryptamine. These observations strongly suggest that in salivary glands from the fly *Calliphora erythrocephala* D-LSD causes stimulation by combining with the same receptor site normally occupied by 5-HT (BERRIDGE and PRINCE, 1973, 1974).

γ) Stimulation of M-Receptors by Ergot Alkaloids

Although experiments with isolated organs from animals have not, so far, suggested an interaction of ergot alkaloids with M-receptors, there is some evidence that in longitudinal muscle strips from human intestine ergot alkaloids may stimulate M-receptors, thus causing release of acetylcholine.

Both circular and longitudinal muscle strips from human ileum contracted in response to 5-HT. On circular muscle strips the calculated $pA_{2(2\,\mathrm{min})}$ values against 5-HT were 8.0 for methysergide and 7.7 for cinanserin, indicating that in this preparation responses to 5-HT might be mediated mainly through D-receptors. On longitudinal muscle strips from human ileum, however, cinanserin was about 100 times less potent in antagonizing 5-HT-induced contractions ($pA_{2(2\,\mathrm{min})}$ value = 5.5), while methysergide enhanced responses to 5-HT, suggesting that in these muscle layers D-receptors are not involved in the response to 5-HT (METCALFE and TURNER, 1969; TURNER, 1973). When high concentrations of methysergide (10–50 µg/ml) were tested on specimens of longitudinal muscles from human intestine, they caused a contraction which was similar in nature and additive to that induced by 5-HT, and both were blocked by the same concentration of atropine (60 ng/ml). Moreover, after inhibition of cholinesterase by eserine, responses to methysergide were enhanced, suggesting the involvement of an indirect cholinergic mechanism in the stimulant activity of methysergide on longitudinal muscle strips from human intestine (METCALFE and TURNER, 1970).

c) Ergot Alkaloids as 5-HT Receptor Blocking Agents

Blocking agents, especially selective blocking agents, are the most important means of characterizing and classifying drug receptors. The use of competitive antagonists for the purpose of defining receptors (by their affinities for these antagonists) was discussed in Section A. Although the use of log dose-respose curves in isolated preparations and the use of competitive antagonists is ideal for classifying receptors, the ideal can frequently not be attained, either because the system does not lend itself to isolated organ work but only to in vivo work where the concentrations of antagonist are not well defined or stable, or because no reversible and competitive antagonists are available for receptor analysis.

In the case of 5-HT antagonists, although highly active and specific compounds have been described, they do not generally behave as competitive antagonists. Typically they produce nonparallel log dose-response curves with progressive lowering of maxima, such as are shown in Figures 9 and 12 for D-LSD and ergotamine, respectively. Frequently curves show both depression of maxima and lateral displacement. In the following discussion we have characterized such antagonists by both their pA_2 values at the 50% response level and their pD'_2 values (from the antagonist concentration, reducing the maximum of the dose-response curve to one-half), regarding both as essentially empirical measurements.

Structure activity relationships of lysergic acid derivatives. Small amide derivatives of lysergic acid, e.g., D-LSD, BOL-148, methysergide, ergometrine, and methylergometrine, are among the most potent and selective 5-HT antagonists, whereas peptide alkaloids, e.g., ergotamine, ergotoxine, and their dihydroderivatives, are usually less selective, showing closely similar affinities to both 5-HT receptors and α-adrenoceptors. Ergot compounds possess the indolealkylamine group of 5-HT as a rigid part of the lysergic acid structure, which might be responsible for the high affinity of these substances to 5-HT receptors. The degree of specifity, i.e., the degree of selective affinity to 5-HT receptors, of an ergot compound will, however, largely depend on the environment of the 5-HT receptor, i.e., on the existence and stereochemical arrangement of accessory receptor areas which may be tissue- and species-dependent. As demonstrated by BACH et al. (1974) the side chain at position 8 in an ergolene is not essential for the antagonistic activity of an ergot compound. Ergolene was found to be only three times less potent than methysergide in antagonizing the constrictor response to 5-HT in isolated rat stomach strips. On the other hand, prolongation of the side chain at position 8 of a lysergic acid derivative seems to enhance the affinity to accessory receptor areas, thus leading to very potent and long-acting 5-HT antagonists like GYKI 32084 (1-methyl-9,10-dihydro-d-lysergyl-nitro-argininol). For antagonism of 5-HT effects by GYKI 32084 a pA_2 value of 9.8 on the isolated rat uterus and a pD'_2 value of 9.7 on the rat stomach strip was calculated (BORSY et al., 1973; PIK and BORSY, 1974). A further potent 5-HT antagonist with a very long-lasting activity is MCE (1-methyl-8β-carbobenzyl-aminomethyl-10α-ergoline), which effectively protected guinea-pigs from 5-HT-induced bronchospasm and which was also found to be about 500 times more potent than methysergide in antagonizing response to 5-HT when tested on the isolated rat uterus (BERETTA et al., 1965a, b).

The affinity to 5-HT receptors of an ergot compound will largely depend on the test organ employed, and data obtained on one tissue of a certain species will often not be applicable to another preparation.

D-*LSD (d-lysergic acid diethylamide)* is a highly potent and selective 5-HT antagonist. Most of the studies investigating the peripheral anti 5-HT activity of D-LSD employed the isolated rat uterus. After 10 min incubation of a rat uterus preparation with D-LSD, a pA_2 value of 8.7 (=2 nM) for antagonism of 5-HT by D-LSD was calculated (GADDUM, 1953; GADDUM and HAMEED, 1954; GADDUM et al., 1955). This antagonism by D-LSD, which appears to be competitive at low concentrations, increases progressively and becomes "unsurmountable" with time of incubation (GADDUM et al., 1955). Prolonged exposure to D-LSD may render the antagonism irreversible. Similar observations have been reported

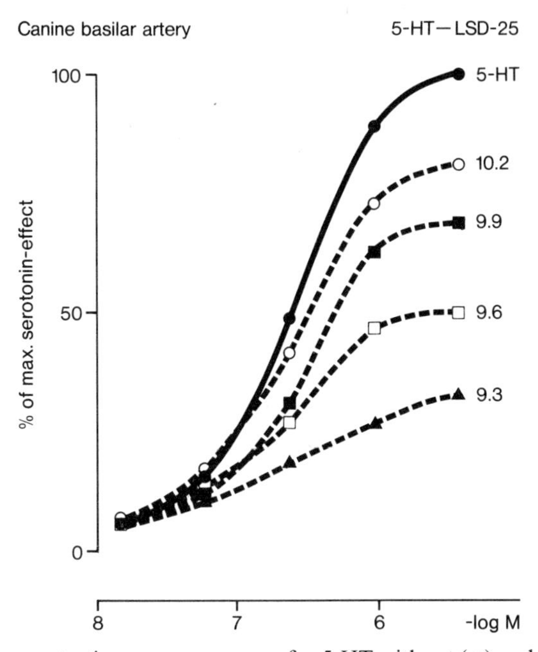

Fig. 9. Cumulative concentration-response curves for 5-HT without (●) and 30 min after D-LSD (LSD-25) in the final concentrations of $10^{-10.2}$ (○), $10^{-9.9}$ (■), $10^{-9.6}$(□) and $10^{-9.3}$M (▲) on spiral strips from canine basilar arteries. (MÜLLER-SCHWEINITZER, unpublished)

concerning intracranial blood vessels from various species. On the isolated circular smooth muscle of the middle cerebral artery from the goat, the vasoconstrictor effect of 5-HT was selectively antagonized by D-LSD. This antagonism by D-LSD was found to progress from surmountable to unsurmountable blockade as the D-LSD concentration was increased. A 10-min incubation with 6 nM D-LSD reduced the maximum response to 5-HT by about 50%. As observed with canine basilar arteries (TODA, 1975), this unsurmountable blockade could be reversed by removal of D-LSD from the bathing fluid (URQUILLA et al., 1974, 1975). Using a 30-min incubation time on spiral strips from canine basilar arteries, D-LSD antagonized responses to 5-HT in a noncompetitive way (Fig. 9). For antagonism of 5-HT by D-LSD a $pD'_{2(30\,min)}$ value of 9.6 (=0.25 nM) was calculated (Table 1).

As has been mentioned, 5-HT stimulates mainly M-receptors in the guinea-pig ileum, causing acetylcholine release. D-receptors are also stimulated but to a lesser extent, and they make only a partial contribution to the stimulant effect. It follows from this that the maximal inhibition of 5-HT effects by ergot compounds (which affect solely D-receptors) is only about 50%. Maximal antagonism of 5-HT effects by D-LSD could be achieved with concentrations of 0.01 to 0.1 µg/ml, whereas higher concentrations caused no further inhibition (GADDUM, 1957; GADDUM and HAMEED, 1954; GADDUM and PICARELLI, 1957; GINZEL, 1957; JAQUES et al., 1956).

Methysergide (1-methyl-d-lysergic acid butanolamide). For several years D-LSD was considered to be the most potent 5-HT antagonist. Studies of structure-activity

Table 1. Antagonism of 5-HT by various ergot alkaloids

	Canine	Bovine
D-LSD	9.6	9.2
Methylergometrine	9.1	
Methysergide	7.7	9.1*
Ergotamine	9.6*	9.2*
α-Ergokryptine	8.6	
Bromocriptine	7.8	
Dihydroergotamine	9.1	8.8*
Dihydroergotoxine mesylate	8.1	7.9
Dihydroergocornine		7.9
Dihydroergocristine		7.9
Dihydro-α-ergokryptine	7.8	7.7
Dihydro-β-ergokryptine	8.4	7.8

Note: pD'_2 values were calculated after an incubation time of 30 and 60 (*) min on spiral strips from canine and bovine basilar arteries (MÜLLER-SCHWEINITZER, unpublished)

relationships of lysergic acid derivatives, however, have shown that the 5-HT receptor blocking activity of these compounds can be increased by substitution of different radicals, mainly in position 1 and 2 of the ring complex of lysergic acid (CERLETTI and DOEPFNER, 1956; 1958a, b; CERLETTI and KONZETT, 1956; FREGNAN and GLÄSSER, 1968; ROTHLIN, 1957a, b; STOLL and HOFMANN, 1956). It was found that the introduction of a methyl group at position 1 of the lysergic acid increased the 5-HT antagonistic activity on the isolated rat uterus of ergometrine by 24 times and enhanced those of D-LSD and methylergometrine by about four times (CERLETTI and DOEPFNER, 1956, 1958a, b).

Methysergide seems to be the most potent 5-HT antagonist on the isolated rat stomach strip showing selective inhibition of 5-HT effects at threshold concentrations of about 1 nM (BAKHLE and SMITH, 1974a; FRANKHUIJZEN and BONTA, 1974b; GÖRLITZ and FREY, 1973; OFFERMEIER and ARIENS, 1966). When investigated on the isolated rat stomach preparation, methysergide shifted the log dose-response curve for 5-HT to the right but also lowered its maximal height, suggesting that methysergide exhibits a dualism in its antagonism of 5-HT consisting of a competitive and a noncompetitive part. As observed with D-LSD the antagonism by methysergide increased with time of incubation.

Figure 10 shows the influence of the time of incubation on the 5-HT antagonism induced by methysergide on the isolated rat fundus. In the presence of 1 nM methysergide the maximum response to 5-HT is progressively diminished by increasing the time of incubation. Thus, the calculated pA_2 values for antagonism of 5-HT by methysergide were found to be 8.9 after 5 min, 9.5 after 30 min and 10.1 after 60 min incubation time (FRANKHUIJZEN and BONTA, 1974b; GÖRLITZ and FREY, 1973), and similarly the calculated pD'_2 values were 8.0, 8.9 and 9.3 after 5, 30 and 60 min, respectively (FRANKHUIJZEN and BONTA, 1974b).

On bovine basilar arteries the $pD'_{2(60\ \mathrm{min})}$ value for antagonism of 5-HT by methysergide was 9.1, indicating that in this vascular tissue methysergide and

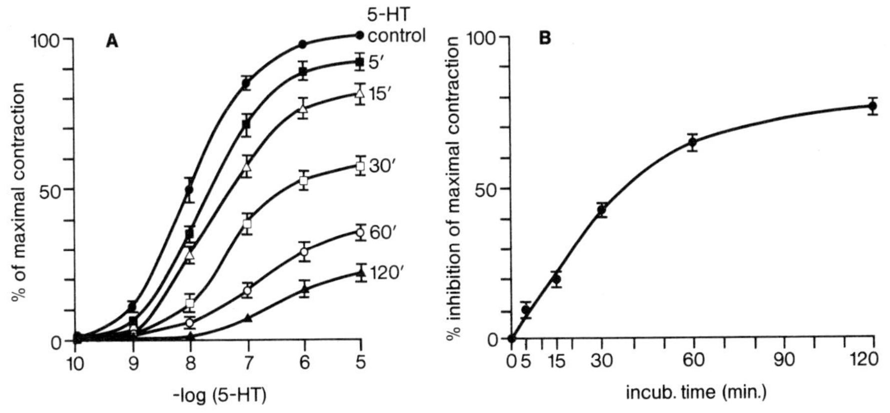

Fig. 10. (A) Dose-response curves for 5-HT without and in the presence of 1 nM methysergide after different incubation times on the rat fundus strip. (B) Dependence of the percentage inhibition of the maximal response to 5-HT on the preincubation time. [From Figure 2, FRANKHUIJZEN, A.L., BONTA, I.L.: Europ. J. Pharmacol. **26**, 223 (1974)]

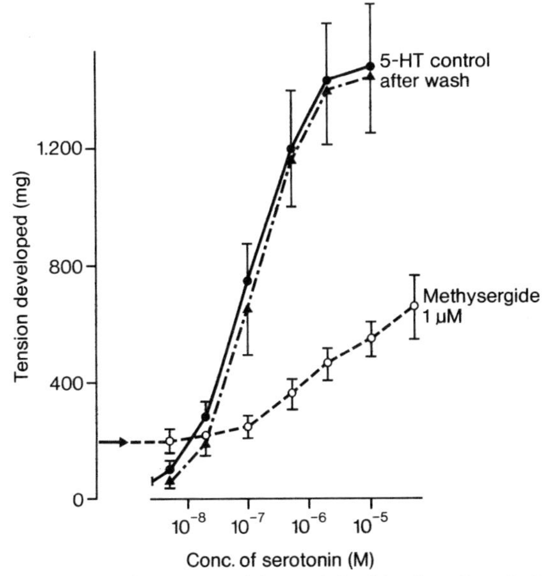

Fig. 11. Dose-response curves for 5-HT without (●), 20 min after 1 μM methysergide (○) and after washout of methysergide (▲) on spiral strips from canine cerebral arteries. [From Figure 2, TODA, N.: J. Pharmacol. exp. Ther. **193**, 387 (1975)]

D-LSD ($pD'_{2(30\ \text{min})}$ value = 9.2) are nearly equipotent in antagonizing responses to 5-HT (Table 1). As observed with D-LSD on canine basilar arteries, the 5-HT antagonism by methysergide could be reversed by removal of the drug from the bathing fluid (TODA, 1975; TODA et al., 1976) (Fig. 11).

On blood vessels from various species methysergide proved to be highly selective in antagonizing the vasoconstrictor responses to 5-HT. For antagonism of 5-HT effects by methysergide the $pA_{2(2\text{ min})}$ value on human saphenous veins was 8.2 (METCALFE and TURNER, 1969; TURNER, 1973), and both the $pA_{2(15\text{ min})}$ value on canine saphenous arteries (MÜLLER-SCHWEINITZER, 1975a) and the $pA_{2(30\text{ min})}$ value on rabbit aortic strips (APPERLEY et al., 1974, 1976) were 8.5, whereas in both preparations about 1000 times higher methysergide concentrations were necessary to antagonize vasoconstrictor responses to noradrenaline to an equal extent.

BOL-148 (2-bromo-d-lysergic acid diethylamide). In some preparations, e.g., isolated rat uterus, the 5-HT antagonism induced by BOL-148 was found to be somewhat stronger than that induced by D-LSD (CERLETTI and DOEPFNER, 1956, 1958a, b; CERLETTI and KONZETT, 1956; CERLETTI and ROTHLIN, 1955; FANCHAMPS et al., 1960; SOLLERO et al., 1956). In most tissues, however, BOL-148 and D-LSD seem to be equipotent in antagonizing responses to 5-HT. On rabbit aortic strips $pA_{2(10\text{ min})}$ values for BOL-148 were 9.0 against 5-HT and 6.4 against noradrenaline (KOHLI, 1968), suggesting that in the rabbit aorta 5-HT and noradrenaline combine with different receptor sites, and indicating that BOL-148 selectively antagonized 5-HT receptors, since for blockade of α-adrenoceptors about 400 times higher concentrations of BOL-148 were necessary. Using helical aortic strips from reserpinized rats the 5-HT antagonism by BOL-148 occurred in similar concentrations ($pA_{2(15\text{ min})}$ value $=8.9$) but was less selective than on rabbit aortic strips, since in the rat aorta only about 10 times higher concentrations of BOL-148 were required to antagonize responses to noradrenaline ($pA_{2(15\text{ min})}$ value $=7.9$) to the same extent (KRISHNAMURTY, 1971).

In the rat aortic strip the antagonism induced by BOL-148 was not influenced by prolongation of the incubation time (KRISHNAMURTY, 1971), while that on the isolated rat fundus strip increased progressively with time of incubation (BARLOW and KHAN, 1959a).

Ergot peptides in most preparations also antagonized responses to 5-HT effectively and essentially irreversibly. On the isolated rat uterus for the antagonism of 5-HT by dihydroergotamine and dihydroergokryptine $pA_{2(10\text{ min})}$ values of 6.9 and 6.8, respectively, were calculated (GADDUM et al., 1955), thus indicating that in this preparation both ergot alkaloids are about 100 times less potent than D-LSD in antagonizing 5-HT effects. Moreover, the 5-HT antagonism by peptide alkaloids is usually much less selective than that induced by amide derivatives of lysergic acid, since ergot peptides besides antagonizing responses to 5-HT also inhibit those to catecholamines in similar concentrations. Furthermore, in doses necessary to inhibit 5-HT effects these ergot alkaloids develop stimulating activity to a greater or lesser extent. This is especially the case for the natural and less so for hydrogenated compounds. Cumulative dose-response curves for 5-HT without and in the presence of ergotamine on spiral strips from canine external carotid arteries are shown in Figure 12. Ergotamine caused a considerable increase in tension on its own and progressively lowered the maximal response to 5-HT, indicating noncompetitive antagonism. Similar curves have been obtained when ergotamine was tested against 5-HT on canine basilar arteries by TODA et al. (1976).

The agonistic and antagonistic activities of ergotamine were investigated in detail on the isolated rat stomach strip by FRANKHUIJZEN (1975). When tested

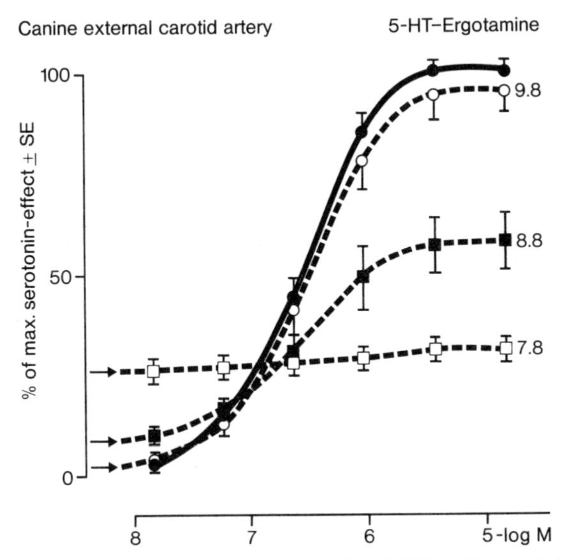

Fig. 12. Cumulative concentration-response curves for 5-HT without (●) and 60 min after ergotamine in the final concentrations of $10^{-9.8}$ (○), $10^{-8.8}$ (■) and $10^{-7.8}$ M (□) on spiral strips from canine external carotid arteries. (MÜLLER-SCHWEINITZER, unpublished)

against 5-HT, ergotamine behaved like a noncompetitive antagonist with considerable intrinsic activity. After an incubation time of 70 min, about 6 nM ergotamine reduced the maximal response to 5-HT by about 50%. Similarly ergotamine acted as a noncompetitive dualist when tested against 5-HT on canine arterial strips. On canine saphenous arteries, ergotamine antagonized 5-HT effects in a noncompetitive way with a $pD'_{2(60\ \mathrm{min})}$ value of 8.9 (=1.3 nM) but showed competitive antagonism against noradrenaline ($pA_{2(60\ \mathrm{min})}$ value = 8.7), thus demonstrating that in this vascular preparation ergotamine has affinity for both α-adrenergic and 5-HT receptor sites. However, as already mentioned, the affinity of an ergot compound to a certain receptor area depends on the type of tissue employed. Using canine arteries from different vascular beds, it has been found that the selectivity of the 5-HT antagonism induced by ergotamine shows considerable differences. While on canine saphenous arterial strips ergotamine antagonized responses to both 5-HT and noradrenaline in similar concentration ranges, it failed to inhibit those to noradrenaline on canine basilar and external carotid arteries but developed the same or even stronger anti-5-HT activity as on saphenous arteries (MÜLLER-SCHWEINITZER, 1976c, d; MÜLLER-SCHWEINITZER and STÜRMER, 1975), thus indicating that in arterial vascular smooth muscle cells from the carotid vascular bed ergotamine has a selective affinity to 5-HT receptor sites.

The pD'_2 values calculated for antagonism of 5-HT by different ergot alkaloids (Table 1) demonstrate the strong 5-HT blocking activity of peptide alkaloids on spiral strips from canine and bovine basilar arteries.

At any rate, in most smooth muscle preparations the 5-HT antagonism by peptide alkaloids is usually much less selective than that induced by amide derivatives of lysergic acid, and it must be considered that peptide alkaloids might also combine with α-adrenoceptors when they are used as 5-HT receptor blocking agents. A number of investigations demonstrating 5-HT receptor blocking activity of ergot alkaloids in various preparations are summarized in Table 2.

Table 2. Methods demonstrating 5-HT antagonism by ergot alkaloids

Preparation, species, references	Observations
Basilar artery – dog (ALLEN et al., 1974; MÜLLER-SCHWEINITZER, 1976c, d; TODA, 1974, 1975; TODA et al., 1974, 1976) – bovine (MÜLLER-SCHWEINITZER, 1975b) – man (MÜLLER-SCHWEINITZER, 1976c, d)	Selective noncompetitive and reversible 5-HT antagonism by both D-LSD and methysergide at concentrations of 0.6–10 nM. Ergotamine behaved like a noncompetitive dualist.
Middle cerebral artery – goat (URQUILLA et al., 1974, 1975) – cat (HARDEBO and EDVINSSON, 1976; NIELSEN and OWMAN, 1971)	
Ear artery (isolated perfused) – rabbit (CARROLL et al., 1972; FINGL and GADDUM, 1953; FOZARD, 1973b; GADDUM, 1954; GADDUM and HAMEED, 1954; SAVINI, 1956)	Perfusion of 1–10 ng/ml D-LSD, BOL-148 or ergometrine antagonized selectively 5-HT-induced vasoconstrictor effects.
Temporal artery – man (CARROLL et al., 1972)	High concentrations of methysergide, ergotamine or 1-methyl-ergotamine inhibited 5-HT effects.
Maxillary and lingual artery – cat (HARDEBO and EDVINSSON, 1976)	Methysergide antagonized 5-HT effects competitively.
Carotid artery – sheep (SHAW and WOOLLEY, 1953; WOOLLEY and SHAW, 1953) – dog (MÜLLER-SCHWEINITZER and STÜRMER, 1975)	Both ergotamine and ergotoxine reduced the vasoconstrictor response to 5-HT. Ergotamine acted as a noncompetitive dualist ($pD'_{2(60\,\mathrm{min})}=8.4$).
External carotid vasculature – dog (SAXENA, 1972a, b, 1974a, b; SAXENA and DE VLAAM SCHLUTER, 1974; VIDRIO and HONG, 1976)	In vivo ergotamine first reduced and at higher doses reversed 5-HT effects. Methysergide antagonized vasodilator response to 5-HT.
Internal carotid vasculature – dog (MCHEDLISHVILI and ORMOTSADZE, 1974; VIDRIO and HONG, 1976). – monkey (KARLSBERG et al., 1962, 1963)	Methysergide and dihydroergotoxine mesylate antagonized selectively vasoconstrictor effects of 5-HT.
Nasal mucosa vessels – dog (CARPI and VIRNO, 1957; SCHÖNBAUM and LAMAR, 1975; SCHÖNBAUM et al., 1974, 1975; VARGAFTIG and LEFORT, 1974)	Methysergide at high concentrations antagonized both 5-HT-induced vasoconstriction and vasodilatation which occurred in the presence of ergotamine.
Aortic strips – rat (KRISHNAMURTY, 1971) – rabbit (APPERLEY et al., 1974, 1976; GARRETT and BROWN, 1970, 1972; KOHLI, 1968; KOHLI and INNES, 1964; WURZEL, 1966)	Selective 5-HT antagonism by BOL-148 and methysergide, both being about equipotent against 5-HT.

Table 2 (continued)

Preparation, species, references	Observations
Coronary artery in situ – dog (MENA and VIDRIO, 1976)	5-HT-induced dilatation was antagonized by pretreatment of the dogs with methysergide.
Cutaneous vasculature (in situ) – rat (CHAHL and LADD, 1976)	Methysergide antagonized 5-HT-induced vasoconstriction.
Saphenous artery – dog (MÜLLER-SCHWEINITZER, 1975a, 1976c, d; MÜLLER-SCHWEINITZER and STÜRMER, 1975)	Highly selective 5-HT antagonism by methysergide ($pA_{2(15\,min)}=8.5$) less selective noncompetitive inhibition by ergotamine.
Peripheral artery – man (MÜLLER-SCHWEINITZER, 1976c, d)	Noncompetitive 5-HT antagonism by ergotamine of similar potency as observed in dog saphenous arteries.
Saphenous vein – man (METCALFE and TURNER, 1969; TURNER, 1973)	Antagonism of 5-HT by methysergide ($pA_{2(2\,min)}=8.2$).
Hand veins in situ – man (COLLIER et al., 1972; DEL BIANCO et al., 1972, 1975; SICUTERI et al., 1964a, b)	Injection of µg doses of D-LSD, BOL-48, methysergide 1-methyl-ergotamine or nicergoline antagonized 5-HT-induced venoconstriction.
Forearm blood flow – man (GLOVER et al., 1957; WALSH, 1967)	
Pulmonary vessels – rat (BAKHLE and SMITH, 1974a, b) – guinea-pig (STARR and WEST, 1966) – dog (JOINER et al., 1974, 1975) – sheep (EYRE, 1975) – cattle (EYRE, 1971)	Selective 5-HT antagonism has been demonstrated for methysergide and for BOL-148.
Lungs, isolated perfused – rat (ALABASTER and BAKHLE, 1976; BAKHLE and SMITH, 1972, 1974b; FOZARD and LEACH, 1968) – rabbit (HAUGE et al., 1966) – cat (GADDUM et al., 1953; GINZEL and KOTTEGODA, 1953) – dog (DAICOFF et al., 1968; ROSE and LAZARO, 1958). – sheep (HALMAGYI and COLEBATCH, 1961)	Methysergide, BOL-148 and ergotamine selectively antagonized 5-HT-induced vasoconstriction and release of spasmogens. D-LSD antagonized 5-HT more selectively than peptide alkaloids. In vivo 5-HT-induced rise in pulmonary arterial pressure was blocked after methysergide, D-LSD and BOL-148.
Mesenteric vessels – rat (HAEUSLER and FINCH, 1972) – dog (HALL and O'CONNOR, 1973; LUDANY et al., 1959; STRONG and BOHR, 1967b) – cattle (HOLROYDE and EYRE, 1975)	Methysergide, D-LSD and BOL-148 were tested as 5-HT antagonists.
Mesenteric vasculature (in situ) – cat (BIBER et al., 1974; CERLETTI, 1955; FARA, 1974)	Dihydroergotamine blocked selectively vasodilator effect of low 5-HT doses. D-LSD reduced selectively vasoconstrictor effect of high 5-HT doses.

Table 2 (continued)

Preparation, species, references	Observations
Ischemic ulcers induced by 5-HT – rat (SCHERBEL, 1960; WILHELMI, 1957; WILHELMI and SCHINDLER, 1959)	Methysergide and D-LSD protected rats from 5-HT-induced gastrointestinal ulcers.
Kidney, isolated perfused – rat (CERLETTI, 1955; CERLETTI and KONZETT, 1956; PASSOW et al., 1960) Renal infarcts – rat (JASMIN and BOIS, 1960)	D-LSD, acetyl-LSD, and BOL-148 inhibited 5-HT-induced vasoconstriction and protected rats from 5-HT-induced renal infarcts.
Antidiuretic action – rat (CHODERA, 1963; DEL GRECO et al., 1956; ERSPAMER, 1952, 1953)	Methysergide, D-LSD, BOL-148, dihydroergotamine, and dihydroergotoxine mesylate antagonized 5-HT-induced antidiuresis.
Umbilical vessels – man (ALTURA et al., 1972; ÅSTRÖM and SAMELIUS, 1957; DYER and GANT, 1973; ELIASSON and ÅSTRÖM, 1955; GOKHALE et al., 1966, GULATI and KELKAR, 1971; PANIGEL, 1959, 1962). – monkey (DYER et al., 1972)	Methysergide and BOL-148 antagonized vasoconstrictor response to 5-HT in similar concentrations (0.05–0.1 μg/ml) and caused small contraction. D-LSD antagonized 5-HT-induced vasoconstriction. Dihydroergotamine was less selective.
– sheep (DYER, 1969, 1970; DYER and GANT, 1973)	BOL-148 selectively antagonized 5-HT effects.
– guinea-pig (NAIR, 1974; NAIR and DYER, 1974)	BOL-148 antagonized responses to noradrenaline more effectively than those to 5-HT or D-LSD.
Foetal death induced by 5-HT – mouse (FLÜCKIGER and SALZMANN, 1961; HARPER and SKARNES, 1972; POULSON and ROBSON, 1963; TERAKI, 1970)	Methysergide and D-LSD effectively protected the litters against the toxic effect of 5-HT.
– rat (BALDRATTI et al., 1965; PFEIFER et al., 1969)	Ergoline derivative MCE was more active than methysergide.
Atrium – guinea-pig (GREEF et al., 1959; LEVY and MICHEL-BER, 1956; MAGISTRETTI and VALZELLI, 1955; POURRIAS, 1975; TARDOS and ADAM, 1974; TRENDELENBURG, 1960) – hamster (GONZALES et al., 1975)	D-LSD and BOL-148 reduced but failed to abolish positive inotropic and chronotropic activity of 5-HT.
– cat (TRENDELENBURG, 1960)	Selective 5-HT antagonism by D-LSD.
– rat (BENFEY et al., 1974)	Inotropic effect of 5-HT was inhibited by 15 μM dihydroergotamine.
Ovarian suspensory ligament – rat (DAVIS, 1976)	Methysergide antagonized 5-HT-induced contraction unmasking a relaxant activity of 5-HT mediated by release of a PGE_2-like substance.
Uterus – rat (ARCARI et al., 1972; BERETTA et al., 1965a; BERNARDI et al., 1975; BORSY et al., 1973; CERLETTI, 1955; CERLETTI and DOEPFNER, 1956, 1958a, b; CERLETTI and KONZETT, 1956; CERLETTI and ROTHLIN, 1955; CHAMBERS and MARSHALL, 1967; COSTA, 1956;	D-LSD at ng concentrations antagonized selectively responses to 5-HT but induced spontaneous contractions at higher concentrations. 5-HT antagonism by methysergide, BOL-148, ergometrine, or methylergometrine was similar in potency to that induced by D-LSD ($pA_{2(10\,min)}=8.7$).

Table 2 (continued)

Preparation, species, references	Observations
DELAY and THUILLIER, 1956; DOEPFNER and CERLETTI, 1957; DYKSTRA et al., 1967, 1973; ENGELHARDT, 1975; ERSPAMER, 1952, 1953; FANCHAMPS et al., 1960; FINGL and GADDUM, 1953; GADDUM, 1953, 1954; GADDUM and HAMEED, 1954; GADDUM et al., 1955; GOGERTY and DILLE, 1957; PIK and BORSY, 1974; SOLLERO et al., 1956; STONE et al., 1961; TOTHILL, 1967; VOTAVA et al., 1957, 1958)	Peptide alkaloids were about 100 times less potent in antagonizing 5-HT effects and produced more or less spontaneous contractions. For antagonism of 5-HT the $pA_{2(10\ min)}$ values were 6.9 and 6.8 for dihydroergotamine and dihydroergokryptine, respectively.
Esophagus – chicken (BARTLET, 1974; BARTLET and HASSAN, 1968)	Methysergide antagonized contractions but not relaxation in response to 5-HT.
Stomach – rat (BACH et al., 1974; BAKHLE and SMITH, 1974a; BARFKNECHT et al., 1973; BARLOW, 1961; BARLOW and KHAN, 1959a, b; BARZAGHI et al., 1973; CASENTINI and GALLI, 1956; FRANKHUIJZEN, 1975; FRANKHUIJZEN and BONTA, 1974a, b; GÖRLITZ and FREY, 1973; HANDSCHUMACHER and VANE, 1967; MARLEY and WHELAN, 1976; OFFERMEIER and ARIENS, 1966; OGLE and WONG, 1971; PIK and BORSY, 1974; VANE, 1957, 1960)	Most ergot compounds antagonized 5-HT effects in a noncompetitive and nearly irreversible way. D-LSD seems to be slightly less potent than both metysergide and BOL-148. Ergotamine acted as a noncompetitive dualist of 5-HT.
– guinea-pig (YAMAGUCHI, 1972)	
– man (FISHLOCK et al., 1965)	D-LSD (0.1 μg/ml) blocked 5-HT.
– fish (GROVE et al., 1974)	Methysergide antagonized 5-HT.
Duodenum – rat (LEVY and MICHEL-BER, 1956; VOTAVA et al., 1958)	D-LSD inhibited responses to 5-HT.
– mouse (DRAKONTIDES and GERSHON, 1968)	Methysergide blocked muscle receptors for 5-HT.
– rabbit (SOLLERO et al., 1956)	BOL-148 reduced 5-HT effects.
Jejunum – rat (HAYASHI, 1975) – cat (BARABE et al., 1975) – dog (LUDANY et al., 1959) – man (FISHLOCK et al., 1965)	Selective inhibition of 5-HT effects has been demonstrated with D-LSD and methysergide.
Ileum – rat (FURUKAWA and NOMOTO, 1974, 1975) – guinea-pig (BELESLIN and VARAGIC, 1958; BERETTA et al., 1965a; BROWNLEE and JOHNSON, 1963; CHAMBERS and MARSHALL, 1967; DAY and VANE, 1963; GADDUM, 1957; GADDUM and HAMEED, 1954; GADDUM and PICARELLI, 1957; GINZEL, 1957; INNES and KOHLI, 1969; JAQUES et al., 1956; SOLLERO et al., 1956)	Maximal inhibition of 5-HT effects (about 50%) could be achieved with 0.01–0.1 μg/ml D-LSD or BOL-148. Higher concentrations induced contractions but no further inhibition. Dihydroergotamine was less potent and less selective, since it antagonized responses to 5-HT and histamine at the same concentration ranges.
– man (BENNETT and STOCKLEY, 1975; FISHLOCK, 1964; METCALFE and TURNER, 1969, 1970; TURNER, 1973)	Methysergide antagonized 5-HT ($pA_{2(2\ min)}=8.0$).

Table 2 (continued)

Preparation, species, references	Observations
Colon – rat (GAGNON, 1972; JAQUES et al., 1956; PARRATT and WEST, 1957b; REGOLI and VANE, 1964)	Selective antagonism of 5-HT by D-LSD or BOL-148 (0.01–0.2 μg/ml) and by methysergide (0.3 μg/ml).
Rectal cecum – fowls (BARTLET, 1974; CLEUGH et al., 1961)	Potent 5-HT antagonism by methysergide.
Rectum – cockroach (BROWN, 1975)	BOL-148 antagonized selectively 5-HT effects.
Intestine – fish (GADDUM and SZERB, 1961)	Methysergide (50 ng/ml) antagonized responses to 5-HT.
Ureter – pig (CIMA and FRESCHI, 1957)	D-LSD at 0.2 μg/ml antagonized 5-HT effects selectively.
Urinary bladder in situ – dog (GYERMEK, 1960, 1962)	BOL-148 antagonized the prolonged contraction mediated by D-receptor stimulation, leaving the first twitch-like phase unchanged.
Trachea – guinea-pig (CHAHL and O'DONNELL, 1971; CONSTANTINE and KNOTT, 1964)	Methysergide (5–50 ng/ml) inhibited 5-HT effects selectively.
Lungs (isolated perfused) – guinea-pig (BHATTACHARYA, 1955; KING 1956, 1957; MARLEY and WHELAN, 1976) – cat (GADDUM et al., 1953)	D-LSD, BOL-148, methysergide, dihydroergotamine, and ergotamine prevented 5-HT-induced bronchospasm.
Bronchospasm, 5-HT-induced, in vivo – guinea-pig (BARZAGHI et al., 1973; BERETTA et al., 1965a, b; BERRY and COLLIER, 1964; CERLETTI, 1955; ENGELHARDT, 1975; HERXHEIMER, 1953, 1955, 1956; HOLGATE and WARNER, 1960; KONZETT, 1956; MARLEY and WHELAN, 1976; SICUTERI et al., 1960) – cat (CERLETTI and KONZETT, 1956; KONZETT, 1956) – rat (CHURCH, 1975)	Selective protection against 5-HT-induced bronchospasm was found with D-LSD BOL-148, and methysergide (1–10 μg/kg). Dihydroergotamine and ergotamine showed only negligible antagonism.
Aggregation, 5-HT-induced	
Platelets – human (BORN et al., 1972; BOULLIN and GREEN, 1975; BOULLIN et al., 1975a; CUMINGS, 1974; CUMINGS and HILTON, 1971; HILTON and CUMINGS, 1971; MICHAL and MOTAMED, 1975, 1976; O'BRIEN, 1964) – sheep (MICHAL, 1969) – pig (DRUMMOND and GORDON, 1974; GORDON and DRUMMOND, 1975) – rat (DRUMMOND and GORDON, 1975a) – duck (BELAMARICH and SIMONEIT, 1973)	5-HT initiates aggregation of platelets by reacting with a receptor similar to the D-receptor of smooth muscle, which can be blocked selectively by D-LSD, BOL-148, methysergide, 1-methyl-ergotamine, and ergotamine at ng concentrations.
Blood cells from various animals (PITZELE and DOBELL, 1973; SWANK and FELLMAN, 1966; SWANK et al., 1963)	

Table 2 (continued)

Preparation, species, references	Observations
Capillary permeability	
Mesenteric vascular bed – rat (MOUTON and DEMAILLE, 1975)	Methysergide inhibited tumoral cell diffusion facilitated by 5HT.
Paw edema – rat (BERDE et al., 1960; BERETTA et al., 1965a; BORSY et al., 1973; CERLETTI and BERDE, 1967; CERLETTI and DOEPFNER, 1958a; CRUNKHORN and MEACOCK, 1971; DOEPFNER and CERLETTI, 1958; ENGELHARDT, 1975; FANCHAMPS et al., 1960; GELFAND and WEST, 1961; MALING et al., 1974; MAWSON and WHITTINGTON, 1970; MÖRSDORF and BODE, 1959; PARRATT and WEST, 1957a, 1958; STONE et al., 1961; VOGEL and MAREK, 1961; VOTAVA and LAMPLOVA, 1959; WEST, 1957)	Methysergide proved to be the most potent ergot compound in antagonizing 5-HT-induced edema of the rat paw. BOL-148 was about four times less potent than D-LSD. The peptide alkaloids, e.g., ergotamine, 1-methyl-ergotamine, and dihydroergotamine, exerted an edema-inhibiting effect only at high concentration ranges.
Skin capillary permeability – mouse (CHURCH and MILLER, 1975) – rat (CRUNKHORN and WILLIS, 1971)	Methysergide inhibited 5-HT-induced inflammation selectively.
Nictitating membrane (in vitro) – cat (THOMPSON, 1958)	D-LSD (1 ng/ml) and dihydroergotamine (10 ng/ml) diminished 5-HT-induced contractions.
Secretion, induced by 5-HT	
Adrenal medulla (in vivo) – cat (MARLEY and WHELAN, 1974, 1976)	5-HT-induced release of adrenaline from adrenal medulla was abolished following intra-arterial injection of methysergide.
Kidney (in vivo) – rat (MEYER et al., 1974)	Methysergide inhibited the stimulation of renin-angiotensin system by 5-HT.
Pancreas (in vitro) – golden hamster (FELDMAN and LEBOVITZ, 1970a, b)	Methysergide antagonized 5-HT-induced inhibition of the insuline release.
Pituitary gland (in vivo)	
– amphibians (BURGERS and IMAI, 1962; BURGERS et al., 1958, 1962; ITURRIZA, 1965; ITURRIZA and KOCH, 1964)	D-LSD prevented the release of intermedin from the pituitary gland induced by 5-HT.
– crustacean (FINGERMAN and RAO, 1970; RAO and FINGERMAN, 1970)	D-LSD and methysergide prevented 5-HT-induced release of red-pigment-dispersing hormone from neuroendocrine system.
Motility of parasites	
– *Fasciola hepatica* (BERETTA and LOCATELLI, 1968; MANSOUR, 1957; MANSOUR et al., 1957)	5-HT-induced motor activity could be antagonized by MCE and BOL-148. Dihydroergotamine exhibited only weak 5-HT antagonism.
– *Schistosoma mansoni* (HILLMAN et al., 1974; TOMOSKY et al., 1974)	BOL-148, MCE, dihydroergotamine, and methysergide, but not D-LSD antagonized 5-HT-induced motor activity.
Byssus retractor muscle – *Mytilus edulis* (STEVENS and BAGUET, 1968)	BOL-148 abolished 5-HT-induced relaxation of the contracted byssus muscle.

Table 2 (continued)

Preparation, species, references	Observations
Hearts of certain molluscs	
– *Venus mercenaria* (CHONG and PHILLIS, 1965; GREENBERG, 1960a; HIGGINS, 1974; WELSH and MCCOY, 1957; WRIGHT et al., 1962)	Longlasting and selective antagonism by methysergide and BOL-148 against responses to 5-HT and D-LSD.
– *Cyprina, Buccinum* (WELSH, 1954b, 1956)	D-LSD antagonized 5-HT without stimulating the hearts by itself.
– *Helix aspersa* (KERKUT and LAVERACK, 1960)	D-LSD acted as a 5-HT antagonist with stimulating activity.
– *Helix pomatia* (ROZSA and GRAUL, 1964)	Only BOL-148 antagonized 5-HT effects.

2. Effects of Ergot Alkaloids on 5-HT Metabolism

a) Effects of Ergot Alkaloids on 5-HT Metabolism in Peripheral Tissues

Following the in vivo administration of ergot compounds, such as D-LSD, methysergide or BOL-148, time-dependent changes in the levels of 5-HT in several tissues have been observed. The injection of D-LSD at doses of 50–500 μg/kg caused an increase in the 5-HT level within 10–15 min in rat blood platelets (TORRE et al., 1974a) and in rabbit blood (SANKAR et al., 1964), while 60 min after the i.v. administration of D-LSD into pregnant rabbits a decrease in the 5-HT content in arterial and venous blood was found (ZHABIN and URAZAEVA, 1975). When assayed 120 min after the administration of methysergide, the 5-HT concentration in rat blood was unchanged (OWEN et al., 1971b).

In tissues from rat intestinal tract maximal increase in the level of 5-HT was found 60 min after the injection of a single dose of methysergide (THOMPSON and CAMPBELL, 1967). Chronic administration of methysergide (5 mg/kg/day) for 4 weeks increased the content of 5-HT but also that of noradrenaline, particularly in the rat lung (MIELKE et al., 1973).

Following the injection of [^{14}C] labeled 5-HTP into rabbits an increase in the levels of 5-HT as well as of the radioactivity in several visceral tissues 15 min after the injection of both D-LSD and BOL-148 was observed (SANKAR et al., 1961, 1962, 1964). However, D-LSD increased not only the incorporation of radioactivity following the administration of labeled 5-HTP but also that after [^{14}C]-histidine and that after [^{14}C]noradrenaline. On the other hand D-LSD decreased the levels of histamine and noradrenaline while increasing that of 5-HT. Thus, it cannot be excluded that changes in 5-HT contents induced by ergot alkaloids may be mediated indirectly by mutual interaction with the levels and/or binding of other biogenic amines (SANKAR et al., 1964).

α) *Biological Inactivation of 5-HT in Peripheral Tissues*

In the isolated perfused rabbit heart 1 μg/ml methysergide enhanced metabolite appearance in the perfusion fluid as assessed by the perfusion of [^{3}H]5-HT (FOZARD and BERRY, 1976; FOZARD and WRIGHT, 1974). Although this observation could suggest that methysergide enhanced the biological inactivation of 5-HT, in vitro studies on suspension of guinea-pig liver and rat fundus showed that neither BOL-148 (BARLOW, 1961) nor methysergide (SEILER and WASSERMANN, 1973) displayed any change of MAO activity.

β) Uptake and Release of 5-HT by Peripheral Tissues

There is good evidence for the existence of at least two different 5-HT receptors on blood platelets from various species: One receptor mediating cellular stimulation (platelet shape change, platelet aggregation) by 5-HT, and the other receptor mediating the uptake of 5-HT (BORN et al., 1972; BOULLIN et al., 1975b; DRUMMOND and GORDON, 1975b; DRUMMOND et al., 1976). Ergot alkaloids were found to be potent antagonists of the stimulatory 5-HT receptors, while causing only weak inhibition of the active transport of 5-HT. Methysergide (BORN et al., 1972; CUMINGS and HILTON, 1971; DRUMMOND and GORDON, 1975a; HILTON and CUMINGS, 1971; MITCHELL and SHARP, 1964; O'BRIEN, 1964; PITZELE and DOBELL, 1973), D-LSD and methergoline (DRUMMOND and GORDON, 1975a; MICHAL, 1969), BOL-148, ergotamine and 1-methyl-ergotamine (CUMINGS and HILTON, 1971) caused about 50% reduction of 5-HT-induced stimulation when used at nM concentrations. However, when tested as inhibitors of the platelet 5-HT transport system, 130–150 μM of D-LSD, BOL-148 or methysergide were necessary to cause a 50% reduction of 5-HT uptake (BORN et al., 1972; CUMINGS and HILTON, 1971; TRENCHARD et al., 1975; STACEY, 1961). The peptide alkaloids ergotamine and dihydroergotamine (LINGJAERDE, 1970; STACEY, 1961) were only two to 10 times more potent than the lysergic acid derivatives in decreasing the 5-HT uptake by blood platelets. Thus, ergot alkaloids were at least 10,000 times less potent as inhibitors of the platelet 5-HT transport system as compared to their blocking activity against the stimulatory 5-HT receptors on blood platelets.

Using chlorprothixene isomers as blocking agents, DRUMMOND et al. (1976) found that cis-chlorprothixene was about 200 times more potent than its trans-isomer as an inhibitor of the 5-HT-induced aggregation, while the latter was twice as inhibitory as its cis-isomer when tested against the active uptake of 5-HT. It was suggested that 5-HT adopts different conformations for binding to its two platelet receptors: A less extended form of its side chain when binding to the stimulatory receptors but an extended form of its side chain when binding at the uptake receptor. It follows from this that the lack of effect of ergot alkaloids on 5-HT uptake might be due to a failure of the rigid ergolene moiety to mimic 5-HT in its extended conformation.

Several in vitro studies seem to support this assumption. In suspension of guinea-pig liver and rat fundus BOL-148 failed to affect the penetration of both tryptamine and 5-HT (BARLOW, 1961; HANDSCHUMACHER and VANE, 1963, 1967). The extraneuronal accumulation of 5-HT into the isolated rabbit ear artery was unaltered after 30 min preincubation with 100 μM methysergide (BUCHAN et al., 1974).

Facilitation of the uptake of [^{3}H]5-HT was observed in the isolated cat spleen perfused with methysergide at 0.3–1 μg/min (OWEN et al., 1971a, b; SALZMANN and KALBERER, 1973) and in the isolated rabbit heart perfused with 1 μg/ml ergotamine (FOZARD and BERRY, 1976; FOZARD and WRIGHT, 1974). Even higher concentrations of ergot alkaloids, such as methysergide, ergotamine, 1-methyl-ergotamine and dihydroergotamine, inhibited the [^{3}H]5-HT uptake into the isolated perfused cat spleen (OWEN et al., 1971a, b; SALZMANN and KALBERER, 1973).

Methysergide has been found to exhibit a dose-dependent protective influence against the 5-HT depleting activity of reserpine in rat blood in vivo (OWEN et al., 1971a, b), but it failed to affect the reserpine-induced reduction of 5-HT content in human blood platelets in vitro (CUMING and HILTON, 1971).

In addition, there is no evidence for an interference of ergot alkaloids with the spontaneous release of 5-HT from blood platelets in vitro. Up to 10 μM, neither D-LSD (CARLSSON et al., 1957) nor the peptide alkaloids ergotamine and dihydroergotamine (LINGJAERDE, 1970) developed any effect on spontaneous efflux of 5-HT from blood platelets.

In conclusion, at concentrations which cause pharmacologic effects ergot alkaloids will not interfere with either uptake or release of 5-HT in peripheral tissues.

b) Effects of Ergot Alkaloids on 5-HT Metabolism in the Central Nervous System

Investigations on the influence of ergot alkaloids on the metabolism of 5-HT in the brain showed that D-LSD produced a small but reproducible increase in the level of 5-HT in the rat brain. About 30 to 120 min following the administration of D-LSD into rats the 5-HT concentration of the brain was elevated (BOGGAN and FREEDMAN, 1973; DIAZ and HUTTUNEN, 1971; DIAZ et al., 1967, 1968; FREEDMAN, 1960, 1961, 1963, 1966; FREEDMAN and AGHAJANIAN, 1967; FREEDMAN and BOGGAN, 1974; FREEDMAN and COQUET, 1965; FREEDMAN and GIARMAN, 1962; FREEDMAN et al., 1970; KING et al., 1974; LOVELL et al., 1967; MATIN and VIJAYVARGIYA, 1967; PETERS, 1974a; RANDIC and PADJEN, 1971; SCHANBERG and GIARMAN, 1962; TONGE and LEONARD, 1969). Only within the first few minutes following the injection of D-LSD could a small decrease of the 5-HT level be observed (LOVELL et al., 1967; TORRE et al., 1974a, b). When assayed 2–4 h after the administration of D-LSD the 5-HT concentration in the brain was usually unchanged (ANDÉN et al., 1968; BOGGAN and FREEDMAN, 1973; FREEDMAN and BOGGAN, 1974; PAASONEN and GIARMAN, 1958; SCHANBERG and GIARMAN, 1962; SCHILDKRAUT et al., 1969; TONGE and LEONARD, 1969).

These observations have been confirmed in mice (CARLSSON and LINDQVIST, 1972; GLOWINSKI et al., 1973; RUCKEBUSCH et al., 1965; SZARA et al., 1967) and in rabbits (BRODIE, 1954; BRODIE et al., 1956; FREEDMAN, 1963; SANKAR et al., 1961, 1962, 1964).

Additional studies demonstrated that after administration of D-LSD the concentration of 5-HIAA in the brain was decreased (AGHAJANIAN and WEISS, 1968; BOGGAN and FREEDMAN, 1973; CARLSSON and LINDQVIST, 1972; DIAZ et al., 1967, 1968; FREEDMAN and AGHAJANIAN, 1967; FREEDMAN and BOGGAN, 1974; FREEDMAN et al., 1970; LOVELL et al., 1967; PETERS, 1974a; RANDIC and PADJEN, 1971; ROSECRANS et al., 1967; SCHILDKRAUT et al., 1969).

Both 1-acetyl-LSD (FREEDMAN, 1961, 1963; FREEDMAN and GIARMAN, 1962) and 1-methyl-LSD (FREEDMAN, 1963; FREEDMAN et al., 1970) showed D-LSD-like activity.

BOL-148 at doses about 10 times higher than D-LSD also increased the 5-HT level in rat brain within the first 30 min following its administration (FREEDMAN, 1960, 1961; FREEDMAN and GIARMAN, 1962), but no change of the levels of either 5-HT or 5-HIAA could be detected at a later time (DIAZ et al., 1967, 1968; FREEDMAN, 1963; FREEDMAN et al., 1970; KING et al., 1974).

Neither methysergide (ANSELL et al., 1969; D'AMICO et al., 1976; FREEDMAN, 1961; FREEDMAN and GIARMAN, 1962; FREEDMAN et al., 1970; JACOBY et al., 1975) nor L-LSD (FREEDMAN, 1961; FREEDMAN and GIARMAN, 1962; FREEDMAN et al., 1970) were found to increase the level of 5-HT or change that of 5-HIAA in brains.

Methergoline (FUXE et al., 1975a) and methysergide (ANSELL et al., 1969; SOFIA and VASSAR, 1975) have been found to cause dose-dependent decreases of the 5-HT levels in brains from rats and guinea-pigs (D'AMICO et al., 1976) when used at doses of 1–5 mg/kg. About 10 times higher doses were required to decrease the 5-HT level in rat brains with ergotamine (SOFIA and VASSAR, 1975).

SNIDER et al. (1975) found that high doses of bromocriptine increased the 5-HT level, whereas CORRODI et al. (1975) observed no change of the 5-HT concentrations in rat brains after the administration of bromocriptine, ergocornine or PTR 17-402 (6-methyl-8β-[4-(p-methoxyphenyl)-1-piperazinyl]methyl-9-ergolene). Bromocriptine (SNIDER et al., 1975) and dihydroergotoxine mesylate (LOEW et al., 1976) decreased the 5-HIAA concentrations only when used at extremely high doses.

Although several ergot compounds have been found to increase the 5-HT level in the rat brain, only D-LSD also consistently decreased the concentration of 5-HIAA and at the same time the rate of synthesis of 5-HT, indicating that D-LSD slowed the turnover of 5-HT in the brain. Various mechanisms, e.g., enhanced vesicular binding, inhibition of 5-HT release, interneuronal feedback inhibition and/or inhibition of firing, were suggested to be involved in the effect of D-LSD in slowing down the 5-HT turnover.

In the rat brain the largest single collection of 5-HT-containing neurones is situated in the raphe nuclei of the midbrain. Projections from the dorsal raphe nucleus supply the principal 5-HT input to the forebrain (ANDÉN et al., 1966). Placement of electrolytic lesions in the rat midbrain raphe nuclei led to a selective fall in the level of 5-HT in the forebrain (KUHAR et al., 1971, 1972b). Electrical stimulation of the 5-HT-containing neurones of the midbrain raphe nuclei led to an increase of the 5-HIAA level and a decrease of the level of 5-HT in the forebrain, indicating that 5-HT can be released via specific axons projecting into the forebrain from 5-HT-containing neurones in the midbrain (AGHAJANIAN et al., 1967). An increase in brain 5-HT turnover associated with an increase in the level of 5-HIAA in the brain could also be induced by exposure of rats to elevated ambient temperature. Moreover, it was found that with rising body temperature there was a concomitant increase in the rate of firing of individual raphe neurones (WEISS and AGHAJANIAN, 1971). Both the stimulation-induced changes in 5-HT levels (KOSTOWSKI and GIACALONE, 1969; RANDIC and PADJEN, 1971) as well as the temperature-induced increase in the level of 5-HIAA (AGHAJANIAN and WEISS, 1968; CURZON and MARSDEN, 1976; WEISS and AGHAJANIAN, 1971) could be prevented by treatment of rats with D-LSD as well as by midbrain raphe lesions (WEISS and AGHAJANIAN, 1971).

There exists a reciprocal relationship between brain 5-HT content and the rate of firing of raphe cells. Elevation of brain 5-HT levels inhibits the firing of raphe neurones (AGHAJANIAN, 1972a, b; AGHAJANIAN et al., 1970b). As described in part 3, a of this section, D-LSD was also found to inhibit the firing of 5-HT-containing neurones. These results suggest, therefore, that the D-LSD-induced decrease in 5-HT turnover could result from an inhibition of firing rate of 5-HT-containing neurones.

α) Synthesis and Biological Inactivation of 5-HT in Neuronal Tissues

The regulation of 5-HT synthesis in serotoninergic neurones involves several processes, such as active transport mechanisms of uptake of tryptophan, its hydroxylation into 5-hydroxytryptophan (5-HTP) by the action of the highly specific enzyme tryptophan hydroxylase, and the decarboxylation of 5-HTP into 5-HT by the 5-hydroxytryptophan decarboxylase. Although there is good evidence for the existence of a negative feedback which controls the synthesis of 5-HT in serotoninergic neurones via intraneuronal levels of 5-HT, little is known about the factors which control the active transport into serotoninergic neurones or about the regulation of tryptophan hydroxylation which may be affected by various factors of environmental conditions and possibly by interneuronal feedback regulations (CARLSSON et al., 1972a, b; GLOWINSKI et al., 1973; HAMON and GLOWINSKI, 1974).

Treatment of animals with low doses of D-LSD was found to increase endogenous tryptophan levels in the mouse (GLOWINSKI et al., 1973) and rat brain (DIAZ and HUTTUNEN, 1971; FREEDMAN and BOGGAN, 1974; HAMON et al., 1974; HALARIS et al., 1975; TONGE and LEONARD, 1970), while both methysergide (JACOBY et al., 1975) and bromocriptine (SNIDER et al., 1975) failed to alter the tryptophan level in rat brains.

Chronic treatment of rats with low doses of D-LSD (20 μg/kg/day) for 1 month increased the rate of [^{3}H]5-HT derived from intracisternally injected [^{3}H]tryptophan (DIAZ and HUTTUNEN, 1971) as well as that derived from i.v. injected [^{3}H]-tryptophan in most brain areas, with the exception of forebrain (PETERS, 1974b). On the other hand, injection of a single dose of D-LSD decreased the conversion of labeled tryptophan into 5-HT in rat (DIAZ and HUTTUNEN, 1971; LIN et al., 1969; SHIELDS and ECCLESTON, 1973) and mouse brains (GLOWINSKI et al., 1973). A decreased synthesis of [^{3}H]5-HT from [^{3}H]tryptophan could also be observed in rat striatal slices even 60 min after the i.p. injection of a single high dose (1 mg/kg) of D-LSD (HAMON et al., 1974).

In contrast to these findings with D-LSD, BOL-148 did not change the rate of conversion of tryptophan into 5-HT in brains from either rats (LIN et al., 1969) or mice (SCHUBERT et al., 1970), and methysergide also failed to change the rise in 5-HT level following the administration of 5-HTP in guinea-pig brains (KLAWANS et al., 1973, 1975).

D-LSD was found to prevent the activation of tryptophan hydroxylase induced by methiothepin in rat brainstem slices. Administration of methiothepin, a potent 5-HT receptor blocking drug (MONACHON et al., 1972), into rats in vivo or to the incubating medium of rat brainstem slices in vitro resulted in a stimulation of the rates of formation of [^{3}H]5-HT and [^{3}H]5-hydroxyindole acetic acid ([^{3}H]5-HIAA) as compared to those in control tissues. This effect was related partly to an enhanced accumulation of [^{3}H]tryptophan in slices; however, it was also due to an activation of the rate of tryptophan hydroxylation, as estimated from the elevated conversion index of tryptophan into 5-hydroxyindoles ([^{3}H]5-hydroxyindoles/tryptophan specific activity). This methiothepin-induced activation of tryptophan hydroxylation could be prevented when brainstem slices were incubated in the presence of both methiothepin (30 μM) and D-LSD (10 μM) (HAMON et al., 1976a, b).

Treatment of mice with l-tryptophan approximately doubled the 5-HTP accumulation in the brain induced by decarboxylase inhibition with Ro 4-4602 (N^1-(DL-seryl)-N^2-(2,3,4-trihydroxybenzyl)hydrazine). This 5-HTP accumulation could be retarded by hydroxylase inhibitors but also by D-LSD (1–6 mg/kg) administered 60 min before death. Since additional experiments on mouse brain slices gave no support for a direct inhibition of tryptophan hydroxylase by D-LSD, it was suggested that synthesis and turnover of 5-HT is regulated by a feedback mechanism operating via changes in the intraneuronal 5-HT levels and/or in the activity of postsynaptic receptors (CARLSSON and LINDQVIST, 1972; CARLSSON et al., 1972a, b). In contrast to these findings with D-LSD, no change of the 5-HTP accumulation in rat brains following decarboxylase inhibition could be induced with bromocriptine (SNIDER et al., 1975).

The active uptake of 5-HTP by rat brain slices was unchanged after pretreatment of the animals with D-LSD (SCHANBERG and GIARMAN, 1960). Following the i.p. administration of labeled 5-HTP into mice, D-LSD, but not BOL-148, increased the levels of radioactive metabolites of 5-HTP in most brain areas (SZARA et al., 1967).

As observed with peripheral tissues, D-LSD had no influence on the biological inactivation of 5-HT. Neither in vitro nor in vivo was D-LSD found to change the destruction of 5-HT in the rat brain when used at pharmacologically active doses (FREEDMAN, 1961; FREEDMAN and AGHAJANIAN, 1967; FREEDMAN and GIARMAN, 1962). Only when used at concentrations higher than 10 μg/ml did D-LSD enhance the enzymatic inactivation of 5-HT in rat brain slices (HAMON et al., 1974).

β) Uptake of Exogenous 5-HT by Neuronal Tissues

5-HT is suggested to function as the main neurotransmitter in several invertebrates. The uptake of [^{3}H]5-HT by subesophageal ganglia of the snail *Helix pomatia* was not affected by D-LSD at concentrations of 10–200 μM (OSBORNE et al., 1975) and in the parasites *Schistosoma mansoni* and *Mesocestoides corti* ergot compounds, such as D-LSD, BOL-148, methysergide and 1-methyl-LSD, also failed to change the uptake of 5-HT (BENNETT and BUEDING, 1973; HARIRI, 1975).

Similar results have been obtained with brain slices and hypothalamic synaptosomes from vertebrates. Up to 10 μM D-LSD failed to affect the uptake of [^{3}H]5-HT into brain slices from mice (ROSS and RENYI, 1967) and rats (ZIEGLER et al., 1973) as well as that by rat hypothalamic synaptosomes (TUOMISTO, 1974).

The uptake of [^{3}H]5-HT into rat brain slices was found to be reduced to 50% by 500 μM methysergide (SHASKAN and SNYDER, 1970), 10 μM methergoline (FUXE et al., 1975a) and 1.6 μM PTR 17–402 (CORRODI et al., 1975). Used at 10 μM, bromocriptine caused 20% inhibition, while ergocornine failed to change the uptake of [^{3}H]5-HT by rat brain slices (CORRODI et al., 1975). In rat hypothalamic synaptosomes, 10 μM ergotamine reduced the accumulation of [^{3}H]5-HT by 50% (TUOMISTO, 1974).

There is evidence for the existence of at least two kinetically distinct 5-HT uptake mechanisms in the rat brain, and it was supposed that 5-HT—even in low doses—may also enter catecholaminergic neurones in significant proportions (SHASKAN and SNYDER, 1970).

γ) Release of 5-HT From Neuronal Tissues

Release of 5-HT From Extragranular Storage Sites

It seems possible that in the rat brain 5-HT is stored in at least two pools receiving amine synthesized by separate pathways. As has been mentioned, the strongest inhibition of [^{3}H]5-HT accumulation into rat brain slices was obtained with the ergolene derivative PTR 17-402 having an ED_{50} of 1.6 μM. This effect, however, seemed to be due to a PTR 17-402-induced 5-HT release from extragranular stores. It has been found that PTR 17-402 increased the spontaneous [^{3}H]5-HT release from cortical slices from nialamide-pretreated rats already in a concentration of 0.1 μM, while there was no releasing effect on slices of untreated animals. Based upon these observations, it was concluded that PTR 17-402 depleted only extragranular 5-HT stores, and that the large granular pool, where in slices of untreated animals most of the [^{3}H]5-HT is probably localized, may not be affected by PTR 17-402 (CORRODI et al., 1975).

Release of 5-HT From Granular Storage Sites

As has been mentioned, there is considerable evidence that 5-HT is formed and stored in presynaptic neuronal structures of special neurones and serves as neurotransmitter in the central nervous system (ANDÉN et al., 1969). In response to stimulation of 5-HT-containing neurones, the amine is released into the extracellular space, where it is partly deaminated by monoamine oxidase and partly taken up again by the nerve terminal. The existence of an inhibitory feedback loop from 5-HT-sensitive units to 5-HT-containing neurones and consequently presynaptic 5-HT-release inhibition as a mode of action of ergot alkaloids, seems therefore plausible.

Using a cerebroventricular perfusion technique to investigate neurochemical changes in the cerebrospinal fluid in rats, D-LSD at doses as low as 75 μg/kg intraperitoneally decreased significantly the efflux of [^{3}H]5-HT formed in vivo from [^{3}H]tryptophan paralleled with a total inhibition of raphe cell firing (GALLAGER and AGHAJANIAN, 1974, 1975). At higher doses, D-LSD inhibited the 5-HT overflow induced by electrical stimulation of midbrain raphe nuclei in rats (RANDIC and PADJEN, 1971) and decreased the overall output of [^{14}C]activity following a 30-min intraventricular infusion of [^{14}C]5-HT, having no discernible action on catecholaminergic pools (SPARBER, 1975; TILSON and SPARBER, 1972). These findings were supported by the observation that the retention of intraventricularly injected [^{3}H]5-HT in the rat brain was increased 60 min after i.p. treatment of the animals with D-LSD (ZIEGLER et al., 1973).

In vitro D-LSD at concentrations of 1–200 μM was found to inhibit 5-HT release from brain slices from guinea-pigs (KAWAI, 1970) and rats induced by electrical stimulation (CHASE et al., 1967, 1969; FARNEBO and HAMBERGER, 1971b; KATZ and KOPIN, 1969; KOPIN, 1970).

Reduction of the 5-HT overflow during electrical stimulation of brain slices has also been found with ergocornine (1 μM) and bromocriptine (10 μM) (CORRODI et al., 1975; FARNEBO and HAMBERGER, 1974) and with 1-acetyl-LSD (200 μM), whereas BOL-148 and L-LSD failed to inhibit the stimulation-evoked 5-HT release (KATZ and KOPIN, 1969; KOPIN, 1970).

In addition, D-LSD reduced the 5-HT overflow in response to depolarization induced by potassium. In rat striatal slices the release of [^{3}H]5-HT, synthesized from [^{3}H]tryptamine or taken up by tissue, was increased when concentrations of potassium in the incubation medium reached 30 or 50 mM. D-LSD administered in vivo (1 mg/kg) or in vitro (1 to 10 μM) effectively prevented the potassium-induced 5-HT release. The inhibitory effect of D-LSD on 5-HT release could be seen as soon as 10 min after the administration in vivo, when [^{3}H]5-HT synthesis was not affected by D-LSD. These observations suggested, therefore, that the inhibitory effect of D-LSD on 5-HT release could be mediated by a local feedback process linked to the stimulating action of the ergot compound on presynaptic 5-HT receptors (HAMON et al., 1974, 1976a).

While several ergot alkaloids reduced stimulation-induced 5-HT overflow, methiothepin, a potent 5-HT receptor blocking agent (MONACHON et al., 1972), significantly increased the 5-HT overflow induced by electrical stimulation of rat brain slices without inhibiting its uptake (FARNEBO and HAMBERGER, 1974).

These observation strongly suggest that 5-HT release can be modified by 5-HT acting on presynaptic 5-HT receptors, and that several ergot compounds may inhibit 5-HT release by stimulating these presynaptic 5-HT receptors.

Effects of Ergot Alkaloids on Drug-Induced Depletion of Neuronal 5-HT Stores

In the rat brain and spinal cord D-LSD markedly reduced the rate of 5-HT depletion due to tryptophan hydroxylase inhibition with either H 22/54 (α-propyl-dopacetamide) or PCPA (p-chlorophenylalanine) (ANDÉN, 1968; ANDÉN et al., 1968; TONGE and LEONARD, 1969) and stimulated the endogenous repletion of 5-HT stores after the administration of reserpine (FREEDMAN, 1960, 1961, 1963; FREEDMAN and GIARMAN, 1962; HALARIS and LOVELL, 1973).

In reserpinized rats 1-acetyl-LSD and BOL-148 showed also a certain activity, while methysergide failed to elevate the brain 5-HT levels (FREEDMAN, 1960; FREEDMAN and GIARMAN, 1962).

It has been suggested that D-LSD acted by either enhanced binding of 5-HT to storage sites (FREEDMAN, 1961, 1963, 1975; HALARIS and LOVELL, 1973; LOVELL et al., 1967; SCHANBERG and GIARMAN, 1962) or by an inhibitory feedback mechanism to presynaptic 5-HT neurones via stimulation of postsynaptic 5-HT receptors (ANDÉN, 1968; ANDÉN et al., 1968).

When the tryptophan hydroxylase was inhibited by H 22/54, only ergocornine and PTR 17-402, in addition to D-LSD, were found to reduce the 5-HT depletion in the rat brain, while bromocriptine (CORRODI et al., 1975), BOL-148 and methysergide (ANDÉN et al., 1968) failed to change the H 22/54-induced 5-HT depletion. On the other hand, methergoline enhanced the H 22/54-induced 5-HT depletion of the whole brain and counteracted the reduction of H 22/54-induced 5-HT depletion caused by D-LSD. The enhancement of the H 22/54-induced 5-HT depletion by methergoline was suggested to be partly due to a 5-HT receptor blocking action of methergoline, which may lead to a compensatory activity of central 5-HT neurones. However, an additional presynaptic action was also assumed (FUXE et al., 1975a).

3. Effects of Ergot Alkaloids on Neuronal 5-HT Receptors

Based upon the observation that D-LSD provided powerful and specific antagonism against 5-HT in smooth muscle preparations, GADDUM (1953, 1954) and WOLLEY and SHAW (1954a, b) already assumed that D-LSD might produce its central actions by interfering with the function of 5-HT in the brain. The subsequent research on the possible interactions of ergot alkaloids with the serotoninergic system in the brain led to conflicting results. Though several reports suggested that ergot alkaloids, e.g., D-LSD, ergometrine, BOL-148 or 1-methyl lysergic acid diethylamide, can antagonize the effects of 5-HT on spontaneous or evoked electrical activity in cat brains recorded via macro-electrodes (BOND and GUTH, 1964; GADDUM and VOGT, 1956; GUTH and SPIRTES, 1958; VOGT, 1954; VOGT et al., 1957), many reports showed either no antagonism or even synergism between different ergot compounds and 5-HT (BRADLEY, 1958; BRADLEY and HANCE, 1956a, b; GADDUM and VOGT, 1956; MARRAZZI, 1957; MARAZZI and HART, 1955a, b; SCHWARZ et al., 1956; VOGT, 1954; VOGT et al., 1957).

Since systemically applied 5-HT is not supposed to cross the blood brain barrier, most of these findings probably resulted from an action of 5-HT on peripheral, e.g., vascular, 5-HT receptors. Much interesting information came from the use of 5-HT precursors and/or monoamine oxidase inhibitors to bypass the blood brain barrier and elevate the endogenous 5-HT levels. In rabbits, methysergide effectively prevented EEG changes due to i.v. injection of 5-HTP but failed to change responses to i.v. injections of 5-HT (NAREBSKI et al., 1963).

In addition, the use of tryptophan hydroxylase inhibitors or amine-releasing agents to deplete endogenous 5-HT stores proved a useful method to study the interaction of drugs with neuronal 5-HT receptors.

The best available method for directly evaluating the qualitative effects of drugs on single neurones is by microiontophoresis. This method permits the application of relatively small amounts of substances directly into the immediate spatial environment of a living neurone, while neuronal responses can be recorded by microelectrodes. The microiontophoresis thus eliminates several of the interpretive uncertainties associated with parenteral or topical methods of pharmacologic analysis.

It has been demonstrated that brain 5-HT is contained primarily within specific neuronal elements located in raphe nuclei of the brainstem (DAHLSTRÖM and FUXE, 1964, 1965). Projections from the dorsal raphe nucleus supply the principal 5-HT input to the forebrain (ANDÉN et al., 1966). 5-HT-containing cell bodies in the caudal raphe nuclei of the brainstem give rise to axons which descend the spinal cord to contact motoneurones (FUXE, 1965). Other postsynaptic areas that receive a dense and uniform 5-HT input are the ventral lateral geniculate, amygdala, optic tectum and subiculum (AGHAJANIAN et al., 1973), the hippocampus and superior colliculus (BLOOM et al., 1972, 1973).

On both the 5-HT-containing raphe neurones as well as on neurones receiving 5-HT input, microiontophoretically applied 5-HT produces inhibition. Neurones receiving little or no 5-HT input, e.g., cells in the reticular formation or neurones of the cerebral cortex, may be either excited or inhibited by 5-HT.

a) Effects of Ergot Alkaloids on 5-HT-Containing Neurones

The histochemical identification and mapping of the location of 5-HT-containing neurones in the rat brain (DAHLSTRÖM and FUXE, 1965) provided the possibility to study the effects of drugs on the activity of single 5-HT-containing neurones directly by means of microelectrode recording. Raphe neurones produce a characteristic spontaneous activity of regular rhythm. Both 5-HT and D-LSD inhibited the firing of raphe neurones when applied microiontophoretically (AGHAJANIAN and HAIGLER, 1974; AGHAJANIAN et al., 1972; BRAMWELL and GONYE, 1973; HAIGLER and AGHAJANIAN, 1973a, b, 1974b), the latter being much more potent than 5-HT (AGHAJANIAN and HAIGLER, 1974). When submaximal amounts of D-LSD and 5-HT were ejected simultaneously, their combined inhibitory effects were additive (AGHAJANIAN et al., 1972). Microiontophoretically applied methysergide and methergoline also mimicked the inhibitory activity of 5-HT (HAIGLER and AGHAJANIAN, 1974a), while BOL-148 was found to have less than 1% of the activity of D-LSD in depressing raphe neurones (AGHAJANIAN and HAIGLER, 1974; AGHAJANIAN et al., 1972). Systemically administered D-LSD produced also a reversible inhibition of raphe cell firing. When injected i.v., D-LSD was active at a dose range of 3–20 μg/kg (AGHAJANIAN et al., 1968, 1970a; BENNETT and AGHAJANIAN, 1976; FOOTE et al., 1969; GALLAGER and AGHAJANIAN, 1974, 1975, 1976, HAIGLER and AGHAJANIAN, 1973a, b, 1974a; MOSKO and JACOBS, 1974; SVENSSON et al., 1974), while BOL-148 at doses about 10 times higher than D-LSD induced only partial inhibition of raphe firing (AGHAJANIAN et al., 1970a).

The failure of both PCPA (p-chlorophenylalanine) (AGHAJANIAN et al., 1970b) and Ro 4-4602 (GALLAGER and AGHAJANIAN, 1976) to alter D-LSD-induced inhibition of raphe firing indicated that these D-LSD effects were not dependent on 5-HT synthesis.

BENNETT and AGHAJANIAN (1976) found that the response of single raphe neurones to i.v. D-LSD was correlated with binding of the drug in the brain. Raphe firing was rapidly decreased by a dose of 3 μg/kg D-LSD i.v., which corresponded to the high-affinity binding of the drug in vitro. Studies on identified neurones within the serotoninergic system showed that presynaptic (5-HT-containing) neurones are more sensitive to the inhibitory activity of D-LSD than are postsynaptic (cells receiving 5-HT input) neurones (Fig. 13). The primary effect of D-LSD at low doses may thus be to inhibit raphe neurones by blocking 5-HT release via stimulation of presynaptic 5-HT receptors (AGHAJANIAN and HAIGLER, 1974).

b) Effects of Ergot Alkaloids on Neurones Receiving Inhibitory 5-HT Input

Neurones receiving a dense 5-HT input are relatively insensitive to D-LSD at ejection currents that are highly effective in the raphe (HAIGLER and AGHAJANIAN, 1973b, 1974b). When administered systemically at low doses, D-LSD has its primary action upon the presynaptic (i.e., raphe) neurones. The postsynaptic (i.e., ventral lateral geniculate nucleus) neurones tend to accelerate at these low doses perhaps due to a release from a tonic inhibitory influence of raphe on postsynaptic cells (AGHAJANIAN, 1972a; AGHAJANIAN and HAIGLER, 1974; HAIGLER and AGHAJANIAN, 1973b) (Fig. 13). No acceleration, but rather depression, of postsynaptic neuronal firing was observed when methysergide or methergoline was administered intravenously (HAIGLER and AGHAJANIAN, 1974a).

The spontaneous discharge of neurones in the lateral geniculate nucleus (LGN) is supposed to depend on the amount of tonic inhibition excerted by 5-HT neurones upon reticular "generator cells." Reduction of brain 5-HT by substances which inhibit storage or synthesis of 5-HT induces the occurrence of ponto-geniculo-occipital (PGO) waves. Drugs increasing the synaptic concentration of 5-HT by inhibiting neuronal uptake or directly stimulating 5-HT receptors reduce or abolish the PGO-waves. PGO-waves are thus a suitable parameter for detecting the possible effect of a drug on central 5-HT receptors. Using this method, evidence has been provided that D-LSD, methysergide and BOL-148 (FROMENT et al., 1971; HAEFELY et al., 1976; JALFRE et al., 1970, 1972, 1974; MONACHON et al., 1972; RUCH-MONACHON et al., 1976a) as well as the peptide alkaloid dihydroergotamine (RUCH-MONACHON et al., 1976b) effectively reduced drug-induced PGO-waves in the cat lateral geniculate body by directly stimulating 5-HT receptors when administered systemically (Fig. 14).

CURTIS and DAVIS (1961, 1962) first applied the technique of microiontophoresis to the study of neuronal responses of the cat LGN. Both 5-HT and D-LSD were found to diminish or block spontaneous activity and orthodromic firing evoked by nerve stimulation. Ergometrine and methylergometrine were two to three times more potent than D-LSD. BOL-148, methysergide and 12-hydroxy-methylergometrine were very weak, and ergotamine was not active in depressing the activity of cat LGN neurones. Thus, only ergot compounds of the amide type were found to mimic the inhibitory activity of 5-HT. Moreover, neither worker found antagonism of 5-HT effects by ergot alkaloids (CURTIS and DAVIS, 1961, 1962; PHILLIS et al., 1967; TEBÉCIS and DIMARIA, 1972).

These findings have been confirmed on neurones in the rat LGN. In these postsynaptic neurones, microiontophoretically applied ergot compounds, such as D-LSD, methysergide and methergoline had inhibitory activity and never antagonized the depression of firing induced by ejection of 5-HT. Moreover, the effects

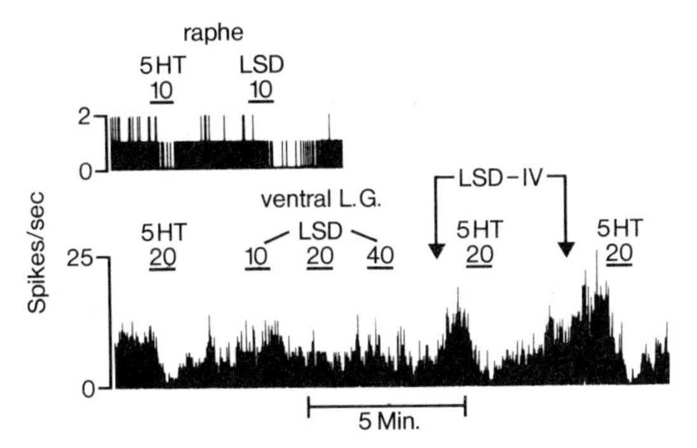

Fig. 13. Effect of 5-HT and D-LSD on the activity of a dorsal raphe neurone and a neurone in the ventral lateral geniculate nucleus (LGN) of the rat. Upper trace: The raphe neurone is inhibited by the microiontophoretic ejection of 5-HT and D-LSD. Lower Trace: The LGN neurone is also inhibited by microiontophoretic 5-HT but is relatively insensitive to D-LSD applied microiontophoretically. D-LSD intravenously (*arrows*) caused acceleration of firing but no 5-HT antagonism. [From Figure 2, AGHAJANIAN, G.K., HAIGLER, H.J.: Adv. Biochem. Psychopharmacol. **10**, 169 (1974)]

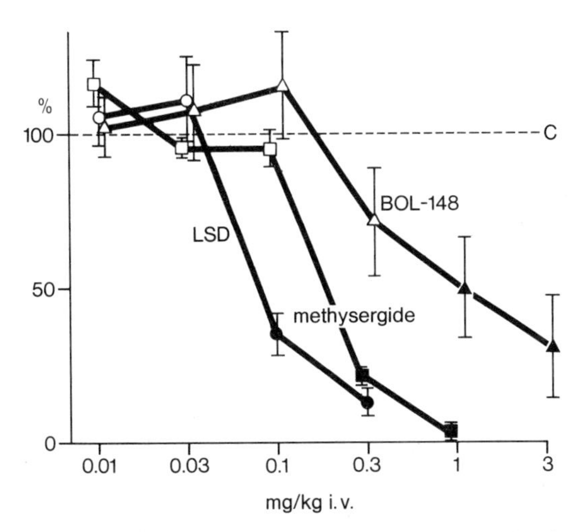

Fig. 14. Reduction of the density of Ro 4-1284-induced PGO-waves in the cat lateral geniculate body by D-LSD, methysergide and BOL-148. [From Figure 4, RUCH-MONACHON, M.A. (et al.): Arch. int. Pharmacodyn. **219**, 274 (1976)]

of combined administration of 5-HT and ergot compounds were often additive and sometimes produced an inhibition lasting much longer than the inhibition produced by 5-HT alone (AGHAJANIAN and HAIGLER, 1974; HAIGLER and AGHAJANIAN, 1973b, 1974a).

Investigating the actions of 5-HT and D-LSD in more detail, two types of dose-dependent depressant actions in the cat LGN have been observed. The depression of orthodromic firing at low concentrations of 5-HT or D-LSD was suggested to be mediated by block of the release or effect of an excitatory transmitter from optic nerve terminals, whereas the depression of chemically and sometimes also of antidromic-evoked firing at higher concentrations of 5-HT or D-LSD was suggested to indicate a direct action on postsynaptic 5-HT receptors of LGN neurones (TEBÉCIS and DIMARIA, 1972). These findings support the notion that D-LSD might have a higher affinity to presynaptic than to postsynaptic 5-HT receptor sites.

In cats, reserpine-induced PGO-like activity could be reduced by injecting both 5-HT and D-LSD into the locus ceruleus, while methysergide increased the frequency of the PGO waves, indicating 5-HT blocking activity (KOSTOWSKI et al., 1975).

5-HT is supposed to act as inhibitory neurotransmitter of the raphe-hippocampal pathway. Stimulation of raphe nuclei as well as iontophoretically applied 5-HT generated a long-lasting inhibition of spontaneous discharges of the hippocampal pyramidal neurones. Responses to 5-HT could be antagonized by iontophoretically administered ergot alkaloids, such as D-LSD, BOL 148 and methysergide (SEGAL and BLOOM, 1974). While methysergide also antagonized responses to raphe stimulation, D-LSD failed to alter these effects (SEGAL, 1975).

Guinea-pig brain slices containing the superior colliculus and incoming optic tract maintained electrical activity and were used for recording of postsynaptic field potentials evoked by optic tract stimulation. In this preparation 5-HT (0.1–1 μM) suppressed the evoked potentials without changing spontaneous activity. Similarly, D-LSD, used at 1000 times lower concentrations, caused a decrease of the postsynaptic field potentials which, however, was less than that induced by 5-HT. When tested against 5-HT both D-LSD and lysergic acid ethylamide (LAE) enhanced the 5-HT-induced suppression at low concentrations (1–10 nM) but antagonized the 5-HT effects when used at higher concentrations. In contrast, BOL-148 and morphine were found to be devoid of antagonistic activity against 5-HT (KAWAI and YAMAMOTO, 1968, 1969).

c) Effects of Ergot Alkaloids on Areas With Neurones Which are Either Excited or Inhibited by 5-HT

Cells in areas which receive little or no 5-HT input, e.g., neurones in the cerebral cortex or reticular formation, may be either excited or inhibited by 5-HT. Microiontophoretical studies provided evidence that in cat cortical neurones two separate receptors for 5-HT might exist: One for excitation and one for depression, showing marked pharmacologic differences in their responses to 5-HT antagonists. While several 5-HT antagonists effectively inhibited 5-HT-induced excitation, the same 5-HT antagonists failed to block 5-HT-induced depression. In the cat's cerebral cortex various kinds of neuronal discharge, including spontaneous firing, responses evoked by afferent nervous stimulation and excitation produced by local application of glutamate, were depressed by 5-HT. A similar but much more prolonged depression could be obtained with ergot compounds, such as D-LSD, methysergide BOL-148, ergometrine or 12-hydroxy-ergometrine (KRNJEVIC and PHILLIS, 1963a, b; LEGGE et al., 1966; ROBERTS and STRAUGHAN, 1967), while methylergometrine had a predominantly excitant activity (KRNJEVIC and PHILLIS, 1963a). D-LSD, methysergide, and BOL-148 failed to antagonize the depressant effect of 5-HT but selectively prevented 5-HT-induced excitation (BEVAN et al., 1974a, b; BRADSHAW et al., 1971; KRNJEVIC and PHILLIS, 1963a; LEGGE et al., 1966; ROBERTS and STRAUGHAN, 1967; SZABADI and BRADSHAW, 1974). Recently, potentiation of responses to 5-HT by low concentrations of methysergide has been reported, and it has been suggested that a selective blockade of masked inhibitory receptors may be the basis for this dose-dependent phenomenon (BEVAN et al., 1974a, b; SZABADI and BRADSHAW, 1974). Low concentrations of methysergide may block the more sensitive masked inhibitory receptors only, causing potentiation of the response, whereas higher concentrations of the same antagonist may block the less sensitive dominant receptors as well, causing antagonism of the observed response to 5-HT (SZABADI and BRADSHAW, 1974).

In rats, microiontophoretic application of 5-HT to cells of the reticular formation (BRIGGS, 1976; HAIGLER and AGHAJANIAN, 1974a) or to pontine raphe neurones originating in the nucleus paragigantocellularis lateralis (COUCH, 1974) induced both inhibition and excitation. D-LSD, methysergide and methergoline antagonized the 5-HT-induced excitation, leaving the inhibitory activity unaffected. Similar results have been obtained with postsynaptic neurones in the cat. In studies where microiontophoretic application of 5-HT to cells in the cat brainstem induced both inhibitory and excitatory responses, D-LSD had only inhibitory activity (BRADLEY and WOLSTENCROFT, 1964, 1965). When tested against 5-HT, D-LSD selectively antagonized the excitatory response to 5-HT but never the inhibitory effect. Methysergide was less potent than D-LSD, and BOL-148 only rarely antagonized responses to 5-HT (BOAKES et al., 1969, 1970a, b).

Stimulation of the reticular formation in the cat depressed some neurones and excited others within the thalamus. When 5-HT was administered microiontophoretically to single thalamic neurones, it depressed the majority of cells in the superficial group but excited a greater proportion of deeper cells. Both D-LSD and methysergide depressed most of the cells on which they were tested. These included neurones which were also depressed by 5-HT and some which were not affected by the latter (PHILLIS et al., 1967).

Serotoninergic neurones in the spinal cord originating in the raphe nuclei in the brainstem are supposed to influence motoneurone excitability by either facilitating or inhibiting transmission. In rabbits and rats, all the 5-HT in the spinal cord is associated with such descending fibers. In cats, high values of 5-HT in the areas of motor outflow to the limbs suggest the existence of additional segmental 5-HT-containing neurones (ANDERSON, 1972).

In the acutely spinalized rat elevation of endogenous 5-HT levels with nialamide plus 5-HTP causes athetoid movements and hyperextension in the hindlegs, tremor in the forelimbs and movements of the head. Similar symptoms could be provoked with D-LSD (ANDÉN, 1968; ANDÉN et al., 1968) and ergocornine (CORRODI et al., 1975) in a dose-dependent manner. D-LSD and ergocornine produced these changes even after depletion of 5-HT stores, suggesting that both ergot compounds directly stimulated 5-HT receptors of postsynaptic neurones.

PTR 17-402 also produced a dose-dependent increase in extensor reflex activity which, however, was abolished by combined reserpine-H 22/54 treatment and increased by prior treatment with the MAO inhibitor nialamide, indicating that this ergolene derivative acted indirectly by releasing 5-HT (CORRODI et al., 1975). Methergoline blocked head twitches and facilitation of reflex activity induced by 5-HTP in both mice (FERRINI and GLASSER, 1965) and rats (CLINESCHMIDT and LOTTI, 1974). Moreover, it caused a dose-dependent reduction of D-LSD-induced increase in extensor reflex activity without having any intrinsic activity (FUXE et al., 1975a). The peptide alkaloid bromocriptine antagonized the enhancement of the extensor reflex by the 5-HT receptor stimulating drug 5-methoxydimethyltryptamine also without showing any intrinsic activity (CORRODI et al., 1975). Neither antagonism of the effects of 5-HTP or D-LSD nor any functional action could be found with BOL-148 and methysergide (ANDÉN et al., 1968).

In both spinal dogs (MARTIN and EADES, 1970) and cats (BELL and MARTIN, 1974) D-LSD, like tryptamine, facilitated the excitability of motoneurones. Both effects could be inhibited by cyproheptadine, indicating the involvement of serotoninergic mechanisms. While in the dog methysergide also induced facilitation of the flexor reflex which could be inhibited by cyproheptadine (MARTIN and EADES, 1970), it induced initial depression of C-fiber reflexes in the cat. Thereafter, methysergide also facilitated the C-fiber reflex in the cat, and this effect again could be inhibited by cyproheptadine (BELL and MARTIN, 1974). In the cat, methysergide also antagonized the effects of tryptamine on the flexor reflex, while phenoxybenzamine and cocaine failed to block these tryptamine effects (MARLEY and VANE, 1967).

These results suggest that ergot compounds, such as D-LSD, methysergide and ergocornine, might increase motoneurone activity by directly stimulating postsynaptic 5-HT receptors. On the other hand, the same ergot compounds, D-LSD and methysergide as well as BOL-148 developed antagonistic properties when the spinal neuronal activity was either increased or inhibited by elevating the endogenous 5-HT level. These latter effects might reflect stimulation of presynaptic 5-HT receptors by ergot compounds, thus leading to inhibition of 5-HT release.

Elevation of the spinal cord level of 5-HT by MAO inhibitors (ANDERSON et al., 1967) or by injection of the 5-HT precursor 5-HTP into a spinal cat produced a number of neuronal potentials and increased the monosynaptic spike amplitudes. The administration of methysergide, D-LSD, BOL-148 as well as of cyproheptadine during the height of action resulted in a reversal of all excitatory effects (ANDERSON et al., 1967; BANNA and ANDERSON, 1968; SHIBUYA and ANDERSON, 1968).

Intact guinea-pigs developed myoclonus within 1 hr after injection of the 5-HT precursor 5-HTP. At this time the whole brain 5-HT level was unchanged. The 5-HTP-induced myoclonus was acutely prevented by methysergide, while chronically pretreatment with methysergide intensified 5-HTP-induced myoclonus again without changing brain 5-HT levels. It was assumed that prolonged methysergide administration can result in pharmacologically induced denervation hypersensitivity of central 5-HT receptors (GOETZ and KLAWANS, 1974; KLAWANS et al., 1973, 1975).

Another function of the descending serotoninergic system—the inhibitory influence on motoneurone excitability, which could be induced by treatment of the acute spinal cat with 5-HTP or reserpine—was found to be antagonized by both methysergide and BOL-148, while phenoxybenzamine failed to reverse the

5-HTP-induced reflex depression (ENGBERG et al., 1966, 1968a, b; PROUDFIT and ANDERSON, 1973).

Activation of the bulbospinal system in the cat by stimulation of the caudal raphe nuclei via implanted electrodes either facilitated or inhibited segmentally monosynaptic reflexes, dependent on the interval between the conditioning brainstem volley and the test stimulus to the dorsal root. Methysergide shifted the brainstem conditioning curve in a facilitatory direction with no change in the shape of the curve (PROUDFIT and ANDERSON, 1972, 1973). An increased facilitation of raphe-evoked monosynaptic reflexes might have been the reason for the previously stated reduction of inhibition of spinal reflexes in response to methysergide, D-LSD and BOL-148 in the same experimental model (CLINESCHMIDT and ANDERSON, 1969, 1970). In rats, electrical stimulation of the nucleus raphe medianus increased the lumbosacral motoneurone excitability. This effect was potentiated by the administration of l-tryptophan, indicating the involvement of serotoninergic neurones. Intravenous injection of both D-LSD (5–15 μg/kg) and methysergide (0.75–1 mg/kg) reduced the effectiveness of nucleus raphe stimulation. Raphe stimulation as well as microiontophoretical application of 5-HT to cells from which potentials were recorded increased the amplitude of extracellular field potential responses. Both effects could be antagonized by microiontophoretically applied methysergide as well as by cinanserine.

The similarity of the responses of lumbar motoneurones to applied 5-HT and the activity within the raphe-spinal pathway suggested that lumbar motoneurone excitability in the rat could be increased by raphe-spinal pathway via release of 5-HT in the ventral horn of the spinal cord, and that both effects could be antagonized by ergot compounds, such as D-LSD and methysergide (BARASI and ROBERTS, 1973, 1974). Further evidence for this was provided by the finding that symptoms such as abduction of the hindpaws and muscular rigidity following the injection of 5-HTP into the lateral ventricle could be prevented by BOL-148 (2 mg/kg), methysergide and D-LSD (1 mg/kg) given i.p. immediately before the 5-HTP administration (REICHENBERG et al., 1975).

In the rabbit olfactory bulb, both D-LSD and BOL-148 appeared to interact with 5-HT as well as with α-adrenergic receptor sites. Electrophoretic administration of both 5-HT and noradrenaline always resulted in slowing of the spontaneous discharge of olfactory neurones. D-LSD and BOL-148 occasionally also slowed the spontaneous rate of discharge by themselves and blocked responses to both 5-HT and noradrenaline being rather more effective against noradrenaline than against 5-HT. On the other hand, phentolamine and dibenamine selectively antagonized responses to noradrenaline without changing those to 5-HT (BLOOM et al., 1964; SALMOIRAGHI et al., 1964).

d) Effects of Ergot Alkaloids on 5-HT Receptors Which Modify Ganglionic Transmission

Studies on the ganglionic transmission in the isolated cat superior cervical ganglion demonstrated that there exist at least two independent receptors for 5-HT mediating opposite physiological effects. In a medium and high dose range (threshold dose

3–10 nmol 5-HT), a short-lasting stimulation and depolarization with facilitation of ganglionic transmission occurred, which was unchanged by low doses of ergot compounds, such as D-LSD or methysergide. Only when doses of 100 nmol and more were used did D-LSD depress the stimulant action of 5-HT.

With extremely low doses (threshold dose approximately 30–100 picomol 5-HT) up to the highest ones there occurred a long-lasting inhibition of ganglionic transmission which seemed to involve both pre- and postsynaptic sites of action. D-LSD and methysergide again showed no blocking activity against 5-HT effects, but both ergot compounds inhibited ganglionic transmission, as did 5-HT. Inhibition of ganglionic transmission with D-LSD occurred at doses of 0.3–1 nmol while 1 μmol induced complete blockade of the ganglionic transmission. A characteristic property of 5-HT, which has been already described for smooth muscle stimulation, was a very marked desensitization of the excitatory but not of the inhibitory 5-HT receptors (HAEFELY, 1971, 1974).

In addition, enhancement of the postsynaptic nerve activity by stimulant doses of 5-HT has been observed in the cat inferior mesenteric ganglion. In this preparation the 5-HT effect again could be prevented only by high doses of ergot compounds, such as BOL-148 (40–200 μg) and D-LSD (200–400 μg), but also by similar high doses of cocaine, atropine or morphine (BINDLER and GYERMEK, 1961; GYERMEK and BINDLER, 1962), indicating the involvement of some indirect actions.

In vitro investigations on the isolated rat superior cervical ganglion demonstrated inhibition of ganglionic transmission by methysergide (5–10 μg/ml) (KALBERMATTEN, 1962) but no antagonism of the stimulant activity of 5-HT by methysergide (WATSON, 1970).

Responses to submaximal preganglionic stimulation in the isolated rat stellate ganglion were increased by 5-HT and BOL-148 as well as by methysergide when used at μg/ml concentrations (HERTZLER, 1961).

To summarize: The effects of ergot compounds, such as D-LSD, methysergide and BOL-148, on 5-HT receptors modifying ganglionic transmission generally resemble those induced by 5-HT. Depending on the concentrations used, both inhibitory and stimulatory effects may be observed, suggesting the involvement of two types of 5-HT receptors. Antagonism of 5-HT effects by ergot alkaloids occurred only when they were used at extremely high concentrations.

The chemoreceptor discharges in the cat carotid body increased in response to both 5-HT (5 μg i.a.) and D-LSD (10 μg i.a.) but were unchanged after methysergide. Moreover, methysergide and D-LSD up to 100 μg/kg failed to change the chemoreceptor stimulant action of 5-HT in cats (NISHI, 1975), as BOL-148 and ergotamine did not prevent the chemoreceptor stimulant action of 5-HT in dogs (SALMOIRAGHI et al., 1957). These observations support the notion that cat's coronary chemoreflex in response to 5-HT was not antagonized but rather increased by D-LSD (ZAKUSOV, 1962). They are further in line with the finding that 5-HT-induced spikes in some afferent fibers of the cat vagus nerve were enhanced by D-LSD (100 μg/kg) (GYERMEK and SUMI, 1963).

In vitro D-LSD, like 5-HT, enhanced spontaneous and light-evoked activity of ganglion cells of the rabbit retina while methysergide caused depression of the activity (AMES and POLLEN, 1969).

e) Effects of Ergot Alkaloids on 5-HT Receptors Which Modify Release of Acetylcholine

The first pharmacologic data on nervous 5-HT receptors distinguishable from those obtained on smooth muscle came from studies of ROCHA E SILVA et al. (1953) and GADDUM and PICARELLI (1957) on the isolated guinea-pig ileum. These authors described nervous receptors in the guinea-pig ileum which could be activated by 5-HT and were markedly influenced by drugs, such as cocaine, atropine and morphine but not by ergot alkaloids.

The classical "M-receptors," described by GADDUM and PICARELLI (1957), are supposed to be localized at the varicose cell processes from which acetylcholine is released towards the muscle. Spike activity in such processes, which can be recorded by extracellular techniques, is increased by 5-HT, and this effect is prevented by morphine (DINGLEDINE et al., 1974).

In contrast, intracellular recordings from single myenteric plexus neurones demonstrated that 5-HT at concentrations of 25 nM to 1 μM reversibly depressed EPSP (excitatory postsynaptic potentials) evoked by single focal stimulation but failed to change responses to acetylcholine. This action of 5-HT could be antagonized by methysergide, D-LSD, and cyproheptadine but was unaffected by morphine. Besides preventing the action of 5-HT, methysergide (1.7 μM) also slightly depressed the EPSP amplitude, indicating some 5-HT-like activity. These findings suggested that 5-HT reduces EPSP in guinea-pig ileum by inhibiting the release of acetylcholine from presynaptic nerve terminals within the myenteric plexus (HENDERSON and NORTH, 1975; NORTH and HENDERSON, 1975).

Using muscle twitch reflexes and intravenous 5-HT, facilitation of flexor reflexes and inhibition of extensor reflexes in the spinal cat have been observed. D-LSD usually augmented the stimulatory effect of 5-HT and prevented the depressor effect of 5-HT (LITTLE et al., 1957; SLATER et al., 1955; WEIDMANN, 1957; WEIDMANN and CERLETTI, 1957).

Since 5-HT is not supposed to cross the blood-brain barrier, the effects probably resulted from an action of 5-HT on peripheral receptors or sensory nerve endings as has been suggested by DEFFENU and MANTEGAZZINI (1966). These authors found that 5-HT was about 10 times more potent when injected intra arterially as compared to intra venous administration. Methysergide and also dibenamine and chlorpromazine prevented the inhibitory effect of 5-HT. These findings were supported by the finding that in the rat nerve-muscle preparation methysergide, like cyproheptadine and chlorpromazine, prevented 5-HT-induced muscle weakness (PATTEN et al., 1974).

DRETCHEN et al. (1972) showed that 5-HT reversed the effects of neuromuscular blocking agents, and that this 5-HT effect could be reduced by methysergide, whereas α-adrenergic blocking agents or M-receptor blockers did not affect the anticurare action of 5-HT. It was suggested that 5-HT acts presynaptically at the neuromuscular junction by increasing the amount of acetylcholine liberated on nerve stimulation.

Bilateral microinjections of 5-HT into the rabbit nucleus amygdalae caused an increase of motor activity as well as arousal of the electroencephalographic activity in the cortex, while i.p. administration of methysergide (5 mg/kg) induced a slight reduction of the electrogenesis. While atropine effectively prevented the changes of electrogenesis evoked by 5-HT, both methysergide and cyproheptadine only slightly reduced the responses to 5-HT which was administered 60 min later. These results suggested that the stimulation induced by injecting 5-HT into the rabbit nucleus amygdalae was mediated mainly through the release of acetylcholine (PRZEWLOCKI, 1975).

To conclude, both facilitation and inhibition of acetylcholine release may be induced by 5-HT. Ergot compounds such as D-LSD and methysergide usually antagonized the effects in response to decreased acetylcholine release. Both ergot alkaloids, however, failed to inhibit 5-HT effects induced by enhanced acetylcholine release, which could be blocked by drugs, such as cocaine, atropine and morphine.

f) Effects of Ergot Alkaloids on Neuronal 5-HT Receptors in Invertebrates

Many neurones of molluscs are accessible, large, well identifiable and highly sensitive to 5-HT, thus being more suitable to study the interaction of drugs with neuronal receptor sites than are neurones of vertebrate species. Moreover, there seem to exist many common properties between the 5-HT receptors of molluscan neurones and those in vertebrates. Both are easily desensitized by high 5-HT concentrations and both may mediate physiologically opposite effects in response to 5-HT, e.g., excitation and inhibition or facilitation and depression of responses to other stimuli. The effects of ergot alkaloids are often mixed agonistic-antagonistic, depending on the concentrations employed. In some molluscs, e.g., *Helix aspersa* and *Aplysia californica,* at least six different types of neuronal responses to 5-HT in terms of their pharmacologic and physiologic properties have been distinguished. Some of these responses to 5-HT were found to be blocked by high concentrations (10 μM) of D-LSD (GERSCHENFELD, 1971; GERSCHENFELD and PAUPARDIN, 1972; GERSCHENFELD and PAUPARDIN-TRITSCH, 1974a, b, c). Cells with inhibition of long duration, the so-called CILDA neurones (GERSCHENFELD and TAUC, 1964), are highly sensitive to both acetylcholine and 5-HT. Depolarization of 2–4 mV could be obtained with 1 nM 5-HT at the receptor level. These 5-HT receptors are blocked by BOL-148 in a selective and competitive way ($pA_2=8.0$) (GERSCHENFELD and STEFANI, 1965), whereas for antagonism of 5-HT by D-LSD much higher concentrations (100 μg/ml) were necessary (GERSCHENFELD and STEFANI, 1965, 1966, 1967, 1968; GERSCHENFELD and TAUC, 1964; SHIMAHARA and TAUC, 1975).

The ciliary activity of an isolated gill-nerve-ganglion preparation from the mussel *Mytilus edulis* is activated by 2–10 Hz electro stimulation of the brachial nerve. This effect was suggested to be mediated by the release of 5-HT. Evidence for this was provided by the observation that reserpine treatment of the mussel significantly diminished the 5-HT content in the gill and also reduced the response to electrical stimulation (AIELLO and GUIDERI, 1966). Responses to electrical stimulation, but not those to exogenous 5-HT, were also significantly decreased by cocaine (AIELLO and GUIDERI, 1964). Moreover, BOL-148 reversibly diminished the effects of both nerve stimulation and exogenous 5-HT. In this preparation BOL-148 itself caused slight stimulation at concentrations about 10 times lower than those required for 5-HT antagonism (AIELLO and GUIDERI, 1966; AIELLO and PAPARO, 1974).

5-HT is also suggested to function as neurotransmitter of the relaxing nerve fibers supplying the anterior byssus retractor muscle of *M. edulis* (WELSH, 1954a; TWAROG, 1954). When contraction of the anterior byssus retractor muscle was induced by nerve stimulation, the following relaxation was much slower in the presence of BOL-148 (10 μg/ml). This action of BOL-148 on tension delay could be partly reversed by 5-HT (BULLARD, 1967).

Antagonism by methysergide of 5-HT-induced increase in spontaneous activity in giant neurones has been found in the subesophageal ganglion of the snail *Achatina fulica* (TAKEUCHI et al., 1974). Responses of the heart of the snail *Helix pomatia* to stimulation of the intestinal nerve were also antagonized by BOL-148 (0.1 μg/ml), while D-LSD at the same concentration enhanced the effects (RÓZSA and GRAUL, 1964).

In *Helix pomatia* 5-HT is suggested to be the transmitter in synaptic connections between giant 5-HT-containing cells and non-amine-containing neurones. Iontophoretic application of 5-HT to the non-amine-containing cells produced a depolarizing potential change. D-LSD (30–300 μM) also elicited depolarization and reduced the responsiveness to 5-HT of these neurones. Methysergide and BOL-148 used at the same concentration ranges evoked less depolarization but similar antagonism of 5-HT effects. Lower concentrations of these ergot alkaloids failed to antagonize responses to 5-HT. Neither D-LSD nor methysergide produced reduction of EPSP resulting from giant 5-HT cell stimulation when used at 1–30 μM. On the contrary, 1 μM D-LSD was found to enhance the EPSP effects, suggesting the involvement of a presynaptic action of D-LSD (COTTRELL, 1970b). Concentrations of D-LSD required to abolish EPSP elicited by giant 5-HT cells resulted in a considerable depolarization and activation of the non-amine-containing cells (COTTRELL, 1970a, b; COTTRELL and MACON, 1974; COTTRELL et al., 1974).

4. Effects of Ergot Alkaloids on 5-HT-Sensitive Enzyme Systems

Various invertebrate systems have proved of value in studying the interaction of drugs with 5-HT receptor sites as well as the intermediate steps following activation of the 5-HT receptor. Some effects in response to stimulation of 5-HT receptor sites are mediated by an increase in the formation of cyclic AMP (3′,5′-adenosine monophosphate).

In salivary glands from the blow-fly *Calliphora erythrocephala,* besides inducing fluid secretion, 5-HT has been shown to cause 2–4 fold increase in cyclic AMP concentrations (PRINCE et al., 1972). A similar stimulation of both fluid secretion and cyclic AMP formation was produced with D-LSD. After 10 min incubation of salivary glands with either 10 nM 5-HT or 10 nM D-LSD, the level of cyclic AMP was increased by about 30% (BERRIDGE and PRINCE, 1974).

The liver fluke *Fasciola hepatica* responds to 5-HT with increased rhythmical movements paralleled with striking increase in the formation of cyclic AMP mainly in the oral end of the fluke. D-LSD at 1 nM, although enhancing the motility, failed to increase the cyclic AMP formation. On the contrary, with 5 nM D-LSD a 50% inhibition of the 5-HT effect on adenylate cyclase was obtained. Only when used at 10 μM did D-LSD slightly increase the formation of cyclic AMP. Based upon the observation that it took about four times more to reverse the D-LSD effect by washout as compared to the 5-HT effect, it was assumed that for activation of the adenylate cyclase system in the liver fluke a certain degree of reversibility of the effector-receptor complex may be required (Abrahams, 1974; Abrahams et al., 1976; Mansour et al., 1960).

In the mollusc *Macrocallista nimbosa* the 5-HT-induced increase in myocardial cyclic AMP could be blocked by 1 μM methysergide (Higgins, 1974).

Adenylate cyclase sensitive to 5-HT has also been found on homogenates from cockroach thoracic ganglia. In this preparation a selective inhibition of 50% of the 5-HT-induced activation of adenylate cyclase could be obtained with BOL-148 and D-LSD at concentrations of 10 and 20 nM, respectively, while for a 50% inhibition by cyproheptadine 200 nM were required. Both D-LSD and BOL-148 stimulated the adenylate cyclase when used at concentrations of 1 μM and higher (Nathanson and Greengard, 1974).

As far as known a 5-HT sensitive adenylate cyclase system in nervous tissues from vertebrates has been found only in brains from young rats. In cell-free preparations from superior and inferior colliculi of 1 to 3 days old rats half maximal stimulation of the adenylate cyclase was produced with 1 μM 5-HT. D-LSD inhibited more than 50% of the 5-HT effect when used at the relatively high concentration of 10 μM, and the 5-HT antagonism induced by BOL-148, methysergide and MCE (1-methyl-8β-carbobenzyloxy-aminomethyl-10 α-ergoline) was still weaker than that caused by D-LSD (Von Hungen et al., 1974a, 1975). In this preparation, 10–100 μM D-LSD were necessary to produce a slight stimulation of adenylate cyclase activity, and BOL-148, methysergide or MCE were devoid of any stimulating activity (Hamon et al., 1976a; Von Hungen et al., 1975).

These findings were supported by experiments on rat brain stem slices where D-LSD at 100 μM raised the concentration of cyclic AMP, but 5-HT failed to change the level of cyclic AMP (Uzunov and Weiss, 1972).

In rat heart slices 5-HT was found to increase cyclic AMP accumulation indirectly by releasing endogenous catecholamines. This effect could be inhibited by high (15 μM) concentrations of dihydroergotamine but not by phenoxybenzamine (Benfey et al., 1974).

Studies on the effects of receptor stimulation on the lipid metabolism have shown that in the isolated guinea-pig ileum stimulation of D-receptors by 5-HT (125 μM) elicited an increase in phosphatidylinositol turnover. This effect could be abolished by 10 μg/ml methysergide (Jafferji and Michell, 1976).

A stereospecific inhibition of an enzymatic activity by ergot compounds in vitro has been demonstrated using a de-acetylase (aryl acylamidase) isolated from rat brains. This enzymatic activity could be inhibited in vitro by 5-HT as well as by pharmacologically active ergot compounds, such as D-LSD, BOL-148 and methysergide at concentrations of 10–100 μM, while L-LSD was inactive as inhibitor of the enzymatic activity (Paul and Halaris, 1976; Paul et al., 1976).

C. Actions of Ergot Alkaloids at Dopamine Receptors

1. Actions of Ergot Alkaloids at Extraneuronal Dopamine Receptors

a) General Description of "Specific Dopamine Receptors"

Until a few years ago, dopamine was known only as the precursor of noradrenaline. However, its unusual distribution as well as the discovery of specific dopaminergic pathways suggested that this amine had also physiological roles. The structure of dopamine is consistent with a multireceptor potential and fits in adrenergic as well as in serotoninergic receptors, both of which also represent binding sites for ergot compounds (Fig. 15). It follows from this that antagonists, especially those containing the ergoline moiety, will often have a narrow range of selectivity.

In vascular smooth muscles both contraction and relaxation in response to dopamine has been demonstrated in arteries and veins. In canine renal arteries (KELLY, 1972; STRANDHOY et al., 1972; ZAROLINSKI and BROWNE, 1971) and in aortic strips from rats (COHEN and BERKOWITZ, 1975) and rabbits (KOHLI, 1969) the dopamine-induced contractions appear to be due, at least in part, to stimulation of α-adrenoceptors. Alpha-adrenergic blocking agents, such as phentolamine and phenoxybenzamine, antagonized responses to both dopamine and noradrenaline in similar concentrations. In canine femoral and carotid arteries, however, the dopamine receptor appears to be related to 5-HT- or tryptamine receptors but not to α-adrenoceptors. In canine femoral and carotid arterial strips the 5-HT receptor blocking agent cyproheptadine produced nearly identical pA_2 values (7.5, 7.6 and 7.4) when tested against dopamine, 5-HT and tryptamine. Moreover, dopamine and 5-HT exerted cross protection on dopamine, 5-HT and tryptamine receptors against blockade by both cyproheptadine as well as by phenoxybenzamine, while noradrenaline failed to protect any of these receptors in canine arteries (GILBERT and GOLDBERG, 1975). When isolated canine renal, mesenteric, coronary, intracerebral or small (<1 mm, outside diameter) femoral arteries were exposed to phenoxybenzamine and contracted with potassium or prostaglandin $F_{2\alpha}$, dopamine caused dose-dependent relaxation (GOLDBERG, 1975; GOLDBERG and TODA,

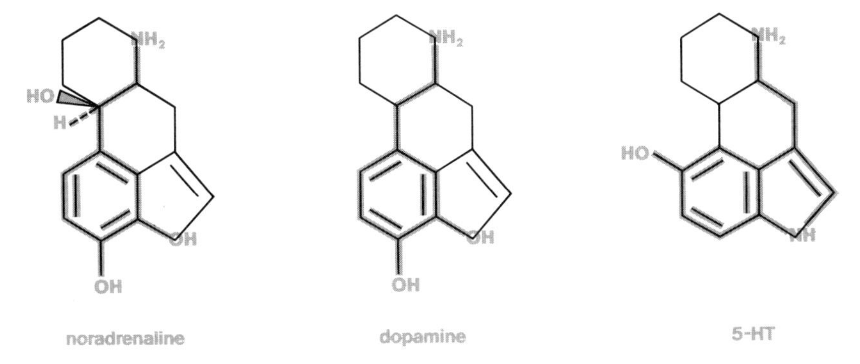

Fig. 15. Common structural conformations of noradrenaline, dopamine and 5-HT with the ergoline moiety

1975; GOLDBERG et al., 1973; TODA and GOLDBERG, 1973, 1975; TODA et al., 1973). Studies of potential dopamine antagonists have demonstrated only partial antagonism of dopamine-induced relaxation, since all the selective dopamine antagonists active in vivo, e.g., haloperidol, chlorpromazine, apomorphine and bulbocapnine, in estimated effective concentrations caused marked relaxation of the isolated canine arteries (GOLDBERG et al., 1973). Attempts to antagonize dopamine-induced relaxation in canine renal and mesenteric arteries with ergometrine have been without success (MÜLLER-SCHWEINITZER, 1975b). Thus, the definite characterization of a peripheral dopamine receptor has not yet been accomplished.

b) Effects of Ergot Alkaloids on Peripheral Dopamine Receptors

Dopamine receptors in the longitudinal musculature of the worm *Schistosoma mansoni* mediate lengthening of the worms in response to dopamine, noradrenaline, adrenaline and apomorphine. The relaxation of the longitudinal musculature induced by these agonists could be antagonized more effectively by dopamine blockers, such as haloperidol, spiroperidol and pimozide, than by α- or β-adrenergic blocking agents, indicating that the lengthening of the worms was mediated by stimulation of dopamine receptors. Responses to the three agonists could also be antagonized by ergot alkaloids, such as ergometrine, dihydroergocristine and dihydroergotamine, suggesting that these ergot compounds combined with the dopamine receptor (TOMOSKY et al., 1974).

2. Interaction of Ergot Alkaloids With Indirect Dopamine Effects

Dopamine in a concentration of 0.1 μM produced contraction of the rat stomach fundus preparation. Repeated exposure to dopamine resulted in tachyphylaxis, but the sensitivity to dopamine could be restored by incubating the tissue with 5-HT. This action of dopamine, which thus might be caused indirectly by release of 5-HT, could be blocked by methysergide (0.1 μM). It remains to be demonstrated, however, whether methysergide antagonized the 5-HT-releasing activity of dopamine or whether it competed with the released amine at the 5-HT receptor site (SONNEVILLE, 1968).

3. Actions of Ergot Alkaloids at Neuronal Dopamine Receptors

a) Effects of Ergot Alkaloids on Neuronal Dopamine Receptors in Invertebrates

Interaction of ergot alkaloids with neuronal dopamine receptors was first investigated on neurones of invertebrates. Although there may be similarities between the dopamine receptors and the 5-HT receptors – which are also binding sites for most ergot compounds – evidence for the existence of separate receptors for dopamine on the one hand and for 5-HT on the other has been provided. WOODRUFF et al. (1971) found that the snail neurones used in their study were all hyperpolarized by dopamine but depolarized by 5-HT. The effects of both agonists could be blocked by ergot compounds, such as D-LSD and methysergide.

It can be further assumed that distinct dopamine receptors and adrenoceptors exist. Structure activity studies suggested that the structural requirements for dopamine-like activity are more specific than those for activity on adrenergic receptors (WOODRUFF and WALKER, 1969).

More detailed studies showed the existence of two types of dopamine receptors mediating physiologically opposite effects in the brain of *Helix aspersa* (STRUYKER BOUDIER and VAN ROSSUM, 1974). Dopamine receptors mediating neuronal excitation (DA_e receptors) are selectively activated by apomorphine and selectively inhibited by neuroleptics, such as haloperidol (STRUYKER BOUDIER et al., 1974), whereas the dopamine receptors mediating neuronal inhibition (DA_i receptors) are selectively activated by (3,4-dihydroxy-phenylamino)-2-imidazoline (DPI) and selectively inhibited by ergot compounds, such as ergometrine (STRUYKER BOUDIER et al., 1975; COOLS and VAN ROSSUM, 1976).

Ergometrine, which has little or no α-adrenergic blocking activity, was the first ergot compound to be described as a potent antagonist of the inhibitory action of dopamine on neurones of the snail *H. aspersa* (WALKER et al., 1968; WOODRUFF et al., 1970). In addition to these findings, long-lasting antagonism of the inhibitory action of dopamine on *Helix* neurones has been found with D-LSD, methysergide (WOODRUFF et al., 1971), and also with the peptide alkaloids ergotoxine, ergotamine and their dihydrogenated derivatives dihydroergotoxine mesylate and dihydroergotamine. As compared to the dopamine blocking activity of ergometrine, the natural ergopeptins were found to be about 10 times less potent, and their dihydrogenated derivatives were at least 100 times less potent in antagonizing the dopamine-induced inhibition of *Helix* neurones (WALKER et al., 1968; STRUYKER BOUDIER et al., 1974).

As observed with *H. aspersa* neurones, the addition of dopamine to identified neurones in ganglia of *Aplysia californica* induced both excitatory and inhibitory postsynaptic responses, but only the latter effect could be antagonized with D-LSD (SATO and SAWADA, 1975), ergometrine, methylergometrine or ergotamine (ASCHER, 1972). The blocking action of both ergometrine and methylergometrine was preceded by a small hyperpolarization, indicating some agonistic activity.

BERRY and COTTRELL (1975), studying the effects of iontophoretically applied dopamine on central neurones of the water snail *Planorbis corneus,* also observed excitatory and inhibitory responses. In this preparation ergometrine again specifically antagonized the inhibitory postsynaptic potentials in response to stimulation of dopamine-containing neurones as well as the inhibitory response to applied dopamine. As observed with *Aplysia* neurones, ergometrine developed some agonistic activity. The addition of ergometrine resulted in a hyperpolarization and reduction or abolition of spontaneous firing in the follower cells (BERRY and COTTRELL, 1975; COTTRELL et al., 1974).

Dopamine receptors sensitive to ergot compounds have been found to mediate inhibition of lateral ciliary activity in the bivalve mollusc *Modiolus demissus.* This effect was antagonized by ergometrine, methysergide and BOL-148 (MALANGA, 1973). A further type of dopamine receptor seems to mediate stimulation of the frontal ciliary activity in bivalve molluscs. This effect was antagonized by ergometrine and BOL-148 but unchanged by methysergide (MALANGA, 1973, 1974).

In addition, ergometrine was found to antagonize the inhibitory action of dopamine in the intestine of the mollusc *Tapes watlingi* (DOUGAN and MCLEAN, 1970).

There was no change of the dopamine uptake into subesophageal ganglia of the snail *Helix pomatia* by D-LSD up to 10–200 μM (OSBORNE et al., 1975).

b) Effects of Ergot Alkaloids on Neuronal Dopamine Receptors in Vertebrates

Investigations on the electrical properties and responses to transmural stimulation in neurones of the submucous plexus of the guinea-pig ileum showed that most neurones received excitatory synaptic input, but an appreciable proportion of neurones also received a single inhibitory input—both being activated by transmural stimulation. BOL-148 (0.1–1 μg/ml) was found to antagonize the inhibitory synaptic potentials in a selective and reversible way (HIRST and MCKIRDY, 1975). Using the technique of iontophoretic application of drugs to neurones of the submucous plexus of guinea-pig small intestine, it could be demonstrated that both dopamine and noradrenaline caused responses which closely resembled those inhibitory synaptic potentials evoked by transmural stimulation, while 5-HT caused excitation of the neurones. Moreover, it was found that methysergide, like BOL-148, antagonized both the inhibitory synaptic potentials and the inhibitory effects of dopamine and noradrenaline but had only little activity when tested against 5-HT potentials (HIRST and SILINSKY, 1975). These findings support the notion that ergometrine at concentrations of 0.03–1 μM reversed the inhibitory action of low concentrations of both dopamine and noradrenaline in the isolated rabbit jejunum (WOODRUFF et al., 1969).

Studies on the canine cardiac sympathetic ganglion demonstrated inhibition of the ganglionic transmission by catecholamines, such as noradrenaline, adrenaline and dopamine, injected into the right subclavian artery during preganglionic nerve stimulation. Dihydroergotamine antagonized responses to both adrenaline and dopamine. Apomorphine and haloperidol selectively antagonized the effects of dopamine, while phentolamine did not significantly affect responses to dopamine. These results suggest that the receptors for dopamine may differ from those for noradrenaline and adrenaline (ICHIMASA et al., 1975).

It has been proposed to use *Helix aspersa* dopamine-sensitive neurones as model for the design of drugs selectively interfering with dopamine-sensitive structures in mammalian brains. Two distinct types of dopamine receptors having electrophysiologic and pharmacologic properties comparable to those of DA_e and DA_i receptors within the snail have been found within the feline caudate nucleus. As observed with *Helix* neurones, evidence has been provided that only DA_i receptors are selectively antagonized by ergot compounds, such as ergometrine, while DA_e receptors can be blocked by neuroleptics, such as haloperidol (COOLS, 1975; COOLS and VAN ROSSUM, 1976; COOLS et al., 1976; VAN ROSSUM et al., 1975). Microiontophoretic studies on the effectiveness of these antagonists within the caudate nucleus of cats are, however, required to prove this hypothesis.

In rats, apparently the dopamine-loaded structures within the brain contain two anatomically-histochemically distinct areas, which are each characterized by their own pharmacologic features: The neostriatum, which is more sensitive to apomorphine than to ergometrine, and the nucleus accumbens, which is more sensitive to ergot alkaloids such as ergometrine than to apomorphine. Administration of ergometrine directly into the nucleus accumbens of rats produced a pattern of enhanced locomotor activity similar to that seen after dopamine injection (PIJNENBURG and VAN ROSSUM, 1973; PIJNENBURG et al., 1973). The locomotor stimulation after ergometrine was blocked by low doses of haloperidol and pimozide, suggesting that dopamine receptors are involved in the action of ergometrine. Depletion of dopamine and noradrenaline in the brain by pretreatment of the rats with α-methyl-p-tyrosine had no influence on the activity of ergometrine, indicating that a presynaptic action is unlikely. Methysergide was ineffective in producing locomotor stimulation (PIJNENBURG et al., 1973). Bromocriptine (2-bromo-α-ergokryptine, CB 154, Parlodel) antagonized the dopamine-induced hyperactivity only at doses considered very large in behavioural terms (COSTALL and NAYLOR, 1976). Moreover, in contrast to that observed with ergometrine, bromocriptine appeared to have affinity to presynaptic dopamine receptors as well. The stimulation-induced release of [^{3}H]dopamine from superfused striatal synaptosomes was significantly inhibited by 0.1 μM bromocriptine (MULDER et al., 1975).

Biochemical studies provided first evidence for the possible existence of dopaminergic neurones in the rat cortex (THIERRY et al., 1973a, b). Using the technique of microiontophoresis on cortical neurones from rats, it was found that the majority of cells tested responded in the same manner to dopamine and ergometrine (CROSSMAN et al., 1973) as well as to agroclavine (STONE, 1974). Moreover, chlorpromazine, an antagonist at central dopamine receptors (YORK, 1972), selectively antagonized responses to both dopamine and agroclavine, leaving those to noradrenaline and 5-HT unchanged. From these results it was suggested that agroclavine and possibly other ergot alkaloids may have an agonistic action at central dopamine receptors (STONE, 1974).

c) Effects of Ergot Alkaloids on Neuronal Dopamine Turnover

Although the levels of dopamine in rat brain were not affected by ergot alkaloids, such as D-LSD (DA PRADA et al., 1975b), methergoline (FUXE et al., 1975a), ergocornine and bromocriptine (CORRODI et al., 1973), these ergot alkaloids caused a clearcut decrease in dopamine turnover as indicated by the retardation of the disappearance of dopamine in the brain following the administration of α-methyl-p-tyrosine (CORRODI et al., 1973; FUXE et al., 1974; HÖKFELT and FUXE, 1972; DA PRADA et al., 1975a, b; SNIDER et al., 1976). Further experiments demonstrated that ergot alkaloids, such as ergocornine, bromocriptine (CORRODI et al., 1973; HÖKFELT and FUXE, 1972) and PTR 17-402 (6-methyl-8β-[4-(p-methoxyphenyl)-1-piperazinyl]methyl-9-ergolene) (FUXE et al., 1975b) mainly reduced dopamine turnover in the subcortical limbic areas and in the neostriatum. The action on dopamine metabolism by these ergot compounds might probably be due to dopamine receptor stimulating activity of these agents. It has been shown that γ-hydroxybutyric acid inhibits neuronal firing in dopaminergic neurones, thus causing several alterations in dopamine metabolism, e.g., increase in dopamine concentration (WALTERS et al., 1973). As observed with various dopamine agonists, both ergocornine and bromocriptine inhibited the rise in dopamine after γ-hydroxybutyric acid, thus providing evidence for the concept of local receptor feedback on dopamine synthesis. Haloperidol, which effectively antagonized the inhibition by apomorphine, failed to block that induced by ergocornine or bromocriptine. These results support the notion that there are at least two types of dopamine receptors (HANDFORTH and SOURKES, 1975).

4. Effects of Ergot Alkaloids on Dopamine-Sensitive Enzyme Systems

Recent evidence has been accumulating which suggests that specific dopamine receptors are involved in the elevation of cyclic AMP (3′,5′-adenosine monophosphate) occurring after addition of dopamine to mammalian brain and retina in vitro. Reports indicating that a number of ergot derivatives exert dopamine-like actions on central neurones in the rat gave rise to investigations of the interaction of ergot alkaloids with dopamine-sensitive adenylate cyclase systems in the rat brain. UZUNOV and WEISS (1972) found that incubation of rat brain stem slices with D-LSD increased the concentration of cyclic AMP, and that this activity of D-LSD was not shared by BOL-148. The inhibition of the D-LSD-induced accumulation of cyclic AMP by the neuroleptic trifluoperazine suggested the involvement of dopamine receptors. Further studies demonstrated that D-LSD may act both as agonist and as antagonist on the dopamine-sensitive adenylate cyclase systems within the rat brain. A significant stimulation of the adenylate cyclase in rat striatal tissue could be obtained with concentrations of D-LSD as low as 0.1 μM and was increased about 30% by 10–20 μM D-LSD (DA PRADA et al., 1975a, b; SPANO et al., 1975a, b; VON HUNGEN et al., 1974b). This was about one-half the activation produced by an equimolar concentration of dopamine. Responses to both dopamine and D-LSD could be abolished by equimolar concentrations of haloperidol, chlorpromazine, BOL-148 and MLD (1-methyl-d-lysergic acid diethylamide), while propranolol failed to antagonize the stimulation of striatal adenylate cyclase by either dopamine or D-LSD. On the other hand, 1 μM D-LSD antagonized the stimulation of cerebral adenylate cyclase activity by dopamine (Fig. 16) (DA PRADA et al., 1975a, b; VON HUNGEN et al., 1974a, b).
Stimulation of striatal adenylate cyclase could also be elicited with ergometrine (ELKHAWAD and WOODRUFF, 1975; ELKHAWAD et al., 1975; MUNDAY et al., 1976), while both MLD (1-methyl-d-lysergic acid diethylamide) and BOL-148 (SPANO et al., 1975a, b; VON HUNGEN et al., 1974a) were devoid of any intrinsic activity. The injection of bromocriptine (0.5–2 mg/kg i.p.) into rats produced a dose-dependent increase of striatal cyclic AMP concentration. In vitro, however, bromocriptine up to 100 μM was inactive in stimulating dopamine sensitive adenylate cyclase in rat striatal homogenates, though it inhibited the dopamine-induced stimulation of the enzyme activity even at concentrations as low as 1 μM (TRABUCCHI et al., 1976). This dopamine antagonism by bromocriptine, however, appears not to be selective. It has been found that bromocriptine is less potent in antagoniz-

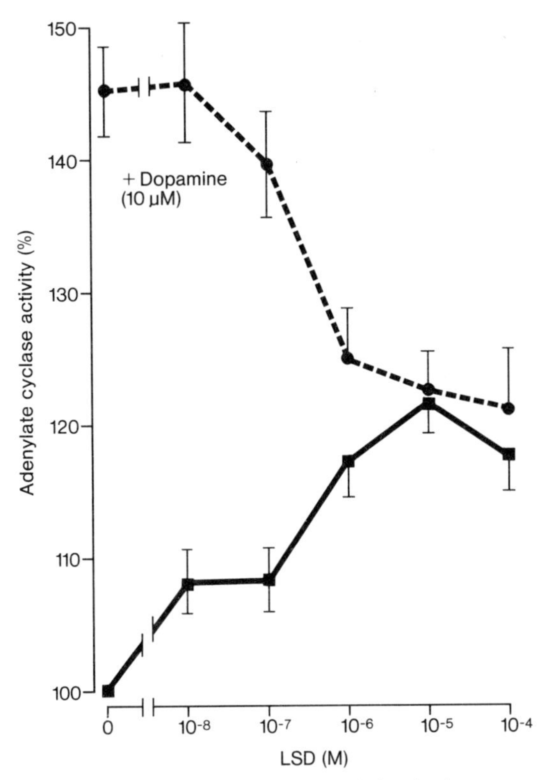

Fig. 16. Effect of D-LSD on the adenylate cyclase activity in homogenates of rat striatum without (■——■) and in the presence of 10 µM dopamine (●---●). Each point indicates a mean value with SEM from 7 experiments. [From Figure 3, DA PRADA, M. (et al.): Brain Res. **94**, 70 (1975)]

ing the activation of striatal adenylate cyclase by dopamine (pA_2 value 5.9) than that induced by noradrenaline (pA_2 value 6.3) (MARKSTEIN et al., unpublished).

The dopamine-sensitive adenylate cyclase in retinae of different animal species could also be activated by D-LSD at a concentration of 1 µM (SPANO et al., 1975a, b). In the isolated rabbit retina significant increases in cyclic AMP concentration were found after incubation with ergometrine, agroclavine or bromocriptine. The increases in cyclic AMP elicited by the three ergot compounds were detectable at 1 µM and comparable to those seen after dopamine or apomorphine when concentrations of 100 µM were used. Moreover, the responses to the ergot alkaloids could be blocked by the dopamine antagonist fluphenazin, suggesting that the three ergot alkaloids stimulated dopamine receptors in the rabbit retina (SCHORDERET, 1976; SCHORDERET and FRANGAKI, 1976).

5. Effects of Ergot Alkaloids on Dopamine Receptors Mediating Hormone Secretion

There is good evidence that dopamine receptors control prolactin secretion from the pituitary gland. Both dopamine and apomorphine were found to inhibit the release of prolactin from the isolated pituitary, while neuroleptics, such as haloperidol and perphenazine, antagonized responses to both agonists (MACLEOD and LEHMEYER, 1972, 1974). Incubation of pituitary glands from female rats with 0.2 μM α-ergokryptine caused a 50% inhibition of prolactin secretion. Responses to both α-ergokryptine and apomorphine could be blocked by the in vitro presence of 0.1 μM haloperidol or perphenazine (HILL-SAMLI and MACLEOD, 1975; MACLEOD and LEHMEYER, 1974). These results suggest that dopamine inhibits prolactin secretion by stimulating dopamine receptors in the pituitary gland, and that this effect can be mimicked by α-ergokryptine.

D. Actions of Ergot Alkaloids at Adrenoceptors

R. SALZMANN and TH. BUCHER

I. Effects of Ergot Alkaloids Mediated by Peripheral α-Adrenoceptors

It is now clear that ergot alkaloids, by virtue of their own complex chemical structure, which includes the lysergic acid group, interact in a complex manner with drug receptors. In earlier times the pharmacologic effects of ergot alkaloids were attributed to a "direct" action on smooth muscle without reference to receptors; this notion was applied particularly to their stimulant effects, since blocking effects of ergot alkaloids on specific receptor sites, such as adrenergic or 5-HT receptors, had been known for a long time. More recently there has been increasing evidence that some, or perhaps all, of the stimulant effects of ergot alkaloids are also exerted at specific receptor sites on which they may act as partial agonists. Ergot alkaloids may also interfere in other ways with neurotransmission processes either peripheral or central, e.g., by promoting or inhibiting transmitter release or by blocking uptake sites.

a) Ergot Alkaloids as α-Adrenoceptor Blocking Agents

DALE's early work on ergot (DALE, 1906) has been the source of most subsequent developments in receptor pharmacology of both ergot and catecholamines (SCHILD, 1976). In his discussion of adrenaline reversal (SOLLMANN and BROWN, 1905; DALE, 1906), DALE does not use the word *receptor* (although he was aware of LANGLEY's postulated *receptive substances*), referring only to *motor* and *inhibitor myoneural junctions* of the sympathetic.

Nevertheless, his work was the first to show clearly that ergot alkaloids could block adrenergic receptors. He also showed that the block by ergot spared the inhibitory effects of adrenaline on smooth muscle as well as its stimulant effect on the heart, thus anticipating AHLQUIST's (1948) subdivision into α- and β-"adrenotropic" receptors.

A number of investigations dealing with α-adrenoceptor block by ergot alkaloids is summarized in Table 3. Certain important test systems on which the antagonism between catecholamines and ergot alkaloids has been investigated are discussed in more detail below.

Table 3. Alpha-adrenoceptor blocking activity of ergot alkaloids in isolated preparations in vitro and in situ
(Abbreviations for agonists: A = adrenaline, NA = noradrenaline, PH = phenylephrine)

Ergot compounds	Preparation and species	Pharmacologic effect of ergot compounds					References
BOL-148 (2-Bromo-D-LSD)	Brain slices (hypothalamus, brain stem), rat	10^{-5} M. Antagonism of elevation in cAMP due to NA					1
	Isolated ear, rabbit	100 μg/l: Reduction of the effects of A and NA					2
	Heart, rabbit	10^{-6} M. Reduction of positive inotropic effects of NA					1
	Aorta, rabbit	Agonist	$pA_{2(10\,min)}$		$pA_{10(10\,min)}$ normal strips	reserpinized strips	3
		NA	6.4		5.6	5.7	
		PH	–		5.8	–	
		Methoxamine	–		5.7	–	
		Nordefrine	–		5.3	–	
		Ephedrine	–		5.0	5.0	
		d-Amphetamine	–		4.6	4.4	
	Aorta, rat	Agonist	$pA_{2(15\,min)}$ normal	reserpinized	$pA_{10(15\,min)}$ normal	reserpinized	4
		NA	7.8	7.9	6.5	6.5	
		Methoxamine	7.7		6.7		
		Nordefrine	7.8		6.6		
	Mesenteric arteries, dog	1×10^{-7} M to 1×10^{-5} M: Reduction of vasoconstrictor responses to NA					1
	Umbilical artery, man	15 μg/0.3 ml: No alteration of the contractions to tyramine or NA					5
	Uterus (primed by isoprenaline), rat	100 ng/ml: Prevention of motor responses to A, NA and PH					6
Dihydroergocornine	Seminal vesicle, guinea-pig	2 to 60×10^{-5}: Inhibition of A-reaction. Relative effectiveness: Ergotamine = 1, dihydroergocornine = 25					7, 8, 9, 10, 11
	Uterus (isolated), rabbit	2 to 3×10^{-5}: Inhibition of excitatory A-effect. Relative effectiveness: Ergotamine = 1, dihydroergocornine = 2.5					8, 9, 10, 11
	Uterus (in situ), rabbit	Inhibition of A-effect by 0.125–0.15 mg/kg i.v.					8
Dihydroergocristine	Aorta thoracalis, rabbit	ED_{50} (Inhibition of NA-effect): 1.2×10^{-7}					12
	Vena palmaris metacarpalis profunda, bovine	ED_{50} (Inhibition of NA-effect): 8.5×10^{-9}					12
	Seminal vesicle, guinea-pig	2 to 60×10^{-5}: Inhibition of A-reaction. Relative effectiveness: Ergotamine = 1, dihydroergocristine = 35					7, 8, 9, 10, 11

Table 3 (continued)

Ergot compounds	Preparation and species	Pharmacologic effect of ergot compounds	References
	Uterus (isolated) rabbit	2 to 30×10^{-5}: Inhibition of excitatory A-effects. Relative effectiveness: Ergotamine = 1, dihydro-ergocristine = 3.5	8, 9, 10, 11
	Uterus (in situ) rabbit	0.15 mg/kg i.v.: Inhibition of A-effect	8
	Hind limb (innervated, perfused), dog	Inhibition of increase in vascular resistance to NA. Intermediate activity between ergotamine and 1-methyl-ergotamine	13, 14, 15
Dihydro-ergo-kryptine	Seminal vesicle, guinea-pig	2 to 60×10^{-5}: Inhibition of A-effect. Relative effectiveness: Ergotamine = 1, dihydro-ergokryptine = 35. Inhibition of A-effect by dihydro-α-ergokryptine and dihydro-β-ergokryptine (0.5–5 μg/l). Relative activity: Dihydro-α-ergokryptine 100%, dihydro-β-ergokryptine 130%	7, 8, 9, 10, 11, 16
	Uterus (isolated) rabbit	2 to 30×10^{-5}: Inhibition of excitatory A-effect. Relative effectiveness: Ergotamine = 1, dihydro-ergokryptine = 5	8, 9, 10, 11
	Uterus (in situ) rabbit	Inhibition of A-effect. 0.15–0.2 mg/kg i.v.	8
Dihydro-ergosine	Seminal vesicle, guinea-pig	Inhibition of A-effect. Relative effectiveness: Ergotamine = 1, dihydroergosine = 6	8, 9
	Uterus (isolated), rabbit	Inhibition of excitatory A-effect. Relative effectiveness: Ergotamine = 1, dihydroergosine = 2	8, 9
	Uterus (in situ), rabbit	Inhibition of A-effect. 0.15–0.2 mg/kg i.v.	8
Dihydro-ergostine	Hind limb (innervated, perfused), dog	Inhibition of increase in vascular resistance to NA. Intermediate activity between that of ergotamine and 1-methylergotamine	13, 14, 15
Dihydro-ergot-amine (DHE-45, Dihyder-got)	Superior cervical ganglion, rabbit	10^{-5} M. Inhibition of depressant action of A	17
	Isolated perfused ear, rabbit	20 μg/l: Greatly diminished response to A	18
	Papillary muscle, cat	3.7–7.4×10^{-5} M. Competitive antagonism against A and NA	19
	Blood vessels		
	a) Arteries		
	Aorta, rabbit	Inhibition of A and NA. Apparent K_I in Mols/Liter: 2×10^{-8} (30 min), 10^{-8} (60 min), 5×10^{-9} (240 min)	20
	Auricular artery, rabbit	pA_2 against NA: 8.0	21
	Saphenous arteries, dog	$pA_{2(15\,min)}$ against NA: 8.4	22
	Umbilical artery, man	9.2 to 23.1 μg/0.3 ml. Total block of constrictor and dilator responses to A and NA	23
		23 μg/0.3 ml. Abolition of contractions to tyramine and NA	5

Table 3 (continued)

Ergot compounds	Preparation and species	Pharmacologic effect of ergot compounds	References
Dihydro-ergot-amine (con-tinued)	*b) Veins*		
	Femoral veins, dog	$pA_{10(15\,min)}$ against NA: 8.4	24, 25
	Saphenous veins, man (normal, varicous), dog	$pA_{10(15\,min)}$ against NA: 5.6 (man), 7.2 (dog)	24, 25
	Intestinal tract		
	Intestinum, dog	0.1–1 mg/kg i.v.: Reduction of inhibitory response to PH	26
	Jejunum, rabbit	5–200 µg/50 ml: Order of decreasing susceptibility to blockade by DHE was methoxamine $\sim$PH > A > NA > isoproterenol	27
	Ileum, cat	2 mg/kg i.v.: Antagonism of the inhibitory effects of A and NA	28
	rabbit	Stronger inhibition of the A-effect than ergotamine	29
	Taenia caecum, guinea-pig	10 µg/ml: Abolition of relaxation to NA	30
	Genital organs		
	Seminal vesicle, guinea-pig	2 to 60×10^{-5}: Inhibition of A-effect. Relative effectiveness: Ergotamine = 1, dihydroergotamine = 7	7, 8, 9, 10, 11
		Inhibition of A-effect. ED_{50}: 2 ng/ml	31
	Vas deferens, guinea-pig	$pA_{2(30\,min)}$ against NA: 8.3	32
	Retractor penis, dog	0.5 mg/kg i.v.: Reduction of the contraction to A and PH	26
	Uterus, dog	Blockade of A-stimulation and reversal to inhibition	33
	guinea-pig	Blockade of A-stimulation	33
	rabbit	2 to 30×10^{-5}. Blockade of A-stimulation. Relative effectiveness: Ergotamine = 1, dihydroergotamine = 2.25	8, 9, 10, 11, 33,
		2×10^{-5}. Antagonism of A-contraction	34
		0.02–0.05 mg/kg i.v.: Inhibition of A-effect	8
	rat	0.01–20 ng/l: Reduction of inhibitory effect to A	35
		10 µg/ml: Prevention of inhibitory responses to A and PH	36
		Blockade of A-inhibition	37,38
		100 ng/ml: Inhibition of the motor responses to A, NA and PH (in two of five instances)	6
	man	Blockade of stimulation, occasional reversal to inhibition	39
		1:3 Mill. to 1:80 Mill.: Inhibition of the excitatory effect of A and NA	40
	Other preparations		
	Hind limb (inner-vated, perfused), dog	Inhibition of increase in vascular resistance to NA. 5 times less active than ergotamine (for a 40% NA-inhibition). Intermediate activity between ergot-amine and 1-methylergotamine	13, 14, 15, 41

Table 3 (continued)

Ergot compounds	Preparation and species	Pharmacologic effect of ergot compounds	References
	Melanophores, lizard (Anolis carolinensis)	Only partial inhibition of MSH-reaction. Dihydroergotamine inhibits α-adrenergic receptor activity of concentrations which do not antagonize MSH-darkening	42
Dihydroergotoxine mesylate (Hydergine)	Seminal vesicle, guinea-pig	ED_{50} (inhibition of A): 0.66 ng/ml	31
	Uterus (in situ), rabbit	1 mg/kg i.v.: Antagonism against A, NA and ergometrine	43
	rat	200 ng/ml: Inhibition of motor effect of A, NA and PH	6
	man	1:3 Mill. to 1:80 Mill.: Inhibition of excitatory effect of A and NA	40
	Jejunum, man	Block of PH-effect; response to isoprenaline only reduced	44
	Taenia coli, man	5 μg/ml: Abolition of NA relaxation 1 μg/ml: Complete block of A-relaxation	45
Ergocornine	Seminal vesicle, guinea-pig	2 to 60×10^{-5}. Inhibition of A-effect. Relative effectiveness: Ergotamine = 1, ergocornine = 2	7, 8, 9, 10, 11,
	Uterus (isolated), rabbit	2 to 30×10^{-5}. Inhibition of A-effect. Relative effectiveness: Ergotamine = 1, ergocornine = 0.5	10, 11
	Uterus (in situ), rabbit	0.025–0.2 mg/kg i.v.: Inhibition of A-effect	8
Ergocristine	Seminal vesicle, guinea-pig	2 to 60×10^{-5}. Inhibition of A-effect. Relative effectiveness: Ergotamine = 1, ergocristine = 4	7, 8, 9, 10, 11
	Uterus (isolated), rabbit	2 to 30×10^{-5}. Inhibition of A-effect. Relative effectiveness: Ergotamine = 1, ergocristine = 1	8, 9, 10, 11
	Uterus (in situ), rabbit	0.1–0.2 mg/kg i.v.: Inhibition of A-effect	8
Ergokryptine	Seminal vesicle, guinea-pig	2 to 60×10^{-5}. Inhibition of A-effect. Relative effectiveness: Ergotamine = 1, ergokryptine = 4 Inhibition of A-effect by α-ergokryptine and β-ergokryptine (1–10 μg/l). Relative activity: α 100%, β 160%	7, 8, 9, 10, 11, 16
	Uterus (isolated), rabbit	2 to 30×10^{-5}. Inhibition of A-effect. Relative effectiveness: Ergotamine = 1, ergokryptine = 1.5	8, 9, 10, 11
	Uterus (in situ), rabbit	0.15–0.2 mg/kg i.v.: Inhibition of A-effect	8
Ergometrine (Ergotocine, Ergobasine)	Ear, rabbit	100 to 1000 μg/l: No definite effect on A and NA. 100 μg/l: No significant effect on the response to A	2 18
	Ventricle, rat	5×10^{-7} and 2×10^{-6} g/ml: Significant reduction of positive inotropic action of tyramine	46
	Ventricle (electrically stimulated), rat	5×10^{-7} g/ml: Potentiation of A 2×10^{-6} g/ml: No significant change of NA	47
	Uterus, rabbit	1:500,000: No inhibition of A-reaction	48

Table 3 (continued)

Ergot compounds	Preparation and species	Pharmacologic effect of ergot compounds	References
Ergosine	Seminal vesicle, guinea-pig	Inhibition of A-effect. Relative effectiveness: Ergotamine = 1, ergosine = 1	8, 9
	Uterus (isolated), rabbit	Inhibition of A-effect. Relative effectiveness: Ergotamine = 1, ergosine = 1	8, 9
	Uterus (in situ), rabbit	0.15–0.2 mg/kg i.v.: Inhibition of A-effect	8
Ergo-stetrine	Uterus (isolated), rabbit	0.2 to 0.4 mg/50 ml: Inhibition of A to only a relatively slight degree	49
Ergostine	Hind limb, dog	Inhibition of increase in vascular resistance to NA	13, 14, 15
	Seminal vesicle, guinea-pig	Approximately three times more active in inhibiting the A-effect than ergotamine	50
Ergot-amine (Gy-nergene)	Dilator iridis, rabbit	$1:10^5$ to $1:8 \times 10^5$: Antagonism against A (reversal of A-effect)	51
	Isolated perfused ear, rabbit	Suppression or reversal of A-constriction M/10 Mill.: Inhibition of A-effect 40 µg/l: Abolition of A-effect	52 53 18
	Nictitating membrane, cat, dog	Fairly regular inversion of A-effect after high doses	54, 55, 56
	Circulatory system		
	Ventricle, rat	1.5×10^{-6} g/ml: Significant reduction of positive inotropic action of tyramine	46
	Papillary muscle, cat	10^{-6} M: Total abolition of the contractile force of methoxamine. Reduction by at least half the contractile force of PH	57
	Blood vessels		
	a) Arteries		
	Basilar artery, dog, man	No change of response to NA	58
	External carotid artery, dog	No inhibition of NA-reaction. Dose response curves for NA were shifted to the left	59
	Arteria coronaris cordis, bovine	Inhibition of dilating action of A	52
	Mesenteric artery, bovine	Inhibition of A-contraction	52
	Saphenous artery, dog	$pA_{2(60\,\text{min})}$ against NA: 8.7	59
	b) Veins		
	Lateral saphenous vein, dog	pA_2 against A and NA: 8.2	60

Table 3 (continued)

Ergot compounds	Preparation and species	Pharmacologic effect of ergot compounds	Ref-er-ences
Ergot-amine (con-tinued)	Femoral vein, dog	pA_2 against NA (competitive antagonism): 9.0	61
		pD'_2 against NA (non-competitive antagonism): 7.6	
		$pA_{2(15\,min)}$ against NA: 8.8	62
	Pulmonary vessels, cat	$>10^{-5}$. Reversal of the action of A and NA	63
	Intestinal tract		
	Stomach, guinea-pig	Preparations with previously increased tone: $2\times10^{-8}-2\times10^{-6}$ M: Enhancement of the inhibitory action of PH 5×10^{-6} M: Antagonism of the effects produced by A, NA and PH Preparations with low (spontaneous) tone: $pA_{2(20\,min)}$ against PH: 8.0. pA_2 against A, NA were not determined because responses were too small and variable that quantitative evaluation was not feasible	64
	Jejunum, rabbit	Weaker inhibition of the A-effect than DHE	29
	Genital organs		
	Vas deferens, guinea-pig	1 mg/200 ml: Inhibition or slight inversion of A-contraction	65
	Seminal vesicle, guinea-pig	2 to 60×10^{-5}. Inhibition of A-contraction	7, 8, 9, 10, 11, 52
		A-inhibitory action approx. 50 times stronger than that of LSD	66
		Approximately three times less active in inhibiting the A-effect than ergostine	50
		$pA_{2(20\,min)}$ against A, NA and PH: 8.1	67
		ED_{50} (inhibition of A-effect): 14 ng/ml	31
	Uterus, guinea-pig	Blockade of A-stimulation and reversal to inhibition. No effect on A-inhibition	68
		Inhibition of A-decrease of tone	52
	rabbit	Inversion or inhibition of A-contraction	52
		1:2 Mill. to 1:4 Mill. Diminution, removal or reversal of the contracting A-reactions	69
		Inhibition of excitatory A-reaction	8, 10, 11
	rat	No effect on A-inhibition	68
	Other preparations		
	Hind limb, dog	Dose-dependent inhibition of the increase in vascular resistance to NA	13,14, 15, 41
	Extremity, frog	Suppression or reversal of A-constriction	52
	Melanophores, lizard (Anolis carolinensis)	10^{-5} M. Prevention from catecholamine (A, NA) lightening of MSH-darkened skins. Increased darkening of skins in response to catecholamines after the skins have been treated with ergotamine	70, 71, 72
	Spleen, cat	ED_{50} (Inhibition of A-effect): 0.02 µg/ml	73
Ergot-aminine	Nictitating membrane, cat	No action on A-contraction after high concentrations	55

Table 3 (continued)

Ergot compounds	Preparation and species	Pharmacologic effect of ergot compounds	References
Ergotoxine	Isolated, perfused ear, rabbit	0.02 μg/ml: Same constriction with a dose of A 10 times greater than initial test dose	53
	Nictitating membrane, cat	Up to 9 mg/kg: Relaxation of A-contraction	74
		Relaxation of A- and NA-contraction	75
		Relaxation after A and NA in the ergotoxine-treated animal	56
	Seminal vesicle, guinea-pig	1 in 4×10^6: Reduction of A-contraction by 75%	76
		1 in 1.5×10^6: Almost complete annulment of the A-action	
	Bladder, rabbit	Abolition of A-excitation. No change of A-inhibition	77
	Uterus, rabbit	Inhibition or abolition of stimulative activity of A and ergostetrine	49
		1:10 Mill.: Inhibition of A-reaction	48
	Spleen, dog, rabbit, cat, buffalo, man	1:100,000: Abolition of A-effect on dog's, rabbit's, cat's or buffalo's splenic capsule	
		1:25,000: Abolition of A-effect in human splenic capsule	78
		0.25–2 μg/50 ml: Inhibition of A-reaction	79
	Hind limb, cat	0.5 mg: Reversal of A-effect	76
D-LSD	Brain slices (hypothalamus, brain stem), rat	10^{-5} M: Antagonism against NA-induced elevation in cyclic AMP	1
	Isolated, perfused ear, rabbit	100 μg/l: Increase of A- and NA effects	2
	Heart, rabbit	10^{-6} M. Reduction of positive inotropic effects of NA	1
	Pulmonary vessels, cat	Little effect on the actions of A and NA	63
	Mesenteric arteries, dog	10^{-6} M. Diminution of NA effect by 25%	1
	Seminal vesicle, guinea-pig	Approximately 50 times weaker than ergotamine (inhibition of A-effect)	66
	Uterus, rat	0.01–20 ng/l: Reduction of inhibitory A-effect	35
	Trachea, guinea-pig, rat	0.3 μg/ml: No NA-antagonism	80
	Hind leg, cat, dog	10^{-6}: Only slight diminution of A-effect	63
1-Methyl-dihydro-ergocristine	Hind limb, dog	Only weak inhibition of increase in vascular resistance to NA	13, 14, 15
5′-Methyl-ergoalanine	Hind limb, dog	Strong α-adrenergic blocking activity of increase in vascular resistance to NA	13, 14, 15
1-Methyl-ergostine	Hind limb, dog	Only weak inhibition of increase in vascular resistance to NA	13, 14, 15

Table 3 (continued)

Ergot compounds	Preparation and species	Pharmacologic effect of ergot compounds	References
1-Methyl-ergotamine	Seminal vesicle, guinea-pig	ED_{50} (Inhibition of A-reaction): 19.6 ng/ml	31
	Hind limb, dog	Only weak inhibition of increase in vascular resistance to NA	13, 14, 15, 41
Methysergide (Deseril)	Isolated organs (general)	No adrenolytic effect in contrast to the ergot alkaloids of the peptid group	81
	Aorta, rabbit	pA_2 against NA: 5.3	82
	Saphenous arteries, dog	$pA_{2(15\,min)}$ against NA: 5.5	22
	Vas deferens, rat	$pA_{2(5\,min)}$ against NA: 5.8	83
	Colon, rat	1 µg/ml: No significant alteration of contractile responses to A	84
		300 ng/ml: Contractions induced by A were reduced by 49% (10 ng), 34% (30 ng) and 22% (100 ng) 500, 1000 ng/ml: merely reduced contractile responses to A ('non-specific antagonism against A')	85
	Stomach, guinea-pig	Up to 10^{-6} M. No antagonistic action against A, NA, PH	64
	rat	No effect on contractions to A, NA and PH	86
Nicergoline (MNE, Sermion)	Ileum, guinea-pig	Reduction of A $ED_{50}=0.007$ µg/ml	87
Sensibamine	Uterus (gravid), rabbit	1:2 to 1:4 Mill.: Diminution, removal or reversal of the contracting A-reaction	69
10-Methoxy-ergoline derivatives	Seminal vesicle, guinea-pig	Among the pyridyl carboxylic esters of 1-methyl-10α-methoxydihydrolysergol, the nicotinates, and notably those having an electron-withdrawing group in position 5, are characterized by a strong alpha adrenergic blocking activity (against adrenaline). Relative activity 120 to 7800, ergotamine = 100 For further detail see original paper	88
6-Methyl-8β-aminomethyl-10α-ergoline (Dihydrolysergamine)	Seminal vesicle, guinea-pig	Structure-activity relationship of carboxylic and carbonic acid derivatives of dihydrolysergamine with regard to α-adrenoceptor-blockade, oxytocic and anti-5-HT-activity is described For details see original paper	89

References: 1. PALMER and BURKS (1971); 2. SAVINI (1956); 3. KOHLI (1968); 4. KRISHNAMURTY (1971); 5. GULATI and KELKAR (1971); 6. TOTHILL (1967); 7. BRÜGGER (1945); 8. ROTHLIN (1946/1947); 9. ROTHLIN and CERLETTI (1949); 10. ROTHLIN and BRÜGGER (1945a); 11. ROTHLIN and BRÜGGER (1945b); 12. FLÜCKIGER and BALTHASAR (1967); 13. AELLIG and

Table 4. Relative values of the adrenaline-antagonistic action of natural and dihydrogenated ergot alkaloids on isolated organs. [From Table 3, ROTHLIN, E.: Bull. Schweiz. Akad. Med. Wissensch. **2**, 262 (1946/47)]

Isolated uterus of rabbit				Isolated seminal vesicle of guinea-pig			
Natural		Hydrogenated		Natural		Hydrogenated	
Ergocornine	0.5	Dihydroergosine	2.0	*Ergotamine*	1	Dihydroergosine	6
Ergotamine	1.0	Dihydroergotamine	2.25	Ergosine	1	Dihydroergotamine	7
Ergosine	1.0	Dihydroergocornine	2.5	Ergocornine	2	Dihydroergocornine	25
Ergocristine	1.0	Dihydroergocristine	3.5	Ergocristine	4	Dihydroergocristine	35
Ergokryptine	1.5	Dihydroergokryptine	5.0	Ergokryptine	4	Dihydroergokryptine	35

Adrenaline-induced contraction of isolated guinea-pig seminal vesicle. In this preparation (BRÜGGER, 1945) ergot alkaloids antagonize adrenaline-induced contractions without exerting a contractile effect of their own. Adrenaline produces a slow rise in tone of the isolated preparation followed by a series of intermittent contractions. The objective of this procedure is to find the dose of ergot which after 20 min incubation reduces adrenaline responses by 50%. The block by ergot alkaloids is reversible so that two alkaloids may be compared in the same preparation by a cross-over procedure. The relative activities of two ergot alkaloids as α-blockers may be compared quantitatively by this method; the data in Table 4 represent average activity ratios, relative to ergotamine, obtained from about 100 determinations each. The dihydrogenated ergot alkaloids were consistently more active by this test than the corresponding natural alkaloids; among the latter ergocristine and ergokryptine were most active.

BERDE (1969); 14. BERDE (1971); 15. BERDE (1972); 16. SCHLIENTZ et al. (1968); 17. CHRIST and NISHI (1971); 18. GADDUM and HAMEED (1954); 19. KIMURA et al. (1970); 20. FURCHGOTT (1955); 21. FOZARD (1973b); 22. MÜLLER-SCHWEINITZER (1975a); 23. GOKHALE et al. (1966); 24. MÜLLER-SCHWEINITZER (1973); 25. MÜLLER-SCHWEINITZER (1974c); 26. LEVY and AHLQUIST (1961); 27. LUM et al. (1966); 28. TÜRKER et al. (1965); 29. ROTHLIN (1946); 30. ÅBERG et al. (1969); 31. PACHA and SALZMANN (1970); 32. BIRMINGHAM and SZOLCSÁNYI (1965); 33. GREEFF and HOLTZ (1951); 34. SCHILD (1960); 35. HOLZBAUER and VOGT (1955); 36. LEVY and TOZZI (1963); 37. WIQVIST (1959); 38. RUDZIK and MILLER (1962); 39. GARRETT (1955); 40. ROTHLIN and BERDE (1954); 41. AELLIG (1967); 42. GOLDMAN and HADLEY (1972); 43. FREGNAN and GLÄSSER (1964); 44. WHITNEY (1965); 45. BUCKNELL and WHITNEY (1964); 46. WENZEL and SU (1966a); 47. WENZEL and SU (1966b); 48. DAVIS et al. (1935); 49. THOMPSON (1935); 50. CERLETTI (1963); 51. SACHS and YONKMAN (1942); 52. ROTHLIN (1925); 53. FLECKENSTEIN (1952); 54. BACQ (1934a); 55. BACQ (1934b); 56. SMITH (1963); 57. PARMLEY et al. (1974); 58. MÜLLER-SCHWEINITZER (1976c); 59. MÜLLER-SCHWEINITZER and STÜRMER (1975); 60. GUIMARÃES and OSSWALD (1969); 61. MÜLLER-SCHWEINITZER and STÜRMER (1972); 62. MÜLLER-SCHWEINITZER and STÜRMER (1974a); 63. GINZEL and KOTTEGODA (1953); 64. GUIMARÃES (1969b); 65. BACQ (1934c); 66. ROTHLIN (1957c); 67. GUIMARÃES (1969a); 68. MENDEZ (1928); 69. RÖSSLER and UNNA (1935); 70. GOLDMAN and HADLEY (1969); 71. GOLDMAN and HADLEY (1970a); 72. GOLDMAN and HADLEY (1970b); 73. BICKERTON et al. (1962); 74. ROSENBLUETH (1932); 75. ACHESON (1940); 76. BROWN and DALE (1935); 77. STREULI (1916); 78. SAAD (1935); 79. GYÖRGY et al. (1958b); 80. FLEISCH et al. (1970); 81. FANCHAMPS et al. (1960); 82. APPERLEY et al. (1974); 83. GÖRLITZ and FREY (1973); 84. BELISLE and GAGNON (1971); 85. GAGNON (1972); 86. OGLE and WONG (1971); 87. ARCARI et al. (1968); 88. ARCARI et al. (1972); 89. FREGNAN and GLÄSSER (1968).

Instead of guinea-pig seminal vesicle, the rat's seminal vesicle may be used (LEITCH et al., 1954).

Adrenaline contraction of isolated rabbit uterus. BROOM and CLARK (1923) introduced a method in which the abolition of the motor action of adrenaline on the rabbit uterus provides a basis for the standardization of ergot. The BROOM-CLARK method is of historical interest, having been the starting point for studies of the antagonism between adrenaline and ergotamine from which some of the early ideas of receptor theory arose (GADDUM, 1926; CLARK's Appendix to MENDEZ, 1928), but it has serious disadvantages as a test method: An unsharp endpoint (complete abolition of the adrenaline response); insufficiently long contact with ergot (5 min followed by washout before adding adrenaline); a frequent stimulant effect of ergot on rabbit uterus; and a frequent relaxant effect of adrenaline preceding its contractile action. ROTHLIN and BRÜGGER (1945a, b) modified the method, obtaining the results of Table 4, which again show greater blocking activity of dihydrogenated compared to natural alkaloids, although the discrepancy is less than in seminal vesicles.

GADDUM (1926) employed the isolated rabbit uterus for a graded response assay. He proved that plotting the adrenaline response on a logarithmic scale in the absence and presence of ergotamine results in two parallel lines (Fig. 17). This was an early demonstration of competitive drug antagonism (although GADDUM did not interpret it thus). The degree of displacement of the parallel lines can be considered as measuring the affinity of ergotamine for catecholamine receptors; the displacement would no doubt have been greater if more than 5 min had been allowed for equilibration with ergotamine.

Adrenaline inhibition of rabbit intestine. It has been shown repeatedly that ergotamine antagonizes the inhibitory effect of adrenaline on the isolated rabbit intestine (NANDA, 1931). Pendulum movements are particularly affected. Hydrated ergot alkaloids are also effective (Fig. 18).

The antagonism by ergot alkaloids is specific for catecholamines; papaverine relaxation of the intestine is not antagonized (ROTHLIN et al., 1954).

This effect of ergot alkaloids seems to contradict DALE's view that only the stimulant actions of adrenaline are antagonized, but it fits readily into the wider hypothesis that ergot alkaloids block α-adrenoceptors, since there is evidence from various species that both α- and β-adrenoceptors contribute to intestinal relaxation (AHLQUIST and LEVY, 1959; FURCHGOTT, 1960). JENKINSON and MORTON (1967a, b, c) analyzed the dual mechanism of catecholamines in producing relaxation in the isolated guinea-pig tenia coli. They showed that two mechanisms are involved: (1) An α-adrenoceptor-mediated ionic mechanism causing increased potassium permeability and hyperpolarization which is antagonized by typical α-adrenoceptor blocking agents such as phentolamine; (2) A β-adrenergic mechanism which can function in the absence of a polarized cell membrane, bringing about relaxation by catecholamines in completely depolarized intestinal muscle (EVANS et al., 1958). This mechanism is antagonized by β-adrenoceptor blocking agents.

Noradrenaline contraction of isolated veins. MÜLLER-SCHWEINITZER (1974c) studied the effect of dihydroergotamine (DHE) on the noradrenaline-induced contraction of isolated veins, recording isometric tension in spiral strips of dog saphenous and femoral veins and human varicose veins. Cumulative log dose-response

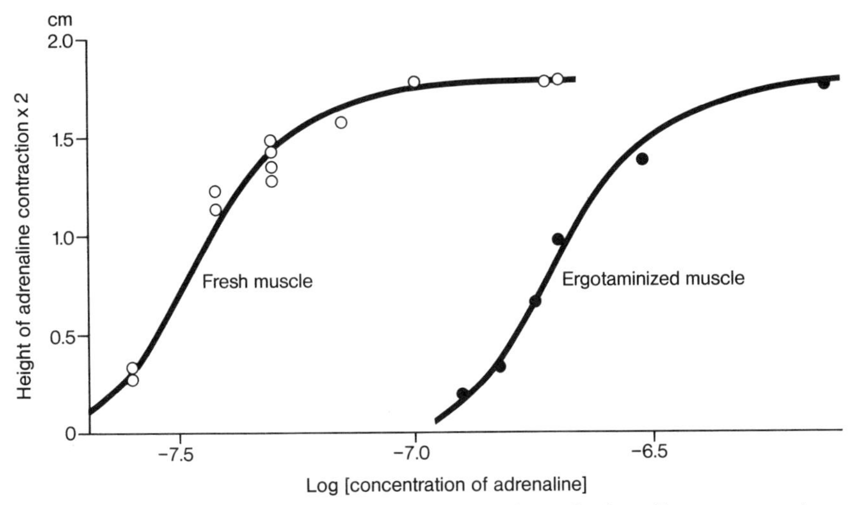

Fig. 17. Contraction of isolated rabbit uterus. Antagonism of adrenaline responses by ergotamine. [From Figure 4, GADDUM, J.H.: J. Physiol. (Lond.) **61**, 144 (1926)]

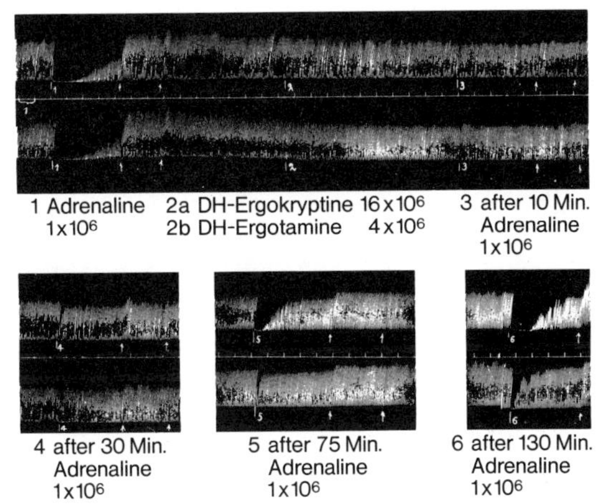

Fig. 18. Record of the isolated small intestine of the rabbit. Inhibition of adrenaline by dihydroergokryptine and dihydroergotamine. [From Figure 10, ROTHLIN, E.: Bull. Schweiz. Akad. Med. Wissensch. **2**, 266 (1946/47)]

curves of noradrenaline exhibited a parallel shift in the presence of dihydroergotamine in all three vein preparations. As shown in Figures 19, 20 and 21, their displacement corresponded approximately to that expected in a simple competitive antagonism (Fig. 22).

Contrary to a simple competitive relationship, however, dihydroergotamine also produced a slight rise in baseline, due to a partial agonist effect, and, with higher concentrations, some reduction of maximum responses. These results are summarized in Table 5, which shows: (1) the $pA_2 - pA_{10}$ differences for dihydroergotamine approximate to the theoretical value of 0.95 expected for competitive

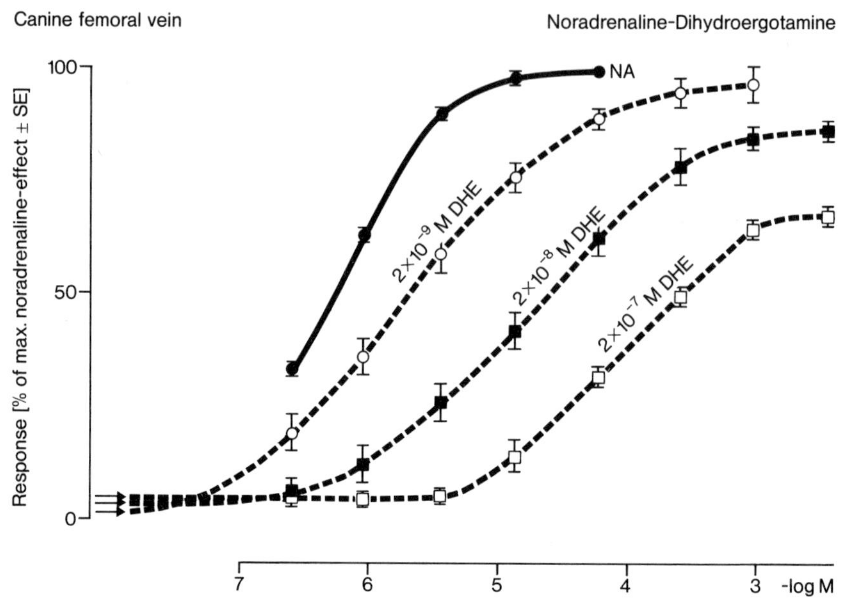

Fig. 19. Cumulative concentration-response curves for noradrenaline without (●) and 15 min after dihydroergotamine in the final concentrations of 2×10^{-9} (○), 2×10^{-8} (■) and 2×10^{-7} M (□) on spiral strips from canine femoral veins. [From Figure 1, MÜLLER-SCHWEINITZER, E.: Europ. J. Pharmacol. **27**, 232 (1974)]

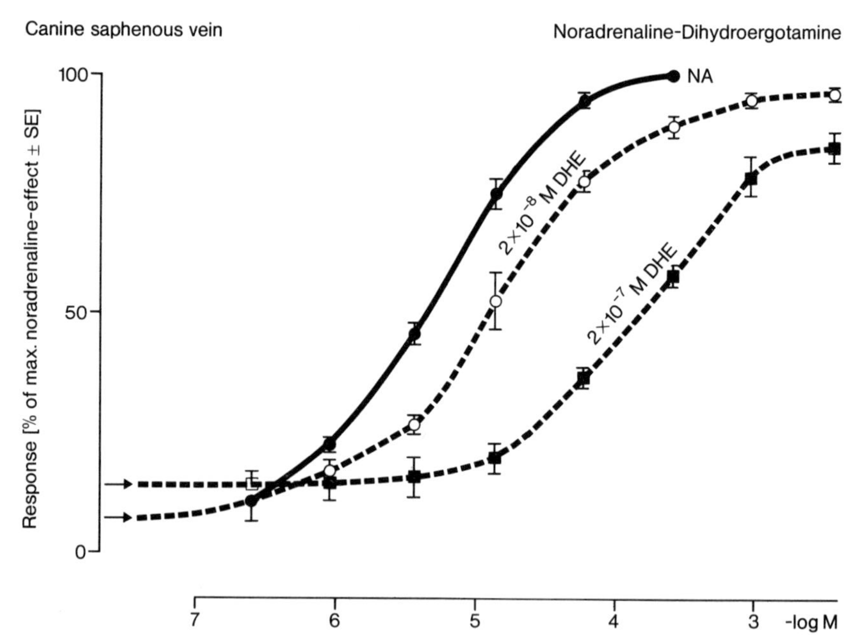

Fig. 20. Cumulative concentration-response curves for noradrenaline without (●) and 15 min after dihydroergotamine in the final concentrations of 2×10^{-8} (○) and 2×10^{-7} M (■) on spiral strips from canine saphenous veins. [From Figure 2, MÜLLER-SCHWEINITZER, E.: Europ. J. Pharmacol. **27**, 232 (1974)]

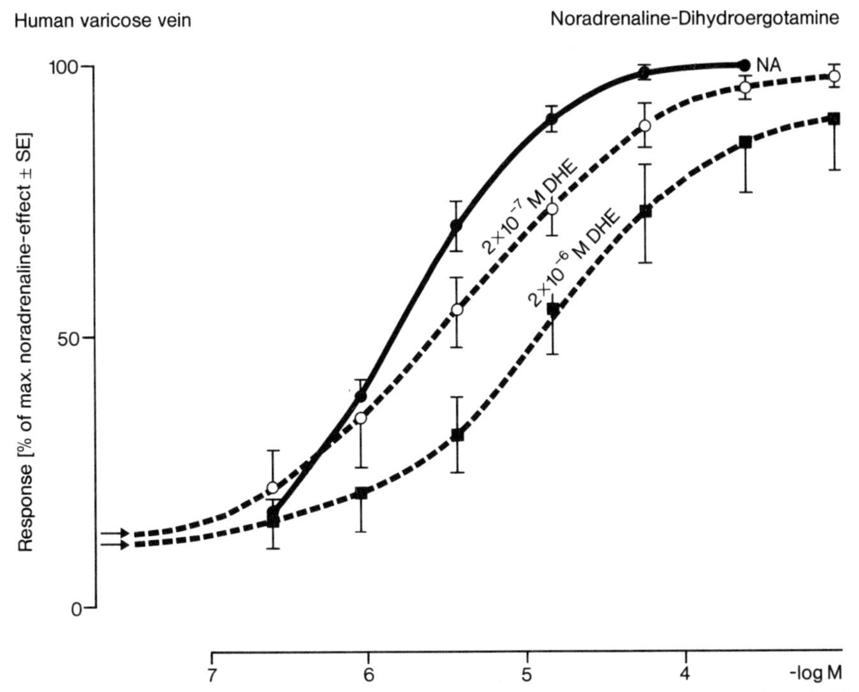

Fig. 21. Cumulative concentration-response curves for noradrenaline without (●) and 15 min after dihydroergotamine in the final concentrations of 2×10^{-7} (○) and 2×10^{-6} M (■) on spiral strips from human varicose veins. [From Figure 3, MÜLLER-SCHWEINITZER, E.: Europ. J. Pharmacol. **27**, 233 (1974)]

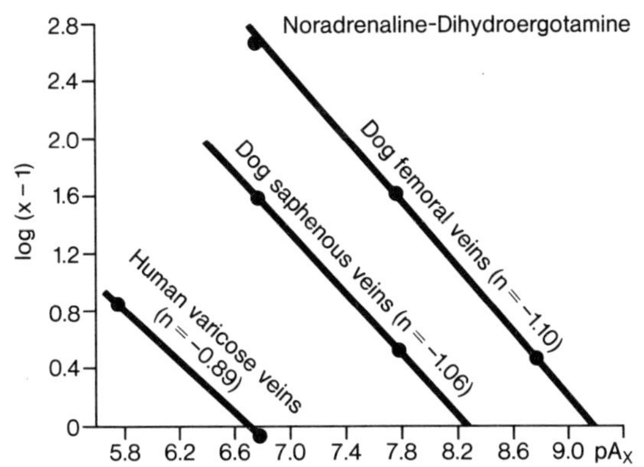

Fig. 22. Plots of the data from Figures 19, 20 and 21 according to ARUNLAKSHANA and SCHILD (1959). The slopes are slightly atypical in terms of a simple competitive antagonism. [From Figure 4, MÜLLER-SCHWEINITZER, E.: Europ. J. Pharmacol. **27**, 233 (1974)]

antagonism; (2) Intrinsic (stimulant) activity or efficacy of dihydroergotamine in terms of the noradrenaline maximum is relatively low; (3) The receptor affinities of dihydroergotamine as expressed by pA_2 values show marked differences in the three vein preparations, although the agonist activities of dihydroergotamine as expressed by pD_2 values appear to be similar. The differences in pA_2 values

Table 5. Antagonist and partial agonist effects of dihydroergotamine on isolated vein strips. [From Table 1, MÜLLER-SCHWEINITZER, E.: Europ. J. Pharmacol. **27**, 234 (1974)]

	pA values against noradrenaline		pD_2 value	Intrinsic activity
	pA_{10}	pA_2		
Human varicose veins	5.6	6.7	7.5	0.3
Dog saphenous veins	7.2	8.0	8.3	0.1
Dog femoral veins	8.4	9.2	8.0	0.16

Table 6. Antagonism of noradrenaline by various ergot alkaloids. pA_2 values were calculated after an incubation time of 15 min on spiral strips from canine femoral veins (MÜLLER-SCHWEINITZER, unpublished)

Ergot type: "peptide"		"amide"	
Ergotamine	8.8	Ergometrine	<5.5
1-Methylergotamine	8.3	Methylergometrine	<5.5
α-Ergokryptine	9.0	Methysergide	5.5
Bromocriptine[a]	8.9	BOL-148	7.1
Ergocornine	8.8		
Dihydroergovaline	8.5		
Dihydroergotamine	9.2		
Dihydro-α-ergokryptine	9.1		

[a] 2-bromo-α-ergokryptine, CB-154, Parlodel.

are puzzling, since they seem to indicate differences in α-adrenoceptors in these preparations; they can possibly be explained by technical considerations, e.g., insufficient time for attainment of full equilibrium of receptors with dihydroergotamine.

Table 6 summarizes pA_2 values obtained by MÜLLER-SCHWEINITZER (1975b) on canine femoral veins, with various ergot alkaloids of the "peptide" and "amide" types, using noradrenaline as agonist. The pA_2 values for various peptides are closely similar; the difference between ergotamine and dihydroergotamine is only 0.4 (log units). Among the amide alkaloids tested only BOL-148 (2-bromo-d-lysergic acid diethylamide, 2-bromo-LSD) had appreciable, if relatively low, activity; ergometrine (ergobasine, ergonovine, ergotocine), methylergometrine (d-lysergic acid L-2-butanolamide, Methergine) and methysergide (1-methyl-lysergic acid-L-2-butanolamide, Deseril) showing little or no α-adrenoceptor blocking activity.

Noradrenaline stimulation of cyclic AMP (cAMP) formation in rat brain slices. PALMER and BURKS (1971) have shown that D-LSD (d-lysergic acid diethylamide, Delyside) and BOL-148 antagonize the stimulant effect of noradrenaline on cAMP formation in rat brain stem and hypothalamus. MARKSTEIN and WAGNER (1975) have shown that dihydroergotoxine mesylate (Hydergine) antagonizes the stimulant effect of noradrenaline in rat brain cortex. Figure 23 shows recent results obtained by these authors in rat brain cortex slices. Dihydroergotoxine mesylate antagonizes

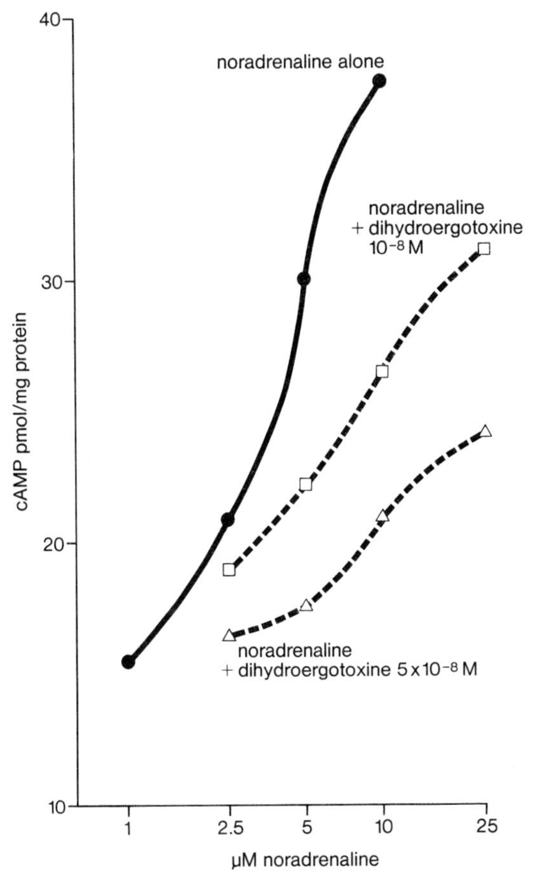

Fig. 23. Cyclic AMP (cAMP) production in rat cerebral cortex slices. Tissue incubated in Ringer (45 min, 37° C) followed by dihydroergotoxine mesylate (15 min) followed by noradrenaline (8 min). Means of two experiments. cAMP was measured by a protein-binding assay using sepharose-bound cAMP-binding protein. [From Figure 5, MARKSTEIN, R., WAGNER, H.: Gerontology **24** (Suppl. I), 101 (1978)]

the effect of noradrenaline on cAMP formation, shifting the response curve to the right. A clear shift of the noradrenaline curve occurs with low concentrations of dihydroergotoxine mesylate (10^{-8}M), indicating a high affinity for catecholamine receptors in the brain. The shift becomes more pronounced with 5×10^{-8}M. The antagonism is of the "noncompetitive" type with progressive depression of maxima. Their evidence suggested that dihydroergotoxine mesylate blocks exclusively α-adrenoceptors; the α-blocker phentolamine produced similar effects. On the other hand, stimulation of cAMP formation by isoprenaline was not antagonized by dihydroergotoxine mesylate, although it was antagonized by β-adrenoceptor blockers. Figure 24 shows evidence that effective concentrations of dihydroergotoxine mesylate accumulate in rat brain if it is fed orally (3 mg/kg/day) over a period of weeks. It was found from the reduction in the noradrenaline effect that the accumulation of dihydroergotoxine mesylate was only marginal after 1 week but obvious after

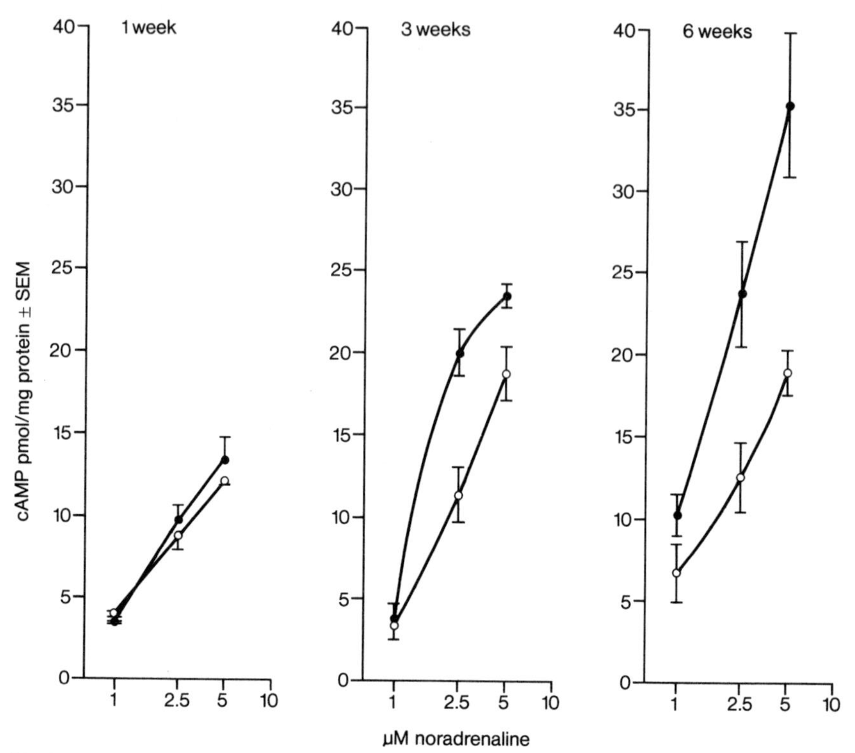

Fig. 24. Accumulation of dihydroergotoxine mesylate in rat brain following oral administration of 3 mg/kg/day for 1, 3 and 6 weeks (○—○). Dihydroergotoxine mesylate content was inferred from inhibition of noradrenaline stimulated cAMP production compared to controls (●—●). Means of four experiments. [From Figure 7, MARKSTEIN, R., WAGNER, H.: Gerontology **24** (Suppl. I), 103 (1978)]

3 and 6 weeks, when the log dose-response curves indicated a concentration of the order of 5×10^{-8}M dihydroergotoxine mesylate present in brain tissue (Fig. 24).

Catecholamine-promoted platelet aggregation. Adrenaline and noradrenaline promote the aggregation of blood platelets in man, rabbit and various other species (MILLS and ROBERTS, 1967; BARTHEL and MARKWARDT, 1974) which effect is antagonized by dihydroergotamine. Both the first and the second phase of aggregation are affected. Similar antagonistic effects are produced by phentolamine, suggesting that α-adrenoceptors are involved. Curiously, dibenamine has been found inactive in blocking adrenaline-promoted platelet aggregation.

b) Ergot Alkaloids as α-Adrenoceptor Stimulating Agents

The mechanism of action of ergot alkaloids in causing smooth muscle contraction is complex and not fully understood; it appears to be different in different types of smooth muscle. As has been mentioned, the older textbook notion (e.g., SOLLMANN, 1948) of a "direct" stimulant effect on smooth muscle has been superseded by the notion that ergot alkaloids activate certain standard drug receptors, such as α-adrenoceptors and receptors for 5-HT and dopamine, the abundance of any particular receptor type varying in different tissues. The section that follows is concerned with evidence of α-adrenoceptor stimulation by ergot alkaloids.

Stimulant effects on α-adrenoceptors. The notion that ergot alkaloids stimulate adrenaline receptors has been around for a long time. BACQ suggested in 1934 that ergotamine augments the tonus of tissues stimulated by adrenaline, observing a close correspondence between the stimulant effects of ergotamine and adrenaline in various tissues (BACQ, 1934a). MALORNY and ORZECHOWSKI (1940) considered that ergotamine and ergometrine had sympathomimetic activity. They suggested that they act on sympathetic receptors, exhibiting stimulation, tachyphylaxis and antagonism. INNES (1962a) carried out receptor protection experiments (FURCHGOTT, 1954) which showed that receptors for ergotamine and ergometrine were "protected" by adrenaline.

Experiments with α-adrenoceptor blockers have demonstrated their antagonism of ergot alkaloids in a variety of preparations. GYÖRGY et al. (1958a) found that dibenamine antagonizes ergotoxine, reducing its pressor effect in the decapitated cat and abolishing its stimulant effect on the nictitating membrane. KONZETT (1960) showed that dibenamine antagonizes ergometrine stimulation of the rabbit uterus in situ. Phenoxybenzamine has been found to antagonize the vasoconstrictor action of ergotamine in the rabbit hindlimb (WEIDMANN and TAESCHLER, 1966) and the action of dihydroergotamine in constricting capacitance vessels in the anesthetized cat (CHU and STÜRMER, 1973; CHU et al., 1976). Phentolamine antagonizes the vasoconstrictor action of dihydroergotamine in human hand veins (AELLIG, 1974) and the effects of ergotamine in decreasing volume and increasing vascular resistance in the perfused cat spleen (SALZMANN et al., 1968).

Although this evidence is suggestive of an action of ergot alkaloids on α-adrenoceptors, it is inconclusive in view of the known unspecific effects of α-blockers, particularly their anti-5-HT-effects. More quantitative evidence is provided by the following experiments.

Dual effect of ergotamine on α-adrenoceptors. MÜLLER-SCHWEINITZER and STÜRMER (1974a, b) have shown that ergotamine acts as both partial agonist and antagonist on α-adrenoceptors in dog femoral and saphenous veins. Their principal findings were as follows: (1) Ergotamine stimulates canine isolated veins, functioning as a slow-acting partial agonist of about one-third the efficacy (intrinsic activity) of noradrenaline (Fig. 4); (2) Phentolamine antagonizes the stimulant effects of both noradrenaline and ergotamine, producing parallel log dose-response curves in both cases. However, whereas the effect of phentolamine on noradrenaline curves was a simple shift to the right, its effect on ergotamine was a shift to the right coupled with a theoretically unexpected progressive increase of the maxima of the curves (Fig. 25). Measurement by the method of ARUNLAKSHANA and SCHILD (1959), based on the degree of parallel shift of the cumulative log dose-response curves, gave the pA_2 values shown in Table 7.

The authors considered that the pA_2 values of phentolamine with noradrenaline and ergotamine as agonists probably indicate that they act on the same receptor, on the theory that agonists acting on the same receptor give similar pA_2 values when tested with the same competitive antagonist (ARUNLAKSHANA and SCHILD, 1959). They considered that irregularities in the ergotamine response may be due

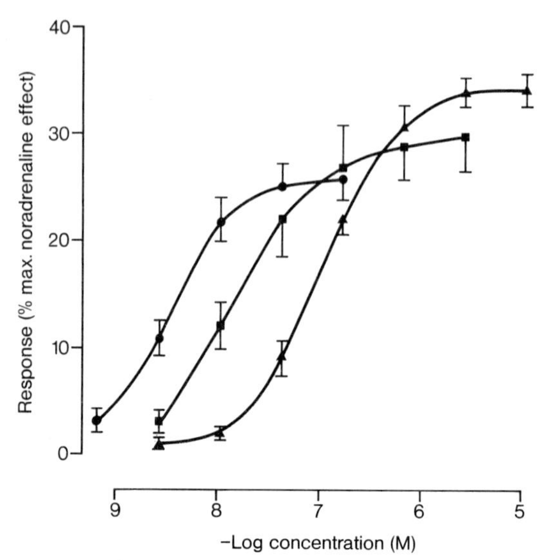

Fig. 25. Cumulative concentration-response curves for ergotamine without (●) and 15 min after phentolamine in the final concentrations of 3.6×10^{-7} (■) and 3.6×10^{-6} M (▲) on spiral strips from canine femoral veins. The bars represent ±SEM. [From Figure 3, MÜLLER-SCHWEINITZER, E., STÜRMER, E.: Brit. J. Pharmacol. **51**, 444 (1974)]

Table 7. Antagonism by phentolamine of responses to ergotamine and noradrenaline of dog saphenous and femoral vein strips. pA_2 values were calculated after an incubation time of 15 min; n refers to slope of ARUNLAKSHANA and SCHILD plot. [From MÜLLER-SCHWEINITZER, E., STÜRMER, E.: Blood Vessels **11**, 183–190 (1974) and Brit. J. Pharmacol. **51**, 441–446 (1974)]

	Ergotamine	Noradrenaline
Saphenous vein	6.9 (n = −0.97)	7.0 (n = −0.83)
Femoral vein	6.8 (n = −0.83)	7.5 (n = −0.95)

to a second action of ergotamine, such as stimulation of 5-HT receptors (cf. Section B, part 1,b), stimulation of prostaglandin synthesis (cf. Section H) as well as the long-lasting and relatively stable drug-receptor bond produced by ergotamine; (3) Ergotamine antagonizes noradrenaline, producing a series of log dose-response curves with progressively increasing base-lines and with parallelism in the upper reaches (Fig. 5), characteristic of the interaction of a partial and full agonist (VAN ROSSUM, 1963). These findings provide evidence that in isolated canine veins ergotamine in low concentrations stimulates α-adrenoceptors while acting as a competitive antagonist of catecholamines in higher concentrations.

Dual effect of ergotamine on melanophores. BACQ (1933) noted that injections of ergotamine in the catfish resulted in melanosome dispersion within innervated melanophores of normal skin but caused melanosome aggregation within denervated melanophores. PARKER (1941) obtained similar results with innervated pigment cells but not on denervated melanophores. GOLDMAN and HADLEY (1970a), working on the noninnervated melanophores of the lizard, found that ergotamine acts both as α-adrenergic agonist and antagonist on the noninnervated melanophores of the lizard: It lightens the skin, which is a characteristic α-adrenergic agonist effect, while subsequently blocking (or reversing) the effects of other α-adrenoceptor stimulants.

2. Depletion of Noradrenaline From Tissues by Ergot Alkaloids

a) Depletion of Noradrenaline From Peripheral Tissues

With but one or two minor exceptions, there is no evidence that ergot alkaloids exert an "indirect" sympathomimetic effect (i.e., release of transmitter substance from sympathetic nerve terminals).

In experiments on the isolated perfused spleen of the cat, no evidence of noradrenaline release into perfusion fluid by ergotamine was seen, in spite of very strong contractions produced by ergotamine (SALZMANN et al., 1967, 1968) (Fig. 26). In the femoral vascular bed of anesthetized dogs, ergotamine caused a marked, long-lasting vasoconstriction when given in μg doses either intravenously or intraarterially, the response being measured as a decrease in femoral artery flow or an increase of the perfusion pressure. This response was antagonized by phentolamine but unaffected by guanethidine or by pretreatment of the animals with reserpine, indicating that ergotamine did not act by releasing noradrenaline (OSSWALD

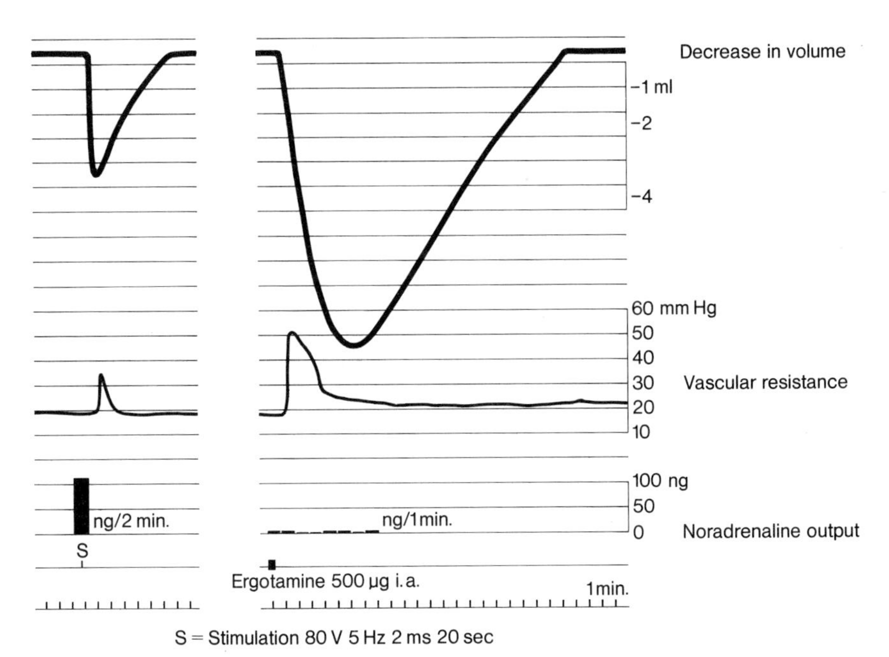

Fig. 26. The effect of ergotamine on the isolated perfused spleen of the cat. Ergotamine, 500 μg i.a., causes strong contraction of the trabecular muscles (volume reduction of the spleen) and vasoconstriction (increase of vascular resistance in the organ). This effect is more pronounced with ergotamine than with supramaximal sympathetic nerve stimulation. In contrast to nerve stimulation, ergotamine causes no noradrenaline release. [From Figure 4, SALZMANN, R. (et al.): Naunyn Schmiedebergs Arch. Pharmacol. **261**, 366 (1968)]

et al., 1970). Likewise, there was no evidence that the vasoconstrictor activity of methysergide in the isolated perfused auricular artery of the rabbit was accompanied by catecholamine release, because here too reserpine pretreatment failed to antagonize the responses (FOZARD, 1973b). In dog saphenous vein strips, 3×10^{-5}M cocaine caused a 6-fold potentiation of the responses to noradrenaline and a ca. 20-fold inhibition of responses to tyramine, whereas dose-response curves for ergotamine were unaffected, thus providing further evidence against noradrenaline release by ergotamine (MÜLLER-SCHWEINITZER, 1974a).

Dihydroergotamine increased plasma concentrations of free fatty acids in normal and adrenalectomized dogs. Pretreatment of dogs with reserpine did not reduce this response to dihydroergotamine (SCRIABINE et al., 1968). Dihydroergotamine had no significant effect on the outflow of [^{3}H]noradrenaline from canine subcutaneous adipose tissue (FREDHOLM and ROSELL, 1970).

There is some indirect evidence that D-LSD can release noradrenaline from sympathetic nerve endings: GILLESPIE and MCGRATH (1974, 1975) showed that contractions of isolated rat anococcygeus muscle and rat vas deferens in response to tyramine, guanethidine and D-LSD were abolished by 6-hydroxydopamine, which destroys sympathetic nerve terminals, while responses to noradrenaline were enhanced. On the other hand, AMBACHE et al. (1975) reported that reserpine pretreatment failed to antagonize D-LSD responses in the rat anococcygeus.

In rabbits some decrease of noradrenaline concentration was found after 150–175 µg/kg i.v. D-LSD in liver, lung, kidney and heart, but not in spleen (SANKAR et al., 1964).

b) Depletion of Noradrenaline From Brain

Effects on the release of central neurotransmitters have been reported for several psychotropic drugs; it is suggested that the release may contribute to the influence of these compounds on behavior. Several authors have described a release of noradrenaline from the brain by D-LSD and related compounds (ANDÉN et al., 1968; FREEDMAN, 1963; LEONARD and LISKA, 1971; SANKAR et al., 1964, 1969; STOLK et al., 1974; SUGRUE, 1969).

Experiments by FREEDMAN (1963) have shown that D-LSD (1.3 mg/kg) decreased noradrenaline concentrations in whole rat brain by about 20%. A fall in noradrenaline concentrations was also observed after 1.6 mg/kg of ALD (1-acetyl-lysergic acid diethylamide). Likewise, noradrenaline levels in rat brains were decreased by 0.2 mg/kg i.p. D-LSD (LEONARD and LISKA, 1971) and 1.3 mg/kg D-LSD (STOLK et al., 1974). After tyrosine hydroxylase inhibition, D-LSD increased the rate of depletion of intraneuronal noradrenaline in the brain of rats (ANDÉN et al., 1968). According to investigations of SUGRUE (1969), administration of 1 mg/kg i.p. D-LSD did not significantly lower the noradrenaline content of the hypothalamus in rats; a significant fall was observed, however, after 2 mg/kg D-LSD. SANKAR et al. (1964) found that D-LSD decreased the noradrenaline concentration in brain tissues of rabbits (cerebrum, cerebellum, stem, rest of brain).

No correlation was demonstrated between the changes in the noradrenaline content of the rat hypothalamus and the alterations in behavior induced by D-LSD (SUGRUE, 1969). According to SUGRUE, excitation induced by D-LSD is not mediated through the release of noradrenaline and may be due to a direct stimulation of central α-adrenoceptors by D-LSD.

No evidence of a noradrenaline depleting action of D-LSD in the central nervous system is provided by findings of NG et al. (1970). D-LSD (10^{-4}M) failed to produce any change in release of [^{3}H]noradrenaline in vitro in rat brain slices. Likewise, BOL-148 was without effect on noradrenaline concentrations in rat brain (FREEDMAN, 1963) and rat hypothalamus (SUGRUE, 1969).

3. Effects of Ergot Alkaloids on Noradrenaline Release and Theories on the Mechanism of Noradrenaline "Overflow"

Many authors have shown that the outflow of neuronally released noradrenaline is increased by α-adrenoceptor blocking agents, including ergot alkaloids.

Spleen. Most investigations of the effect of ergot compounds on the release of noradrenaline from sympathetic nerve terminals were carried out on the cat spleen in situ or the isolated perfused cat spleen. The early observation by BROWN and GILLESPIE (1957) that phenoxybenzamine elevated the output of transmitter was extended to dihydroergotoxine mesylate and other α-blocking agents by BROWN et al. (1961). An increased noradrenaline content in the cat spleen perfusate after nerve stimulation was also described for ergotamine (BERDE, 1971, 1972; PACHA and SALZMANN, 1970; SALZMANN et al., 1967, 1968; SALZMANN and PACHA, 1968, 1976) (Fig. 27), dihydroergotamine (BERDE, 1971, 1972; PACHA and SALZMANN, 1970; SALZMANN and PACHA, 1968, 1976), 1-methyl-ergotamine (BERDE, 1971, 1972;

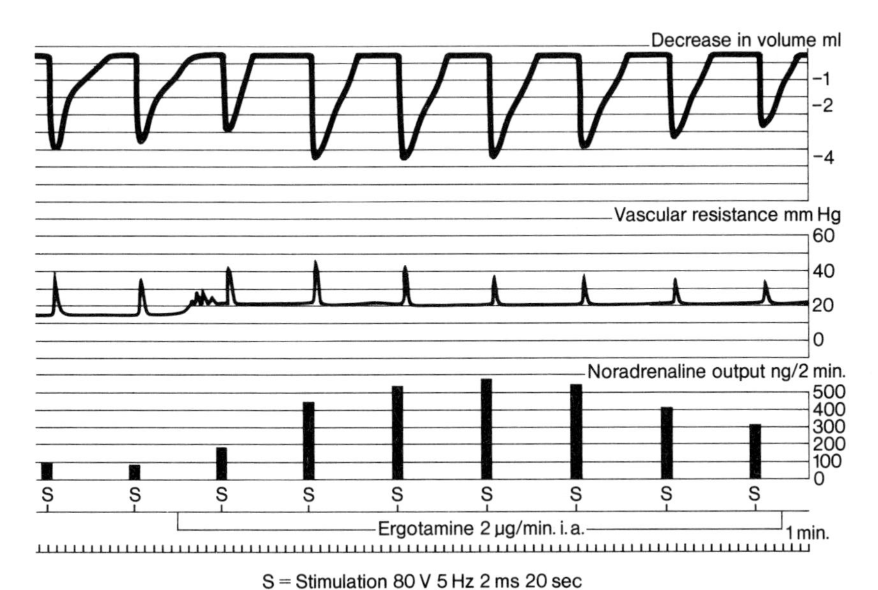

Fig. 27. The effect of ergotamine on the response of the isolated perfused spleen of the cat to sympathetic nerve stimulation. Ergotamine (2 µg/min), reinforces volume contraction and vasoconstriction of the spleen and distinctly increases noradrenaline release in the venous output consequent to sympathetic nerve stimulation. [From Figure 6, SALZMANN, R. (et al.): Naunyn Schmiedebergs Arch. Pharmacol. **261**, 370 (1968)]

PACHA and SALZMANN, 1970; SALZMANN and PACHA, 1976), methysergide (SALZMANN and PACHA, 1976) and dihydroergotoxine mesylate (BERDE, 1971, 1972; BLAKELEY et al., 1963; BROWN, 1965; CRIPPS and DEARNALEY, 1971, 1972; PACHA and SALZMANN, 1970). The most pronounced increases were found with drug infusion rates between 0.5 and 10 μg/min. Quantitatively, dihydroergotamine, 1-methylergotamine and dihydroergotoxine mesylate caused a larger increase of noradrenaline release than ergotamine (BERDE, 1971, 1972; SALZMANN and PACHA, 1968; PACHA and SALZMANN, 1970).

The individual components of dihydroergotoxine mesylate, namely dihydroergocornine, dihydroergocristine and dihydroergokryptine, show the same effects (increase of noradrenaline outflow and α-adrenoceptor blockade) as dihydroergotoxine mesylate (PACHA and SALZMANN, 1970).

There is also evidence from other isolated organs, such as heart and vas deferens, that an increased outflow of neuronally liberated noradrenaline is brought about by ergot compounds.

Heart. STARKE (1972) found that noradrenaline release from the isolated rabbit heart following sympathetic nerve stimulation was enhanced by dihydroergotamine (2×10^{-7}), although the uptake of exogenous noradrenaline was not affected up to 6×10^{-6} of dihydroergotamine. In experiments with isolated guinea-pig atria the [^{3}H]noradrenaline efflux in response to sympathetic nerve stimulation was increased more than 2-fold by 10^{-5}M dihydroergotamine (MCCULLOCH et al., 1972). According to RAND et al. (1975), this concentration of dihydroergotamine is optimal for increasing stimulation-induced efflux. Dihydroergotamine was, however, less effective than either phenoxybenzamine or phentolamine. It is interesting that dihydroergotoxine mesylate (3×10^{-7}) further enhanced the effect of cocaine and desipramine on nerve stimulation-induced noradrenaline efflux in the isolated rabbit heart (STJÄRNE and WENNMALM, 1971; WENNMALM, 1971a, b).

Vas deferens. Dihydroergotoxine mesylate (10^{-7}) increased the efflux of [^{3}H]-noradrenaline from the electrically stimulated vas deferens of the guinea-pig by 125%. After pharmacologic blockade of neuronal and extraneuronal uptake of noradrenaline, and after inhibition of local prostaglandin formation, dihydroergotoxine mesylate remained effective in increasing outflow of [^{3}H]noradrenaline in response to transmural stimulation (HEDQVIST, 1973, 1974).

Different explanations have been given for the effects of ergot compounds on the release and overflow of noradrenaline.

a) Occupation of α-Adrenoceptors

In 1957, BROWN and GILLESPIE studied the output of noradrenaline resulting from postganglionic sympathetic nerve stimulation in the venous blood of the spleen of anesthetized cats. They showed that at frequencies of stimulation below 10/sec no noradrenaline could be detected; with increasing frequency of stimulation the output per stimulus increased, reaching a maximum at about 30/sec. The amount of transmitter in the venous blood was not affected by substances inhibiting monoamine oxidase, such as iproniazid (isopropylisonicotinyl hydrazine, Marsilid) at either frequency. The noradrenaline overflow in the venous blood could be altered

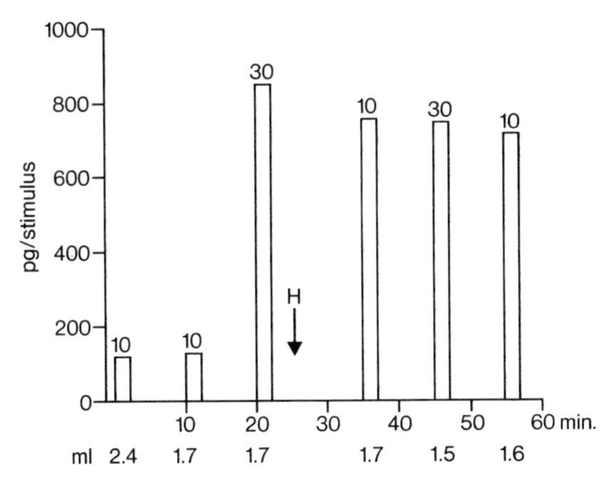

Fig. 28. Output of noradrenaline from the spleen of the cat in response to trains of 200 stimuli to the splenic nerve. The figures at the top of each block indicate the frequency of stimulation. The plasma volume of each sample is given below the abscissa. Between the third and fourth samples dihydroergotoxine mesylate (0.5 mg/kg) was given by intravenous injection. [From Figure 3, BROWN, G.L. (et al.): J. Physiol. (Lond.) **159**, 369 (1961)]

by administering the α-adrenoceptor blocking agents dibenamine and phenoxybenzamine; these drugs greatly increased the output of transmitter.

The authors suggested that noradrenaline liberated from nerve endings is inactivated after combination with α-adrenoceptors. According to this hypothesis, only small quantities of noradrenaline appear in the circulation with low stimulation rates, because the receptor is capable of combining with and/or destroying most of it; at high frequencies of stimulation increasing amounts of noradrenaline overflow into the circulation, because the receptor mechanism is saturated. A similar effect, namely increased noradrenaline release, results from blockade of tissue receptors by α-adrenoceptor blocking agents. The findings of BROWN et al. (1961) that dihydroergotoxine mesylate (0.5 mg/kg i.v.) raised the output of noradrenaline in the venous blood at 10 Hz to that of 30 Hz (Fig. 28) was explained by this theory of receptor occupation, namely that α-adrenoceptors are involved in the inactivation of the neuronally released transmitter from spleen (BROWN and GILLESPIE, 1957; KIRPEKAR and CERVONI, 1963). With dihydroergotoxine mesylate (0.5 mg/kg i.v.), recoveries of infused noradrenaline into the arterial blood supply of the cat spleen increased from 29% (controls) to 61% (GILLESPIE and KIRPEKAR, 1965a, b). The authors assumed that reincorporation of transmitter into the nerve endings might be the most important mechanism removing noradrenaline; they suggest that tissue receptors may play an important part in the reincorporation of transmitter into the nerve endings, acting as a "brake" on the diffusion away from the nerve endings.

Later, THOENEN et al. (1964a, b) found that the ability of the α-adrenoceptor blocking agents phenoxybenzamine, phentolamine and azapetine to increase the noradrenaline outflow after electrical stimulation of the splenic nerves of cats varied considerably from drug to drug. There was no correlation between the intensity of the α-adrenoceptor blocking effect and the increase in noradrenaline output. Likewise, results with ergotamine, dihydroergotamine, 1-methylergotamine and dihydroergotoxine mesylate on the isolated perfused cat spleen showed that a marked increase of the release of neuronally liberated noradrenaline can be produced by ergot alkaloids, which possess relatively little postsynaptic α-blocking activity (BERDE, 1971, 1972; PACHA and SALZMANN, 1970). These findings are evidence against the view of BROWN and GILLESPIE (1957) that the increased noradrenaline output is caused by blockade of post-synaptic α-adrenergic receptors. THOENEN et al. (1964a, b) postulated a dual site of action of α-adrenergic blocking agents at the peripheral sympathetic synapse of the cat's spleen: Blockade of α-adrenergic receptors and inhibition of re-uptake of neuronally released noradrenaline.

b) Inhibition of Noradrenaline and Adrenaline Uptake

Uptake mechanisms. The major mechanism of physiological inactivation of noradrenaline is an uptake process of noradrenaline either into the postganglionic sympathetic neurones or into extraneuronal sites. The neuronal uptake of noradrenaline has been referred to as $uptake_1$ (IVERSEN, 1965, 1967, 1973). This uptake and inactivation process involves a transport of noradrenaline and related amines from the extracellular space through the axonal membrane of sympathetic nerves and from the axoplasm into storage vesicles. The $uptake_1$ process is saturable and has a very high affinity for noradrenaline. Other amines related to noradrenaline can also act as substrates for this uptake. It is known that 75–80% of the released transmitter noradrenaline is normally removed by the $uptake_1$ mechanism into the sympathetic nerve endings (IVERSEN, 1973).

A second uptake process for catecholamines in the isolated perfused rat heart was discovered by IVERSEN (1965) and was called $uptake_2$. In this process catecholamines are taken up by a different transport system into various extraneuronal peripheral tissues. $Uptake_2$ operates mainly at high perfusion concentrations of noradrenaline, but it can also operate at low concentrations of catecholamines together with $uptake_1$. Physiologically, $uptake_2$ may play some role in terminating the actions of noradrenaline in sympathetically innervated tissues, but it seems to play a minor role compared with $uptake_1$.

$Uptake_1$ is inhibited by structural analogues of noradrenaline and by many other drugs, such as tricyclic antidepressants, local anesthetics, adrenoceptor blocking agents, etc. (IVERSEN, 1967). Inhibitors of $uptake_2$ are in part different from those of $uptake_1$, including for instance steroids, phenoxybenzamine and metanephrine (IVERSEN, 1973). An inhibition of noradrenaline uptake has also been described for ergot alkaloids.

Spleen. In slices of cat spleen incubated with dl-noradrenaline-7[^{3}H], ergotamine (10^{-6}M) inhibited the uptake of noradrenaline by 30% (DENGLER et al., 1961). The increased outflow of neuronally liberated noradrenaline in the perfusate of the isolated cat spleen during infusions of ergotamine, dihydroergotamine, 1-methylergotamine and dihydroergotoxine mesylate (SALZMANN et al., 1967; SALZMANN and PACHA, 1968; SALZMANN et al., 1968; PACHA and SALZMANN, 1970; BERDE, 1971, 1972; SALZMANN and PACHA, 1976) was explained by inhibition of re-uptake of noradrenaline into the nerve endings. The finding that the enzymatic breakdown of noradrenaline was not inhibited by ergotamine (SALZMANN et al.,

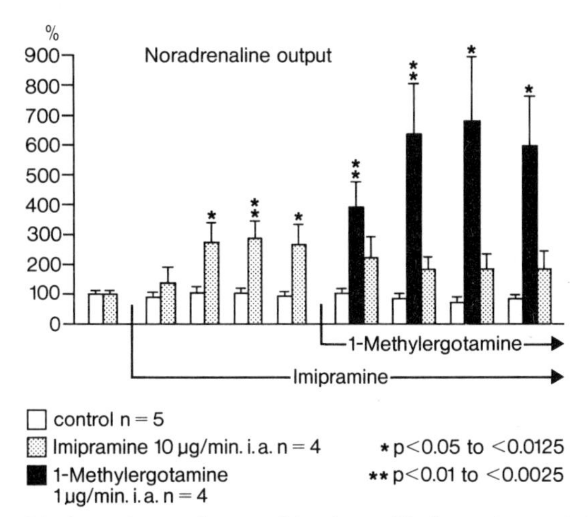

Fig. 29. The effect of imipramine and a combination of imipramine and 1-methylergotamine on noradrenaline output after nerve stimulation in the isolated perfused cat spleen. The heights of the columns indicate the values (mean + SEM) attained by a parameter on nerve stimulation, expressed as a percentage of the response to the first stimulation (first stimulation = 100%). The column groups show the responses of control and test preparations to successive stimulus trains given at 10 min intervals. [From Figure 8, SALZMANN, R., PACHA, W.: Postgrad. Med. J. **52** (Suppl. 1), 30 (1976)]

1968) further supported this interpretation. However, more recent results have shown that inhibition of catecholamine uptake cannot fully explain the action of ergot alkaloids on noradrenaline output from the spleen. When noradrenaline outflow from the spleen was maximally increased by blocking noradrenaline re-uptake by imipramine or desmethylimipramine, dihydroergotamine and 1-methylergotamine were able to raise the noradrenaline overflow still further (SALZMANN and PACHA, 1976) (Fig. 29). Thus, a further mechanism may be involved in the increase of noradrenaline outflow by ergot compounds.

During studies in the isolated blood-perfused cat spleen CRIPPS and DEARNALEY (1972) found that dihydroergotoxine mesylate (ca. 10^{-5}M) raised the noradrenaline output in response to electrical stimulation of the splenic nerve. When uptake processes 1 and 2 were blocked in cat spleen with cocaine (2×10^{-5}M) and normetanephrine (10^{-4}M), a further increase in noradrenaline overflow occurred with 10^{-5}M dihydroergotoxine mesylate (CRIPPS and DAERNALEY, 1971, 1972) (Fig. 30). The authors consider it improbable that any of the known uptake mechanisms in the spleen [uptake$_1$ and uptake$_2$, uptake processes into collagen and connective tissue, uptake into endothelial cells (GILLESPIE et al., 1970)] could be responsible for the effect of dihydroergotoxine mesylate. Two possible explanations given of the increased noradrenaline overflow after application of dihydroergotoxine mesylate were that a further site of uptake of noradrenaline which is blocked by dihydroergotoxine mesylate might exist and/or that α-adrenoceptor blocking agents may facilitate the release of transmitter from the nerve endings.

Splenic nerve granules. An interaction of ergot alkaloids with uptake of noradrenaline in bovine splenic nerve granules has been observed by EULER and

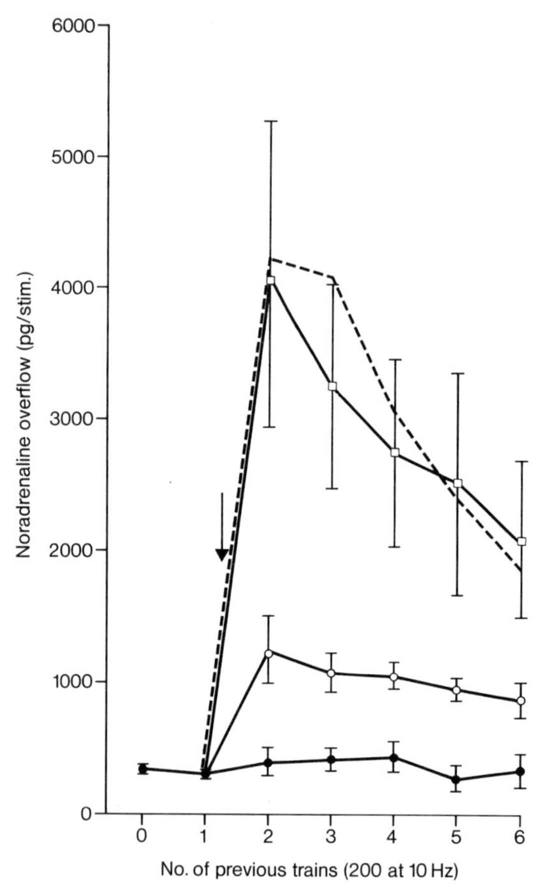

Fig. 30. Effect of blocking α-adrenoceptors and uptake processes. Mean noradrenaline overflow from the isolated spleen at successive trains of 200 stimuli at 10 Hz given at 10 min intervals. ● = no drug; ○ = cocaine (1 mg) + normetanephrine (2 mg); □ = cocaine (1 mg) + normetanephrine (2 mg) + dihydroergotoxine mesylate (0.6 mg); --- = phenoxybenzamine (5 mg). Drugs were given at the arrow. Bars = SEM, n = 4. The SEM after phenoxybenzamine were (in order) ± 737, 137, 156, 326 and 227 pg/stim. (n = 4). [From Figure 7, CRIPPS, H., DAERNALEY, D.P.: J. Physiol. (Lond.) **227**, 656 (1972)]

LISHAJKO (1966, 1968), STJÄRNE and LISHAJKO (1966) and EULER (1970, 1972). Dihydroergotoxine mesylate (2×10^{-5} M) inhibited the uptake of noradrenaline in partially depleted bovine splenic nerve granules in the presence of ATP-Mg (EULER and LISHAJKO, 1966). Dihydroergotoxine mesylate (3×10^{-5} M) and dihydroergotamine (3×10^{-5} M to 3×10^{-4} M) exerted an inhibitory action on the reuptake of [^{3}H]labeled noradrenaline (EULER and LISHAJKO, 1968). The highest activity among several α-blocking agents was shown by dihydroergotamine (EULER and LISHAJKO, 1968; EULER, 1970). STJÄRNE and LISHAJKO (1966) found that dihydroergotoxine mesylate at a concentration sufficient to inhibit strongly the transport mechanism responsible for spontaneous noradrenaline release during incubation in vitro, blocked noradrenaline uptake only moderately and did not affect the mechanism transporting dopamine to the β-hydroxylation site.

Heart. Dihydroergotamine, in concentrations of up to 6×10^{-5}, did not interfere with the uptake of exogenous noradrenaline in the isolated rabbit heart (STARKE, 1972) but enhanced the output of noradrenaline in response to sympathetic nerve stimulation at a concentration of 2×10^{-7}. The results were explained by an α-adrenoceptor-mediated feedback inhibition of noradrenaline liberation (STARKE, 1972; cf. part 3,c of this section).

Brain. D-LSD (10^{-8} to 10^{-6}M) did not cause inhibition of the uptake of radioactively labeled noradrenaline in slices of cat cortex (DENGLER et al., 1961). D-LSD (10^{-5}M) did not inhibit noradrenaline uptake into rat striatal, cortical, and hypothalamic synaptosomes, whereas ergotamine ($1\text{–}2 \times 10^{-5}$M) inhibited the uptake noncompetitively (TUOMISTO, 1974).

Reflex vasodilatation. WELLENS et al. (1970) found no modification of noradrenaline uptake in the dog hind leg after ergotamine and suggested that the inhibition of reflex vasodilatation by ergotamine occurs in the absence of an inhibitory effect on noradrenaline uptake in tissues.

Blood platelets, erythrocytes. BORN (1967) and BORN and SMITH (1970) demonstrated that the immediate uptake of [^{3}H]adrenaline in human blood platelets was partly inhibited by dihydroergotamine. This drug inhibited adrenaline-induced aggregation and the adrenaline potentiating effect on ADP aggregation in human blood platelets (BORN et al., 1967a). In search of a possible correlation between adrenaline-induced aggregation of rabbit blood platelets and uptake of adrenaline by platelets, BARTHEL and MARKWARDT (1975) studied the effects of dihydroergotamine (10^{-11} M) and BOL 148 (3×10^{-6} M) on these reactions. While adrenaline-induced aggregation of blood platelets was completely inhibited by dihydroergotamine and BOL-148 (BARTHEL and MARKWARDT, 1974, 1975) (Fig. 31), there were no significant differences in [^{14}C]adrenaline uptake of the experimental samples compared with nontreated controls. BARTHEL and MARKWARDT (1975) drew the conclusion that the adrenaline-induced aggregation of rabbit blood platelets is not associated with the uptake of this amine.

In human erythrocytes, noradrenaline was taken up at slow rates proportional to the concentration of the amine in the medium up to 1.6×10^{-5}. BOL-148 did not diminish the uptake of noradrenaline (BORN et al., 1967b).

c) Blockade of Prejunctional α-Adrenoceptors

Several authors have postulated the presence of α-adrenoceptors in adrenergic nerve endings, suggesting that noradrenaline released by nerve stimulation acts on these presynaptic or prejunctional α-adrenoceptors to inhibit its own release. These receptors thus mediate an endogenous negative feedback mechanism (FARNEBO and HAMBERGER, 1971a; KIRPEKAR and PUIG, 1971; STARKE, 1972; STARKE and MONTEL, 1973; RAND et al., 1975; LANGER et al., 1975). Alpha-adrenoceptor blocking drugs enhance noradrenaline release from stimulated tissues, because the presynaptic α-adrenoceptors are occupied and the feedback mechanism blocked.

Facilitation of noradrenaline release by blockade of presynaptic α-adrenoceptors was considered for the interpretation of the increased noradrenaline outflow after

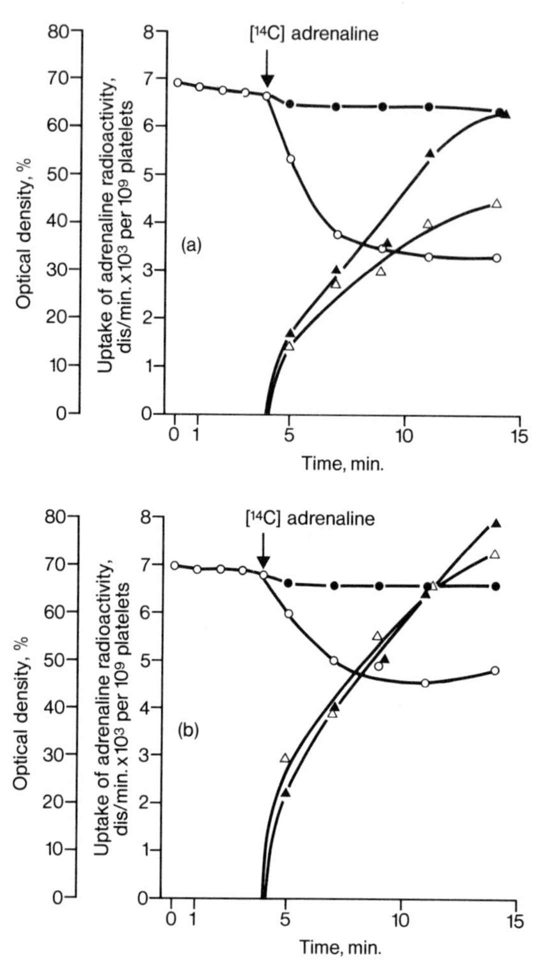

Fig. 31. Aggregation of rabbit blood platelets in TRIS-buffered Tyrode's solution (pH 7.4, 22–24°) by 5×10^{-6} M [^{14}C]adrenaline and its uptake under the influence of (a) 10^{-11} M DHE; (b) 3×10^{-6} M BOL-148. Aggregation and [^{14}C]adrenaline uptake, resp., of the blood platelets in the absence (○, △) and in the presence of inhibitor (●, ▲). Each value represents the mean from five to eight experiments. For the sake of clarity standard deviations of the means have been omitted. [From Figure 1, BARTHEL, W., MARKWARDT, F.: Biochem. Pharmacol. **24**, 1903 (1975)]

the administration of dihydroergotamine in the isolated rabbit heart (STARKE, 1972) and in isolated guinea-pig atria (MCCULLOCH et al., 1972; RAND et al., 1975). Since inhibition of catecholamine uptake is insufficient to explain fully the action of ergot alkaloids on noradrenaline overflow from the isolated cat spleen (as previously explained), it seems likely that a blockade of presynaptic α-adrenoceptors is at least partly responsible for it (CRIPPS and DEARNALEY, 1972; SALZMANN and PACHA, 1976). HEDQVIST (1973, 1974) suggested that blockade of presynaptic α-adrenoceptors by dihydroergotoxine mesylate can remove a feedback mechanism for noradrenaline-release in the isolated guinea-pig vas deferens not mediated by prostaglandins. This was postulated, since both re-uptake of released noradrenaline and generation of prostaglandin were inhibited by prior administration of desmethylimipramine, normetanephrine, and 5, 8, 11, 14-eicosatetranoic acid.

d) Other Possible Mechanisms of Stimulation of "Overflow" by Ergot Alkaloids

The finding that noradrenaline release is inhibited by prostaglandins of the E series (BRUNDIN, 1968; HEDQVIST, 1969; HEDQVIST and BRUNDIN, 1969; EULER and HEDQVIST, 1969; HEDQVIST et al., 1970; HEDQVIST and EULER, 1972) has led to the speculation that prostaglandins liberated during nerve stimulation play a role in a physiological feedback mechanism which modulates the release of noradrenaline from nerve endings (HEDQVIST and BRUNDIN, 1969; HEDQVIST 1970a, b). Substances which inhibit prostaglandin synthesis can therefore be expected to block the feedback mechanism, leading to increased noradrenaline release.

SALZMANN and PACHA (1976) studied the effects of ergotamine, dihydroergotamine, 1-methylergotamine and methysergide on the responses of the isolated per-

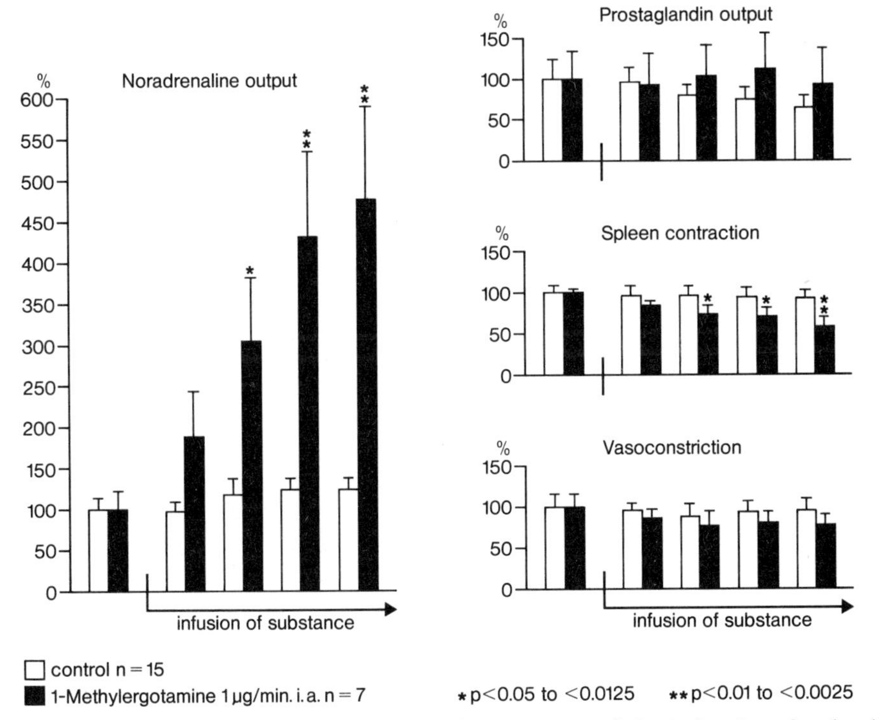

Fig. 32. The effect of 1-methylergotamine on the responses of the isolated perfused spleen of the cat to postganglionic sympathetic stimulation. The heights of the columns indicate the values (mean+SEM) attained by a parameter on nerve stimulation, expressed as a percentage of the response to the first stimulation (first stimulation=100%). The column pairs show the responses of control and test preparations to successive stimulus trains given at 10 min intervals. [From Figure 3, SALZMANN, R., PACHA, W.: Postgrad. Med. J. **52** (Suppl. 1), 27 (1976)]

fused cat spleen (noradrenaline and prostaglandin efflux, spleen contraction and vasoconstriction) after postganglionic sympathetic nerve stimulation. The ergot alkaloids increased noradrenaline efflux while only slightly affecting prostaglandin outflow (Fig. 32), suggesting that antagonism of prostaglandin-mediated feedback-inhibition of noradrenaline release is probably not involved in the increased noradrenaline overflow brought about by ergot alkaloids.

Anticholinesterase activity. An alternative hypothesis to explain the increase of transmitter release was proposed by BOYD et al. (1960), who described anticholinesterase activity for adrenergic blocking agents. It was suggested that their effect in increasing noradrenaline release might be due to their action upon a cholinergic link in the sympathetic post-ganglionic nerves; but BLAKELEY et al. (1963) considered that the effect of dihydroergotoxine mesylate in increasing transmitter overflow in cat spleen cannot be attributed to an anticholinesterase action.

4. Effects of Ergot Alkaloids on the Responses of Organs to Stimulation of Their Sympathetic Innervation

The critical finding reported by DALE in his classical paper of 1906 was not simply the reversal by ergot alkaloids of the pressor response to adrenaline in the anesthetized cat but the parallelism between the effects of ergot on the responses to injected adrenaline and to stimulation of the sympathetic nerves of a whole variety of organs in situ. These organs comprised mainly a number of different smooth muscle preparations, and DALE's finding was that where the response to sympathetic nerve stimulation was a contraction, adrenaline mimicked these effects, and both responses were abolished or reversed by ergot alkaloids. Conversely, where the response to nerve stimulation was inhibitory, adrenaline also relaxed the smooth muscle, and neither effect was antagonized by ergot. Thus, although it was to be 20 years before the true nature of the events occurring at sympathetic nerve terminals was established, and over 40 years passed before AHLQUIST (1948) proposed the classification of α- and β-adrenoceptors, DALE had seen not only the effects of the blockade of α-adrenoceptors on responses to adrenaline but also on the responses of organs to stimulation of their sympathetic innervation.

To a very large extent, antagonism by ergot alkaloids of responses of organs to stimulation of their sympathetic innervation is adequately explained in terms of α-adrenoceptor blockade. There are however some qualifications of this statement which must be made. A disparity between observations of α-adrenoceptor blockade, as seen when exogenous catecholamines are used to stimulate α-adrenoceptors, and the blockade of responses to sympathetic nerve stimulation, lies in the finding that considerably higher concentrations of the blocking agent may be required to abolish the response to nerve stimulation. This is true as much for other types of α-adrenoceptor blocking drugs as for ergot derivatives. For example, BIRMINGHAM and WILSON (1963) found that in the isolated guinea-pig vas deferens preparation, the concentrations of dihydroergotamine (3×10^{-4}) and phentolamine (2×10^{-4}) necessary to abolish responses to field stimulation of the nervous elements, in addition to abolishing responses to noradrenaline, also reduced those to added acetylcholine and potassium chloride almost to zero. Similar results were reported for ergotamine by BOYD et al. (1960). In cases such as this it is not justifiable to state categorically that the effect on the response to stimulation was due to blockade of α-adrenoceptors and not to a nonspecific depressive action. This resistance to blockade exhibited by nervously mediated stimuli when compared to exogenously administered neurotransmitters is not an uncommon phenomenon and is possibly accounted for by high local concentrations of the transmitter substance occurring in the junctional cleft between the nerve ending and the effector cell, and overcoming the block.

The historical importance of α-adrenoceptor blockade in the pharmacology of ergot has perhaps obscured some of the more subtle properties of ergot alkaloids and related compounds which have a bearing on adrenergic neuronal transmission. Inhibition by ergot alkaloids of responses to stimulation of adrenergic nerves is conveniently accounted for as being due to "α-block," and the possibility that other mechanisms may be involved in some situations has been understandably ignored. Recent publications have shown that some ergot-related compounds can indeed in certain circumstances inhibit adrenergic transmission by impairing the release of noradrenaline.

Vas deferens. D-LSD, which is practically devoid of α-adrenoceptor blocking activity, inhibits responses to electrical field stimulation of postganglionic nerves in desheathed (i.e., ganglion-free) vas deferens preparations from rats, mice, guinea-pigs, rabbits and gerbils (meriones shawii) without antagonizing motor responses to noradrenaline (AMBACHE et al., 1971, 1973a; HUGHES, 1973; GILLESPIE and MCGRATH, 1975). The effect of D-LSD is dose-dependent up to a maximally effective concentration of 10^{-7} g/ml (Fig. 33), rapid in onset (2–8 min) and slowly reversible on washing out the drug (recovery time >1 h). The recovery time was prolonged by lengthening the contact time or raising the D-LSD concentration. The possibility that a tryptaminergic motor transmission might be involved was excluded by the findings of AMBACHE and ZAR (1971) that 5-HT failed to contract the guinea-pig vas deferens, and that the inhibitory effect of D-LSD was not shared by BOL-148 or by methysergide, both of which are more potent 5-HT-receptor blocking agents than D-LSD (CERLETTI and DOEPFNER, 1958b). In the guinea-pig and mouse vas deferens, the inhibitory effect of D-LSD was itself antagonized by the α-adrenoceptor blocking agent phentolamine and also by phenoxybenzamine, although the latter was considerably less effective (AMBACHE et al., 1973a; HUGHES, 1973; HUGHES et al., 1975). Both HUGHES (1973) and AMBACHE et al. (1973a) concluded that D-LSD might act by stimulating prejunctional α-adrenoceptors, thereby reducing the output of the sympathetic transmitter. This idea was supported by the demonstration that D-LSD inhibited the overflow of [^{3}H] label from the guinea-pig vas deferens on field stimulation after incubating the tissue with [^{3}H]noradrenaline or [^{3}H]tyrosine, an effect which was also antagonized by phentolamine (HUGHES, 1973) (Fig. 34).

The existence of a D-LSD resistant component of concentrations of the guinea-pig vas deferens evoked by field stimulation was reported by AMBACHE et al. (1973a). These authors found that the inhibitory effect of D-LSD was greater for short train lengths (<10 pulses), and when the tissue was stimulated with trains of 20 pulses (10 Hz) there was practically no reduction of the response by D-LSD. GILLESPIE and MCGRATH (1975), using the vas deferens of the rat, confirmed

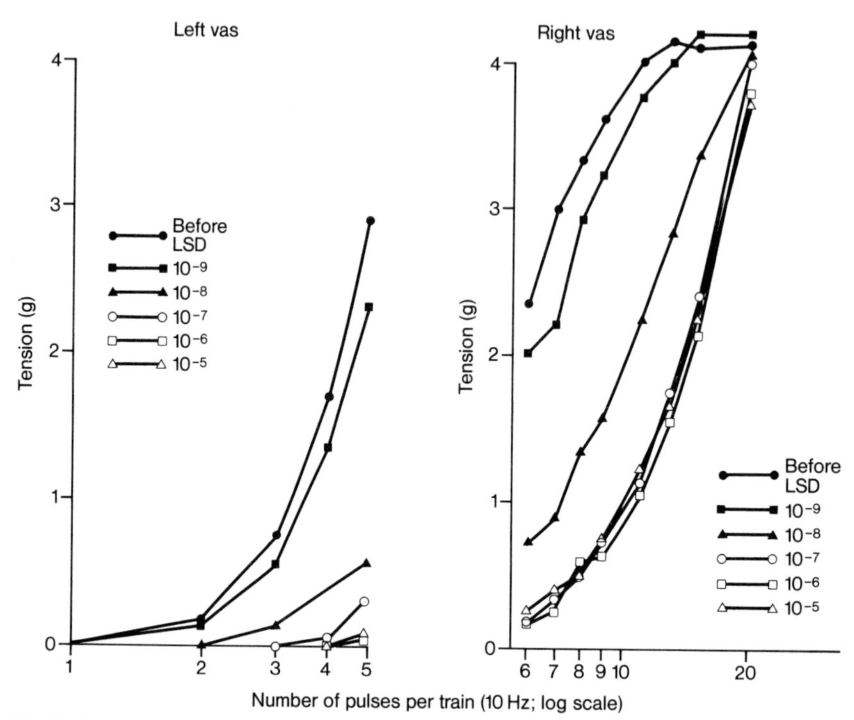

Fig. 33. Relationship between the concentration of D-LSD and the degree of inhibition of the susceptible component in the motor response to field stimulation of intramural nerves. Vasa deferentia from the same guinea-pig stimulated at 1 min intervals with trains of 1 msec pulses. Note increasing inhibition in the concentration range 10^{-9} to 10^{-7}g/ml with no further deepening of inhibition at 10^{-5} g/ml. The contribution of the D-LSD-resistant component to the motor response is insignificant with trains of <5 pulses but grows spectacularly between 5 and 20 pulses. [From Figure 3, AMBACHE, N. (et al.): J. Physiol. (Lond.) **231**, 257 (1973)]

that the motor response to nerve stimulation comprises two components: An initial twitch followed by a slow contraction. The twitch, which occurs at all train lengths—including sometimes even single pulse stimuli, is the component of the response which was inhibited by D-LSD. Longer train lengths (>20 pulses) evoke, in addition, the secondary slow contraction which was not affected by D-LSD in some experiments and in others was slightly potentiated. These effects were also seen in the vas deferens in situ in the pithed rat on i.v. injection of D-LSD.

In addition to D-LSD, ergometrine, methylergometrine, ergotamine, dihydroergotamine and ergocristine have all been reported to inhibit motor responses of the isolated guinea-pig vas deferens to sympathetic nerve stimulation (BOYD et al., 1960; BIRMINGHAM and WILSON, 1963; AMBACHE et al., 1973a). In the isolated vas deferens of the mouse, BENNETT and MIDDLETON (1975) described a significant decrease in the amplitude of the excitatory junction potential after 10^{-5} dihydroergocornine or dihydroergocristine. A comprehensive explanation of these effects in terms of simple α-adrenoceptor blockade is not tenable, since ergometrine and methylergometrine are only weak antagonists at α-adrenoceptors (Table 3). Further-

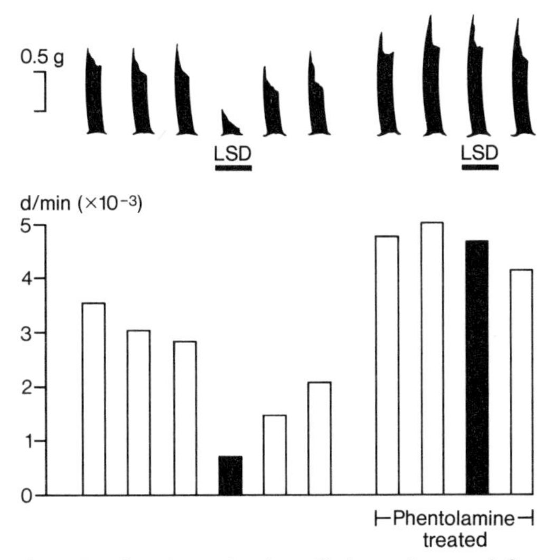

Fig. 34. Antagonism of D-LSD by phentolamine. Guinea-pig vas deferens labeled with [^{3}H]-noradrenaline and field-stimulated. Upper part: tension in the vas deferens during periods of stimulation. Lower part: increased levels of [^{3}H]-labeled material released into the bath during periods of stimulation in the absence (*white columns*) and presence (*black columns*) of D-LSD (50 ng/ml). For the experiments on the right-hand side, phentolamine (2 μg/ml) was present in the bathing solution. [From Figure 1, HUGHES, J.: Brit. J. Pharmacol. **49**, 707 (1973)]

more, AMBACHE et al. (1973a) reported that the inhibitory effect of dihydroergotamine was prevented by phentolamine. Therefore, it may be that dihydroergotamine, and possibly other ergot alkaloids, can inhibit the effects of sympathetic nerve stimulation in two ways, namely by exciting prejunctional α-adrenoceptors as well as by blocking postjunctional α-adrenoceptors.

Anococcygeus muscle. D-LSD inhibits responses to motor sympathetic nerve stimulation in rat and cat anococcygeus muscles without depressing noradrenaline contractions (AMBACHE et al., 1973b, 1975; GILLESPIE and MCGRATH, 1975). As is the case in the vas deferens, the inhibition by D-LSD was maximal with short trains and declined with longer trains of stimuli, indicating the existence of a D-LSD resistant component of the response. The D-LSD effect was dose-dependent and was antagonized by phentolamine. Unlike the guinea-pig vas deferens, the rat anococcygeus was contracted by 5-HT. However, the possible involvement of 5-HT as a transmitter substance would not explain the effect of D-LSD, because methysergide was considerably weaker than D-LSD in inhibiting motor transmission. Methysergide also suppressed contractions evoked by noradrenaline and acetylcholine in doses which did not block motor transmission. BOL-148 slightly inhibited the responses to nerve stimulation but also depressed noradrenaline contractions, indicating that it blocked α-adrenoceptors. Responses to acetylcholine were at the same time potentiated. Raising the concentration of BOL-148 slightly potentiated motor transmission, possibly by blocking prejunctional α-adrenoceptors. These results obtained by AMBACHE et al. (1975) using the rat anococcygeus are similar to those reported for the vas deferens of the guinea-pig (above), so that the antagonism by D-LSD of motor transmission in both preparations may be due to the same mechanism, namely a reduction in transmitter output brought about by stimulation of prejunctional α-adrenoceptors. The possibility that prostaglandin release might be involved was excluded by experiments using indomethacin, which failed to reduce the effect of D-LSD. GILLESPIE and MCGRATH (1975) compared the action of D-LSD in the anococcygeus muscle of the cat with that of the adrenergic neurone blocking agent guanethidine, both of which not only inhibited motor responses to nerve stimulation but also contracted the muscle. Phentolamine antagonized this contractile response in both instances, but it was also prevented by pretreatment of the tissue with 6-hydroxydopamine, which destroys sympathetic nerve terminals. The contractile response is therefore probably due to release of sympathetic transmitter from the nerve terminals. The authors drew particular attention to the similarities between D-LSD and guanethidine, but it is as yet too early to be able to say whether these two drugs share a common site or mode of action on sympathetic motor nerves.

Other organs. AMBACHE et al. (1975) investigated the effects of D-LSD at a number of autonomic nerve-muscle junctions. Using electrical field stimulation to excite selectively the nervous elements in the tissues studied, they found that inhibition of transmission by an agonist action of D-LSD at prejunctional α-adrenoceptors was confined to the sympathetic junctions (rat anococcygeus, dog retractor penis and dog splenic capsule strips). In four of six experiments using the dog splenic capsule, however, D-LSD antagonized not only the responses to field stimulation but also those to administered noradrenaline, revealing a blocking action at postjunctional α-adrenoceptors in this preparation. The dog splenic capsule also was distinguished from the other two preparations in that it did not respond to high concentrations of D-LSD with outright contractions [an action attributed to release of noradrenaline from sympathetic nerve endings (GILLESPIE and MCGRATH, 1975)]. The absence of this response in the dog splenic capsule would be accounted for by the blocking action of D-LSD at postjunctional α-adrenoceptors in this preparation, although it was not established whether or not noradrenaline release was inhibited. At a parasympathetic nerve-muscle junction (longitudinal muscle of the guinea-pig ileum), no inhibition by D-LSD of responses to electrical field stimulation was observed. On the contrary, D-LSD, especially in high concentrations, potentiated the motor responses to electrical stimulation and to administered acetylcholine. This potentiation was attributed by the authors to blockade of prejunctional α-adrenoceptors. Evidence for the existence of such receptors on parasympathetic nerve endings was obtained using propranolol-treated guinea-pig ileum preparations in which noradrenaline powerfully antagonized responses to field stimulation without inhibiting contractions evoked by administered acetylcholine. Furthermore, this effect was antagonized by D-LSD, thus supporting the idea that both substances act at prejunctional α-adrenoceptors. At another parasympathetic nerve-muscle junction (rabbit rectococcygeus) (AMBACHE et al., 1975), both potentiation by D-LSD and inhibition by noradrenaline of the twitches evoked by field stimulation were observed. However, D-LSD did not antagonize the effect of noradrenaline, which was also obtained in the presence of propranolol. This finding contrasts with that made in the guinea-pig ileum and suggests that potentiation of transmission by D-LSD in the rabbit rectococcygeus might be mediated by a site other than the prejunctional α-adrenoceptor. Such an alternative might be provided by a 5-HT receptor, in which case the potentiation might be regarded as a purely physical phenomenon (i.e., an increase in muscle tone without visible contraction, due to a partial agonist effect of D-LSD).

Effects on responses to nerve stimulation in whole animals. DREW (1976) recently published a method which allows a comparison of the effects of drugs on pre- and postjunctional α-adrenoceptors in a single preparation. The method is an extension of that described by GILLESPIE and MUIR (1967) and involves selective electrical stimulation of the cardiac sympathetic outflow in the pithed rat. Heart rate was maintained constantly elevated by continuous stimulation, while blood pressure was hardly affected. Agonist effects on postjunctional α-adrenoceptors were measured as elevations of blood pressure and actions on the prejunctional receptors by means of the fall in heart rate. The ratio of doses required to produce given magnitudes of effect on blood pressure and heart rate was determined for each of a number of substances. The results indicated D-LSD to be a highly selective stimulant of prejunctional α-adrenoceptors, more selective in fact than clonidine. The reduction in heart rate induced by D-LSD was antagonized by phentolamine but not by cyproheptadine. While such experiments are possessed of a certain elegance insofar as the comparison is drawn between two independent effects in the same preparation at the same time, the results cannot be regarded as furnishing a general rule; affinities of drugs to both pre- and postjunctional receptors must be expected to vary from one organ to another [cf. the blockade of postjunctional α-adrenoceptors by D-LSD in dog splenic capsule and of the prejunctional α-adrenoceptors in the guinea-pig ileum (AMBACHE et al., 1975)]. Furthermore, it is questionable whether the assumption that vasoconstrictor activity is due solely to postjunctional α-adrenoceptor stimulation is entirely justifiable, even in the pithed animal. In pithed cats an agonist effect of dihydroergotoxine mesylate at prejunctional α-adrenoceptors has been shown by SCHOLTYSIK (1975). Small i.v. doses of dihydroergotoxine mesylate dose-dependently inhibited the increases in heart rate evoked by electrical stimulation of spinal segments C_7 and T_1, and the effect was partly prevented by phenoxybenzamine. The same stimulus simultaneously contracted the nictitating membrane but here dihydroergotoxine mesylate did not affect the responses to stimulation up to a dose of 3.5 μg/kg i.v.

A number of papers not mentioned in this text, in which effects of ergot alkaloids on responses to nerve stimulation have been described are summarized in Table 8.

Table 8. Miscellaneous observations on the effects of ergot alkaloids on responses to nerve stimulation in various organ systems

Preparation, species, nerve stimulated	Observations, references. (The response to stimulation is muscle contraction except where otherwise stated)
Aorta (spiral strips) in vitro – rabbit, field stimulation	Dihydroergotamine (2×10^{-6}): 70% reduction in response. Dihydroergotoxine mesylate (2×10^{-6}): 50% reduction in response. Result complicated in both cases by partial agonist effect (1).

Table 8 (continued)

Preparation, species, nerve stimulated	Observations, references. (The response to stimulation is muscle contraction except where otherwise stated)
Penile artery (spiral strips) in vitro – bull, field stimulation	This preparation commonly possesses high spontaneous tone and relaxes in response to field stimulation. The relaxation is not affected by methysergide (10^{-7} to 5×10^{-6}), which itself induces contractions (2).
Portal vein (longitudinal strips) in vitro – rabbit, field stimulation	Ergotamine (5×10^{-7} to 5×10^{-6}) blocks contractions and raises tone, exposing a relaxant response (3,4). BOL-148 (10^{-7}) affects neither contractile nor relaxant responses (3).
Spleen (perfused) in vitro – cat, splenic nerve	Spleen contractions are only weakly antagonized by ergotamine infusions (>1 μg/min i.a.) (5,6); more strongly by dihydroergotamine (0.1 to 100 μg/min i.a.) (7). Dihydroergotoxine mesylate (approx. 10^{-5} M) can also block the response (8). Order of potency for inhibition of contractions: dihydroergotamine > dihydroergotoxine mesylate > ergotamine > 1-methylergotamine (9).
Seminal vesicle in vitro – guinea-pig, hypogastric nerve	Dihydroergotoxine mesylate (3×10^{-6}) reduces responses by up to 40%. The same concentration of dihydroergotoxine mesylate abolishes responses to noradrenaline and partially antagonizes responses to ATP (10). A purinergic innervation has been postulated (11).
Retractor penis in vitro – bull, field stimulation	Ergotamine (5×10^{-6}) and methysergide (10^{-7} to 1.3×10^{-6}) evoke contractions, thereby revealing relaxation in response to stimulation (2).
Nictitating membrane in vivo – cat, cervical sympathetic nerve	Small doses of ergotamine (1 μg/kg i.v.) potentiate pre- and postganglionic stimulation; larger doses (>5 μg/kg i.v.) inhibit (12). Ergotaminine is without effect (13). Ergotoxine antagonizes the response (14).
Submaxillary gland in vivo – rat, cervical sympathetic nerve	Duct constriction is abolished and secretion reduced by dihydroergotamine (0.5 to 1 mg/kg i.v.) (15).
Parotid gland in vivo – cat, cervical sympathetic nerve	Duct constriction is abolished by dihydroergotamine (0.5 to 1.5 mg/kg i.v.) but secretion is only slightly reduced (16).
Esophagus in vitro – chicken, vagus nerve	Contractions are not antagonized by methysergide (10^{-8}) (17).
Rectum in vitro – chicken, Remak nerve	Contractions are not antagonized by methysergide (10^{-8}) (17).
Swim bladder in vitro – cod (gadus morhua), field stimulation	Dihydroergotamine (10^{-5}) blocks contractions of the radial muscle (18).

References: 1. PATERSON (1965); 2. KLINGE and SJÖSTRAND (1974); 3. HUGHES and VANE (1967); 4. HUGHES and VANE (1970); 5. SALZMANN et al. (1967); 6. SALZMANN et al. (1968); 7. SALZMANN and PACHA (1968); 8. CRIPPS and DEARNALEY (1972); 9. PACHA and SALZMANN (1970); 10. NAKANISHI and TAKEDA (1973b); 11. NAKANISHI and TAKEDA (1973a); 12. SALZMANN and WEIDMANN (1966); 13. BACQ (1934b); 14. CANNON and ROSENBLUETH (1937); 15. THULIN (1974); 16. THULIN (1975); 17. BARTLET (1974); 18. NILSSON (1971).

5. Actions of Ergot Alkaloids at β-Adrenoceptors

There is no evidence for either stimulation or block of β-adrenoceptors by ergot compounds. In studies on the vascular bed of the anesthetized dog, ergotamine had no detectable agonistic or antagonistic actions on β-adrenoceptors, as shown by the absence of positive inotropic and chronotropic effects as well as by the failure of ergotamine to block the cardiostimulant, vasodilator and retractor penis-relaxing actions of isoprenaline (GUIMARÃES and OSSWALD, 1969; OSSWALD et al., 1970). These in vivo observations correlate well with those found in vitro, where ergotamine failed to block β-adrenoceptors in canine saphenous veins (GUIMARÃES and OSSWALD, 1969) and in isolated guinea-pig atria (OSSWALD and GUIMARÃES, 1962). Pretreatment of the isolated guinea-pig trachea with 1.5–15 μM dihydroergotamine diminished the maximum relaxation in response to isoprenaline, indicating that the antagonism by dihydroergotamine was noncompetitive and nonspecific (LEVY and WILKENFELD, 1970). In cultured rat astrocytoma cells an increase in the content of cAMP induced by both noradrenaline and isoprenaline can be blocked by β- but not by α-adrenoceptor blocking drugs. Preincubation of confluent cultures with 50 nM dihydroergotamine inhibited the stimulatory effect of noradrenaline on cAMP level, suggesting that in this experimental model dihydroergotamine presumably has some action at β-adrenoceptors (MAURER and GRIEDER, 1975).

The frog erythrocyte adenylate cyclase can also be activated by isoprenaline, adrenaline and noradrenaline in descending order of potency. Propranolol (5 μM) inhibited the isoprenaline effect, indicating the involvement of β-adrenoceptors. When dihydroergotamine was tested as antagonist, extremely high concentrations (50–500 μM) were necessary to inhibit the isoprenaline-induced stimulation of the frog adenylate cyclase. The inhibition by dihydroergotamine was of the noncompetitive type, suggesting an unspecific effect (CHAN and ELLENBOGEN, 1974). These findings are supported by the observation that in rat cerebral cortex slices, dihydroergotoxine mesylate antagonized stimulation of cAMP formation caused by noradrenaline but failed to inhibit that induced by isoprenaline (MARKSTEIN and WAGNER, 1975).

E. The Shape of Ergotamine and Dihydroergotamine in Relation to Their Interaction With α-Adrenoceptors

H.P. WEBER and T.J. PETCHER

From crystal structure determinations of a number of ergopeptins and *iso*ergopeptins (WEBER and PETCHER, 1976), certain conclusions may be drawn as to the preferred conformation of biologically active ergopeptins in solution and, by extension, at the biological receptor. The observed conformations of the potent molecules ergotamine and dihydroergotamine are presented in Figure 35, from which it is clear that, with the single exception of the D-ring conformation, the shapes of the two molecules are practically identical. This minor conformational difference between the molecules, although of negligible effect on the gross topography,

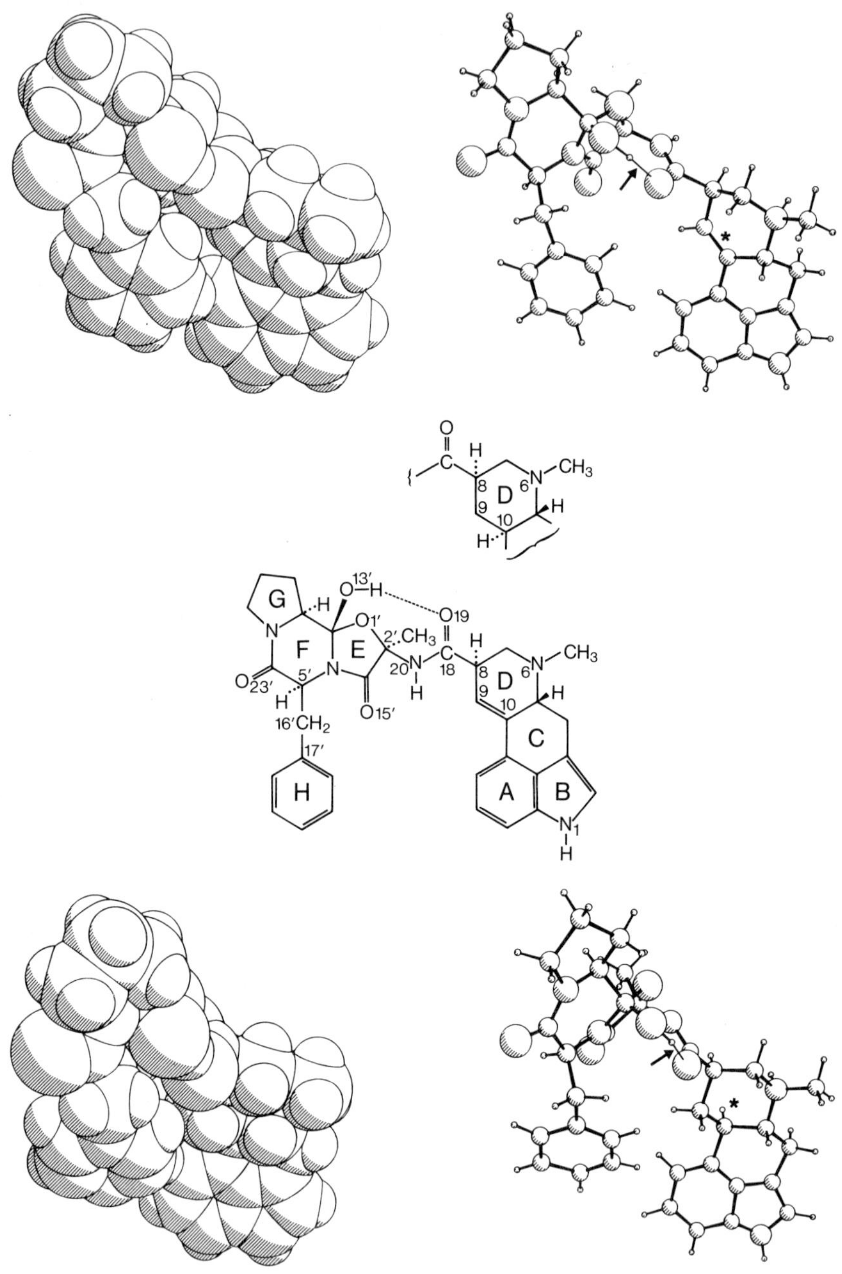

Fig. 35. Molecules of ergotamine and dihydroergotamine in the conformation observed in crystal structure determinations of their *para*bromobenzoate and hydrobromide salts respectively. Each molecule is shown in two representations, a space-filling, and a "ball and stick" model, respectively. The upper pair of diagrams are of ergotamine, the lower of dihydroergotamine. The *intra*molecular hydrogen bond discussed in the text is arrowed in both molecules, and the structural formula carries atom and ring labeling where mention is made of specific *intra*molecular rotations about single bonds. The double bond of ergotamine and the C(10) hydrogen atom of dihydroergotamine, discussed in the section on receptor binding, are labeled with asterisks for easy reference

must be responsible for the existing differences in biological activity between ergotamine and dihydroergotamine, namely: In α-adrenergic systems, dihydroergotamine has slightly greater affinity than ergotamine, but this latter is a more efficacious partial agonist. In the following paragraphs, an attempt is made to correlate these differences in the phenomenologic parameters "affinity" and "efficacy" with the observed structural differences and to explain the mode of interaction of biologically potent ergopeptins with the α-adrenergic receptor in physico-chemical terms.

Molecular flexibility of ergopeptins. It is clear from the molecular formulae of ergopeptins that the A/B/C- and the E/F-ring system (Fig. 35) each form a rigid molecular fragment. Apart from these fixed fragments, the molecules have in principle a fairly large number of degrees of conformational freedom, mainly rotations about formal single bonds, such as C(8)–C(18), N(20)–C(2′), C(5′)–C(16′), and C(16)–C(17′), together with pseudorotations in the two saturated rings D and G. From crystallographic studies of ergopeptins one may infer that much of this apparent flexibility is limited by various *intra*molecular forces. Prominent among these internal interactions is a strong *hydrogen bond* (Fig. 35) between the cyclol hydroxyl O(13′) and carboxyl oxygen O(19). Together with the invariably observed *trans* peptide bond C(18)–N(20), this hydrogen bond fixes the torsion angles around the single bond N(20)–C(2′) within a narrow range.

The proline ring G shows minor conformational variations in the different structures. The flexible benzyl group H, however, appears to be restricted to a certain orientation in four of the investigated structures, while another orientation is adopted in two other structures. It may be assumed that steric hindrance between neighboring atoms is responsible for this reduced flexibility. The major structural determinant is, however, the D-ring conformation, which is shown in Figure 36,

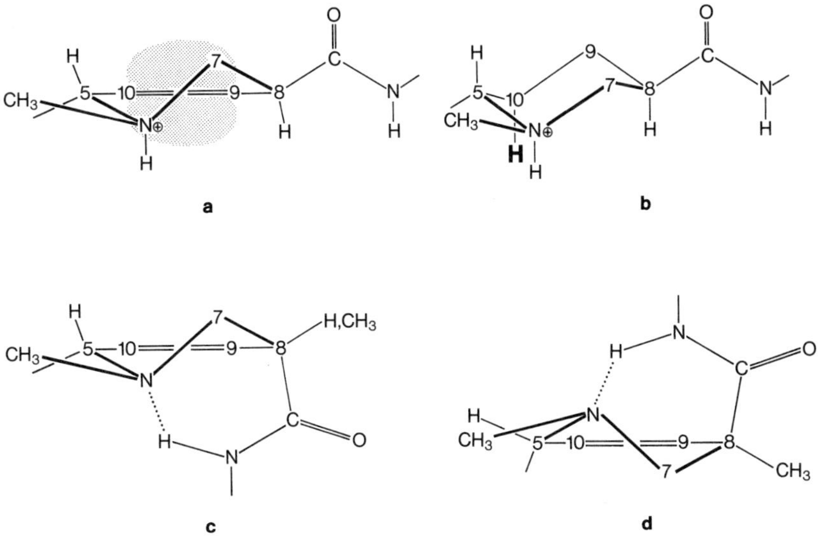

Fig. 36. The D-ring partial conformations of (a) ergotamine, (b) dihydroergotamine, (c) *iso*ergotamine and 8-methyl-*iso*-ergotamine, and (d) 8-methyl-ergotamine. The π-electron density cloud of the double bond is indicated in (a) and the C(10) hydrogen atom appears bold in (b). Note the entirely different conformations of (c) and (d) in comparison to (a) and (b)

for various ergopeptins. It may be seen that in the biologically active compounds ergotamine and dihydroergotamine, the amide group is *equatorial* to the D-ring, while in the biologically inactive forms this group is *axial* (and stabilized in this position by an internal hydrogen bond N(20)–H..N(6)). The torsion angles around C(8)–C(18) in the structures of ergotamine and dihydroergotamine fall in a rather narrow range, such that the plane of the amide group is roughly normal to the mean plane of the D-ring. This restricted rotation may be attributed to Van der Waals contacts between the atoms adjacent to the C(8)–C(18) bond.

Preferred conformation and receptor binding. The various factors discussed above, and the fact that one always observes the same conformational features in various *X*-ray crystal structure determinations in which the environments of the molecules studied are quite different, leads one to suggest that biologically active ergopeptins possess a preferred conformation which is faithfully represented in Figure 35. This conformation is likely to dominate the ensemble of solution conformers; in other words, this is the most likely shape of the molecule at the moment of approach to its receptor. The further passage of events at the receptor, such as mutual conformational change and production of the biological response, must, in the absence of direct evidence, remain matters for conjecture. A knowledge of the drug conformation, however, does enable one to speculate as to the nature of the interaction.

The structural differences between ergotamine and dihydroergotamine causing the known differences in biological activity must be sought in electronic and steric differences in the D-ring. The differences are small but obviously significant: Dihydroergotamine has a hydrogen atom projecting below the plane of the ring at C(10) in the same direction as the proton on N(6) where ergotamine has none; ergotamine has π-electron density at C(9)–C(10) where dihydroergotamine has none (Fig. 36).

It seems clear that the pharmacophore, or effector group of ergopeptins, is contained in the lysergic acid moiety, this molecular fragment exhibiting as it does "buried" catecholamine-like and 5HT-like segments (Fig. 37), which may explain why ergotamine and dihydroergotamine can react with both α-adrenoreceptors and 5-HT receptors. One may thus postulate the following binding areas for the pharmacophore, common to both ergotamine and dihydroergotamine:

(1) the indole nucleus
  - hydrogen bonding N(1)–H... receptor
  - π–π or hydrophobic interaction

(2) N(6), which is protonated at physiological pH
  - hydrogen bonding $N(6)^+$–H... receptor

One of these hydrogen bonds, N(6)–H..., is then directed below the plane of the lysergic acid fragment as drawn, while one, N(1)–H... is parallel to this plane.

Additionally, the peptide moiety seems intimately involved in α-antagonist activity: ergolines, for example, are not good α-blockers. Both ergotamine and dihydroergotamine exhibit high receptor affinity and both are long-acting. This has been thought to indicate "auxiliary binding"—which might loosely be attributed to the peptide part of ergot alkaloids. One obvious candidate to take part in a stereospecific binding of the peptide fragment to the receptor is the N(20)–H group, which maintains a constant orientation with respect to the lysergyl moiety,

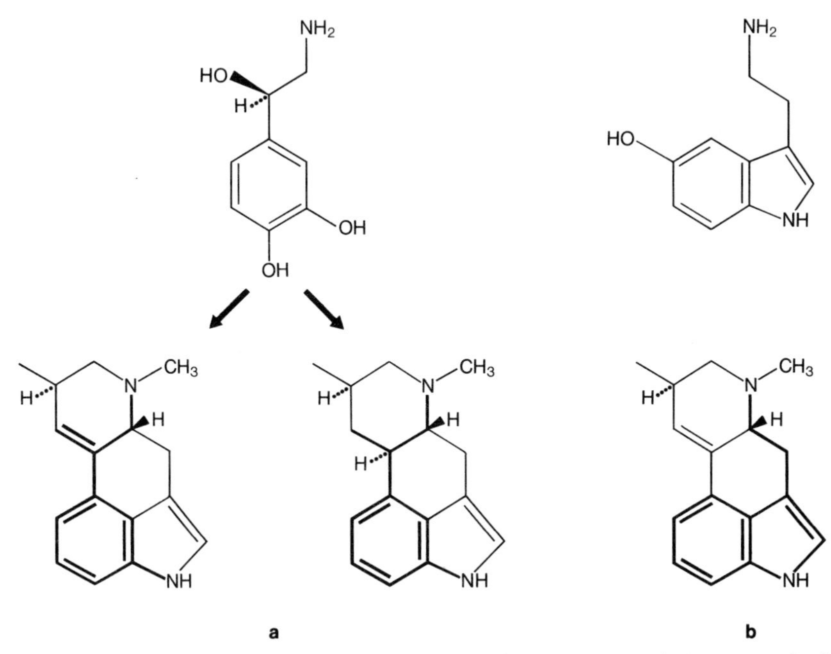

Fig. 37. The "buried" structural fragments of (a) noradrenaline and (b) serotonin in the lysergic acid skeleton. It may be seen that the important *meta*-hydroxyl group of the catecholamines comes into coincidence with N(1), an isosteric group, and that the absolute stereochemistry at the side chain α-carbon of noradrenaline is identical to that at C(10) of dihydroergotamine

and, like N(6)–H, is directed below the plane of this group. Whether one can, in fact, separate part of the total binding of a drug to its receptor and conveniently label this "auxiliary binding" is a moot point. Since, however, the peptide moiety is common to both ergotamine and dihydroergotamine and is in a similar spatial relationship to the lysergyl residue in both molecules, "auxiliary binding" sites are unlikely to contribute to *differences* in biological potency.

The differences between ergotamine and dihydroergotamine binding must therefore occur at the C(9)–C(10) position. In this area, the two molecules differ in both electronic structure and in conformation. If one superposes (–)-noradrenaline on the lysergic acid skeleton, one finds that the side chain hydroxyl group is approximately coincident with the double bond in ergotamine, and that the α-hydrogen atom of (–)-noradrenaline corresponds in position and absolute configuration to that of the C(10) hydrogen atom of dihydroergotamine. One may thus postulate that the greater efficacy of ergotamine is due to the presence of π-electron density of the C(9)–C(10) double bond, which mimics the lone pair electron density of the side chain hydroxyl group of (–)-noradrenaline. The greater affinity of dihydroergotamine might then be attributed to the presence of the C(10) hydrogen atom, which fits optimally into a receptor niche available for the corresponding hydrogen atom of (–)-noradrenaline.

F. Actions of Ergot Alkaloids at Acetylcholine Receptors

As far as is known, ergot alkaloids neither stimulate nor block receptors for acetylcholine. Observations suggesting that methysergide may cause release of acetylcholine by stimulating M-receptors in longitudinal muscle strips from human intestine are discussed in Section B, part 1, b, γ. Most reports describe enhancement of responses to cholinomimetic agents by ergot compounds. These experimental data are discussed in Section J.

G. Actions of Ergot Alkaloids at Histamine Receptors

There is no evidence that ergot alkaloids interact with histamine receptors at concentrations which elicit therapeutic effects. In the isolated guinea-pig ileum ergot compounds, such as ergotamine, dihydroergotamine, dihydroergocristine, dihydroergokryptine and dihydroergocornine, inhibit responses to histamine only when used at extremely high concentration (4–500 μM) (BIRCHER and SCHALCH, 1948; GADDUM and HAMEED, 1954; GADDUM and PICARELLI, 1957). Similarly high concentrations of dihydroergotoxine mesylate or ergotamine are required to antagonize the vasoconstrictor effect of histamine in bovine arteries (PICHLER et al., 1953) and in rabbit cerebral arteries (POLITOFF and MACRI, 1966), respectively. Compared to their α-adrenoceptor and 5-HT receptor blocking activities, these ergot alkaloids are more than 10,000 times less potent in antagonizing responses to histamine, and it can be assumed that this effect is nonspecific. Ergotamine (up to 650 ng/ml) does not prevent the histamine-induced rise in perfusion pressure in isolated rat lungs (BAKHLE and SMITH, 1972) or the histamine-induced bronchospasm in guinea-pigs (LOEW et al., 1946). Neither D-LSD nor methysergide inhibit histamine-induced bronchospasm (CERLETTI, 1955; HOLGATE and WARNER, 1960; KONZETT, 1956; SICUTERI et al., 1960). Absence of histamine antagonism has been further reported for D-LSD on isolated guinea-pig atria (TRENDELENBURG, 1960), for both D-LSD (KRIVOY, 1957) and methylergometrine (BIRCHER and SCHALCH, 1948) on the isolated guinea-pig ileum, for BOL-148 on isolated strips from rat stomach (VANE, 1957) and cat spleen (INNES, 1962b) and for methysergide on the guinea-pig vas deferens (KATSURAGI and SUZUKI, 1974). In man, methysergide does not antagonize the hypertensive action of histamine on the cerebrospinal fluid, though it effectively reduces the action of the histamine liberator 48/80 (SICUTERI et al., 1959).

H. Interaction of Ergot Alkaloids With Prostaglandins

I. Interference of Ergot Alkaloids With Endogenous Prostaglandin Synthesis

In certain canine veins peptide alkaloids, such as ergotamine and dihydroergotamine, have been shown to enhance endogenous prostaglandin synthesis. Evidence for this was provided by the observation that a canine vein strip, contracted by ergotamine or dihydroergotamine, required for its complete relaxation the com-

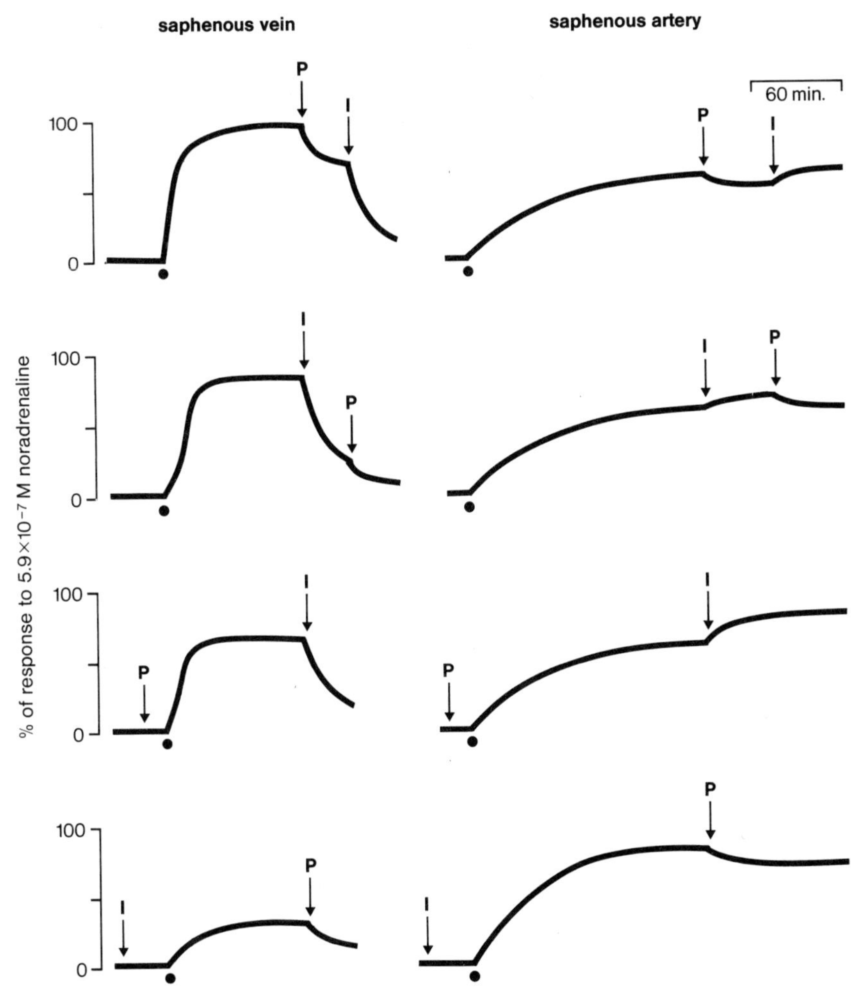

Fig. 38. Influence of phentolamine (*P*) and indomethacin (*I*) on dihydroergotamine-induced contractions in spiral strips from canine blood vessels. [From Figure 1, MÜLLER-SCHWEINITZER, E., BRUNDELL, J.: Europ. J. Pharmacol. **34**, 199 (1975)]

bined action of an α-adrenoceptor antagonist, phentolamine, and a drug which blocks endogenous prostaglandin synthesis, such as indomethacin (Fig. 38). Moreover, arachidonic acid, a prostaglandin precursor, was more effective in contracting vein strips in the presence of ergotamine or dihydroergotamine than in the presence of noradrenaline or potassium chloride or in control strips (MÜLLER-SCHWEINITZER, 1973, 1974a, b, c; MÜLLER-SCHWEINITZER and BRUNDELL, 1975a, b). Although a significant increase in the level of prostaglandin E-like activity in the bathing fluid occurred with both noradrenaline- and ergotamine-induced contractions, only the latter were decreased by indomethacin (MÜLLER-SCHWEINITZER and BRUNDELL, 1975a, b), indicating that in dogs the venoconstrictor responses to ergotamine and to dihydroergotamine are mediated at least partly by enhanced formation of a vasoactive prostaglandin-like substance, possibly an intermediate of prostaglandin synthesis.

Enhancement of endogenous prostaglandin synthesis in venous smooth muscle cells by ergot alkaloids seems to be species-dependent, since it was not possible to repeat these observations either on human or on feline vein strips (MÜLLER-SCHWEINITZER, unpublished).

Contractions of canine saphenous arteries were also accompanied by formation of a prostaglandin-like material which, however, had opposite physiological effects. In arteries, indomethacin *enhanced* dihydroergotamine-induced contractions (Fig. 38) and arachidonic acid had *relaxant* activity. In contrast to the findings in veins, in canine arterial vascular smooth muscles endogenous prostaglandin synthesis was *not* significantly enhanced by dihydroergotamine (MÜLLER-SCHWEINITZER, 1974b; MÜLLER-SCHWEINITZER and BRUNDELL, 1975b). Ergotamine, dihydroergotamine, 1-methyl ergotamine and methysergide (1 μg/min) also failed to affect the prostaglandin output from the isolated perfused cat spleen induced by sympathetic nerve stimulation, and only a relatively high concentration (10 μg/min) of methysergide increased the prostaglandin output during sympathetic nerve stimulation (SALZMANN and PACHA, 1976). In isolated perfused rat lungs, where 5-HT has been shown to release prostaglandin-like material, methysergide (5–200 ng/ml) and ergotamine (650 ng/ml) alone failed to modify prostaglandin release (ALABASTER and BAKHLE, 1976; BAKHLE and SMITH, 1972, 1974a). In vitro, D-LSD slightly inhibited the conversion of 8,11,14-eicosatrienoic acid into prostaglandin E_1 by bovine seminal vesicles only when used at extremely high concentrations (372 μM) (BURNSTEIN et al., 1973).

In vivo, D-LSD (0.2 mg/kg i.p.) failed to induce changes in the level of prostaglandins in rat cerebral cortex (ZATZ and ROTH, 1975). These observations have been largely confirmed in cats using methysergide. In unanesthetized cats, injection of 5-HT into the rostral hypothalamus produced a biphasic response of body temperature of which the delayed and long-lasting hyperthermic phase could be abolished by pretreatment with indomethacin, indicating the involvement of endogenous prostaglandin synthesis. Methysergide attenuated the initial temperature increase but failed to reduce the secondary, by a sustained release of prostaglandin mediated, hyperthermia (KOMISKEY and RUDY, 1975).

2. Interference of Ergot Alkaloids With Prostaglandin Effects

On isolated canine saphenous veins, the potency of exogenous prostaglandin E_2 was significantly increased in the presence of dihydroergotamine, whereas on isolated canine saphenous arteries dihydroergotamine did not change the responses to prostaglandin E_2 (MÜLLER-SCHWEINITZER and BRUNDELL, 1975b). Methysergide failed to change the vasoconstrictor activity of prostaglandin $F_{2\alpha}$ on canine basilar arteries in vitro (ALLEN et al., 1974) and in vivo in dogs (NAKANO, 1968) and monkeys (WHITE et al., 1971a, b) and failed to prevent death induced by prostaglandin $F_{2\alpha}$ in mice (HARPER and SKARNES, 1972). D-LSD also failed to affect responses to both prostaglandin A_2 in the isolated guinea-pig ileum (STRACZOWSKI et al., 1974) and prostaglandin E_1 on isolated canine mesenteric arteries (STRONG and BOHR, 1967a, b).

In addition to various mediators, e.g., biogenic amines such as histamine and 5-HT, prostaglandins are involved in changes of vascular permeability during inflammation. In rats, inflammatory effects of locally injected prostaglandins E_1 and E_2 were partially reduced by pretreatment of the animals with methysergide (RICO et al., 1973; GYIRES and KNOLL, 1975; CRUNCKHORN and WILLIS, 1971). Since methysergide is a potent 5-HT antagonist, it is likely that its effect in these experiments was due to inhibition of responses to 5-HT released by prostaglandins (CHAHL and LADD, 1976).

There is evidence that in some tissues prostaglandin E_1 interacts with structures of the cell membrane functionally related to the 5-HT D-receptors. Thus, when canine tracheal rings were made to contract by 5-HT, 8 ng/ml prostaglandin E_1 caused complete relaxation, whereas 64-times-higher prostaglandin E_1 concentrations induced only partial relaxation of tracheal rings contracted by acetylcholine. Methysergide (1–10 µg/ml) antagonized this relaxant activity of prostaglandin E_1 dose-dependently in the presence of acetylcholine, whereas dihydroergotamine showed no inhibitory effect. It was concluded that in dog tracheal smooth muscle, prostaglandin E_1 acts at the membrane surface at or close to the specific 5-HT receptor (TÜRKER and KHAIRALLAH, 1969). A further demonstration of an interaction between prostaglandin E_1 and 5-HT receptor sites was provided on the isolated duodenum from reserpinized rats. In this preparation, prostaglandin E_1-induced contractions, which are presumably mediated by some mechanisms other than release of 5-HT, could be antagonized by BOL-148 (20–40 ng/ml) but were unchanged after atropine or dihydroergotamine (KHAIRALLAH et al., 1967).

Binding studies with D-[^{3}H]LSD have suggested that the affinity of D-LSD to synaptosomes of rat cerebral cortical gray matter is increased by prostaglandin E_1 (FARROW and VUNAKIS, 1973).

In conclusion: (1) Interaction of ergot alkaloids with prostaglandin synthesis has been shown only in the smooth muscle cells of canine veins where both ergotamine and dihydroergotamine induced enhanced formation of a prostaglandin-like substance with venoconstrictor activity; (2) Interaction of ergot alkaloids with prostaglandin effects has been demonstrated in certain smooth muscles, like canine trachea and rat duodenum, where prostaglandin E_1 seems to act at or close to the 5-HT D-receptor and can be antagonized by methysergide or BOL-148, respectively.

J. Stimulation of Smooth Muscle by Ergot Alkaloids Mediated by Miscellaneous Mechanisms

In addition to interaction of ergot alkaloids with defined receptor sites of endogenous agents, as described in the preceding sections of this chapter, there exists the phenomenon of potentation of responses to other agonists by ergot alkaloids. This phenomenon, which concerns the effects of various endogenous amines, acetylcholine and other agents, such as angiotensin and vasopressin, appears to be mediated by different mechanisms.

1. Enhancement of Responses to Biogenic Amines by Ergot Alkaloids in Vascular Smooth Muscles

There exist arteries, predominantly branches from the external carotid vascular bed, where low concentrations of ergot derivatives cause enhancement of responses to biogenic amines, such as catecholamines, histamine and 5-HT. Potentiation of responses to biogenic amines has also been observed when these were tested after perfusion of an isolated rabbit ear artery with a high concentration of 5-HT or tryptamine (GINZEL and KOTTEGODA, 1953) or when catecholamines were tested during perfusion of an isolated rabbit ear or human temporal artery with 5-HT (CARROLL and GLOVER, 1973; CARROLL et al., 1974; DE LA LANDE and RAND, 1965; DE LA LANDE et al., 1966; SAVINI, 1956).

The most frequently used in vitro preparation showing enhanced responses to biogenic amines in the presence of ergot compounds is the isolated rabbit ear artery. In this preparation sensitization to the vasoconstrictor activity of catecholamines and also to that of histamine could be induced with 5-HT as well as with low concentrations of D-LSD (GADDUM, 1954; GADDUM and HAMEED, 1954; SAVINI, 1956), ergometrine (CARROLL and GLOVER, 1973), methysergide (APPERLEY et al., 1976; CARROLL and GLOVER, 1973; CARROLL et al., 1972, 1974; DE LA LANDE et al., 1966; FOZARD, 1973a, b, 1976a, b), and with low concentrations of peptide alkaloids, such as ergotoxin (JANG, 1941), ergotamine, 1-methyl-ergotamine and dihydroergotamine (CARROLL and GLOVER, 1973; CARROLL et al., 1972, 1974; OSSWALD and GUIMARÃES, 1962).

Contrary to these observations, BOL-148 (10–100 ng/ml) did not consistently sensitize the isolated rabbit ear artery to the vasoconstrictor activity of noradrenaline. BOL-148 enhanced the vasoconstrictor response to 5-HT at the 20 ng/ml concentration level and above (FOZARD, 1973b), but it markedly reduced the degree of sensitization produced by 5–10 ng/ml 5-HT (DE LA LANDE et al., 1966).

The responsiveness of the isolated perfused human temporal artery resembles that of the rabbit ear artery. Methysergide, injected at concentrations of 1–10 ng and 5-HT in the same concentration range enhanced responses to noradrenaline and histamine. The same phenomenon could be observed with dihydroergotamine or ergotamine (0.1–5 ng) and with 1-methyl-ergotamine (1–10 ng). Compared to the potentiation caused by 5-HT or methysergide, however, that induced by the ergot peptides did not occur immediately, but it was more prolonged (CARROLL and GLOVER, 1973; CARROLL et al., 1972, 1974). These in vitro findings were confirmed by clinical studies. In human subjects ergotamine (0.5 mg i.v.) caused constriction of the temporal artery, and this effect was enhanced in response to "cold pressure" and noradrenaline (PICHLER et al., 1956).

On spiral strips from dog external carotid arteries ergotamine shifted the dose-response curve for noradrenaline to the left. The maximum sensitization to the vasoconstrictor effects of noradrenaline (ca. 4-fold) was induced with about 2 nM ergotamine added 60 min previously to the bathing fluid, a concentration which in saphenous arteries from the same dogs had considerable α-adrenergic blocking activity (MÜLLER-SCHWEINITZER and STÜRMER, 1975). In canine nasal mucosa vessels ergotamine at low doses potentiated also 5-HT-induced vasoconstriction as assessed by volume (pressure) changes in the closed nasal cavity (SCHÖNBAUM et al., 1974).

The most consistent enhancement of responses to noradrenaline, tyramine, histamine, 5-HT, tryptamine and vasopressin in arteries from the external carotid vasculature was observed with methysergide. Besides potentiating effects of various biogenic amines in arterial preparations from the rabbit ear and human temporal artery in vitro (APPERLEY et al., 1976; CARROLL and GLOVER, 1973; CARROLL et al., 1972, 1974; DE LA LANDE et al., 1966; FOZARD, 1973a, b, 1976a, b), it enhanced vasoconstrictor responses to noradrenaline in the external carotid vascular bed from dogs (SAXENA, 1972a, b, 1975) and those to 5-HT in the vessels of canine nasal mucosa (SCHÖNBAUM and LAMAR, 1975; SCHÖNBAUM et al., 1975).

Besides the external carotid vasculature from different species, enhancement of the vasoconstrictor activity of catecholamines by an ergolene derivative has also been demonstrated in the isolated perfused rat kidney, where D-LSD even in large doses failed to inhibit the action of adrenaline or noradrenaline. On the contrary, D-LSD (0.1 μg) increased the vasoconstriction caused by adrenaline, while a comparable 5-HT vasoconstriction was diminished (CERLETTI, 1955).

In man, potentiation of the stimulating activity of adrenaline by D-LSD has been demonstrated in the venoconstriction test (DEL BIANCO et al., 1972). This finding was confirmed by the recent observation that in the same test responses to 5-HT were also potentiated by ng concentrations of D-LSD, methysergide and ergotamine (FANCIULLACCI et al., 1975; SICUTERI et al., 1975).

The mechanism by which ergot alkaloids sensitize vascular smooth muscle cells is still unclear. Based upon the observation that in rabbit ear and human temporal arteries neither cyproheptadine and pizotifen, which are very potent 5-HT antagonists, nor morphine prevented sensitization of smooth muscle cells by both 5-HT and ergot compounds, it has been assumed that potentiation is mediated by separate receptors which are not identical with the 5-HT receptor mediating vasoconstriction (CARROLL and GLOVER, 1973; CARROLL et al., 1974). Separate 5-HT vasoconstrictor and dilator receptors have been proposed to exist also in the dog carotid vasculature (SCHÖNBAUM et al., 1974; VARGAFTIG and LEFORT, 1974). Studies on common 5-HT antagonists suggested that in the carotid vascular bed of dogs receptors for 5-HT are of a "special" type that differ from the usual musculotropic D-receptors present in other vascular and nonvascular smooth muscles (SAXENA et al., 1971; SAXENA, 1972a, 1974a, b; SAXENA and DE VLAAM SCHLUTER, 1974).

An alternative explanation might be that ergot compounds cause potentiation by noradrenaline uptake inhibition. However, this would preclude potentiation of those agents which are not taken up by storage sites. Moreover, there is no evidence that ergot alkaloids at pharmacologically active concentrations block the amine-uptake by vascular tissue.

Findings that 5-HT enhanced vasoconstrictor responses not only to noradrenaline but also those to histamine and angiotensin, and that sensitization could also occur in the phenoxybenzamine-treated artery as well as in the chronically sympathectomized artery, indicated that the sensitization resulted from a nonspecific interaction (DE LA LANDE and RAND, 1965; DE LA LANDE et al., 1966). On the other hand, no experimental data exist suggesting that 5-HT or ergot alkaloids interfere with a later step in the chain of events following the receptor stimulation by an agonist.

FOZARD (1973b, 1976a, b) suggested that sensitization of the rabbit ear artery results from a subthreshold vasoconstriction achieving threshold or greater levels in the presence of other vasoconstrictor agents. This would imply that only compounds with intrinsic activity will enhance the effects of other vasoconstrictor agents, and that the potentiating compound develops its stimulating activity via receptors or mechanisms which differ from those activated by the potentiated drug. This suggestion was supported by the observation that sensitization of the rabbit ear artery could be prevented if steps were undertaken to eliminate the vasoconstrictor properties of the potentiating drug and by the fact that other compounds, for example histamine, produced a similar degree of sensitization at concentrations producing comparable vasoconstriction (FOZARD, 1976a, b).

In spiral strips from canine external carotid arteries ergotamine caused constriction by stimulating 5-HT receptors (MÜLLER-SCHWEINITZER, 1976a). At the same time, ergotamine enhanced responses to noradrenaline while blocking those to 5-HT (MÜLLER-SCHWEINITZER and STÜRMER, 1975). In this preparation, responses to noradrenaline were also enhanced after treatment with cocaine (33 μM) as well as after inhibition of endogenous prostaglandin synthesis with indomethacin (0.3 μM). Both cocaine and indomethacin caused a slight increase in tension by themselves, indicating some (indirect) stimulating activity (MÜLLER-SCHWEINITZER, unpublished 1975b).

These results thus support the notion that the phenomenon of potentiation of responses to other vasoconstrictor agents is a nonspecific effect of compounds with intrinsic vasoconstrictor activity (FOZARD, 1976b).

2. Enhancement of Responses to Biogenic Agents by Ergot Alkaloids in Nonvascular Smooth Muscles

Investigations on the amine potentiating effect of ergot compounds on the nictitating membrane of the cat demonstrated that most ergolene derivatives of the amide type, such as methysergide (DALESSIO et al., 1962), D-LSD, ALD-52 (1-acetyl-lysergic acid diethylamide), LAE-32 (d-lysergic acid ethylamide) and LSM (d-lysergic acid morpholide) at threshold doses of about 2 μg/kg i.v. effectively enhanced responses to catecholamines. BOL-148 was about 100 times less potent than D-LSD (COSTA and ZETLER, 1959). As observed with blood vessels from the carotid bed, responses to adrenaline in the cat nictitating membrane could be also enhanced by 5-HT (LECOMTE, 1953).

By contrast the amine potentiation induced by ergot alkaloids of the peptide type, such as ergotamine, dihydroergotamine, 1-methylergotamine and ergostine could be observed only within a limited dose range because of an α-adrenoceptor blocking activity becoming manifest at doses of 50 μg/kg i.v. (COSTA and ZETLER, 1959; DA GRACA FERNANDES and OSSWALD, 1967; SALZMANN and PACHA, 1968; SALZMANN et al., 1967, 1968; SALZMANN and WEIDMANN, 1966; WEIDMANN and TAESCHLER, 1966).

Further studies demonstrated that in the cat nictitating membrane ergot compounds, besides potentiating responses to catecholamines, also augmented those to 5-HT. When combined with 5-HT, however, the ergot alkaloids of the peptide type, e.g., ergotamine, dihydroergotamine and 1-methyl ergotamine, proved to be more potent than the ergolene derivative methysergide (SALZMANN and KALBERER, 1973; SALZMANN and WEIDMANN, 1966; WEIDMANN and TAESCHLER, 1966).

Besides potentiating the effect of various amines, ergot compounds, such as D-LSD, BOL-148, ergotamine and dihydroergotamine, produced gradually increasing contractions of the cat nictitating membrane in vitro, indicating intrinsic activity (THOMPSON, 1958). In vivo the ergotoxine-induced contraction of the cat nictitating membrane could be blocked by chlorpromazine, which has 5-HT receptor blocking activity (GYERMEK, 1966), as well as by the α-adrenoceptor blocking agents dibenamine and phentolamine (GYÖRGY et al., 1958a). Moreover, it has been demonstrated that the presence of sympathetic tonus or that of a physiological transmitter is not necessary, indicating that ergot compounds stimulate the cat nictitating membrane by acting directly at the periphery. WEIDMANN and TAESCHLER (1966) mentioned that the ergot compounds used in their studies caused amine potentiation in the cat nictitating membrane as well as vasoconstriction at the same dose ranges. The authors concluded that the same mechanisms might be involved in both potentiation and vasoconstriction. It seems likely, therefore, that in the cat nictitating membrane the amine potentiating activity of ergot alkaloids is mediated by the same mechanism as in the vessels of the carotid bed, i.e., by subthreshold stimulation.

D-LSD potentiated contractions elicited by noradrenaline in the isolated rabbit uterus (VALDECASA et al., 1956) and in isolated vasa deferentia from rats (AREFOLOV et al., 1975) and guinea-pigs, though it produced no observable effect by itself (HITNER and DI GREGORIO, 1974; HUGHES, 1973). Similarly, ergometrine, which alone had no stimulating activity, increased the maximum response to cumulative doses of noradrenaline in the isolated guinea-pig vas deferens. In the same preparation ergometrine decreased the maximum response to cumulative doses of dopamine, with some potentiation of the effects of low concentrations of the agonist (WOODRUFF et al., 1969, 1970).

The mechanism by which both D-LSD and ergometrine sensitize these preparations to the constrictor activity of noradrenaline appears to be different from that proposed for the amine potentiation in carotid vessels and cat nictitating membrane, since neither D-LSD nor ergometrine developed any stimulating activity. In addition, the possibility of motor transmission by 5-HT in the guinea-pig vas deferens has been excluded (AMBACHE and ZAR, 1971). Thus, it can be assumed that there exist no postjunctional 5-HT receptors which could function as binding sites for ergolene derivatives. However, D-LSD has been shown to interact with prejunctional α-adrenoceptors in the isolated guinea-pig vas deferens (HUGHES, 1973). Moreover, inhibition of noradrenaline uptake by various ergot alkaloids has been demonstrated in different extravascular tissues (cf. Section D, part 3 of this chapter). It seems possible, therefore, that both D-LSD and ergometrine potentiate noradrenaline effects in the guinea-pig vas deferens by $uptake_1$ inhibition via stimulation of prejunctional α-adrenoceptors.

There exist only a small number of reports concerning enhancement of 5-HT in extravascular smooth muscles. Using extremely low concentrations of D-LSD

(0.005–0.2 ng/ml), enhancement of 5-HT effects on the isolated rat uterus has been described (COSTA, 1956; DELAY and THUILLIER, 1956), an observation which, however, could not be confirmed by CERLETTI and DOEPFNER (1958b). Some enhancement of 5-HT effects has also been observed with relatively high concentrations of ergotamine (2.5–25 μg/ml) in the isolated rat duodenum (LEVY and MICHEL-BER, 1956) and with both ergotamine and BOL-148 in the gastric longitudinal muscles from the fish *Pleuronectes platessa* (GROVE et al., 1974). In the isolated heart from the snail *Helix pomatia*, 0.1 μg/ml D-LSD caused enhancement and prolongation of the effects of both 5-HT and intestinal nerve stimulation (RÓZSA and GRAUL, 1964).

Potentiation of smooth muscle stimulating effects of acetylcholine by methysergide has been observed in the isolated guinea-pig vas deferens (KATSURAGI and SUZUKI, 1974), human intestine (GLEGG and TURNER, 1971; METCALFE and TURNER, 1969, 1970; TURNER, 1973) and in the isolated dog trachea (TÜRKER and KHAIRALLAH, 1969). D-LSD appeared to enhance the bronchospasm induced by acetylcholine in anesthetized guinea-pigs while preventing that evoked by 5-HT (HOLGATE and WARNER, 1960). BOL-148 (0.2–1 μg/ml) enhanced responses to acetylcholine in the isolated rat stomach strip (VANE, 1957), while both methysergide (1 nM) and ergotamine (10 nM) failed to change responses to acetylcholine in this preparation (FRANKHUIJZEN, 1975; FRANKHUIJZEN and BONTA, 1974b). Within a small concentration range (0.1–1 μg/ml), however, ergotamine potentiated responses to acetylcholine in the isolated guinea-pig vas deferens (BOYD et al., 1960) and more consistently in the isolated rabbit uterus (BRÜGGER, 1938). Enhancement of the stimulatory activity of acetylcholine by dihydroergotoxine mesylate has been observed in the toad rectus abdominis muscle (BURN and NG, 1964).

Several authors attributed the mechanism by which ergot alkaloids enhance acetylcholine effects in smooth muscles to an anticholinesterase activity. In fact, inhibition of cholinesterase could be demonstrated with most ergot derivatives when used at sufficiently high concentrations (AMMON, 1935; BOYD et al., 1960; BRÜGGER, 1938; GAUTRELET and SCHEINER, 1939; GLEGG and TURNER, 1971; LOEWI and NAVRATIL, 1926; MATTHES, 1930; NAVRATIL, 1937; SIMON and WINTER, 1976; THOMPSON et al., 1954, 1955). However, several observations contradict the assumption that potentiation of acetylcholine effects by ergot alkaloids is caused by cholinesterase inhibition. BRÜGGER (1938) already mentioned that the mode of action of the ergot alkaloids ergotamine and ergometrine differed from that of physostigmine. While physostigmine potentiated acetylcholine effects in both rabbit uterus and guinea-pig vas deferens, the ergot alkaloids consistently enhanced acetylcholine effects only in the rabbit uterus. Both ergot alkaloids developed intrinsic activity, while physostigmine failed to stimulate the rabbit uterus. On the other hand, physostigmine proved to be about 100 times more potent than the ergot alkaloids when tested as cholinesterase inhibitor (BRÜGGER, 1938). In the guinea-pig vas deferens, methysergide potentiated not only responses to acetylcholine but also those to arecoline which were unchanged after cholinesterase inhibition by neostigmine (KATSURAGI and SUZUKI, 1974). Together these observations indicate that ergot alkaloids act quite differently from a cholinesterase inhibitor.

In conclusion, the most consistent enhancement of effects of biogenic agents induced by ergot alkaloids has been observed in vascular smooth muscles and seems to be a characteristic property of the external carotid bed.

K. Biochemical Identification of Specific Binding Sites for Ergot Alkaloids

D. HAUSER

It is generally accepted that the first event in drug action is the formation of a reversible complex between the drug (D) and a specific receptor (R) following second order reaction kinetics:

$$R + D \underset{k_d}{\overset{k_a}{\rightleftarrows}} RD$$

Under steady-state conditions the affinity constant K_A is given by

$$K_A = \frac{1}{K_D} = \frac{k_a}{k_d} = \frac{[RD]}{[R][D]}$$

where K_D is the dissociation constant, k_a and k_d are the rate constants of association and dissociation, and $[RD]$, $[R]$ and $[D]$ are the concentrations of drug-receptor complex, unoccupied receptor and free drug, respectively.

During the past few years considerable progress has been made in the identification and purification of a variety of specific membrane and intracellular binding sites, the binding characteristics of which are consistent with those expected of a receptor.

It is now generally agreed that the term "receptor" refers to a molecule or molecular complex, which is capable of recognizing and selectively interacting with an endogenous compound or a drug, and which, after binding it, is capable of generating some signal that leads ultimately to a biological response (EHRENPREIS et al., 1969; BIRNBAUMER et al., 1974; KAHN, 1976). Since receptors have not yet been identified as pure chemical entities, KAHN (1976) has defined a receptor as "a cellular component which has the ability to selectively recognize and bind an endogenous molecule or a drug and which has binding characteristics consistent with a potential for signal generation."

Cytoplasmic receptors are the prime target of steroid hormones (LIAO, 1975; O'MALLEY and HARDMAN, 1975), whereas receptors for other hormones, neurotransmitters, and antigens are associated with the cell surface (CUATRECASAS and GREAVES, 1976).

In the early 1960's radioactively labeled ligands were already being used to study directly the interaction of endogenous compounds or drugs with their specific receptors, but the problem of nonspecific adsorption tended to complicate these studies. Most radioactive compounds bind to biological membranes and to many other surfaces besides. Since the number of such nonspecific sites is virtually infinite by comparison with the small number of hormone or neurotransmitter receptors, it seemed impossible to identify specific sites in the presence of a vast majority of nonspecific sites.

"Specific binding" usually refers to that portion of bound radioactivity, which is displaced in the presence of an excess of structurally and stereochemically specific ligands. A typical example of the relationship between specific and nonspecific binding is given in Figure 39. Nonspecific binding of [^{3}H]dihydroergotamine to brain membranes, measured in the presence of a large excess of nonradioactive dihydroergotamine, increases by contrast with total binding linearly with [^{3}H]dihydroergotamine concentration (CLOSSE and HAUSER, 1976). At 0.2 nM [^{3}H]dihydroergotamine nonspecific binding represents only about 20% of total binding. In

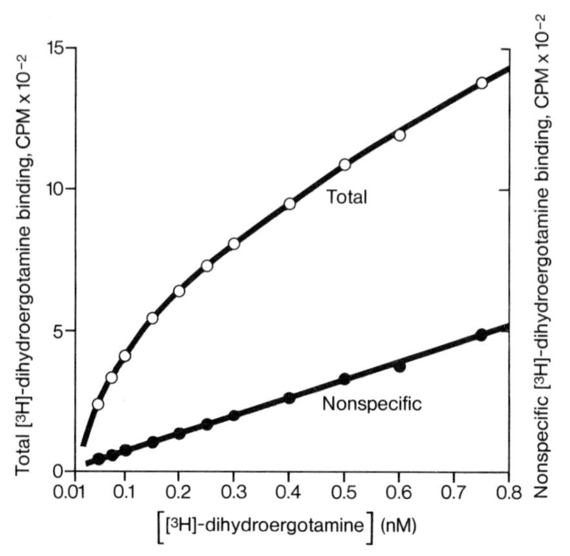

Fig. 39. Saturation of [^{3}H]dihydroergotamine binding. Increasing concentrations of [^{3}H]dihydroergotamine were incubated with rat brain membranes in the presence (nonspecific) or absence (total) of 10 μM unlabeled dihydroergotamine. Incubation was terminated by cooling to 0° C, and bound and free [^{3}H]dihydroergotamine were separated by centrifugation. (CLOSSE and HAUSER, unpublished)

order to perform binding studies at such low concentrations, a specific radioactivity of more than 15 Ci/mmole is desirable.

The problem of nonspecific binding was overcome by using ligands of high pharmacologic potency and labeled to high specific radioactivity. This method was first used successfully with the peptide hormones ACTH and angiotensin (ROTH, 1973). Since then numerous analogous studies have been undertaken in order to identify specific hormone and neurotransmitter binding sites (SNYDER and BENNETT, 1976).

Such binding measurements are supposed to reflect the interaction with a pharmacologic receptor, if a number of criteria is satisfied: (1) The labeled ligand used as a membrane probe must be fully active biologically, so as to mimic the activity of the parent endogenous compound. The binding must demonstrate (2) strict structural and steric specificity and (3) saturability, which indicates a finite and limited number of binding sites. (4) The presence of the binding should be restricted to tissues known to be physiologically sensitive to the parent agonist. (5) The binding should in most cases demonstrate reversibility, which is kinetically consistent with the physiological effects of the parent compound (CUATRECASAS et al., 1975; HOLLENBERG and CUATRECASAS, 1975).

1. Interaction of Ergot Compounds With Specific Sites in the Central Nervous System

D-LSD is a highly potent 5-HT antagonist in smooth muscle preparations (cf. Section B, part 1,c), and it has been assumed that the hallucinogenic effects of D-LSD are mediated by an interaction with 5-HT receptors. It is therefore not surprising that most of the earlier studies dealing with the biochemical identification of 5-HT receptors employed D-LSD and other ergot compounds as inhibitors of 5-HT binding.

Using [^{14}C]5-HT of low specific radioactivity MARCHBANKS et al. (1964) and MARCHBANKS (1966) identified three binding sites in nerve ending particles obtained from rat brain. [^{14}C]5-HT binding at the "high" affinity site ($K_D = 5 \cdot 10^{-7}$ M) was inhibited by both D-LSD and the pharmacologically inactive antipode L-LSD (MARCHBANKS, 1967). This binding site therefore lacked the stereospecificity expected of a receptor binding site. In analogous studies with [^{14}C]5-HT, binding was partially inhibited not only by D-LSD (WISE and RUELIUS, 1968; DETTE and WESEMANN, 1975) but also by morphine and D-tubocurarine (UNGAR et al., 1976). Stereospecificity was not determined in any of these studies.

With the availability of D-[^{3}H]LSD of higher specific radioactivity (>1 Ci/mmole), it became possible to identify low concentrations of high affinity binding sites (dissociation constant $K_D < 10^{-8}$M). FARROW and VAN VUNAKIS (1972, 1973), using equilibrium dialysis, characterized high ($K_D = 9$ nM) as well as medium ($K_D = 1{,}2$ μM) affinity binding of D-[^{3}H]LSD to subcellular fractions of grey matter in rat cerebral cortex. Bound D-[^{3}H]LSD was displaced by 5-HT, certain other hallucinogenic drugs, and the D-LSD antagonist L-methyl-1,2,5,6-tetrahydropyridine-N,N-diethylcarboxamide (CHRISTIAN et al., 1975) but not by L-LSD, the unnatural antipode. In other words, the binding was found to be stereospecific by contrast with earlier findings. DIAB et al. (1971) demonstrated by autoradiography of freeze-dried sections, binding of D-[^{3}H]LSD in vivo to specific neurones in the caudate nucleus, midbrain, medulla, and cortex of rats.

Using either centrifugation or the more efficient and rapid filtration technique of PERT and SNYDER (1973), saturable, stereospecific D-[^{3}H]LSD binding of high affinity ($K_D = 4$–10 nM) has been confirmed in several rat brain regions (BENNETT and AGHAJANIAN, 1974; BENNET and SNYDER, 1975; LOVELL and FREEDMAN, 1976). The highest concentrations of D-[^{3}H]LSD binding sites are found in the corpus striatum, cerebral cortex, and hippocampus. The association and dissociation rates of binding are temperature dependent, equilibrium being reached most rapidly at 37° C (Fig. 40).

Lesion in the midbrain raphé nuclei, which results in degeneration of the serotoninergic input to the forebrain (KUHAR et al., 1972a), does not affect D-[^{3}H]LSD binding (BENNETT and AGHAJANIAN, 1974; BENNETT and SNYDER, 1975). Hence D-LSD binding is probably not associated with presynaptic sites.

D-LSD (but not L-LSD), BOL-148, D-isolysergic acid amide, and methysergide are potent inhibitors of specific [^{3}H]5-HT binding to rat brain membranes (BENNETT and SNYDER, 1976; FILLION et al., 1976). In fact, D-[^{3}H]LSD and [^{3}H]5-HT binding sites have a close resemblance (BENNETT and SNYDER, 1976). The regional and developmental patterns are similar for both sites. Furthermore, BENNETT and AGHAJANIAN (1976) have shown that the concentration required for half-saturation of specific D-LSD binding in vitro corresponds to the concentration in vivo, at which the activity of raphé neurones containing 5-HT are inhibited by D-LSD.

Dihydroergotamine, which has been found to antagonize 5-HT effects in basilar arteries (Table 1), binds saturably, reversibly, and with high affinity ($K_D = 0.2$ nM) to rat brain membranes (CLOSSE and HAUSER, 1976).

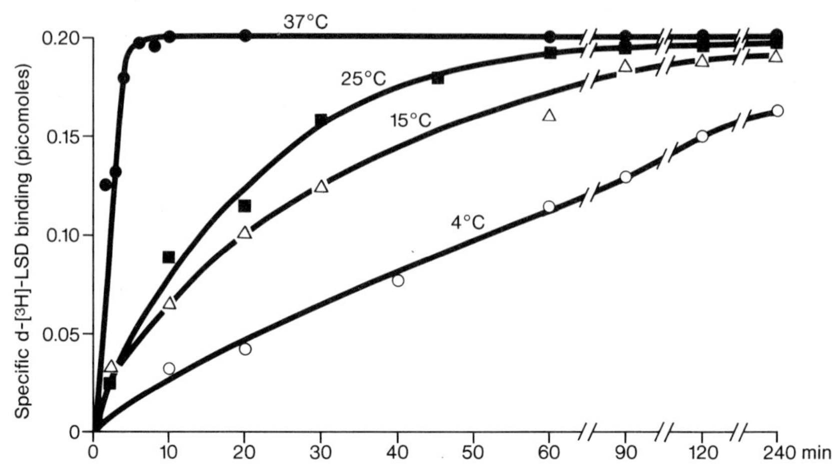

Fig. 40. Association rates of D-[^{3}H]LSD binding at different temperatures. Aliquots of cerebral cortex P3 membranes were incubated with 3 nM D-[^{3}H]LSD at various temperatures for varying lengths of time in 50 mM TRIS·HCl buffer with 0.1% ascorbic acid. The samples were then filtered and specific D-[^{3}H]LSD binding was counted after the addition of 15 ml scintillation liquid. [From Figure 2, BENNETT, J.P., SNYDER, S.H.: Brain Res. **94**, 523 (1975)]

Specific [^{3}H]dihydroergotamine binding, which is defined as the difference between binding in the absence (total binding) and presence (nonspecific binding) of a large excess of unlabeled dihydroergotamine, is saturable, half-maximal saturation occurring at approximately 0.2 nM (Fig. 41, *inset*). Scatchard analysis of the same data gives a curve with upward concavity (Fig. 41), which can be interpreted as negative cooperativity of a single class or the existence of multiple classes of binding sites.

The dissociation constant K_D of the high affinity site under steady-state conditions is 0.23 nM, which agrees well with the value obtained independently from kinetic analysis of [^{3}H]dihydroergotamine binding. Both the association and dissociation rates of [^{3}H]dihydroergotamine binding are comparatively slow. In the forward reaction at 37° C, equilibrium is reached in 30 min, whereas in the dissociation reaction the half-life is approximately 20 min (Fig. 42, *inset*).

The regional and subcellular distribution of specific [^{3}H]dihydroergotamine binding (CLOSSE and HAUSER, 1976) resembles the localization of [^{3}H]5-HT binding in rat brain (BENNETT and SNYDER, 1976). In both cases the concentration of specific binding sites is highest in the hippocampus and the corpus striatum and lowest in the cerebellum. At the subcellular level specific binding sites are most numerous in the "synaptosomal" fraction.

[^{3}H]Dihydroergotamine binding is stereospecific, the pharmacologically inactive antipode of dihydroergotamine (STADLER and STÜRMER, 1970) being more than 2000 times less potent than dihydroergotamine in inhibiting specific [^{3}H]dihydroergotamine binding. Assay of membranes from the whole rat brain reveals that 5-HT is the only neurotransmitter capable of inhibiting specific [^{3}H]dihydroergotamine binding (CLOSSE and HAUSER, 1976). l- and d-noradrenaline in particular,

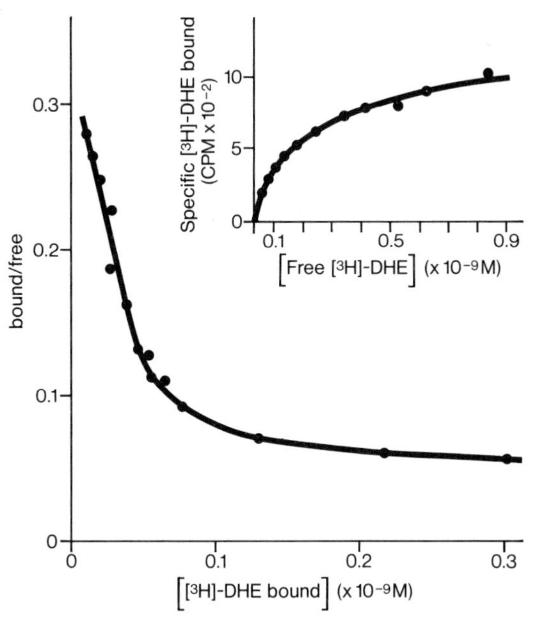

Fig. 41. Binding of [^{3}H]dihydroergotamine to rat brain membranes as a function of [^{3}H]dihydroergotamine concentration. Increasing concentrations of [^{3}H]dihydroergotamine were incubated with rat brain membranes in the presence (nonspecific) and absence (total) of 10 μM nonradioactive dihydroergotamine. Values of total [^{3}H]dihydroergotamine binding are plotted according to SCATCHARD. Inset: Saturation of specific [^{3}H]dihydroergotamine binding. [From Figure 4, CLOSSE, A., HAUSER, D.: Life Sci. **19**, 1857 (1976)]

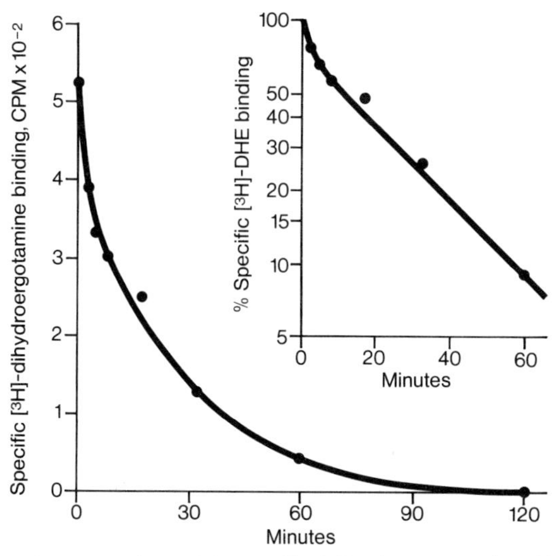

Fig. 42. Time course of dissociation of bound [^{3}H]dihydroergotamine. Rat brain membranes were incubated with [^{3}H]dihydroergotamine (nM) for 30 min at 37° C. Nonradioactive dihydroergotamine (20 μM final concentration) was added and [^{3}H]dihydroergotamine binding was assayed at various times. Inset: Semilogarithmic plot of the same data. [From Figure 3, CLOSSE, A., HAUSER, D.: Life Sci. **19**, 1856 (1976)]

and a variety of α-adrenergic agonists and antagonists, are very weak inhibitors of specific [^{3}H]dihydroergotamine binding (Closse and Hauser, 1976).

The characteristic of D-LSD binding suggest (Bennett and Aghajanian, 1974; Bennett and Snyder, 1976) that in most brain regions specific D-LSD binding sites are related to postsynaptic 5-HT receptors. The differential ligand specificity at D-[^{3}H]LSD and [^{3}H]5-HT binding sites is consistent with a two-state receptor model as proposed by Snyder and Bennett (1976). Thus [^{3}H]5-HT would bind with 5-HT receptors in the "agonist state," while D-LSD, a mixed agonist-antagonist, binds with equal affinity to both the "agonist" and "antagonist states."

With dihydroergotamine the available evidence is less conclusive.

In some regions of the brain D-[^{3}H]LSD binding appears to involve other than 5-HT receptor sites. In calf caudate nucleus D-[^{3}H]LSD binding has been linked, in part at least, with postsynaptic dopamine receptors (Burt et al., 1976a). Ergotamine, ergocornine, ergocristine, α-ergokryptine, ergometrine and bromocriptine have substantial affinity for specific dopamine binding sites as well (Cresse et al., 1976; Burt et al., 1976b), which is compatible with many of the known pharmacologic effects of these drugs (cf. Section C).

Several ergot compounds, including dihydroergotamine, are very potent inhibitors at binding sites of both the α-adrenoceptor agonist [^{3}H]clonidine and the α-adrenoceptor antagonist [^{3}H]WB-4101 (Greenberg et al., 1976; S.H. Snyder, personal communication). Whether these central α-adrenoceptor binding sites are relevant to the action of ergot compounds remains to be seen.

2. Peripheral Binding Sites for Ergot Compounds

Recently, a specific binding site for [^{3}H]dihydroergokryptine has been identified on cell membranes of the rabbit uterus (Williams and Lefkowitz, 1976). The characteristics of this site differ from those of the binding site for the closely related [^{3}H]dihydroergotamine identified in the rat brain (Closse and Hauser, 1976). In the peripheral tissue preparation, steady-state binding is reached much more rapidly, and ligand specificity satisfies the criteria that must be fulfilled for the identification of α-adrenoceptors. Binding of [^{3}H]dihydroergokryptine is rapid and stereospecific; α-adrenoceptor agonists and antagonists have binding affinities that parallel their potencies in eliciting or blocking physiological α-adrenergic responses.

L. References

Åberg, G., Andersson, R., Welin-Fogelberg, I.: Inhibition of tone in the taenia of the guinea pig caecum. Europ. J. Pharmacol. **7**, 296–299 (1969)

Abrahams, S.L.: Effect of serotonin, LSD, and other indoleamines on adenyl cyclase in the liver fluke. Fed. Proc. **33**, 1249 (1974)

Abrahams, S.L., Northup, J.K., Mansour, T.E.: Adenosine cyclic 3', 5'-monophosphate in the liver fluke, *Fasciola hepatica*. I. Activation of adenylate cyclase by 5-hydroxyptamine. Molec. Pharmacol. **12**, 49–58 (1976)

Acheson, G.H.: The responses of the nictitating membrane of the cat to certain stimulants after ergotoxine. Amer. J. Physiol. **128**, 695–702 (1940)

Aellig, W.H.: Periphere Kreislaufwirkungen von Ergotamin, Dihydroergotamin und l-Methylergotamin an der innervierten, perfundierten Hinterextremität des Hundes. Helv. physiol. Pharmacol. Acta **25**, 374–396 (1967)

Aellig, W.H.: Venoconstrictor effect of dihydroergotamine in superficial hand veins. Europ. J. clin. Pharmacol. **7**, 137–139 (1974)

Aellig, W.H., Berde, B.: Studies of the effect of natural and synthetic polypeptide type ergot compounds on a peripheral vascular bed. Brit. J. Pharmacol. **36**, 561–570 (1969)

Aghajanian, G.K.: Influence of drugs on the firing of serotonin-containing neurons in brain. Fed. Proc. **31**, 91–96 (1972a)

Aghajanian, G.K.: Chemical feedback regulation of serotonin-containing neurons in brain. Ann. N.Y. Acad. Sci. **193**, 86–94 (1972b)

Aghajanian, G.K., Haigler, H.J.: Mode of action of LSD on serotonergic neurons. Adv. Biochem. Psychopharmacol. **10**, 167–177 (1974)

Aghajanian, G.K., Weiss, B.L.: Block by LSD of the increase in brain serotonin turnover induced by elevated ambient temperature. Nature (Lond.) **220**, 795–796 (1968)

Aghajanian, G.K., Rosecrans, J.A., Sheard, M.H.: Serotonin: release in the forebrain by stimulation of midbrain raphe. Science **156**, 402–403 (1967)

Aghajanian, G.K., Foote, W.E., Sheard, M.H.: Lysergic acid diethylamide: sensitive neuronal units in the midbrain raphe. Science **161**, 706–708 (1968)

Aghajanian, G.K., Foote, W.E., Sheard, M.H.: Action of psychotogenic drugs on single midbrain raphe neurons. J. Pharmacol. exp. Ther. **171**, 178–187 (1970a)

Aghajanian, G.K., Graham, A.W., Sheard, M.H.: Serotonin-containing neurons in brain: depression of firing by monoamine oxidase inhibitors. Science **169**, 1100–1102 (1970b)

Aghajanian, G.K., Haigler, H.J., Bloom, F.E.: Lysergic acid diethylamide and serotonin: direct actions on serotonin-containing neurons in rat brain. Life Sci. **11(I)**, 615–622 (1972)

Aghajanian, G.K., Kuhar, M.J., Roth, R.H.: Serotonin-containing neuronal perikarya and terminals: differential effects of p-chlorophenylalanine. Brain Res. **54**, 85–101 (1973)

Ahlquist, R.P.: A study of the adrenotropic receptors. Amer. J. Physiol. **153**, 586–600 (1948)

Ahlquist, R.P., Levy, B.: Adrenergic receptive mechanism of canine ileum. J. Pharmacol. exp. Ther. **127**, 146–149 (1959)

Aiello, E., Guideri, G.: Nervous control of ciliary activity. Science **146**, 1692–1693 (1964)

Aiello, E., Guideri, G.: Relationship between 5-hydroxytryptamine and nerve stimulation of ciliary activity. J. Pharmacol. exp. Ther. **154**, 517–523 (1966)

Aiello, E., Paparo, A.: A role for acetylcholine in the regulation of ciliary activity. Comp. gen. Pharmacol. **5**, 285–297 (1974)

Alabaster, V.A., Bakhle, Y.S.: Release of smooth muscle-contracting substances from isolated perfused lungs. Europ. J. Pharmacol. **35**, 349–360 (1976)

Allen, G.S., Henderson, L.M., Chou, S.N., French, L.A.: Cerebral arterial spasm. Part 2: In vitro contractile activity of serotonin in human serum and CSF on the canine basilar artery, and its blockage by methylsergide and phenoxybenzamine. J. Neurosurg. **40**, 442–450 (1974)

Altura, B.M., Malaviya, D., Reich, C.F., Orkin, L.R.: Effects of vasoactive agents on isolated human umbilical arteries and veins. Amer. J. Physiol. **222**, 345–355 (1972)

Ambache, N., Zar, M.A.: Evidence against adrenergic motor transmission in the guinea-pig vas deferens. J. Physiol. (Lond.) **216**, 359–389 (1971)

Ambache, N., Dunk, L.P., Miall, P., Zar, M.A.: Unexplained inhibitory action of D-lysergic acid diethylamide (LSD) on postganglionic motor transmission in the guinea-pig vas deferens. Brit. J. Pharmacol. **42**, 659P–660P (1971)

Ambache, N., Dunk, L.P., Verney, J., Zar, M.A.: An inhibition of post-ganglionic motor transmission in the mammalian vas deferens by D-lysergic acid diethylamide. J. Physiol. (Lond.) **231**, 251–270 (1973a)

Ambache, N., Killick, S.W., Srinivasan, V., Zar, M.A.: Presynaptic inhibition of adrenergic motor transmission in rat anococcygeus muscle by D-lysergic acid diethylamide (LSD). J. Physiol. (Lond.) **233**, 35P–37P (1973b)

Ambache, N., Killick, S.W., Srinivasan, V., Zar, M.A.: Effects of lysergic acid diethylamide on autonomic postganglionic transmission. J. Physiol. (Lond.) **246**, 571–593 (1975)

Ames, A. III, Pollen, D.A.: Neurotransmission in central nervous tissue: A study of isolated rabbit retina. J. Neurophysiol. **32**, 424–442 (1969)

Ammon, R.: Die Cholinesterase. Ergebn. Enzymforsch. **4**, 102–110 (1935)
Andén, N.-E.: Changes in the impulse flow of central monoamine nerves by drugs affecting monoamine receptors. Acta pharmacol. (Kbh.) **25**, 5–6 (1968)
Andén, N.-E., Dahlström, A., Fuxe, K., Larsson, K., Olson, L., Ungerstedt, U.: Ascending monoamine neurons to the telencephalon and diencephalon. Acta physiol. scand. **67**, 313–326 (1966)
Andén, N.-E., Corrodi, H., Fuxe, K., Hökfelt, T.: Evidence for a central 5-hydroxytryptamine receptor stimulation by lysergic acid diethylamide. Brit. J. Pharmacol. **34**, 1–7 (1968)
Andén, N.-E., Carlsson, A., Häggendal, J.: Adrenergic mechanisms. Annu. Rev. Pharmacol. **9**, 119–134 (1969)
Anderson, E.G.: Bulbospinal serotonin-containing neurons and motor control. Fed. Proc. **31**, 107–112 (1972)
Anderson, E.G., Baker, R.G., Banna, N.R.: The effects of monoamine oxidase inhibitors on spinal synaptic activity. J. Pharmacol. exp. Ther. **158**, 405–415 (1967)
Ansell, G.B., Beeson, M.F., Bradley, P.B.: The effects of stressful stimuli and drugs on the concentrations and turnover rates of monoamines in rat brain. In: The Present Status of Psychotropic Drugs. Cerletti, A., Bové, F.J. (eds.), pp. 299–301. Amsterdam: Exerpta Medica Foundation 1969
Apperley, E., Humphrey, P.P.A., Levy, G.P.: Receptors for 5-hydroxytryptamine and noradrenaline in rabbit aorta and central ear artery. Brit. J. Pharmacol. **52**, 131P–132P (1974)
Apperley, E., Humphrey, P.P.A., Levy, G.P.: Receptors for 5-hydroxytryptamine and noradrenaline in rabbit isolated ear artery and aorta. Brit. J. Pharmacol. **58**, 211–221 (1976)
Arcari, G., Dorigotti, L., Fregnan, G.B., Glässer, A.H.: Vasodilating and alpha-receptor blocking activity of a new ergoline derivative. Brit. J. Pharmacol. **34**, 700P (1968)
Arcari, G., Bernardi, L., Bosisio, G., Coda, S., Fregnan, G.B., Glässer, A.H.: 10-Methoxyergoline derivatives as α-adrenergic blocking agents. Experientia (Basel) **28**, 819–820 (1972)
Arefolov, V.A., Pidevich, I.N., Panasyuk, L.V., Firsov, V.K.: Pharmacological analysis of some adrenomimetic effects of serotonin. Byul. éksp. Biol. Med. **80**, 45–48 (1975)
Ariens, E.J.: Affinity and intrinsic activity in the theory of competitive inhibition. Part I: Problems and theory. Arch. int. Pharmacodyn. **99**, 32–49 (1954)
Ariens, E.J., Van Rossum, J.M., Simonis, A.M.: A theoretical basis of molecular pharmacology. Part II: Interactions of one or two compounds with two interdependent receptor systems. Arzneimittel-Forsch. **6**, 611–621 (1956)
Arunlakshana, O., Schild, H.O.: Some quantitative uses of drug antagonists. Brit. J. Pharmacol. **14**, 48–58 (1959)
Ascher, P.: Inhibitory and excitatory effects of dopamine on *Aplysia* neurones. J. Physiol. (Lond.) **225**, 173–209 (1972)
Åström, A., Samelius, U.: The action of 5-hydroxytryptamine and some of its antagonists on the umbilical vessels of the human placenta. Brit. J. Pharmacol. **12**, 410–414 (1957)
Bach, N.J., Hall, D.A., Kornfeld, E.C.: Descarboxylysergic acid (9,10-didehydro-6-methylergoline). J. med. Chem. **17**, 312–314 (1974)
Bacq, Z.M.: The action of ergotamine on the chromatophores of the catfish (*Ameiurus nebulosus*). Biol. Bull. **65**, 387–388 (1933)
Bacq, Z.M.: La pharmacologie du système nerveux autonome, et particulièrement du sympathique, d'après la théorie neurohumorale. Ann. Physiol. **10**, 468–528 (1934a)
Bacq, Z.M.: Action de l'ergotamine et de l'ergotaminine sur la membrane nictitante. C.R. Soc. Biol. (Paris) **116**, 341–342 (1934b)
Bacq, Z.M.: Recherches sur la physiologie du système nerveux autonome. IV. Réactions de la vésicule séminale et du canal déférent du cobaye à l'adrénaline, à l'acéthylcholine et aux ions Ca et K. Arch. int. Pharmacodyn. **47**, 123–129 (1934c)
Bakhle, Y.S., Smith, T.W.: Release of spasmogenic substances induced by vasoactive amines from isolated lungs. Brit. J. Pharmacol. **46**, 543P–544P (1972)
Bakhle, Y.S., Smith, T.W.: The nature of the tryptamine receptor mediating spasmogen release from rat isolated lungs. Brit. J. Pharmacol. **50**, 463P (1974a)
Bakhle, Y.S., Smith, T.W.: Tryptamine receptors in rat pulmonary artery. Brit. J. Pharmacol. **51**, 459–461 (1974b)
Baldratti, G., Arcari, G., Suchowsky, G.K.: Studies on a compound antagonistic to 5-hydroxytryptamine. Experientia (Basel) **21**, 396–397 (1965)

Banna, N.R., Anderson, E.G.: The effects of 5-hydroxytryptamine antagonists on spinal neuronal activity. J. Pharmacol. exp. Ther. **162**, 319–325 (1968)
Barabé, J., Park, W.K., Regoli, D.: Application of drug receptor theories to the analysis of the myotropic effects of bradykinin. Canad. J. Physiol. Pharmacol. **53**, 345–353 (1975)
Barasi, S., Roberts, M.H.T.: The action of 5-hydroxytryptamine antagonists and precursors on bulbospinal facilitation of spinal reflexes. Brain Res. **52**, 385–388 (1973)
Barasi, S., Roberts, M.H.T.: The modification of lumbar motoneurone excitability by stimulation of a putative 5-hydroxy-tryptamine pathway. Brit. J. Pharmacol. **52**, 339–348 (1974)
Barfknecht, C.F., Nichols, D.E., Rusterholz, D.B., Long, J.P., Engelbrecht, J.A., Beaton, J.M., Bradley, R.J., Dyer, D.C.: Potential psychotomimetics. 2-amino-1,2,3,4-tetrahydronaphthalene analogs. J. med. Chem. **16**, 804–808 (1973)
Barlow, R.B.: Effects on amine oxydase of substances which antagonize 5-hydroxytryptamine more than tryptamine on the rat fundus strip preparation. Brit. J. Pharmacol. **16**, 153–162 (1961)
Barlow, R.B., Khan, I.: Actions of some analogues of tryptamine on the rat uterus and on the isolated rat fundus strip preparation. Brit. J. Pharmacol. **14**, 99–107 (1959a)
Barlow, R.B., Khan, I.: Actions of some analogues of 5-hydroxy-tryptamine on the isolated rat uterus and the rat fundus strip preparations. Brit. J. Pharmacol. **14**, 265–272 (1959b)
Barthel, W., Markwardt, F.: Aggregation of blood platelets by biogenic amines and its inhibition by antiadrenergic and antiserotoninergic agents. Biochem. Pharmacol. **23**, 37–45 (1974)
Barthel, W., Markwardt, F.: Aggregation of blood platelets by adrenaline and its uptake. Biochem. Pharmacol. **24**, 1903–1904 (1975)
Bartlet, A.L.: Actions of putative transmitters in the chicken vagus nerve/oesophagus and Remak nerve/rectum preparations. Brit. J. Pharmacol. **51**, 549–558 (1974)
Bartlet, A.L., Hassan, T.: Some actions of histamine and 5-hydroxytryptamine on isolated chicken oesophagus. Brit. J. Pharmacol. **32**, 156–163 (1968)
Barzaghi, F., Baumgartner, H.R., Carruba, M., Mantegazza, P., Pletscher, A.: The 5-hydroxytryptamine-like actions of 5,6-dihydroxytryptamine. Brit. J. Pharmacol. **48**, 245–254 (1973)
Beernink, K.D., Nelson, S.D., Mansour, T.E.: Effect of lysergic acid derivatives on the liver fluke *Fasciola hepatica*. Int. J. Neuropharmacol. **2**, 105–112 (1963)
Belamarich, F.A., Simoneit, L.W.: Aggregation of duck thrombocytes by 5-hydroxytryptamine. Microvasc. Res. **6**, 229–234 (1973)
Beleslin, D., Varagić, V.: The effect of cooling and of 5-hydroxytryptamine on the peristaltic reflex of the isolated guinea-pig ileum. Brit. J. Pharmacol. **13**, 266–270 (1958)
Belisle, S., Gagnon, D.J.: Stimulating action of catecholamines on isolated preparations of the rat colon and human and rabbit taeniae coli. Brit. J. Pharmacol. **41**, 361–366 (1971)
Bell, J.A., Martin, W.R.: Studies of tryptamine and lysergic acid diethylamide (LSD) on cutaneous C-fiber and polysynaptic reflexes in the cat. J. Pharmacol. exp. Ther. **190**, 492–500 (1974)
Benfey, B.G., Cohen, J., Kunos, G., Vermes-Kunos, I.: Dissociation of 5-hydroxytryptamine effects on myocardial contractility and cyclic AMP accumulation. Brit. J. Pharmacol. **50**, 581–585 (1974)
Bennett, A., Stockley, H.L.: The intrinsic innervation of the human alimentary tract and its relation to function. Gut **16**, 443–453 (1975)
Bennett, J.L., Aghajanian, G.K.: D-LSD binding to brain homogenates: Possible relationship to serotonin receptors. Life Sci. **15**, 1935–1944 (1974)
Bennett, J.L., Aghajanian, G.K.: Response of single raphe neurons to (+)-LSD: Correlation with (+)-LSD binding in brain. J. Pharm. Pharmacol. **28**, 516–518 (1976)
Bennett, J.L., Bueding, E.: Uptake of 5-hydroxytryptamine by *Schistosoma mansoni*. Molec. Pharmacol. **9**, 311–319 (1973)
Bennett, J.P., Snyder, S.H.: Stereospecific binding of D-lysergic acid diethylamide (LSD) to brain membranes: relationship to serotonin receptors. Brain Res. **94**, 523–544 (1975)
Bennett, J.P., Snyder, S.H.: Serotonin and lysergic acid diethylamide binding in rat brain membranes: relationship to postsynaptic serotonin receptors. Molec. Pharmacol. **12**, 373–389 (1976)
Bennett, M.R., Middleton, J.: An electrophysiological analysis of the effects of amine-uptake blockers and α-adrenoceptor blockers on adrenergic neuromuscular transmission. Brit. J. Pharmacol. **55**, 87–95 (1975)

Berde, B.: New studies on the circulatory effects of ergot compounds with implications to migraine. In: Background to Migraine. Cumings, J.N. (ed.), pp. 66–75. London: William Heinemann Medical Books 1971

Berde, B.: Some new vascular and biochemical aspects of the mechanism of action of ergot compounds. Headache **11**, 139–147 (1972)

Berde, B., Cerletti, A.: Über den Melanophoreneffekt von D-Lysergsäure-diäthylamid und verwandten Verbindungen. Helv. physiol. pharmacol. Acta **14**, 325–333 (1956)

Berde, B., Cerletti, A.: Über den Angriffspunkt von D-Lysergsäure-diäthylamid und 5-Hydroxytryptamin im Melanophorentest. Z. ges. exp. Med. **129**, 149–153 (1957)

Berde, B., Doepfner, W., Cerletti, A.: Über die Wirkungsdauer einiger Serotoninantagonisten. Helv. physiol. pharmacol. Acta **18**, 537–544 (1960)

Beretta, C., Locatelli, A.: Inhibitory activity of 8β-carbobenzyloxyaminomethyl-1,6-dimethyl-10α-ergoline towards stimulant effects by 5-hydroxytryptamine and amphetamine on liver fluke, *Fasciola hepatica,* in vitro. J. Pharm. Pharmacol. **20**, 744–748 (1968)

Beretta, C., Ferrini, R., Glässer, A.H.: 1-Methyl-8β-carbobenzyloxy-aminomethyl-10α-ergoline, a potent and long-lasting 5-hydroxytryptamine antagonist. Nature (Lond.) **207**, 421–422 (1965a)

Beretta, C., Glässer, A.H., Nobili, M.B., Silvestri, R.: Antagonism of 5-hydroxytryptamine-induced bronchospasm in guinea-pigs by 8β-carbobenzyloxyaminomethyl-1,6-dimethyl-10α-ergoline. J. Pharm. Pharmacol. **17**, 423–428 (1965b)

Bernardi, L., Bosisio, G., Elli, C., Patelli, B., Temperilli, A., Arcari, G., Glässer, H.A.: Ergoline derivatives. Note XIII. α-adrenergic blocking drugs. Farmaco [Sci.] **30**, 789–801 (1975)

Berridge, M.J., Prince, W.T.: Mode of action of hallucinogenic molecules. Nature (Lond.) New Biol. **243**, 283–284 (1973)

Berridge, M.J., Prince, W.T.: The nature of the binding between LSD and a 5-HT receptor: A possible explanation for hallucinogenic activity. Brit. J. Pharmacol. **51**, 269–278 (1974)

Berry, P.A., Collier, H.O.J.: Bronchoconstrictor action and antagonism of a slow-reacting substance from anaphylaxis of guinea-pig isolated lung. Brit. J. Pharmacol. **23**, 201–216 (1964)

Berry, M.S., Cottrell, G.A.: Excitatory, inhibitory and biphasic synaptic potentials mediated by an identified dopamine-containing neurone. J. Physiol. (Lond.) **244**, 589–612 (1975)

Bevan, P., Bradshaw, C.M., Roberts, M.H.T., Szabadi, E.: The effect of microelectrophoretically applied mescaline on cortical neurones. Neuropharmacology **13**, 1033–1045 (1974a)

Bevan, P., Bradshaw, C.M., Szabadi, E.: Potentiation and antagonism of neuronal responses to monoamines by methysergide and sotalol. Brit. J. Pharmacol. **50**, 445P (1974b)

Bhattacharya, B.K.: A pharmacological study on the effect of 5-hydroxytryptamine and its antagonists on the bronchial musculature. Arch. int. Pharmacodyn. **103**, 357–367 (1955)

Biber, B., Fara, J., Lundgren, O.: A pharmacological study of intestinal vasodilator mechanisms in the cat. Acta physiol. scand. **90**, 673–683 (1974)

Bickerton, R.K., Rockhold, W.T., Micalizzi, E.R.: Use of isolated strips of cat spleen for the assay of α-adrenergic blocking compounds. J. Pharm. Sci. **51**, 837–840 (1962)

Bindler, E.H., Gyermek, L.: Influence of 5-HT antagonists on the ganglionic stimulant action of 5-HT and DMPP. Fed. Proc. **20**, 319 (1961)

Bircher, R., Schalch, W.R.: Über die Wirkung von Mutterkornalkaloiden bei histaminergischen Reaktionen. Helv. physiol. pharmacol. Acta **6**, 813–820 (1948)

Birmingham, A.T., Szolcsányi, J.: Competitive blockade of adrenergic α-receptors and histamine receptors by thymoxamine. J. Pharm. Pharmacol. **17**, 449–458 (1965)

Birmingham, A.T., Wilson, A.B.: Preganglionic and postganglionic stimulation of the guinea-pig isolated vas deferens preparation. Brit. J. Pharmacol. **21**, 569–580 (1963)

Birnbaumer, L., Pohl, S.L., Kaumann, A.J.: Receptors and acceptors: A necessary distinction in hormone binding studies. Adv. Cyclic Nucleotide Res. **4**, 239–281 (1974)

Blakeley, A.G.H., Brown, G.L., Ferry, C.B.: Pharmacological experiments on the release of the sympathetic transmitter. J. Physiol. (Lond.) **167**, 505–514 (1963)

Bloom, F.E., Costa, E., Salmoiraghi, G.C.: Analysis of individual rabbit olfactory bulb neuron responses to the microelectrophoresis of acetylcholine, norepinephrine and serotonin synergists and antagonists. J. Pharmacol. exp. Ther. **146**, 16–23 (1964)

Bloom, F.E., Hoffer, B.J., Siggins, G.R., Barker, J.L., Nicoll, R.A.: Effects of serotonin on central neurons: Microiontophoretic administration. Fed. Proc. **31**, 97–106 (1972)
Bloom, F.E., Hoffer, B.J., Nelson, C., Sheu, Y., Siggins, G.R.: The physiology and pharmacology of serotonin mediated synapses. In: Serotonin and Behavior. Barchas, J., Usdin, E. (eds.), pp. 249–261. New York: Academic Press 1973
Boakes, R.J., Bradley, P.B., Briggs, I., Dray, A.: Antagonism by LSD to effects of 5-HT on single neurones. Brain Res. **15**, 529–531 (1969)
Boakes, R.J., Bradley, P.B., Briggs, I., Dray, A.: Effects of lysergic acid derivatives on 5-hydroxytryptamine excitation of brain stem neurones. Brit. J. Pharmacol. **38**, 453P-454P (1970a)
Boakes, R.J., Bradley, P.B., Briggs, I., Dray, A.: Antagonism of 5-hydroxytryptamine by LSD-25 in the central nervous system: A possible neuronal basis for the actions of LSD-25. Brit. J. Pharmacol. **40**, 202–218 (1970b)
Boggan, W.O., Freedman, D.X.: LSD tolerance and brain serotonin metabolism. Fed. Proc. **32**, 694 (1973)
Bond, H.W., Guth, P.S.: Interaction of 5-hydroxytryptamine and lysergic acid diethylamide in the central nervous system. Pharmacologist **6**, 171 (1964)
Born, G.V.R.: The uptake of adrenaline by human blood platelets. Naunyn-Schmiedebergs Arch. Pharmacol. **259**, 155–156 (1967)
Born, G.V.R., Smith, J.B.: Uptake, metabolism and release of [^{3}H]-adrenaline by human platelets. Brit. J. Pharmacol. **39**, 765–778 (1970)
Born, G.V.R., Mills, D.C.B., Roberts, G.C.K.: Potentiation of platelet aggregation by adrenaline. J. Physiol. (Lond.) **191**, 43P–44P (1967a)
Born, G.V.R., Day, M., Stockbridge, A.: The uptake of amines by human erythrocytes in vitro. J. Physiol. (Lond.) **193**, 405–418 (1967b)
Born, G.V.R., Juengjaroen, K., Michal, F.: Relative activities on and uptake by human blood platelets of 5-hydroxytryptamine and several analogues. Brit. J. Pharmacol. **44**, 117–139 (1972)
Borsy, J., Magó-Karacsony, E., Balogh, T., Pik, K.: Preparation new semi-synthetic lysergic acid derivatives: Investigation into the correlation of molecular structure and antiserotonin activity II. Acta pharm. hung. **43**, 207–217 (1973)
Boullin, D.J., Green, A.R.: Effect of brain 5-HT agonists and antagonists on platelet aggregation. Sixth Internat. Congr. Pharmacol., Helsinki, 1975. Abstract 695
Boullin, D.J., Green, A.R., Grimes, R.P.J.: Human blood platelet aggregation induced by dopamine, 5-hydroxytryptamine and analogues. J. Physiol. (Lond.) **252**, 46P–47P (1975a)
Boullin, D.J., Grimes, R.P.J., Orr, M.W.: The actions of flupethixol upon 5-hydroxytryptamine-induced aggregation and the uptake of 5-hydroxytryptamine and dopamine by human blood platelets. Brit. J. Pharmacol. **55**, 555–557 (1975b)
Boyd, H., Chang, V., Rand, M.J.: The anticholinesterase activity of some antiadrenaline agents. Brit. J. Pharmacol. **15**, 525–531 (1960)
Bradley, P.B.: The effects of 5-hydroxytryptamine on the electrical activity of the brain and on behaviour in the conscious cat. In: 5-Hydroxytryptamine. Lewis, G.P. (ed.), pp. 214–220. London: Pergamon Press 1958
Bradley, P.B., Hance, A.J.: The effects of intraventricular injections of D-lysergic acid diethylamide (LSD 25) and 5-hydroxytryptamine (serotonin) on the electrical activity of the brain of the conscious cat. J. Physiol. (Lond.) **132**, 50P–51P (1956a)
Bradley, P.B., Hance, A.J.: The effects of intraventricular injections of drugs on the electrical activity of the brain of the conscious cat. Electroenceph. clin. Neurophysiol. **8**, 699–700 (1956b)
Bradley, P.B., Wolstencroft, J.H.: The action of drugs on single neurones in the brain stem. In: Neuro-Psychopharmacology. Bradley, P.B., Fluegel, F., Hoch, P.H. (eds.), pp. 237–240. Amsterdam: Elsevier 1964
Bradley, P.B., Wolstencroft, J.H.: Actions of drugs on single neurones in the brain stem. Brit. med. Bull. **21**, 15–18 (1965)
Bradshaw, C.M., Roberts, M.H.T., Szabadi, E.: Effect of mescaline on single cortical neurones. Brit. J. Pharmacol. **43**, 871–873 (1971)
Bramwell, G.J., Gonye, T.: Responses of midbrain neurones to iontophoretically applied 5-hydroxytryptamine. Brit. J. Pharmacol. **48**, 357P-358P (1973)

Briggs, I.: Excitatory responses to raphe stimulation in the rat bulbar reticular formation. J. Physiol. (Lond.) **256**, 111P (1976)
Brodie, B.B.: Storage and release of 5-hydroxytryptamine (HT). Possible significance in chemical mediation in brain. In: Ciba Symposium on Hypertension, pp. 64–83. London: Churchill 1954
Brodie, B., Shore, P.A., Pletscher, A.: Serotonin-releasing activity limited to Rauwolfia alkaloids with tranquilizing action. Science **123**, 992–993 (1956)
Broom, W.A., Clark, A.J.: The standardisation of ergot preparations. J. Pharmacol. exp. Ther. **22**, 59–74 (1923)
Brown, B.E.: Proctolin: A peptide transmitter candidate in insects. Life Sci. **17**, 1241–1252 (1975)
Brown, L.: The release and fate of the transmitter liberated by adrenergic nerves. Proc. roy. Soc. B **162**, 1–19 (1965)
Brown, G.L., Dale, H.: The pharmacology of ergometrine. Proc. roy. Soc. B **118**, 446–477 (1935)
Brown, G.L., Gillespie, J.S.: The output of sympathetic transmitter from the spleen of the cat. J. Physiol. (Lond.) **138**, 81–102 (1957)
Brown, G.L., Davies, B.N., Ferry, C.B.: The effect of neuronal rest on the output of sympathetic transmitter from the spleen. J. Physiol. (Lond.) **159**, 365–380 (1961)
Brownlee, G., Johnson, E.S.: The site of the 5-hydroxytryptamine receptor on the intramural nervous plexus of the guinea-pig isolated ileum. Brit. J. Pharmacol. **21**, 306–322 (1963)
Brügger, I.: Experimenteller Beitrag zur Wirkungsweise vegetativer Pharmaka. Arch. int. Pharmacodyn. **59**, 43–60 (1938)
Brügger, J.: Die isolierte Samenblase des Meerschweinchens als biologisches Testobjekt zur quantitativen Differenzierung der sympathikolytischen Wirkung der genuinen Mutterkornalkaloide und ihrer Dihydroderivate. Helv. physiol. pharmacol. Acta **3**, 117–134 (1945)
Brundin, J.: The effect of prostaglandin E_1 on the response of the rabbit oviduct to hypogastric nerve stimulation. Acta physiol. scand. **73**, 54–57 (1968)
Buchan, P., Lewis, A.J., Sugrue, M.F.: A comparison of the accumulation of noradrenaline and 5-hydroxytryptamine into arterial smooth muscle. Brit. J. Pharmacol. **52**, 132P–133P (1974)
Bucknell, A., Whitney, B.: A preliminary investigation of the pharmacology of the human isolated taenia coli preparation. Brit. J. Pharmacol. **23**, 164–175 (1964)
Bullard, B.: The nervous control of the anterior byssus retractor muscle of *Mytilus edulis*. Comp. Biochem. Physiol. **23**, 749–759 (1967)
Burgers, A.C.J., Imai, K.: The melanophore-stimulating potency of single pituitary glands of normal and of D-lysergic acid diethylamide (D-LSD)-treated *Xenopus laevis*. Gen. comp. Endocr. **2**, 603–604 (1962)
Burgers, A.C.J., Leemreis, W., Dominiczak, T., Van Oordt, G.J.: Inhibition of the secretion of intermedine by D-lysergic acid diethylamide (LSD-25) in the toad, *Xenopus laevis*. Acta endocr. (Kbh.) **29**, 191–200 (1958)
Burgers, A.C.J., Zandee, D.I., Van Bakel, J.M.M., Hillemans, G.M.L., Van Oordt, G.J.: The effect of LSD-derivatives and serotonin on the melanophores of the toad, *Xenopus laevis*. Acta physiol. pharmacol. neerl. **11**, 341–342 (1962)
Burn, J.H., Ng, K.K.F.: The action of Hydergine at postganglionic sympathetic terminations. J. Physiol. (Lond.) **175**, 66P (1964)
Burnstein, S., Levin, E., Varanelli, C.: Prostaglandins and cannabis—II. Inhibition of biosynthesis by the naturally occurring cannabinoids. Biochem. Pharmacol. **22**, 2908–2910 (1973)
Burt, D.R., Creese, I., Snyder, S.H.: Binding interaction of lysergic acid diethylamide and related agents with dopamine receptors in the brain. Molec. Pharmacol. **12**, 631–638 (1976a)
Burt, D.R., Creese, I., Snyder, S.H.: Properties of [^{3}H] haloperidol and [^{3}H]dopamine binding associated with dopamine receptors in calf brain membranes. Molec. Pharmacol. **12**, 800–812 (1976b)
Cambridge, G.W., Holgate, J.A.: Superfusion as a method for the study of drug antagonism. Brit. J. Pharmacol. **10**, 326–334 (1955)
Cannon, W.B., Rosenblueth, A.: Autonomic neuro-effector systems. Experimental Biology Monographs. New York: MacMillan 1937

Carlsson, A., Lindqvist, M.: The effect of L-tryptophan and some psychotropic drugs on the formation of 5-hydroxytryptophan in the mouse brain in vivo. J. Neural Transm. **33**, 23–43 (1972)
Carlsson, A., Shore, P.A., Brodie, B.B.: Release of serotonin from blood platelets by reserpine in vitro. J. Pharmacol. exp. Ther. **120**, 334–339 (1957)
Carlsson, A., Bédard, P., Lindqvist, M., Magnusson, T.: The influence of nerve-impulse flow on the synthesis and metabolism of 5-hydroxytryptamine. Biochem. J. **128**, 70P–71P (1972a)
Carlsson, A., Bédard, P., Lindqvist, M., Magnusson, T.: The influence of nerve-impulse flow on the synthesis and metabolism of 5-hydroxytryptamine in the central nervous system. In: Neurotransmitters and Metabolic Regulation. Smellie, R.M.S. (ed.), pp. 17–32. London: The Biochemical Society 1972b
Carpi, A., Virno, M.: The action of ergotamine on the intracranial venous pressure and on the cerebral venous outflow of the dog. Brit. J. Pharmacol. **12**, 232–239 (1957)
Carroll, P.R., Glover, W.E.: Independence of the vasoconstrictor and the potentiating effects of 5-hydroxytryptamine and some ergot derivatives. Proc. Aust. physiol. pharmacol. Soc. **4**, 40 (1973)
Carroll, P.R., Ebeling, P.W., Glover, W.E.: Vascular responses to some drugs used in the treatment of migraine. Abstracts, Australasian Society for Clinical and Experimental Pharmacologists, November 1972
Carroll, P.R., Ebeling, P.W., Glover, W.E.: The responses of the human temporal and rabbit ear artery to 5-hydroxytryptamine and some of its antagonists. Ajebak **52**, 813–823 (1974)
Casentini, S., Galli, G.: Serotonina, antiserotoninici e motilita gastrica. Boll. Soc. ital. Biol. sper. **32**, 1640–1642 (1956)
Cerletti, A.: Lysergic acid diethylamide (LSD) and related compounds. In: Neuropharmacology. Abramson, H.A. (ed.), pp. 9–84. Trans. Second Conf. Princeton: Josiah Macy, Jr., Foundation 1955
Cerletti, A.: Ergostin—Neue Perspektiven der Chemie und Pharmakologie des Mutterkorns. Med. exp. (Basel) **8**, 278–286 (1963)
Cerletti, A., Berde, B.: Die Wirkung von D-Lysergsäure-diäthylamid (LSD 25) und 5-Oxytryptamin auf die Chromatophoren von *Poecilia reticulatus*. Experientia (Basel) **11**, 312–313 (1955)
Cerletti, A., Berde, B.: New approaches in the development of compounds from ergot with potential therapeutic use in migraine. In: Background to Migraine. Smith, R. (ed.), pp. 53–64. London: William Heinemann Medical Books 1967
Cerletti, A., Doepfner, W.: Über die 5-Oxytryptamin-hemmende Wirkung von LSD-Derivaten und andern Lysergsäureamiden am isolierten Rattenuterus. 20th Intern. Physiol. Congress Bruxelles, 1956, Abstr. Comm., pp. 165–166
Cerletti, A., Doepfner, W.: Spezifische Steigerung der serotonin-antagonistischen Wirkung von Lysergsäurederivaten durch Methylierung des Indolstickstoffes der Lysergsäure. Helv. physiol. pharmacol. Acta **16**, C55–C57 (1958a)
Cerletti, A., Doepfner, W.: Comparative study on the serotonin antagonism of amide derivatives of lysergic acid and of ergot alkaloids. J. Pharmacol. exp. Ther. **122**, 124–136 (1958b)
Cerletti, A., Konzett, H.: Spezifische Hemmung von 5-Oxytryptamin-Effekten durch Lysergsäurediäthylamid und ähnliche Körper. Naunyn-Schmiedebergs Arch. Pharmacol. **228**, 146–148 (1956)
Cerletti, A., Rothlin, E.: Role of 5-hydroxytryptamine in mental diseases and its antagonism to lysergic acid derivatives. Nature (Lond.) **176**, 785–786 (1955)
Chahl, L.A., Ladd, R.J.: The effects of prostaglandins E_1, E_2 and $F_{2\alpha}$ on the cutaneous vasculature of the rat. Brit. J. Pharmacol. **56**, 317–322 (1976)
Chahl, L.A., O'Donnell, S.R.: The effects on some receptors of guinea-pig trachea of a series of sympathomimetic amines. Europ. J. Pharmacol. **16**, 201–208 (1971)
Chambers, P.N., Marshall, P.B.: Similar pharmacological properties of ergometrine and methysergide. J. Pharm. Pharmacol. **19**, 65 (1967)
Chan, P.S., Ellenbogen, L.: New evidence for the β-adrenergic receptor blocking activity of dihydroergotamine. Arch. int. Pharmacodyn. **209**, 204–213 (1974)
Chase, T.N., Breese, G.R., Kopin, I.J.: Serotonin release from brain slices by electrical stimulation: Regional differences and effect of LSD. Science **157**, 1461–1463 (1967)

Chase, T.N., Katz, R.I., Kopin, I.J.: Release of [^{3}H] serotonin from brain slices. J. Neurochem. **16**, 607–615 (1969)
Chodera, A.: Blockade of 5-hydroxytryptamine antidiuresis in rats by 2-bromlysergic acid diethylamide tartrate and 1-methyl-lysergic acid butanolamide. J. Pharm. Pharmacol. **15**, 386–389 (1963)
Chong, G.C., Phillis, J.W.: Pharmacological studies on the heart of *Tapes watlingi:* A mollusc of the family Veneridae. Brit. J. Pharmacol. **25**, 481–496 (1965)
Christ, D.D., Nishi, S.: Site of adrenaline blockade in the superior cervical ganglion of the rabbit. J. Physiol. (Lond.) **213**, 107–117 (1971)
Christian, S.T., McClain, L.D., Morin, R.D., Benington, F.: Blockage of LSD binding at its high affinity site on synaptosomal membranes by 1-methyl-1,2,5,6-tetrahydropyridine-N,N-diethyl-carboxamide. Experientia (Basel) **31**, 910–911 (1975)
Chu, D., Stürmer, E.: Studies on the mechanism of action of dihydroergotamine (DHE) on the vascular bed of cat skeletal muscle. Brit. J. Pharmacol. **48**, 331P–332P (1973)
Chu, D., Owen, D.A.A., Stürmer, E.: Effects of ergotamine and dihydroergotamine on the resistance and capacitance vessels of skin and skeletal muscle in the cat. Postgrad. med. J. **52** (Suppl. 1), 32–36 (1976)
Church, M.K.: Response of rat lung to humoral mediators of anaphylaxis and its modification by drugs and sensitization. Brit. J. Pharmacol. **55**, 423–430 (1975)
Church, M.K., Miller, P.: Simple models of anaphylaxis and of histamine and 5-hydroxytryptamine induced inflammation using the mouse pinna. Brit. J. Pharmacol. **55**, 315P (1975)
Cima, G., Freschi, C.: Attivitá della serotonina e dei suoi antagonisti sull'uretere isolato. Boll. Soc. ital. Biol. sper. **33**, 867–869 (1957)
Cleugh, J., Gaddum, J.H., Holton, P., Leach, E.: Assay of substance P on the fowl rectal caecum. Brit. J. Pharmacol. **17**, 144–158 (1961)
Clineschmidt, B.V., Anderson, E.G.: Lysergic acid diethylamide: antagonism of supraspinal inhibiton of spinal reflexes. Brain Res. **16**, 296–300 (1969)
Clineschmidt, B.V., Anderson, E.G.: The blockade of bulbospinal inhibition by 5-hydroxytryptamine antagonists. Exp. Brain Res. **11**, 175–186 (1970)
Clineschmidt, B.V., Lotti, V.J.: Indoleamine antagonists: relative potencies as inhibitors of tryptamine- and 5-hydroxytryptophan-evoked responses. Brit. J. Pharmacol. **50**, 311–313 (1974)
Closse, A., Hauser, D.: Dihydroergotamine binding to rat brain membranes. Life Sci. **19**, 1851–1864 (1976)
Cohen, M.L., Berkowitz, B.A.: Differences between the effects of dopamine and apomorphine on rat aortic strips. Europ. J. Pharmacol. **34**, 49–58 (1975)
Collier, J.G., Nachev, C., Robinson, B.F.: Effect of catecholamines and other vasoactive substances on superficial hand veins in man. Clin. Sci. **43**, 455–467 (1972)
Constantine, J.W., Knott, C.: Benzquinamide and the 5-hydroxytryptamine receptors in guinea pig trachea. J. Pharmacol. exp. Ther. **146**, 400–403 (1964)
Cools, A.R.: Two topographically, functionally and pharmacologically distinct dopamine-sensitive sites within the cat brain. Sixth Internat. Congr. Pharmacol., Helsinki, 1975, Abstract 1149
Cools, A.R., Van Rossum, J.M.: Excitation-mediating and inhibition-mediating dopamine-receptors: A new concept towards a better understanding of electrophysiological, biochemical, pharmacological, functional and clinical data. Psychopharmacologia **45**, 243–254 (1976)
Cools, A.R., Struyker Boudier, H.A.J., Van Rossum, J.M.: Depamine receptors: Selective agonists and antagonists of functionally distinct types within the feline brain. Europ. J. Pharmacol. **37**, 283–293 (1976)
Corrodi, H., Fuxe, K., Hökfelt, T., Lidbrink, P., Ungerstedt, U.: Effect of ergot drugs on central catecholamine neurons: evidence for a stimulation of central dopamine neurons. J. Pharm. Pharmacol. **25**, 409–412 (1973)
Corrodi, H., Farnebo, L.O., Fuxe, K., Hamberger, B.: Effect of ergot drugs on central 5-hydroxytryptamine neurons: evidence for 5-hydroxytryptamine release or 5-hydroxytryptamine receptor stimulation. Europ. J. Pharmacol. **30**, 172–181 (1975)
Costa, E.: Effects of hallucinogenic and tranquilizing drugs on serotonin evoked uterine contractions. Proc. Soc. exp. Biol. (N.Y.) **91**, 39–41 (1956)

Costa, E., Zetler, G.: Interactions between epinephrine and some psychotomimetic drugs. J. Pharmacol. exp. Ther. **125**, 230–236 (1959)
Costall, B., Naylor, R.J.: Apomorphine as an antagonist of the dopamine response from the nucleus accumbens. J. Pharm. Pharmacol. **28**, 592–595 (1976)
Cottrell, G.A.: Direct post-synaptic responses to stimulation of serotonin-containing neurons. Nature (Lond.) **225**, 1060–1062 (1970a)
Cottrell, G.A.: Actions of LSD-25 and reserpine on a serotonergic synapse. J. Physiol. (Lond.) **208**, 28P–29P (1970b)
Cottrell, G.A., Macon, J.B.: Synaptic connexions of two symmetrically placed giant serotonin-containing neurones. J. Physiol. (Lond.) **236**, 435–464 (1974)
Cottrell, G.A., Berry, M.S., Macon, J.B.: Synapses of a giant serotonin neurone and a giant dopamine neurone: studies using antagonists. Neuropharmacology **13**, 431–439 (1974)
Couch, J.R.: Blockade of excitatory 5-HT synapse by LSD. Pharmacologist **16**, 244 (1974)
Creese, I., Burt, D.R., Snyder, S.H.: The dopamine receptor: differential binding of D-LSD and related agents to agonist and antagonist states. Life Sci. **17**, 1715–1720 (1976)
Cripps, H., Dearnaley, D.P.: Evidence suggesting uptake of noradrenaline at adrenergic receptors in the isolated blood-perfused cat spleen. J. Physiol. (Lond.) **216**, 55P-56P (1971)
Cripps, H., Dearnaley, D.P.: Vascular responses and noradrenaline overflow in the isolated blood-perfused cat spleen: some effects of cocaine, normetanephrine and α-blocking agents. J. Physiol. (Lond.) **227**, 647–664 (1972)
Crossman, A.R., ElKhawad, A.O.A., Walker, R.J., Woodruff, G.N.: Effects of ergometrine on dopamine receptors. J. Physiol. (Lond.) **232**, 59P (1973)
Crunkhorn, P., Meacock, S.C.R.: Mediators of the inflammation induced in the rat paw by carrageenin. Brit. J. Pharmacol. **42**, 392–402 (1971)
Crunkhorn, P., Willis, A.L.: Cutaneous reactions to intradermal prostaglandins. Brit. J. Pharmacol. **41**, 49–56 (1971)
Cuatrecasas, P., Greaves, M.F.: Receptors and recognition. Series A, Vol. I. London: Chapman and Hall; New York: Wiley 1976
Cuatrecasas, P., Hollenberg, M.D., Chang, K.-J., Bennett, V.: Hormone receptor complexes and their modulation of membrane function. Recent Progr. Hormone Res. **31**, 37–94 (1975)
Cumings, J.N.: The relationship of serotonin and platelets in migraine. Arch. Neurobiol. **37** (Suppl.), 67–75, 77–84 (1974)
Cumings, J.N., Hilton, B.P.: Effects of methysergide on platelets incubated with reserpine. Brit. J. Pharmacol. **42**, 611–619 (1971)
Curtis, D.R., Davis, R.: A central action of 5-hydroxytryptamine and noradrenaline. Nature (Lond.) **192**, 1083–1084 (1961)
Curtis, D.R., Davis, R.: Pharmacological studies upon neurons of the lateral geniculate nucleus of the cat. Brit. J. Pharmacol. **18**, 217–246 (1962)
Curzon, G., Marsden, C.A.: Effect of LSD on rat brain 5-hydroxytryptamine metabolism at elevated environmental temperature. Brit. J. Pharmacol. **56**, 368P–369P (1976)
Dahlström, A., Fuxe, K.: Evidence for the existence of mono-amine neurons in the central nervous system. I. Demonstration of monoamines in the cell bodies of brain stem neurons. Acta physiol. scand. **62** (Suppl. 232), 5–55 (1964)
Dahlström, A., Fuxe, K.: Evidence for the existence of mono-amine neurons in the central nervous system. II. Experimentally induced changes in the intraneuronal amine levels of bulbospinal neuron systems. Acta physiol. scand. **64** (Suppl. 247), 7–36 (1965)
Daicoff, G.R., Chavez, F.R., Anton, A.H., Swenson, E.W.: Serotonin-induced pulmonary venous hypertension in pulmonary embolism. Thorac. cardiovasc. Surg. **56**, 810–815 (1968)
Dale, H.H.: On some physiological actions of ergot. J. Physiol. (Lond.) **34**, 163–206 (1906)
Dalessio, D.J., Camp, W.A., Goodell, H., Chapman, L.F., Zileli, T., Ramos, A.O., Ehrlich, R., Fortuin, F., McCattell, K., Wolff, H.C.: Studies on headache: the relevance of the prophylactic action of UML-491 in vascular headache of the migraine type to the pathophysiology of this syndrome. Wld Neurol. **3**, 66–72 (1962)
Da Graca-Fernandez, M., Osswald, W.: Einfluss von Ergotamin und Pentobarbital auf die Blutdruck- und Nickhautwirkungen von Noradrenalin und Tyramin. Med. Pharmacol. exp. **17**, 65–71 (1967)

D'Amico, D.J., Patel, B.C., Klawans, H.L.: The effect of methysergide on 5-hydroxytryptamine turnover in whole brain. J. Pharm. Pharmacol. **28**, 454–456 (1976)
Da Prada, M., Saner, A., Burkhard, W.P., Bartholini, G., Pletscher, A.: Evidence for stimulation of cerebral dopamine receptors by LSD. Sixth Internat. Congr. Pharmacol., Helsinki, 1975a, Abstract 187
Da Prada, M., Saner, A., Burkard, W.P., Bartholini, G., Pletscher, A.: Lysergic acid diethylamide: evidence for stimulation of cerebral dopamine receptors. Brain Res. **94**, 67–73 (1975b)
Davis, M.E., Adair, F.L., Chen, K.K., Swanson, E.E.: The pharmacologic action of ergotocin, a new ergot principle. J. Pharmacol. exp. Ther. **54**, 398–407 (1935)
Davis, W.G.: A dual action of 5-hydroxytryptamine on the ovarian suspensory ligament of the rat. J. Pharm. Pharmacol. **28**, 502–504 (1976)
Day, M., Vane, J.R.: An analysis of the direct and indirect actions of drugs on the isolated guinea-pig ileum. Brit. J. Pharmacol. **20**, 150–170 (1963)
Deffenu, G., Mantegazzini, P.: Effects of 5-hydroxytryptamine on spinal reflexes of the cat. Psychopharmacologia **10**, 96–102 (1966)
De La Lande, I.S., Cannel, V.A., Waterson, J.G.: The interaction of serotonin and noradrenaline on the perfused artery. Brit. J. Pharmacol. **28**, 255–272 (1966)
De La Lande, I.S., Rand, M.J.: A simple isolated nerve-blood vessel preparation. Aust. J. exp. Biol. med. Sci. **43**, 639–656 (1965)
Delay, J., Thuillier, J.: Dualité d'action du diéthylamide de l'acide lysergique sur la contraction uterine provoquée par la 5-hydroxytryptamine (sérotonine). C.R. Soc. Biol. (Paris) **150**, 1335–1336 (1956)
Del Bianco, P.L., Fanciullacci, M., Franchi, G., Sicuteri, F.: Human 5-hydroxytryptamine venomotor receptors. Pharmacol. Res. Commun. **7**, 395–408 (1975)
Del Bianco, P.L., Franchi, G., Fanciullacci, M., Sicuteri, F.: Clinical pharmacology of 5-hydroxytryptamine and catecholamines venomotor receptors. Arch. int. Pharmacodyn. **196** (Suppl.), 113–116 (1972)
Del Greco, F., Masson, G.M.C., Corcoran, A.C.: Renal and arterial effects of serotonin in the anesthetized rat. Amer. J. Physiol. **187**, 509–514 (1956)
Dengler, H.J., Spiegel, H.E., Titus, E.O.: Effects of drugs on uptake of isotopic norepinephrine by cat tissues. Nature (Lond.) **191**, 816–817 (1961)
Dette, G.A., Wesemann, W.: Studies on serotonin binding proteins of nerve ending membranes. J. Neural Transm. **37**, 281–295 (1975)
Diab, I.M., Freedman, D.X., Roth, L.J.: [^{3}H] Lysergic acid diethylamide: cellular autoradiographic localization in rat brain. Science **173**, 1022–1024 (1971)
Díaz, J.-L., Huttunen, M.O.: Persistent increase in brain serotonin turnover after chronic administration of LSD in the rat. Science **174**, 62–64 (1971)
Diaz, P., Ngai, S.H., Costa, E.: The effect of LSD on the metabolism of rat brain serotonin (5-HT). Pharmacologist **9**, 251 (1967)
Diaz, P.M., Ngai, S.H., Costa, E.: Factors modulating brain serotonin turnover. Adv. Pharmacol. Chemother. **6B**, 75–92 (1968)
Dingledine, R., Goldstein, A., Kendig, J.: Effects of narcotic opiates and serotonin on the electrical behaviour of neurons in the guinea-pig myenteric plexus. Life Sci. **14**, 2299–2309 (1974)
Doepfner, W., Cerletti, A.: Über den Serotonin-Antagonismus einiger Antihistaminika unter Berücksichtigung ihrer chemischen Struktur. Int. Arch. Allergy **10**, 348–354 (1957)
Doepfner, W., Cerletti, A.: Comparison of lysergic acid derivatives and antihistamines as inhibitors of the edema provoked in the rat's paw by serotonin. Int. Arch. Allergy **12**, 89–97 (1958)
Dougan, D.F.H., McLean, J.R.: Evidence for the presence of dopaminergic nerves and receptors in the intestine of a mollusc, *Tapes watlingi*. Comp. gen. Pharmacol. **1**, 33–46 (1970)
Drakontides, A.B., Gershon, M.D.: 5-Hydroxytryptamine receptors in the mouse duodenum. Brit. J. Pharmacol. **33**, 480–492 (1968)
Dretchen, K., Ghoneim, M.M., Long, J.P.: Interactions of serotonin with neuromuscular blocking agents. Europ. J. Pharmacol. **18**, 121–127 (1972)
Drew, G.M.: Effects of α-adrenoceptor agonists and antagonists on pre- and postsynaptically located α-adrenoceptors. Europ. J. Pharmacol. **36**, 313–320 (1976)

Drummond, A.H., Gordon, J.L.: Platelet release reaction induced by 5-hydroxytryptamine. J. Physiol. (Lond.) **240**, 39P–40P (1974)
Drummond, A.H., Gordon, J.L.: Inhibition of 5-hydroxy-[^{3}H]-tryptamine binding to rat blood platelets by 5-HT antagonists and uptake inhibitors. Brit. J. Pharmacol. **55**, 257–258 (1975a)
Drummond, A.H., Gordon, J.L.: Specific binding sites for 5-hydroxytryptamine on rat blood platelets. Biochem. J. **150**, 129–132 (1975b)
Drummond, A.H., Whigham, K.A.E., Prentice, C.R.M.: Effects of chlorprothixene isomers on platelet 5-hydroxytryptamine receptors: evidence for different 5-hydroxytryptamine conformations at uptake and stimulatory sites. Europ. J. Pharmacol. **37**, 385–388 (1976)
Dyer, D.C.: The pharmacology of spirally-cut sheep umbilical blood vessels. Pharmacologist **11**, 230 (1969)
Dyer, D.C.: The pharmacology of isolated sheep umbilical blood vessels. J. Pharmacol. exp. Ther. **175**, 565–570 (1970)
Dyer, D.C.: Evidence for the action of D-lysergic acid diethylamide, mescaline and bufotenine on 5-hydroxytryptamine receptors in umbilical vasculature. J. Pharmacol. exp. Ther. **188**, 336–341 (1974)
Dyer, D.C., Gant, D.W.: Vasoconstriction produced by hallucinogens on isolated human and sheep umbilical vasculature. J. Pharmacol. exp. Ther. **184**, 366–375 (1973)
Dyer, D.C., Ueland, K., Eng, M.: Responses of isolated monkey umbilical veins to biogenic amines and polypeptides. Arch. int. Pharmacodyn. **200**, 213–221 (1972)
Dykstra, S.L., Berdahl, J.M., Campbell, K.N., Combs, C.M., Lankin, D.G.: Phenylindenes and phenylindans with antireserpine activity. J. med. Chem. **10**, 418–428 (1967)
Dykstra, S.J., Minielli, J.L., Lawson, J.E., Ferguson, H.C., Dungan, K.W.: Lysergic acid and quinidine analogs. 2-(O-acylamino-phenethyl) piperidines. J. med. Chem. **16**, 1015–1020 (1973)
Ehrenpreis, S., Fleisch, J.H., Mittag, T.W.: Approaches to the molecular nature of pharmacological receptors. Pharmacol. Rev. **21**, 131–181 (1969)
Eliasson, R., Åström, A.: Pharmacological studies on the perfused human placenta. Acta pharmacol. (Kbh.) **11**, 254–264 (1955)
ElKhawad, A.O., Woodruff, G.N.: Evidence for direct stimulation of dopamine receptors by ergometrine in mice and rats. Sixth Internat. Congr. Pharmacol., Helsinki, 1975, Abstract 1147
ElKhawad, A.O., Munday, K.A., Poat, J.A., Woodruff, G.N.: The effect of dopamine receptor stimulants on locomotor activity and cyclic AMP levels in the rat striatum. Brit. J. Pharmacol. **53**, 456P–457P (1975)
Engberg, I., Lundberg, A., Ryall, R.W.: The effect of reserpine on transmission from the flexor reflex afferents. Acta physiol. scand. **68** (Suppl. 277), 45 (1966)
Engberg, I., Lundberg, A., Ryall, R.W.: The effect of reserpine on transmission in the spinal cord. Acta physiol. scand. **72**, 115–122 (1968a)
Engberg, I., Lundberg, A., Ryall, R.W.: Is the tonic decerebrate inhibition of reflex paths mediated by monoaminergic pathways? Acta physiol. scand. **72**, 123–133 (1968b)
Engelhardt, G.: Zur Pharmakologie des 9,10-Dihydro-10-(1-methyl-4-piperidyliden)-9-anthrol (WA 335), eines Histamin- und Serotoninantagonisten. Arzneimittel-Forsch. **25**, 1723–1737 (1975)
Erspamer, V.: Modificazioni delle azioni dell enteramina ad opera di farmaci simpaticomimetici e di farmaci simpaticolitici. Ricerca Sci. **22**, 1568–1577 (1952)
Erspamer, V.: Pharmacological studies on enteramine (5-Hydroxytryptamine). Arch. int. Pharmacodyn. **93**, 293–316 (1953)
Euler, U.S.v.: Effect of some metabolic factors and drugs on uptake and release of catecholamines in vitro and in vivo. In: New Aspects of Storage and Release Mechanisms of Catecholamines. Schümann, H.J., Kroneberg, G. (eds.), pp. 144–158. Berlin-Heidelberg-New York: Springer 1970
Euler, U.S.v.: Adrenergic nerve particles in relation to uptake and release of neurotransmitter. J. Endocr. **55**, 2–9 (1972)
Euler, U.S.v., Hedqvist, P.: Inhibitory action of prostaglandins E_1 and E_2 on the neuromuscular transmission in the guinea-pig vas deferens. Acta physiol. scand. **77**, 510–512 (1969)

Euler, U.S.v., Lishajko, F.: Inhibitory action of adrenergic blocking agents on catecholamine release and uptake in isolated nerve granules. Acta physiol. scand. **68**, 257–262 (1966)
Euler, U.S.v., Lishajko, F.: Inhibitory action of adrenergic blocking agents on reuptake and net uptake of noradrenaline in nerve granules. Acta physiol. scand. **74**, 501–506 (1968)
Evans, D.H.L., Schild, H.O., Thesleff, S.: Effects of drugs on depolarized plain muscle. J. Physiol. (Lond.) **143**, 474–485 (1958)
Eyre, P.: Pharmacology of bovine pulmonary vein anaphylaxis in vitro. Brit. J. Pharmacol. **43**, 302–311 (1971)
Eyre, P.: Atypical tryptamine receptors in sheep pulmonary vein. Brit. J. Pharmacol. **55**, 329–333 (1975)
Fanchamps, A., Doepfner, W., Weidmann, H., Cerletti, A.: Pharmakologische Charakterisierung von Deseril, einem Serotonin-Antagonisten. Schweiz. med. Wschr. **90**, 1040–1046 (1960)
Fanciullacci, M., Franchi, G., Sicuteri, F.: Facilitazione dell' azione venocostrittrice della 5-idrossitriptamina da ergotamina, metisergide e LSD-25 nell'uomo. Boll. Soc. ital. Biol. sper. **51**, 517–522 (1975)
Fara, J.: Mesenteric vasodilator responses to 5-hydroxytryptamine. Gastroenterology **66**, 689 (1974)
Farnebo, L.-O., Hamberger, B.: Drug-induced changes in the release of [^{3}H]-noradrenaline from field stimulated rat iris. Brit. J. Pharmacol. **43**, 97–106 (1971a)
Farnebo, L.-O., Hamberger, B.: Drug-induced changes in the release of ^{3}H-monoamines from field stimulated rat brain slices. Acta physiol. scand. (Suppl.) **371**, 35–44 (1971b)
Farnebo, L.-O., Hamberger, B.: Regulation of [^{3}H] 5-hydroxytryptamine release from rat brain slices. J. Pharm. Pharmacol. **26**, 642–644 (1974)
Farrow, J.T., Van Vunakis, H.: Binding of D-lysergic acid diethylamide to subcellular fractions from rat brain. Nature (Lond.) **237**, 164–165 (1972)
Farrow, J.T., Van Vunakis, H.: Characteristics of D-lysergic acid diethylamide binding to subcellular fractions derived from rat brain. Biochem. Pharmacol. **22**, 1103–1113 (1973)
Feldman, J.M., Lebovitz, H.E.: Specificity of serotonin inhibition of insulin release from golden hamster pancreas. Diabetes **19**, 475–479 (1970a)
Feldman, J.M., Lebovitz, H.E.: Mechanism of epinephrine and serotonin inhibition of insulin release in the golden hamster in vitro. Diabetes **19**, 480–486 (1970b)
Ferrini, R., Glässer, A.: Antagonism of central effects of tryptamine and 5-hydroxytryptophan by 1,6-dimethyl-8β-carbo-benzyloxyaminomethyl-10α-ergoline). Psychopharmacologia **8**, 271–276 (1965)
Fillion, G., Fillion, M.-P., Spirakis, Ch., Bahers, J.-M., Jacob, J.: 5-Hydroxytryptamine binding to synaptic membranes from rat brain. Life Sci. **18**, 65–74 (1976)
Fingerman, M., Rao, K.R.: Action of biogenic amines on crustacean chromatophores. Comp. gen. Pharmacol. **1**, 341–348 (1970)
Fingl, E., Gaddum, J.H.: Hydroxytryptamine blockade by dihydroergotamine in vitro. Fed. Proc. **12**, 320 (1953)
Fishlock, D.J.: The action of 5-hydroxytryptamine on the circular muscle of the human ileum and colon in vitro. J. Physiol. (Lond.) **170**, 11P–12P (1964)
Fishlock, D.J., Parks, A.G., Dewell, J.V.: Action of 5-hydroxytryptamine on the human stomach, duodenum and jejunum in vitro. Gut **6**, 338–342 (1965)
Fleckenstein, A.: A quantitative study of antagonists of adrenaline on the vessels of the rabbit's ear. Brit. J. Pharmacol. **7**, 553–562 (1952)
Fleisch, J.H., Maling, H.M., Brodie, B.B.: Evidence for existence of alpha-adrenergic receptors in the mammalian trachea. Amer. J. Physiol. **218**, 596–599 (1970)
Flückiger, E., Balthasar, H.U.: Dihydroergocristin: Unterschiedliche Wirkungen an venösem und arteriellem Gewebe. Arzneimittel-Forsch. **17**, 6–9 (1967)
Flückiger, E., Salzmann, R.: Serotoninantagonismus an der Placenta. Experientia (Basel) **17**, 131 (1961)
Foote, W.E., Sheard, M.H., Aghajanian, G.K.: Comparison of effects of LSD and amphetamine on midbrain raphe units. Nature (Lond.) **222**, 567–569 (1969)
Fozard, J.R.: Clonidine and methysergide: effects on an isolated artery. Naunyn-Schmiedebergs Arch. Pharmacol. **279** (Suppl.), R21 (1973a)

Fozard, J.R.: Drug interactions on an isolated artery. In: Background to Migraine. Cumings, J.N. (ed.), pp. 150–169. London: William Heinemann Medical Books 1973b
Fozard, J.R.: The mechanisms by which migraine prophylactic drugs modify vascular reactivity in vitro. "Headache '76", Joint Meeting of the Italian Headache and the Scandinavian Migraine Societies, Florence, 1976a, Abstract, pp. 7–8
Fozard, J.R.: Comparative effects of four migraine prophylactic drugs on an isolated extracranial artery. Europ. J. Pharmacol. **36**, 127–139 (1976b)
Fozard, J.R., Berry, J.L.: Interactions between antimigraine drugs and a high affinity uptake and storage machanism for 5-hydroxytryptamine. Pharmacology **14**, 357–361 (1976)
Fozard, J.R., Leach, G.D.H.: The hypotensive action of 5-hydroxytryptamine (5-HT) in anaesthetised and pithed rats. Europ. J. Pharmacol. **2**, 239–249 (1968)
Fozard, J.R., Wright, J.L.: Interaction between antimigraine drugs and a high affinity uptake and storage mechanism for 5-hydroxytryptamine. Sixth Migraine Symposium, London, 1974, Abstract, pp. 9–10
Frankhuijzen, A.L.: Analysis of ergotamine-5-HT interaction on the isolated rat stomach preparation. Europ. J. Pharmacol. **30**, 205–212 (1975)
Frankhuijzen, A.L., Bonta, I.L.: Effect of mianserin, a potent anti-serotonin agent, on the isolated rat stomach fundus preparation. Europ. J. Pharmacol. **25**, 40–50 (1974a)
Frankhuijzen, A.L., Bonta, I.L.: Receptors involved in the action of 5-HT and tryptamine on the isolated rat stomach fundus preparation. Europ. J. Pharmacol. **26**, 220–230 (1974b)
Fredholm, B.B., Rosell, S.: Fate of ^{3}H-noradrenaline in canine subcutaneous adipose tissue. Acta physiol. scand. **80**, 404–411 (1970)
Freedman, D.X.: LSD-25 and brain serotonin in reserpinized rat. Fed. Proc. **19**, 266 (1960)
Freedman, D.X.: Effects of LSD-25 on brain serotonin. J. Pharmacol. exp. Ther. **134**, 160–166 (1961)
Freedman, D.X.: Psychotomimetic drugs and brain biogenic amines. Amer. J. Psychiat. **119**, 843–850 (1963)
Freedman, D.X.: Aspects of the biochemical pharmacology of psychotropic drugs. In: Psychiatric Drugs. Solomon, P. (ed.), pp. 32–57. New York: Grune and Stratton 1966
Freedman, D.X.: LSD, psychotogenic procedures and brain neuro-humors. Psychopharmacol. Bull. **11**, 42–43 (1975)
Freedman, D.X., Aghajanian, G.K.: Approaches to the pharmacology of LSD-25. Lloydia **29**, 309–314 (1967)
Freedman, D.X., Boggan, W.O.: Brain serotonin metabolism after tolerance dosage of LSD. Adv. Biochem. Psychopharmacol. **10**, 151–157 (1974)
Freedman, D.X., Coquet, C.A.: Regional and subcellular distribution of LSD and effects on 5-HT levels. Pharmacologist **7**, 183 (1965)
Freedman, D.X., Giarman, N.J.: LSD-25 and the status and level of brain serotonin. Ann. N.Y. Acad. Sci. **96**, 98–106 (1962)
Freedman, D.X., Gottlieb, R., Lovell, R.A.: Psychotomimetic drugs and brain 5-hydroxytryptamine metabolism. Biochem. Pharmacol. **19**, 1181–1188 (1970)
Fregnan, G.B., Glässer, A.H.: Activity of eledoisin, other polypeptides and ergometrine on the uterus in situ of rabbit and other animal species. J. Pharm. Pharmacol. **16**, 744–750 (1964)
Fregnan, G.B., Glässer, A.H.: Structure-activity relationship of various acyl derivatives of 6-methyl-8β-aminomethyl-10α-ergoline (dihydrolysergamine). Experientia (Basel) **24**, 150–151 (1968)
Froment, J.L., Eskazan, E., Jouvet, M.: Effets du LSD et du méthysergide sur les pointes ponto géniculo occipitales. C.R. Soc. Biol. (Paris) **165**, 2153–2157 (1971)
Furchgott, R.F.: Dibenamine blockade in strips of rabbit aorta and its use in differentiating receptors. J. Pharmacol. exp. Ther. **111**, 265–284 (1954)
Furchgott, R.F.: The pharmacology of vascular smooth muscle. Pharmacol. Rev. **7**, 183–265 (1955)
Furchgott, R.F.: Receptors for sympathomimetic amines. In: Ciba Foundation Symposium on Adrenergic Mechanisms. Wolstenholme, G.E.W., O'Connor, M. (eds.), pp. 246–252. London: J. and A. Churchill 1960
Furchgott, R.F.: The pharmacological differentiation of adrenergic receptors. Ann. N.Y. Acad. Sci. **139**, 553–570 (1967)

Furchgott, R.F.: The classification of adrenoceptors (adrenergic receptors). An evaluation from the standpoint of receptor theory. In: Handbook of Experimental Pharmacology. Catecholamines. Blaschko, H., Muscholl, E. (eds.), Vol. XXXIII, pp. 283–335. Berlin-Heidelberg-New York: Springer 1972

Furukawa, K., Nomoto, T.: 5-Hydroxytryptamine receptors in isolated rat ileum. Jap. J. Pharmacol. **24** (Suppl.), 95 (1974)

Furukawa, K., Nomoto, T.: Changes in the response to ACh, nicotine and 5-hydroxytryptamine in chemical sympathectomized rat ileum. Jap. J. Pharmacol. **25** (Suppl.), 29P (1975)

Fuxe, K.: Evidence for the existence of monoamine neurons in the central nervous system. IV. Distribution of monoamine terminals in the central nervous system. Acta physiol. scand. **64** (Suppl. 247), 37–85 (1965)

Fuxe, K., Corrodi, H., Hökfelt, T., Lidbrink, P., Ungerstedt, U.: Ergocornine and 2-Br-α-ergocryptine. Evidence for prolonged dopamine receptor stimulation. Med. Biol. **52**, 121–132 (1974)

Fuxe, K., Agnati, L., Everitt, B.: Effects of methergoline on central monoamine neurones. Evidence for a selective blockade of central 5-HT receptors. Neurosci. Lett. **1**, 283–290 (1975a)

Fuxe, K., Agnati, L.F., Hökfelt, T., Jonsson, G., Lidbrink, P., Ljungdahl, A., Lofstrom, A., Ungerstedt, U.: The effect of dopamine receptor stimulating and blocking agents on the activity of supersensitive dopamine receptors and on the amine turnover in various dopamine nerve terminal systems in the rat brain. J. Pharmacol. (Paris) **6**, 117–129 (1975b)

Gaddum, J.H.: The action of adrenalin and ergotamine on the uterus of the rabbit. J. Physiol. (Lond.) **61**, 141–150 (1926)

Gaddum, J.H.: Antagonism between lysergic acid diethylamide and 5-hydroxytryptamine. J. Physiol. (Lond.) **121**, 15P (1953)

Gaddum, J.H.: Drugs antagonistic to 5-hydroxytryptamine. In: Ciba Symposium on Hypertension. Wolstenholme, G.E.W., Cameron, M.P. (eds.), pp. 75–77. London: J. and A. Churchill 1954

Gaddum, J.H.: Drugs which antagonize the actions of 5-hydroxytryptamine on peripheral tissues. In: 5-Hydroxytryptamine. Lewis, G.P. (ed.), pp. 195–205. New York: Pergamon Press 1957

Gaddum, J.H., Hameed, K.A.: Drugs which antagonize 5-hydroxytryptamine. Brit. J. Pharmacol. **9**, 240–248 (1954)

Gaddum, J.H., Paasonen, M.K.: The use of some molluscan hearts for the estimation of 5-hydroxytryptamine. Brit. J. Pharmacol. **10**, 474–483 (1955)

Gaddum, J.H., Picarelli, Z.P.: Two kinds of tryptamine receptor. Brit. J. Pharmacol. **12**, 323–328 (1957)

Gaddum, J.H., Szerb, J.C.: Assay of substance P on goldfish intestine in a microbath. Brit. J. Pharmacol. **17**, 451–463 (1961)

Gaddum, J.H., Vogt, M.: Some central actions of 5-hydroxytryptamine and various antagonists. Brit. J. Pharmacol. **11**, 175–179 (1956)

Gaddum, J.H., Hebb, C.O., Silver, A., Swan, A.A.B.: 5-Hydroxytryptamine. Pharmacological action and destruction in perfused lungs. Quart. J. exp. Physiol. **38**, 255–262 (1953)

Gaddum, J.H., Hameed, K.A., Hathway, D.E., Stephens, F.F.: Quantitative studies of antagonists for 5-hydroxytryptamine. Quart. J. exp. Physiol. **40**, 49–74 (1955)

Gagnon, D.J.: Contraction of the rat colon by sympathomimetic amines: effect of methysergide and 5-HT desensitization. Europ. J. Pharmacol. **17**, 319–324 (1972)

Gallager, D.W., Aghajanian, G.K.: Chlorimipramine and LSD: differential effects on the in vivo release of ^{3}H-5HT. Pharmacologist **16**, 244 (1974)

Gallager, D.W., Aghajanian, G.K.: Effects of chlorimipramine and lysergic acid diethylamide on efflux of precursor-formed ^{3}H-serotonin: correlations with serotonergic impulse flow. J. Pharmacol. exp. Ther. **193**, 785–795 (1975)

Gallager, D.W., Aghajanian, G.K.: Inhibition of firing of raphe neurones by tryptophan and 5-hydroxytryptophan: blockade by inhibiting serotonin synthesis with Ro-4-4602. Neuropharmacology **15**, 149–156 (1976)

Gant, D.W., Dyer, D.C.: D-Lysergic acid diethylamide (LSD-25): a constrictor of human umbilical vein. Life Sci. **10**, 235–240 (1971)

Garrett, R.L., Brown, J.H.: Bradykinin-potentiated contractions induced by serotonin (5-HT), norepinephrine (NE) and potassium (K^+) in rabbit aortic strips. Pharmacologist **12**, 263 (1970)
Garrett, R.L., Brown, J.H.: Bradykinin interaction with 5-hydroxytryptamine, norepinephrine and potassium chloride in rabbit aorta. Proc. Soc. exp. Biol. (N.Y.) **139**, 1344–1348 (1972)
Garrett, W.J.: The effects of adrenaline, noradrenaline and dihydroergotamine on excised human myometrium. Brit. J. Pharmacol. **10**, 39–44 (1955)
Gautrelet, J., Scheiner, H.: Détermination du pouvoir anticholinesterasique de différentes substances par la méthode de la décontraction du muscle droit de l'abdomen de la grenouille contracté par l'acétylcholine. C.R. Soc. Biol. (Paris) **131**, 738–740 (1939)
Gelfand, M.D., West, G.B.: Experimental studies with the butanolamide and propanolamide of 1-methyl-lysergic acid. Int. Arch. Allergy **18**, 286–291 (1961)
Gerschenfeld, H.M.: Serotonin: Two different inhibitory actions on snail neurons. Science **171**, 1252–1254 (1971)
Gerschenfeld, H.M., Paupardin, D.: Actions of 5-hydroxytryptamine on mulluscan neuronal membranes. In: Drug Receptors. Rang, H.P. (ed.), pp. 45–61. London: Macmillan 1972
Gerschenfeld, H.M., Paupardin-Tritsch, D.: Ionic mechanisms and receptor properties underlying the responses of molluscan neurones to 5-hydroxytryptamine. J. Physiol. (Lond.) **243**, 427–456 (1974a)
Gerschenfeld, H.M., Paupardin-Tritsch, D.: On the transmitter function of 5-hydroxytryptamine at excitatory and inhibitory monosynaptic junctions. J. Physiol. (Lond.) **243**, 457–481 (1974b)
Gerschenfeld, H.M., Paupardin-Tritsch, D.: Excitatory and inhibitory monosynaptic actions mediated by a serotonin ccntaining neuron in *Aplysia californica*. J. Physiol. (Lond.) **243**, 28P-29P (1974c)
Gerschenfeld, H.M., Stefani, E.: 5-Hydroxytryptamine receptors and synaptic transmission in molluscan neurones. Nature (Lond.) **205**, 1216–1218 (1965)
Gerschenfeld, H.M., Stefani, E.: An electrophysiological study of 5-hydroxytryptamine receptors of neurones in the molluscan nervous system. J. Physiol. (Lond.) **185**, 684–700 (1966)
Gerschenfeld, H.M., Stefani, E.: Acetylcholine and 5-hydroxytryptamine receptors in neurones of the land-snail *Cryptomphallus aspersa*. J. Physiol. (Lond.) **191**, 14P–15P (1967)
Gerschenfeld, H.M., Stefani, E.: Evidence for an excitatory transmitter role of serotonin in molluscan central synapses. In: Advances in Pharmacology. Garattini, S., Shore, P.A. (eds.), pp. 369–392. New York-London: Academic Press 1968
Gerschenfeld, H.M., Tauc, L.: Différents aspects de la pharmacologie des synapses dans le système nerveux central des mollusques. J. Physiol. (Paris) **56**, 360–361 (1964)
Gilbert, J.-C., Goldberg, L.I.: Characterization by cyproheptadine of the dopamine-induced contraction in canine isolated arteries. J. Pharmacol. exp. Ther. **193**, 435–442 (1975)
Gillespie, J.S., Kirpekar, S.M.: Uptake and release of H^3-noradrenaline by the splenic nerves. J. Physiol. (Lond.) **178**, 44P–45P (1965a)
Gillespie, J.S., Kirpekar, S.M.: The inactivation of infused noradrenaline by the cat spleen. J. Physiol. (Lond.) **176**, 205–227 (1965b)
Gillespie, J.S., McGrath, J.C.: The effect of lysergic acid diethylamide (LSD) on the vas deferens and anococcygeus muscle. Brit. J. Pharmacol. **52**, 128P (1974)
Gillespie, J.S., McGrath, J.C.: The effects of lysergic acid diethylamide on the response to field stimulation of the rat vas deferens and the rat and cat anococcygeus muscles. Brit. J. Pharmacol. **54**, 481–488 (1975)
Gillespie, J.S., Muir, T.C.: A method of stimulating the complete sympathetic outflow from the spinal cord to blood vessels in the pithed rat. Brit. J. Pharmacol. **30**, 78–87 (1967)
Gillespie, J.S., Hamilton, D.N.H., Hosie, R.J.A.: The extraneuronal uptake and localization of noradrenaline in the cat spleen and the effect on this of some drugs, of cold and of denervation. J. Physiol. (Lond.) **206**, 563–590 (1970)
Ginzel, K.H.: The action of lysergic acid diethylamide (LSD 25), its 2-brom derivative (BOL 148) and of 5-hydroxytryptamine (5-HT) on the peristaltic reflex of the guinea-pig ileum. J. Physiol. (Lond.) **137**, 62P–63P (1957)
Ginzel, K.H., Kottegoda, S.R.: A study of the vascular actions of 5-hydroxytryptamine, tryptamine, adrenaline and nor-adrenaline. Quart. J. exp. Physiol. **38**, 225–231 (1953)

Glegg, A.M., Turner, P.: Cholinergic interactions of methysergide and cinanserin on isolated human smooth muscle. Arch. int. Pharmacodyn. **191**, 301–309 (1971)

Glover, W.E., Marshall, R.J., Whelan, R.F.: The antagonism of the vascular effects of 5-hydroxytryptamine by BOL 148 and sodium salicylate in the human subject. Brit. J. Pharmacol. **12**, 498–503 (1957)

Glowinski, J., Hamon, M., Hery, F.: Regulation of 5-HT synthesis in central serotoninergic neurons. In: New Concepts in Neurotransmitter Regulation. Mandell, A.J. (ed.), pp. 239–257. New York: Plenum Press 1973

Görlitz, B.D., Frey, H.H.: Comparison of the blocking effects of antagonists of adrenaline and 5-hydroxytryptamine on their mutual receptors. J. Pharm. Pharmacol. **25**, 651–653 (1973)

Goetz, C.G., Klawans, H.L.: Myoclonus, methysergide, and serotonin. Lancet **1974/I**, 1284–1285

Gogerty, J.H., Dille, J.M.: Pharmacology of D-lysergic acid morpholide (LSM). J. Pharmacol. exp. Ther. **120**, 340–348 (1957)

Gokhale, S.D., Gulati, O.D., Kelkar, L.V., Kelkar, V.V.: Effect of some drugs on human umbilical artery in vitro. Brit. J. Pharmacol. **27**, 332–346 (1966)

Goldberg, L.I.: Comparison of putative dopamine receptors in blood vessels and the central nervous system. Adv. Neurol. **9**, 53–56 (1975)

Goldberg, L.I., Toda, N.: Dopamine induced relaxation of isolated canine renal, mesenteric and femoral arteries contracted with prostaglandin $F_{2\alpha}$. Circulat. Res. **36** (Suppl. I), 97–102 (1975)

Goldberg, L.I., Tjandramaga, T.B., Anton, A.H., Toda, N.: New investigations of the cardiovascular actions of dopamine. In: Frontiers in Catecholamine Research. Usdin, E., Snyder, S. (eds.), pp. 513–521. New York: Pergamon Press 1973

Goldman, J.M., Hadley, M.E.: In vitro demonstration of adrenergic receptors controlling melanophore responses of the lizard, *Anolis carolinensis*. J. Pharmacol. exp. Ther. **166**, 1–7 (1969)

Goldman, J.M., Hadley, M.E.: Direct agonistic and antagonistic effects of ergotamine on vertebrate melanophores. Arch. int. Pharmacodyn. **183**, 239–246 (1970a)

Goldman, J.M., Hadley, M.E.: Cyclic AMP and adrenergic receptors in melanophore responses to methylxanthines. Europ. J. Pharmacol. **12**, 365–370 (1970b)

Goldman, J.M., Hadley, M.E.: Sulfhydryl requirement for *alpha* adrenergic receptor activity and melanophore stimulating hormone (MSH) action on melanophores. J. Pharmacol. exp. Ther. **182**, 93–100 (1972)

Gonzáles, R., Garcia, M., Rojas, R.: The mode of action of serotonin on the isolated atrium of hamsters. Sixth Internat. Congr. Pharmacol., Helsinki, 1975, Abstract 1433

Gordon, J.L., Drummond, A.H.: Irreversible aggregation of pig platelets and release of intracellular constituents induced by 5-hydroxytryptamine. Biochem. Pharmacol. **24**, 33–36 (1975)

Greeff, K., Holtz, P.: Über die Uteruswirkung des Adrenalins und Arterenols. Ein Beitrag zum Problem der Uterusinnervation Arch. int. Pharmacodyn. **88**, 228–252 (1951)

Greeff, K., Benfey, B.G., Bokelmann, A.: Anaphylaktische Reaktionen am isolierten Herzvorhofpräparat des Meerschweinchens und ihre Beeinflussung durch Antihistaminica, BOL, Dihydroergotamin und Reserpin. Naunyn-Schmiedebergs Arch. Pharmacol. **236**, 421–434 (1959)

Greenberg, D.A., U'Prichard, D.C., Snyder, S.H.: Alpha-noradrenergic receptor binding in mammalian brain: differential labeling of agonist and antagonist states. Life Sci. **19**, 69–76 (1976)

Greenberg, M.J.: The responses of the *venus* heart to catecholamines and high concentrations of 5-hydroxytryptamine. Brit. J. Pharmacol. **15**, 365–374 (1960a)

Greenberg, M.J.: Structure-activity relationship of tryptamine analogues on the heart of *Venus mercenaria*. Brit. J. Pharmacol. **15**, 375–388 (1960b)

Grove, D.J., O'Neill, J.G., Spillett, P.B.: The action of 5-hydroxytryptamine on longitudinal gastric smooth muscle of the plaice, *Pleuronectes platessa*. Comp. gen. Pharmacol. **5**, 229–238 (1974)

Guimarães, S.: Reversal by pronethalol of dibenamine blockade: A study on the seminal vesicle of the guinea-pig. Brit. J. Pharmacol. **36**, 594–601 (1969a)

Guimarães, S.: *Alpha* excitatory, *alpha* inhibitory and *beta* inhibitory adrenergic receptors in the guinea-pig stomach. Arch. int. Pharmacodyn. **179**, 188–201 (1969b)
Guimarães, S., Osswald, W.: Adrenergic receptors in the veins of the dog. Europ. J. Pharmacol. **5**, 133–140 (1969)
Gulati, O.D., Kelkar, V.V.: Effect of tyramine on human umbilical artery in vitro. Brit. J. Pharmacol. **42**, 155–158 (1971)
Guth, P.S., Spirtes, M.A.: Interaction in the central nervous system between serotonin and lysergic acid derivatives. In: Neuropsychopharmacology. Proc. 1st. Intern. Congr. Neuropharmacol., Rome, Bradley, P.B., Deniker, P., Radouco-Thomas, C. (eds.), pp. 319–323. London: Elsevier 1958
Gyermek, L.: The action of 5-hydroxytryptamine on the urinary bladder of the dog. Pharmacologist **2**, 89 (1960)
Gyermek, L.: Action of 5-hydroxytryptamine on the urinary bladder of the dog. Arch. int. Pharmacodyn. **137**, 137–144 (1962)
Gyermek, L.: Drugs which antagonize 5-hydroxytryptamine and related indolealkylamines. In: 5-Hydroxytryptamine and Related Indolealkylamines. Handbook of Experimental Pharmacology. Eichler, O., Farah, A. (eds.), Vol. XIX, pp. 471–528. Berlin-Heidelberg-New York: Springer 1966
Gyermek, L., Bindler, E.: Blockade of the ganglionic stimulant action of 5-hydroxytryptamine. J. Pharmacol. exp. Ther. **135**, 344–348 (1962)
Gyermek, L., Sumi, T.: Potentiating actions of indolealkylamines and lysergic acid diethylamide on reflexes elicited by 5-hydroxytryptamine. Proc. Soc. exp. Biol. (N.Y.) **114**, 436–439 (1963)
Gyires, K., Knoll, J.: Inflammation and writhing syndrome inducing effect of PGE_1, PGE_2 and the inhibition of these actions. Pol. J. Pharmacol. Pharm. **27**, 257–264 (1975)
György, L., Borbély, L., Kelemen, B., Somkúti, T.: Über die adrenerg-erregenden Eigenschaften des Ergotoxins. Acta physiol. Acad. Sci. hung. **14**, 391–398 (1958a)
György, L., Somkúti, T., Kelemen, B., Borbély, L.: The problem of ergotoxin-adrenaline synergism and antagonism: the effect of general anaesthesia. Acta physiol. Acad. Sci. hung. **14**, 287–300 (1958b)
Haefely, W.: Effects of serotonin (5-HT) and some related indole compounds in a mammalian sympathetic ganglion. Experientia (Basel) **27**, 1112 (1971)
Haefely, W.: The effects of 5-hydroxytryptamine and some related compounds on the cat superior cervical ganglion in situ. Naunyn-Schmiedebergs Arch. Pharmacol. **281**, 145–165 (1974)
Haefely, W., Ruch-Monachon, M.A., Jalfre, M.: Interaction of psychotropic agents with central neurotransmitters as revealed by their effects on PGO waves in the cat. Arzneimittel-Forsch. **26**, 1036–1039 (1976)
Haeusler, G., Finch, L.: Vascular reactivity to 5-hydroxytryptamine and hypertension in the rat. Naunyn-Schmiedebergs Arch. Pharmacol. **272**, 101–116 (1972)
Haigler, H.J., Aghajanian, G.K.: Mescaline and LSD: Direct and indirect effects on serotonin-containing neurons in brain. Europ. J. Pharmacol. **21**, 53–60 (1973a)
Haigler, H.J., Aghajanian, G.K.: A comparison of effects of D-lysergic acid diethylamide (LSD) and serotonin on pre- and postsynaptic cells in the serotonin system. Fed. Proc. **32**, 303 (1973b)
Haigler, H.J., Aghajanian, G.K.: Peripheral serotonin antagonists: failure to antagonize serotonin in brain areas receiving a prominent serotonergic input. J. Neural Transm. **35**, 257–273 (1974a)
Haigler, H.J., Aghajanian, G.K.: Lysergic acid diethylamide and serotonin: a comparison of effects on serotonergic neurons and neurons receiving serotonergic input. J. Pharmacol. exp. Ther. **188**, 688–699 (1974b)
Halaris, A.E., Lovell, R.A.: On the nature of the serotonin binding after LSD. Fed. Proc. **32**, 694 (1973)
Halaris, A.E., Freedman, D.X., Fang, V.S.: Plasma corticoids and brain tryptophan after acute and tolerance dosage of LSD. Life Sci. **17**, 1467–1472 (1975)
Hall, W.J., O'Connor, P.C.: The action of vasoactive drugs on longitudinal and circular muscle of dog mesenteric vein. J. Pharm. Pharmacol. **25**, 109–118 (1973)

Halmagyi, D.F.J., Colebatch, H.J.H.: Serotonin-like cardiorespiratory effects of a serotonin antagonist. J. Pharmacol. exp. Ther. **134**, 47–52 (1961)
Hamon, M., Glowinski, J.: Regulation of serotonin synthesis. Life Sci. **15**, 1533–1548 (1974)
Hamon, M., Bourgoin, S., Jagger, J., Glowinski, J.: Effects of LSD on synthesis and release of 5-HT in rat brain slices. Brain Res. **69**, 265–280 (1974)
Hamon, M., Bourgoin, S., Enjalbert, A., Bockaert, J., Hery, F., Ternaux, J.P., Glowinski, J.: The effect of quipazine on 5-HT metabolism in the rat brain. Naunyn-Schmiedebergs Arch. Pharmacol. **294**, 99–108 (1976a)
Hamon, M., Bourgoin, S., Hery, F., Ternaux, J.P.: In vivo and in vitro activation of soluble tryptophan hydroxylase from rat brainstem. Nature (Lond.) **260**, 61–63 (1976b)
Handforth, A., Sourkes, T.L.: Inhibition by dopamine agonists of dopamine accumulation following γ-hydroxybutyrate treatment. Europ. J. Pharmacol. **34**, 311–319 (1975)
Handschumacher, R.E., Vane, J.R.: Studies relating constrictions to entrance of 5-hydroxytryptamine (5-HT) and tryptamine (T) in smooth muscle. Fed. Proc. **22**, 167 (1963)
Handschumacher, R.E., Vane, J.R.: The relationship between the penetration of tryptamine and 5-hydroxytryptamine into smooth muscle and the associated contractions. Brit. J. Pharmacol. **29**, 105–118 (1967)
Hardebo, J.E., Edvinsson, L.: Mechanical actions of serotonin and the effect of related inhibitors in intracranial and extracranial vessels. "Headache '76", Joint Meeting of the Italian Headache and the Scandinavian Migraine Societies, Florence, 1976, Abstract, pp. 11–13
Hariri, M.: Uptake of 5-hydroxytryptamine by *Mesocestoides corti* (Cestoda). J. Parasit. **61**, 440–448 (1975)
Harper, M.J.K., Skarnes, R.C.: Inhibition of abortion and fetal death produced by endotoxin or prostaglandin $F_{2\alpha}$. Prostaglandins **2**, 295–309 (1972)
Hauge, A., Lunde, P.K.M., Waaler, B.A.: The effect of bradykinin, kallidin and eledoisin upon the pulmonary vascular bed of an isolated blood-perfused rabbit lung preparation. Acta physiol. scand. **66**, 269–277 (1966)
Hayashi, A.: Receptors for phenylephrine and 5-hydroxytryptamine in the rat jejunum. Fukushima J. med. Sci. **21**, 59–68 (1975)
Hedqvist, P.: Modulating effect of prostaglandin E_2 on noradrenaline release from the isolated cat spleen. Acta physiol. scand. **75**, 511–512 (1969)
Hedqvist, P.: Studies on the effect of prostaglandins E_1 and E_2 on the sympathetic neuromuscular transmission in some animal tissues. Acta physiol. scand. (Suppl.) **345**, 1–40 (1970a)
Hedqvist, P.: Control by prostaglandin E_2 of sympathetic neurotransmission in the spleen. Life Sci. **9**, 269–278 (1970b)
Hedqvist, P.: Dissociation of prostaglandin and α-receptor mediated control of adrenergic transmitter release. Acta physiol. scand. **87**, 42A–43A (1973)
Hedqvist, P.: Role of the α-receptor in the control of noradrenaline release from sympathetic nerves. Acta physiol. scand. **90**, 158–165 (1974)
Hedqvist, P., Brundin, J.: Inhibition by prostaglandin E_1 of noradrenaline release and of effector response to nerve stimulation in the cat spleen. Life Sci. **8**, 389–395 (1969)
Hedqvist, P., von Euler, U.S.: Prostaglandin-induced neurotransmission failure in the field-stimulated, isolated vas deferens. Neuropharmacology **11**, 177–187 (1972)
Hedqvist, P., Stjärne, L., Wennmalm, Å.: Inhibition by prostaglandin E_2 of sympathetic neurotransmission in the rabbit heart. Acta physiol. scand. **79**, 139–141 (1970)
Henderson, G., North, R.A.: Presynaptic action of 5-hydroxytryptamine in the myenteric plexus of the guinea-pig ileum. Brit. J. Pharmacol. **54**, 265 (1975)
Hertzler, E.C.: 5-Hydroxytryptamine and transmission in sympathetic ganglia. Brit. J. Pharmacol. **17**, 406–413 (1961)
Herxheimer, H.: Further observations on the influence of 5-hydroxytryptamine on bronchial function. J. Physiol. (Lond.) **122**, 49P–50P (1953)
Herxheimer, H.: The 5-hydroxytryptamine shock in the guinea-pig. J. Physiol. (Lond.) **128**, 435–445 (1955)
Herxheimer, H.: Bronchoconstrictor agents and their antagonists in the intact guinea-pig. Arch. int. Pharmacodyn. **106**, 371–380 (1956)
Higgins, W.J.: Intracellular actions of 5-hydroxytryptamine on the bivalve myocardium. J. exp. Zool. **190**, 99–109 (1974)

Hillman, G.R., Olsen, N.J., Senft, A.W.: Effect of methysergide and dihydroergotamine on *Schistosoma mansoni*. J. Pharmacol. exp. Ther. **188**, 529–535 (1974)
Hill-Samli, M., MacLeod, R.M.: Thyrotropin-releasing hormone blockade of the ergocryptine and apomorphine inhibition of prolactin release in vitro. Proc. Soc. exp. Biol. (N.Y.) **149**, 511–514 (1975)
Hilton, B.P., Cumings, J.N.: An assessment of platelet aggregation induced by 5-hydroxytryptamine. J. clin. Path. **24**, 250–258 (1971)
Hirst, G.D.S., McKirdy, H.C.: Synaptic potentials recorded from neurones of the submucous plexus of guinea-pig intestine. J. Physiol. (Lond.) **249**, 369–385 (1975)
Hirst, G.D.S., Silinsky, E.M.: Some effects of 5-hydroxytryptamine, dopamine and noradrenaline on neurones in the submucous plexus of guinea-pig small intestine. J. Physiol. (Lond.) **251**, 817–832 (1975)
Hitner, H., Di Gregorio, G.J.: Preliminary investigation of the peripheral sympathomimetic effects of phencyclidine. Arch. int. Pharmacodyn. **212**, 36–42 (1974)
Hökfelt, T., Fuxe, K.: On the morphology and the neuroendocrine role of the hypothalamic catecholamine neurons. In: Brain-Endocrine Interaction. Median Eminence: Structure and Function, Knigge, K.M., Scott, D.F., Weindt, A. (eds.), pp. 181–223. Basle: Karger 1972
Holgate, J.A., Warner, B.T.: Evaluation of antagonists of histamine, 5-hydroxytryptamine and acetylcholine in the guinea-pig. Brit. J. Pharmacol. **15**, 561–566 (1960)
Hollenberg, M.D., Cuatrecasas, P.: Studies on the interaction of hormones with plasma membrane receptors. Biochem. Actions Horm. **3**, 41–85 (1975)
Holroyde, M.C., Eyre, P.: Reactivity of isolated bovine mesenteric and hepatic veins to vasoactive agents and specific antigen. Europ. J. Pharmacol. **30**, 36–42 (1975)
Holzbauer, M., Vogt, M.: Modification by drugs of the response of the rat's uterus to adrenaline. Brit. J. Pharmacol. **10**, 186–190 (1955)
Hughes, J.: Inhibition of noradrenaline release by lysergic acid diethylamide. Brit. J. Pharmacol. **49**, 706–708 (1973)
Hughes, J., Vane, J.R.: An analysis of the responses of the isolated portal vein of the rabbit to electrical stimulation and to drugs. Brit. J. Pharmacol. **30**, 46–66 (1967)
Hughes, J., Vane, J.R.: Relaxations of the isolated portal vein of the rabbit induced by nicotine and electrical stimulation. Brit. J. Pharmacol. **39**, 476–489 (1970)
Hughes, J., Kosterlitz, H.W., Leslie, F.M.: Effect of morphine on adrenergic transmission in the mouse vas deferens. Assessment of agonist and antagonist potencies of narcotic analgesics. Brit. J. Pharmacol. **53**, 371–381 (1975)
Ichimasa, S., Kushiku, K., Furukawa, T.: Pharmacological studies on ganglionic transmission: Influence of antagonists on the catecholamine-induced ganglionic inhibition in the cardiac sympathetic ganglia. Jap. J. Pharmacol. **25** (Suppl.), 20 (1975)
Innes, I.R.: Identification of the smooth muscle excitatory receptors for ergot alkaloids. Brit. J. Pharmacol. **19**, 120–128 (1962a)
Innes, I.R.: An action of 5-hydroxytryptamine on adrenaline receptors. Brit. J. Pharmacol. **19**, 427–441 (1962b)
Innes, I.R., Kohli, J.D.: Excitatory action of sympathomimetic amines on 5-hydroxytryptamine receptors of gut. Brit. J. Pharmacol. **35**, 383–393 (1969)
Iturriza, F.C.: The effect of D-lysergic acid diethylamide on the melanophores of the toad *Bufo arenarum* under different experimental conditions. Acta endocr. (Kbh.) **48**, 322–328 (1965)
Iturriza, F.C., Koch, O.R.: Effect of administration of lysergic acid diethylamide (LSD) on the colloid vesicles of the pars intermedia of the toad pituitary. Endocrinology **75**, 615–616 (1964)
Iversen, L.L.: The inhibition of noradrenaline uptake by drugs. In: Advances in Drug Research. Harper, N.J., Simmonds, A.B. (eds.), pp. 1–46. London-New York: Academic Press 1965
Iversen, L.L.: The uptake and storage of noradrenaline in sympathetic nerves. Cambridge: University Press 1967
Iversen, L.L.: Catecholamine uptake processes. Brit. med. Bull. **29**, 130–135 (1973)
Jacoby, J.H., Shabshelowitz, H., Fernstrom, J.D., Wurtman, R.J.: The mechanism by which methiothepin, a putative serotonin receptor antagonist, increases brain 5-hydroxyindole levels. J. Pharmacol. exp. Ther. **195**, 257–264 (1975)

Jafferji, S.S., Michell, R.H.: Stimulation of phosphatidylinositol turnover by histamine, 5-hydroxytryptamine and adrenaline in the longitudinal smooth muscle of guinea-pig ileum. Biochem. Pharmacol. **25**, 1429–1430 (1976)

Jalfre, M., Monachon, M.-A., Haefely, W.: Pharmacological modifications of benzoquinolizine-induced geniculate spikes. Experientia (Basel) **26**, 691 (1970)

Jalfre, M., Monachon, M.A., Haefely, W.: Drugs and PGO waves in the cat. In: First Can. Int. Symposium of Sleep. McClure, D.J. (ed.), pp. 155–185. Montreal: Roche Scientific Service 1972

Jalfre, M., Ruch-Monachon, M.-A., Haefely, W.: Methods for assessing the interaction of agents with 5-hydroxytryptamine neurons and receptors in the brain. Adv. Biochem. Psychopharmacol. **10**, 121–134 (1974)

Jang, C.S.: The potentiation and paralysis of adrenergic effects by ergotoxine and other substances. J. Pharmacol. exp. Ther. **71**, 87–94 (1941)

Jaques, R., Bein, H.J., Meier, R.: 5-Hydroxytryptamine antagonists, with special reference to the importance of sympathomimetic amines and isopropyl-noradrenaline. Helv. physiol. pharmacol. Acta **14**, 269–278 (1956)

Jasmin, G., Bois, P.: Effect of various agents on the development of kidney infarcts in rats treated with serotonin. Lab. Invest. **9**, 503–513 (1960)

Jenkinson, D.H., Morton, I.K.M.: Adrenergic blocking drugs as tools in the study of the actions of catecholamines on the smooth muscle membrane. Ann. N.Y. Acad. Sci. **139**, 762–771 (1967a)

Jenkinson, D.H., Morton, I.K.M.: The effect of noradrenaline on the permeability of depolarized intestinal smooth muscle to inorganic ions. J. Physiol. (Lond.) **188**, 373–386 (1967b)

Jenkinson, D.H., Morton, I.K.M.: The role of α- and β-adrenergic receptors in some actions of catecholamines on intestinal smooth muscle. J. Physiol. (Lond.) **188**, 387–402 (1967c)

Joiner, P.D., Kadowitz, P.J., Davis, L.B., Hyman, A.L.: Contractile responses of canine isolated intrapulmonary arteries (IPA) and veins (IPV) to norepinephrine (NE), serotonin (5-HT) and tyramine (TYR). Pharmacologist **16**, 299 (1974)

Joiner, P.D., Kadowitz, P.J., Davis, L.B., Hyman, A.L.: Contractile responses of canine isolated pulmonary lobar arteries and veins to norepinephrine, serotonin and tyramine. Canad. J. Physiol. Pharmacol. **53**, 830–838 (1975)

Kahn, C.R.: Membrane receptors for hormones and neurotransmitters. J. Cell Biol. **70**, 261–286 (1976)

Kahr, H., Fischer, W.: Die Wirkung des 5-Oxtryptamins auf das Pigmentsystem der Haut. Klin. Wschr. **35**, 41–44 (1957)

Kalbermatten, J.P. de: Effet de la sérotonine sur l'hypersensibilité de dénervation du ganglion sympathique cervical isolé du rat. Helv. physiol. pharmacol. Acta **20**, 294–315 (1962)

Karlsberg, P., Adams, J.E., Elliott, H.W.: Inhibition and reversal of serotonin-induced cerebral vasospasm. Surg. Forum **13**, 425–427 (1962)

Karlsberg, P., Elliott, H.W., Adams, J.E.: Effects of various pharmacologic agents on cerebral arteries. Neurology (Minneap.) **13**, 772–778 (1963)

Katsuragi, T., Suzuki, T.: Methysergide-induced potentiation of the cholinergic response of the guinea-pig vas deferens. Jap. J. Pharmacol. **24** (Suppl.), 145 (1974)

Katz, R.I., Kopin, I.J.: Effect of D-LSD and related compounds on release of norepinephrine-H^3 and serotonin-H^3 evoked from brain slices by electrical stimulation. Pharmacol. Res. Commun. **1**, 54–62 (1969)

Kawai, N.: Release of 5-hydroxytryptamine from slices of superior colliculus by optic tract stimulation. Neuropharmacology **9**, 395–397 (1970)

Kawai, N., Yamamoto, C.: Antagonism between serotonin and LSD studied in vitro in thin sections from the superior colliculus of guinea-pig. Brain Res. **7**, 325–328 (1968)

Kawai, N., Yamamoto, C.: Effects of 5-hydroxytryptamine, LSD and related compounds on electrical activities evoked in vitro in thin sections from the superior colliculus. Int. J. Neuropharmacol. **8**, 437–449 (1969)

Kelly, M.J.: Receptors for dopamine in some isolated vascular tissues of the dog. Brit. J. Pharmacol. **46**, 575P–577P (1972)

Kerkut, G.A., Laverack, M.S.: A cardio-accelerator present in tissue extracts of the snail *Helix aspersa*. Comp. Biochem. Physiol. **1**, 62–71 (1960)

Khairallah, P.A., Page, I.H., Türker, R.K.: Some properties of prostaglandin E_1 action on muscle. Arch. int. Pharmacodyn. **169**, 328–341 (1967)
Kimura, M., Waki, I., Tamura, H.: Actions of dibenamine on adrenergic β-receptors in cat's papillary muscle (Molecular pharmacological studies on drug-receptor interaction systems in drug action IX). Jap. J. Pharmacol. **20**, 16–22 (1970)
King, T.O.: Hydroxytryptamine. The antagonism of its broncho-constrictor action. Int. Physiologenkongress, Brüssel, August 1956, p. 499
King, T.O.: The antagonism of 5-hydroxytryptamine pneumoconstriction. Arch. int. Pharmacodyn. **110**, 71–76 (1957)
King, A.R., Martin, I.L., Melville, K.A.: Reversal learning enhanced by lysergic acid diethylamide (LSD): concomitant rise in brain 5-hydroxytryptamine levels. Brit. J. Pharmacol. **52**, 419–425 (1974)
Kirpekar, S.M., Cervoni, P.: Effect of cocaine, phenoxybenzamine and phentolamine on the catecholamine output from spleen and adrenal medulla. J. Pharmacol. exp. Ther. **142**, 59–70 (1963)
Kirpekar, S.M., Puig, M.: Effect of flow-stop on noradrenaline release from normal spleens and spleens treated with cocain, phentolamine or phenoxybenzamine. Brit. J. Pharmacol. **43**, 359–369 (1971)
Klawans, Jr., H.L., Goetz, C., Weiner, W.J.: 5-Hydroxytryptophan-induced myoclonus in guinea-pigs and the possible role of serotonin in infantile myoclonus. Neurology (Minneap.) **23**, 1234–1240 (1973)
Klawans, H.L., D'Amico, D.J., Patel, B.C.: Behavioral supersensitivity to 5-hydroxytryptophan induced by chronic methysergide pretreatment. Psychopharmacologia **44**, 297–300 (1975)
Klinge, E., Sjöstrand, N.O.: Contraction and relaxation of the retractor penis muscle and the penile artery of the bull. Acta physiol. scand. (Suppl.) **420**, 1–88 (1974)
Kohli, J.D.: Receptors for sympathomimetic amines in the rabbit aorta: Differentiation by specific antagonists. Brit. J. Pharmacol. **32**, 273–279 (1968)
Kohli, J.D.: A comparative study of dopamine and noradrenaline on the rabbit aorta. Canad. J. Physiol. Pharmacol. **47**, 171–174 (1969)
Kohli, J.D., Innes, I.R.: Differentiation between norepinephrine (NE) and 5-hydroxytryptamine (5-HT) receptors in vascular smooth muscle with 2-bromo-lysergic acid diethylamide (BOL). Pharmacologist **6**, 207 (1964)
Komiskey, H.L., Rudy, T.A.: The involvement of methysergide-sensitive receptors and prostaglandins in the hyperthermia evoked by 5-HT in the cat. Res. Commun. Chem. Path. Pharmacol. **11**, 195–208 (1975)
Konzett, H.: The effects of 5-hydroxytryptamine and its antagonists on tidal air. Brit. J. Pharmacol. **11**, 289–294 (1956)
Konzett, H.: Specific antagonism of dibenamine to ergometrine. In: Ciba Foundation Symposium on Adrenergic Mechanisms. Wolstenholme, G.E.W., O'Connor, M. (eds.), pp. 463–465. London: J. and A. Churchill 1960
Kopin, I.J.: V. Interaction between the drugs and brain amines. Neurosci. Res. Prog. Bull. **8**, 27–32 (1970)
Kostowski, W., Giacalone, E.: Effect of psychotropic drugs on the release of serotonin induced by electrical stimulation of midbrain raphe in rats. In: The Present Status of Psychotropic Drugs. Cerletti, A., Bové, F.J. (eds.), pp. 289–291. Amsterdam: Excerpta Medica Foundation 1969
Kostowski, W., Gumulka, W., Jerlicz, M.: The effects of serotonin injections into the locus coeruleus on ponto geniculo occipital (PGO) waves and cortical EEG pattern in cats. Pol. J. Pharmacol. Pharm. **27**, 127–137 (1975)
Krishnamurty, V.S.R.: Receptors for sympathomimetic amines and 5-hydroxytryptamine in the rat aorta. Arch. int. Pharmacodyn. **189**, 90–99 (1971)
Krivoy, W.A.: The preservation of substance P by lysergic acid diethylamide. Brit. J. Pharmacol. **12**, 361–364 (1957)
Krnjević, K., Phillis, J.W.: Actions of certain amines on cerebral cortical neurones. Brit. J. Pharmacol. **20**, 471–490 (1963a)
Krnjević, K., Phillis, J.W.: Iontophoretic studies of neurones in the mammalian cerebral cortex. J. Physiol. (Lond.) **165**, 274–304 (1963b)

Kuhar, M.J., Roth, R.H., Aghajanian, G.K.: Selective reduction of tryptophan hydroxylase activity in rat forebrain after midbrain raphe lesions. Brain Res. **35**, 167–176 (1971)
Kuhar, M.J., Aghajanian, G.K., Roth, R.H.: Tryptophan hydroxylase activity and synaptosomal uptake of serotonin in discrete brain regions after midbrain lesions: correlations with serotonin levels and histochemical fluorescence. Brain Res. **44**, 165–176 (1972a)
Kuhar, M.J., Roth, R.H., Aghajanian, G.K.: Synaptosomes from forebrains of rats with midbrain raphe lesions: selective reductions of serotonin uptake. J. Pharmacol. exp. Ther. **181**, 36–45 (1972b)
Langer, S.Z., Enero, M.A., Adler-Graschinsky, E., Dubocovich, M.L., Celuchi, S.M.: Presynaptic regulatory mechanisms for noradrenaline release by nerve stimulation. In: Central Action of Drugs in Blood Pressure Regulation. Davies, D.S., Reid, J.L. (eds.), pp. 133–150. Kent: Pitman Medical Publishing 1975
Lecomte, J.: Sensibilisation à l'adrénaline par la 5-hydroxytryptamine. Arch. int. Physiol. Biochim. **61**, 84–85 (1953)
Legge, K.F., Randic, M., Straughan, D.W.: The pharmacology of neurones in the pyriform cortex. Brit. J. Pharmacol. **26**, 87–107 (1966)
Leitch, J.L., Liebig, C.S., Haley, T.J.: The use of the rat's isolated seminal vesicle for the assay of sympatholytic drugs. Brit. J. Pharmacol. **9**, 236–239 (1954)
Leonard, B.E., Liska, K.J.: Effects of morpholino-, pyrrolidino-, piperizino-, and cyclooctyl-derivatives of beta-alanine on brain amines and amino acids. Life Sci. **10**, 93–104 (1971)
Levy, B., Ahlquist, R.P.: An analysis of adrenergic blocking activity. J. Pharmacol. exp. Ther. **133**, 202–210 (1961)
Levy, B., Tozzi, S.: The adrenergic receptive mechanism of the rat uterus. J. Pharmacol. exp. Ther. **142**, 178–184 (1963)
Levy, B., Wilkenfeld, E.: The actions of selective β-receptor antagonists on the guinea-pig trachea. Europ. J. Pharmacol. **11**, 67–74 (1970)
Lévy, J., Michel-Ber, E.: Contribution à l'action pharmacologique exercée par la sérotonine sur quelques organes isolés (intestine et oreillette). J. Physiol. (Paris) **48**, 1051–1084 (1956)
Liao, S.: Cellular receptors and mechanisms of action of steroid hormones. Int. Rev. Cytol. **41**, 87–172 (1975)
Liebeswar, G., Goldman, J.E., Koester, J., Mayeri, E.: Neural control of circulation in Aplysia. III. Neurotransmitters. J. Neurophysiol. **38**, 767–779 (1975)
Lin, R.C., Ngai, S.H., Costa, E.: Lysergic acid diethylamide: role in conversion of plasma tryptophan to brain serotonin (5-hydroxytryptamine). Science **166**, 237–239 (1969)
Lingjaerde, O. Jr.: Effects of ergotamine and dihydroergotamine on uptake of 5-hydroxytryptamine in blood platelets. Europ. J. Pharmacol. **13**, 76–82 (1970)
Little, K.D., DiStefano, V., Leary, D.E.: LSD and serotonin effects on spinal reflexes in the cat. J. Pharm. exp. Ther. **119**, 161 (1957)
Loew, D.M., Depoortere, H., Buerki, H.R.: Effects of dihydrogenated ergot alkaloids on the sleep-wakefulness cycle and on brain biogenic amines in the rat. Arzneimittel-Forsch. **26**, 1080–1083 (1976)
Loew, E.R., Kaiser, M.E., Moore, V.: Effect of various drugs on experimental asthma produced in guinea-pig by exposure to atomized histamine. J. Pharm. exp. Ther. **86**, 1–6 (1946)
Loewi, O., Navratil, E.: Über humorale Übertragbarkeit der Herznervenwirkung. XI. Über den Mechanismus der Vaguswirkung von Physostigmin und Ergotamin. Pflügers Arch. **214**, 689–696 (1926)
Lovell, R.A., Freedman, D.X.: Stereospecific receptor sites for D-lysergic acid diethylamide in rat brain: Effects of neurotransmitters, amine antagonists, and other psychotropic drugs. Molec. Pharmacol. **12**, 620–630 (1976)
Lovell, R.A., Rosecrans, J.A., Freedman, D.X.: Effects of LSD on rat brain serotonin metabolism. Fed. Proc. **26**, 708 (1967)
Ludány, G., Gáti, T., Szabó, St., Hideg, J.: 5-Hydroxytryptamin (Enteramin, Serotonin) und die Darmzottenbewegung. Arch. int. Pharmacodyn. **118**, 62–69 (1959)
Lum, B.K.B., Kermani, M.H., Heilman, R.D.: Intestinal relaxation produced by sympathomimetic amines in the isolated rabbit jejunum: selective inhibition by adrenergic blocking agents and by cold storage. J. Pharmacol. exp. Ther. **154**, 463–471 (1966)
McCulloch, M.W., Rand, M.J., Story, D.F.: Inhibition of ^{3}H-noradrenaline release from

sympathetic nerves of guinea-pig atria by a presynaptic α-adrenoceptor mechanism. Brit. J. Pharmacol. **46**, 523P–524P (1972)
MacLeod, R.M., Lehmeyer, J.E.: Regulation of the synthesis and release of prolactin. In: Lactogenic Hormones. Wolstenholme, G.E.W., Knight, J. (eds.). A Ciba Foundation Symposium, pp. 53–76. Edinburgh-London: Churchill Livingstone 1972
MacLeod, R.M., Lehmeyer, J.E.: Studies on the mechanism of the dopamine-mediated inhibition of prolactin secretion. Endocrinology **94**, 1077–1085 (1974)
Magistretti, M., Valzelli, L.: Ricerche sulla attività inotropa della serotonina sull'orecchietta e sul cuore isolati. Boll. Soc. ital. Biol. sper. **31**, 1035–1037 (1955)
Malanga, C.J.: Dopaminergic responses by gill cilia of bivalve molluscs. Fed. Proc. **32**, 691 (1973)
Malanga, C.J.: Dopaminergic stimulation of ciliary activity in the gill of the bivalve mollusc, *Mytilus edulis*. Fed. Proc. **33**, 551 (1974)
Maling, H.M., Webster, M.E., Williams, M.A., Saul, W., Anderson, W., Jr.: Inflammation induced by histamine, serotonin, bradykinin and compound 48/80 in the rat: antagonists and mechanisms of action. J. Pharmacol. exp. Ther. **191**, 300–310 (1974)
Malorny, G., Orzechowski, G.: Untersuchungen über die Wirkungsweise der Sympathicomimetica. III. Über die ephedrinähnliche Wirkung der Secalealkaloide Ergotamin und Ergometrin. Naunyn-Schmiedebergs Arch. Pharmacol. **196**, 253–259 (1940)
Mansour, T.E.: Effect of lysergic acid diethylamide, serotonin and related compounds on a parasitic trematode, *Fasciola hepatica*. Fed. Proc. **15**, 454–455 (1956)
Mansour, T.E.: The effect of lysergic acid diethylamide, 5-hydroxytryptamine, and related compounds on the liver fluke, *Fasciola hepatica*. Brit. J. Pharmacol. **12**, 406–409 (1957)
Mansour, T.E., Lago, A.D., Hawkins, J.L.: Occurrence and possible role of serotonin in *Fasciola hepatica*. Fed. Proc. **16**, 319 (1957)
Mansour, T.E., Sutherland, E.W., Rall, T.W., Bueding , E.: The effect of serotonin (5-hydroxytryptamine) on the formation of adenosine 3′,5′-phosphate by tissue particles from the liver fluke, *Fasciola hepatica*. J. biol. Chem. **235**, 466–470 (1960)
Marchbanks, R.M.: Serotonin binding to nerve ending particles and other preparations from rat brain. J. Neurochem. **13**, 1481–1493 (1966)
Marchbanks, R.M.: Inhibitory effects of lysergic acid derivatives and reserpine on 5-HT binding to nerve ending particles. Biochem. Pharmacol. **16**, 1971–1979 (1967)
Marchbanks, R.M., Rosenblatt, F., O'Brien, R.D.: Serotonin binding to nerve-ending particles of the rat brain and its inhibition by lysergic acid diethylamide. Science **144**, 1135–1137 (1964)
Markstein, R., Wagner, H.: The effect of dihydroergotoxin, phentolamine and pindolol on catecholamine-stimulated adenylcyclase in rat cerebral cortex. F.E.B.S. Lett. **55**, 275–277 (1975)
Markstein, R., Wagner, H.: Effect of dihydroergotoxine on cyclic AMP generating systems in rat cerebral cortex slices. Gerontology **24** (Suppl. I), 94–105 (1978)
Markstein, R. et al.: unpublished results 1976
Marley, E., Vane, J.R.: Tryptamines and spinal cord reflexes in cats. Brit. J. Pharmacol. **31**, 447–465 (1967)
Marley, E., Whelan, J.E.: Some unexpected pharmacological effects of p-chlorophenylalanine methyl ester (PCPA methyl ester). Brit. J. Pharmacol. **52**, 133P–134P (1974)
Marley, E., Whelan, J.E.: Some pharmacological effects of p-chlorphenylalanine unrelated to tryptophan hydroxylase inhibition. Brit. J. Pharmacol. **56**, 133–144 (1976)
Marrazzi, A.S.: The effects of certain drugs on cerebral synapses. Ann. N.Y. Acad. Sci. **66**, 496–507 (1957)
Marrazzi, A.S., Hart, E.R.: Evoked cortical responses under the influence of hallucinogens and related drugs. Electroencephalogr. Clin. Neurophysiol. **7**, 146 (1955a)
Marrazzi, A.S., Hart, E.R.: Relationship of hallucinogens to adrenergic cerebral neurohumors. Science **121**, 365–367 (1955b)
Martin, W.R., Eades, C.G.: The action of tryptamine on the dog spinal cord and its relationship to the agonistic actions of LSD-like psychotogens. Psychopharmacologia **17**, 242–257 (1970)
Matin, M.A., Vijayvargiya, R.: Chlorpromazine-lysergic acid diethylamide antagonism. J. Pharm. Pharmacol. **19**, 192–193 (1967)

Matthes, K.: The action of blood on acetylcholine. J. Physiol. (Lond.) **70**, 338–348 (1930)
Maurer, R., Grieder, A.: Effects of dihydroergotamine on cAMP content in cultured glial cells. Experientia (Basel) **31**, 730–731 (1975)
Mawson, C., Whittington, H.: Evaluation of the peripheral and central antagonistic activities against 5-hydroxytryptamine of some new agents. Brit. J. Pharmacol. **39**, 223P (1970)
Mchedlishvili, G.I., Ormotsadze, L.G.: Experimental models of spasm of the internal carotid artery. Pat. Fiziol. éksp. Ter. **5**, 79–81 (1974)
Mena, M.A., Vidrio, H.: On the mechanism of the coronary dilator effect of serotonin in the dog. Europ. J. Pharmacol. **36**, 1–5 (1976)
Mendez, R.: Antagonism of adrenaline by ergotamine. J. Pharmacol. **32**, 451–464 (1928)
Metcalfe, H.L., Turner, P.: Pharmacological studies of cinanserin in human isolated smooth muscle. Brit. J. Pharmacol. **37**, 519P (1969)
Metcalfe, H.L., Turner, P.: A comparison of the effects of cinanserin and methysergide on responses of isolated smooth muscle to acetylcholine. Arch. int. Pharmacodyn. **183**, 148–158 (1970)
Meyer, D.K., Abele, M., Hertting, G.: Influence of serotonin on water intake and the renin-angiotensin system in the rat. Arch. int. Pharmacodyn. **212**, 130–140 (1974)
Michal, F.: D-receptor for serotonin on blood platelets. Nature (Lond.) **221**, 1253–1254 (1969)
Michal, F., Motamed, M.: Time-dependent potentiation and inhibition by 5-hydroxytryptamine of platelet aggregation induced by ADP. Brit. J. Pharmacol. **54**, 221–222 (1975)
Michal, F., Motamed, M.: Shape change and aggregation of blood platelets: interaction between the effects of adenosine diphosphate, 5-hydroxytryptamine and adrenaline. Brit. J. Pharmacol. **56**, 209–218 (1976)
Mielke, H., Seiler, K.-U., Stumpf, U., Wassermann, O.: Über eine Beziehung zwischen dem Serotoninstoffwechsel und der pulmonalen Hypertonie bei Ratten nach Gabe verschiedener Anorektika. Z. Kardiol. **62**, 1090–1098 (1973)
Mills, D.C.B., Roberts, G.C.K.: Effects of adrenaline on human blood platelets. J. Physiol. (Lond.) **193**, 443–453 (1967)
Mitchell, J.R.A., Sharp, A.A.: Platelet clumping in vitro. Brit. J. Haematol. **10**, 78–93 (1964)
Mörsdorf, K., Bode, H.H.: Zur Beeinflussung der Permeabilitätssteigernden Wirkung des Serotonins durch verschiedenartige Pharmaka. Arch. int. Pharmacodyn. **118**, 292–297 (1959)
Monachon, M.-A., Burkhard, W.P., Jalfre, M., Haefely, W.: Blockade of central 5-hydroxytryptamine receptors by methiothepin. Naunyn-Schmiedebergs Arch. Pharmacol. **274**, 192–197 (1972)
Mosko, S., Jacobs, B.L.: Effect of peripherally administered serotonin on the neuronal activity of midbrain raphe neurons. Brain Res. **79**, 315–320 (1974)
Mouton, Y., Demaille, A.: La barrière capillaire du mésentère de rat ayant reçu une injection intravasculaire d'hepatome ascitique de Zajdela. III. Influence de la sérotonine et de l'histamine sur l'extravasation tumorale. C. R. Soc. Biol. (Paris) **169**, 974–978 (1975)
Müller-Schweinitzer, E.: Investigations on the mode of action of dihydroergotamine in human saphenous and dog saphenous and femoral veins. Naunyn-Schmiedebergs Arch. Pharmacol. **279** (Suppl.), R44 (1973)
Müller-Schweinitzer, E.: Further studies on the mode of action of ergotamine on canine vein strips. Naunyn-Schmiedebergs Arch. Pharmacol. **282** (Suppl.), R68 (1974a)
Müller-Schweinitzer, E.: Enhanced synthesis of prostaglandin-like substance(s) contributes to the mode of action of dihydroergotamine. Naunyn-Schmiedebergs Arch. Pharmacol. **285** (Suppl.), R57 (1974b)
Müller-Schweinitzer, E.: Studies on the peripheral mode of action of dihydroergotamine in human and canine veins. Europ. J. Pharmacol. **27**, 231–237 (1974c)
Müller-Schweinitzer, E.: Differentiation between serotonin- and alpha-adrenoceptor blocking agents in isolated canine saphenous arteries. Naunyn-Schmiedebergs Arch. Pharmacol. **287** (Suppl.), R21 (1975a)
Müller-Schweinitzer, E.: unpublished results 1975b
Müller-Schweinitzer, E.: Responsiveness of isolated canine cerebral and peripheral arteries to ergotamine. Naunyn-Schmiedebergs Arch. Pharmacol. **292**, 113–118 (1976a)
Müller-Schweinitzer, E.: Evidence for stimulation of 5-HT receptors in canine saphenous arteries by ergotamine. Naunyn-Schmiedebergs Arch. Pharmacol. **295**, 41–44 (1976b)

Müller-Schweinitzer, E.: Comparative studies on the mode of action of ergotamine in canine and human arteries. "Headache '76", Joint Meeting of the Italian Headache and the Scandinavian Migraine Societies, Florence, 1976c, Abstract, pp. 22–23
Müller-Schweinitzer, E.: Comparative studies on the mode of action of ergotamine in canine and human arteries. In: Proceedings of "Headache '76". Torino: C.G. Edizioni Medico-Scientifico 1976d (in press)
Müller-Schweinitzer, E., Brundell, J.: Enhanced prostaglandin synthesis contributes to the venoconstrictor activity of ergotamine. Blood Vessels **12**, 193–205 (1975a)
Müller-Schweinitzer, E., Brundell, J.: Modification of canine vascular smooth muscle responses to dihydroergotamine by endogenous prostaglandin synthesis. Europ. J. Pharmacol. **34**, 197–206 (1975b)
Müller-Schweinitzer, E., Stürmer, E.: Investigations on the mode of action of ergotamine in the isolated femoral vein of the dog. Experientia (Basel) **28**, 743 (1972)
Müller-Schweinitzer, E., Stürmer, E.: Investigations on the mode of action of ergotamine in the isolated femoral vein of the dog. Brit. J. Pharmacol. **51**, 441–446 (1974a)
Müller-Schweinitzer, E., Stürmer, E.: Studies on the mechanism of the venoconstrictor activity of ergotamine on isolated canine saphenous veins. Blood Vessels **11**, 183–190 (1974b)
Müller-Schweinitzer, E., Stürmer, E.: Effects of ergotamine on the responses of isolated saphenous and external carotid arteries of the dog to noradrenaline and serotonin: Sixth Internat. Congress Pharmacol., Helsinki, 1975, Abstract 1555
Mulder, A.H., Stoof, J.C., Tilders, F.J.H.: Depolarization-induced release of central neurotransmitters from rat brain synaptosomes embedded in sephadex G-15 in a superfusion system. Sixth Internat. Congress Pharmacol., Helsinki, 1975, Abstract 1118
Munday, K.A., Poat, J.A., Woodruff, G.N.: Structure activity studies on dopamine receptors, a comparison between rat striatal adenylate cyclase and *Helix aspersa* neurones. Brit. J. Pharmacol. **57**, 452P–453P (1976)
Nair, X.: Contractile responses of guinea-pig umbilical arteries to various hallucinogenic agents. Res. Commun. Chem. Path. Pharmacol. **9**, 535–542 (1974)
Nair, X., Dyer, D.C.: Responses of guinea-pig umbilical vasculature to vasoactive drugs. Europ. J. Pharmacol. **27**, 294–304 (1974)
Nakanishi, H., Takeda, H.: The possible role of adenosine triphosphate in chemical transmission between the hypogastric nerve ending and seminal vesicle in the guinea-pig. Jap. J. Pharmacol. **23** (Suppl.), 19 (1973a)
Nakanishi, H., Takeda, H.: The possible role of adenosine triphosphate in chemical transmission between the hypogastric nerve terminal and seminal vesicle in the guinea-pig. Jap. J. Pharmacol. **23**, 479–490 (1973b)
Nakano, J.: Effects of prostaglandins E_1, A_1 and $F_{2\alpha}$ on the coronary and peripheral circulations. Proc. Soc. exp. Biol. (N.Y.) **127**, 1160–1163 (1968)
Nanda, T.C.: The action of ergotamine on the response of the rabbit's gut to adrenaline. J. Pharmacol. exp. Ther. **42**, 9–16 (1931)
Narebski, J., Romanowski, W., Kadziella, W.: Effect of 1-methyl-d-lysergic butanolamide (Deseril) on EEG changes due to 5-hydroxytryptamine and 5-hydroxytryptophane. Acta physiol. pol. **14**, 157–170 (1963)
Nathanson, J.A., Greengard, P.: Serotonin-sensitive adenylate cyclase in neural tissue and its similarity to the serotonin receptor: a possible site of action of lysergic acid diethylamide. Proc. natl. Acad. Sci. (Wash.) **71**, (3) 797–801 (1974)
Navratil, E.: Über die Beeinflussung der Cholinesterase durch Ergobasin. Klin. Wschr. **2**, 64–65 (1937)
Ng, K.Y., Chase, T.N., Kopin, I.J.: Drug-induced release of ^{3}H-norepinephrine and ^{3}H-serotonin from brain slices. Nature (Lond.) **228**, 468–469 (1970)
Nielsen, K.C., Owman, C.: Contractile response and amine receptor mechanisms in isolated middle cerebral artery of the cat. Brain Res. **27**, 33–42 (1971)
Nilsson, S.: Adrenergic innervation and drug responses of the oval sphincter in the swimbladder of the cod *Gadus morhua*. Acta physiol. scand. **83**, 446–453 (1971)
Nishi, K.: The action of 5-hydroxytryptamine on chemoreceptor discharges of the cat's carotid body. Brit. J. Pharmacol. **55**, 27–40 (1975)
North, R.A., Henderson, G.: Action of morphine on guinea-pig myenteric plexus and mouse vas deferens studied by intracellular recording. Life Sci. **17**, 63–66 (1975)

O'Brien, J.R.: A comparison of platelet aggregation produced by seven compounds and a comparison of their inhibitors. J. clin. Path. **17**, 275–281 (1964)
Offermeier, J., Ariens, E.J.: Serotonin. I. Receptors involved in its action. Arch. int. Pharmacodyn. **164**, 192–215 (1966)
Ogle, C.W., Wong, C.Y.: The inhibitory and excitatory properties of alpha adrenoceptors in the rat stomach. Life Sci. **10**, 153–159 (1971)
O'Malley, B.W., Hardman, J.G.: Hormon action, part A: steroid hormones. Methods Enzymol. **36**, 135–411 (1975)
Osborne, N.N., Hiripi, L., Neuhoff, V.: The in vitro uptake of biogenic amines by snail *Helix pomatia* nervous tissue. Biochem. Pharmacol. **24**, 2141–2148 (1975)
Osswald, W., Guimarães, S.: Über den Mechanismus der Isoprenalinumkehr. Naunyn-Schmiedebergs Arch. Pharmacol. **243**, 1–15 (1962)
Osswald, W., Guimarães, S., Garret, J.: Influence of propranolol and ICI 50.172 on the cardiovascular actions of catecholamines as modified by ergotamine. J. Pharmacol. exp. Ther. **174**, 315–322 (1970)
Owen, D.A.A., Herd, J.K., Kalberer, F., Pacha, W., Salzmann, R.: The influence of ergotamine and methysergide on the storage of biogenic amines. Headache **11**, 91–92 (1971a)
Owen, D.A.A., Herd, J.K.,, Kalberer, F., Pacha, W., Salzmann, R.: The influence of ergotamine and methysergide on the storage of biogenic amines. In: Proc. Intern. Headache Symposium, Elsinore, Denmark. Dalessio, D.J., Dalsgaard-Nielson, T., Diamond, S. (eds.), pp. 153–161. Basle: Sandoz 1971b
Paasonen, M.K., Giarman, N.J.: Brain levels of 5-hydroxytryptamine after various agents. Arch. int. Pharmacodyn. **114**, 189–200 (1958)
Pacha, W., Salzmann, R.: Inhibition of the re-uptake of neuronally liberated noradrenaline and α-receptor blocking action of some ergot alkaloids. Brit. J. Pharmacol. **38**, 439P–440P (1970)
Palmer, G.C., Burks, T.F.: Central and peripheral adrenergic blocking actions of LSD and BOL. Europ. J. Pharmacol. **16**, 113–116 (1971)
Panigel, M.: Contribution à la physiologie de la circulation foeto-placentaire. I. Etude de la vaso-motricité des artères du cordon ombilical humain. J. Physiol. (Paris) **51**, 941–969 (1959)
Panigel, M.: Placental perfusion experiments. Amer. J. Obstet. Gynec. **84**, 1664–1683 (1962)
Parker, G.H.: The responses of catfish melanophores to ergotamine. Biol. Bull. **81**, 163–167 (1941)
Parmley, W.W., Rabinowitz, B., Chuck, L.: The role of alpha adrenergic receptors in mediating positive inotropic effects in ventricular myocardium. Amer. J. Cardiol. **33**, 161 (1974)
Parratt, J.R., West, G.B.: Inhibition of oedema production in the rat. J. Physiol. (Lond.) **135**, 24P–25P (1957a)
Parratt, J.R., West, G.B.: 5-Hydroxytryptamine and the anaphylactoid reaction in the rat. J. Physiol. (Lond.) **139**, 27–41 (1957b)
Parratt, J.R., West, G.B.: Inhibition by various substances of oedema formation in the hind-paw of the rat induced by 5-hydroxytryptamine, histamine, dextran, eggwhite and compound 48/80. Brit. J. Pharmacol. **13**, 65–70 (1958)
Passow, H., Schniewind, H., Weiss, C.: Die Wirkung von 5-Hydroxytryptamin auf das Gefäßsystem der isolierten Rattenniere. Naunyn-Schmiedebergs Arch. Pharmacol. **240**, 179–186 (1960)
Paterson, G.: The response to transmural stimulation of isolated arterial strips and its modification by drugs. J. Pharm. Pharmacol. **17**, 341–349 (1965)
Patten, B.M., Oliver, K.L., Engel, W.K.: Serotonin-induced muscle weakness. Arch. Neurol. (Chic.) **31**, 347–349 (1974)
Paul, S.M., Halaris, A.E.: Rat brain de-acetylating activity: Stereospecific inhibition by LSD and serotonin-related compounds. Biochem. biophys. Res. Commun. **70**, 207–211 (1976)
Paul, S.M., Halaris, A.E., Freedman, D.X., Hsu, L.L.: Rat brain aryl acylamidase: Stereospecific inhibition by LSD and serotonin-related compounds. J. Neurochem. **27**, 625–627 (1976)
Pert, C.B., Snyder, S.H.: Properties of opiate-receptor binding in rat brain. Proc. natl. Acad. Sci. (Wash.) **70**, 2243–2247 (1973)

Peters, D.A.V.: Comparison of the chronic and acute effects of D-lysergic acid diethylamide (LSD) treatment on rat brain serotonin and norepinephrine. Biochem. Pharmacol. **23**, 231–237 (1974a)

Peters, D.A.V.: Chronic lysergic acid diethylamide administration and serotonin turnover in various regions of rat brain. J. Neurochem. **23**, 625–628 (1974b)

Pfeifer, Y., Sadowsky, E., Sulman, F.G.: Prevention of serotonin abortion in pregnant rats by five serotonin antagonists. Obstet. Gynecol. **33**, 709–714 (1969)

Phillis, J.W., Tebecis, A.K., York, D.H.: The inhibitory action of monoamines on lateral geniculate neurones. J. Physiol. (Lond.) **190**, 563–581 (1967)

Pichler, E., Lazarini, W., Filippi, R.: Über schraubenförmige Struktur von Arterien. II. Mitteilung: Pharmakologische Strukturanalyse von Hirnarterien. Naunyn-Schmiedebergs Arch. Pharmacol. **219**, 420–439 (1953)

Pichler, E., Ostfeld, A.M., Goodell, H., Wolff, H.G.: Studies on headache: Central versus peripheral action of ergotamine tartrate and its relevance to the therapy of migraine headache. Arch. Neurol. Psychiat. (Chic.) **76**, 571–577 (1956)

Pijnenburg, A.J.J., van Rossum, J.M.: Stimulation of locomotor activity following injection of dopamine into the nucleus accumbens. J. Pharm. Pharmacol. **25**, 1003–1004 (1973)

Pijnenburg, A.J.J., Woodruff, G.N., van Rossum, J.M.: Ergometrine induced locomotor activity following intracerebral injection into the nucleus accumbens. Brain Res. **59**, 289–302 (1973)

Pik, K., Borsy, J.: The mechanism of action of GYKI-32084, a new antiserotonin agent. Naunyn-Schmiedebergs Arch. Pharmacol. **284** (Suppl.), R62 (1974)

Pitzele, S., Dobell, A.R.C.: Inhibition of serotonin-induced blood cell aggregation in the dog. Surgery **73**, 416–422 (1973)

Politoff, A., Macri, F.: Pharmacologic differences between isolated, perfused arteries of the choroid plexus and of the brain parenchyma. Int. J. Neuropharmacol. **5**, 155–162 (1966)

Poulson, E., Robson, J.M.: Prevention by antagonists of the toxic action of 5-hydroxytryptamine on pregnancy. Brit. J. Pharmacol. **21**, 150–154 (1963)

Pourrias, B.: Analyse des effets tensionels et cardiaques de la tryptine. J. Pharmacol. (Paris) **6**, 153–164 (1975)

Prince, W.T., Berridge, J., Rasmussen, H.: Role of calcium and adenosine-3′,5′-cyclic monophosphate in controlling fly salivary gland secretion. Proc. natl. Acad. Sci. (Wash.) **69**, 553–557 (1972)

Proudfit, K., Anderson, E.G.: Alteration by serotonin antagonists of the effects of bulbospinal stimulation on spinal reflex pathways. Fed. Proc. **31**, 270 (1972)

Proudfit, H.K., Anderson, E.G.: Influence of serotonin antagonists on bulbospinal systems. Brain Res. **61**, 331–341 (1973)

Przewlocki, R.: The effect of serotonin microinjections into the nuclei amygdale on EEG and behaviour in the rabbit. Pol. J. Pharmacol. Pharm. **27** (Suppl.), 209–216 (1975)

Rand, M.J., McCulloch, M.W., Story, D.F.: Pre-junctional modulation of noradrenergic transmission by noradrenaline, dopamine and acetylcholine. In: Central Action of Drugs in Blood Pressure Regulation. Davies, D.S., Reid, J.L. (eds.), pp. 94–132. Kent: Pitman Medical Publishing 1975

Randic, M., Padjen, A.: Effect of N,N-dimethyltryptamine and D-lysergic acid diethylamide on the release of 5-hydroxy-indoles in rat forebrain. Nature (Lond.) **230**, 532–533 (1971)

Rao, K.R., Fingerman, M.: Action of biogenic amines on crustacean chromatophores. II. Analysis of the responses of erythrophores in the fiddler crab, *Uca pugilator,* to indolealkylamines and an eyestalk hormone. Comp. gen. Pharmacol. **1**, 117–126 (1970)

Regoli, D., Vane, J.R.: A sensitive method for the assay of angiotensin. Brit. J. Pharmacol. **23**, 351–359 (1964)

Reichenberg, K., Wiszniowska, G., Marchaj, J.: The influence of 5-hydroxytryptophan (5-HTP) administered into the lateral brain ventricle on the behavior and body temperature in rats. Pol. J. Pharmacol. Pharm. **27** (Suppl.), 217–222 (1975)

Rico, J.M.G.T., Rico, J.T., Ferreira, J.M.C., Cravo, A.C.: L'effet des prostaglandines PGE_1, PGE_2 et $PGF_{2\alpha}$ sur la perméabilité vasculaire chez le rat. C.R. Soc. Biol. (Paris) **167**, 1315–1318 (1973)

Roberts, M.H., Straughan, D.W.: Excitation and depression of cortical neurones by 5-hydroxytryptamine. J. Physiol. (Lond.) **193**, 269–294 (1967)
Rocha e Silva, M., Valle, J.R., Picarelli, Z.P.: A pharmacological analysis of the mode of action of serotonin (5-hydroxytryptamine) upon the guinea-pig ileum. Brit. J. Pharmacol. **8**, 378–388 (1953)
Rössler, R., Unna, K.: Zur Pharmakologie des neuen Mutterkornalkaloides Sensibamin. Naunyn-Schmiedebergs Arch. Pharmacol. **179**, 115–126 (1935)
Rose, J.C., Lazaro, E.J.: Pulmonary vascular responses to serotonin and effects of certain serotonin antagonists. Circulat. Res. **6**, 283–288 (1958)
Rosecrans, J.A., Lovell, R.A., Freedman, D.X.: Effects of lysergic acid diethylamide on the metabolism of brain 5-hydroxytryptamine. Biochem. Pharmacol. **16**, 2011–2021 (1967)
Rosenblueth, A.: The action of certain drugs on the nictitating membrane. Amer. J. Physiol. **100**, 443–446 (1932)
Ross, S.B., Renyi, A.L.: Accumulation of tritiated 5-hydroxytryptamine in brain slices. Life Sci. **6**, 1407–1415 (1967)
Roth, J.: Peptide hormone binding to receptors: a review of direct studies in vitro. Metabolism **22**, 1059–1073 (1973)
Rothlin, E.: Über die pharmakologische und therapeutische Wirkung des Ergotamins auf den Sympathicus. Klin. Wschr. **4**, 1437–1443 (1925)
Rothlin, E.: Zur Pharmakologie des Sympathicolyticums Dihydroergotamin DHE 45. Schweiz. med. Wschr. **76**, 1254–1259 (1946)
Rothlin, E.: The pharmacology of the natural and dihydrogenated alkaloids of ergot. Bull. schweiz. Akad. med. Wiss. **2**, 249–273 (1946/47)
Rothlin, E.: Pharmacology of lysergic acid diethylamide (LSD) and some of its related compounds. In: Psychotropic drugs. Garattini, S., Ghetti, V. (eds.), pp. 36–47. Amsterdam: Elsevier Press 1957a
Rothlin, E.: Lysergic acid diethylamide and related substances. Ann. N.Y. Acad. Sci. **66**, 668–676 (1957b)
Rothlin, E.: Pharmacology of lysergic acid diethylamide and some of its related compounds. J. Pharm. Pharmacol. **9**, 569–587 (1957c)
Rothlin, E., Berde, B.: Über die Wirkung hydrierter Mutterkornalkaloide auf isolierte Muskelstreifen des menschlichen Uterus nahe am Termin, am Termin und während der Geburt. Helv. physiol. pharmacol. Acta **12**, 191–205 (1954)
Rothlin, E., Brügger, J.: Quantitative Differenzierung von 4 genuinen und hydrierten Mutterkornalkaloiden am isolierten Kaninchen-Uterus und an der isolierten Samenblase des Meerschweinchens. Helv. physiol. pharmacol. Acta **3**, C43–C44 (1945a)
Rothlin, E., Brügger, J.: Quantitative Untersuchungen der sympathikolytischen Wirkung genuiner Mutterkornalkaloide und derer Dihydroderivate am isolierten Uterus des Kaninchens. Helv. physiol. pharmacol. Acta **3**, 519–535 (1945b)
Rothlin, E., Cerletti, A.: Pharmakologie des Hochdrucks. Verh. dtsch. Ges. Kreisl.-Forsch. **15**, 158–185 (1949)
Rothlin, E., Konzett, H., Cerletti, A.: The antagonism of ergot alkaloids towards the inhibitory response of the isolated rabbit intestine to epinephrine and norepinephrine. J. Pharmacol. exp. Ther. **112**, 185–190 (1954)
Rózsa, K.S., Graul, C.: Is serotonin responsible for the stimulative effect of the extracardiac nerve in *Helix pomatia?* Ann. Biol. Tihany **31**, 85–96 (1964)
Ruch-Monachon, M.-A., Jalfre, M., Haefely, W.: Drugs and PGO waves in the lateral geniculate body of the curarized cat. II. PGO wave activity and brain 5-hydroxytryptamine. Arch. int. Pharmacodyn. **219**, 269–286 (1976a)
Ruch-Monachon, M.-A., Jalfre, M., Haefely, W.: Drugs and PGO waves in the lateral geniculate body of the curarized cat. V. Miscellaneous compounds. Synopsis of the role of central neurotransmitters on PGO wave activity. Arch. int. Pharmacodyn. **219**, 326–346 (1976b)
Ruckebusch, Y., Roche, M., Schurch, D.: Parallélisme des effets des psychodysleptiques majeurs sur la toxicité de groupe et de taux cérébral en sérotonine. C.R. Soc. Biol. (Paris) **159**, 1745–1748 (1965)
Rudzik, A.D., Miller, J.W.: The mechanism of uterine inhibitory action of relaxin-containing ovarian extracts. J. Pharmacol. exp. Ther. **138**, 82–87 (1962)

Saad, K.: The effect of drugs on the isolated splenic capsule of man and other animals. Quart. J. Pharm. Pharmacol. **8**, 31–38 (1935)
Sachs, E., Yonkman, F.F.: The pharmacological behavior of the intraocular muscles. V. The action of yohimbine and ergotamine on the dilator iridis. J. Pharmacol. exp. Ther. **75**, 105–110 (1942)
Salmoiraghi, G.C., McCubbin, J.W., Page, I.H.: Effects of D-lysergic acid diethylamide and its brom derivative on cardiovascular responses to serotonin and on arterial pressure. J. Pharmacol. exp. Ther. **119**, 240–247 (1957)
Salmoiraghi, G.C., Bloom, F.E., Costa, E.: Adrenergic mechanisms in rabbit olfactory bulb. Amer. J. Physiol. **207**, 1417–1424 (1964)
Salzmann, R., Kalberer, F.: Antimigraine drugs and storage of serotonin. In: Background to Migraine. Cumings, J.N. (ed.), pp. 63–72. London: William Heinemann Medical Books 1973
Salzmann, R., Pacha, W.: Vergleichende Untersuchungen über die Beeinflussung adrenerger Reaktionen durch Ergotamin und Dihydroergotamin an verschiedenen Versuchsmodellen. Helv. physiol. pharmacol. Acta **26**, CR246–CR248 (1968)
Salzmann, R., Pacha, W.: The effects of ergot compounds on the release of noradrenaline and prostaglandins from the isolated perfused cat spleen during nerve stimulation. Postgrad. med. J. **52** (Suppl. 1), 24–31 (1976)
Salzmann, R., Weidmann, H.: Die Wirkung von Ergotamin auf humorale und neuronale Effekte an der Nickhaut der Katze. Helv. physiol. pharmacol. Acta **24**, C117 (1966)
Salzmann, R., Pacha, W., Weidmann, H.: Der Einfluß von Ergotamin auf humorale und neuronale Wirkungen an der Nickhaut und an der Milz der Katze. Helv. physiol. pharmacol. Acta **25**, CR433–CR435 (1967)
Salzmann, R., Pacha, W., Taeschler, M., Weidmann, H.: The effect of ergotamine on humoral and neuronal actions in the nictitating membrane and the spleen of the cat. Naunyn-Schmiedebergs Arch. Pharmacol. **261**, 360–378 (1968)
Sankar, D.V.S., Sankar, D.B., Phipps, E., Gold, E.: Effect of administration of lysergic acid diethylamide on serotonin levels in the body. Nature (Lond.) **191**, 499–500 (1961)
Sankar, D.V.S., Phipps, E., Gold, E., Sankar, D.B.: Effect of LSD, BOL, and chlorpromazine on „Neurohormone“ metabolism. Ann. N.Y. Acad. Sci. **96**, 93–97 (1962)
Sankar, D.V.S., Broer, H.H., Cates, N., Sankar, D.B.: Studies on biogenic amines and psychoactive drug actions, with special reference to lysergic acid diethyl amide. Trans. N.Y. Acad. Sci. **26**, 369–379 (1964)
Sankar, D.V.S., Cates, N.R., Domjan, M.: Comparative biochemical pharmacology of psychoactive drugs. Clin. Res. **17**, 395 (1969)
Sato, M., Sawada, M.: Selective blocking action of LSD on inhibitory dopamine receptors. Neuropharmacology **14**, 883–886 (1975)
Savini, E.C.: The antagonism between 5-hydroxytryptamine and certain derivatives of lysergic acid. Brit. J. Pharmacol. **11**, 313–317 (1956)
Saxena, P.R.: The effects of antimigraine drugs on the vascular responses by 5-hydroxytryptamine and related biogenic substances on the external carotid bed of dogs: possible pharmacological implications to their antimigraine action. Headache **12**, 44–45 (1972a)
Saxena, P.R.: The effects of some antimigraine drugs on the vascular resistance in the external carotid bed of the dog. In: Vascular Smooth Muscle. Betz, E. (ed.), pp. 93–95. Berlin-Heidelberg-New York: Springer 1972b
Saxena, P.R.: Selective carotid vasoconstriction by ergotamine as a relevant mechanism in its antimigraine action. Arch. Neurobiol. **37** (Suppl.), 301–315 (1974a)
Saxena, P.R.: Selective vasoconstriction in carotid vascular bed by methysergide: possible relevance to its antimigraine effect. Europ. J. Pharmacol. **27**, 99–105 (1974b)
Saxena, P.R.: On the mechanism of action of methysergide in vascular headaches of migraine type. In: Headache, II. Biochemical Bases and Drug Therapy. Münch. Med. Wochenschr. (ed.), pp. 91–100, 137–138. München: O. Spatz 1975
Saxena, P.R., De Vlaam-Schluter, G.M.: Role of some biogenic substances in migraine and relevant mechanism in antimigraine action of ergotamine-studies in an experimental model for migraine. Headache **13**, 142–163 (1974)
Saxena, P.R., van Houwelingen, P., Bonta, I.L.: The effects of mianserin hydrochloride on

the vascular responses evoked by 5-hydroxytryptamine and related vasoactive substances. Europ. J. Pharmacol. **13**, 295–305 (1971)
Schanberg, S.M., Giarman, N.J.: Uptake of serotonin (5-HT) and 5-hydroxytryptophan (5-HTP) by brain slices. Pharmacologist **2**, 67 (1960)
Schanberg, S.M., Giarman, N.J.: Drug-induced alterations in the sub-cellular distribution of 5-hydroxytryptamine in rat's brain. Biochem. Pharmacol. **11**, 187–194 (1962)
Scherbel, A.: Pharmacodynamic effects of UML-491 in animal and man. Wiss. Ausstellung, 6. Int. Kongress Inn. Med., Basel, August 1960, Abstract
Schild, H.O.: pA, a new scale for the measurement of drug antagonism. Brit. J. Pharmacol. **2**, 189–206 (1947)
Schild, H.O.: Non-competitive antagonism. J. Physiol. (Lond.) **124**, 33P–34P (1954)
Schild, H.O.: Effect of adrenaline on depolarized smooth muscle. In: Ciba Foundation Symposium on Adrenergic Mechanisms. Wolstenholme, G.E.W., O'Connor, M. (eds.), pp. 288–294. London: J. and A. Churchill 1960
Schild, H.O.: Parallelism of log dose-response curves in competitive antagonism. Pharmacol. Res. Commun. **1**, 1–2 (1969)
Schild, H.O.: Some aspects of receptor pharmacology of ergotamine. Postgrad. med. J. **52** (Suppl. 1), 9–11 (1976)
Schildkraut, J.J., Schanberg, S.M., Breese, G.R., Kopin, I.J.: Effects of psychoactive drugs on the metabolism of intracisternally administered serotonin in rat brain. Biochem. Pharmacol. **18**, 1971–1978 (1969)
Schlientz, W., Brunner, R., Rüegger, A., Berde, B., Stürmer, E., Hofmann, A.: β-Ergokryptin, ein neues Alkaloid der Ergotoxin-Gruppe. Pharm. Acta Helv. **43**, 497–509 (1968)
Schönbaum, E., Lamar, J.-C.: Anti-serotonin drugs in nasal vessels. Sixth Internat. Congress Pharmacology, Helsinki, 1975, Abstract 698
Schönbaum, E., Vargaftig, B.B., Lefort, J.: Nasal vessels and serotonin. Pharmacologist **16**, 243 (1974)
Schönbaum, E., Vargaftig, B.B., Lefort, J., Lamar, J.C., Hasenack, T.: An unexpected effect of serotonin antagonists on the canine nasal circulation. Headache **15**, 180–187 (1975)
Scholtysik, G.: Inhibition of accelerator nerve stimulation in cats by dihydroergotoxine. Sixth Internat. Congress Pharmacology, Helsinki, 1975, Abstract 742
Schorderet, M.: Direct evidence for the stimulation of rabbit retina dopamine receptors by ergot alkaloids. Neurosci. Lett. **2**, 87–91 (1976)
Schorderet, M., Frangaki, A.: Effects of antiparkinsonian drugs on cAMP accumulation in rabbit retina. Experientia (Basel) **32**, 782 (1976)
Schubert, J., Nybäck, H., Sedvall, G.: Accumulation and disappearance of ^{3}H-5-hydroxytryptamine formed from ^{3}H-tryptophan in mouse brain: effect of LSD 25. Europ. J. Pharmacol. **10**, 215–224 (1970)
Schwarz, B.E., Wakim, K.G., Bickford, R.G., Lichtenheld, F.R.: Behavioural and electroencephalographic effects of hallucinogenic drugs. Arch. Neurol. Psychiat. (Chic.) **75**, 83–90 (1956)
Scriabine, A., Bellet, S., Kershbaum, A., Feinberg, L.J.: Effect of dihydroergotamine on plasma free fatty acids (FFA) in dogs. Life Sci. **7**, 453–463 (1968)
Segal, M.: Physiological and pharmacological evidence for a serotonergic projection to the hippocampus. Brain Res. **94**, 115–131 (1975)
Segal, M., Bloom, F.E.: The projection of midline raphe nuclei to the hippocampus of the rat. Fed. Proc. **33**, 299 (1974)
Seiler, K.-U., Wassermann, O.: MAO-inhibitory properties of anorectic drugs. J. Pharm. Pharmacol. **25**, 576–578 (1973)
Shaskan, E.G., Snyder, S.H.: Kinetics of serotonin accumulation into slices from rat brain: relationship to catecholamine uptake. J. Pharm. exp. Ther. **175**, 404–418 (1970)
Shaw, E., Woolley, D.W.: Yohimbine and ergot alkaloids as naturally occurring antimetabolites of serotonin. J. biol. Chem. **203**, 978–989 (1953)
Shaw, E., Woolley, D.W.: Some serotoninlike activities of lysergic acid diethylamide. Science **124**, 121–122 (1956)
Shibuya, T., Anderson, E.G.: The influence of chronic cord transection on the effects of 5-hydroxytryptophan, L-tryptophan and pargyline on spinal neuronal activity. J. Pharmacol. exp. Ther. **164**, 185–190 (1968)

Shields, P.J., Eccleston, D.: Evidence for the synthesis and storage of 5-hydroxytryptamine in two separate pools in the brain. J. Neurochem. **20**, 881–888 (1973)
Shimahara, T., Tauc, L.: Heterosynaptic facilitation in the giant cell of Aplysia. J. Physiol. (Lond.) **247**, 321–342 (1975)
Sicuteri, F., Michelacci, S., Franchi, G.: Antagonism between an antiserotonin – the butanolamide of 1-methyl-lysergic acid – and the effects of a histamine-liberating substance 48/80 B.W. in man. Int. Arch. Allergy **15**, 291–299 (1959)
Sicuteri, F., Franchi, G., Michelacci, S.: Inhibition by lysergic acid derivatives of bronchospasm induced in guinea-pigs by serotonin aerosol. Med. Exp. **3**, 89–94 (1960)
Sicuteri, F., Del Bianco, P.L., Fanciullacci, M., Franchi, G.: Il test della venocostrizione per la misura della sensibilità alla 5-idossitriptamina e alle catecolamine nell'uomo. Boll. Soc. ital. Biol. sper. **40**, 1148–1150 (1964a)
Sicuteri, F., Fanciullacci, M., Del Bianco, P.L., Franchi, G.: Inibizione della venocostrizione da 5-idrossitriptamina nell'uomo da parte del metisergide (UML-491) e di altri antiserotoninici. Boll. Soc. ital. Biol. sper. **40**, 1151–1152 (1964b)
Sicuteri, F., Franchi, G., Fanciullacci, M.: Serotonin potentiation of methysergide, LSD 25 and ergotamine in man: An informal approach to migraine pharmacology. In: Headache, II. Biochemical Bases and Drug Therapy. Münch. Med. Wochenschr. (ed.), pp. 101–104, 137–138. München: O. Spatz 1975
Simon, G., Winter, M.: The effect of sympatholytic and sympathomimetic agents on acetylcholinesterase and cholinesterase activity in vitro. Biochem. Pharmacol. **25**, 881–882 (1976)
Slater, I.H., Davis, K.H., Leary, D.E., Boyd, E.S.: The action of serotonin and lysergic acid diethylamide on spinal reflexes. J. Pharmacol. exp. Ther. **113**, 48–49 (1955)
Smith, C.B.: Relaxation of the nictitating membrane of the spinal cat by sympathomimetic amines. J. Pharmacol. exp. Ther. **142**, 163–170 (1963)
Snider, S.R., Hutt, C., Stein, B., Fahn, S.: Increase in brain serotonin produced by bromocryptine. Neurosci. Lett. **1**, 237–241 (1975)
Snider, S.R., Hutt, C., Stein, B., Prasad, A.L.N., Fahn, S.: Correlation of behavioural inhibition or excitation produced by bromocriptine with changes in brain catecholamine turnover. J. Pharm. Pharmacol. **28**, 563–566 (1976)
Snyder, S.H., Bennett, J.P.: Neurotransmitter receptors in the brain: biochemical identification. Annu. Rev. Physiol. **38**, 153–175 (1976)
Sofia, R.D., Vassar, H.B.: The effects of ergotamine and methysergide on serotonin metabolism in the rat brain. Arch. int. Pharmacodyn. **216**, 40–50 (1975)
Sollero, L., Page, I.H., Salmoiraghi, G.C.: Brom-lysergic acid diethylamide: A highly potent serotonin antagonist. J. Pharmacol. exp. Ther. **117**, 10–15 (1956)
Sollmann, T.: A Manual of Pharmacology and its Applications to Therapeutics and Toxicology, 7th ed. Philadelphia-London: W.B. Saunders 1948
Sollmann, T., Brown, E.D.: Intravenous injection of ergot. J. Amer. med. Ass. **45**, 229–240 (1905)
Sonneville, P.F.: An indirect action of dopamine on the rat fundus strip mediated by 5-hydroxytryptamine. Europ. J. Pharmacol. **2**, 367–370 (1968)
Spano, P.F., Cattabeni, F., Govoni, S., Trabucchi, M.: Selective stimulation by d-LSD of dopamine-sensitive adenylate cyclase in various rat brain areas. Sixth Internat. Congress Pharmacol., Helsinki, 1975a, Abstract 186
Spano, P.F., Kumakura, K., Tonon, G.C., Govoni, S., Trabucchi, M.: LSD and dopamine-sensitive adenylate cyclase in various rat brain areas. Brain Res. **93**, 164–167 (1975b)
Sparber, S.B.: Neurochemical changes associated with schedule controlled behavior. Fed. Proc. **34**, 1802–1812 (1975)
Stacey, R.S.: Uptake of 5-hydroxytryptamine by platelets. Brit. J. Pharmacol. **16**, 284–295 (1961)
Stadler, P.A., Stürmer, E.: Comparative studies on the pharmacological properties of stereoisomers of ergotamine and dihydroergotamine. Naunyn-Schmiedebergs Arch. Pharmacol. **266**, 457–458 (1970)
Starke, K.: α-Sympathomimetic inhibition of adrenergic and cholinergic transmission in the rabbit heart. Naunyn-Schmiedebergs Arch. Pharmacol. **274**, 18–45 (1972)
Starke, K., Montel, H.: Sympathomimetic inhibition of noradrenaline release: mediated by prostaglandins? Naunyn-Schmiedebergs Arch. Pharmacol. **278**, 111–116 (1973)

Starr, M.S., West, G.B.: The effect of bradykinin and anti-inflammatory agents on isolated arteries. J. Pharm. Pharmacol. **18**, 838–840 (1966)
Stephenson, R.P.: A modification of receptor theory. Brit. J. Pharmacol. **11**, 379–393 (1956)
Stevens, B., Baguet, F.: Action de l'acide bromolysergique diéthylamide (BOL 148) sur les propriétés mécaniques d'un muscle lisse de Lamellibranche. Arch. int. Physiol. Biochim. **76**, 552–554 (1968)
Stjärne, L., Lishajko, F.: Drug-induced inhibition of noradrenaline synthesis in vitro in bovine splenic nerve tissue. Brit. J. Pharmacol. **27**, 398–404 (1966)
Stjärne, L., Wennmalm, A.: Quantitative estimation of secretion and reuptake of adrenergic transmitter in the rabbit heart. Acta physiol. scand. **81**, 286–288 (1971)
Stolk, J.M., Barchas, J.D., Goldstein, M., Boggan, W., Freedman, D.X.: A comparison of psychotomimetic drug effects on rat brain norepinephrine metabolism. J. Pharmacol. exp. Ther. **189**, 42–50 (1974)
Stoll, A., Hofmann, A.: The ergot alkaloids. In: The Alkaloids. Manske, R.H.F. (ed.), Chap. 21, Vol. VIII. New York: Academic Press 1965
Stone, C.A., Wenger, H.C., Ludden, C.T., Stavorski, J.M., Ross, C.A.: Antiserotonin-antihistaminic properties of cyproheptadine. J. Pharmacol. exp. Ther. **131**, 73–84 (1961)
Stone, T.W.: Further evidence for a dopamine receptor stimulating action of an ergot alkaloid. Brain Res. **72**, 177–180 (1974)
Straczowski, W., Kalicinski, A., Nowak, W., Malofiejew, M.: The effects of prostaglandin A_2 (PGA_2) on the guinea-pig isolated ileum. Pol. J. Pharmacol. Pharm. **26**, 253–255 (1974)
Strandhoy, J.W., Cronnelly, R., Long, J.P., Williamson, H.E.: Effects of vasoactive agents and diuretics on isolated superfused interlobar renal arteries. Proc. Soc. exp. Biol. (N.Y.) **141**, 336–339 (1972)
Streuli, H.: Die Wechselwirkung von inneren Sekreten und die Beziehung dieser Wirkung zum Problem der Erregung und Hemmung. Z. Biol. **66**, 167–228 (1916)
Strong, C.G., Bohr, D.F.: Effects of Prostaglandins E_1, E_2, A_1 and $F_{1\alpha}$ on isolated vascular smooth muscle. Circulation **36** (Suppl. 2), II 244–II 245 (1967a)
Strong, C.G., Bohr, D.F.: Effects of prostaglandins E_1, E_2, A_1 and $F_{1\alpha}$ on isolated vascular smooth muscle. Amer. J. Physiol. **213**, 725–733 (1967b)
Struyker Boudier, H., Van Rossum, J.M.: Dopamine-induced inhibition and excitation of neurones of the snail *Helix aspersa*. Arch. int. Pharmacodyn. **209**, 314–324 (1974)
Struyker Boudier, H.A.J., Gielen, W., Cools, A.R., Van Rossum, J.M.: Pharmacological analysis of dopamine-induced inhibition and excitation of neurones of the snail *Helix aspersa*. Arch. int. Pharmacodyn. **209**, 324–331 (1974)
Struyker Boudier, H., Teppema, L., Cools, A., Van Rossum, J.M.: (3,4-dihydroxy-phenylamino)-2-imidazoline (DPI), a new potent agonist at dopamine receptors mediating neuronal inhibition. J. Pharm. Pharmacol. **27**, 882–883 (1975)
Sugrue, M.F.: A study of the role of noradrenaline in behavioural changes produced in the rat by psychotomimetic drugs. Brit. J. Pharmacol. **35**, 243–252 (1969)
Svensson, T.H., Bunney, B.S., Aghajanian, G.K.: Noradrenergic regulation of brain serotonergic neurons: Evidence from single unit studies with clonidine. Pharmacologist **16**, 244 (1974)
Swank, R.L., Fellman, J.H.: Blood cell aggregation and biological agents. Bibl. anat. (Basel) **8–9**, 98–103 (1966)
Swank, R.L., Fellman, J.H., Hissen, W.W.: Aggregation of blood cells by 5-hydroxytryptamine (serotonin). Circulat. Res. **13**, 392–400 (1963)
Szabadi, E., Bradshaw, C.M.: The role of physical and biological factors in determining the time course of neuronal responses. Neuropharmacology **13**, 537–545 (1974)
Szara, S., Morton, D.M., Aikens, A.: Comparison of hallucinogenic and nonhallucinogenic congeners on regional serotonin metabolism in brain. Pharmacologist **9**, 250 (1967)
Takeuchi, H., Mori, A., Kohsaka, M.: Effets des indolamines et de leurs analogues sur l'activité électrique d'un neurone géant identifié d'*Achatina fulica* Ferussac. C.R. Soc. Biol. (Paris) **186**, 658–663 (1974)
Tardos, L., Adam, V.: The chronotropic activity of serotonin. Naunyn-Schmiedebergs Arch. Pharmacol. **248** (Suppl.), R81 (1974)

Tebécis, A.K., DiMaria, A.: A re-evaluation of the mode of action of 5-hydroxytryptamine on lateral geniculate neurones: Comparison with catecholamines and LSD. Exp. Brain Res. **14**, 480–493 (1972)
Teraki, Y.: A study on the action mechanism of foetal death with 5-HT and the influence of its antagonists. Acta obstet. gynaec. Jap. **17**, 142 (1970)
Thierry, A.M., Blanc, G., Sobel, A., Stinus, L., Glowinski, J.: Dopaminergic terminals in rat cortex. Science **182**, 499–501 (1973a)
Thierry, A.M., Stinus, L., Blanc, G., Glowinski, J.: Some evidence for the existence of dopaminergic neurones in the rat cortex. Brain Res. **50**, 230–234 (1973b)
Thoenen, H., Hürlimann, A., Haefely, W.: Dual site of action of phenoxybenzamine in the cat's spleen: Blockade of α-adrenergic receptors and inhibition of re-uptake of neurally released norepinephrine. Experientia (Basel) **20**, 272–273 (1964a)
Thoenen, H., Hürlimann, A., Haefely, W.: Wirkungen von Phenoxybenzamin, Phentolamin und Azapetin auf adrenergische Synapsen der Katzenmilz. Helv. physiol. pharmacol. Acta **22**, 148–161 (1964b)
Thompson, J.H., Campbell, L.B.: The influence of 1-methyl-d-lysergic acid butanolamide on gastrointestinal serotonin in the Sprague-Dawley rat. Biochem. Pharmacol. **16**, 1377–1380 (1967)
Thompson, J.W.: Studies on the responses of the isolated nictitating membrane of the cat. J. Physiol. (Lond.) **141**, 46–72 (1958)
Thompson, M.R.: Some properties of ergostetrine. J. Amer. Pharm. Ass. **24**, 748–753 (1935)
Thompson, R.H.S., Tickner, A., Webster, G.R.: Cholinesterase inhibition by lysergic acid diethylamide. Biochem. J. **58**, XIX-XX (1954)
Thompson, R.H.S., Tickner, A., Webster, G.R.: The action of lysergic acid diethylamide on mammalian cholinesterases. Brit. J. Pharmacol. **10**, 61–65 (1955)
Thulin, A.: Motor and secretory effects of autonomic nerves and drugs in the rat submaxillary gland. Acta physiol. scand. **92**, 217–223 (1974)
Thulin, A.: Influence of autonomic nerves and drugs on myoepithelial cells in parotid gland of cat. Acta physiol. scand. **93**, 477–482 (1975)
Tilson, H.A., Sparber, S.B.: Studies on the concurrent behavioral and neurochemical effects of psychoactive drugs using the push-pull cannula. J. Pharmacol. exp. Ther. **181**, 387–398 (1972)
Toda, N.: Influence of 5-hydroxykynurenamine, a new serotonin metabolite, on isolated cerebral arteries. Jap. J. Pharmacol. **24** (Suppl.), 68 (1974)
Toda, N.: Analysis of the effect of 5-hydroxykynurenamine, a serotonin metabolite, on isolated cerebral arteries, aortas and atria. J. Pharmacol. exp. Ther. **193**, 385–392 (1975)
Toda, N., Goldberg, L.I.: Dopamine-induced relaxation of isolated arterial strips. J. Pharm. Pharmacol. **25**, 587–589 (1973)
Toda, N., Goldberg, L.I.: Effects of dopamine on isolated canine coronary arteries. Cardiovasc. Res. **9**, 384–389 (1975)
Toda, N., Goldberg, L.I., Fujiwara, M.: Dopamine-induced relaxation of isolated blood vessels. Jap. J. Pharmacol. **23** (Suppl.), 45 (1973)
Toda, N., Tokuyama, T., Senoh, S., Hirata, F., Hayaishi, O.: Effects of 5-hydroxykynurenamine, a new serotonin metabolite, on isolated dog basilar arteries. Proc. natl. Acad. Sci. (Wash.) **71**, 122–124 (1974)
Toda, N., Hayashi, S., Fu, W.L.H., Nagasaka, Y.: Serotonin antagonism in isolated canine cerebral arteries. Jap. J. Pharmacol. **26**, 57–63 (1976)
Tomosky, T.K., Bennett, J.L., Bueding, E.: Tryptaminergic and dopaminergic responses of Schistosoma mansoni. J. Pharmacol. exp. Ther. **190**, 260–271 (1974)
Tonge, S.R., Leonard, B.E.: The effects of some hallucinogenic drugs upon the metabolism of 5-hydroxy-tryptamine in the brain. Life Sci. **8 (I)**, 805–814 (1969)
Tonge, S.R., Leonard, B.E.: The effect of some hallucinogenic drugs on the amino acid precursors of brain monoamines. Life Sci. **9 (I)**, 1327–1335 (1970)
Torre, M., Bogetto, F., Torre, E.: Effect of LSD-25 and 1-methyl-d-lysergic acid butanolamide on rat brain and platelet serotonin levels. Psychopharmacologia **36**, 117–122 (1974a)
Torre, M., Torre, E., Bogetto, F.: Somministrazione di etanolo a varie dosi: livelli di serotonina cerebrale nel ratto. Somministrazione contemporanea di LSD-25 e UML: Livelli di serotonina cerebrale e comportamento condizionato nel ratto. Boll. Soc. ital. Biol. sper. **50**, 1639–1645 (1974b)

Tothill, A.: Investigation of adrenaline reversal in the rat uterus by the induction of resistance to isoprenaline. Brit. J. Pharmacol. **29**, 291–301 (1967)
Trabucchi, M., Spano, P.F., Tonon, G.C., Frattola, L.: Effects of bromocriptine on central dopaminergic receptors. Life Sci. **19**, 225–232 (1976)
Trenchard, A., Turner, P., Pare, C.M.B., Hills, M.: The effects of protryptiline and clomipramine in vitro on the uptake of 5-hydroxytryptamine and dopamine in human platelet-rich plasma. Psychopharmacologia **43**, 89–93 (1975)
Trendelenburg, U.: The action of histamine and 5-hydroxytryptamine on isolated mammalian atria. J. Pharmacol. exp. Ther. **130**, 450–460 (1960)
Türker, K., Kiran, B.K., Kaymakcalan, S.: Distribution of adrenergic receptors in the cat ileum. Arch. int. Pharmacodyn. **156**, 130–142 (1965)
Türker, R.K., Khairallah, P.A.: Prostaglandin E_1 action on canine isolated tracheal muscle. J. Pharm. Pharmacol. **21**, 498–501 (1969)
Tuomisto, J.: Inhibition of noradrenaline (NA), dopamine (DA) and 5-HT uptake in synaptosomes by reserpine, 6-hydroxy-1,2,3,4-tetrahydroharmane (6HTH), LSD and ergotamine. J. Pharmacol. (Paris) **5** (Suppl. 2), 100 (1974)
Turner, P.: Some pharmacological studies on drugs used in the prophylactic treatment of migraine. In: Background to Migraine. Cumings, J.N. (ed.), pp. 170–173. London: William Heinemann Medical Books 1973
Twarog, B.M.: Responses of a molluscan smooth muscle to acetylcholine and 5-hydroxytryptamine. J. cell. comp. Physiol. **44**, 141–164 (1954)
Ungar, F., Hitri, A., Alivisatos, S.G.A.: Drug antagonism and reversibility of the binding of indole amines in brain. Europ. J. Pharmacol. **36**, 115–125 (1976)
Urquilla, P.R., Marco, E., Lluch, S.: Pharmacological receptors of the cerebral blood vessels of the goat. Fed. Proc. **33**, 568 (1974)
Urquilla, P.R., Marco, E.J., Lluch, S.: Pharmacological receptors of the cerebral arteries of the goat. Blood Vessels **12**, 53–67 (1975)
Uzunov, P., Weiss, B.: Psychopharmacological agents and the cyclic AMP system of rat brain. Adv. Cyclic Nucleotide Res. **1**, 435–451 (1972)
Valdecasas, F.G., Calvet, F., Cuenca, E., Salvá, J.A.: Die potenzierende Wirkung verschiedener psychoaktiver Substanzen auf Adrenalin und Serotonin. Arzneimittel-Forsch. **6**, 594–596 (1956)
Vane, J.R.: A sensitive method for the assay of 5-hydroxytryptamine. Brit. J. Pharmacol. **12**, 344–349 (1957)
Vane, J.R.: The actions of sympathomimetic amines on tryptamine receptors. In: Ciba Foundation Symposium on Adrenergic Mechanisms, pp. 356–372. London: J. and A. Churchill 1960
Van Rossum, J.M.: Cumulative dose-response curves. II. Technique for the making of dose-response curves in isolated organs and the evaluation of drug parameters. Arch. int. Pharmacodyn. **143**, 299–330 (1963)
Van Rossum, J.M., Pijnenburg, A.J.J., Cools, A.R., Broekkamp, C.L.E., Struyker Boudier, H.A.J.: Behavioural pharmacology of the neostriatum and the limbic striatum. In: Neuropharmacology. Excerpta Medica Int. Congress Series No. 359, pp. 505–516. Amsterdam 1975
Vargaftig, B.B., Lefort, J.: Pharmacological evidence for a vasodilator receptor to serotonin in the nasal vessels of the dog. Europ. J. Pharmacol. **25**, 216–225 (1974)
Vidrio, H., Hong, E.: Vascular tone and reactivity to serotonin in the internal and external carotid vascular beds of the dog. J. Pharmacol. exp. Ther. **197**, 49–56 (1976)
Vogel, G., Marek, M.L.: Über die Hemmung verschiedener Rattenpfoten-Oedeme durch Serotonin-Antagonisten. Arzneimittel-Forsch. **11**, 1051–1054 (1961)
Vogt, M.: Drugs interfering with central actions of 5-hydroxytryptamine. In: Ciba Foundation Symposium on Hypertension, pp. 209–213. London: J. and A. Churchill 1954
Vogt, M., Gunn, C.G., Sawyer, Ch.: Electroencephalographic effects of intraventricular 5-HT and LSD in the cat. Neurology (Minneap.) **7**, 559–566 (1957)
Von Hungen, K., Roberts, S., Hill, D.F.: Serotonin and catecholamine activation of brain adenylate cyclase: Effects of psychoactive drugs. Trans. Amer. Soc. Neurochem. **5**, 150 (1974a)

Von Hungen, K., Roberts, S., Hill, D.F.: LSD as an antagonist at central dopamine receptors. Nature (Lond.) **252**, 588–589 (1974b)

Von Hungen, K., Roberts, S., Hill, D.F.: Serotonin-sensitive adenylate cyclase activity in immature rat brain. Brain Res. **84**, 257–267 (1975)

Votava, Z., Lamplová, I.: Antiserotonin effect of derivatives of d-lysergic acid (cycloalkylamides, LSD, ergometrine) and chlorpromazine in rats. Activ. nerv. sup. (Praha) **1**, 269–275 (1959)

Votava, Z., Podvalová, I., Semonský, M.: Oxytocic effect of some d-lysergic acid cycloalkylamides. Nature (Lond.) **179**, 474–475 (1957)

Votava, Z., Podvalová, I., Semonský, M.: Studies on the pharmacology of d-lysergic acid cycloalkylamides. Arch. int. Pharmacodyn. **115**, 114–130 (1958)

Walker, R.J., Woodruff, G.N., Glaizner, B., Sedden, C.B., Kerkut, G.A.: The pharmacology of *Helix* dopamine receptor of specific neurones in the snail, *Helix aspersa*. Comp. Biochem. Physiol. **24**, 455–469 (1968)

Walsh, J.A.: Antagonism by methysergide of vascular effects of 5-hydroxytryptamine in man. Brit. J. Pharmacol. **30**, 518–530 (1967)

Walters, J.R., Roth, R.H., Aghajanian, G.K.: Dopaminergic neurons, similar biochemical and histochemical effects of γ-hydroxybutyrate and acute lesions of the nigro-striatal pathway. J. Pharmacol. exp. Ther. **186**, 630–639 (1973)

Watson, P.J.: Drug receptor sites in the isolated superior cervical ganglion of the rat. Europ. J. Pharmacol. **12**, 183–193 (1970)

Weber, H.P., Petcher, T.J.: unpublished observations 1976

Weidmann, H.: Die Wirkung von D-Lysergsäure-diäthylamid und 5-Hydroxytryptamin auf spinale Reflexe. Helv. physiol. pharmacol. Acta **15**, C43–C44 (1957)

Weidmann, H., Cerletti, A.: Die Wirkung von D-Lysergsäurediäthylamid und 5-Hydroxytryptamin (Serotonin) auf spinale Reflexe der Katze. Helv. physiol. pharmacol. Acta **15**, 376–383 (1957)

Weidmann, H., Taeschler, M.: Influence des substances antimigraineuses sur les effets des catécholamines, de la sérotonine et de la stimulation des nerfs sympathiques. Extrait du Symposium International sur les Céphalées vasculaires, pp. 33–40. St-Germain-en-Laye 1966

Weiss, B.L., Aghajanian, G.K.: Activation of brain serotonin metabolism by heat: Role of midbrain raphe neurons. Brain Res. **26**, 37–48 (1971)

Wellens, D., Szigetvari, E., Wauters, E.: Reflex vasodilation, ergotamine and uptake of circulating norepinephrine. Arch. int. Pharmacodyn. **183**, 412–415 (1970)

Welsh, J.H.: Excitation of the heart of *Venus mercenaria*. Naunyn-Schmiedebergs Arch. Pharmacol. **219**, 23–29 (1953)

Welsh, J.H.: Hydroxytryptamine: A neurohormone in the invertebrates. Fed. Proc. **13**, 162–163 (1954a)

Welsh, J.H.: Marine invertebrate preparations useful in the bioassay of acetylcholine and 5-hydroxytryptamine. Nature (Lond.) **173**, 955–956 (1954b)

Welsh, J.H.: Neurohormones. In: The Hormones. Pincus, G., Thimann, K.V. (eds.), Chap. 3. New York: Academic Press 1955

Welsh, J.H.: Neurohormones of invertebrates. 1. Cardioregulators of *Cyprina* and *Buccinum*. J. Marine Biol. Assoc. United Kingdom **35**, 193–201 (1956)

Welsh, J.H.: Serotonin as a possible neurohumoral agent: Evidence obtained in lower animals. Ann. N.Y. Acad. Sci. **66**, 618–630 (1957)

Welsh, J.H., McCoy, A.C.: Actions of d-lysergic acid diethylamide and its 2-bromo derivative on heart of *Venus mercenaria*. Science **125**, 348 (1957 I)

Wennmalm, Å.: Quantitative evaluation of release and reuptake of adrenergic transmitter in the rabbit heart. Acta physiol. scand. **82**, 532–538 (1971a)

Wennmalm, Å.: Studies on mechanisms controlling the secretion of neurotransmitters in the rabbit heart. Acta physiol. scand. (Suppl.) **365**, 1–36 (1971b)

Wenzel, D.G., Su, J.L.: Interactions of nicotine and tyramine with adrenergic blocking agents on ventricle strips. Arch. int. Pharmacodyn. **162**, 180–185 (1966a)

Wenzel, D.G., Su, J.L.: Interactions between sympathomimetic amines and blocking agents on the rat ventricle strip. Arch. int. Pharmacodyn. **160**, 379–389 (1966b)

West, G.B.: 5-Hydroxytryptamine, tissue mast cells and skin oedema. Int. Arch. Allergy **10**, 257–275 (1957)
White, R.P., Denton, I.C., Robertson, J.T.: Differential effects of prostaglandins A_1, E_1 and $F_{2\alpha}$ on cerebrovascular tone in dogs and rhesus monkeys. Fed. Proc. **30**, 625 (1971a)
White, R.P., Heaton, J.A., Denton, I.C.: Pharmacological comparison of prostaglandin $F_{2\alpha}$, serotonin and norepinephrine on cerebrovascular tone of monkey. Europ. J. Pharmacol. **15**, 300–309 (1971b)
Whitney, B.: A preliminary investigation of the pharmacology of longitudinal muscle strips from human isolated jejunum. J. Pharm. Pharmacol. **17**, 465–473 (1965)
Wilhelmi, G.: Ueber die ulcerogene Wirkung von 5-Hydroxytryptamin am Rattenmagen und deren Beeinflussung durch verschiedene Pharmaka. Helv. physiol. pharmacol. Acta **15**, C83–C84 (1957)
Wilhelmi, G., Schindler, W.: Über die gastrotrope Wirkung von 5-Hydroxytryptamin (HTA), seiner Vorstufen und der entsprechenden Isomeren bei der Ratte. Naunyn-Schmiedebergs Arch. Pharmacol. **236**, 49–51 (1959)
Williams, L.T., Lefkowitz, R.J.: Alpha-adrenergic receptor identification by [^{3}H]dihydroergocryptine binding. Science **192**, 791–793 (1976)
Wiqvist, N.: Immediate and prolonged effects of relaxin on the spontaneous activity of the mouse and rat uterus. Acta endocr. (Kbh.) **32** (Suppl. 46), 3–32 (1959)
Wise, C.D., Ruelius, H.W.: The binding of serotonin in brain: A study in vitro of the influence of physicochemical factors and drugs. Biochem. Pharmacol. **17**, 617–631 (1968)
Woodruff, G.N., Agar, J., Albani, M.J., Allen, K.A., Folkard, J.: Observations on some actions of ergometrine, noradrenaline and dopamine on the guinea-pig vas deferens and on the rabbit jejunum. J. Pharm. Pharmacol. **21**, 860–861 (1969)
Woodruff, G.N., Walker, R.J.: The effect of dopamine and other compounds on the activity of neurones of *Helix aspersa*. Structure-activity relationships. Int. J. Neuropharmacol. **8**, 279–289 (1969)
Woodruff, G.N., Walker, J.R., Kerkut, G.A.: Actions of ergometrine on catecholamine receptors in the guinea-pig vas deferens and in the snail brain. Comp. gen. Pharmacol. **1**, 54–60 (1970)
Woodruff, G.N., Walker, R.J., Kerkut, G.A.: Antagonism by derivatives of lysergic acid of the effect of dopamine on *Helix* neurones. Europ. J. Pharmacol. **14**, 77–80 (1971)
Woolley, D.W., Shaw, E.: Yohimbine and ergotoxin as naturally occurring antimetabolites of serotonin. Fed. Proc. **12**, 293 (1953)
Woolley, D.W., Shaw, E.: A biochemical and pharmacological suggestion about certain mental disorders. Science **119**, 587 (1954a)
Woolley, D.W., Shaw, E.: Some neurophysiological aspects of serotonin. Brit. med. J. **2**, 122–126 (1954b)
Wright, A.M., Moorehead, M., Welsh, J.H.: Actions of derivatives of lysergic acid on the heart of *Venus mercenaria*. Brit. J. Pharmacol. **18**, 440–450 (1962)
Wurzel, M.: Serotonin receptor in rabbit artery. Amer. J. Physiol. **211**, 1424–1428 (1966)
Yamaguchi, T.: Effects of 5-hydroxytryptamine on isolated strips of the guinea-pig stomach. Brit. J. Pharmacol. **44**, 100–108 (1972)
York, D.H.: Dopamine receptor blockade—a central action of chlorpromazine on striatal neurones. Brain Res. **37**, 91–100 (1972)
Zakusov, V.V.: Principles of pharmacological influence on coronary chemoreflexes. Arch. int. Pharmacodyn. **140**, 646–654 (1962)
Zarolinski, J.F., Browne, R.K.: Effects of dopamine on canine renal artery. Pharmacologist **13**, 22 (1971)
Zatz, M., Roth, R.H.: Electroconvulsive shock raises prostaglandins F in rat cerebral cortex. Biochem. Pharmacol. **24**, 2101–2103 (1975)
Zhabin, Y.M., Urazaeva, Z.V.: Influence of intravenous administration to pregnant rabbits of the diethylamide of lysergic acid on the content of serotonin, histamine and acetyl choline in mothers and young. Farmakol.i Toksikol. **38**, 93–95 (1975)
Ziegler, M.G., Lovell, R.A., Freedman, D.X.: Effects of lysergic acid diethylamide on the uptake and retention of brain 5-hydroxytryptamine in vivo and in vitro. Biochem. Pharmacol. **22**, 2183–2193 (1973)

CHAPTER IV

Effects on the Uterus

K. SAAMELI

A. Introduction

"The obstetrician bids, and the uterus contracts" was the title of Chassar MOIR's Sandoz Foundation lecture given in 1964 (MOIR, 1964). With this categorical statement he pointed to the great reliability of some drugs, and in particular of ergot, in causing the uterus to contract, thereby diminishing or preventing postpartum haemorrhage and reducing maternal mortality in childbirth.

In this chapter the reader will indeed find much evidence, from both animal and human studies, for predictable, powerful uterotonic actions of ergot alkaloids, but at the same time note that great differences in quality and quantity of the effects exist between compounds from the three structural classes of ergot alkaloids which are of interest in this respect (peptide alkaloids, dihydrogenated peptide alkaloids and lysergic acid-amides), and to some extent also between the individual substances within one of these classes. The reader will furthermore become aware of distinct variations of the responses obtained in different species in vitro and in situ, as well as of findings which have little to do with the obstetric use of the drugs, but are essential for elucidating their mechanism of action and for their general pharmacologic characterization. α-Adrenoceptor- and 5-HT receptor-blockade are discussed extensively in the preceding chapter "Basic Pharmacologic Properties." In order to avoid duplication these aspects will not be covered in a synoptical way. In many instances, however, information on interactions with α-adrenoceptors of the uterus is included—without aiming at any degree of completeness—whenever it is thought to be essential for the understanding of the effects of ergot alkaloids on uterine motor activity.

The material extracted from the relevant literature of the last 40 years—and on some occasions also from earlier times—is presented in six comprehensive tables and is discussed in the corresponding parts of the text. This dual approach is intended to be complementary, but according to his specific needs, the reader may use the two lines of information independently from each other. The tables provide essential data from individual studies with one compound in one species and make reference to the particular experimental conditions, to drug concentrations used in vitro, and to the doses and routes of drug administration in situ. Within one table the first principle of order is given by the various compounds (e.g., in Table 1 ergotamine followed by ergosine, ergosinine, ergotoxine, ergocornine), and for each compound the data is arranged according to the different species in which experiments have been reported. The sequence used consistently throughout the tables for the various species is the following: rat, hamster, guinea pig, rabbit, cat, dog, pig, sheep, monkey, human. Not all of these species, however, appear in all tables. Within one species the material is presented chronologically.

According to the basic principles of this book, the chapter on the uterine effects of ergot alkaloids is confined only to experimental work. Having worked himself as an obstetrician, the author was tempted to include also some of the results published on the clinical use of ergot alkaloids and their invaluable contribution to obstetrics. In view of the enormous amount of clinical literature he was able, however, to resist.

B. Actions on Uterine Motor Activity

In reviewing the pharmacologic actions of ergot alkaloids on the uterus, one must distinguish between experiments which are designed to demonstrate and quantify the stimulatory effects on uterine motor activity (usually called the oxytocic or uterotonic action) and those in which the uterus serves as a test organ for measuring various drug-receptor interactions such as antagonism against either adrenoceptor stimulants or 5-HT.

This chapter deals with the first type of experiments, the one which has definite therapeutic significance for obstetric practice.

The characteristics of the uterine response to an ergot alkaloid with high oxytocic activity are seen in Figure 1. The contractions of the human uterus were recorded on the sixth day of puerperium using the intrauterine bag method. At the arrow 0.5 mg of ergometrine were given by mouth simultaneously with the occurrence of an isolated spontaneous contraction. After a delay of 8 min another contraction, with increased amplitude, was observed, and this was followed by a long period of irregular contractions which, in the initial phase, followed each other at very short intervals of less than 30 s. Relaxation between contractions was incomplete and resting tone was markedly increased. According to MOIR (1932a) "... the rise in base line may be regarded as a measure of the tonicity of the uterus. It may mean that the whole uterus has gone into a long-sustained contraction, or that waves of contraction pass through the muscle substance so frequently that they overlap and cause the organ as a whole to compress its cavity." In the tracing shown the maximal increase in resting tone and the highest frequency of contractions were observed about 15 min after drug administration. At this time the amplitude of the contractions was small, but it increased continuously

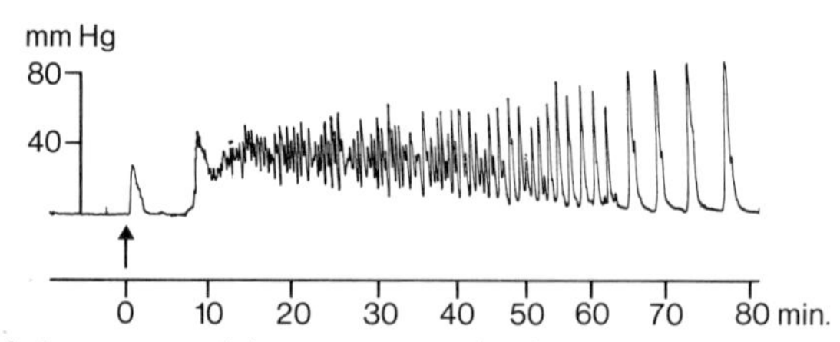

Fig. 1. Response of the puerperal human uterus in situ to ergometrine (0.5 mg given orally at the arrow). Intrauterine pressure recording by means of a transcervically inserted bag. (From DUDLEY and MOIR, 1935)

during the following 60 min while the contractile rhythm slowed down considerably and resting tone gradually decreased to almost the preexisting level. It is interesting to note that in the last part of the tracing the contractions show a striking similarity to the pattern of uterine contractility seen during advanced labor, with respect to resting tone, amplitude, duration, frequency and regularity.

Though the example of ergometrine discussed above seems suitable for demonstrating the principal features of the uterotonic effect of ergot alkaloids, it would be wrong to assume that all compounds of this structural class behave similarly. They show in fact great differences not only in potency, but also in the time required for the onset of action, in their duration of action and in their effectiveness when given orally. Their actions may also vary from one experimental procedure to another and—more important—from one species to another.

1. Peptide Alkaloids

a) Studies on the Isolated Uterus

With the exception of studies designed for the quantification of antagonistic properties against adrenoceptor stimulants or 5-HT, in vitro methods on the isolated uterus have not been used extensively for the pharmacologic testing of this group of ergot alkaloids. The reasons are manifold: great variability of the response to one and the same compound within one species; marked tachyphylaxis, so that as a rule the second application of the same dose gives a smaller response (ROTHLIN, 1938a); difficulty in "washing out" the effects; interactions between various alkaloids, e.g., inhibition by ergotoxine of the contractile action of ergometrine on the rabbit uterus and potentiation by ergotoxine of the contractile action of ergometrine on the guinea pig uterus (MILLER and DE BEER, 1952); poor predictability with regard to the actions in vivo. It is therefore not surprising that the information given in the literature is relatively scanty. The available data on peptide alkaloids are summarized in Table 1, from which the following points emerge:

The *compounds tested* were ergotamine, ergosine, ergosinine (the 8α-isomer of ergosine), ergotoxine (the naturally occurring mixture of ergocornine, ergocristine and ergokryptine), and ergocornine.

Species: The uteri used (as the whole horn or as a strip) were from the rat, hamster, guinea pig, rabbit, cat or human.

All of the compounds proved to be oxytocic in one or more species, but the *pattern of response* (change in resting tone, amplitude, rhythm) varied with different compounds and their bath concentrations, the species, and the experimental conditions. An example in which, using the isolated rabbit uterus, ergotamine at a concentration of 0.2 μg/ml produced an immediate increase in amplitude and rate of contractions with only minimal rise of resting tone is shown in Figure 2. A completely different type of response was, however, observed with ergotamine and ergotoxine at a concentration of 0.4 μg/ml in the isolated uterine horns of a virgin cat, as illustrated in Figure 3. In this species both drugs increased the tone of the almost quiescent organ without augmenting rhythmic activity. The same illustration demonstrates the striking qualitative and quantitative similarity of the effects of ergotamine and ergotoxine in the isolated cat uterus. This is

Table 1. Oxytocic action of peptide alkaloids in vitro

Compound	Species/state	Experimental condition	Drug concentration in bath (µg/ml)	Characteristics of effect	Special observations/ remarks	Ref.
Ergotamine	Rat	Both horns of same uterus	0.08	Relatively short (approx. 15 min) increase in resting tone; similarity with ergotoxine		1
Ergotamine	Rat			Inhibition		2, 3
Ergotamine	Rat	Influence on electrically evoked contraction; uterine horn in toto, isotonic or isometric recording, preload 1 or 2 g; Tyrode solution, O_2/CO_2	0.3	Long-lasting potentiation of electrically induced contraction by 30–50% without change of resting tone, reduction of electrical threshold; similarity with methylergometrine		4
Ergotamine	Guinea pig			Contraction		2, 3
Ergotamine	Guinea pig; virgin	Both horns of same uterus	0.008	Marked and long-lasting increase in amplitude with only a short rise in resting tone; equipotent with ergotoxine	Similarity of contractile pattern with that of ergotoxine	1
Ergotamine	Guinea pig	Oxygenated Locke-Ringer solution		Increase in resting tone, amplitude and rate		5
Ergotamine	Rabbit		0.1	Increase in resting tone, amplitude and rate with a slow onset of action	Persistent effect, not readily washed out	3
Ergotamine	Rabbit	Myometrial strip, Magnus-Kehrer preparation; oxygenated solution according to Fleisch	0.033	Slight increase in tone; ergometrine at same concentration ineffective	Marked and long-lasting potentiation of acetylcholin-induced contraction	6
Ergotamine	Rabbit		0.2	Rapidly occurring increase in amplitude and rate with only minimal rise of resting tone	Long-lasting effect interrupted by addition of adrenaline	7

Table 1 (continuation)

Compound	Species/state	Experimental condition	Drug concentration in bath (µg/ml)	Characteristics of effect	Special observations/ remarks	Ref.
Ergotamine	Rabbit	Myometrial strip, 1 cm in length, preload 3–5 g; oxygenated Ringer solution	0.05	Strong and long-lasting (2–3 h) increase in contractility combined with irregular rise in resting tone	duration of oxytocic effect coincides with duration of adrenolytic action	8
Ergotamine	Rabbit; ovariecto-mized, estrogen-treated	Influence on electrically evoked contraction; myometrial strip, 1 cm in length, isotonic or isometric recording, preload 3–5 g; Tyrode solution O_2/CO_2	0.3	Long-lasting potentiation of electrically induced contraction by 30–50% without change of resting tone; similarity with methylergometrine		4
Ergotamine	Cat; virgin	Both horns of same uterus	0.4	Long-lasting tonic response without rhythmic activity	Similarity with response to ergo-toxine	1
Ergotamine	Human; myomatosis	Longitudinal myometrial strip, 10 × 3–5 mm, Magnus-Kehrer preparation; oxygenated Tyrode solution	1	Increase in tone, contractions more regular		9
Ergosine	Guinea pig Rabbit		0.33 0.17	Uterotonic action, similar to that of ergotoxine		10
Ergosine	Rabbit		0.033	Increase in amplitude and some rise in resting tone, slow onset of action		3
Ergosinine	Rabbit		0.1	Similar to the effects of ergosine, but slightly weaker; onset of action slower		3

Table 1 (continuation)

Compound	Species/state	Experimental condition	Drug concentration in bath (μg/ml)	Characteristics of effect	Special observations/ remarks	Ref.
Ergotoxine	Hamster	Horn, suspended in oxygenated warm Locke solution	13	Persistent increase in tone with only little rhythmic activity, in contrast to ergometrine, which at the same concentration greatly augments rhythm		11
Ergotoxine	Guinea pig; virgin	Both horns of same uterus	0.008	Marked and long-lasting increase in amplitude with only a short rise in resting tone; equipotent with ergotamine	Similarity of contractile pattern with that of ergotamine	1
Ergotoxine	Guinea pig; virgin	Horn, suspended in oxygenated warm Locke solution	0.66 (0.001 with particularly sensitive preparations)	Increase in tone, followed by superimposed rhythmic contractions of small amplitude; qualitative and quantitative similarity with ergometrine	Immediate onset of action with both ergotoxine and ergometrine, but ergotoxine slower to reach maximal tone	11
Ergotoxine	Guinea pig; virgin	Horn, suspended in Van Dyke-Hastings solution, 37.5° C, O_2/CO_2	2	No contraction; potentiation of ergometrine induced contraction		12
Ergotoxine	Rabbit; multiparous	Strip from junction of horn with broad ligament; oxygenated warm Locke solution	1.1	No oxytocic effect for about 10 min, then a short group of contractions (caused by the drug?); in contrast, ergometrine (1.3 μg/ml) elicited strong rhythmic contractions		11

Table 1 (continuation)

Compound	Species/state	Experimental condition	Drug concentration in bath (μg/ml)	Characteristics of effect	Special observations/ remarks	Ref.
Ergotoxine	Rabbit; virgin	Myometrial strip, isotonic recording, preload 0.1–0.3 g; Van Dyke-Hastings solution, 37.5° C, O_2/CO_2	2	No contraction; inhibition of effects of subsequent doses of ergometrine		12
			1	Relaxation of ergometrine-induced contraction		
Ergotoxine	Cat; virgin	Both horns of same uterus	0.4	Long-lasting tonic response without rhythmic activity; similarity with the response to ergotamine		1
Ergotoxine	Human; pregnant	Longitudinal strips removed at surgery; Locke-Ringer solution, 37° C	0.7–1	No oxytocic effect except in 2 out of 12 preparations which responded to even lower concentrations (0.05 μg/ml)	The 2 exceptionally sensitive preparations were also highly sensitive to oxytocin	13
	In labor		0.3–0.1	Marked and sustained rise in resting tone with increase in rate, but little influence on amplitude	Effect cannot easily be washed out; increase in resting tone continues after changing bath	
Ergocornine	Rabbit	Myometrial strip, 1 cm in length, preload 3–5 g; oxygenated Ringer solution	0.04	No oxytocic effect		8

References: 1. Dale and Spiro (1922); 2. Rothlin (1935b); 3. Rothlin (1938b); 4. Härtfelder et al. (1953); 5. Orth and Ritchie (1947); 6. Brügger (1938); 7. Rothlin (1925); 8. Rothlin and Brügger (1945); 9. Flury (1924); 10. Barger (1938); 11. Brown and Dale (1935); 12. Miller and De Beer (1952); 13. Robson (1933).

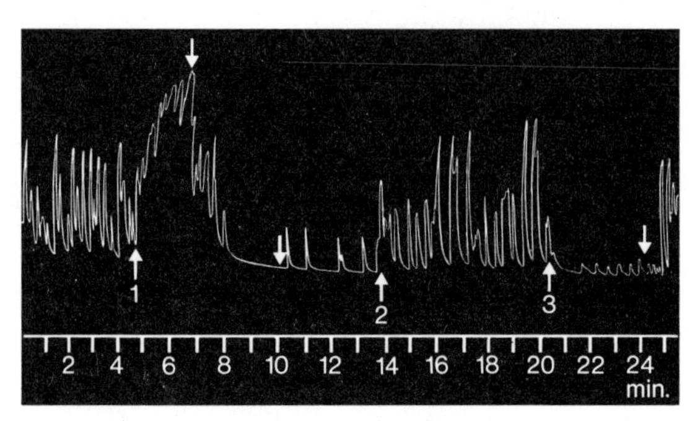

Fig. 2. Effects of ergotamine (and adrenaline) on the isolated rabbit uterus; pattern of the oxytocic effects and inhibition of ergotamine by adrenaline (adrenaline reversal). At 1 and 3 adrenaline 0.2 μg/ml; at 2 ergotamine 0.2 μg/ml; at ↓ wash. (From ROTHLIN, 1925)

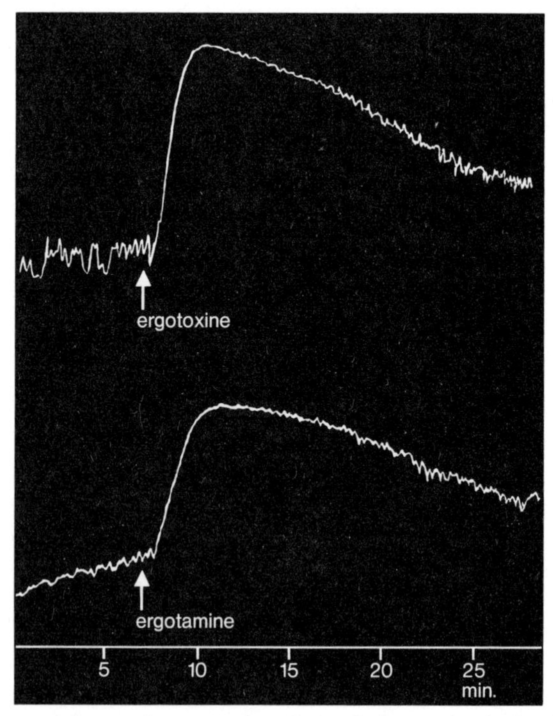

Fig. 3. Effects of ergotoxine and ergotamine (0.4 μg/ml) on the isolated uterine horns of a virgin cat. (From DALE and SPIRO, 1922)

in agreement with observations on the isolated uterus of the virgin guinea pig, but is in sharp contrast to results obtained with the isolated rabbit uterus, where, of the two, only ergotamine showed considerable oxytocic activity.

Irrespective of the pattern of response, the *duration of action* was found to be long, e.g., 2–3 h in the case of ergotamine on the rabbit uterus (ROTHLIN and BRÜGGER, 1945), and the effects persisted after removal of the drug from

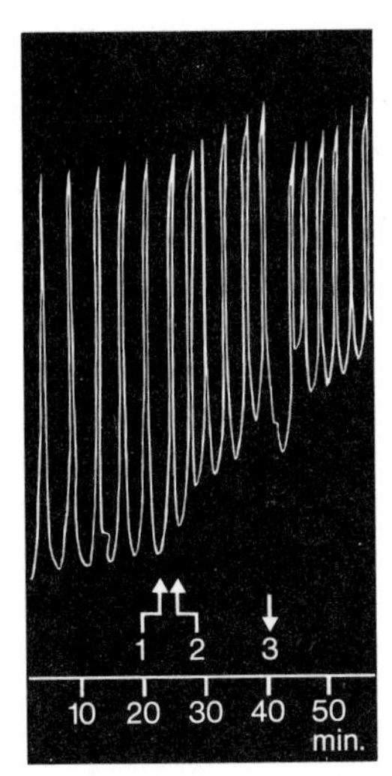

Fig. 4. Effect of ergotoxine on an exceptionally sensitive human uterine strip obtained at caesarian section during the 37th week of pregnancy. At 1 ergotoxine 0.025 μg/ml; at 2 increase to 0.05 μg/ml; at 3 wash. (From ROBSON, 1933)

the bath by flushing. This can be seen in Figure 4, which illustrates the response of a strip of pregnant human uterus to ergotoxine at a concentration of 0.05 μg/ml. When the solution in the bath was changed, there was no reversal of the oxytocic effect and the progressive increase in resting tone progressed further, suggesting that at the time of flushing a certain amount of the drug was fixed to the organ and continued to exert its action.

Potency: When different concentrations of the same drug were tested under the same experimental conditions, the effects were in general dose dependent. However, data which would permit accurate quantitative comparison of the oxytocic potencies of various drugs and of species-related organ sensitivity are lacking. The drug concentrations given in Table 1 are those published as being either effective or ineffective in stimulating uterine activity. It is not usually known where the effective concentrations would be located on a dose response curve.

The effective concentrations are remarkably low. They vary from 0.001 μg/ml (ergotoxine on a particularly sensitive preparation from the virgin guinea pig) to 13 μg/ml (ergotoxine on the hamster uterus), but most observations of uterotonic effects were made at concentrations between 0.03 and 0.3 μg/ml. There is no firm evidence that, on an overall basis, any one of the peptide alkaloids is definitely stronger or weaker than the others. Even with ergosinine (the 8α-isomer of ergosine), which is known to be very weak in other biologic systems, the difference from the uterotonic potency of the parent compound appears to be small (approximately factor 3). In some experiments on the uterus of the guinea pig and rabbit ergotoxine was found to be ineffective at the relatively high concentrations of 1.1 or 2 μg/ml; in other studies, however, in which the guinea pig uterus was used as well as in experiments performed on the cat uterus and the human uterus, the effective concentrations with ergotoxine were similar to those reported for ergotamine.

Species differences: The uterus of the virgin guinea pig may be regarded as the most sensitive preparation for demonstrating the oxytocic effects of ergot compounds. DAVIS et al. (1935b) found it to be approximately 10 times as sensitive as the rabbit uterus to ergometrine, and the figures given in Table 1 on effective concentrations suggest that the same holds true for ergotamine and ergotoxine. From the sparse information available on effects in the hamster, cat and human, one must conclude that the isolated uteri from these species are less sensitive than those of the guinea pig and rabbit, with the exception of strips from the human uterus in labor, which were highly sensitive to ergotoxine.

b) Studies in situ

Studies in which the oxytocic actions of peptide alkaloids (ergotamine, ergosine, ergostine, ergotoxine, ergokryptine, 2-bromo-α-ergokryptine) in various species (guinea pig, rabbit, cat, dog, monkey, human) have been evaluated are summarized in Table 2. The following aspects deserve special attention:

Methods: Most of the animal experiments were done in anesthetized rabbits in estrus. In contrast to the in vitro preparation the phenomenon of tachyphylaxis is not a great problem in the rabbit uterus in situ. This experimental procedure therefore permits repeated administration of the same drug and comparison of different drugs in the same animal. This is illustrated in Figure 5 which also demonstrates that measuring the area under the curve is a possible way of quantifying the time integral of the oxytocic response. ROTHLIN (1938a) considered the rabbit uterus in situ to be the "test organ of choice" for quantitative differentiation of ergot alkaloids. On the other hand, impressive recordings of intrauterine pressure curves from the puerperal dog, resembling those obtained in puerperal women, have been published by SWANSON and HARGREAVES (1934) and DAVIS et al. (1935a). It is surprising that this model never became widely used; the reason is, that already in the early years of ergot research a relatively reliable and practicable method using an intrauterine bag was developed for the evaluation of oxytocic drugs in parturient women by BOURNE and BURN (1927) and was modified for the puerperal human uterus by MOIR (1932a) in order to meet the special features of ergot compounds.

Characteristics of effects: With the exception of the semi-synthetic alkaloid 2-bromo-α-ergokryptine, all the compounds listed in Table 2 showed a clear stimulatory action on the uterus in situ. A typical example of an experiment with ergotamine in the rabbit is shown in Figure 6. The intravenous injection of 0.1 mg/kg body wt. of the drug caused an immediate rise in tone which gradually declined to the base line during the following 10 min and was superimposed with frequent rhythmic contractions of small amplitude. Simultaneous recording of intravaginal pressure changes revealed a similar picture, indicating that the smooth muscle layer of the vagina also possesses a high sensitivity to ergot compounds. During the period of elevated uterine tone mean arterial blood pressure was markedly increased. The similarity in the time course of the changes in blood pressure and uterine motor activity might suggest that the increase in blood pressure is a consequence of the rise in uterine tone and the resulting temporary augmentation of the circulating blood volume. This possibility, however, is excluded. The blood

Table 2. Oxytocic action of peptide alkaloids in situ

Compound	Species/state	Experimental condition	Dose/route of administration	Characteristics of effect	Special observations/ remarks	Ref.
Ergotamine	Rabbit; ovariecto-mized, estrogen-treated	Urethane anesthesia, laparotomy; isotonic recording from exteriorized uterine horn of which the distal end is sutured to the abdominal wall, kept in a moist funnel; in some experiments simultaneous recording of vaginal motility	0.05–0.2 mg/kg i.v.	Immediate rise of tone, reaching maximum within 1–2 min, followed by superimposed rhythmic contractions and decline to base line within approx. 10 min; increased vaginal motility (mainly rhythmic); uterine activity qualitatively and quantitatively similar to that of ergometrine	Concomitant increase in arterial blood pressure	1–4
Ergotamine	Rabbit; estrus	Isometric recording; measurement of the area under the curve	0.1 mg/kg i.v.	As described above (Ref. 1); somewhat stronger than ergostine	Response of same animal to a given dose is reproducible	5
Ergotamine	Cat; puerperal	Transvaginally introduced fluidfilled balloon, closed recording system	0.5–2 mg/kg i.m.	In most animals no or minimal oxytocic effect; much less effective than ergometrine		6
Ergotamine	Dog; day 3–6 postpartum	Transvaginally introduced intrauterine balloon, closed system; ether anesthesia	0.1 mg/kg i.v.	Strong contractions after 1.5 min, lasting for 35 min	Method suitable for pharmacologic testing of active principles of ergot	7, 8
			0.1–0.5 mg/kg p.o.	No or weak response		
			0.6–1 mg/kg p.o.	Strong contractions within 45–55 min, lasting for 50–70 min		
				Results similar to those with ergotoxine, but in contrast to those with various fluid extracts of ergot which, by the oral route, showed a more rapid onset of action		

Table 2 (continuation)

Compound	Species/state	Experimental condition	Dose/route of administration	Characteristics of effect	Special observations/ remarks	Ref.
Ergotamine	Monkey; prior to delivery and postpartum	Visual observation of uterus, or recording from intrauterine double balloon (fundus and cervix) in laparotomized animals under ether anesthesia	Not mentioned	Temporary augmentation of rate and amplitude of contractions; effect less pronounced than that of pituitrine; no spasm, no disturbance of coordinated character of contractions		9
Ergotamine	Human; parturient	Transcervically inserted waterfilled rubber bag, 20 cm above the os, between membranes and uterine wall	0.25–1 mg s.c.	Delayed onset of action (20–30 min), followed by strongly elevated tone (e.g., 50 mm Hg), little relaxation between contractions and little progress in dilatation of the os; very prolonged action, > 16 h after 1 mg	Ergotamine has no therapeutic place in labor, but is an ideal agent for use after delivery	10
Ergotamine	Human; late puerperium (day 6–8 postpartum)	Waterfilled intrauterine bag	0.25 or 0.5 mg i.v. 0.25–1 mg i.m.	Oxytocic effect (rise in base line and rhythmic contractions at intervals of about 1 min with smaller waves superimposed on larger ones) 4–10 min after i.v. and 15–45 min after i.m. injection, lasting ≫ 3 h	Optimum dosage for i.m. injection is 0.5 mg	11, 12
			1.5–3 mg p.o.	Erratic effect (small contractions) 35–≧60 min after administration Ergotamine qualitatively and quantitatively indistinguishable from ergotoxine	Only a very small fraction is absorbed during the 2 or 3 h following oral administration	

Table 2 (continuation)

Compound	Species/state	Experimental condition	Dose/route of administration	Characteristics of effect	Special observations/ remarks	Ref.
Ergotamine	Human; in labor and postpartum	Transcervically inserted balloon in upper or lower uterine segment	0.5 mg i.m. Oral doses	No effect on contractions or muscle tone Some effect demonstrated		13
Ergotamine	Human; mostly multiparas, day 6–8 postpartum	Transcervically inserted waterfilled intrauterine balloon	3 mg p.o.	No oxytocic effect during the following 35–45 min, whereas in the same patients the "alkaloid-free active principle" (water extract of ergot) provoked a prompt response within 10 min	"It is best to give only one drug to each patient, thereby avoiding confusing reactions"	8
Ergotamine	Human; day 5 or 6 postpartum	Transcervically inserted waterfilled intrauterine bag	0.6 mg i.v. 1 or 2 mg i.m.	Gradual onset of oxytocic response within 8–14 min, initial strong and intermittent contractions followed by a period of tetany lasting for 20–65 min	Good clinical effect with 2 mg i.m., occasionally associated with side effects	14
			2 or 6 mg p.o.	Onset of action within 25–55 min, contractions weak and irregular, no increase in tone	Given orally ergotamine (and ergotoxine) are of no clinical value in the puerperium	
				Ergotamine not distinguishable from ergotoxine; aequeous ergot preparations much more active	"Ergot contains an unidentified active principle"	
Ergotamine	Human; postabortum	Simultaneous pressure recording using small rubber balloons in upper and lower uterine segment	0.5 mg i.m. or i.v.	No influence on uterine tone or motility; in contrast to methylergometrine, which caused a rise in base line and increased the rate of contractions		15

Table 2 (continuation)

Compound	Species/state	Experimental condition	Dose/route of administration	Characteristics of effect	Special observations/ remarks	Ref.
Ergotamine	Human; postpartum	External tocography using an electromechanical recorder	0.25–0.75 mg i.m.	0.25 mg often ineffective, in other cases and with higher doses a long-lasting slight oxytocic effect (increase in tone and amplitude, but not in frequency) occurred after 20–30 min; ergometrine and methylergometrine more powerful and act more rapidly, but with shorter duration of action		16
Ergotamine	Human; nonpregnant, at various stages of cycle	Waterfilled intrauterine balloon	0.5 or 0.6 mg i.m.	In first half of cycle, only a slight increase in amplitude of the characteristic A-waves with some delayed rise in tone; in second half of cycle (dominated by B-waves) a slow rise in tone and increased rate of the contractions, but contractile pattern irregular; responses to ergometrine more pronounced than those to ergotamine	Nonpregnant human uterus is much less sensitive to ergotamine (and ergometrine) than puerperal uterus	1
Ergosine	Rabbit; ovariectomized, estrogen-treated	As described above (Ref. 1) for ergotamine	Not mentioned	Slightly more active than ergotamine or ergometrine	Lowering of arterial blood pressure	1

Table 2 (continuation)

Compound	Species/state	Experimental condition	Dose/route of administration	Characteristics of effect	Special observations/ remarks	Ref.
Ergostine	Rabbit; estrus	Isometric recording; measurement of the area under the curve	0.1 mg/kg i.v.	As described above (Ref. 1) for ergotamine; somewhat weaker than ergotamine		5
Ergotoxine	Guinea pig; 12 h postpartum	In situ recording under urethane anesthesia	10 µg i.v.	Series of increasing contractions after a latent period of about 10 min, with diminishing relaxation resulting in a long-lasting ($\gg$2 h) condition of strongly elevated tone with little rhythmic activity; marked difference to effect of ergometrine, for which short latency and predominance of rhythmic over tonic activity are typical		18
Ergotoxine	Rabbit; nonpregnant	In situ recording under urethane anesthesia	0.2–0.4 mg/kg i.v.	Questionable increase in tone and rhythmic activity 12 min after injection; preceding injection of similar dose of ergometrine caused prompt contraction followed by increased rhythmic activity	Immediate long-lasting fall of arterial blood pressure	18, 2
Ergotoxine	Rabbit; ovariectomized, estrogen-treated	As described above (Ref. 1) for ergotamine	0.3 mg/kg i.v.	Immediate rise of tone, maximum reached within 2 min, back to base line 10 min after injection; about 3 times less potent than ergotamine and ergometrine		1, 2

Table 2 (continuation)

Compound	Species/state	Experimental condition	Dose/route of administration	Characteristics of effect	Special observations/ remarks	Ref.
Ergotoxine	Dog; day 3–6 postpartum	Transvaginally introduced intrauterine balloon, closed system; ether anesthesia	0.2 mg/kg i.v.	Strong contractions after 1 min, lasting for 30 min		7, 8
			0.2 mg/kg p.o.	No response		
			0.5–1 mg/kg p.o.	Weak or strong contractions occurring within 30–60 min, lasting for 30–60 min (in one experiment for 120 min)		
				Similarity of responses to those obtained with ergotamine		
Ergotoxine	Human; late puerperium (day 6–8 postpartum)	Waterfilled intrauterine bag	0.25 mg i.v. 0.25–1 mg i.m. 1–2.5 mg p.o.	As described above (Ref. 11) for ergotamine		11, 12
Ergotoxine	Human; mostly multiparas, day 6–8 postpartum	Transcervically inserted waterfilled intrauterine balloon	3 mg p.o.	As described above (Ref. 8) for ergotamine		8
Ergotoxine	Human; day 5 or 6 postpartum	Transcervically inserted waterfilled intrauterine bag	0.6 mg i.v. 1–3 mg i.m.	Gradual onset of oxytocic response within 12–32 min, tetany lasting for 30–60 min	See remarks made above (Ref. 14) for ergotamine	14
			1–3 mg p.o.	Onset of action within 38–56 min, no or only transitory tetany		

Table 2 (continuation)

Compound	Species/state	Experimental condition	Dose/route of administration	Characteristics of effect	Special observations/ remarks	Ref.
Ergokryptine	Rabbit; ovariectomized, estrogen-treated	As described above (Ref. 1) for ergotamine	0.4 mg/kg i.v.	Slight effect, weaker and shorter than the response to a 4 times smaller dose of ergotamine	Long-lasting reduction of arterial blood pressure	4
2-Bromo-α-ergokryptine	Rabbit; spontaneous estrus	Urethane anesthesia, laparotomy; isometric recording from 4 cm segment of a uterine horn fixed in plexiglass chamber; tension adjusted to give maximal responses to 0.25 μg/kg adrenaline i.v.	0.05–0.5 mg/kg i.v.	No oxytocic effect	Inhibition of methylergometrine-induced contractions	19

References: 1. Rothlin (1938a); 2. Rothlin (1938b); 3. Rothlin (1946); 4. Rothlin (1946/47); 5. Berde and Saameli (1966); 6. Oettel and Bachmann (1937); 7. Swanson and Hargreaves (1934); 8. Davis et al. (1935a); 9. Ivy et al. (1931); 10. Bourne and Burn (1927); 11. Moir (1932a); 12. Moir (1932b); 13. Adair and Davis (1934); 14. Koff (1935); 15. Eschbach and Hanke (1953); 16. Huber (1956); 17. Garrett and Moir (1958); 18. Brown and Dale (1935); 19. Stürmer and Flückiger (1974).

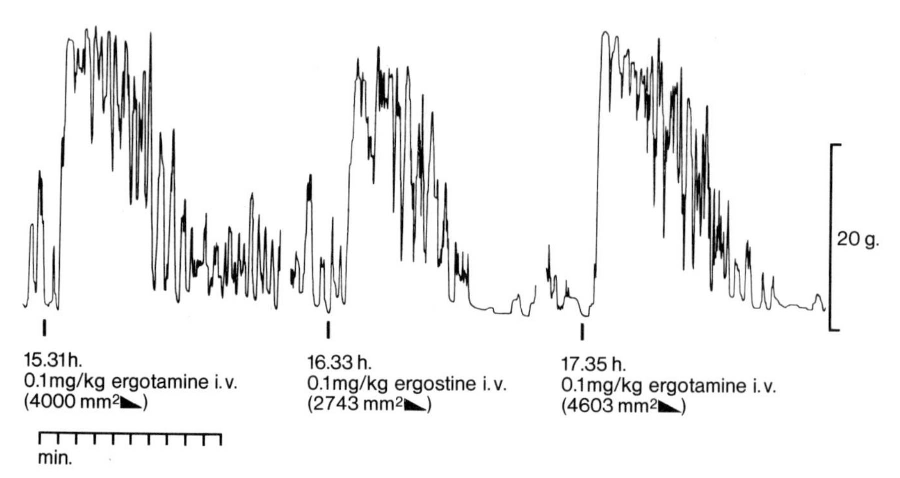

Fig. 5. Isometric recording of the uterotonic effect of ergostine and ergotamine on the estrous rabbit in situ. Evaluation by the "triangle-method": the areas under the curves are expressed in mm^2 of the original tracing. (From BERDE and SAAMELI, 1966)

pressure increase has to be attributed to the well-known vasoconstrictor action of this drug, because of results obtained with other ergot alkaloids. Using the same experimental procedure, ergometrine was found to exert its oxytocic effect without any influence on arterial blood pressure (ROTHLIN, 1938a), and ergosine as well as ergokryptine (one of the constituents of ergotoxine) often cause a reduction in blood pressure at clearly oxytocic doses (ROTHLIN, 1938a; ROTHLIN, 1946/47).

The time required for the onset and full development of an oxytocic effect in vivo varies to some extent from one drug to another; it may also depend on the species and be a function of the dose. The decisive criterion, however, is the route by which the drug is given to the experimental animal or human subject. Most observations indicate that by the *intravenous* and *intramuscular* route the effect occurs in animals almost immediately or within a few minutes of the injection, and that in human subjects it takes usually not longer than 5–15 min to appear. Much longer delays in the onset of action have been reported for the *oral* administration of peptide alkaloids. The values given for ergotamine and ergotoxine in the puerperal dog and in puerperal women range from 25–60 and more min. The marked difference between the parenteral and oral routes obviously points to a relatively poor absorption of peptide alkaloids from the gastrointestinal tract. In this respect the compounds belonging to this class of alkaloids are at variance with the rapidly absorbed drugs ergometrine and methylergometrine, which are members of the nonpeptide (lysergic acid-amide) class of alkaloids.

In the experiment illustrated in Figure 5 the durations of action of ergotamine and ergostine on the rabbit uterus in situ were rather short (approximately 10 min). A somewhat different picture is seen in Figure 6 where the immediate strong oxytocic response to ergotamine also lasted for about 10 min, but was followed by a series of smaller contractions. Considerably longer responses were reported from studies in the dog in which the effects of parenteral or oral doses of ergotamine

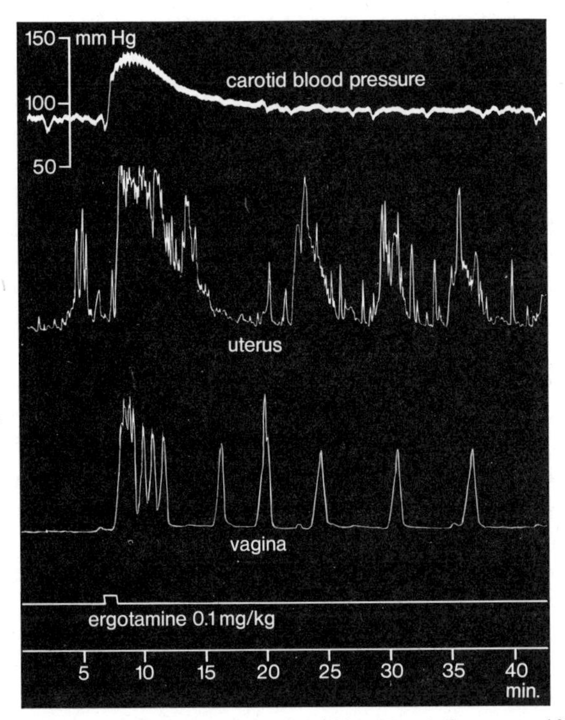

Fig. 6. Effects of ergotamine in the anesthetized rabbit. (From ROTHLIN, 1946/47)

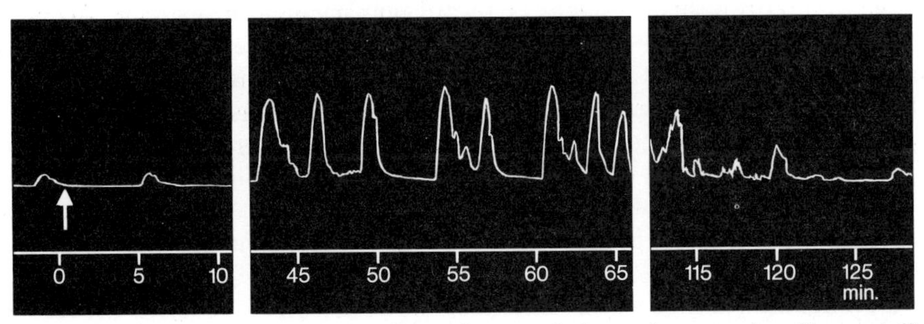

Fig. 7. Time course of the oxytocic effect of an oral dose of ergotamine (6 mg at ↑) on the puerperal human uterus in situ. Recording of intrauterine pressure using a transcervically inserted fluidfilled bag. (From KOFF, 1935; by permission of Surg. Gynec. Obstet.)

and ergotoxine persisted over a period of 30–70 min. A still longer duration of action of these two drugs, in the range of several hours, was observed in puerperal women. An example of such an experiment is depicted in Figure 7.

Effective doses: As with studies on the isolated uterus, the information from published results obtained in situ does not permit an accurate assessment of the individual drug potencies. The picture is further complicated by the fact that the doses required for a measurable oxytocic effect depend greatly on the route of administration. Details concerning effective or ineffective doses are contained in Table 2. With some simplification it can be said that, in order to obtain an effect orally, doses have to be 5–10 times higher than by the parenteral route, whereas the appropriate doses for intramuscular or subcutaneous injections are only slightly higher than those for intravenous administration.

Differences between drugs: On comparing published tracings of uterine motility and accurate descriptions of the effects of various peptide alkaloids, no evidence can be found for any marked differences in the basic response. An exception is 2-bromo-α-ergokryptine which, when tested in the rabbit, did not stimulate uterine motor activity, but—similarly to alkaloids of the dihydrogenated type—inhibited contractions induced by methylergometrine (STÜRMER and FLÜCKIGER, 1974).

Some differences, however, have been claimed concerning quantitative aspects. In contrast to MOIR (1932a), who found ergotamine in puerperal women to be indistinguishable from ergotoxine, the results obtained by ROTHLIN (1938a) in the rabbit indicate a three times higher potency of ergotamine compared with ergotoxine. The same investigator found ergosine to be slightly more active (1938a) and ergokryptine to be more than four times weaker (1946/47) than ergotamine. In Figure 5, published by BERDE and SAAMELI (1966) it can be seen that, again in the rabbit, ergostine is somewhat less potent than ergotamine.

Species differences: As was the case with studies on the isolated uterus, the guinea pig appears to be particularly sensitive also under in situ conditions. In an experiment described by BROWN and DALE (1935) 10 μg of ergotoxine given intravenously 12 h postpartum evoked a very strong and long-lasting uterine response.

The cat uterus postpartum may be regarded as the opposite extreme. According to OETTEL and BACHMANN (1937) intramuscular doses of ergotamine as high as 2 mg/kg body wt. proved to be ineffective in most experiments. This poor sensitivity is probably one of the reasons why ROTHLIN (1938a) considered the cat uterus in situ to be an unsatisfactory method for the quantitative analysis of ergot action.

The in situ uterus of the rabbit in estrus and of the puerperal dog are in an intermediate position with regard to their sensitivity. In general they respond to intravenous doses of ergotamine, ergotoxine and other members of the peptide alkaloids within the range of 0.05–0.5 mg/kg body wt.

A pronounced difference in sensitivity, however, seems to exist between the various animal species tested and man. An intramuscular dose of 0.5 mg of ergotamine or ergotoxine has been said to be the optimum dosage in puerperal women (MOIR, 1932a) and was active also in nonpregnant women (GARRETT and MOIR, 1958). This amounts to less than 0.01 mg/kg body wt. which is appreciably lower than, for example, the doses found to be effective in the rabbit.

2. Dihydrogenated Peptide Alkaloids

From their work on the pharmacologic properties of dihydrogenated peptide alkaloids ROTHLIN (1944, 1946/47) and ROTHLIN and BRÜGGER (1945) concluded that selective saturation of one of the double bonds (C9 to C10) of the lysergic acid moiety resulted in compounds which differ considerably from the natural alkaloids. One of the most prominent divergencies was found in respect to the uterine effects: "The action of the dihydrogenated alkaloids on the uterus is entirely different from that of the natural alkaloids. Not only have these (the dihydrogenated alkaloids) lost the excitatory effect on the uterus, but they are indeed able to inhibit in vitro and in situ the powerful stimulative action of the natural alkaloids such as ergotamine and ergotoxine" (ROTHLIN, 1946/47). The following sections, dealing with the effects on the uterus in vitro and in situ, will show that the early results obtained by these authors in animals were subsequently confirmed by many investigators, whereas in man the situation is equivocal.

a) Studies on the Isolated Uterus

Many of the reported in vitro experiments with dihydrogenated peptide alkaloids were performed in order to demonstrate and quantify their α-adrenoceptor blocking activity; they are discussed in the preceding chapter. The studies mainly concerning effects on uterine motor activity, and in some cases interference with compounds other than catecholamines, are listed in Table 3. The available information is limited to dihydroergotamine, dihydroergotoxine and its constituents (with quantitative data only for dihydroergokryptine). These drugs have been tested in preparations from the rat, guinea pig, rabbit and human.

α) Uterus From Animals

In agreement with ROTHLIN's statement (1946/47) all the compounds were found to lack oxytocic activity on animal uteri, even though in some experiments the drug concentrations were considerably higher than those used in similar studies with nondihydrogenated alkaloids (see Table 1). So far only one exception has been found in the literature: from an illustration published by CLEGG (1963) it is evident that dihydroergotamine at a relatively high concentration (10 μg/ml) caused small regular contractions in the virgin uterus of the guinea pig, a preparation which is known to be particularly sensitive to the oxytocic effect of ergot alkaloids. This is in contrast to observations made by VENKATASUBBU and GOPALA KRISHNAMURTHY (1959) who, in the same species, found dihydroergotamine and also dihydroergotoxine to cause either no effect or slight relaxation of the virgin uterus, and marked relaxation associated with inhibition of rhythmic contractions in preparations from pregnant animals. An inhibitory action of dihydroergotamine was also reported for the rat uterus by RUDZIK and MILLER (1962). In their experiments the drug exerted no effect at concentrations up to 24 μg/ml, but at still higher doses it produced uterine inhibition. Since this effect could be blocked by adrenergic neurone blockade and was not obtained in uteri from reserpine-treated animals it was concluded that dihydroergotamine produced uterine inhibition through the action of endogenous adrenergic stubstances which, under the given conditions, were not blocked by dihydroergotamine. This is readily understood for the uterus of the rat in estrus in which noradrenaline, similarly to adrenaline and isoproterenol, inhibits spontaneous motor activity (DEIS and PICKFORD, 1964; TOTHILL, 1967). For other species, in which stimulation of α-adrenoceptors results in an oxytocic effect, the uterine inhibitory effects of dihydrogenated alkaloids can be explained partly on the basis of their powerful α-adrenoceptor

Table 3. Uterine action of dihydrogenated peptide alkaloids in vitro

Compound	Species/state	Experimental condition	Drug concentration in bath (μg/ml)	Characteristics of effect	Special observations/ remarks	Ref.
Dihydro-ergotamine	Rat; natural estrus	Isotonic recording	10	No oxytocic effect	Inhibition of inhibitory effect of adrenaline, but not of relaxine	1
Dihydro-ergotamine	Rat; virgin or nongravid	Uterine segment, 25 mm in length; oxygenated Ringer solution	1 (?)*	No appreciable effect		2
Dihydro-ergotamine	Rat; induced estrus	Isotonic recording; Locke solution, 37° C, O_2/CO_2	5–24 >24	No oxytocic effect Inhibitory action	Inhibitory action blocked by adrenergic neuron blockade (bretylium); conclusion: uterine inhibition by dihydroergotamine is due to release of adrenergic substances	3
Dihydro-ergotamine	Guinea pig; virgin	Oxygenated Locke–Ringer solution	Not mentioned	No influence on rate or strength of contractions		4
Dihydro-ergotamine	Guinea pig; virgin or gravid	Uterine segment, 25 mm in length; oxygenated Ringer solution	1 (?)* 1 (?)*	Virgin: slight relaxation without inhibition of contractions Gravid: marked relaxation and inhibition of rhythmic contractions for >20 min		2
Dihydro-ergotamine	Guinea pig; virgin	Isotonic recording; Krebs solution, O_2/CO_2	10	Regular small contractions in previously quiescent uterus	Reversal of inhibitory effect of increased $CaCl_2$ concentration leading to a strong uterotonic effect	5
Dihydro-ergotamine	Rabbit	Isotonic recording, Ringer solution	0.1	No oxytocic effect	Inhibition of the marked oxytocic effect of ergometrine (0.4 μg/ml)	6

Table 3 (continuation)

Compound	Species/state	Experimental condition	Drug concentration in bath (μg/ml)	Characteristics of effect	Special observations/ remarks	Ref.
Dihydro-ergotamine	Rabbit		0.33	No oxytocic effect	Inhibition of the excitatory effects of ergotamine, ergometrine and sparteine if given prior to these drugs	7
Dihydro-ergotamine	Rabbit; ovariectomized, estrogen-treated	Influence on electrically evoked contraction; myometrial strip, 1 cm in length, isotonic or isometric recording, preload 3–5 g; Tyrode solution, O_2/CO_2	Cumulative dosage: from 1 to 6 to 11 μg/ml	No potentiation of electrically induced contractions		8
Dihydro-ergotamine	Human; nonpregnant		0.5	Ineffective		9
			1–5	Slight oxytocic effect		
			10	Decrease in tone (questionable)		
	Pregnant		> 2.5 (e.g. 5)	Marked increase in resting tone and rate		
Dihydro-ergotamine	Human; pregnant (caesarian section), near term, at term or during labor	Strips, 8–20 × 2–5 × 1–2 mm, isotonic recording, preload 0.5 g; oxygenated Tyrode solution, 37.5° C	2–5 (threshold)	Enhancement of spontaneous motility in 6 out of 30 uteri; in remainder no evidence for relaxation or inhibition of motility	Effects cannot be repeated on the same organ; qualitatively similar to those observed with oxytocin or methylergometrine; previous dose of oxytocin does not impair sensitivity to dihydroergotamine	10

Table 3 (continuation)

Compound	Species/state	Experimental condition	Drug concentration in bath (µg/ml)	Characteristics of effect	Special observations/ remarks	Ref.
Dihydro-ergotamine	Human; nonpregnant (hysterectomy) at various phases of cycle; pregnant (caesarian section)	Myometrial strip, isotonic recording; Locke-Ringer solution, 37 °C	0.01–5	Usually no influence on spontaneously contracting myometrium; occasionally contractions inhibited in nonpregnant specimens, and stimulated in pregnant specimens		11
Dihydro-ergotamine	Human; nonpregnant (hysterectomy) at various phases of cycle; pregnant (caesarian section)	Strips from upper or lower segment, isotonic recording; modified Tyrode solution, 37.5 °C, O_2/CO_2	2.5–20	Effects were mainly inhibitory, the most prominent response being reduced frequency of spontaneous contractions	No differences in sensitivity between strips from corpus and isthmus, and between strips from pregnant and nonpregnant uteri	12
Dihydro-ergotamine	Human; nonpregnant (hysterectomy); pregnant (caesarian section)	Myometrial strips, 22 × 2 mm; oxygenated Tyrode solution, 37 °C	0.5	Relaxation	Some potentiation of the rate-increasing effect and inhibition of the tone-increasing effect of sparteine	13
Dihydro-ergotoxine	Rat; virgin or nongravid	As described above (Ref. 2) for dihydroergotamine	1 (?)*	No appreciable effect		2
	Guinea pig; virgin		1 (?)*	No effect		
	Gravid			Gradual reduction in uterine tone and amplitude of contractions		

Table 3 (continuation)

Compound	Species/state	Experimental condition	Drug concentration in bath (μg/ml)	Characteristics of effect	Special observations/ remarks	Ref.
Dihydro-ergotoxine	Human; pregnant (caesarian section), near term, at term or during labor	As described above (Ref. 10) for dihydroergotamine	2–4 (threshold)	Enhancement of spontaneous uterine motility in 5 out of 30 uteri; in remainder no relaxation or inhibition of motility	See comment given above (Ref. 10) concerning dihydroergotamine	10
Dihydro-ergokryptine	Rabbit	Myometrial strip, 1 cm in length, preload 3–5 g; oxygenated Ringer solution	0.01–0.1	No oxytocic effect	At 0.1 μg/ml inhibition of oxytocic response to ergometrine	14, 15

* The original publication gives a 1000 times higher concentration; it is assumed that this is an error.

References: 1. WIQVIST (1959); 2. VENKATASUBBU and GOPALA KRISHNAMURTHY (1959); 3. RUDZIK and MILLER (1962); 4. ORTH and RITCHIE (1947); 5. CLEGG (1963); 6. ROTHLIN (1946); 7. DE BOER and VAN DONGEN (1948); 8. HÄRTFELDER et al. (1953); 9. PEREIRA MARTINEZ et al. (1954); 10. ROTHLIN and BERDE (1954); 11. GARRETT (1955); 12. SANDBERG et al. (1961); 13. GARG et al. (1973); 14. ROTHLIN and BRÜGGER (1945); 15. ROTHLIN (1946/47).

blocking activity. For this situation it may be assumed that endogenous catecholamines are prevented from stimulating uterine α-adrenoceptors, an action which is thought to contribute to maintaining physiologic uterine tone and motility, whilst they are still capable of stimulating uterine β-adrenoceptors, an action known to cause relaxation. The inhibitory effect of dihydrogenated alkaloids may then be the result of the unopposed β-sympathomimetic activity of catecholamines. This view is compatible with findings reported by ROTHLIN and BRÜGGER (1945), ROTHLIN (1946, 1946/47), and DE BOER and VAN DONGEN (1948), according to which the oxytocic effects of either ergotamine, ergotoxine, or ergometrine on the isolated rabbit uterus were inhibited by dihydroergotamine and other dihydrogenated peptide alkaloids. This effect can be explained by competition of the dihydrogenated and natural ergot alkaloids for the same receptors. Ergotamine and dihydroergotamine are both powerful α-adrenoceptor blocking agents and both have in addition intrinsic α-stimulant activity, but the latter effect, their "efficacy," is greater with ergotamine relative to which dihydroergotamine can be considered a partial agonist. The total effect of dihydroergotamine on the uterus would thus be expected to result from the interaction of several factors including a weak agonist effect on α-receptors and in higher concentrations complete α-block and a consequent unopposed action on β-adrenoceptors of endogenous catecholamines.

β) Human Uterus

Whereas the results obtained with dihydrogenated alkaloids on isolated uterine tissue from animals are rather uniform, indicating either no effect or inhibition of uterine activity, those reported from experiments on human uterine strips show considerable discrepancies.

ROTHLIN and BERDE (1954) investigated the actions of dihydroergotamine and dihydroergotoxine over a wide dose range in more than 400 strips obtained from uteri at caesarian section, and compared them with the effects of oxytocin and methylergometrine. With dihydroergotamine or dihydroergotoxine they found either no effect (neither stimulant nor inhibitory) or, as shown in Figure 8, a clear oxytocic action. The latter was seen with dihydroergotamine at threshold concentrations of 2–5 μg/ml in 6 out of 30 uteri, and with dihydroergotoxine at similar concentrations in 5 out of the same 30 uteri. A response to methylergometrine occurred in 12 out of these uteri. It may therefore be concluded that the dihydrogenated alkaloids do have an oxytocic action on the human uterus in vitro, but that this preparation is less sensitive to these drugs than to methylergometrine.

Contrarily, dihydroergotamine proved to act mainly in an inhibitory way in the studies reported by SANDBERG et al. (1961). The predominant response of strips from nonpregnant as well as from pregnant human uteri to drug concentrations of 2.5–20 μg/ml consisted in a reduced frequency of spontaneous contractions.

In trying to explain the divergent results, BERDE (1961) pointed to technical differences between the two investigations. In his experiments, the myometrial strips were from the lower uterine segment only, and all were obtained at caesarian section, whereas the Swedish authors worked with tissue from both the lower and upper segment, and two third of their specimens were from nonpregnant

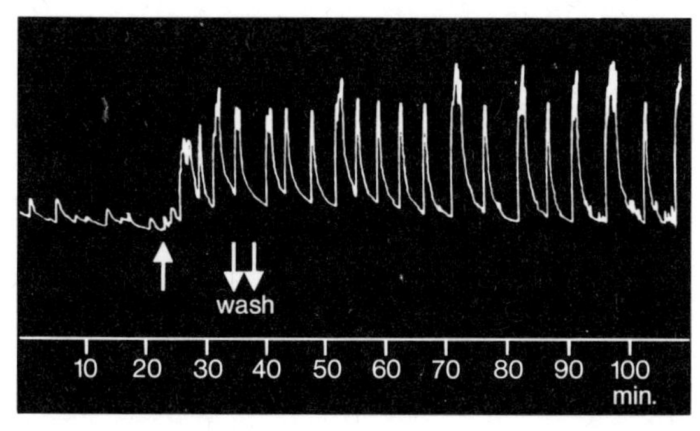

Fig. 8. Effect of dihydroergotoxine (at ↑ 2.5 μg/ml) on the human uterus in vitro. Isotonic recording from a strip obtained at caesarian section. (From ROTHLIN and BERDE, 1954)

uteri. Furthermore, the time during which the drug was left in contact with the tissue was much shorter in the experiments described by ROTHLIN and BERDE (1954).

Relaxation of human myometrial strips by dihydroergotamine at a low concentration (0.5 μg/ml) was also observed by GARG et al. (1973) when the drug was used alone. In combination with sparteine it reversed the increase in tone caused by this oxytocic drug and thereby prevented uterine spasm but enhanced at the same time the stimulant action of sparteine on the contractile rhythm. This finding may reflect a latent stimulant action of dihydroergotamine and suggests that dihydrogenated alkaloids are ambivalent in their influences on the uterus, a view which received further support from results published by PEREIRA MARTINEZ et al. (1954) and GARRETT (1955) who found dihydroergotamine to be either ineffective, inhibitory or excitatory, depending on the dose and/or the hormonal state of the uterus.

b) Studies in situ

The relevant data from studies in which the uterine actions of dihydrogenated peptide alkaloids have been investigated in animals (rat, rabbit, cat, dog) and in women are compiled in Table 4. Most of the reports deal with the effects of dihydroergotamine and dihydroergotoxine, the two drugs which are commercially available, whereas only sporadic information was found in the literature on other compounds of the same structural class, such as dihydroergocornine, dihydroergocristine and dihydroergokryptine (the three constituents of dihydroergotoxine) and the 6-nor-6-isopropyl derivatives of dihydroergotamine and dihydroergocristine.

α) Animal Experiments

The results obtained with dihydrogenated alkaloids in the *rabbit* in situ, which may be regarded as the classical preparation, are in general consistent with the in vitro findings, in that they did not reveal any oxytocic effect either in the nonpregnant or in the pregnant or puerperal state. Several observations even indicate relaxation of the myometrium, inhibition of spontaneous contractions and

Table 4. Uterine action of dihydrogenated peptide alkaloids in situ

Compound	Species/state	Experimental condition	Dose/route of administration	Characteristics of effect	Special observations/ remarks	Ref.
Dihydro-ergotamine	Rat; pregnant	Observations on course of pregnancy, on litters, and on nursing behavior	5 or 10 mg/kg i.v., daily injections during the entire gestation period	Normal course of pregnancy, normal litters, normal nursing behavior	Conclusion: no oxytocic effect	1, 2
Dihydro-ergotamine	Rat 150–300 g; diestrus and first half of pregnancy	Pentobarbitone anesthesia, laparotomy; isotonic or isometric recording from exteriorized segment, kept moist and warm (37.5–38.5° C) by dripping Tyrode solution	0.1 mg i.v. (0.3–0.7 mg/kg)	Enhancement of spontaneous contractions (increase in amplitude) and potentiation of response to oxytocin	Improvement in strength and regularity of uterine contractions interpreted as result of "sympathetic blocking activity"	3
	Estrus and late pregnancy			Very little change of spontaneous or oxytocin-induced contractions		
Dihydro-ergotamine	Rabbit; nonpregnant		Up to 10 times an effective oxytocic dose of ergotamine	No oxytocic effect; relaxation and inhibition of preexisting contractility	Results with dihydro-ergotamine apply also to other dihydrogenated alkaloids	4
Dihydro-ergotamine	Rabbit; nonpregnant	Urethane anesthesia; simultaneous recording of uterine and vaginal contractions and of arterial blood pressure	0.2 mg/kg i.v.	Immediate, complete and long-lasting inhibition of ergotamine-induced uterine and vaginal contractions	Uterine inhibition associated with sharp fall in blood pressure	5
Dihydro-ergotamine	Rabbit; late pregnancy, during labor or puerperal	Urethane anesthesia, laparotomy; isotonic recording from exteriorized uterine horn; in some experiments simultaneous recording of pressure within the other horn and/or vaginal motility (balloon)	0.01–0.4 mg/kg i.v.	No oxytocic effect; in more than half of the experiments spontaneous contractions were reduced or abolished, in some cases tone was decreased; oxytocic action of methylergometrine often weakened or completely suppressed by preceding dose of dihydrogenated alkaloid	Results are similar to those reported for the nonpregnant animal	6

Table 4 (continuation)

Compound	Species/state	Experimental condition	Dose/route of administration	Characteristics of effect	Special observations/ remarks	Ref.
Dihydro-ergotamine	Rabbit 2.7–3 kg; virgin, estrogen-treated or puerperal	Barbiturate anesthesia, laparotomy; isometric recording from segment of uterine horn	0.5 or 1 mg i.v. (0.17–0.37 mg/kg)	In 9 of 10 experiments in the virgin animal no oxytocic effect, in 2 of them some inhibition of spontaneous activity, and in only 1 a slight oxytocic effect was observed following 1 mg; uterine inhibition in one of several experiments in the puerperal animal	No influence on oxytocin-induced contractility, whether given before or after oxytocin	7
Dihydro-ergotamine	Cat; nonpregnant, pregnant or puerperal	Urethane-chloralose anesthesia, spinalization in some nonpregnant animals; otherwise similar to above (Ref. 6) for the rabbit	0.1–0.6 mg/kg i.v., in puerperal animals up to 1 mg/kg	Of 28 nonpregnant or pregnant animals 15 responded with pronounced and 5 with slight oxytocic effect, only 1 of 9 puerperal animals showed a (questionable) oxytocic effect; in no instance there was evidence for inhibition of spontaneous uterine activity	If an oxytocic effect occurred, it could not be repeated in the same experiment, even at 4 times the dose	6
Dihydro-ergotamine	Dog, 10–12 kg; nonpregnant	Ether or paraldehyde anesthesia; intrauterine and intravaginal pressure recording	0.8 mg i.v. (0.07–0.08 mg/kg)	Slight inhibition of uterine movements without affecting the vagina		8
	Pregnant		0.4 mg i.v. (0.03–0.04 mg/kg)	Marked relaxation of uterine musculature and inhibition of spontaneous contractions for 15 min		

Table 4 (continuation)

Compound	Species/state	Experimental condition	Dose/route of administration	Characteristics of effect	Special observations/ remarks	Ref.
Dihydro-ergotamine	Human; first stage of labor	External tocography according to Frey	0.25 or 0.5 mg i.m.	Fall of resting tone, increased amplitude of contractions	Reversal of increased tone caused by i.v. calcium	9
	Shortly after delivery of placenta			No effect on spontaneous or methylergometrine-induced activity		
Dihydro-ergotamine	Human; pregnant at term or in labor	External tocography using two-channel tocodynamometer	Continuous i.v. infusion at 6 µg/min for 2–4 h	Occasionally relaxation (including the lower uterine segment), but in most cases a clear stimulatory effect (increase in amplitude and rate of contractions) was observed	Unfavorable side effects in the mothers, high incidence of fetal distress	10
Dihydro-ergotamine	Human; during labor or at induction of labor	External tocography using three-channel strain-gauge tocodynamometer; in one case amniotic pressure recording (transcervically inserted open-tip catheter)	Continuous i.v. infusion at 1.0–0.5 mg per 30 min, or single i.v. injection of 0.25–1 mg	At low concentrations initial transitory decrease in uterine activity, followed by steady increase; at higher doses marked increase in contractility; rise of resting tone from 8 to 28 mm Hg and marked increase in contraction rate following 1 mg i.v.	No evidence for relaxation of the cervix; dosage for i.v. infusion should not exceed 0.1 mg/30 min	11
Dihydro-ergotamine	Human; day 6 or 7 postpartum	Intrauterine bag method	0.25 and 0.5 mg i.v.	Usually little effect on uterine contractions, but in some cases marked stimulation without increase in resting tone	Pretreatment with dihydroergotamine inhibits oxytocic effect of ergometrine and methylergometrine for several hours, but if these drugs are given first, their oxytocic actions are not affected	12

Table 4 (continuation)

Compound	Species/state	Experimental condition	Dose/route of administration	Characteristics of effect	Special observations/ remarks	Ref.
Dihydro-ergotamine	Human; sub partu	Amniotic pressure recording (transcervically inserted open-tip catheter)	0.25 mg i.m.	Slight increase in resting tone (by 2–3 mm Hg)		13
			0.1–0.25 mg i.v.	Marked increase in resting tone (by 10 mm Hg), in one case dangerous uterine hyperactivity		
Dihydro-ergotamine	Human; puerperal	External tocography (Dodek's apparatus modified) or intra-uterine balloon	0.25–1 mg i.m. or i.v.	Clear-cut, dose dependent increase in uterine activity in almost all cases; lower doses produced increase in frequency and amplitude, higher doses also raised resting tone	Speed of onset slower than with ergometrine	14
Dihydro-ergotamine	Human; pregnant at term or in labor	External tocography according to Jaquet	0.25 or 1 mg i.m.	In 6 of 10 cases marked increase in resting tone with frequent and small contractions; tetanic response in another case	The use of the drug in labor is considered to be dangerous	15
Dihydro-ergotamine	Human; late pregnancy and in labor	Amniotic pressure recording (transabdominally inserted open-tip catheter)	E.g. 0.3 mg i.v. by slow injection	Strong oxytocic response, characterized by rise in tone from 13 to 23 mm Hg, and an increase in frequency from 2.6 to 6.6 contractions per 10 min; loss of the well-coordinated pattern of contractions		16

Table 4 (continuation)

Compound	Species/state	Experimental condition	Dose/route of administration	Characteristics of effect	Special observations/ remarks	Ref.
Dihydro-ergotamine	Human; normal labor or uterine inertia	External tocography according to Jaquet or Lorand	0.25 mg i.m.	In most cases clear oxytocic effect (increase in amplitude and rate, but not in resting tone); most pronounced in patients with uterine inertia in which contractions also became more regular	In some cases severe fetal distress	17
Dihydro-ergotoxine	Rabbit; late pregnancy or during labor	As described above (Ref. 6) for dihydro-ergotamine	0.01–1 mg/kg i.v.	No oxytocic effect; in 4 of 8 experiments clear inhibition of spontaneous uterine activity; in one complete, in another one partial inhibition of oxytocic effect of a subsequent dose of methylergo-metrine	Results are similar to those reported for nonpregnant rabbits	6
Dihydro-ergotoxine	Cat; nonpregnant, pregnant or puerperal	As described above (Ref. 6) for dihydro-ergotamine	0.25–0.8 mg/kg i.v.	Of 14 nonpregnant or pregnant animals 6 responded with clear and 2 with questionable oxytocic effects, whereas in 2 puerperal animals no response occurred	In none of the experiments was there any evidence for uterine relaxation or inhibition of spontaneous activity; oxytocic responses could not be repeated in the same animal	6

Table 4 (continuation)

Compound	Species/state	Experimental condition	Dose/route of administration	Characteristics of effect	Special observations/ remarks	Ref.
Dihydro-ergotoxine	Cat, 1–1.5 kg; nonpregnant	Chloralose anesthesia; intrauterine and intra-vaginal pressure recording	0.12 mg i.v. (0.08–0.12 mg/kg)	Marked relaxation of uterine musculature, no effect on vagina		8
Dihydro-ergotoxine	Dog, 10–12 kg; nonpregnant	Ether or paraldehyde anesthesia; intra-uterine and intravaginal pressure recording	0.06 mg i.v. (0.005–0.006 mg/kg)	Variable results, in a few cases inhibition of uterine motility without effect on the vagina		8
	Pregnant		0.12 mg i.v. (0.01–0.012 mg/kg)	Marked relaxation and inhibition of sponta-neous contractions for 15 min		
Dihydro-ergotoxine	Human; first stage of labor	External tocography according to Crodel	0.15 or 0.3 mg i.m., 0.15 mg i.v.	Enhancement of uterine activity (rise in resting tone, increase in amplitude and rate) reaching in some cases the stage of uterine tetany	Effect mainly inter-preted as result of sympathetic blockade and consecutive un-opposed parasympathetic activity, but a "direct" oxytocic action was not excluded	18
Dihydro-ergotoxine	Human; primiparas during first stage of labor	External tocography according to Crodel	0.3 mg i.m. or i.v. by single administration, 0.075 mg i.m. by repeated administration	Clear oxytocic effect (increase in resting tone, amplitude and rate), enhancement of dilatation of the os (particularly if in an oedematous condition), shortening of labor	Repeated i.m. injections of small doses are the most suitable way of administration	19

Table 4 (continuation)

Compound	Species/state	Experimental condition	Dose/route of administration	Characteristics of effect	Special observations/ remarks	Ref.
Dihydro-ergotoxine	Human; induction of labor in a case of intra-uterine fetal death	Amniotic pressure recording (transabdominally inserted open-tip catheter)	i.v. infusion, 4.3 μg/min during 140 min (0.6 mg total dose)	Little influence on resting tone and amplitude of contractions, but marked and long-lasting increase in frequency (from 1.3 to 5 per 10 min) with a slow onset of action	No change in arterial blood pressure; with a live fetus the high frequency of contractions would be dangerous	20
Dihydro-ergotoxine	Human; early and late puerperium	External tocography (Dodek's apparatus modified) or intrauterine balloon	0.5–3 mg i.v.	Increase in uterine activity, in some cases associated with a rise in base line; $2\frac{1}{2}$ times less potent than dihydroergotamine; relatively slow onset of action (5–20 min with doses up to 1.5 mg, 1–8 min with higher doses); duration of action varying from 16 to >60 min	Effects not always predictable; in some cases an alarming response has followed a small dose of the drug, which therefore is thought to be contraindicated during labor	21
Dihydro-ergotoxine	Human; pregnant at term or in labor	External tocography according to Jaquet	0.3 mg i.m.	In 10 of 16 cases clear increase in rate of contractions and some rise in resting tone; in no instance any evidence for uterine relaxation or inhibition of contractions	Drug (in contrast to dihydroergotamine) considered to be safe for the enhancement of labor	15

Compound	Species/state	Experimental condition	Dose/route of administration	Characteristics of effect	Special observations/ remarks	Ref.
Dihydro-ergotoxine	Human; pregnant at term or in labor, preeclampsia in 19 of the 28 patients	External tocography according to Reynolds, or amniotic pressure recording	0.3 mg as single i.v. injection, or continuous i.v. infusion at a rate of 3.3 or 10 μg/min	Significant, dose-related increase in frequency of contractions with little or no change in intensity; amniotic pressure recording revealed substantial rise in base line pressure	No evidence for a therapeutic effect in preeclampsia; mild to moderate side effects (mainly nausea) in 20% of patients	22
Dihydro-ergotoxine	Human; first stage of labor	External tocography according to Frey	0.75–1 mg p.o. (drops or sublingual tablet)	Mild oxytocic effect (increase in rate and amplitude, contractions more regular) associated with marked relaxation of cervix 15–20 min after the drug; shortening of labor	Beneficial (antihypertensive) effect in preeclampsia	23
Dihydro-ergotoxine	Human; normal labor or uterine inertia	External tocography according to Jaquet or Lorand	0.15 mg i.m.	Slight oxytocic effect (increase in amplitude and rate of contractions without change in resting tone); in patients with uterine inertia the contractions became more regular	Drug (in contrast to dihydroergotamine) is said to be safe in management of uterine inertia in the first stage of labor	17
Dihydro-ergocornine (in the original paper erroneously designated dihydroergotoxine)	Human; early and late puerperium	External tocography (Dodek's apparatus modified) or intrauterine balloon	0.25–1 mg i.v. 1 mg i.m.	Increase in uterine activity, in 9 of 16 cases associated with a rise in base line; same potency as dihydroergotamine; slow onset of action (2–14 min i.v.; 15–72 min i.m.), long duration (30–> 70 min)	See remarks made above (Ref. 21) for dihydro-ergotoxine	21

Table 4 (continuation)

Compound	Species/state	Experimental condition	Dose/route of administration	Characteristics of effect	Special observations/ remarks	Ref.
Dihydro-ergocristine	Rabbit; nonpregnant	Urethane anesthesia; simultaneous recording of uterine and vaginal contractions and arterial blood pressure	0.15 mg/kg i.v.	Inhibition of uterine and vaginal motility; if given simultaneously with 0.45 mg/kg of ergometrine, oxytocic effect of the latter markedly reduced		24
Dihydro-ergocristine	Human; first stage of labor, uterine inertia	External tocography using three-channel strain-gauge tocodynamometer	1 mg i.m.	Spontaneous contractions, simultaneously recorded from the upper, middle and lower uterine segment, not inhibited, but showed a slight increase in frequency	The drug was used here as an "adrenolytic substance"	25
Dihydro-ergocristine	Human; early and late puerperium	External tocography (Dodek's apparatus modified) or intrauterine balloon	1–3 mg i.v.	Increase in uterine activity, in 3 of 6 cases associated with a rise in base line; $2\frac{1}{2}$ times less potent than dihydroergotamine; slow onset of action (4–19 min), long duration (> 40–> 60 min)		21
Dihydro-ergokryptine				Increase in uterine activity, in 2 of 6 experiments associated with a rise in base line; $2\frac{1}{2}$ times less potent than dihydroergotamine; slow onset of action (3–32 min), long duration (> 33–> 53 min)		

Table 4 (continuation)

Compound	Species/state	Experimental condition	Dose/route of administration	Characteristics of effect	Special observations/ remarks	Ref.
6-Nor-6-isopropyl dihydro-ergotamine	Rabbit; spontaneous estrus	Urethane anesthesia, laparotomy; isometric recording from 4 cm uterine segment fixed in plexiglass chamber; tension adjusted in order to give maximal responses to 0.25 μg/kg adrenaline i.v.	0.2–0.6 mg/kg i.v.	Dose-related reproducible uterotonic effect; 3 times less potent than methylergometrine, 2 times less potent than ergotamine	Concomitant dose-related increase in arterial blood pressure; both effects (uterus and blood pressure) were abolished by phentolamine or phenoxybenzamine	26
6-Nor-6-isopropyl dihydro-ergocristine			0.06–1 mg/kg i.v.	Qualitatively similar to 6-nor-6-isopropyl-dihydroergotamine, but about twice as potent		

References: 1. ORTH (1946); 2. ORTH and RITCHIE (1947); 3. DEIS and PICKFORD (1964); 4. ROTHLIN (1944); 5. ROTHLIN (1946); 6. BERDE and ROTHLIN (1953); 7. FUCHS and FUCHS (1960); 8. VENKATASUBBU and GOPALA KRISHNAMURTHY (1959); 9. SAUTER (1948); 10. ALTMAN et al. (1952); 11. BRUNS et al. (1953); 12. GILL (1953); 13. BÖSCH (1954); 14. EMBREY and GARRETT (1955); 15. KREMER and NARIK (1955); 16. ALVAREZ (1961); 17. SHAABAN and YOUSSEF (1959); 18. FEGERL and NARIK (1951); 19. WILHELM (1951); 20. ALVAREZ et al. (1954/55); 21. GARRETT and EMBREY (1955); 22. SNOW et al. (1955); 23. JELINEK (1957); 24. ROTHLIN (1946/47); 25. REYNOLDS et al. (1954); 26. HOOL-ZULAUF and STÜRMER (1976).

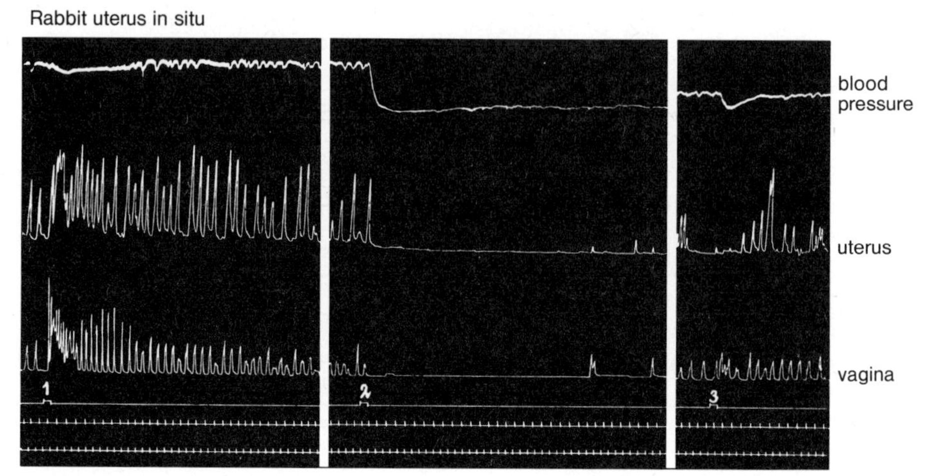

Fig. 9. Inhibition of ergotamine-induced uterine and vaginal contractions by dihydroergotamine in the anesthetized rabbit. At 1 and 3 ergotamine 0.15 mg/kg i.v.; at 2 dihydroergotamine 0.2 mg/kg i.v. Scale at bottom: time in minutes. (From ROTHLIN, 1946)

antagonism against the oxytocic action of ergotamine, ergometrine or methylergometrine. An example of such an experiment is illustrated in Figure 9.

Two recently described exceptions, however, deserve special attention: 6-nor-6-isopropyl-dihydroergotamine and the corresponding derivative of dihydroergocristine proved to be potent oxytocics in the estrous rabbit (HOOL-ZULAUF and STÜRMER, 1976, 1977). In general pharmacologic characterization, which includes evaluation of effects on blood vessels, both compounds were found to possess high α-adrenoceptor stimulating activity.

Since their uterotonic effect in the rabbit can be abolished by α-adrenoceptor blockade (phentolamine or phenoxybenzamine) it may be assumed that they act as partial agonists in which—in contrast to the other dihydrogenated alkaloids—the agonistic properties predominate over the antagonistic action.

In the experiments performed by VENKATASUBBU and GOPALA KRISHNAMURTHY (1959) in *dogs*—similarly to the rabbit—, dihydroergotamine and dihydroergotoxine were slightly inhibitory in nonpregnant animals and caused a marked relaxation and inhibition of spontaneous contractions in pregnant animals. The same paper also describes marked uterine relaxation following dihydroergotoxine in the nonpregnant *cat*. This, however, is in distinct contrast to the result obtained by BERDE and ROTHLIN (1953). In a large series of experiments with dihydroergotamine and dihydroergotoxine, these authors were unable to demonstrate any inhibitory action, but found that both drugs exerted a clear oxytocic effect in the majority of nonpregnant and pregnant cats, whereas puerperal animals were remarkably insensitive. When in a given animal an oxytocic effect was achieved by either drug, it could not be repeated by giving similar or up to 4 times higher doses. This observation of a very pronounced *tachyphylaxis* is not only of considerable methodologic significance; it should also be seen in the light of modern receptor theory. If the drugs exert their oxytocic effects as partial agonists by stimulation of specific receptors in the uterus, the refractoriness of this organ to subsequent doses may be due to receptor blockade brought about by the same drug.

The only study in which the action of a dihydrogenated alkaloid (dihydroergotamine) on uterine motility was directly recorded in the *rat* in situ (DEIS and PICKFORD, 1964) revealed an enhancement of spontaneous contractions with an increase in amplitude and an improvement in regularity, and also indicated some potentiation of the response to oxytocin. These effects occurred quite regularly in diestrus and during the first half of pregnancy. Similar results were obtained with ganglion blocking agents and an adrenergic neurone blocking agent (bretylium), suggesting that in the diestrous and early pregnant rat sympathetic block leads to more regular uterine activity. In rats in estrus or late pregnancy dihydroergotamine only occasionally led to improvement in strength or regularity of uterine contractions. The authors suggested that estrogens and progesterone may play a special part in regulating the relation between sympathetic nerves and the uterine muscle, producing some sort of a sympathetic block of their own, which might explain why in estrus and late pregnancy the adrenergic blocking effects of dihydroergotamine are obviated or reduced. No evidence for an oxytocic effect of dihydroergotamine in pregnant rats was found by ORTH (1946) and ORTH and RITCHIE (1947). Their conclusion, however, was not derived from direct measurement of uterine motility, but was based on the observation that daily treatment with high doses of the drug over the entire period of pregnancy had no influence on the course of pregnancy and on the litters.

β) Human Uterus

Some 20–30 years ago, great attention was paid by many obstetricians to the problem of prolonged labor due to dysrhythmic, incoordinate uterine contractions and cervical spasm. "Hyperactivity of the sympathetic nervous system" was thought to be a main causative factor for this condition. From the fundamental work of ROTHLIN (1944, 1946, 1946/47) it was known at that time that dihydroergotamine and other dihydrogenated alkaloids are strong inhibitors of various pharmacodynamic effects of adrenaline, including its stimulatory action on the uterus, and that in the rabbit these compounds are not only devoid of an oxytocic effect, but may even cause uterine relaxation. It was therefore an obvious step to investigate their therapeutic potential in obstetrics.

The first report on such a study was presented by SAUTER (1948). Combining clinical observations with results obtained by external tocography, he found that dihydroergotamine safely reduced resting tone, increased the amplitude of contractions and caused relaxation of the cervix during labor. These beneficial effects were attributed to the "sympathicolytic" action of the drug which, according to this investigator (1949a) involved not only the musculature, but also the vessels of the uterus, the latter resulting in vasodilatation. In tocographic experiments performed on the postpartum uterus shortly after delivery of the placenta, dihydroergotamine did not lower the high resting tone achieved by an intravenous injection of methylergometrine. This was in contrast to papaverine which, under the same conditions, acting as a true spasmolytic, effectively reduced the elevated tone. It was concluded that the relaxant effect of dihydroergotamine on the uterus

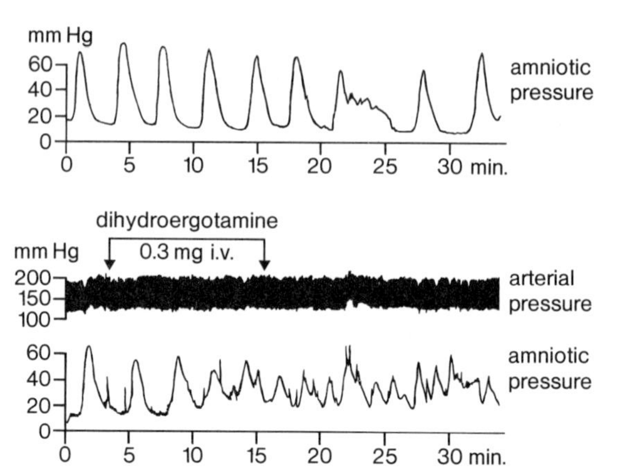

Fig. 10. Effects of dihydroergotamine on intraamniotically recorded uterine contractions and arterial blood pressure in a preeclamptic patient at 36 weeks of pregnancy. Labor was induced with an intracervical bougie. Dihydroergotamine caused an abnormal rise in uterine tone and in the frequency of the contractions which became incoordinated. The elevated blood pressure was not changed. (From ALVAREZ, 1961)

observed during the first stage of labor was not due to a papaverine-like spasmolytic action, but was indeed the consequence of its sympathicolytic (in modern terminology "α-adrenoceptor blocking") properties.

In the following years the favorable actions of dihydroergotamine in the treatment of cervical spasm and prolonged labor, claimed by SAUTER, were in general confirmed by various authors (REIST, 1949; BASKIN and CREALOCK, 1950; GILL and FARRAR, 1951; GILL, 1953), based on clinical observations. However, when an attempt was made to characterize the effects on uterine activity by external tocography or continuous measurement of intrauterine pressure, results were different from those reported by SAUTER. A great variety of experimental conditions were studied (e.g., induction of labor, active labor at various stages of cervical dilatation, uterine inertia, early and late puerperium; administration of the drug at various doses by intramuscular or intravenous injections or by continuous intravenous infusion, and, in one study with dihydroergotoxine, also by the oral route). Dihydroergotamine, as well as dihydroergotoxine and its constituents, were usually found to increase not only the amplitude, but also the frequency of contractions, and in several studies also to raise resting tone. For details and references the reader is referred to Table 4.

An example of an experiment in which a strong and purely oxytocic effect of dihydroergotamine was demonstrated by intra-amniotic pressure recording, an accurate and objective method, is shown in Figure 10. The author of this illustration (ALVAREZ, 1961) pointed out that the hypertonicity and the high frequency of contractions might endanger the fetus, and recommended that dihydroergotamine should not be employed in pregnant women. This view had already been expressed and was extended to dihydroergotoxine and its constituents by EMBREY and GARRETT (1955) (see also GARRETT and EMBREY, 1955; GARRETT, 1960), whereas other investigators were of the opinion that the drugs might have a place in the management of labor, provided that they are used with caution and at low doses (FEGERL and NARIK, 1951; WILHELM, 1951; ALTMAN et al., 1952; BRUNS et al., 1953; GILL, 1953; PEREIRA MARTINEZ et al., 1954). KREMER and NARIK (1955) considered dihydroergotamine even at low doses to be very dangerous, but recommended the administration of dihydroergotoxine at small doses in combination with oxytocin. Safety and efficiency of dihydroergotoxine in reducing cervical tone and in shortening labor was also claimed by JELINEK (1957), who gave the drug orally. However, JEFFCOATE and WILSON (1955) had made clear that in their own tocographic investigations the only demonstrable effect of dihydroergotoxine was an oxytocic one. Although they felt that the oxytocic action was not so strong or dangerous as that of dihydroergotamine, they did not recommend the use of dihydroergotoxine in parturient women.

These somewhat controversial discussions concerning the use of dihydrogenated peptide alkaloids in the management of labor took place between 1948 and about 1960. Since then the interest of obstetricians in these compounds has greatly declined. Although dihydroergotamine and dihydroergotoxine are commercially available and are widely used for other therapeutic purposes, they do not play a significant role in obstetric practice today.

3. Lysergic Acid-Amides

The term "lysergic acid-amides" is used for ergot compounds which, in contrast to the peptide alkaloids and their dihydrogenated derivatives, have a simple amine group linked to the lysergic acid moiety instead of a complex tripeptide moiety. They are of considerably lower molecular weight than the peptide alkaloids. Two members of the group of lysergic acid-amides are important drugs in obstetrics: *ergometrine* as the naturally occurring alkaloid and *methylergometrine*, its semisynthetic derivative.

The fascinating history of the discovery of the "water soluble uterotonic principle of ergot" by MOIR (1932b) and all further chemical, pharmacologic and clinical developments in this field during the few years following MOIR's publication (e.g., SWANSON and HARGREAVES, 1934; ADAIR et al., 1935; BROWN and DALE, 1935; DAVIS et al., 1935a, 1935b; DUDLEY and MOIR, 1935; KOFF, 1935; ROTHLIN, 1935a, 1935b; STOLL and BURCKHARDT, 1935; THOMPSON, 1935; TUCK, 1935) are comprehensively reviewed by BARGER (1938), NELSON and CALVERY (1938) and SMITH (1938). At that time, the question of priority of discovery, the problem of chemical identity of the compounds described almost simultaneously by four working groups in Europe and America, and the different naming of the compounds, caused much discussion and confusion. DALE (1935) was probably the first to suggest that the four names, ergobasine, ergometrine, ergostetrine and ergotocine were different terms for the same substance. An exchange of samples among the four laboratories resulted then in a mutual publication by KHARASCH, KING (in place of DUDLEY et al., then deceased), STOLL and THOMPSON (1936) indicating their agreement that the alkaloids obtained in the four laboratories were the same substance and that the four names were synonymous. The British Pharmacopoeia has adopted the term ergometrine—and only this name is used in this chapter—, whereas a fifth name, ergonovine, became the official term in the United States' Pharmacopoeia.

a) Studies on the Isolated Uterus

The actions of ergometrine and methylergometrine have been studied quite extensively in uterine horns or strips from the rat, guinea pig, rabbit, cat, dog, and human. Ergometrine has also been tested in the hamster, and for methylergometrine additional information is available from in vitro studies in the uterus of the pig and the sheep. For other members of the lysergic acid-amide group (ergometrinine, LSD, 2-bromo-LSD and 2,13-dibromodihydrolysergic acid glycinamide) information is extremely scarce and concerns usually only one species. The data derived from the literature are summarized in Table 5.

From results obtained with ergometrine and methylergometrine in the same study and by comparing the characteristics of their actions in different studies, one can conclude that no appreciable differences exist in vitro between the two drugs. It is therefore justified to discuss their properties together. Another point should be made before going into some details: The therapeutically important advantages of ergometrine and methylergometrine over uterotonic peptide alkaloids such as ergotamine and ergotoxine consist in their more rapid onset of action (particularly by the oral route) and in the higher specificity of their oxytocic action in relation to the vascular effects. Obviously, these features can only be demonstrated in situ, and will be discussed later.

From the purely pharmacologic point of view, there are, however, also in vitro a few distinct differences between the uterine actions of lysergic acid-amides and those of peptide alkaloids:

Compared with ergotamine and ergotoxine, the oxytocic effects of ergometrine and methylergometrine are more easily abolished (or at least greatly attenuated) by rinsing out the bath. This can be seen in Figures 11 and 12 which should be compared with Figure 4.

Tachyphylaxis is in general less marked with the lysergic acid-amides than with the peptide alkaloids. Repeated administration of the drugs in the same preparation has therefore been used for assaying purposes. In the case of the isolated rat uterus, there was even evidence for an increase in sensitivity with the first few applications of ergometrine (PENNEFATHER, 1961). The human uterus, however, was found in most instances to be unresponsive to repeated doses of methylergometrine (ROTHLIN and BERDE, 1954).

On comparing the effects of ergometrine and ergotoxine on the uterine horns from the same virgin guinea pig, BROWN and DALE (1935) observed a striking similarity between the drugs, but they noted that ergometrine acted somewhat more rapidly than ergotoxine. Although both drugs provided a strong contraction immediately after administration to the bath, maximal tone was reached with ergometrine within about half the time required for ergotoxine. This may indicate an easier access of the compound with lower molecular weight to the specific receptors.

In contrast to ergotamine and ergotoxine, ergometrine and methylergometrine possess very little inhibitory activity against the uterine motor action of adrenaline, as shown in Figure 12.

In other respects the characteristics of the uterine actions in vitro of ergometrine and methylergometrine resemble very much those previously described for the

Table 5. Oxytocic action of lysergic acid-amides in vitro

Compound	Species/state	Experimental condition	Drug concentration in bath (μg/ml)	Characteristics of effect	Special observations/ remarks	Ref.
Ergometrine	Rat		Not mentioned	Inhibition		1
Ergometrine	Rat	Isotonic recording; Locke solution, 37.5° C, oxygenated	Not mentioned	Preparation unresponsive to ergometrine (and methylergometrine) even at high concentrations; evidence for relaxation (less than after adrenaline)		2
Ergometrine	Rat		0.05	Oxytocic effect (increase in resting tone and rate), inhibited by a preceding dose of dihydroergotamine (0.34 μg/ml)		3
Ergometrine	Rat; virgin or nongravid	Uterine segment, 25 mm in length; oxygenated Ringer solution	1 (?)*	Slight increase in frequency of contractions, no rise of resting tone		4
Ergometrine	Rat; induced estrus	Isotonic recording from a horn suspended in Gaddum solution, 29° C, oxygenated	0.001 or 0.002	Immediate contraction, prompt relaxation upon washing at the time of the contraction peak	Preparations relatively refractory to the first few applications of the drug; later the height of contraction is dose dependent and can be used for assay purposes (4 × 4 latin square, doses given at 3–4 min intervals)	5
Ergometrine	Rat; induced estrus	Semiisotonic recording (1 g preload) according to Holton	0.01–0.04 in the presence of oxytocin	Variable oxytocic response superimposed on effect elicited by oxytocin	Isolated rat uterus not suitable for: – assaying ergometrine, – assaying oxytocin in the presence of ergometrine	6

Table 5 (continuation)

Compound	Species/state	Experimental condition	Drug concentration in bath (μg/ml)	Characteristics of effect	Special observations/remarks	Ref.
Ergometrine	Rat; spontaneous or induced estrus	Semiisotonic recording from horn suspended in a solution with or without magnesium	0.002–0.04 in the presence of oxytocin	Oxytocic effect often weak and very variable, poor dose response relationship, tachyphylaxis	Presence of magnesium chloride diminishes oxytocic response to ergometrine; at 2 m*M* of $MgCl_2$ preparation suitable for assaying oxytocin in the presence of ergometrine	7, 8
Ergometrine	Hamster; nonpregnant	Horn, suspended in warm Locke solution	0.013	Pronounced increase of tone, followed by relaxation and greatly augmented rhythm		9
Ergometrine	Guinea pig; virgin	Horn, suspended in warm Locke solution	0.66 (0.001 with particularly sensitive preparations)	Increase in tone, followed by superimposed rhythmic contractions of small amplitude; qualitative and quantitative similarity to ergotoxine	Immediate onset of action with both ergometrine and ergotoxine, but less time needed with ergometrine to reach maximal tone	9
Ergometrine	Guinea pig; virgin		0.05	Tetanic contraction, recovery on washing	Preparation about 10 times more sensitive than isolated rabbit uterus, but less suitable for assaying purposes because of great variations	10
Ergometrine	Guinea pig; immature, virgin		Not mentioned	Strong contractions	Preparation much more sensitive to ergometrine than rabbit uterus	11
Ergometrine	Guinea pig	Horn, suspended in Van Dyke-Hastings solution, with or without additional $MgCl_2$	1	Reproducible contractions	Amplitude of contraction reduced by increasing $MgCl_2$ content of the bath	12

Table 5 (continuation)

Compound	Species/state	Experimental condition	Drug concentration in bath (μg/ml)	Characteristics of effect	Special observations/remarks	Ref.
Ergometrine	Guinea pig; virgin and puerperal	Isotonic recording; Locke solution, 37.5° C, oxygenated	7	Immediate very strong long-lasting increase in tone; at lower concentrations tetanic effect less pronounced and response mainly increased rhythm and amplitude; qualitatively and quantitatively similar to methylergometrine	Uteri either sensitive to both ergometrine and methylergometrine, or neither	2
Ergometrine	Guinea pig; virgin	Horn, suspended in Van Dyke-Hastings solution, 37.5° C, O_2/CO_2	1	Small, reproducible contraction, greatly potentiated by a nonoxytocic dose (2 μg/ml) of ergotoxine	Degree of potentiation by ergotoxine (often >100%) correlated neither with the ratio of ergotoxine to ergometrine nor with the height of initial ergometrine contraction	13
Ergometrine	Guinea pig; virgin or gravid	Uterine segment, 25 mm long; oxygenated Ringer solution	1 (?)*	Virgin: marked rise in tone, lasting >10 min Gravid: long-lasting rise in tone with increased rhythmic activity	Similar effects with methylergometrine	4
Ergometrine	Rabbit; multiparous	Strip, suspended in oxygenated warm Locke solution	1.3	Pronounced rhythmic activity without increased tone	After washing out ergometrine, uterotonic response to adrenaline (0.33 μg/ml) enhanced	9
Ergometrine	Rabbit		0.5	Long-lasting rhythmic activity with rise in resting tone	For assaying purposes the height of contractions was taken as the index of activity	10

Table 5 (continuation)

Compound	Species/state	Experimental condition	Drug concentration in bath (μg/ml)	Characteristics of effect	Special observations/ remarks	Ref.
Ergometrine	Rabbit		Not mentioned	Oxytocic effect, twice as potent as ergotamine		1, 14
Ergometrine	Rabbit	Strips, used at intervals up to 3rd day after removal	0.33–20	Strong rhythmic contractions with increased resting tone; in the most sensitive strips threshold concentration was 0.33 μg/ml, in others 2 μg/ml was necessary to produce definite stimulation; effects could be washed out and were inhibited by ergotoxine	Uteri used immediately after removal from the animal were the most sensitive; the isolated rabbit uterus was found to be suitable for assaying different lots of ergometrine, since repeated doses produced satisfactorily constant and dose-related responses	11
Ergometrine	Rabbit	Myometrial strip, Magnus-Kehrer preparation; oxygenated solution according to Fleisch	0.01–0.1	Oxytocic effect absent or minimal; ergometrine weaker than ergotamine	Potentiation of acetylcholine-induced contraction as with ergotamine, but less regular and less persistent	15
Ergometrine	Rabbit; spontaneous or induced estrus	Strip, 20 mm long; Van Dyke-Hastings solution, 37.5° C, O_2/CO_2	0.16–0.2	Contraction after a latent period of 2–5 min, can be washed out	Large doses of ergometrine stimulate contraction more promptly than small doses; latent period used for assaying purposes, more precise than other parameters	16

Table 5 (continuation)

Compound	Species/state	Experimental condition	Drug concentration in bath (μg/ml)	Characteristics of effect	Special observations/ remarks	Ref.
Ergometrine	Rabbit; nonpregnant	Isotonic recording; Locke solution, 37.5° C, oxygenated	0.32–6.7	At low concentration some increase in frequency and amplitude of contractions, at higher concentrations sustained increase in tone with diminished amplitude	When drug effectiveness determined by promptness, height, duration and rate of contraction, no differences between ergometrine and methylergometrine	2
Ergometrine	Rabbit; induced estrus	Strip, 20 mm long; Van Dyke-Hastings solution, 37° C, O_2/CO_2	0.25–1	Contraction (reversible upon washing) occurring after a latent period of 1–3 min	Same approach as above (Ref. 16)	17
Ergometrine	Rabbit; virgin	Strip, isotonic recording, preload 0.1–0.3 g; Van Dyke-Hastings solution, 37.5° C, O_2/CO_2	4–200	Strong contraction e.g., at 20 μg/ml with full recovery after washing; complete inhibition by preceding nonoxytocic dose (2 μg/ml) of ergotoxine	Ergotoxine, added at height of contraction, promptly relaxed the muscle	13
Ergometrine	Cat; puerperal	Longitudinal strip, suspended in warm Locke solution	0.013	Immediate rhythmic activity (in previously quiescent organ) without increase of resting tone, rising to a maximum within about 10 min, continuing with great regularity for several hours	In the cat, as in the guinea pig, the puerperal uterus gives the most striking demonstrations of the action of ergometrine	9
Ergometrine	Cat		Not mentioned	Oxytocic effect questionable		1
Ergometrine	Dog; virgin	Isotonic recording; Locke solution, 37.5° C, oxygenated	Not mentioned	No effect		2

Table 5 (continuation)

Compound	Species/state	Experimental condition	Drug concentration in bath (μg/ml)	Characteristics of effect	Special observations/ remarks	Ref.
Ergometrine	Human; nonpregnant; at various phases of cycle (hysterectomy); pregnant (hysterectomy in early pregnancy or caesarian section at term and during labor)	Strips, isotonic recording; Locke-Ringer solution, 37.5° C, oxygenated	0.4–2	Nonpregnant: 6 of 29 strips from proliferative phase, but none of 18 strips from secretory phase responded with increased activity Pregnant: no response in 6 strips from early pregnancy, but 3 of 9 strips from uteri in labor and 11 of 23 strips from uteri at term (but not in labor) showed an oxytocic response	Pattern of response mainly tonic and similar to that observed with adrenaline, oxytocin or vasopressin	18
Ergometrin*ine*	Rabbit; induced estrus	As above (Ref. 17) for ergometrine	Not mentioned	3.9 (3.5 to 4.5)% of oxytocic activity of ergometrine	Same approach as above (Ref. 16)	17
Metabolites of ergometrine	Guinea pig		Not mentioned	Mixture of 2 metabolites (extracted from bile collected from rats after intravenous ergometrine) contracted the uterus similarly to ergometrine		19
Methylergometrine	Rat	Similar to the experiments described above (Ref. 2) for ergometrine in the rat uterus				2
Methylergometrine	Rat	Influence on electrically-evoked contraction; uterine horn in toto, isotonic or isometric recording, Tyrode solution, O_2/CO_2	0.3	Long-lasting potentiation of electrically induced contraction by 30%–50% without change of resting tone, reduction of electrical threshold; similarity to ergotamine		20

Table 5 (continuation)

Compound	Species/state	Experimental condition	Drug concentration in bath (μg/ml)	Characteristics of effect	Special observations/ remarks	Ref.
Methylergometrine	Rat	Uterine horn, isotonic recording; Tyrode solution, 37° C, oxygenated	0.1–1	Oxytocic effect, large amplitude of contractions (similar to sparteine)	Some of the preparations, for unknown reasons, very insensitive	21
Methylergometrine	Rat; virgin or nongravid	Similar to the experiments described above (Ref. 4) for ergometrine in the rat uterus				4
Methylergometrine	Guinea pig; virgin and puerperal	Similar to the experiments described above (Ref. 2) for ergometrine in the guinea pig uterus				2
Methylergometrine	Guinea pig; nonpregnant (various states) and pregnant	Uterine horn, isotonic recording; Tyrode solution, O_2/CO_2	0.02–1	Oxytocic response very variable, almost absent in preestrus preparations, highest in the pregnant uterus		21
Methylergometrine	Guinea pig; virgin or gravid	Similar to the experiments described above (Ref. 4) for ergometrine in the guinea pig uterus				4
Methylergometrine	Rabbit; nonpregnant	Similar to the experiments described above (Ref. 2) for ergometrine in the nonpregnant rabbit uterus				2
	pregnant		0.24	Long-lasting (>2 h) increase in resting tone of spontaneously contracting uterus		
Methylergometrine	Rabbit; ovariectomized, estrogen-treated	Similar to the experiments described above (Ref. 20) for methylergometrine in the rat uterus				20
Methylergometrine	Rabbit		100	Progressive contracture, superimposed with rhythmic contractions		21

Table 5 (continuation)

Compound	Species/state	Experimental condition	Drug concentration in bath (μg/ml)	Characteristics of effect	Special observations/ remarks	Ref.
Methylergometrine	Rabbit	Vaginal strip	10	Rhythmic contractions with slow increase in resting tone and amplitude	Effect completely inhibited by subsequent dose of α-adrenoceptor blocking agent (dihydroergotamine, phentolamine)	22, 23
Methylergometrine	Dog; virgin	Similar to the experiments described above (Ref. 2) for ergometrine in the dog uterus				2
Methylergometrine	Pig Sheep	Longitudinal strips from outer muscle layer	0.1–1	Strong, mainly tonic response	Inhibition of oxytoxic effect by dihydroergotamine and other α-adrenoceptor blocking agents	23
Methylergometrine	Human; pregnant (caesarian section), near term, at term or during labor	Strips, 8–20 × 2–5 × 1–2 mm, isotonic recording, preload 0.5 g; oxygenated Tyrode solution, 37.5° C	1–5 (threshold)	In 12 out of 30 uteri enhancement of spontaneous uterine motility (increase in amplitude, rate or resting tone), or induction of rhythmic contractions in quiescent strips	Effects can usually not be repeated in the same organ; qualitatively similar to those observed with dihydrogenated amino acid alkaloids or oxytocin	24
Methylergometrine	Human; myomatous uterus (hysterectomy)	Strips, 20 × 2 × 2 mm, cut from uterine fibroids; modified Tyrode solution, O_2/CO_2	2.5	Enhancement of spontaneous motility	Musculature of uterine myomata behaves similarly as normal myometrium	25
Methylergometrine	Human; pregnant (caesarian section)	Strips, 20 × 2 × 2 mm, cut from various parts of the uterus, isotonic recording; modified Tyrode solution, 37.5° C, O_2/CO_2	0.25–1	Rise in resting tone and increased frequency and amplitude of contraction; evidence for higher responsiveness of lower uterine segment compared with corpus	Effects could be washed out	26, 27

Table 5 (continuation)

Compound	Species/state	Experimental condition	Drug concentration in bath (μg/ml)	Characteristics of effect	Special observations/ remarks	Ref.
LSD (*d*-lysergic acid diethylamide)	Rabbit		Not mentioned	Contracting effect, 1.5 times weaker than ergometrine		28
2-bromo-LSD	Rat; induced estrus	Horn, isotonic recording, load 2 g, Locke-Ringer solution, 37° C	0.1–0.5	Increase in frequency of contractions		29
2,13-dibromo-dihydro-lysergic acid glycinamide	Rabbit; estrus		Not mentioned	Strong oxytocic effect, several times more potent than methylergometrine		30
	Human; pregnant (caesarian section) near term or at term		100	Complete inhibition of spontaneous contractions		

* The original publication gives a 1000 times higher concentration; it is assumed that this is an error.

References: 1. ROTHLIN (1935b); 2. KIRCHHOF et al. (1944); 3. DE BOER and VAN DONGEN (1948); 4. VENKATASUBBU and GOPALA KRISHNAMURTHY (1959); 5. PENNEFATHER (1961); 6. BERDE and STÜRMER (1962); 7. SUND (1963a); 8. SUND (1963b); 9. BROWN and DALE (1935); 10. DAVIS et al. (1935b); 11. THOMPSON (1935); 12. FRASER (1939); 13. MILLER and DE BEER (1952); 14. ROTHLIN (1935a); 15. BRÜGGER (1938); 16. VOS (1943); 17. FOSTER and STEWART (1948); 18. ADAIR and HAUGEN (1939); 19. SLAYTOR et al. (1959); 20. HÄRTFELDER et al. (1953); 21. MAYER et al. (1955); 22. WELLHÖNER (1959a); 23. WELLHÖNER (1959b); 24. ROTHLIN and BERDE (1954); 25. INGELMAN-SUNDBERG et al. (1957); 26. SANDBERG et al. (1959); 27. SANDBERG et al. (1961); 28. ROTHLIN (1957); 29. TOTHILL (1967); 30. BERDE and SAAMELI (1966).

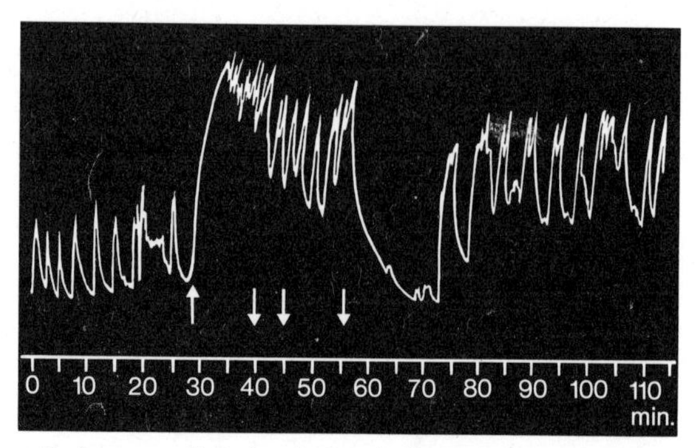

Fig. 11. Effect of methylergometrine (at ↑ 4 μg/ml) on human myometrium in vitro. Strip obtained at caesarian section in a 43 years old preeclamptic primipara at term; isotonic recording. Washing of the bath at ↓ reduces the oxytocic response. (From ROTHLIN and BERDE, 1954)

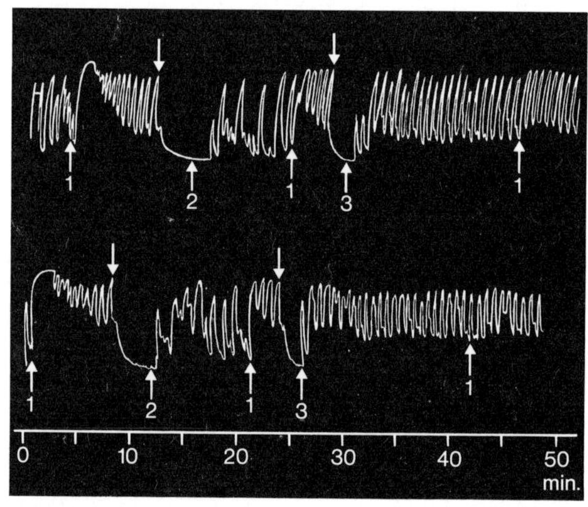

Fig. 12. Actions of ergometrine on isolated strips from rabbit uterus. Oxytocic effect and—only at the high concentration—inhibition of the response to adrenaline. 1. adrenaline 1 μg/ml; 2. ergometrine 8 μg/ml; 3. ergometrine 20 μg/ml; ↓ washing. (From THOMPSON, 1935; by permission of J. Amer. pharm. Ass.)

peptide alkaloids. This applies not only to the similarity in potency (in terms of threshold or effective concentrations in the bath), but also to the fact that the pattern of response (characterized by changes in resting tone, amplitude and rhythm) varies considerably from one species to another and depends on the dose and the experimental conditions, e.g., the hormonal state. An example of the latter was given by ADAIR and HAUGEN (1939) who found that strips from the nonpregnant *human uterus* during the secretory phase of the menstrual cycle and strips from uteri in early pregnancy were insensitive to ergometrine, whereas one fifth of the preparations obtained in the proliferative phase and more than one third of those obtained at term or during labor showed a clear oxytocic effect. The action of methylergometrine on the human myometrium in late pregnancy is depicted in Figure 11. Differences in the experimental conditions may also be responsible for the divergent results obtained in the isolated *rat uterus*. ROTHLIN (1935b) reported ergometrine to be inhibitory in this species, and KIRCHHOF et al. (1944) came to the same conclusion for methylergometrine, pointing out that the relaxant effect was not as marked as that after adrenaline. All other investigators, however, observed an oxytocic action with either one or both of the drugs. According to PENNEFATHER (1961) the isolated rat uterus can even be employed for a bioassay in which, based on the dose related height of contractions, ergometrine concentrations as low as 0.1 μg/ml were estimated. An oxytocic effect of ergometrine in the rat uterus was also found by BERDE and STÜRMER (1962) who, dealing with a drug combination of synthetic oxytocin and ergometrine, were faced with the problem of finding a suitable bioassay for oxytocin in the presence of ergometrine. When ergometrine was present in low concentrations (0.01–0.04 μg/ml) it was liable to elicit contractions or to potentiate contractions due to oxytocin, thereby yielding erroneously high values for the oxytocin content. Since in their experience the sensitivity of the rat uterus to ergometrine fluctuated and the dose response relationship was not always satisfactory, they considered this preparation to be unsuitable for quantitative work with ergometrine and for the estimation of oxytocin in the presence of ergometrine. This view was primarily shared by SUND (1963a), but in a subsequent publication the same author (1963b) showed how the difficulty in assaying oxytocin in the presence of ergometrine could be overcome. He found that adding magnesium chloride to the bath solution abolished the oxytocic effect of ergometrine. A dose dependent inhibitory action of magnesium ions in the bath on the oxytocic effect of ergometrine has previously been demonstrated in the isolated guinea pig uterus by FRASER (1939).

Methods for the estimation of ergometrine have also been elaborated in the isolated *rabbit uterus*. Unlike ergotoxine, ergotamine and other peptide alkaloids which can be assayed by their antagonism to adrenaline, as described by BROOM and CLARK (1923), ergometrine and methylergometrine are virtually devoid of such action. On the other hand, they exert their uterine motor activity in the isolated rabbit uterus quite consistently so that, in one way or another, this action can be used for assaying purposes. DAVIS et al. (1935b) took the height of contraction as the index of activity and found the rabbit uterus to be more suitable than the guinea pig uterus because it showed less variation with different strips. THOMPSON (1935) pointed out a considerable variation in sensitivity of different uteri to ergometrine, but was nevertheless of the opinion that the isolated rabbit uterus provides an excellent method for assaying different lots of ergometrine, since repeated doses produce satisfactorily constant and dose related responses. An improvement of the method—not in specificity but in precision—was achieved by VOS (1943), who found that large doses of ergometrine stimulated the contractions of the isolated rabbit uterus more promptly than small doses. The latent period was therefore used as a criterion of potency, and the doses were adjusted to give latencies between 2 and 5 min. The usefulness of this approach was confirmed by FOSTER and STEWART (1948) who employed it, with some minor modifications, for stability tests with tablets and ampules of ergometrine. They also found that ergometrinine, the 8α-isomer of ergometrine, possessed only 3.9% of the activity of the parent compound.

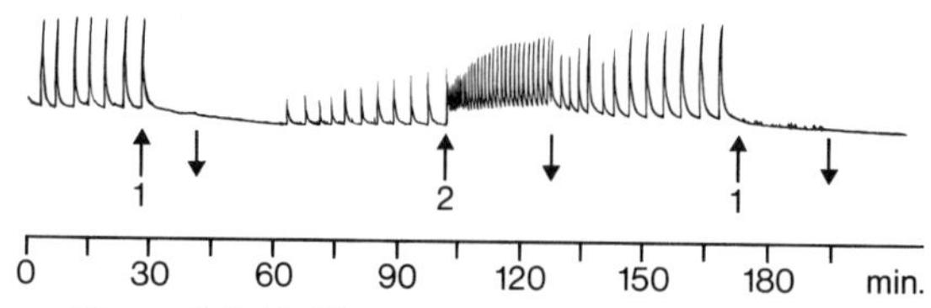

Fig. 13. Inhibitory effect of 2,13-dibromodihydrolysergic acid glycinamide (DDLG) on the motility of human myometrium in vitro. 1. DDLG 0.1 mg/ml; 2. methylergometrine 0.02 mg/ml; ↓ washing. (From BERDE and SAAMELI, 1966)

The low potency of ergometrinine in this study supports the general view that the "-inine derivatives" of ergot alkaloids are relatively inactive in biologic systems. Other compounds which are chemically related to ergometrine showed, however, considerable oxytocic activities. Thus LSD (*d*-lysergic acid diethylamide) in the isolated rabbit uterus was only 1.5 times weaker than ergometrine (ROTHLIN, 1957), and 2-bromo-LSD, a powerful 5-HT antagonist, according to TOTHILL (1967) increased the frequency of contractions in the isolated rat uterus at remarkably low concentrations. Of merely theoretic interest are results reported by SLAYTOR et al. (1959) concerning the oxytocic effects obtained in the isolated guinea pig uterus with unidentified metabolites of ergometrine extracted from rat bile, as well as the observations made with 2,13-dibromodihydrolysergic acid glycinamide (BERDE and SAAMELI, 1966). This compound proved to be several times more potent as an oxytocic than methylergometrine in the isolated rabbit uterus, but was an inhibitor of uterine motor activity on the isolated human myometrium near or at term, as is evident from Figure 13.

b) Studies in situ

The pertinent information on published results obtained with ergometrine, methylergometrine and other nonpeptide alkaloids (1-methyl-lysergic acid L-2-butanolamide, methysergide, Deseril; *d*-lysergic acid diethylamide, LSD; 2-bromo-*d*-lysergic acid diethylamide, 2-bromo-LSD) is compiled in Table 6. Although for therapeutic purposes human experimental data obviously deserve the greatest attention and are abundantly available—it may be recalled that ergometrine was discovered by its action on the human puerperal uterus—many of the characteristic uterine properties of ergometrine and the closely related methylergometrine have been investigated in a variety of animal species, such as the rat, guinea pig, rabbit, cat and dog. As with the in vitro studies no great differences were found between the two drugs with regard to their basic pharmacologic actions. It seems therefore appropriate to discuss them together, whereas the scanty information available for other lysergic acid-amides will be dealt with at the end of this section.

α) Methods

With the exception of human studies most experiments were done under anesthesia. This, to some extent, may have depressed the animals' sensitivity to the oxytocic drug. Indirect evidence for an inhibitory influence of anesthesia can be obtained

Table 6. Uterine action of lysergic acid-amides in situ

Compound	Species/state	Experimental condition	Dose/route of administration	Characteristics of effect	Special observations/remarks	Ref.
Ergometrine	Rat; ovariectomized, with or without estrogen pretreatment	Barbiturate anesthesia or pithed; isotonic recording from horn dissected free from ovarian and mesenteric attachments	0.1–0.5 mg/kg i.v.	Prompt and powerful contractions, rise in tone, lasting 30–40 min		1
Ergometrine	Guinea pig; parous, neither pregnant nor puerperal	Urethane anesthesia; isotonic recording from a uterine segment, animal immersed in warm bath	0.01 mg i.v.	Nonpregnant: small increase in tone, little effect on preexisting high rhythm		2
	Puerperal (day 1 or 2 postpartum)			Puerperal: rapidly (<1 min) occurring strong and regular contractions in the quiescent organ, lasting for several hours, with full relaxation in between	Marked contrast to effect of ergotoxine which takes 10 min for onset of action and leads to sustained rise in tone	
Ergometrine	Guinea pig; parous, nonpregnant, pregnant, puerperal, or estrogen-treated	Urethane anesthesia; ovarian and cervical ends of uterine horn fixed on a rod, movements recorded isotonically from center of uterus (in pregnant animals feti removed)	0.01 mg i.v.	Oxytocic effect; confirmation of results described above (Ref. 2)		1
Ergometrine	Rabbit; nonpregnant	As described above (Ref. 2) for guinea pig	0.2 mg/kg i.v.	Prompt contraction with increased rhythmic activity and elevated tone for about 10 min	Oxytocic effect associated with slight increase in arterial blood pressure	2

Table 6 (continuation)

Compound	Species/state	Experimental condition	Dose/route of administration	Characteristics of effect	Special observations/remarks	Ref.
Ergometrine	Rabbit; ovariectomized, estrogen-treated	Urethane anesthesia, laparotomy; isotonic recording from exteriorized uterine horn of which the distal end is sutured to the abdominal wall, kept in a moist funnel; in some experiments recording of vaginal motility	0.1 mg/kg i.v.	Immediate rise in tone, reaching maximum within 1–2 min, followed by superimposed rhythmic contractions of small amplitude; decline to base line within 10 min; increased vaginal motility (shorter than uterine effect)	Similar to effects of ergotamine, except that ergometrine did not influence blood pressure and did not inhibit the actions of adrenaline; ergometrine also effective by the enteral route	3–6
Ergometrine	Rabbit; puerperal	Unanesthetized; pressure recording from large intrauterine balloon inserted through surgical fistula	0.075 or 0.1 mg i.m.	Long-lasting oxytocic effect (increased amplitude and rate of contraction)	Results comparable with those in puerperal cats	7
Ergometrine	Rabbit; multiparous, nonpregnant	Unanesthetized; intrauterine balloon inserted through previously prepared fistula	0.12 mg i.v.	Relatively weak and short (5 min) oxytocic response with increased rate of contraction and elevated tone	Similar to effects of methylergometrine	8
Ergometrine	Rabbit	Urethane anesthesia, laparotomy; method according to Ref. 5	0.1 mg/kg i.v.	Based on comparison of triangle surface (height of maximal contraction on ordinate, duration of oxytocic action on abscissa) ergometrine had about 70% of the activity of methylergometrine	Great variation of results (range of error 30%–40%)	9
Ergometrine	Rabbit; parous, nonpregnant	As described above (Ref. 1) for guinea pig	0.1 mg/kg i.v. (threshold sometimes 0.01)	Rhythmic and powerful contractions	Effect inhibited by α-adrenoceptor blocking agents (incl. dihydroergotoxine)	1

Table 6 (continuation)

Compound	Species/state	Experimental condition	Dose/route of administration	Characteristics of effect	Special observations/remarks	Ref.
Ergometrine	Cat; nonpregnant (virgin or parous), or in early pregnancy	As described above (Ref. 2) for guinea pig	Not mentioned	Oxytocic effects similar to those of ergotamine and ergotoxine		2
	Puerperal	Spinal	0.07 mg/kg i.v.	Immediate powerful contractions with slowly rising resting tone, lasting >1 h	Increased arterial blood pressure during initial phase of oxytocic effect	
		Decerebrate	0.17 mg/kg intragastric	No perceptible effect; subsequent similar dose given intravenously was very effective		
Ergometrine	Cat		Enteral or intravenous administration	Increase in tone and rhythm		4
Ergometrine	Cat; pregnant		0.25–0.5 mg/kg p.o. or s.c.	Abortion		6
Ergometrine	Cat; puerperal	Slightly anesthetized; transvaginally inserted large intrauterine balloon, closed recording system	0.075–0.1 mg i.m. (e.g. 0.048 mg/kg)	Strong oxytocic effect on previously quiescent uterus (rise in resting tone, lasting >20 min, associated with persistent high rhythmic activity)		7
Ergometrine	Cat, 1–1,5 kg; nonpregnant	Chloralose anesthesia; intrauterine and intravaginal pressure recording	0.1–0.4 mg i.v. (0.07–0.4 mg/kg)	Marked rise in uterine tone for 15 min; no effect on vagina	Similar to methylergometrine	10

Table 6 (continuation)

Compound	Species/state	Experimental condition	Dose/route of administration	Characteristics of effect	Special observations/remarks	Ref.
Ergometrine	Cat; late pregnancy or puerperal	As described above (Ref. 1) for guinea pig	0.2–0.5 mg/kg i.v.	Increase in basal tone, little effect on already maximal contractions		1
Ergometrine	Dog; puerperal	Intrauterine balloon	0.005–0.05 mg/kg i.v.	Oxytocic effect within 1–1.5 min	Results similar to those in puerperal women; dog method suitable for bioassay of ergometrine	11 12
			0.5 mg/kg p.o.	Rhythmic contractions with increase in tone		
Ergometrine	Dog; 10–12 kg; nonpregnant	Ether or paraldehyde anesthesia; intrauterine and intravaginal pressure recording	0.1–0.4 mg i.v. (0.009–0.04 mg/kg)	Slight and only short (5 min) rise in tone; no effect on vagina	Similar to methylergometrine	10
	Pregnant			Marked rise in tone		
Ergometrine	Human; late puerperium (day 6–8 postpartum)	Transcervically inserted intrauterine balloon	0.05–0.25 mg i.v.	Immediate powerful contraction, reaching maximum within 15–20 sec, followed by vigorous rhythmic activity (high rate, small amplitude) superimposed on elevated resting tone, lasting several hours	No change of blood pressure	11–14
			0.3–0.4 mg i.m., p.o. or sublingual	Small contractions and gradual increase in tone, starting 7–12 min after administration, reaching maximum within 5–10 min, gradually declining over several hours	Preceding oral administration of ergotamine or ergotoxine ineffective	

Table 6 (continuation)

Compound	Species/state	Experimental condition	Dose/route of administration	Characteristics of effect	Special observations/remarks	Ref.
Ergometrine	Human; early or advanced puerperium	Transcervically inserted intrauterine balloon or external tocography	0.05–0.1 mg i.v. 0.25–0.5 mg i.m. 0.5–1 mg p.o.	Similar observations as described above (Ref. 11–14); strong contractions 1–2 min after i.v., 3.5–4.5 min after i.m. and 6.5–8 min after oral administration	Rapid onset of action in contrast to ergotamine and ergotoxine, which act slowly, even when given by injection (20 min i.m., 6–7 min i.v.); less side effects than with ergotamine and ergotoxine	15
Ergometrine	Human; late puerperium (day 6–8 postpartum)	Transcervically inserted intrauterine balloon	0.1 mg i.v.	Confirmation of results described above (Ref. 11–15); onset of action within 35–78 sec (mean 55 sec)		16
Ergometrine	Human; therapeutic abortion in first or second trimester	Premedicated, sometimes anesthetized; pressure recording from various sites within the uterus (upper and/or middle and lower segment) using small rubber balloons attached to multichannel catheter	0.2–0.5 mg i.v.	Ergometrine (and methylergometrine) act preferentially on cervix (pressure waves start in cervix and do not always reach corpus), whereas oxytocin activates primarily corpus	Evidence for marked dissociation of corpus and cervix activity	17
Ergometrine	Human; postpartum	External tocography using an electromechanical device	0.05–0.4 mg i.v. or i.m.	Rise in resting tone and increase in frequency of contraction 8 min after i.m. injection; oxytocic effect begins to decline after 90 min		18

Table 6 (continuation)

Compond	Species/state	Experimental condition	Dose/route of administration	Characteristics of effect	Special observations/remarks	Ref.
Ergometrine	Human; early puerperium	External tocography ("Oxford" tocograph) or intrauterine balloon method	0.25–0.5 mg i.v. or i.m., or 0.5 mg i.m. combined with hyaluronidase	Latent period (from injection to onset of oxytocic effect): – ergometrine: i.v. 41″ ± 8″; i.m. 7′ ± 2′33″ – ergometrine + hyaluronidase: i.m. 4′47″ ± 56″	Hyaluronidase speeds action of i.m. ergometrine; therapeutic advantage questionable	19
Ergometrine	Human; various phases of menstrual cycle	Unanesthetized; intrauterine balloon method	0.25–0.5 mg i.v. 0.5–0.75 mg i.m.	First half of cycle: very slight rise in tone with or without increase in amplitude, greater response to i.v. than i.m. injection Second half of cycle and during menstruation: mild oxytocic effect after i.m. injection, strong effect (rise in tone, increased frequency with reduced amplitude) after i.v. administration	During anovulatory cycles, ergometrine had no significant oxytocic effect; nonpregnant uterus much less sensitive to ergometrine (and ergotamine) than puerperal uterus; therapeutic value of ergometrine in dysfunctional haemorrhage appears doubtful	20, 21
Ergometrine	Human; early puerperium (day 1–4 postpartum)	External tocography (strain-gauge instrument according to Smyth); measurement of the area between tracing of uterine motility and base line for 20 min period after injecting drug	0.015, 0.03 or 0.06 mg i.v.	Dose-related oxytocic effects; based on an assay (designed as incomplete randomized blocks of two) ergometrine was 1.5 (at 5% fiducial limits 0.96–2.7) times more active than methylergometrine	Effects of ergometrine and methylergometrine qualitatively similar	22, 23

Table 6 (continuation)

Compound	Species/state	Experimental condition	Dose/route of administration	Characteristics of effect	Special observations/remarks	Ref.
Ergometrine	Human; puerperal (day 2–9 postpartum)	External tocography ("Oxford" tocograph) or intrauterine balloon method	0.25 or 0.5 mg i.m. combined with oxytocin (2.5 or 5 I.U.)	Rapid onset of oxytocic effect (within 2.5 min, as with oxytocin alone) followed by sustained tetanic contraction due to ergometrine	A valuable tool for prevention or treatment of postpartum haemorrhage in circumstances where i.v. injections cannot be given	24
Ergometrine	Human; therapeutic abortion (10–20 weeks gestation)	Intrauterine balloon	0.1–0.5 mg i.v. or continuous i.v. infusion at 3–6 μg/min	Fast rhythm superimposed on tonic contraction of fundus, often associated with tonic contractions of cervix	Compared with oxytoxin, ergometrine is more liable to cause very fast and usually irregular rhythm of contraction and of raising tone; stimulation of uncoordinated activity?	25
	Induction of labor for intrauterine death (30–40 weeks gestation)	External tocography (guard-ring electromanometer)				
	Puerperal (day 2–4 postpartum)	External tocography	0.02–0.06 mg i.v.	Less increase in rate of contractions than in the pregnant uterus, no rise in tone		
Ergometrine	Human; postpartum	Intrauterine pressure recording through transabdominally inserted open-tip catheter	1.4 μg/min for 1 h	Previously well-coordinated postpartum contractions changed into bizarre pattern of uterine motility, characterized by frequent small contractions between and superimposed on irregular large contractions	Similar to effects of sparteine	26

Table 6 (continuation)

Compound	Species/state	Experimental condition	Dose/route of administration	Characteristics of effect	Special observations/remarks	Ref.
Ergometrine	Human; therapeutic abortion, induction of labor	Intrauterine pressure recording through transabdominally inserted open-tip catheter	repeated i.m. or i.v. injections of small doses (5–40 μg) or continuous i.v. infusion (0.6–1.2μg/min)	Uterine response increases throughout pregnancy, reaching maximum during labor and in early postpartum period; characteristic features are high frequency, small amplitude, hypertonus, disturbed coordination	Should never be used with a live fetus in utero	27
Ergometrine	Human; postpartum, normal blood pressure	Intrauterine pressure recording through transabdominally inserted open-tip catheter, combined with continuous intraarterial blood pressure recording	0.2 mg i.v.	Strong, long-lasting oxytocic effect within 2 min: initial tetanic-like contraction followed by frequent rhythmic activity with slightly elevated resting tone	Uterine response associated with persistent increase in arterial blood pressure from 110/50 to 130/70 mmHg	28
Ergometrine	Human; proliferative or secretory phase of cycle	Intrauterine pressure recording from transcervically inserted balloon; simultaneous recording of fallopian tube motility from catheter inserted inside tube during preceding laparotomy	0.001–0.2 mg i.v. or p.o.	Long-lasting increase in tone and motility of tubes at doses ineffective on uterus	Increased motility may impair transport function of tubes and therefore reduce fertility	29
Ergometrine	Human; induction of labor for intrauterine death	Intraamniotic pressure recording with transabdominally inserted open-tip catheter	Continuous intravenous infusion, 0.6–4.8 μg/min	At 0.6 μg/min increased frequency of contraction from 2 to 8 per 10 min; at higher doses further increase of frequency, but resting tone and amplitude uninfluenced	Response to ergometrine differs from that to oxytocin or prostaglandin $F_{2\alpha}$	30

Table 6 (continuation)

Compound	Species/state	Experimental condition	Dose/route of administration	Characteristics of effect	Special observations/remarks	Ref.
Methyl-ergometrine	Rabbit; multiparous, nonpregnant	Similar to the experiments described above (Ref. 8) for ergometrine in the rabbit uterus				8
Methyl-ergometrine	Rabbit; late pregnancy, parturient or puerperal	Urethane anesthesia, laparotomy; isotonic recording from exteriorized uterine horn; in some experiments simultaneous recording of vaginal motility (balloon)	0.15–0.4 mg/kg i.v.	Immediate uterine and vaginal contraction; elevated tone for about 10 min, much longer increase in rhythm	Oxytocic effect of methylergometrine often inhibited by preceding administration of dihydroergotamine or dihydroergotoxine	31
Methyl-ergometrine	Rabbit	Similar to the experiments described above (Ref. 9) for ergometrine in the rabbit uterus				9
Methyl-ergometrine	Rabbit; 31st day of pregnancy	Induction of labor	1–1.3 mg/kg i.m.	Successful induction of labor in about 50% of animals, but only at doses already within toxic range	Method more suitable for testing oxytocin	32, 33
Methyl-ergometrine	Rabbit, 2.7–3 kg; virgin (estrogen-treated) or puerperal	Barbiturate anesthesia, laparotomy; isometric recording from segment of uterine horn	0.1–4 mg i.v. (0.03–1.5 mg/kg)	Difficulty in establishing oxytocic threshold dose, no differences between estrogen-treated virgin and puerperal animals; steep dose response curve (much steeper than with oxytocin), reproducible effect with 1 mg, contracture for 5–10 min with 4 mg	In several experiments spontaneous uterine activity not enhanced, but inhibited by methylergometrine; in other cases previous administration of oxytocin increased sensitivity to methylergometrine, while large doses of methylergometrine reduced sensitivity to oxytocin	34

Table 6 (continuation)

Compound	Species/state	Experimental condition	Dose/route of administration	Characteristics of effect	Special observations/remarks	Ref.
Methyl-ergometrine	Rabbit; estrus	Isometric recording; measurement of the area under the curve	0.025–0.8 mg/kg i.v.	Dose-related oxytocic effects, using up to 6 different doses in one animal		33
Methyl-ergometrine	Cat; pregnant	Urethane-chloralose anesthesia; isotonic recording from exteriorized uterine horn, simultaneous pressure recording (balloon) from other horn	0.5 mg/kg i.v.	Oxytocic effect similar to that produced in the same animal by dihydroergotoxine or oxytocin: transient rise in resting tone with increased frequency of contraction		31
Methyl-ergometrine	Cat, 1–1.5 kg; nonpregnant	Chloralose anesthesia; intrauterine and intravaginal pressure recording	0.04–0.16 mg i.v. (0.03–0.16 mg/kg)	Marked rise in uterine tone for 15 min; no effect on vagina	Similar to ergometrine	10
Methyl-ergometrine	Dog, 10–12 kg; nonpregnant	Ether or paraldehyde anesthesia; intrauterine and intravaginal pressure recording	0.04–0.16 mg i.v. (0.003–0.016 mg/kg)	Slight and only short (5 min) rise in tone; no effect on vagina	Similar to ergometrine	10
	Pregnant			Marked rise in tone		
Methyl-ergometrine	Human; late pregnancy, induction of labor at term, sub partu, early puerperium	External tocography according to Crodel	0.2 mg i.v. or i.m., 0.025–0.17 mg p.o.	Clear oxytocic effects with fast onset and long duration of action; at low doses increase in rate, at high doses marked elevation of tone	Uterine sensitivity to the drug increases towards term and is maximal during labor; careful dosage is essential	35
Methyl-ergometrine	Human; late puerperium (day 6–8 postpartum)	Transcervically inserted intrauterine balloon	0.07–0.1 mg i.v., 0.2 mg p.o.	Qualitatively similar oxytocic effects as with ergometrine, 1.5–2 times more potent than ergometrine, slightly longer duration of action	Well tolerated	16

Table 6 (continuation)

Compound	Species/state	Experimental condition	Dose/route of administration	Characteristics of effect	Special observations/remarks	Ref.
Methyl-ergometrine	Human; therapeutic abortion in first or second trimester	Similar to the experiments described above (Ref. 17) for ergometrine in the human uterus				17
Methyl-ergometrine	Human; third stage of labor	Continuous measurement of intrauterine pressure from umbilical vein with placenta still in utero	0.2 mg i.v.	Marked rise in resting tone (to 33–51 mmHg) and increase in rate of contraction (to 8–19 per 10 min), resulting in considerable shortening of 3rd stage and reduction of blood loss	Effects very similar to those of ergometrine	36
Methyl-ergometrine	Human; postpartum	External tocography using an electromechanical device	0.05–0.4 mg i.v. or i.m.	Onset of oxytocic effect (increase in tone and rate of contraction) within 2–5 min following i.m. administration (slightly shorter than with ergometrine)	Qualitatively similar to ergometrine, somewhat more potent and longer duration of action than ergometrine	18
Methyl-ergometrine	Human; early puerperium (day 1–4 postpartum)	Similar to the experiments described above (Ref. 22) for ergometrine in the human uterus				22, 23
Methyl-ergometrine	Human; postpartum	External tocography using strain-gauge tocodynamometer	0.2 mg i.v., i.m. or s.c.	Long-lasting increase in rate and amplitude of contraction, with i.v. application initial rise of resting tone	Uterus after the first dose refractory to a second dose for several hours	37

Table 6 (continuation)

Compound	Species/state	Experimental condition	Dose/route of administration	Characteristics of effect	Special observations/remarks	Ref.
Methyl-ergometrine	Human; therapeutic abortion, induction of labor	Similar to the experiments described above (Ref. 27) for ergometrine in the human uterus				27
Methyl-ergometrine	Human; nonpregnant, toward end of monophasic cycle	Intrauterine pressure recording with trans-cervically inserted catheter	0.2 mg i.m.	Clear oxytocic effect, starting 7 min after injection		38
Methyl-ergometrine	Human; therapeutic abor-tion during first and second trimester	Intrauterine recording (microballoon between membranes and uterine wall, or intraamniotic open-end catheter)	0.2 mg i.v.	Small but very long-lasting rise in tone, superimposed by rapid, incoordinated contractions of low intensity	Pattern of response differs from that to oxytocin or prosta-glandin E_1, which act more drastically but have a much shorter duration of action	39
Methyl-ergometrine	Human; puerperal (day 6 postpartum)	Intrauterine pressure recording using trans-cervically inserted two-channel open-end catheter	0.2 mg i.v.	Clear oxytocic effect (rise in tone and increase in rate of contraction) on a uterus in which oxytocin-stimulated motor activity was depressed by a β-sym-pathicomimetic drug		40
Methyl-ergometrine	Human; nonpregnant	Intrauterine pressure recording with trans-cervically inserted two-channel open-end catheter	0.2 mg i.v.	Gradual increase of tone, starting 3 min after injec-tion, with return to base line usually within 20 min, but sometimes requiring >60 min	Uterine response present not only in biphasic, but also in monophasic cycles and independent of day of cycle	41
1-methyl-lysergic acid *L*-2-butanol-amide (methysergide, [illegible]	Rabbit; estrus	Urethane anesthesia; simultaneous recording of uterine and vaginal contractions	4 mg/kg i.v.	Small and short uterine and vaginal contraction; effect considerably weaker than that caused by 0.25 mg/kg methylergo-metrine	At high doses inhibition of the oxytocic effect of methylergometrine	42

Table 6 (continuation)

Compound	Species/state	Experimental condition	Dose/route of administration	Characteristics of effect	Special observations/remarks	Ref.
1-methyl-lysergic acid *L*-2-butanol-amide (methysergide, Deseril)	Cat; pregnant	Urethane-chloralose anesthesia; isotonic recording	1 mg/kg i.v.	Clear oxytocic effect, qualitatively similar to that of 0.125 mg/kg methyl-ergometrine, but considerably weaker		42
1-methyl-lysergic acid *L*-2-butanol-amide (methysergide, Deseril)	Human; pregnancy near term, in labor or postpartum		Not specified	Oxytocic effect with delayed onset of action (15–25 min); 8–32 times weaker than methylergometrine		42
d-lysergic acid diethylamide (LSD)	Rabbit	Urethane anesthesia; simultaneous recording of uterine and vaginal contractions	Not mentioned	Oxytocic effect, about 1.5 times weaker than ergometrine		43
2-bromo-*d*-lysergic acid diethylamide (2-bromo-LSD)	Rabbit	Urethane anesthesia; simultaneous recording of uterine and vaginal contractions	Not mentioned	No contraction; in high doses inhibition of spontaneous rhythm and relaxation		43

References: 1. Fregnan and Glässer (1964); 2. Brown and Dale (1935); 3. Rothlin (1935a); 4. Rothlin (1935b); 5. Rothlin (1938a); 6. Rothlin (1938b); 7. Oettel and Bachmann (1937); 8. Kirchhof et al. (1944); 9. Votava and Podvalova (1957); 10. Venkatasubbu and Gopala Krishnamurthy (1959); 11. Davis et al. (1935a); 12. Davis et al. (1935b); 13. Adair et al. (1935); 14. Davis et al. (1936); 15. Dudley and Moir (1935); 16. Gill (1947); 17. Schild et al. (1951); 18. Huber (1956); 19. Embrey and Garrett (1958); 20. Garrett and Moir (1958); 21. Garrett (1959); 22. Myerscough and Schild (1958); 23. Schild (1959); 24. Embrey (1961); 25. Smyth (1961); 26. Hendricks et al. (1965); 27. Cibils and Hendricks (1969); 28. Hendricks and Brenner (1970); 29. Coutinho (1971)[a]; 30. de Koning Gans et al. (1975); 31. Berde and Rothlin (1953); 32. Berde and Cerletti (1958); 33. Berde and Saameli (1966); 34. Fuchs and Fuchs (1960); 35. Bachbauer (1944); 36. Carballo et al. (1953); 37. Müller and Ströker (1959); 38. Baumgarten (1970); 39. Roth-Brandel et al. (1970); 40. Baumgarten et al. (1971); 41. Fröhlich (1974); 42. Fanchamps et al. (1960); 43. Rothlin (1957).

[a] See also Coutinho et al. (1976)

by comparing the low doses of ergometrine used by OETTEL and BACHMANN (1937) for the puerperal rabbit in the unanesthetized condition with those reported by BERDE and ROTHLIN (1953) for methylergometrine—which is about equipotent to ergometrine—in the puerperal rabbit under urethane anesthesia. In the first case intramuscular doses as low as 0.075 mg per animal (body weight not indicated) proved to be strongly oxytocic, whereas in the latter the effective intravenous doses were within the range of 0.15–0.4 mg/kg. There is, on the other hand, no indication that the type of the anesthetic (usually urethane in the guinea pig and rabbit, chloralose or a combination of urethane and chloralose in the cat) is important for interpreting the results.

In *animal experiments* the following basic procedures can be distinguished:

Isotonic, semiisotonic or isometric recording of the contractions occurring in one or both uterine horns in laparotomized animals.

Measuring intrauterine pressure with a transvaginally or transabdominally inserted fluid-filled balloon.

Administration of the compounds under test to pregnant animals with the aim of inducing abortion (cat) or parturition (rabbit).

In contrast to the first and second techniques which, with some variations in details, are still widely used as standard procedures in many laboratories, the "induction of labor-test" was found to be suitable for investigating oxytocin and related substances, but not for ergot alkaloids (BERDE and SAAMELI, 1966); the necessary doses of methylergometrine to induce labor in about 50% of the rabbits near term were already within the toxic range (BERDE and CERLETTI, 1958).

In *human studies* most of the fundamental achievements in the characterization of ergometrine and methylergometrine actions on the uterus were made using *balloons* for continuous intrauterine pressure recording. Indeed, this procedure—described by BOURNE and BURN (1927, 1928, 1930)—was successfully employed by MOIR (1932b) in his work leading to the discovery of the water soluble oxytocic principle of ergot and by ADAIR et al. (1935), DAVIS et al. (1935b), and DUDLEY and MOIR (1935) in their classical investigations of the pure substance ergometrine. From a practical point of view one would expect that the most suitable conditions for inserting balloons are found in the early postpartum phase. A number of such studies were, however, performed during the advanced puerperium (e.g., on the 6th to 8th day after delivery); furthermore there are reports on investigations in which small balloons were used in nonpregnant women (GARRETT and MOIR, 1958; COUTINHO, 1971) and in pregnant women in the course of therapeutic abortion during the first and second trimester (SCHILD et al., 1951; SMYTH, 1961; ROTH-BRANDEL et al., 1970).

Balloon methods have the disadvantage that the presence of a relatively large foreign body within the uterine cavity may induce artefacts in the pressure curve due to local stimulation of the myometrium; moreover the existence of an elastic membrane between the pressure pool and the fluid-filled recording system leads to a complex physical situation which is difficult to define. These drawbacks are absent or at least less pronounced if the pressure measurement is done using thin *open-end catheters* which can be inserted either through the cervix or by transabdominal puncture of the amniotic cavity. The open-end catheter method was first described by ALVAREZ and CALDEYRO (1950) and has since then been favored by other investigators—often with modifications—for studying the uterine effects of various drugs, including ergot alkaloids (HENDRICKS et al., 1965; CIBILS and HENDRICKS, 1969; BAUMGARTEN, 1970; HENDRICKS and BRENNER, 1970; FRÖHLICH, 1974; DE KONING GANS et al., 1975) in the nonpregnant, pregnant and postpartum human uterus. A tracing obtained by intraamniotic recording with a transabdominally inserted open-end catheter is depicted in Figure 10.

Both of the intrauterine pressure measuring techniques carry a small but not completely negligible risk to the patient, and require sterile working conditions. It is therefore not surprising that various methods of *external tocography,* though less accurate, gained much popularity in clinical pharmacology, particularly if relatively large series of experiments were envisaged. The instruments used for this procedure are applied to the abdomen at a point where the pregnant or postpartum uterus comes in contact with the abdominal wall, the patient lying in a supine position. They can be held in position by hand or by an elastic belt passed round the patient. The sensitive part of such a tocometer consists of a bolt or piston which acts as an intermediate transmitter between the contracting uterus and the measuring device—usually nowadays a strain-gauge or a photoelectric cell. Examples of investigations in which ergometrine and/or methylergometrine have been studied by external tocography were given by BACHBAUER (1944), HUBER (1956), EMBREY and GARRETT (1958), MYERSCOUGH and SCHILD (1958), MÜLLER and STRÖKER (1959), EMBREY (1961) and SMYTH (1961).

β) Factors Determining the Oxytocic Response

Species: The data given in Table 6 concerning the doses used (and found effective) in all these experiments point to considerable differences in responsiveness between various species. As with the peptide alkaloids, the guinea pig, a species in which intravenous doses of a few microgram per kilogram were effective (BROWN and DALE, 1935; FREGNAN and GLÄSSER, 1964) appears to be particularly sensitive to nonpeptide alkaloids. High sensitivity with clearly oxytocic doses in the range of about 0.005–0.05 mg/kg i.v. was also observed in the dog, particularly in the puerperal (DAVIS et al., 1935b) or gravid stage (VENKATASUBBU and GOPALA KRISHNAMURTHY, 1959). For the rat, rabbit and cat approximately 10 times higher intravenous doses (0.05–0.5 mg/kg) of ergometrine or methylergometrine were given to elicit or enhance uterine contractions (for references see Table 6). This suggests a somewhat lower sensitivity inherent to these species—of which the nonpregnant, anesthetized rabbit was the most widely used test model—in comparison with the guinea pig and dog.

Responses to even lower doses than those in the guinea pig and dog were, however, demonstrated in the many experiments performed in the human. Assuming an average body weight of 60 kg the effective intravenous doses given to nonpregnant women (GARRETT and MOIR, 1958; GARRETT, 1959; FRÖHLICH, 1974) or given during pregnancy in the course of therapeutic abortion (SCHILD et al., 1951; SMYTH, 1961; ROTH-BRANDEL et al., 1970) and for induction or enhancement of labor near term (BACHBAUER, 1944) amount to 0.002–0.008 mg/kg. Lower doses, ranging approximately from 0.001–0.01 mg/kg i.v., also proved to have an oxytocic effect in women during the third stage of labor (CARBALLO et al., 1953), immediately postpartum, and in the early or advanced puerperium (for references see Table 6). Using a strain-gauge instrument for external tocography in the early puerperium for the purpose of comparing ergometrine with methylergometrine in a strictly quantitative assay, MYERSCOUGH and SCHILD (1958) found the two drugs to be active at intravenous doses as low as 0.015, 0.03, and 0.06 mg, which are equivalent to about 0.25 to 1 µg/kg. Similar results were reported by SMYTH (1961). In the light of these very low threshold doses the amount of 0.2 mg of the drugs contained in commercially available ampules for intravenous or intramuscular injection after delivery represents a rather massive dose which, under many clinical circumstances, could probably be reduced without appreciable loss of therapeutic efficacy.

Hormonal Conditions: In comparing the data given in the literature on the oxytocic responses for ergometrine and methylergometrine one has to pay attention to the actual conditions under which the studies have been performed with regard to the hormonal state of the animal or human patient.

In *animals* a great variety of such conditions exists in experiments in nonpregnant virgin or parous subjects, sometimes ovariectomized, with or without estrogen treatment, as well as in studies done during the various phases of pregnancy, sub partu or in the puerperium. In general, there is clear evidence for a stronger and longer-lasting response of pregnant and particularly of puerperal animals compared with the nonpregnant state (BROWN and DALE, 1935, for the guinea pig and cat; VENKATASUBBU and GOPALA KRISHNAMURTHY, 1959, for the dog), but it should be emphasized that the nonpregnant rabbit in estrus (for references see Table 6) provides very satisfactory results at doses similar to those used in pregnant or puerperal animals. According to FUCHS and FUCHS (1960) the threshold dose for methylergometrine was not lower in puerperal rabbits than in the nonpregnant, estrogen-treated animals, but the response to the same dose was stronger and lasted much longer. This was in contrast to oxytocin, for which (in terms of threshold doses) the sensitivity of the rabbit uterus was much increased immediately after delivery. The authors concluded that methylergometrine is more like histamine or adrenaline, to which the sensitivity of the uterus is not influenced by the ovarian hormones.

This view may hold true in the rabbit, but is not fully supported by the results obtained in other species, and particularly not in *women* where there is strong evidence for an influence of the hormonal situation on the response of the nonpregnant, pregnant, parturient or puerperal uterus to the alkaloids. GARRETT and MOIR (1958) and GARRETT (1959) found ergometrine to be only slightly active when given during the first half of the menstrual cycle or at any time in a monophasic (anovulatory) cycle, the effect being a small increase in base line; however, much more definite responses resembling those seen in the puerperal uterus occurred if the drug was given after ovulation or during menstruation. On an overall basis they concluded that the nonpregnant human uterus is much less sensitive to ergometrine (and ergotamine) than the puerperal uterus, and they cast serious doubts as to the usefulness of such drugs in the treatment of dysfunctional uterine haemorrhage. A therapeutic effect could only be expected in the presence of spontaneously occurring B-waves (MOIR, 1944), which are characteristic of the secretory phase following ovulation. However, the common type of dysfunctional haemorrhage is thought to occur in anovulatory cycles, during which these authors could not find a significant oxytocic action of ergometrine. This is not quite in agreement with results published by BAUMGARTEN (1970) and by FRÖHLICH (1974), who in a few patients, demonstrated a clear oxytocic response to an intravenous dose of methylergometrine during anovulatory cycles. Further evidence for the existence of hormonal influences on the uterine action of low-molecular alkaloids comes from studies in pregnant women, in which a considerable increase in sensitivity takes place throughout pregnancy, reaching its maximum — as with oxytocin — during labor and immediately postpartum (BACHBAUER, 1944; CIBILS and HENDRICKS, 1969). The same conclusion can be drawn from the results of SMYTH (1961). He had to give intravenous doses of ergometrine in the range 0.1–0.5 mg in order to increase uterine motor activity at 10–20 weeks gestation, whereas 0.1 mg doses were sufficient at 30–40 weeks gestation and 0.02–0.06 mg doses during the first few days of puerperium.

Dose: Information on the *dose response relationship* in a strictly pharmacologic sense is rare. This shortcoming may find its explanation in the fact that under most experimental conditions the duration of the oxytocic response is long and some degree of tachyphylaxis to subsequent doses is likely to occur, so that repeated administration of the drug in the same experiment is hardly feasible. An exception is found in the estrous rabbit, for which FUCHS and FUCHS (1960) in the case of methylergometrine were able to demonstrate a clear dose response relationship — with a much steeper dose response curve than for oxytocin — using isometric recording and taking tension developed in excess to that of spontaneous contractions as the parameter. Results indicating an unquestionable dose response relationship in the rabbit were also reported by BERDE and SAAMELI (1966). In these experiments, of which tracings are shown in Figure 8 of Chapter I (page 11) up to six doses of methylergometrine were given to the same animal and were found to cause relatively short-lasting increases in isometrically recorded uterine tension. By quantifying the time integral of the oxytocic effect a satisfactory dose response relationship could be established. In studies performed in puerperal women the difficulties caused by the long duration of action, the reduction of responses to repeated doses on the same day, and the rapid involution of the puerperal uterus, can be overcome in the quantitative assay described by MYERSCOUGH and SCHILD (1958). In a balanced design (incomplete randomized blocks of two) ergometrine and methylergometrine were given intravenously on the second and third day postpartum; the effects were recorded by external tocography and quantified by measuring the area enclosed between the base line and the tracing over a period of 20 min following the injection. Figure 14 illustrates the results from a series of experiments in which only one drug (ergometrine) was used on the same subject. Clearly, in each individual case the greater dose produced the greater effect.

Route of Administration (with reference to the time required for the onset of action): In almost all the *animal experiments* the drugs have been given by *intravenous injection,* and the onset of increased uterine motor activity was then very rapid, usually taking less than 1 min. A relatively fast action by the intravenous route has also been described for peptide alkaloids such as ergotamine or ergotoxine, but evidence was given by BROWN and DALE (1935) in a study on the puerperal guinea pig that ergometrine acts still faster than ergotoxine. Whenever ergometrine or methylergometrine have been given to animals as *intramuscular* or *subcutaneous*

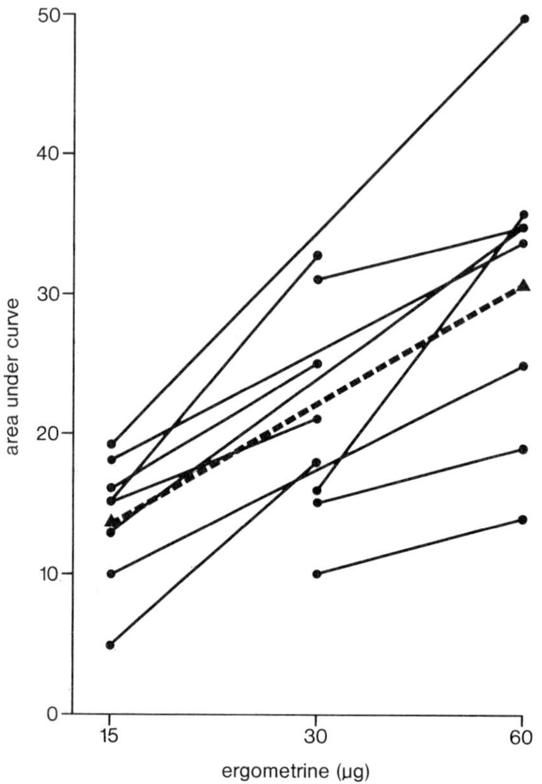

Fig. 14. Dose response curves of ergometrine in puerperal women. External tocography. Points joined by a solid line refer to effects in the same patient on successive days. The broken line is the best-fitting straight line. (From MYERSCOUGH and SCHILD, 1958)

injections they were found to be effective (ROTHLIN, 1938b; BERDE and CERLETTI, 1958) and also to have a fast onset of action (OETTEL and BACHMANN, 1937). Good absorption by the *oral route* is one of the prominent pharmacologic and therapeutic features of the lysergic acid-amides, allowing a clear differentiation from the uterotonic peptide alkaloids. Although this aspect has been investigated to a much greater extent in human studies, results reported by DAVIS et al. (1935b) for the dog should be mentioned. They found that ergometrine elicited a distinct response in the puerperal uterus within $1-1^{1}/_{2}$ min at doses varying from 0.005 to 0.05 mg/kg injected intravenously. When given by mouth, a dose of 0.5 mg/kg produced rhythmic contractions with increase in tone within 6 min. In the rabbit an oxytocic action of intragastrically administered ergometrine has been reported by ROTHLIN (1935a), but given by the same route to the cat the drug was found to be ineffective (BROWN and DALE, 1935).

The intravenous, intramuscular, subcutaneous and oral (including sublingual) route of administration have also been used in the experimental work in *women*. The effectiveness of the various ways of drug administation and the time required for the onset of action is not very different from that in animals. The classical

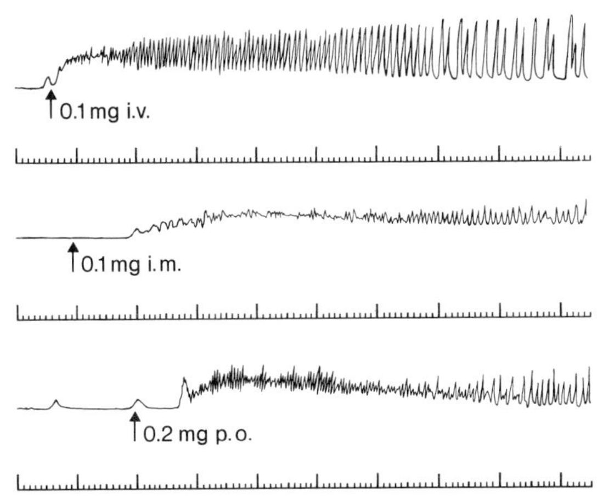

Fig. 15. Effects of methylergometrine given by various routes of administration to puerperal women. Intrauterine balloon method. Time scales in minutes. (From GILL, 1947; by permission of J. Obstet. Gynaec. Brit. Emp.)

results described by DUDLEY and MOIR (1935) for ergometrine in puerperal women indicate strong oxytocic responses occurring within 1–2 min after intravenous injections (0.05 or 0.1 mg), within $3^1/_2$–$4^1/_2$ min after intramuscular injections (0.25–0.5 mg) and within $6^1/_2$–8 min following oral doses (0.5–1 mg). In their experience it took 6–7 min for the effects of ergotamine or ergotoxine to occur when given intravenously at a dose of 0.25 mg and about 20 min when given intramuscularly at twice this dose.

Similar observations—with a tendency for somewhat longer delays by the intramuscular route—have been made by many other investigators not only for ergometrine, but also for methylergometrine. Characteristic tracings published by GILL (1947) for the effects of methylergometrine are shown in Figure 15. Accurate figures with mean values and standard deviations of the time of onset of the oxytocic response to ergometrine have been reported by EMBREY and GARRETT (1958). By the intravenous route with doses of 0.25 or 0.5 mg the drug produced its first effect after 41 ± 8 s, whereas an interval of 7 min $\pm$ 2 min and 33 s was observed with intramuscular injections of 0.5 mg. When—following the advice of KIMBELL (1954)—hyaluronidase, acting as a "spreading factor", was added to the intramuscular injections the latent period was shortened to 4 min and 47 s $\pm$ 56 s. Although this combination clearly offers some advantages for the clinical use of ergometrine by midwives it has not gained popularity, probably because of the high cost of hyaluronidase. Another—apparently more feasible—approach for obtaining a rapidly occurring, but nevertheless long-lasting uterotonic effect after intramuscular injection consists in the combination of the ergot alkaloid with oxytocin, as described by EMBREY (1961). In his investigation the onset of the oxytocic response took about two and a half min with both oxytocin alone and ergometrine plus oxytocin.

Much emphasis has been placed, particularly in the early human studies (DAVIS et al., 1935b; DUDLEY and MOIR, 1935; DAVIS et al., 1936; BACHBAUER, 1944;

GILL, 1947) on demonstrating the high *oral effectiveness* of the lysergic acid-amides, which is in distinct contrast to the rather unsatisfactory results obtained with peptide alkaloids (e.g., ADAIR et al., 1935).

Oral administration of ergometrine and methylergometrine has found a definite place in the prevention and treatment of delayed involution of the puerperal uterus which is often associated with retention of lochia, but the value of such therapy has been debated by MOIR and RUSSEL (1943) and by GARRETT (1960).

In the more recent literature the *parenteral use* of the uterotonic lysergic acid-amides plays the dominant role. This is easily explained by the clinical circumstances under which these drugs are most often used in modern obstetric practice. Their most important and well-established therapeutic domain is prophylaxis and treatment of uterine haemorrhage, a condition for which the very fast onset of action inherent to parenteral, and especially to intravenous injections, is obviously essential.

Familiarity with the method and merits of *continuous intravenous infusion* of oxytocin in the management of labor has probably been one of the reasons why several investigators wanted to try out this mode of administration with nonpeptide ergot alkaloids. Such studies have been performed under varying conditions (therapeutic abortion, induction of labor for intrauterine death, normal labor at term, early postpartum period) by SMYTH (1961), HENDRICKS et al. (1965), CIBILS and HENDRICKS (1969) and DE KONING GANS et al. (1975). None of these experiments yielded any evidence for a particular usefulness of this approach. The rational basis for continuous infusion of oxytocin, namely its short biologic halflife which allows achievement of steady-state conditions within a short time and thereby provides the possibility of flexible adjustment of the infusion speed to the actual needs, does not apply to the ergot compounds. The marked differences between the effects of continuous intravenous infusion of synthetic oxytocin and those observed in the same patient during and after continuous infusion of ergometrine are illustrated in Figure 16.

An attempt to stimulate uterine activity has also been made by injecting methylergometrine intraamniotically. The only response to large amounts of the drug (0.2 and 0.4 mg) in a case of polyhydramnios at 37 weeks of pregnancy was a marginal increase in the preexisting high rate of contractions (CIBILS and HENDRICKS, 1969). This is in contrast to uterotonic prostaglandins which are known to be very active when given intraamniotically.

Concomitant Medication: Some changes of the uterine response to lysergic acid-amides caused by concomitant medication (e.g., possible depression of sensitivity by anesthetics, shortening of the latent period by hyaluronidase) have already been mentioned; a few others remain to be discussed briefly. In the rabbit, a species in which dihydroergotamine and dihydroergotoxine do not stimulate uterine motor activity, the two drugs were shown to reduce or completely inhibit the effects of methylergometrine (BERDE and ROTHLIN, 1953). In agreement with these results FREGNAN and GLÄSSER (1964) found in the same species a strong antagonism of dihydroergotoxine against the oxytocic action of ergometrine, and also against that of adrenaline and noradrenaline. Since similar antagonistic effects were obtained with piperoxane and phenoxybenzamine, but not with hexamethonium or atropine, one may conclude that α-adrenoceptor blockade is the underlying mecha-

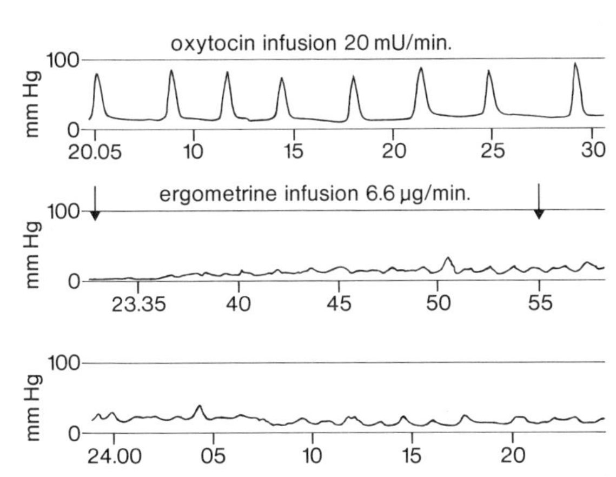

Fig. 16. Effects of continuous intravenous infusion of synthetic oxytocin and ergometrine on uterine contractility in early third trimester. Intrauterine fetal demise. The top tracing shows stable activity induced by 20 mU/min of oxytocin. Three hours later, after the effect of oxytocin had disappeared, an ergometrine infusion (6.6 µg/min for 22 min) was given between the arrows of the middle tracing. This continues at the bottom, illustrating a low, but very incoordinated response with elevated resting tone. Time in minutes. (From CIBILS and HENDRICKS, 1969)

nism of the inhibitory action. Blockade of the effects of ergometrine on the rabbit uterus in situ by dibenamine or phentolamine was first reported and taken as evidence for a peripheral "sympathomimetic" type of action of this drug by KONZETT (1960).

So far, no information is available regarding influences of β-adrenoceptor blockade on the uterine action of ergot compounds, and the few results obtained with β-adrenoceptor stimulants, which are clinically used for depressing premature labor, are controversial. According to STOLTE et al. (1963) Cc25, a derivative of adrenaline, was effective in suppressing ergometrine-induced uterine activity in pregnant women, but BAUMGARTEN et al. (1971) demonstrated clear oxytocic effects of methylergometrine in puerperal women in which oxytocin-induced contractions were strongly inhibited by the β-adrenoceptor stimulant ritodrine.

From a practical point of view, knowledge of interactions between the uterotonic lysergic acid-amides and oxytocin would be of considerable interest, but it seems that this question has never been submitted to a thorough investigation. In their work on the rabbit uterus in situ FUCHS and FUCHS (1960) found that oxytocin, if given before methylergometrine, augmented the sensitivity to the latter, whereas the sensitivity to oxytocin was often for some time reduced by a preceding dose of the ergot drug. In women no major interference occurs; this can be deduced from an observation reported by CIBILS and HENDRICKS (1969) according to which intravenously infused oxytocin was effective in increasing the amplitude of contractions during advanced first stage of labor, but was unable to correct hypertonicity and marked incoordination caused by the previous administration of ergometrine. Further evidence for the two drugs being compatible and even complementary was given by EMBREY (1961) in his tocographic study on the simultaneous intramuscular injection of oxytocin and ergometrine.

γ) *Characteristics of the Oxytocic Effect*

Ample evidence for unquestionable oxytocic effects of ergometrine and methylergometrine in experimental animals and in women has already been given in the preceding parts of this section. This is also shown in Figure 8 of Chapter I (page 11) illustrating the action in the estrous rabbit and in Figures 1, 15 and 16 which are tracings obtained in women. For further details the reader is referred to the survey given in Table 6. For the sake of completeness it should be mentioned that in several cases out of a series of experiments performed by FUCHS and FUCHS (1960) in the estrogen-treated nonpregnant rabbit, methylergometrine at fairly low doses (0.2 or 0.4 mg per animal) failed to stimulate contractions and instead stopped spontaneous activity. No such observations could be found in any other report on animal experiments, but paradoxical effects of methylergometrine in doses higher than 0.05 mg and of ergometrine at even lower doses were described by SAUTER (1948, 1949b, 1950) in women postpartum. Using an externally applied tocographic instrument (FREY's hysterotonograph) he observed immediately occurring reductions in resting tone following the injection of the drug. This change was reversed by spasmolytic agents, which was one reason why it was attributed to a constrictor activity of the ergot drugs within the vascular bed of the uterus, the assumption being that reduced blood flow and consequent hypoxia impaired contractile performance. HUBER (1956), however, could not confirm these findings of a paradoxical effect and was probably right in his suspicion that the special technique employed by SAUTER with FREY's instrument was responsible for erroneous results.

Taking into consideration not only the experimental work discussed in this chapter, but also the vast literature on clinical experience, it is safe to say that ergometrine and methylergometrine have a very high predictability as to their oxytocic effect in women immediately postpartum and during puerperium, irrespective of low or higher doses. This, on the other hand, does not exclude the possibility of tachyphylaxis occurring with repeated administration. Refractoriness to a second dose of methylergometrine—but not to oxytocin—lasting several hours, has been observed by MÜLLER and STRÖKER (1959) in women during the first few hours after delivery, and by GILL (1947) during the advanced puerperium.

The *pattern of uterine response* has been described at the beginning of this chapter (page 234) and shown in Figure 1. Comparison of this tracing (obtained with oral administration of 0.5 mg ergometrine) with that shown at the bottom of Figure 15 (the effect of 0.2 mg methylergometrine) suggests a striking qualitative similarity of the two drugs. The low dose of methylergometrine was almost as effective as the two and a half times higher dose of ergometrine, but this should not be taken as evidence of a greater potency of methylergometrine. Since only minor differences—not always going in the same direction—were found between the two drugs whenever they were submitted to a quantitative comparison within the same study (see page 310), the discrepancy in effective dosage is more likely to reflect an interpatient difference in sensitivity. Considerable quantitative interpatient variations of externally recorded responses to either ergometrine or methylergometrine given to puerperal women on two consecutive days—but reasonably consistent effects in one and the same patient—were observed by MYERSCOUGH and SCHILD (1958).

Similarity in the response to the two drugs was also recognized in animal experiments, particularly in the rabbit (KIRCHHOF et al., 1944). In this species the usual pattern of the oxytocic effect (ROTHLIN, 1938a, 1938b; BERDE and ROTHLIN, 1953; VOTAVA and PODVALOVA, 1957) differs clearly from the one observed in puerperal women, in that the duration of action is much shorter and the strong initial increase in tone is, in contrast to the human uterus, not followed by a period of sustained rhythmic activity with full relaxation between contractions. It must be pointed out, however, that the experiments in rabbits were done in the nonpregnant state, so that the conditions are hardly comparable with those in the human studies. So far, no published tracings of ergometrine- or methylergometrine-stimulated uterine activity have been found from the puerperal rabbit, but those described for the puerperal cat (BROWN and DALE, 1935) or dog (DAVIS et al., 1935a) reveal a definite resemblance to curves obtained in postpartum or puerperal women by intrauterine pressure recording (ADAIR et al., 1935; DAVIS et al., 1935b; DUDLEY and MOIR, 1935; GILL, 1947; EMBREY and GARRETT, 1958; HENDRICKS and BRENNER, 1970; BAUMGARTEN et al., 1971) or by external tocography (DUDLEY and MOIR, 1935; BACHBAUER, 1944; HUBER, 1956; MÜLLER and STRÖKER, 1959).

The *duration of action,* being of a similar order of magnitude for both ergometrine and methylergometrine, appears to vary to some extent from one species to another and depends, of course, on the doses used, but the decisive factor is undoubtedly given by the functional state of the uterus. Although precise figures are often missing in publications—obvious reasons are the limited time allowed for an experiment and, due to variations in spontaneous uterine activity, difficulties in defining the endpoint of an effect—the following much simplified survey may serve as tentative information: in nonpregnant rats (FREGNAN and GLÄSSER, 1964), rabbits (e.g., BROWN and DALE, 1935; ROTHLIN, 1938a; BERDE and SAAMELI, 1966), cats and dogs (VENKATASUBBU and GOPALA KRISHNAMURTHY, 1959), the observed durations of action were rather short, ranging from 5–10 min in the rabbit and the dog, to between 15 and 40 min in the rat and cat. Considerably longer effects were seen in puerperal guinea pigs, rabbits, cats and dogs (BROWN and DALE, 1935; DAVIS et al., 1935a, 1935b; OETTEL and BACHMANN, 1937), lasting for several hours in the guinea pig.

Much the same situation, with a tendency for longer actions than in animals, was found in the human. In the nonpregnant state the decline of elevated tone to base line values after methylergometrine occurred usually within 20, occasionally within 60 min (FRÖHLICH, 1974), which contrasts to the much longer effects observed in pregnant, postpartum and puerperal women. Increased uterine tone and small, rapid, incoordinated contractions lasting for several hours after intravenous injections of methylergometrine were reported by ROTH-BRANDEL et al. (1970) from a study performed during therapeutic abortion in the first and second trimester of pregnancy. Similarly, SMYTH (1961) found ergometrine to be still active and causing slightly elevated resting tone and fast rhythmic contractions 9 h after intravenous injection in a patient with a dead fetus at 29 weeks of pregnancy. However, in view of the therapeutic use of the drugs for prevention and therapy of uterine haemorrhage and of delayed uterine involution, the most relevant clinical findings emerge from those studies which were done in women during the early postpartum period or in the puerperium (references were given above in discussing the "pattern of uterine response"). Under these conditions, both ergometrine and methylergometrine were consistently shown to have a very long duration of action, usually described as lasting for several, occasionally even for up to 12 h.

Comparison between Ergometrine and Methylergometrine: Slight and inconsistent differences in the time of onset and duration of action in women (GILL, 1947; HUBER, 1956) may be disregarded, and it is safe to say that no real qualitative differences of the uterine effects exist between the two drugs if they are compared in the rabbit (KIRCHHOF et al., 1944), in the cat and dog (VENKATASUBBU and GOPALA KRISHNAMURTHY, 1959) and in women (CARBALLO et al., 1953; MYERSCOUGH and SCHILD, 1958). A few publications, however, point to a difference in potency. According to VOTAVA and PODVALOVA (1957) methylergometrine is somewhat more potent than ergometrine in the nonpregnant rabbit. A higher potency of methylergometrine (by a factor of 1.5 to 2) was also reported by GILL (1947) for the human puerperal uterus, but this could not be confirmed by MYERSCOUGH and SCHILD (1958), who in a quantitative assay in puerperal women found methylergometrine to be about 1.5 times less active than ergometrine. The doses used in their study (0.015–0.06 mg) were considerably below the common therapeutic dose (0.1 or 0.2 mg). Since the latter probably represents in most clinical situations a supramaximal dose, it is very unlikely that relatively small differences in potency of the two drugs would be of any practical significance.

Comparison of the Lysergic Acid-Amides with other Oxytocic Agents: Apart from differences in the time required for the onset of action, the in situ uterus preparation in animals is not very suitable for demonstrating qualitative differences of various oxytocic compounds. This general view is supported by comparing the tracings shown in Figure 8 of Chapter I (page 11) and Figures 5 and 6. Similarity of the responses to ergometrine, *ergotamine, ergotoxine*—and in one study on the cat also to *dihydroergotamine, dihydroergotoxine* and even to *oxytocin* (BERDE and ROTHLIN, 1953)—has been reported for the rabbit (ROTHLIN, 1938a, 1938b) and the cat (BROWN and DALE, 1935). The only exception concerns comparative experiments in the puerperal guinea pig, in which intravenous injection of the same dose of ergometrine not only showed a much shorter latent period, but also differed sometimes from ergotoxine in that its stimulant action on rhythm dominated its tonic effect, whereas the opposite was often observed with ergotoxine (BROWN and DALE, 1935).

More clearly differentiated results with various oxytocic drugs were obtained in human studies, but as in most animal experiments the outstanding differences between the lysergic acid-amides ergometrine and methylergometrine and the peptide alkaloids *ergotamine* and *ergotoxine* were confined to the time course of the uterine effects. This conclusion is based on the investigations reported by HUBER (1956) on the externally recorded tocographic effects of ergometrine, methylergometrine and ergotamine in postpartum women and also on the comparison of tracings published by MOIR (1932a) for the action of ergotamine and ergotoxine in puerperal women with those obtained under similar experimental conditions by DAVIS et al. (1935b) in the case of ergometrine and by GILL (1947) in the case of methylergometrine.

When ergometrine or methylergometrine were compared with *sparteine,* a drug from an entirely different chemical group which sometime ago enjoyed a certain popularity for induction and enhancement of labor, HENDRICKS et al. (1965) and

Cibils and Hendricks (1969) found great resemblance of their intrauterine pressure curves recorded in late human pregnancy in labor as well as in the early puerperium.

Little similarity, however, exists in women between the actions of the lysergic acid-amides and *oxytocin*. This has been emphasized by Smyth (1961) in describing tocographic observations made with intravenous administration of ergometrine and oxytocin in patients undergoing therapeutic abortion for induction of labor or intrauterine death, and during the early puerperium. Oxytocin produced good generalized contractions with full relaxation between them, unless the dose was too large. Ergometrine, on the other hand, caused a very fast and usually irregular rhythm of contractions and raised uterine resting tone. An increase in the rate at which oxytocin was infused led to a rise in the rate of contractions, whereas an increase in the rate of infusion of ergometrine enhanced the strength of contractions while the average frequency remained constant. The very pronounced differences in the response of the pregnant human uterus to the two drugs are illustrated in Figure 16, which among several aspects demonstrates a high degree of *incoordination* of ergometrine-induced contractility. This is characteristic for the uterus in late pregnancy (Smyth, 1961; Cibils and Hendricks, 1969), but has also been observed and described as "bizarre changes in the pattern of uterine activity" by Hendricks et al. (1965) in women postpartum. Smyth (1961) assumed that oxytocin promotes the spread of contraction from cell to cell (probably by facilitating conduction of the action potential), thereby "organizing" the whole uterus, or most of it, to contract at the same time, whereas ergometrine was thought to have a local effect on muscle cells and to stimulate many parts of the uterine muscle at different times, thereby causing incoordinated activity. These ideas, though they have never been fully substantiated by clinical physiologists or pharmacologists, may still be regarded as a valuable hypothesis.

Another difference between the lysergic acid-amides and oxytocin was observed by Schild et al. (1951) in patients whose pregnancy was being terminated in the first or second trimester. Simultaneous pressure recordings from various sites within the uterus revealed sometimes a marked dissociation of corpus activity and of cervix activity. The most characteristic effect of ergometrine or methylergometrine was to stimulate small cervical contractions with or without corresponding stimulation of the corpus, whereas oxytocin induced a powerful contraction of the corpus without apparent constrictor effect on the cervix. It is important to note that these results were obtained at early stages of pregnancy. If they are also representative for those in advanced pregnancy or during early labor, they may explain the inefficiency of ergometrine-induced uterine activity and the lack of progress in cervical dilatation during the first stage of labor, as reported by Cibils and Hendricks (1969). The situation, however, is different in those conditions for which the therapeutic use of ergot compounds is recommended. When they are injected at the end of the second stage of labor (at the time of crowning of the head or with the appearance of the anterior shoulder) or immediately after delivery of either the baby or the placenta, their rapidly occurring uterotonic effect is very similar to that produced by the injection of a high dose of oxytocin. It consists of a sustained strong contraction of the entire organ which, depending on the timing of the injection, promotes the delivery of the baby, facilitates the separation and expulsion of the placenta and reduces blood loss.

From studies in pregnant women (therapeutic abortion, intrauterine fetal death), in which ergometrine or methylergometrine were compared not only with oxytocin but also with *prostaglandin* E_1 or with *prostaglandin* $F_{2\alpha}$ it is evident that a greater similarity of the uterine response patterns exists between oxytocin and the prostaglandins than between the ergot drugs and the nonergot compounds. When given by single intravenous injection at midpregnancy, both oxytocin and PGE_1 caused a rapid and very marked rise in tone which gradually returned to a normal level (within about 20 min in the case of oxytocin and 40–50 min in the case of the prostaglandin) and was associated with the occurrence of relatively well coordinated rhythmic contractions of increasing amplitude. In contrast to these compounds, methylergometrine produced only a modest and slowly developing rise in resting tone, but this change lasted for several hours and was paralleled by small, rapid and incoordinated contractions (ROTH-BRANDEL et al., 1970). These results were in essence confirmed by DE KONING GANS et al. (1975). They gave ergometrine and oxytocin by continuous intravenous infusion and $PGF_{2\alpha}$ by intraamniotic injections to women with a dead fetus and observed regular, coordinated contractions with the nonergot drugs, but were unable to produce an efficient type of labor with ergometrine. The only effect obtained with the latter consisted in an increased rate of small, irregular contractions.

Based on a theory derived by DAELS (1974) from diverging in vitro effects of adrenaline and oxytocin on human myometrial strips from the embryologically old inner layer and the younger outer layer of the uterus, DE KONING GANS et al. (1975) assumed that ergometrine preferentially affects the inner layer (archemyometrium), which in the pregnant uterus is less developed than the outer zones. In contrast oxytocin and prostaglandin $F_{2\alpha}$ have a prevalent action on the outer muscle layer (paramyometrium). This interesting way of explaining the qualitative differences between ergot compounds and other oxytocic drugs finds support in DAELS' observations, that adrenaline in the postpartum uterus exerted a powerful contracting effect on tissue from the inner zone, but produced relaxation of strips from the outer layer. Oxytocin, on the other hand, caused only weak and inconsistent contractions in strips obtained from the inner zone, but was very active in stimulating the outer layer tissue. These results in conjunction with the abovementioned considerations are well compatible with the concept that the oxytocic effects of ergot alkaloids and of adrenaline (or noradrenaline) are due to stimulation of the same type of receptors (α-adrenoceptors), whereas a different type of receptor is involved in the uterine response to oxytocin.

δ) *Specificity of the Oxytocic Action*

The problem of specificity can be seen from various aspects. Of considerable importance for the clinical use of the drugs is the question of whether and to what extent they cause *changes in blood pressure* at effective oxytocic doses. In the previous sections of this chapter, dealing with the uterine actions of peptide alkaloids and their dihydrogenated derivatives (see also Figures 6 and 9, and Tables 2 and 4) reference was made to marked increases of arterial blood pressure in the rabbit following the injection of ergotamine or of the 6-nor-6-isopropyl derivatives of dihydroergotamine and dihydroergocristine, as well as to the pronounced hypotensive effects of ergosine, ergotoxine, ergokryptine, dihydroergotamine and dihydroergotoxine or its constituents, occurring in the same species. It is one of the characteristic and clinically most useful features of ergometrine and methylergometrine that they have very little influence on blood pressure. This was first shown for ergometrine by ROTHLIN (1938a, 1938b) in the rabbit and by ADAIR et al. (1935) in both normotensive and hypertensive puerperal women, and has subsequently been confirmed, also in the case of methylergometrine, by many experimental and particularly by clinical investigations. Considering that α-adrenoceptor blockade not only inhibits the oxytocic effects of ergot alkaloids (KONZETT, 1960), but also antagonizes the rise in blood pressure occurring with some compounds (HOOL-ZULAUF and STÜRMER, 1976), one may perhaps conclude that the lack of a hypertensive action which is characteristic for the lysergic acid-amides, is due to a much higher affinity of these compounds for the α-adrenoceptors of the uterus than for those of the peripheral vasculature. The fact that, on the other hand, unlike other alkaloids, ergometrine and methylergometrine do not lower blood pressure, may be explained by the absence of α-adrenoceptor blocking activity, and possibly also on the basis of particularly weak actions on vasomotor centers in the brain.

Another aspect of specificity concerns stimulation of motor activity in the *vagina* and in the *fallopian tubes*. In this respect, as with peptide alkaloids, no claims for specificity of the uterine action of ergometrine and methylergometrine can be made. ROTHLIN (1938a, 1946/47) found ergometrine to cause strong vaginal contractions during the period of uterine activation in the nonpregnant rabbit in situ, and VENKATASUBBU and GOPALA KRISHNAMURTHY (1959) observed an increase in vaginal tone in dogs during pregnancy (but not in the nonpregnant state) following injection of ergometrine or methylergometrine. Special attention should be paid to results described by COUTINHO (1971) and COUTINHO et al. (1976) concerning the action of ergometrine and methylergometrine on the fallopian tube motility in nonpregnant women at various stages of the cycle. These authors observed by direct recording of intratubal, and in some experiments also of intrauterine pressure, strong and long-lasting stimulation of tubal motor activity at oral and parenteral doses of the drugs which had very little effect on the uterus and were well tolerated. They assumed that increased motility may impair the transport of the ovum through the tube and hence prevent its normal development, and that by this mechanism the drugs could exert a *contraceptive effect*. Studies now in progress suggest that ergometrine significantly reduces the conception rate in women when administered immediately postcoitum (COUTINHO et al., 1976).

ε) *Various Lysergic Acid-Amides*

Only sporadic information exists on the uterine actions in situ of lysergic acid-amides other than ergometrine and methylergometrine. *D-lysergic acid diethylamide* (*LSD*), being chemically closely related to ergometrine, is only about 1.5 times weaker than ergometrine in stimulating uterine and vaginal motor activity in the anesthetized, nonpregnant rabbit. Its 2-bromo derivative (*BOL 148*), however, was found to be devoid of oxytocic activity, and at high doses it even caused inhibition of spontaneous rhythm and relaxation of the rabbit uterus (ROTHLIN, 1957). *1-*

Methyl-lysergic acid L-2-butanol-amide (methysergide, Deseril), another closely related drug, showed clear oxytocic effects, qualitatively similar to those obtained with methylergometrine, at rather high doses in the nonpregnant rabbit (4 mg/kg i.v.) and in the pregnant cat (1 mg/kg i.v.). Weight for weight Deseril was approximately 16–30 times weaker than methylergometrine, and at still higher doses than those mentioned, it was capable of inhibiting the uterine effects of methylergometrine in the rabbit. The oxytocic properties of Deseril were confirmed in pregnant and puerperal women, but again, in terms of absolute activity, the drug was 8–32 times weaker than methylergometrine (Fanchamps et al., 1960).

C. References

Adair, F.L., Haugen, J.A.: A study of suspended human uterine muscle strips in vitro. Amer. J. Obstet. Gynec. **37**, 753–762 (1939)

Adair, F.L., Davis, M.E.: A study of human uterine motility. Amer. J. Obstet. Gynec. **27**, 383–394 (1934)

Adair, F.L., Davis, M.E., Kharasch, M.S., Legault, R.R.: A study of a new potent ergot derivative, ergotocin. Amer. J. Obstet. Gynec. **30**, 466–480 (1935)

Altman, S.G., Waltman, R., Lubin, S., Reynolds, S.R.M.: Oxytocic and toxic actions of dihydroergotamine-45. Amer. J. Obstet. Gynec. **64**, 101–109 (1952)

Alvarez, H.: Discussion: motility of parts of human uterus. In: Oxytocin. Caldeyro-Barcia, R., Heller, H. (eds.), pp. 309–311. Oxford: Pergamon Press 1961

Alvarez, H., Caldeyro, R.: Contractility of the human uterus recorded by new methods. Surg. Gynec. Obstet. **91**, 1–13 (1950)

Alvarez, H., Mendez-Bauer, C., Sica Blanco, Y.: Acción de la hydergina sobre la contractilidad del útero humano grávido. An. Ginecotocol. **2**, 67–72 (1954–55)

Bachbauer, A.: Über die Wirkung eines halbsynthetischen Sekalealkaloids als Wehenmittel auf tokometrischer Grundlage. Geburtsh. u. Frauenheilk. **6**, 278–289 (1944)

Barger, G.: The alcaloids of ergot. In: Handbuch der experimentellen Pharmakologie, Vol. VI, Heubner, W., Schüller, J. (eds.), pp. 130–134, 177–179, 185–190. Berlin-Heidelberg-New York: Springer 1938

Baskin, M.J., Crealock, F.W.: The management of cervical spasm with dihydroergotamine methanesulfonate (DHE-45). West. J. Surg. **58**, 302–307 (1950)

Baumgarten, K.: Die Uterusmotilität beim weiblichen Zyklus. Geburtsh. u. Frauenheilk. **30**, 921–933 (1970)

Baumgarten, K., Fröhlich, H., Seidl, A., Sokol, K., Lim-Rachmat, F., Hager, R.: A new β-sympathomimetic preparation for intravenous and oral inhibition of uterine contractions. Europ. J. Obstet. Gynec. **1**, 69–83 (1971)

Berde, B.: Discussion: motility of parts of human uterus. In: Oxytocin. Caldeyro-Barcia, R., Heller, H. (eds.), p. 309. Oxford: Pergamon Press 1961

Berde, B., Cerletti, A.: Quantitative comparison of substances related to oxytocin: a new test. Acta endocr. (Kbh.) **27**, 314–324 (1958)

Berde, B., Rothlin, E.: Über die Uteruswirkung hydrierter Mutterkornalkaloide an Kaninchen und Katzen vor, während und nach der Geburt. Helv. physiol. pharmacol. Acta **11**, 274–282 (1953)

Berde, B., Saameli, K.: Evaluation of substances acting on the uterus. In: Methods in Drug Evaluation. Mantegazza, P., Piccinini, F. (eds.), pp. 481–514. Amsterdam: North-Holland Publishing Company 1966

Berde, B., Stürmer, E.: The biological assay of oxytocin in the presence of ergometrine. J. Pharm. Pharmacol. **14**, 169–171 (1962)

Bösch, K.: Über die Entwicklung, Technik und Resultate der kontinuierlichen Amniondruckmessung und ihrer Kombination mit simultaner externer Tokographie sub partu. Schweiz. med. Wschr. **84**, 850–855 (1954)

Bourne, A., Burn, J.H.: The dosage and action of pituitary extract and of the ergot alkaloids on the uterus in labour, with a note on the action of adrenalin. J. Obstet. Gynaec. Brit. Emp. **34**, 249–268 (1927)
Bourne, A.W., Burn, J.H.: Oxytocin and vasopressin on the uterus in labour. Lancet **1928 II**, 694–695
Bourne, A.W., Burn, J.H.: Action on the human uterus of anaesthetics and other drugs commonly used in labour. Brit. med. J. **2**, 87–89 (1930)
Broom, A.W., Clark, A.J.: The standardisation of ergot preparations. J. Pharmacol. exp. Ther. **22**, 59–74 (1923)
Brown, G.L., Dale, H.: The pharmacology of ergometrine. Proc. roy. Soc. **B118**, 446–477 (1935)
Brügger, I.: Experimenteller Beitrag zur Wirkungsweise vegetativer Pharmaka. Arch. int. Pharmacodyn. **59**, 43–60 (1938)
Bruns, P.D., Snow, R.H., Drose, V.E.: Effect of dihydroergotamine on human uterine contractility. Obstet. and Gynec. **1**, 188–196 (1953)
Carballo, M.A., Caldeyro Barcia, R., Alvarez, H., Agüero, O., Mendy, J.C.: Accion de la metilergonovina sobre la contractilidad uterina durante el alumbramiento. Bol. Soc. chil. Obstet. Ginec. **18**, 252–263 (1953)
Cibils, L.A., Hendricks, C.H.: Effect of ergot derivatives and sparteine sulfate upon the human uterus. J. Reprod. Med. **2**, 147–167 (1969)
Clegg, P.C.: The effect of adrenergic blocking agents on the guinea-pig uterus in vitro, and a study of the histology of the intrinsic myometrial nerves. J. Physiol. (Lond.) **169**, 73–90 (1963)
Coutinho, E.M.: Tubal and uterine motility. In: Proceedings of the 15th Nobel Symposium 1970, Sweden. Diczfalusy, E., Borell, U. (eds.), pp. 97–115. New York-London-Sydney: Wiley 1971
Coutinho, E.M., Maia, H., Nascimento, L.: The response of the human Fallopian tube to ergonovine and methyl-ergonovine in vivo. Amer. J. Obstet. Gynec. **126**, 48–54 (1976)
Daels, J.: Uterine contractility patterns of the outer and inner zones of the myometrium. Obstet. and Gynec. **44**, 315–326 (1974)
Dale, H.H.: The new ergot alkaloid. Science **82**, 99–101 (1935)
Dale, H.H., Spiro, K.: Die wirksamen Alkaloide des Mutterkorns. Naunyn-Schmiedebergs Arch. exp. Path. Pharmak. **95**, 337–350 (1922)
Davis, M.E., Adair, F.L., Rogers, G., Kharasch, M.S., Legault, R.R.: A new active principle in ergot and its effects on uterine motility. Amer. J. Obstet. Gynec. **29**, 155–167 (1935a)
Davis, M.E., Adair, F.L., Chen, K.K., Swanson, E.E.: The pharmacologic action of ergotoxin, a new ergot principle. J. Pharmacol. exp. Ther. **54**, 398–407 (1935b)
Davis, M.E., Adair, F.L., Pearl, S.: The present status of oxytocics in obstetrics. J. Amer. med. Ass. **107**, 261–267 (1936)
De Boer, J., Van Dongen, K.: Experiments with dihydroergotamine. Arch. int. Pharmacodyn. **77**, 434–441 (1948)
Deis, R.P., Pickford, M.: The effect of autonomic blocking agents on uterine contractions of the rat and the guinea-pig. J. Physiol. (Lond.) **173**, 215–225 (1964)
De Koning Gans, H.J., Martinez, A.A.V., Eskes, T.K.A.B.: Intermittent low-dose administration of prostaglandins intra-amniotically in pathological pregnancies. Europ. J. Obstet. Gynec. Reprod. Biol. **5/6**, 307–315 (1975)
Dudley, H.W., Moir, C.: The substance responsible for the traditional clinical effect of ergot. Brit. med. J. **1**, 520–523 (1935)
Embrey, M.P.: Simultaneous intramuscular injection of oxytocin and ergometrine: a tocographic study. Brit. med. J. **1**, 1737–1738 (1961)
Embrey, M.P., Garrett, W.J.: A study of the effects of dihydroergotamine on the intact human uterus. J. Obstet. Gynaec. Brit. Emp. **62**, 150–154 (1955)
Embrey, M.P., Garrett, W.J.: Ergometrine with hyaluronidase: speed of action. Brit. med. J. **2**, 138–139 (1958)
Eschbach, W., Hanke, R.: Uterusmotilität post abortum. Zbl. Gynäk. **75**, 481–489 (1953)
Fanchamps, A., Doepfner, W., Weidmann, H., Cerletti, A.: Pharmakologische Charakterisierung von Deseril®, einem Serotonin-Antagonisten. Schweiz. med. Wschr. **90**, 1040–1046 (1960)

Fegerl, H., Narik, G.: Die Beeinflussung der Wehentätigkeit durch das sympathische und parasympathische Nervensystem. Geburtsh. u. Frauenheilk. **11**, 822–834 (1951)
Flury, F.: Pharmakologische Untersuchungen am ausgeschnittenen menschlichen Uterus. Z. Geburtsh. Gynäk. **87**, 291–300 (1924)
Foster, G.E., Stewart, G.A.: The stability of ergometrine preparations, chemical and biological studies. Quart. J. Pharmacol. **21**, 211–218 (1948)
Fraser, A.M.: The effect of magnesium on the response of the uterus to posterior pituitary hormones. J. Pharmacol. exp. Ther. **66**, 85–94 (1939)
Fregnan, G.B., Glässer, A.H.: Activity of eledoisin, other polypeptides and ergometrine on the uterus in situ of rabbit and other animal species. J. Pharm. Pharmacol. **16**, 744–750 (1964)
Fröhlich, H.: Steuermechanismen der Motilität des nichtgraviden Uterus in situ. Wien. klin. Wschr. **86** (Suppl. 24), 3–28 (1974)
Fuchs, A.-R., Fuchs, F.: The effect of oxytocic substances upon the rabbit uterus in situ. Acta physiol. scand. **49**, 103–113 (1960)
Garg, K.N., Sharma, S., Bala, S.: Experimental studies of sparteine sulphate on strips of human uterus. Jap. J. Pharmacol. **23**, 195–200 (1973)
Garrett, W.J.: The effects of adrenaline, noradrenaline and dihydroergotamine on excised human myometrium. Brit. J. Pharmacol. **10**, 39–44 (1955)
Garrett, W.J.: A theory of uterine action. J. Obstet. Gynaec. Brit. Emp. **66**, 927–938 (1959)
Garrett, W.J.: Why ergometrine? A review of ergot in practice today. Med. J. Aust. **47/I**, 677–680 (1960)
Garrett, W.J., Embrey, M.P.: The effect of the hydrogenated ergotoxine-group alkaloids on the intact human uterus. J. Obstet. Gynaec. Brit. Emp. **62**, 523–529 (1955)
Garrett, W.J., Moir, J.C.: Ergot and the non-pregnant uterus. J. Obstet. Gynaec. Brit. Emp. **65**, 583–587 (1958)
Gill, R.C.: The effect of methyl-ergometrine on the human puerperal uterus. J. Obstet. Gynaec. Brit. Emp. **54**, 482–488 (1947)
Gill, R.C.: Further observations on the effect of dihydroergotamine upon human uterine action. J. Obstet. Gynaec. Brit. Emp. **60**, 103–109 (1953)
Gill, R.C., Farrar, J.M.: Experiences with di-hydro-ergotamine in the treatment of primary uterine inertia. J. Obstet. Gynaec. Brit. Emp. **58**, 79–91 (1951)
Härtfelder, G., Kuschinsky, G., Mosler, H.K.: Über pharmakologische Wirkungen an elektrisch gereizten glatten Muskeln. Naunyn-Schmiedebergs Arch. exp. Path. Pharmak. **234**, 66–78 (1953)
Hendricks, C.H., Brenner, W.E.: Cardiovascular effects of oxytocic drugs used post partum. Amer. J. Obstet. Gynec. **108**, 751–760 (1970)
Hendricks, C.H., Reid, D.W.J., Van Fraagh, I., Cibils, L.A.: Effect of sparteine sulfate upon uterine activity in human pregnancy. Amer. J. Obstet. Gynec. **91**, 1–9 (1965)
Hool-Zulauf, B., Stürmer, E.: Oxytocic activity of two dihydro-ergot peptide alkaloids on the rabbit uterus in situ. Abstr. of the 17th Spring Meeting, March 23–26, 1976, Mainz. Naunyn-Schmiedebergs Arch. Pharmacol. **293** (Suppl.), 139 (1976)
Hool-Zulauf, B., Stürmer, E.: Oxytocic activity of two dihydrogenated ergot peptide alkaloids on the rabbit uterus in situ. Arzneimittel-Forsch. **27**, 2323–2325 (1977)
Huber, R.: Tokographische Kontrolle einiger gebräuchlicher Sekale-Rein-Alkaloide am menschlichen Uterus post partum. Zbl. Gynäk. **78**, 748–756 (1956)
Ingelman-Sundberg, A., Lindgren, L., Ryden, G., Sandberg, F.: The spontaneous motility of uterine fibromyomata and their responses to pharmacological stimuli. Acta obstet. gynec. scand. **36**, 263–269 (1957)
Ivy, A.C., Hartman, C.G., Koff, A.: The contractions of the monkey uterus at term. Amer. J. Obstet. Gynec. **22**, 388–399 (1931)
Jeffcoate, T.N.A., Wilson, J.K.: The effect of hydergine on uterine action. Lancet **1955 I**, 1187–1190
Jelinek, E.: Resultate der oralen Anwendung von Hydergin während der 1. Geburtsphase. Gynaecologia (Basel) **143**, 414–425 (1957)
Kharasch, M.S., King, H., Stoll, A., Thompson, M.R.: The new ergot alkaloid. Science **83**, 206–207 (1936)

Kimbell, N.: Intramuscular ergometrine and hyaluronidase in prevention of post-partum haemorrhage. Brit. med. J. **2**, 130–131 (1954)
Kirchhof, A.C., Racely, C.A., Wilson, W.M., David, N.A.: An ergonovine-like oxytocic synthetized from lysergic acid. West. J. Surg. **52**, 197–208 (1944)
Koff, A.K.: A study of the action of ergot on the human puerperal uterus. Surg. Gynec. Obstet. **60**, 190–202 (1935)
Konzett, H.: Specific antagonism of dibenamine to ergometrine. In: Ciba Foundation Symposium on Adrenergic Mechanism. Wolstenholme, G.E.W., O'Connor, M. (eds.), pp. 463–465. London: Churchill 1960
Kremer, H., Narik, G.: Die pharmakodynamische Beeinflußbarkeit der Uterusmotorik sub partu. Geburtsh. u. Frauenheilk. **15**, 433–443 (1955)
Mayer, M., Halpern, B., Nogueira, I.: Accouchement – Délivrance; étude pharmacodynamique de certaines substances utéro-sédatives et utéro-contracturantes. Bull. Féd. Soc. Gynéc. Obstét. franç. **7**, 591–604 (1955)
Miller, G.B., De Beer, E.J.: The ability of ergotoxine to modify the contractile action of ergonovine on the isolated uterus. J. Pharmacol. exp. Ther. **104**, 412–415 (1952)
Moir, C.: Clinical comparison of ergotoxine and ergotamine. Brit. med. J. **1**, 1022–1024 (1932a)
Moir, C.: The action of ergot preparations on the puerperal uterus. Brit. med. J. **1**, 1119–1122 (1932b)
Moir, C.: The effect of posterior lobe pituitary gland fractions on the intact human uterus. J. Obstet. Gynaec. Brit. Emp. **51**, 181–197 (1944)
Moir, C., Russel, C.S.: An investigation of the effect of ergot alkaloids in promoting involution of the postpartum uterus. J. Obstet. Gynaec. Brit. Emp. **50**, 94–104 (1943)
Moir, J.C.: The obstetrician bids, and the uterus contracts. Brit. med. J. **2**, 1025–1029 (1964)
Müller, H.A., Ströker, W.: Studien über die Uterusmotilität. Die spontane Motilität in der Postplacentarperiode und Metherginwirkung. Arch. Gynäk. **191**, 369–376 (1959)
Myerscough, P.R., Schild, H.O.: Quantitative assays of oxytocic drugs on the human postpartum uterus. Brit. J. Pharmacol. **13**, 207–212 (1958)
Nelson, E.E., Calvery, H.O.: Present status of the ergot question. Physiol. Rev. **18**, 297–327 (1938)
Oettel, H., Bachmann, H.: Untersuchungen am puerperalen Säugeruterus über Hypophysin, Ergometrin und Mutterkornextrakte. Naunyn-Schmiedebergs Arch. exp. Path. Pharmak. **185**, 242–258 (1937)
Orth, O.S.: Studies of the sympathicolytic drug dihydroergotamine (D.H.E. 45). Fed. Proc. **5**, 196 (1946)
Orth, O.S., Ritchie, G.: A pharmacological evaluation of dihydroergotamine methanesulfonate (D.H.E. 45). J. Pharmacol. exp. Ther. **90**, 166–173 (1947)
Pennefather, J.N.: The estimation of ergometrine on the rat uterus. J. Pharm. Pharmacol. **13**, 60–61 (1961)
Pereira Martinez, A., Del Sol, J.R., Slocker, Castro, C.: Los alcaloides dihydrogenados del cornezuelo de centeno en obstetricia. Acta ginec. (Madr.) **1**, 7–18 (1954)
Reist, A.: Neuere Auffassungen über Wesen und Behandlung von geburtsstörenden Anomalien des Weichteilweges. In: Schweizerisches Medizinisches Jahrbuch, pp. XLI–LVII. Basel: Schwabe 1949
Reynolds, S.R.M., Harris, J.S., Kaiser, I.H.: Effects of adrenalin and noradrenalin on uterine contractions. In: Clinical Measurements of Uterine Forces in Pregnancy and Labor, p. 221. Springfield Ill.: Thomas 1954
Robson, J.M.: The reactivity and activity of the human uterus at various stages of pregnancy and at parturition. J. Physiol. (Lond.) **79**, 83–93 (1933)
Roth-Brandel, U., Bygdeman, M., Wiqvist, N.: A comparative study on the influence of prostaglandin E_1, oxytocin and ergometrin on the pregnant human uterus. Acta obstet. gynec. scand. **49** (Suppl. 5), 1–7 (1970)
Rothlin, E.: Über die pharmakologische und therapeutische Wirkung des Ergotamins auf den Sympathicus. Klin. Wschr. **30**, 1437–1443 (1925)
Rothlin, E.: Sur les propriétés pharmacologiques d'un nouvel alcaloïde de l'ergot de seigle, l'ergobasine. C.R. Soc. Biol. (Paris) **119**, 1302–1311 (1935a)

Rothlin, E.: Über ein neues Mutterkornalkaloid. Schweiz. med. Wschr. **65**, 947–949 (1935b)
Rothlin, E.: Beitrag zur differenzierenden Analyse der Mutterkornalkaloide. Schweiz. med. Wschr. **68**, 971–975 (1938a)
Rothlin, E.: Chemisch-pharmakologische Stellungnahme zum Mutterkornproblem. Arch. Gynäk. **166**, 88–105 (1938b)
Rothlin, E.: Zur Pharmakologie der hydrierten natürlichen Mutterkornalkaloide. Helv. physiol. pharmacol. Acta **2**, C48–C49 (1944)
Rothlin, E.: Zur Pharmakologie des Sympathicolyticums Dihydroergotamin DHE 45. Schweiz. med. Wschr. **76**, 1254–1259 (1946)
Rothlin, E.: The pharmacology of the natural and dihydrogenated alkaloids of ergot. Bull. schweiz. Akad. med. Wiss. **2**, 249–273 (1946/47)
Rothlin, E.: Pharmacology of lysergic acid diethylamide and some of its related compounds. J. Pharm. Pharmacol. **9**, 569–587 (1957)
Rothlin, E., Berde, B.: Über die Wirkung hydrierter Mutterkornalkaloide auf isolierte Muskelstreifen des menschlichen Uterus nahe am Termin, am Termin und während der Geburt. Helv. physiol. pharmacol. Acta **12**, 191–205 (1954)
Rothlin, E., Brügger, J.: Quantitative Untersuchungen der sympathikolytischen Wirkung genuiner Mutterkornalkaloide und derer Dihydroderivate am isolierten Uterus des Kaninchens. Helv. physiol. pharmacol. Acta **3**, 519–535 (1945)
Rudzik, A.D., Miller, J.W.: The mechanism of uterine inhibitory action of relaxin-containing ovarian extracts. J. Pharmacol. exp. Ther. **138**, 82–87 (1962)
Sandberg, F., Ingelman-Sundberg, A., Lindgren, L., Rydén, G.: Comparison of in vitro and in vivo effects of four synthetic oxytocics on pregnant human uterus. Arzneimittel-Forsch. **9**, 544–548 (1959)
Sandberg, F., Ingelman-Sundberg, A., Lindgren, L., Rydén, G.: The effect of oxytocin on the motility of different parts of the pregnant and non-pregnant human uterus in vitro as compared with other oxytocic drugs. In: Oxytocin. Caldeyro-Barcia, R., Heller, H. (eds.), pp. 295–312. Oxford: Pergamon Press 1961
Sauter, H.: Verwendung von Dihydroergotamin (DHE 45) in der Geburtshilfe. Schweiz. med. Wschr. **78**, 475–480 (1948)
Sauter, H.: Gefäßwirkung verschiedener Pharmaka, insbesondere von Adrenalin und der dihydrierten Secalealkaloide beim postpartalen menschlichen Uterus. Schweiz. med. Wschr. **79**, 572–576 (1949a)
Sauter, H.: Die konstriktorische Wirkung verschiedener Wehenmittel auf die Uterusgefäße. Gynaecologia (Basel) **127**, 302–324 (1949b)
Sauter, H.: Beziehungen zwischen Uterustonus und Uterusdurchblutung. Schweiz. med. Wschr. **80**, 1306–1309 (1950)
Schild, H.O.: The use of incomplete randomized blocks in an oxytocic assay. In: Quantitative Methods in Human Pharmacology and Therapeutics: Proceedings of a Symposium Held in London, March, 1958. Laurence, D.R. (ed.), pp. 154–159. London: Pergamon Press 1959
Schild, H.O., Fitzpatrick, R.J., Nixon, W.C.W.: Activity of the human cervic and corpus uteri. Lancet **1951 I**, 250–253
Shaaban, A.H., Youssef, A.F.: Effect of autonomic drugs on uterine action in labour. Gaz. Egypt. Soc. Gynaec. Obstet. **9**, 107–132 (1959)
Slaytor, M., Pennefather, J.N., Wright, S.E.: Metabolites of LSD and ergometrine. Experientia (Basel) **15**, 111 (1959)
Smith, R.G.: The present status of ergonovine. J. Amer. med. Ass. **111**, 2201–2209 (1938)
Smyth, C.N.: A comparison of the effects of oxytocin and ergometrine on the human uterus. In: Oxytocin. Caldeyro-Barcia, R., Heller, H. (eds.), pp. 281–294. Oxford: Pergamon Press 1961
Snow, R.H., Bruns, P.D., Drose, V.E.: Effect of hydergine (dihydrogenated ergot) on preeclampsia and uterine contractility. Amer. J. Obstet. Gynec. **70**, 302–307 (1955)
Stoll, A., Burckhardt, E.: L'ergobasine, un nouvel alcaloïde de l'ergot de seigle, soluble dans l'eau. C.R. Acad. Sci. (Paris) **200**, 1680–1682 (1935)
Stolte, L.A.M., Eskes, T.K.A.B., Seelen, J.C.: Uterine activity and adrenaline derivatives. Acta physiol. pharmacol. neerl. **12**, 179–180 (1963)

Stürmer, E., Flückiger, E.: In vivo smooth muscle stimulant activity of 2-bromo-α-ergokryptine mesylate (CB 154) as compared with that of ergotamine. IRCS med. Sci. **2**, 1591 (1974)
Sund, R.B.: On the actions of ergometrine on isolated rat uterus in absence and presence of magnesium ions. Medd. norske farm. Selsk. **25**, 89–96 (1963a)
Sund, R.B.: Assay of oxytocin in pharmaceutical solutions containing both oxytocin and ergometrine, by the isolated rat uterus method. Medd. norske farm. Selsk. **25**, 101–114 (1963b)
Swanson, E.E., Hargreaves, C.C.: The action of ergot and its alkaloids on the puerperal uteri of dogs. J. Amer. pharm. Ass. sci. Ed. **23**, 867–872 (1934)
Thompson, M.R.: Some properties of ergostetrine. J. Amer. pharm. Ass. **24**, 748–753 (1935)
Tothill, A.: Investigation of adrenaline reversal in the rat uterus by the induction of resistance to isoprenaline. Brit. J. Pharmacol. **29**, 291–301 (1967)
Tuck, V.L.: A clinical test of the newly recognized oxytocic principle of ergot and a new method of administration. Amer. J. Obstet. Gynecol. **5**, 718–723 (1935)
Venkatasubbu, V.S., Gopala Krishnamurthy, L.B.: Pharmacological and clinical evaluation of the action of hydrogenated ergot alkaloids on the uterus. Curr. Med. Pract. **3**, 629–638 (1959)
Vos, Jr., B.J.: Use of the latent period in the assay of ergonovine on the isolated rabbit uterus. J. Amer. pharm. Ass. sci. Ed. **32**, 138–141 (1943)
Votava, Z., Podvalova, I.: Pharmacological studies of ergometrine and methylergometrine. Acta pharmacol. (Kbh.) **13**, 309–318 (1957)
Wellhöner, H.-H.: Wirkung von Pharmaka auf die glatte Muskulatur der Scheide. Naunyn-Schmiedebergs Arch. exp. Path. Pharmak. **236**, 167 (1959a)
Wellhöner, H.-H.: Antagonistische Beeinflussung der Methylergobasinwirkung an Uterus und Vagina durch einige Sympathicolytika und Adrenolytika. Med. exp. (Basel) **1**, 138–145 (1959b)
Wilhelm, F.: Verwendungsmöglichkeiten des Hydergin in der Geburtshilfe. Klin. Med. (Wien) **6**, 414–421 (1951)
Wiqvist, N.: Desensitizing effect of exo- and endogenous relaxin on the immediate uterine response to relaxin. Acta endocr. (Kbh.) **46** (Suppl.), 3–14 (1959)

CHAPTER V

Actions on the Heart and Circulation

BARBARA J. CLARK, D. CHU, and W.H. AELLIG

A. Actions on Systemic Blood Pressure

1. Nature of the Effect

a) Peptide Alkaloids

Numerous publications have confirmed DALE's initial observation that the effect of ergotoxine on blood pressure in normotensive or spinal animals is universally pressor (DALE, 1906; BARGER and DALE, 1907). The substance is considerably more potent than might appear from the experiments of early workers, who consistently used doses which must be regarded as toxic. A marked pressor effect can be obtained in the anesthetised cat with an intravenous dose as low as 50 µg/kg (LANDS et al., 1950). Blood pressure increases in response to each of the components of ergotoxine (23, 24, 25, 26)* (ROTHLIN, 1946; SCHLIENTZ et al., 1968).

Pressor activity is a property shared by ergotamine (20) (ROTHLIN, 1923). Threshold effects can be obtained in the dog from an intravenous dose of 1 µg/kg (SAXENA, 1974). The effect following a dose of 50 µg/kg in the cat is relatively short, lasting only 10–15 min, although the rise in pressure may be as great as 120 mmHg. The brevity of the response is of interest in that associated increases in tone in the nictitating membrane persist for up to 3 h (INNES, 1962). In the dog, cat, and fowl, tachyphylaxis occurs. Responses to successive doses diminish both in magnitude and duration until the response is finally depressor (ROTHLIN, 1923; HARVEY et al., 1954; INNES, 1962). The nature of the primary response to ergotamine is largely dependent upon pre-existing blood pressure levels. In rats with renal hypertension (VAN PROOSDIJ-HARTZEMA and DE JONGH, 1955) and in dogs with neurogenic hypertension (HEYMANS and BOUCKAERT, 1933; KRAUSE et al., 1971), blood pressure is depressed. Increases and decreases in blood pressure also occur in response to ergotamine in man. Normotensive subjects respond to parenteral administration of 0.25–0.5 mg with increases in systolic and diastolic pressure of up to 20 mmHg lasting approximately 1 h (POOL et al., 1936; LENNOX, 1938; STEINMANN et al., 1948), whereas reductions occur in hypertensive patients (BARÁTH, 1926; IMMERWAHR, 1927; LENNOX, 1938).

b) Derivatives of Peptide Alkaloids

Reduction of the double bond at position 9,10 in the lysergic acid moiety of the peptide alkaloids to yield the corresponding 9,10-dihydro derivatives results

* The numbers in brackets refer to specific compounds described in Chapter II.

in compounds which differ considerably in pharmacologic activity from the natural alkaloids. Vasoconstrictor and uterotonic actions and interference with blood pressure control mechanisms are greatly attenuated, whereas antagonism at α-adrenoceptor sites is enhanced.

The effects of dihydroergotamine (102b) on blood pressure in normotensive animals vary from one laboratory to another, depending neither on species, dose, nor anesthetic used. Like ergotamine, dihydroergotamine may induce pressor responses, transient at doses below 50 μg/kg (de Vleeschhower, 1949), but long-lasting at higher doses, sometimes followed by a prolonged reduction in pressure (Schmitt and Fenard, 1970; Schmitt et al., 1971). Hypotensive effects in the absence of an initial pressor response have also been reported (Rothlin, 1946; Logaras, 1947; Fahim et al., 1974; Schmitt, 1958), which are particularly pronounced in hypertensive animals (van Proosdij-Hartzema and de Jongh, 1955; Ripa et al., 1967). Such effects are not observed in man. Blood pressure usually rises in response to dihydroergotamine in both normotensive and hypertensive subjects (Werkö and Lagerlöf, 1949; Hammerschmidt and Odenthal, 1950; Mellander and Nordenfelt, 1970; Ulrich and Siggaard-Andersen, 1971; Echt and Lange, 1974; Boismare et al., 1975a; Lohmann et al., 1975). Increases, when they occur, do not exceed 15 mmHg.

Dihydroergocornine (102d), dihydroergocristine (102c), dihydroergokryptine (102e, f) alone or in combination (dihydroergotoxine) evoke depressor effects more consistently in experimental animals than does dihydroergotamine (Rothlin, 1946; Bluntschli et al., 1949; Bálint, 1965; Lockett and Wadley, 1969; Rothman and Drury, 1957). A pronounced fall in blood pressure (−30 mmHg) lasting for more than 2 h has been obtained with an intravenous dose of only 5 μg/kg of dihydroergotoxine in the anesthetized cat (Bircher and Cerletti, 1949). The response is reversed to pressor if small doses are repeated (Taeschler et al., 1952) or high doses are given (Sherif et al., 1956; Schmitt and Fenard, 1970; Schmitt et al., 1971). In hypertensive animals, the effect of dihydroergotoxine is depressor at both low and high doses (Oyen, 1956; Rothlin et al., 1956; Taeschler, 1965), but tachyphylaxis occurs when a very high dose (1 mg/kg) is given over a period of several days (Taeschler, 1965).

Unlike dihydroergotamine, dihydroergotoxine and its components exert long-lasting (3–5 h) depressor effects in man, in both normotensive and hypertensive subjects. The magnitude of the response depends largely on pre-existing blood pressure (Goetz, 1949; Kappert, 1949b; Barcroft et al., 1951; Duret, 1951; Heimdal and Nordenfelt, 1953; McCall et al., 1953; Marques and Rato, 1954; Sherif et al., 1956). The effects of the individual components of dihydroergotoxine do not differ greatly one from another (Kappert, 1949b). A comparison of reductions in systolic pressure produced by an intravenous dose of 0.5 mg of each component and 0.3 mg dihydroergotamine showed the following order of efficacy: dihydroergotoxine = dihydroergocornine > dihydroergocristine > dihydroergokryptine. Kappert compared the hypotensive effects of a single intravenous dose of dihydroergocornine in healthy individuals and patients with either essential or renal hypertension. The greatest effect was observed in the latter, but he also observed that initial blood pressure was considerably higher in this group than in the patients with essential hypertension. He suggested that the intensity of the response to the drug in hypertensive patients is dependent on the initial level of blood pressure rather than on the nature of the disease. This supposition is doubtful in the light of results obtained by SHERIF et al. (1956) with dihydroergotoxine. In accordance with KAPPERT's findings, blood pressure reductions in response to the drug in patients with renal hypertension exceeded those in patients with essential hypertension. In this study, however, initial blood pressures were lower in the renal than in the essential hypertension group. Not only was the mean blood pressure fall in the renal hypertensive patients more pronounced, but the response was somewhat longer in duration. One possible explanation is that elimination of the drug might be delayed in patients with impaired renal function. This is unlikely, since urinary excretion of peptide ergot alkaloids after intravenous administration is only about 10%; excretion in the bile is the most important route of elimination (NIMMERFALL and ROSENTHALER, 1976; AELLIG and NÜESCH, 1977). An alternative explanation is that dihydroergotoxine increases renal plasma flow and sodium excretion, and this might enhance its antihypertensive effect in patients with renal disease (DEUTSCH and MARKOFF, 1953; LASCH, 1954; HANDLEY and MOYER, 1954; MOYER et al., 1955).

A bromine atom in position 2 of the lysergic acid moiety as in α-ergokryptine (2-bromo-α-ergokryptine; bromocriptine) (38) leads to a fundamental change in biological activity. The major effect of bromocriptine on the cardiovascular system and in the central nervous system is stimulation of dopamine receptors. Long-lasting, dose-dependent reductions in blood pressure are obtained in anesthetized dogs from a dose of 6 μg/kg given intravenously, but at high doses, the depressor effect diminishes (CLARK, 1977). Postural falls in blood pressure have been reported in patients undergoing therapy with high doses (30–50 mg daily) of the drug for Parkinson's disease or acromegaly (THORNER et al., 1975; TEYCHENNE et al., 1975; GREENACRE et al., 1976). Reports have appeared indicating that the drug may lower blood pressure in hypertensive patients (KAYE et al., 1976; STUMPE et al., 1977).

c) Simple Amides of Lysergic Acid and Their Derivatives

The activity spectrum of the naturally-occurring alkaloid ergometrine is quite different from that of the peptide alkaloids. It exerts practically no α-adrenoceptor blocking activity but retains considerable blocking activity at 5-HT receptor sites. Its predominant effect is to stimulate uterine contractions and for this reason, it is used exclusively in obstetrics. Ergometrine (19) has minimal effects on the cardiovascular system. In the dog and cat, small doses (0.5–2 mg) induce slight increases or no change in blood pressure, but at higher doses the effect is depressor (DAVIS et al., 1935; GLÄSSER, 1961; BELL et al., 1974). When the *L*-2-aminopropanol side chain of ergometrine is replaced by an *L*-2-aminobutanol residue (methylergometrine) (73a), oxytocic activity is retained, but a further loss in activity on the cardiovascular system in animals occurs (DAVID and KIRCHOF, 1947). Comparisons between the effects of parenteral administration of methylergometrine and ergometrine (0.2 mg i.v.) in obstetric patients have produced equivocal results. In studies comprising 200 patients for each drug, increases in blood pressure of more than

20 mm Hg were recorded in 10–15% of patients receiving methylergometrine compared with 30% of the patients given ergometrine (SCHADE, 1951; LAKE, 1954). On the other hand, other investigators have found no significant alterations in systolic or diastolic pressure with either drug (FITZGERALD, 1956; LIPTON et al., 1960).

When the hydrogen atom on the indole nitrogen of non-peptide ergot compounds is replaced by a methyl group, 5-HT antagonistic activity predominates. One of the most potent 5-HT antagonists is 1-methyl-lysergic acid *L*-butanolamide (methysergide) (34a). Some workers have reported prolonged reductions in blood pressure in the anesthetized cat or monkey in response to low doses (from 50 μg/kg) (FANCHAMPS et al., 1960; KARLSBERG et al., 1963). Others have been unable to reproduce such an effect in the cat, dog, sheep, monkey, or man (HALMÁGYI and COLEBATCH, 1961; DALESSIO, 1963; SAXENA, 1972, 1974; ANTONACCIO et al., 1975; SPIRA et al., 1976). Doses of methysergide in excess of 1 mg/kg are, however, clearly depressor both in dogs and hypertensive rats (ANTONACCIO et al., 1975; ANTONACCIO and COTÉ, 1976).

D-Lysergic acid diethylamide (*d*-LSD) (73b), which differs from ergometrine only in having a diethylamide instead of an isopropanolamide side chain, induces prolonged hypotension in the anesthetized cat and dog (CERLETTI and ROTHLIN, 1955; SHAW and WOOLLEY, 1956; ROTHLIN, 1957; GINZEL, 1958; TAUBERGER and KLIMMER, 1968), sometimes preceded by a transient pressor effect (SHAW and WOOLLEY, 1956). In the fowl (BUÑAG and WALASZEK, 1962), the rat (SALMOIRAGHI et al., 1957; SUGAAR et al., 1961) and in man (GRAHAM and KHALIDI, 1954; SOKOLOFF et al., 1956), the effect is pressor. The compound does not always lower blood pressure in hypertensive animals, although it may induce quite dramatic falls at very high doses (SALMOIRAGHI et al., 1957; SUGAAR et al., 1961). *D*-Lysergic acid methylcarbinolamide (12), one of the active principles present in the seeds of *rivea* and a strain of *Claviceps paspali, corymbosa* (ololiuqui), is structurally related to *d*-LSD. The slight difference in structure is responsible for qualitative and quantitative differences in activity. It has only weak hallucinogenic activity (HOFMANN, 1972) and unlike *d*-LSD exerts an oxytocic effect on the uterus equivalent to that of ergometrine (GLÄSSER, 1961). Although the compound has negligible effects on blood pressure in the rabbit, it induces sustained hypotension in the cat at high doses (GLÄSSER, 1961).

d) Other Derivatives

α) Derivatives of 10-Methoxyergoline

A number of nicotinic esters of 1-methyl-10α-ethoxydihydrolysergol bearing various substituents in the pyridine nucleus are potent blocking agents at α-adrenoceptor and 5-HT receptor sites. Nicergoline (1-methyl-10α-methoxydihydrolysergol 5-bromo-nicotinate) (104e), although approximately 10 times more active in inhibiting responses to adrenaline than dihydroergotoxine in vitro, has only moderate depressor activity in anesthetized animals. In conscious animals, blood pressure is not influenced at all at doses up to 600 μg/kg i.v. (ARCARI et al., 1968, 1972).

β) Urea Derivatives of 8 β-Aminomethyl-6-methyl-ergolene

These compounds are effective in reducing blood pressure in hypertensive rats. Of a series of 28 derivatives, 19 induced significant reductions in blood pressure. The most potent was 1,1-dimethyl-3-[6-methyl-8β-(9-ergolenyl)-methyl] urea (88h). Blood pressure was still depressed after 24 h after a dose of 50 μg/kg s.c. (FEHR et al., 1974).

2. Effects on Blood Pressure Control Mechanisms

a) Natural Ergot Alkaloids

Evidence that ergot alkaloids may influence the function of certain regions in the central nervous system concerned with the control of blood pressure was first provided by ROTHLIN's experiments with ergotamine in anesthetized rabbits and cats (ROTHLIN, 1923, 1925). He showed that this compound, while augmenting depressor responses to stimulation of the peripheral vagus, inhibited or abolished reductions in blood pressure resulting from stimulation of the central end of the vagus. The possibility that this inhibitory effect could be interpreted as evidence for an action within the central nervous system was dismissed. Later, GANTER (1926) demonstrated that small doses of ergotamine inhibited pressor responses to bilateral occlusion of the common carotid arteries, asphyxia, and hypercapnea. These effects were all considered to be due to peripheral blockade of excitatory sympathetic nerve impulses.

α) Baroreceptor Reflexes

The concept of a central action being at least in part responsible for the actions of ergotamine on sinus baroreceptor reflexes was introduced by HEYMANS and REGNIERS (1929). Ergotamine was shown to inhibit depressor responses to mechanical and electrical stimulation of the carotid sinus region and pressor responses to carotid occlusion in the cat. In the dog, reflexes elicited in response to raising or lowering pressure in an isolated sinus were also inhibited, ruling out an effect of the drug at the sinus itself. Although it seemed that the inhibitory effect of ergotamine on reflex depressor responses must occur within the central nervous system, the mechanism underlying the effect of the drug on pressor responses was less clear. A peripheral effect on α-adrenoceptors in vascular smooth muscle could not be discounted since the dose used (0.25 mg/kg i.v.) also inhibited the pressor response to adrenaline. Nevertheless, the response to carotid occlusion could be abolished by a large dose of ergotamine (1 mg) injected into the cerebral ventricles, suggesting that a central action might also be involved (HEYMANS et al., 1930). Doubt was cast on the relevance of this latter finding in the light of experiments using a technique whereby the head of a dog was perfused with blood from a donor dog. The cephalic ends of the common carotid arteries and jugular veins of the recipient dog were anastomosed with the cardiac ends of the corresponding vessels of the donor dog. The head of the recipient was connected to its trunk by the spinal cord alone. Injections of ergotamine (0.25 mg/kg) into the cephalic circulation of the recipient dog had only a moderate inhibitory effect on the sinus vasomotor reflex (relayed via the vasomotor center and spinal cord to the trunk). Conversely, the same dose injected into the circulation of the trunk abolished the reflex. As in their earlier experiments, the dose of ergotamine used also abolished the pressor response to adrenaline but not that to cerebral hypoxia (HEYMANS et al., 1930).

VON EULER and SCHMITERLÖW (1944) observed that a small rise in blood pressure often occurs during occlusion of the carotid arteries in the presence of ergotamine. It might be argued that this effect is due to incomplete inhibition of the sinus baroreceptor reflex by the dose of ergotamine used. This is not the case, however, since it was shown that the effect completely disappears (except for the mechanical blood pressure rise) when the animal is allowed to breathe oxygen (Fig. 1). Whether or not an occlusion pressor effect occurs after ergotamine during ventilation with air depends on the adequacy of ventilation and the level of systemic blood pressure. This may well explain the discordance between the findings of HEYMANS et al. (1930) and KRAUSE (1954). KRAUSE used the same cross-perfusion technique as the former authors and obtained conclusive evidence that the action of ergotamine on sinus baroreceptor reflexes was entirely central. Injections of smaller doses of ergotamine than those used by HEYMANS and his colleagues into the perfused cerebral circulation of the recipient dog not only abolished baroreceptor reflexes, but also lowered blood pressure. Injections into the trunk induced only minor changes in responses to raising or lowering pressure in the carotid sinus and tended to potentiate pressor responses to catecholamines. SCHMITT (1958) obtained similar results in intact dogs.

The conclusion drawn by HEYMANS et al. that inhibition of pressor responses to carotid occlusion by ergotamine was due to a peripheral block of α-adrenoceptors was based on the fact that ergotamine (0.25 mg/kg) abolished adrenaline-induced blood pressure rises. SCHMITT (1958) on the other hand found that a dose of 0.5 mg/kg potentiated the effects of both adrenaline and noradrenaline. GERNANDT and ZOTTERMAN (1946) showed that inhibition of pressor responses to injected adrenaline and endogenous catecholamines released by splanchnic nerve stimulation occurred simultaneously, and that a very large dose (2 mg/kg) was necessary to abolish responses to both stimuli. The minimum effective doses inhibiting sino-aortic reflexes in cats and dogs lie between 0.01 and 0.05 mg/kg i.v. (HEYMANS et al., 1930; WRIGHT, 1930; VON EULER and SCHMITERLÖW, 1944; SUTTON et al., 1950; KRAUSE et al., 1971). Since these doses do not inhibit pressor responses to injected catecholamines, an effect of ergotamine at some site within the reflex arc other than the effector cell must be invoked.

The elegant experiments of WRIGHT (1930) on the effects of ergotamine on sino-aortic reflex mechanisms in cats deserve particular attention. His findings demonstrated clearly that the effects of the alkaloid are due almost entirely to an action within the central nervous system. Intravenous administration of doses of ergotamine as small as 0.01 mg/kg decreased the magnitude of the fall in blood pressure in response to stimulation of the central end of the cut vagus. Pressor reflexes to bilateral carotid occlusion and afferent (peroneal) nerve trunk stimulation were inhibited at higher doses (from 0.1 mg/kg). He ruled out the possibility of peripheral blockade of the stimulant effects of endogenous catecholamines by showing that splanchnic nerve stimulation and acute cerebral ischemia (produced by compressing carotid and vertebral arteries) still produced marked increases in blood pressure. The possibility that ergotamine had interfered with nerve conduction was also excluded by showing that neither apnea nor bradycardia elicited by central vagal stimulation, nor flexor and crossed extensor reflexes in decerebrate animals were inhibited following doses which depressed pressor reflexes. WRIGHT proposed that ergotamine inhibited pressor reflexes by blocking central transmission of excitatory impulses in the neighborhood of the termination of the afferent side of the reflex arc, since he had demonstrated the integrity of the efferent limb of the reflex arc. He considered that the inhibitory action of ergotamine on depressor responses could be accounted for by assuming that ergotamine either depressed the formation of a central inhibitory agent, or altered the cell membrane in such a manner as to prevent access of the inhibitory agent.

β) Chemoreceptor Reflexes

Two factors are responsible for the rise in blood pressure following occlusion of the common carotid arteries. One is a reduction in baroreceptor impulses, resulting from reduced pressure in the sinus region. The vasomotor centers, normally inhibited by baroreceptor impulse traffic, escape this inhibition and as a result, efferent nerve activity is increased. The second factor is an increase in chemoreceptor impulse activity resulting from the hypoxic condition which develops within the carotid body when blood flow is reduced by clamping. In an adequately ventilated animal, the chemoreceptor component of the blood pressure rise is rather small (EYZAGUIRRE and LEWIN, 1961) and can be eliminated completely by ventilating with pure oxygen (VON EULER and LILJESTRAND, 1943; LANDGREN and NEIL, 1951). If the oxygen content in the inspired air is reduced, the chemoreceptor component of the carotid occlusion response is greatly exaggerated (von EULER and LILJESTRAND, 1943).

Hypoxia

VON EULER and SCHMITERLÖW (1944) found that under hypoxic conditions the inhibitory effect of ergotamine on the response to carotid occlusion in the cat appeared very weak (Fig. 1). When the ventilation mixture was replaced by pure oxygen, however, the response was completely eliminated. This strongly suggested that ergotamine selectively blocked baroreceptor mechanisms, leaving chemoreceptor mechanisms intact.

Not only does ergotamine fail to block the pressor effects of local hypoxia in the carotid sinus region, but it also has no inhibitory effect on the blood pressure rise induced by oxygen lack (VON EULER and LILJESTRAND, 1946; SUTTON et al., 1950). Acute hypoxia in the cat causes a rise in blood pressure which is almost entirely due to chemoreceptor stimulation (BOUCKAERT et al., 1941). The pressor response to hypoxia is greatly enhanced after selective denervation of the baroreceptors, but is reversed to a fall after complete denervation of the reflexogenic zones. At doses up to 0.2 mg/kg, ergotamine produces what can be regarded as selective baroreceptor denervation. The normal compensatory mecha-

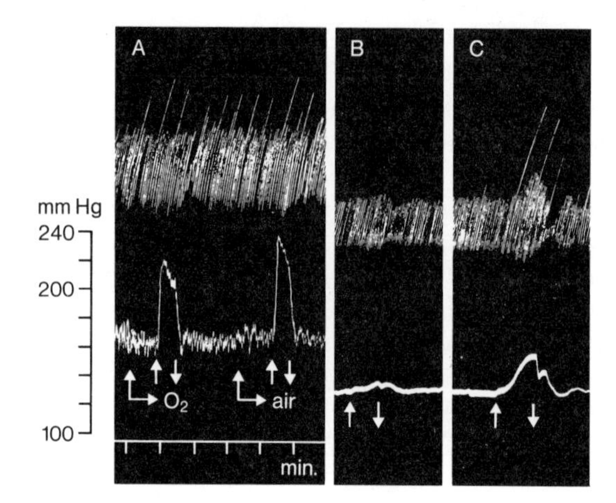

Fig. 1 A–C. Effects of ergotamine on the pressor response to carotid occlusion in the anesthetized cat (chloralose). Upper curve respiration, lower curve blood pressure. A. Occlusion during ventilation with oxygen (1st response) and air (2nd response). B and C. Occlusion during ventilation with oxygen (B) and air (C) after intravenous administration of ergotamine 0.1 mg/kg (VON EULER and SCHMITERLÖW, 1944)

nism which minimizes the effects of oxygen want on blood pressure is removed by the drug, and the blood pressure rise is accentuated (VON EULER and LILJESTRAND, 1946).

MARSH and VAN LIERE (1948) showed that a reversal of hypoxia-induced rises in blood pressure could be obtained with a high dose of ergotamine (1 mg/kg), although the response to adrenaline and ephedrine remained pressor. This was in contrast to the results they obtained with the α-adrenoceptor blocking drugs yohimbine, piperoxan (933 F), and α-naphthylmethyl-β-chloroethylamine hydrochloride (SY-14) which blocked pressor responses to adrenaline at doses equal to or less than those found necessary to reverse responses to hypoxia.

Chemical Stimulation of Chemoreceptors

Reflex respiratory and vasomotor responses to stimulation of chemoreceptors by potassium cyanide and nicotine (HEYMANS et al., 1931; HEYMANS et al., 1932b) are also not suppressed by doses of ergotamine up to 0.1 mg/kg despite the fact that these doses abolish reflexes evoked by pressure changes in the sinus (VON EULER and SCHMITERLÖW, 1944; SUTTON et al., 1950). As in hypoxia, it is possible to reduce the reflex response to these agents using higher doses of ergotamine before any blocking effect on the action of adrenaline can be demonstrated (VON EULER and SCHMITERLÖW, 1944).

Carbon Dioxide Accumulation

In contrast to its lack of effect in hypoxia, ergotamine causes a profound change in the vasomotor responses to asphyxia, hypoventilation, and inhalation of carbon dioxide, the normal rise in blood pressure being replaced by a marked reduction

(GANTER, 1926; KOHN, 1932; HEYMANS and BOUCKAERT, 1933; VON EULER and LILJESTRAND, 1946; GERNANDT and ZOTTERMANN, 1946; VON EULER and HESSER, 1947; LILJESTRAND, 1948).

Carbon dioxide, like hypoxia, also stimulates chemoreceptors but, unlike hypoxia, also has a direct influence on central nervous structures which contributes to the blood pressure rise. If normal blood pressure regulation is eliminated by total sympathectomy or destruction of the spinal cord, carbon dioxide induces an appreciable fall in pressure (BACQ et al., 1934, 1939; VON EULER and LILJESTRAND, 1946). This is due to an unmasking of its local vasodilator action (LILJESTRAND, 1948). Relatively low tensions of carbon dioxide in the intact animal cause a decrease in blood pressure, which is accentuated in animals in which sinus and vagus nerves have been cut. Higher carbon dioxide tensions cause an increase. In the former case, the peripheral effect predominates; in the latter, the central effect is dominant (VON EULER and LILJESTRAND, 1946).

VON EULER and LILJESTRAND (1946) found that the reductions in blood pressure induced by inhalation of increasing concentrations of carbon dioxide in the inhaled gas mixture were considerably greater after administration of a small dose of ergotamine than the reductions observed after denervating baroreceptors and chemoreceptors. An even greater blood pressure fall occurred after ergotamine administration in debuffered animals, which suggested that ergotamine was not blocking that part of the pressor response which runs over the chemoreceptor reflex arc. The main action of ergotamine in hypercapnea is therefore that of blocking the vasomotor center to the action of carbon dioxide, which then exerts its local vasodilating action revealed by a fall in blood pressure. It is noteworthy that in these experiments, although the stimulating effect of carbon dioxide on blood pressure was abolished, the effect of oxygen lack was still present. An additional observation of some interest is that although ergotamine does not affect the respiratory response to hypoxia or potassium cyanide, it clearly diminishes the respiratory response to carbon dioxide (LILJESTRAND, 1948). This further emphasises that ergotamine acts on the central nervous system in a very selective way.

Asphyxia

In asphyxia, oxygen lack is combined with carbon dioxide accumulation and antagonistic factors come into play. Stimulation of sino-aortic chemoreceptors by hypoxia and carbon dioxide and stimulation of the vasomotor center by carbon dioxide will both result in an increase in pressure. The local vasodilator effect of carbon dioxide will tend to diminish or overcome the pressor effect. The net result may be little change (LILJESTRAND, 1948) or a rise in blood pressure accompanied by a gradual increase in the efferent discharge of action potentials in the splanchnic nerve (GERNANDT et al., 1946).

GERNANDT and ZOTTERMAN (1946) found that ergotamine (0.05–0.1 mg/kg) reversed the rise in blood pressure due to asphyxia to a fall but did not diminish and sometimes even accentuated splanchnic nerve activity. For the latter they could find no satisfactory explanation and assumed a peripheral block of α-adrenoceptors. According to LILJESTRAND (1948), the importance of the splanchnic nerves in the regulation of blood pressure in hypercapnea should not be overestimated.

Table 1. Blood pressure changes in response to stimulation of baroreceptors and chemoreceptors in anesthetized cats. ↑=rise, ↓=fall, ↔=no change in blood pressure

Stimulus	Sino-aortic receptors involved	Intact animals	Denervation of reflexogenic zones	Destruction of brain and spinal cord	Pretreatment with ergotamine (0.05–0.2 mg/kg i.v.)	Reference
Carotid occlusion	Baroreceptors	↑	↔		↔	1
Potassium cyanide	Chemoreceptors	↑	↔		↑	1
Hypoxia (<20% oxygen)	Mostly chemoreceptors	↑	↓	↓	↑	2
Hypercapnea (>20% CO_2)	Chemoreceptors	↑	↑	↓	↓	2
Asphyxia (hypoxia + hypercapnea	Mostly chemoreceptors	↑			↓	3

References: 1. VON EULER and SCHMITTERLÖW (1944); 2. VON EULER and LILJESTRAND (1946); 3. GERNANDT and ZOTTERMAN (1946).

He showed that severing the splanchnics does not significantly alter the blood pressure changes due to asphyxia or inhalation of carbon dioxide. If carbon dioxide causes a fall in blood pressure, the fall is accentuated by ergotamine. This is so regardless of whether the splanchnic nerves are intact or not. The increased splanchnic nerve discharge seen in the experiments of GERNANDT and ZOTTERMAN was probably the result of chemoreceptor stimulation by hypoxia and carbon dioxide which was not blocked by ergotamine. The local effect of carbon dioxide on vascular smooth muscle, exerted in the absence of an opposing central effect, was sufficient to overcome the effect of increased sympathetic nerve activity.

The effects of ergotamine on central blood pressure control mechanisms are summarized in Table 1.

b) Hydrogenated Ergot Alkaloids

There is no evidence that dihydroergotamine possesses inhibitory effects of any significance on baroreceptor or chemoreceptor reflex mechanisms at intravenous doses below those which inhibit pressor responses to injected adrenaline (VON EULER and HESSER, 1947; DE VLEESCHHOUWER, 1949; SUTTON et al., 1950; SCHMITT, 1958). Although increases in systemic blood pressure due to decreased intrasinusal pressure may be inhibited, depressor responses to raised intrasinusal pressure are potentiated (VON EULER and HESSER, 1947). It is of interest that a dose of 50 µg/kg of dihydroergotamine, which reverses adrenaline responses, does not influence reflex increases in blood pressure; doses at least three times greater are required to obtain an inhibitory effect (VON EULER and HESSER, 1947; DE VLEESCHHOUWER,

1949). Administration of dihydroergotamine into the cerebral ventricles inhibits responses to chemoreceptor stimulation (GINZEL, 1958) and electrical stimulation of pressor areas in the hypothalamus and medulla (SCHMITT and SCHMITT, 1964) but fails to influence baroreceptor reflexes (SCHMITT and SCHMITT, 1960).

Hydrogenation of ergotamine, therefore, has resulted not only in a reduction in vasoconstrictor activity but also in a significant reduction in ability to inhibit blood pressure control mechanisms. A similar loss of potency is seen in the hydrogenated forms of two of the components of ergotoxine, i.e., dihydroergokryptine and dihydroergocornine. Dihydroergocristine appears to represent an exception. Substantial inhibition of pressor responses to carotid occlusion can be obtained with both the natural and the hydrogenated forms at doses below 10 μg/kg i.v. in the absence of evidence of α-adrenoceptor blockade (PROCHNIK et al., 1950; SUTTON et al., 1950; KRAUSE et al., 1971). The mixture of all three compounds, i.e., dihydroergotoxine, exerts a demonstrable depression of blood pressure regulatory mechanisms when injected directly into the cerebral circulation or into the cerebral ventricles (KRAUSE, 1954; SHARE, 1973; TADEPALLI et al., 1976). Results obtained using the intravenous route are equivocal; doses which inhibit the response to carotid occlusion invariably exert a blocking action on peripheral α-adrenoceptors (KRAUSE, 1954; SUTTON et al., 1950; SCHMITT, 1958; KRAUSE et al., 1971). All the dihydro ergot alkaloids have been shown to lower blood pressure in normotensive animals. It is not always appreciated that any influence, whether chemical or physical, which lowers blood pressure will, of necessity, reduce the response to carotid occlusion (see HEYMANS and NEIL, 1958).

c) Lysergic Acid Derivatives

D-LSD, like ergotamine, inhibits pressor responses to carotid occlusion. A fundamental difference between the two compounds, however, lies in the fact that the action of *d*-LSD appears to be mainly confined to an action on the chemoreceptor component of the reflex in contrast to ergotamine which predominantly affects the baroreceptor component (GINZEL, 1958).

GINZEL showed that intracerebroventricular (50–200 μg) or intravenous (50–100 μg/kg) administration of *d*-LSD in anesthetised cats abolished the difference in the magnitude of the blood pressure increases in response to carotid occlusion during ventilation with air and with oxygen (Fig. 2). The difference is a measure of the extent to which chemoreceptor stimulation contributes to the response at the time (LANDGREN and NEIL, 1951). In accordance with the finding of VON EULER and SCHMITERLÖW (1944), the pressor response to occlusion remaining after elimination of the chemoreceptor component by *d*-LSD disappeared when ergotamine was given. Unlike ergotamine, *d*-LSD also inhibits chemoreceptor pressor reflexes elicited by potassium cyanide, sebacinyl-bis-choline (Fig. 2), asphyxia, and selective stimulation of sinus nerve chemoreceptor fibers but fails to inhibit depressor responses to stimulation of baroreceptor fibers (GINZEL, 1958). In view of the latter, it is probable that depression in the response to carotid occlusion sometimes observed following *d*-LSD administration in animals in which the chemoreceptor component of the response has been eliminated by ventilating with oxygen resulted from a reduction in blood pressure rather than an inhibitory

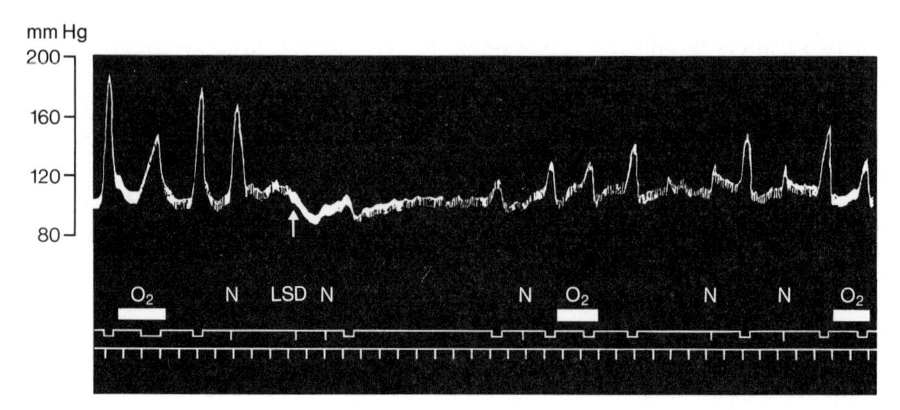

Fig. 2. Effects of *d*-LSD on blood pressure responses to chemoreceptor stimulation in the anesthetized cat (chloralose). White bars indicate ventilation with oxygen (O_2). Long signal indicates carotid occlusion; brief signal indicates injections of 10 µg sebacinyl-bis-choline (N) into the lingual artery or 200 µg of *d*-LSD into the lateral ventricle. Time, 30 sec (GINZEL, 1958)

effect of the drug itself on the baroreceptor reflex (WEIDMANN and CERLETTI, 1958; GINZEL, 1958). No reduction in the effects of adrenaline or noradrenaline was observed during the chemoreceptor reflex blockade induced by *d*-LSD, neither was the response of the nictitating membrane to preganglionic nerve stimulation affected. From these findings, it was concluded that *d*-LSD did not block impulse transmission through junctional regions within the peripheral efferent pathway of the reflex.

GINZEL considered the possibility that the central blocking effect of *d*-LSD on chemoreceptor reflexes might be correlated with the psychotropic activity of the compound. No correlation could be established. Lysergic acid pyrrolidide (73f) is equiactive with *d*-LSD, and 2-bromo-LSD (37a) half as active in blocking the reflexes, but neither have psychotropic activity (CERLETTI and ROTHLIN, 1955; SANKAR, 1975). Lysergic acid monoethylamide (73h) on the other hand, which has one tenth of the psychotropic activity of *d*-LSD (CERLETTI, 1956), is 2–5 times more active than *d*-LSD in blocking chemoreceptor reflexes; 1-acetyl LSD (36f), which has psychotropic activity equivalent to that of *d*-LSD (SANKAR, 1975), is inactive.

Methysergide (1-methyl-lysergic acid *L*-2-butanolamide) has been shown to inhibit pressor responses to carotid occlusion (FANCHAMPS et al., 1960; DALESSIO, 1963; SAXENA, 1974) and stimulation of the hypothalamic pressor area (DALESSIO, 1963), but no detailed analysis of its action on blood pressure control mechanisms has been undertaken.

The contrasting results obtained with *d*-LSD and ergotamine are of particular interest in that they demonstrate that two members of one chemical group can distinguish by their actions between two pathways concerned in blood pressure control mechanisms, namely, those derived from baroreceptors and chemoreceptors. The fact that *d*-LSD does not block the respiratory chemoreceptor reflex evoked by cyanide and nicotine also implies a pharmacologic differentiation between two centers within the central nervous system (respiratory and vasomotor) receiving afferent impulses from sino-aortic chemoreceptors.

d) Effects on Cardiovascular Reflexes in Man

α) *Pressor Reflexes*

The reflex rise in blood pressure which occurs when an extremity is immersed in cold water (cold pressor test) or during the Valsalva maneuver is inhibited by dihydroergotoxine and dihydroergocornine but not by ergotamine or dihydroergotamine (Kappert, 1949a; Athanasiou, 1949; Freis et al., 1949; Duret, 1951; Niesel et al., 1953, Pichler et al., 1956). However, inhibitory effects occur at doses which exert substantial α-adrenoceptor blockade, from which it must be concluded that they are most likely due to a peripheral rather than a central action (Kappert, 1949a; Duret, 1951). On the other hand, the response to the cold pressor test is progressively diminished with time in patients under treatment with methysergide. This drug, unlike the dihydro ergot alkaloids, enhances the pressor response to noradrenaline. The inhibitory effect, therefore, must be attributed to a central block of a reflex vasomotor mechanism (Dalessio, 1963).

β) *Depressor reflexes*

Congestion of a limb by means of a proximally applied occlusion cuff produces a fall in blood pressure in hypertensive patients. After administration of dihydroergocornine, which itself reduces blood pressure, limb congestion can lead to circulatory collapse. Freis et al. (1951) showed that this was not due to excessive blood pooling (measured plethysmographically and by dye injections) and considered it due to a failure of a compensatory reflex vasoconstrictor mechanism. In this study also, a peripheral block of α-adrenoceptors cannot be excluded.

In patients with hypertension and in particular those with primary arteriosclerosis without hypertension, firm pressure over the carotid sinus may give rise to a profound fall in pressure and/or bradycardia. Hyper-reactive patients may complain of spontaneous attacks of dizziness and fainting. Sinus compression in these patients can induce partial or complete heart block. This type of reaction is termed the "carotid sinus syndrome". Both dihydroergotamine and dihydroergotoxine enhance the carotid sinus reflex in patients with the cardiac form of the carotid sinus syndrome; only heart rate responses were reported (Franke, 1950). The degree of cardiac slowing which occurred during compression of the sclerosed sinus was markedly increased, whereas compression of the unaffected sinus had little effect. Atropine inhibited compression-induced bradycardia in control studies but only partially inhibited the augmented response of the patients given dihydroergotoxine. It would seem that the effect of dihydroergotoxine was due to a depressant effect on cardiac sympathetic nerve activity rather than due to vagal excitation (Franke, 1950). In patients responding normally to carotid sinus compression, neither ergotamine, dihydroergotamine, nor dihydroergotoxine altered the depressor effect or the bradycardia (CORSI and DOHRN, 1946; FRANKE, 1950; LOTTENBACH, 1953; PICHLER et al., 1956).

3. Effects on the Carotid Sinus and Impulse Transmission in Sino-Aortic Nerves

Reflex regulation of blood pressure occurs by the action of arterial pressure itself on receptors located in the vascular walls of the sino-aortic areas. Arterial pressure does not act directly on the receptors but by stretching the walls of the arteries where the receptors are located. Drugs which modify the distensibility of the wall or the active tension in the wall will, in turn, indirectly modify baroreceptor activity (HEYMANS and NEIL, 1958). An increase in impulse activity of the baroreceptor fibers, a profound fall in blood pressure, and suppression of the pressor response to carotid occlusion can be provoked by topical application of vasoconstrictor substances to the carotid sinus wall (HEYMANS and VAN DEN HEUVEL-HEYMANS, 1950). Topical application of ergotamine and dihydroergotoxine have no such action (DELAUNIS and MARTINI, 1953). Hydergine, on the other hand, induces a reduction in the pressor response to carotid occlusion and a small increase in blood pressure (DELAUNIS and MARTINI, 1953; MAZZELLA, 1958). This is difficult to reconcile with the response to intracarotid administration of the compounds when a diminution of the pressor reflex is accompanied by a blood pressure fall (KRAUSE, 1954).

A number of less direct studies have shown that it is improbable that an action on the sinus itself can be involved in the effects of the ergot alkaloids on blood pressure or vasomotor reflexes. In cross-circulation studies, blood pressure falls when the head of an animal is perfused via the carotid artery with blood from a donor animal treated with ergotamine or dihydroergotoxine. Blood pressure still falls after dividing the sinus nerves (KRAUSE, 1954). Blood pressure responses to alterations in pressure in the carotid sinus are inhibited by ergotamine and dihydroergotamine just as effectively when the sinus is isolated from the circulation as when the carotid circulation is intact (HEYMANS and REGNIERS, 1929; VON EULER and HESSER, 1947). In addition, impulse activity in nerve fibers arising from either baroreceptors or chemoreceptors is not altered by an intravenous dose of ergotamine 25 times greater than that which inhibits pressor responses to lowered intracarotid pressure (VON EULER and SCHMITERLÖW, 1944). Intracarotid injection of a small dose (10 μg) of *d*-LSD, on the other hand, induces an increase in chemoreceptor discharges in the cat (NISHI, 1975), but doses up to 10 times greater, given by the same route, do not alter the size of reflex responses arising from these receptors (GINZEL, 1958). Falls in blood pressure in this species are obtained when *d*-LSD is given intravenously, when injected into the cerebral ventricles (GINZEL, 1958), and after excision of the carotid bifurcation (CERVONI et al., 1963). With methysergide, depressor effects obtained in the dog are enhanced after denervating the sino-aortic areas (ANTONACCIO et al., 1975).

There is sufficient evidence to conclude that the inhibitory effects of ergot alkaloids on vasomotor reflexes and reductions in blood pressure neither involve a direct effect on sino-aortic baro- or chemoreceptors nor blockade of impulse transmission within the peripheral afferent pathway of the reflex.

4. Effects on Responses to Catecholamines and 5-Hydroxytryptamine

a) Noradrenaline and Adrenaline

Many ergot alkaloids antagonize the pressor and vasoconstrictor actions of noradrenaline and adrenaline. *D*-LSD and brom-LSD are only slightly active (GINZEL and KOTTEGODA, 1953; GINZEL, 1958), whereas ergometrine, methylergometrine, and methysergide are not only devoid of α-adrenoceptor blocking activity but may enhance the stimulant effects of catecholamines (DAVIS et al., 1935; DAVID and KIRCHOF, 1947; FANCHAMPS et al., 1960; DALESSIO et al., 1961; DALESSIO, 1963; SAXENA, 1972; ANTONACCIO et al., 1975; ANTONACCIO and COTÉ, 1976).

Only limited data are available concerning the relative potencies of those alkaloids with antagonistic activity (Table 2). When their local effects are compared in the femoral vascular bed using the intra-arterial route of administration, the natural alkaloids appear more potent than the hydrogenated derivatives. When their effects on blood pressure responses to adrenaline are compared by the intravenous route, the reverse is true. Much larger doses are required to obtain an inhibitory effect following intravenous administration. This is partly due to the fact that the doses given intra-arterially are based on total body weight rather than

Table 2. α-Adrenoceptor blockade: approximate minimal doses of ergot alkaloids (mg/kg) required to inhibit the pressor or vasoconstrictor effects of noradrenaline (NA) or adrenaline (A). *Dose protecting 50% of animals against the lethal effect of adrenaline

Species	Dog	Dog	Dog	Dog	Cat	Rabbit	Fowl	Rat*
Agonist	NA	NA	A	A	A	A	A	A
Dose of agonist	0.1 µg/min	1 µg	1 µg	5 µg	1 µg/kg	5 µg/kg	2 µg/kg	200 µg/kg
Route of administration of ergot alkaloid	i.a.	i.a.	i.a.	i.v.	i.v.	i.v.	i.v.	i.v.
Ergotamine	0.001	0.01	0.001	1	0.7	2	3–10	
Ergostine	0.001							
5′-Methyl-ergoalanine	0.001							
Dihydroergotamine	0.025			0.5	0.2	1	2–6	
Dihydroergostine	0.025							
Dihydroergocristine	0.025							
Dihydroergokryptine						0.3		0.5
Dihydroergocornine					0.03	0.4	3–5	
Dihydroergotoxine		0.02	0.002	0.1		0.4	3–8	0.05
1-Methyl-ergotamine	>0.125							
1-Methyl-ergostine	>0.125							
1-Methyl-dihydro-ergocristine	>0.125							
Nicergoline								0.02
Reference	1	2	2	3	4	5	6	7

References: 1. AELLIG and BERDE (1969); 2. HALEY and McCORMICK (1956); 3. SCHMITT (1958); 4. HARVEY et al. (1952); 5. HARVEY and NICKERSON (1953); 6. HARVEY et al. (1954); 7. ARCARI et al. (1972).

on the weight of the region studied. Nevertheless, it has been observed that small intravenous doses of the alkaloids diminish or abolish catecholamine-induced vasoconstriction in the renal or intestinal bed while exerting no inhibitory effect on pressor responses (Woods et al., 1932; Longo and Santa, 1968).

In other studies not included in the table, marked inhibition of pressor responses to adrenaline, noradrenaline, or angiotensin has been obtained with doses of the hydrogenated alkaloids ranging from 1 to 100 μg/kg i.v. (de Boer and van Dongen, 1948; Sutton et al., 1950; Gyermek et al., 1950; Cotten et al., 1957; Levy and Ahlquist, 1961; Schmitt and Petillot, 1969; Morpugo et al., 1975), whereas doses of between 0.25 and 2 mg/kg i.v. of ergotamine are necessary to demonstrate a similar effect (Rothlin, 1923; Heymans et al., 1930; Gernandt and Zotterman, 1946; Marsh and van Liere, 1948; Gyermek et al., 1950). The doses of agonist were different in each study which would account for the wide variability in the doses of the alkaloids found effective.

Some pharmacologists have been unable to demonstrate α-adrenoceptor blockade with these drugs, but it seems that the choice of anesthetic used can markedly influence the results obtained. Blockade is evident in animals anesthetised with chloralose or urethane, whereas under barbiturate anesthesia (pentobarbitone, pentothal, dial/urethane, amytal) the alkaloids generally enhance the pressor responses to catecholamines, despite the fact that their local vasoconstrictor effects may be abolished. This problem does not arise with non-ergot α-adrenoceptor blocking agents (Herwick et al., 1939; Cotten et al., 1957).

A frequent observation has been that pressor responses to adrenaline are inhibited with greater facility than those to noradrenaline or electrical stimulation of sympathetic nerves (Gyermek et al., 1950; Sutton et al., 1950; Haley and McCormick, 1956; Cotten et al., 1957; Schmitt, 1958; Longo and Santa, 1968; Osswald et al., 1970; Morpugo et al., 1975). Ariëns and Simonis (1976) have suggested that α-adrenoceptors for adrenaline and noradrenaline may not be identical. If this hypothesis can be substantiated, it could be that the ergot alkaloids display a certain selectivity for receptors for adrenaline. A more likely explanation for the apparent greater potency of the ergot alkaloids on adrenaline-induced responses is suggested by data presented by Nickerson et al. (1953). They showed that the pressor response to small doses of adrenaline is reversed to a depressor response when only 50% or less of the vasoconstrictor activity has been inhibited. The remaining effect is masked by the vasodilator action of the amine resulting from activation of vascular β-adrenoceptors. This means that the reversal of an adrenaline response does not necessarily imply that stimulation of α-adrenoceptors is completely abolished. Reversal will only be apparent, however, if the stimulant effect of adrenaline on cardiac β-adrenoceptors does not in turn mask its effects on vascular β-adrenoceptors (*vide infra*).

The effects of therapeutic doses of the ergot alkaloids on the increases in pressure due to injections or infusions of catecholamines in man are unpredictable. Ergotamine and dihydroergotamine either enhance pressor effects or have no effect (Youmans et al., 1933; Gatzek et al., 1949). Dihydroergotoxine and dihydroergocornine sometimes attenuate or block adrenaline-induced responses (Kappert, 1949a; Kappert et al., 1950; Duret, 1951; Corsi, 1952; Goetz and Katz, 1949; Sherif et al., 1956; Härich et al., 1975) but sometimes have no effect (Gatzek et al., 1949; BARCROFT et al., 1951; FREIS et al., 1951; BERNSMEIER, 1954). Nevertheless, although YOUMANS et al. failed to demonstrate an inhibitory effect on the blood pressure rise induced by adrenaline, the dose of ergotamine given inhibited the associated hyperglycemia and increase in metabolic rate. BARCROFT and his colleagues likewise found no direct evidence for α-adrenoceptor blockade with dihydroergotoxine, but an infusion of the drug into the brachial artery induced vasodilation in the ipselateral limb, whereas the contralateral limb was unaffected. This might be regarded as indirect evidence for blockade of the effects of endogenous noradrenaline.

b) Isoprenaline

Small doses of ergotamine (20–30 µg/kg i.v.) enhance the pressor actions of adrenaline and noradrenaline in the dog but diminish the depressor action of isoprenaline or convert the usual fall in blood pressure to a rise. Although the heart is slowed by the alkaloid, the acceleration due to isoprenaline and adrenaline is not diminished and may be potentiated. The blood pressure rise is clearly not the result of vasoconstriction. Although ergotamine causes marked vasoconstriction itself lasting for more than 2 h, isoprenaline still induces dilation in femoral and mesenteric vessels (LANDS et al., 1950; LEVY and AHLQUIST, 1961; WELLENS and WAUTERS, 1966a, 1968; OSSWALD et al., 1970). Both the tachycardia and the rise in blood pressure observed in response to isoprenaline and adrenaline after ergotamine can be abolished with the β-adrenoceptor blocking agents propranolol, dichloroisoprenaline, and practolol (LEVY and AHLQUIST, 1961; OSSWALD et al., 1970; MOUILLÉ, 1970). The ability of ergotamine to produce isoprenaline "reversal" and to potentiate the pressor actions of adrenaline has been unanimously attributed to a manifestation of the cardiac stimulant action of the amines in the presence of a constricted vascular bed. Increases in heart rate, contractility, and particularly cardiac output induced by isoprenaline have all been shown to be greatly enhanced by ergotamine (WELLENS and WAUTERS, 1968). The action of ergotamine in reversing responses to isoprenaline can be eliminated if the vasoconstrictor action of the drug is prevented by the α-adrenoceptor blocking drugs yohimbine, phentolamine, or phenoxybenzamine (HAZARD et al., 1963; MOUILLÉ, 1970).

c) Dopamine

Ergometrine is an effective antagonist of the effects of dopamine in the ganglia of *Helix aspersa* (WALKER et al., 1968). This prompted BELL and his colleagues (1974, 1975) to examine the drug for dopamine antagonism in the dog. Administration of ergometrine (0.5 mg) into the aorta abolishes or attenuates renal and femoral dilator responses to intra-aortic injections of dopamine. The effect is relatively short-lasting (15 min) but is selective. Dilator responses to acetylcholine, isoprenaline, histamine, bradykinin, and 5-HT are not inhibited. Methylergometrine has similar effects. Selective blockade of the effects of dopamine receptor stimulation (by dopamine and bromocriptine) can be obtained following intravenous administration of 50 µg/kg. The blocking effect of this dose lasts for approximately 1 h (CLARK, unpublished).

d) 5-Hydroxytryptamine

The circulatory response to 5-HT in intact animals is modified by many complicating factors, and there are marked species variations in the nature of the response. Intravenous administration results in an initial pressor phase due to vasoconstriction and cardiac stimulation, but reflex hypotension and bradycardia and peripheral and ganglionic inhibition of vasoconstrictor nerve tone may overcome the rise in blood pressure. The pressor component is best revealed in ganglion-blocked or spinal animals. When given by close-arterial administration into a selected vascular bed, it produces net constriction when the bed is dilated but dilation if the vessels are constricted. This bidirectional response derives from the fact that 5-HT produces small vessel dilation at the same time that it constricts large vessels (HADDY et al., 1959).

D-LSD and its brominated derivative are effective antagonists of the stimulant action of 5-HT in several smooth muscle preparations, but their activity against cardiovascular responses to 5-HT has received less attention. SALMOIRAGHI and his colleagues (1957) have shown that there are prominent species differences not only in the cardiovascular responses to 5-HT but also in the ability of brom-LSD or *d*-LSD to prevent them. Both compounds inhibit the pressor and the depressor components of the response to 5-HT over long periods in rats, but in dogs and cats neither drug has any pronounced effect (PAGE and MCCUBBIN, 1953; SALMOIRAGHI et al., 1957). The blocking action of brom-LSD is also insignificant on the perfused vascular bed of the dog hind limb. When antagonistic activity is present, it is usually nonspecific in that responses to noradrenaline are reduced more effectively and for a longer period than are those to 5-HT (SALMOIRAGHI et al., 1957). In contrast, *d*-LSD prevents the vasoconstrictor actions of 5-HT in the hind limb of both cat and dog and the perfused pulmonary vessels of the cat without greatly modifying responses to adrenaline or noradrenaline (GINZEL and KOTTEGODA, 1953).

Several ergot alkaloids have been shown to inhibit the fall in blood pressure induced by 5-HT in the anesthetized fowl (BUÑAG and WALASZEK, 1962). The depressor effect in this species is mainly due to the release of endogenous histamine by 5-HT. Of the drugs tested, methysergide was the most specific and also the most potent, i.e., methysergide > ergometrine > brom-LSD > *d*-LSD > dihydroergotamine > ergotamine. This order of potency is rather different from that which CERLETTI and DOEPFNER (1958) and FANCHAMPS et al. (1960) found in the rat uterus, i.e., methysergide > *d*-LSD = brom-LSD > ergometrine > dihydroergotamine > ergotamine.

Surprisingly, although the least active in the rat uterus and the fowl, ergotamine is considerably more potent than methysergide in antagonizing the cardiovascular actions of 5-HT in the dog. Increases in blood pressure and resistance in femoral, renal, and carotid vessels induced by 5-HT are reduced or abolished from a dose of 1 μg/kg i.v. (PAGE and MCCUBBIN, 1953; SALMOIRAGHI et al., 1957; WELLENS and WAUTERS, 1966a, b; SAXENA, 1972); 5-HT antagonism occurs at doses which have no effect or enhance responses to noradrenaline and adrenaline.

Methysergide is potent in inhibiting 5-HT-induced increases in blood pressure and renal and femoral vascular resistance in dogs (FANCHAMPS et al., 1960) and increases in resistance in forearm veins in man (methysergide = nicergoline > *d*-LSD > 1-methyl ergotamine > brom-LSD) (DEL BIANCO et al., 1975). In comparison with ergotamine, however, it appears rather weakly active in the carotid vascular bed (KARLSBERG et al., 1963; SAXENA, 1972; WELCH et al., 1974b; VARGAFTIG and LEFORT, 1974; SPIRA et al., 1976).

SAXENA (1972) has suggested that the apparent potency of ergotamine may be due to the enormous increase in vascular tone which the drug produces, which would favor a dilator response to 5-HT (HADDY et al., 1959). On the other hand, VARGAFTIG and LEFORT (1974) found that reversal of the 5-HT effect from constriction to dilation induced by ergotamine in nasal vessels of the dog did not subside when the constriction evoked by ergotamine had faded. Methysergide not only reduced the constriction induced by 5-HT (at comparatively high doses) but also the dilator response revealed by treatment with ergotamine. The results obtained by VARGAFTIG and LEFORT are consistent with the hypothesis that separate receptors for 5-HT-induced constriction and dilation of nasal vessels are present. Ergotamine blocks constriction and unmasks dilation. Mianserin and cyproheptadine block only the dilator response, whereas methysergide inhibits both the vasoconstriction and vasodilation.

Interaction between ergot alkaloids and 5-HT receptors in blood vessels is clearly complex and still poorly understood (see Chapter III). It is of importance to realize that antagonism of the effects of 5-HT by the alkaloids may not be relevant for their beneficial effects in migraine (Section E 4). Small doses, closer to those used in therapy, enhance the vasoconstrictor effects of 5-HT (VARGAFTIG and LEFORT, 1974; SCHÖNBAUM et al., 1975; SICUTERI et al., 1975).

5. Mechanisms Involved in the Hypotensive Action

Despite the fact that some ergot alkaloids have a modulating effect on central blood pressure control mechanisms, there is no direct evidence that their blood pressure lowering effects are due to a depression of sympathetic nerve activity. SCHMITT and FENARD (1970) found that ergotamine, dihydroergotamine, and dihydroergotoxine provoked a reduction in recorded action potentials in preganglionic splanchnic nerves only during the pressor phase of the blood pressure response; occasionally activity was augmented. In some experiments, high doses of the dihydro derivatives induced a progressive diminution of electrical activity. This was not seen with ergotamine (GERNANDT and ZOTTERMAN, 1946; SCHMITT and FENARD, 1970), for which there is much firmer evidence for a central inhibitory effect on baroreceptor reflexes than for the other two drugs. Ergotamine is a very powerful vasoconstrictor substance, and reductions in blood pressure are not commonly seen following intravenous administration unless resting blood pressure is high (BARÁTH, 1926; IMMERWAHR, 1927; HEYMANS and BOUCKAERT, 1933; LENNOX, 1938; PROOSDIJ-HARTZEMA and DE JONGH, 1955; KRAUSE et al., 1971). This would probably account for the reported absence of effects on sympathetic nerve activity.

KRAUSE and his colleagues (1971) showed that ergotamine lowered blood pressure by about 80 mmHg in dogs made hypertensive by denervating sino-aortic reflexogenic zones. After decapitation, blood pressure was restored to hypertensive levels by infusing noradrenaline. Subsequent administration of ergotamine had

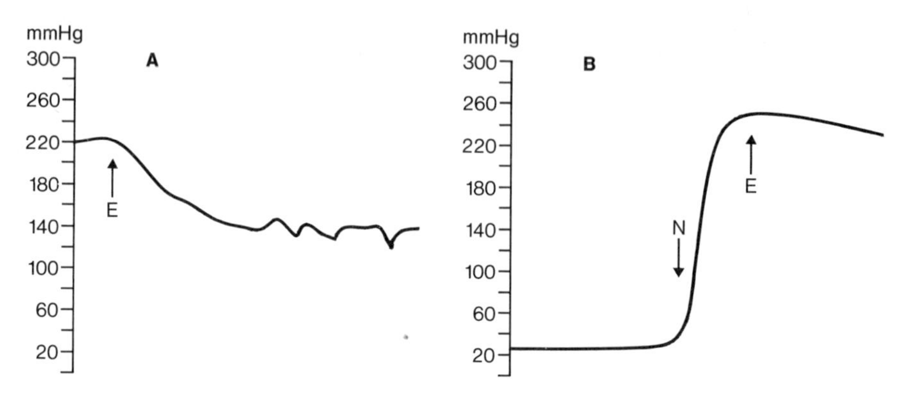

Fig. 3A and B. Effect of ergotamine 25 µg/kg i.v. (E) on blood pressure in an anesthetized dog after division of the sinus nerves and vagi (A) and in the same animal after decapitation (B). Intravenous infusion of noradrenaline begun at N (after KRAUSE et al., 1971)

no significant effect on the level of blood pressure (Fig. 3). This excluded blockade of α-adrenoceptors as the cause of the blood pressure fall before decapitation and was considered by the authors as indirect evidence for a centrally mediated effect. This supported an earlier finding, that administration of the drug into the vascularly isolated head of a dog in cross-circulation studies not only inhibited baroreceptor reflexes in the trunk but also lowered blood pressure (KRAUSE, 1954).

Very small doses of ergotamine (from 10 ng/kg) injected directly into the cerebral ventricles have no effect on systemic blood pressure but induce considerable reductions in resistance in the femoral vascular bed (RETTORI and HALEY, 1967). The assumption was made that the vasodilation reflected central depression of noradrenergic sympathetic nerve activity. An alternative explanation is activation of cholinergic sympathetic vasodilator nerves to skeletal muscle (FOLKOW and UVNÄS, 1950; ELIASSON et al., 1951, 1952). CHU and STÜRMER (1973) have shown that vasodilation taking place in skeletal muscle in response to dihydroergotamine can be inhibited by atropine and potentiated by a cholinesterase inhibitor. It is conceivable that ergotamine might have a similar action. Such a mechanism is clearly not the major cause of the hypotensive action of the ergot alkaloids, as will be discussed later, but it may be a contributory factor.

After elimination of tonic noradrenergic nerve activity (pithing, high spinal section, reserpine), blood pressure rises in response to all the peptide alkaloids. If vasoconstrictor tone is then restored to normotensive levels with an intravenous infusion of adrenaline or noradrenaline, the natural alkaloids and the 1-methyl derivative of ergotamine increase blood pressure further, whereas the hydrogenated derivatives of ergotamine and ergotoxine all decrease blood pressure (ROTHLIN, 1949; SCHMITT and SCHMITT, 1959, 1960; SCHLIENTZ et al., 1968; CERLETTI and BERDE, 1969; MORPUGO et al., 1975). There is no doubt that ergotamine possesses α-adrenoceptor blocking activity, but it would appear that this component of the drug's action is not sufficiently dominant to counteract the effect of its strong agonist activity at α-adrenoceptor and 5-HT receptor sites. These experiments provide additional support for the hypothesis that the vasodepressor action of ergotamine is centrally mediated. They also emphasize that blockade of vascular α-adrenoceptors probably makes an important contribution to the vasodepressor actions of the hydrogenated alkaloids.

It has long been assumed that all hydrogenated peptide alkaloids induce blood pressure lowering effects largely as a result of an action on central nervous structures (ROTHLIN, 1946; KONZETT and ROTHLIN, 1953). This concept needs to be revised. KONZETT and ROTHLIN attempted to locate the site of action of these drugs by sectioning the brain and spinal cord of the cat at different levels, thereby determining which structures were essential for the hypotensive action. They did this in the belief that blockade of peripheral α-adrenoceptors was of only minor importance, and the major effect of the alkaloids was to enhance the outflow of vasodilator impulses. The possibility that depression of vasoconstrictor impulses might also be involved was considered but not discussed. They found that the compounds always caused a fall in blood pressure provided that the medulla oblongata and the spinal cord down to the level of the seventh thoracic segment (T7) were intact. The presence or absence of the cerebrum and diencephalon was not of importance. Transections of the spinal cord at levels above T7 increased the incidence of pressor effects. Responses were all pressor in the spinal cat or the intact cat treated with a ganglion blocking agent. These results, which were in accordance with those obtained by BLUNTSCHLI (1948), were claimed to confirm a central action of the drug. The fundamental misconception made in this study was the assumption that the hydrogenated alkaloids reduced blood pressure by enhancing the vasodilator outflow from the central nervous system. Experimental evidence available today suggests that the medullary control of vasomotor tone is effected solely by variations in vasoconstrictor discharge. Alterations in vasodilator nerve activity appear to be entirely unassociated with blood pressure regulating mechanisms (LINDGREN and UVNÄS, 1954, 1955). KONZETT and ROTHLIN's results, therefore, could be explained just as well in terms of peripheral inhibition of a diminishing level of resting vasomotor tone.

Administration of dihydroergotoxine into the cerebral circulation of the dog in cross-circulation studies, as with ergotamine, causes a fall in blood pressure in the vascularly isolated trunk (KRAUSE, 1954). MURRAY and his colleagues (1959) described a similar effect for dihydroergotamine, but no experimental details were given. On the other hand, although intracerebroventricular injections of dihydroergotoxine have been shown to induce mild reductions in blood pressure, which may be associated with a reduction in splanchnic nerve activity (SHARE, 1973; TADEPALLI et al., 1976), dihydroergotamine has no effect or may induce a slight pressure rise. When a fall occurs, it parallels antagonism of the pressor effects of catecholamines and can be attributed to overflow of the drug into the peripheral circulation and therefore to α-adrenoceptor blockade (SCHMITT and SCHMITT, 1960). It must be concluded that the contribution made by a central inhibiting action on vasomotor tone in the hypotensive action of the hydrogenated ergot alkaloids is of relatively little importance. It is of interest to compare the antihypertensive effects of ergotamine and dihydroergotamine. Despite the fact that dihydroergotamine is a more powerful α-adrenoceptor antagonist than is ergotamine, it is less effective in lowering blood pressure in rats with experimental hypertension (Fig. 4).

There is now considerable evidence suggesting that bromocriptine stimulates dopamine receptors within the central nervous system (HÖKFELT and FUXE, 1972;

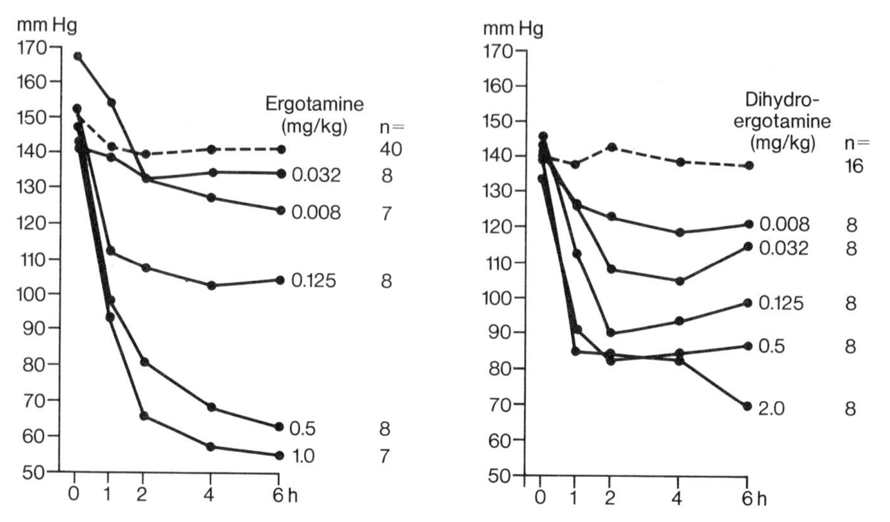

Fig. 4. Effects of intramuscular injections of ergotamine and dihydroergotamine on blood pressure in rats with renal hypertension. Mean results obtained in groups of 7–40 animals (VAN PROOSDIJ-HARTZEMA and DE JONG, 1955)

CORRODI et al., 1973; JOHNSON et al., 1976). This prompted VOLKMAN and GOLDBERG (1976) to examine the drug's effects on peripheral dopamine receptors in the dog. Dopamine receptors are considered to be present in several vascular beds but principally in the renal and mesenteric vessels. Stimulation of these receptors by dopamine elicits vasodilation in these beds with a consequent fall in systemic blood pressure (for review, see GOLDBERG, 1972). VOLKMAN and GOLDBERG injected doses of bromocriptine up to 1000 times the minimal effective dose of dopamine into the renal artery but were unable to demonstrate a dilator effect. CLARK (1977) confirmed this result but found that if the drug was administered slowly by the intravenous route, dose-dependent falls in blood pressure could be obtained from a dose of only 6 μg/kg. Resistance in the superior mesenteric and renal vessels was decreased, whereas that in the carotid vascular bed was not changed. The effects of bromocriptine on blood pressure and resistance were abolished by pretreatment with the dopamine receptor blocking agents haloperidol (YEH et al., 1969), ergometrine (BELL et al., 1974), and methylergometrine (CLARK, unpublished). An action on dopamine receptors was confirmed by showing that the drug had no effect on blood pressure in animals in which the celiac, mesenteric, and renal vessels were ligated, thereby excluding from the circulation the major beds considered to possess dopamine receptors.

Administration of dopamine and apomorphine into the cerebral ventricles of the cat induces dose-dependent reductions in blood pressure, which can be inhibited dose-dependently by haloperidol and pimozide but not by phentolamine. This indicates the existence of dopamine receptors within the central nervous system, mediating hypotensive responses (HEISE, 1976). CLARK et al. (1978) have shown that bromocriptine lowers blood pressure in the cat following intracerebroventricular administration. This occurs at a dose which is ineffective by the intravenous route. It is probable that stimulant effects of bromocriptine on both central and peripheral dopamine receptors are involved in the hypotensive action of the drug. An observation of interest in this respect is that in acromegalic patients undergoing treatment with bromocriptine, there was a marked decrease in the noradrenaline levels in plasma and urine. This suggests a reduction in sympathetic nerve activity (NILSSON and HÖKFELT, 1977).

An additional mechanism which might be considered as possibly being involved in the blood pressure lowering (or antihypertensive) effect of some ergot alkaloids is stimulation of prejunctional α-adrenoceptors or dopamine receptors in noradrenergic nerves, thereby causing a diminished release of transmitter. The evidence supporting the hypothesis that transmitter release is modulated by stimulation or blockade of these receptors is discussed in Section D. Both α-adrenoceptor and dopamine receptor agonists inhibit noradrenaline efflux in response to nerve stimulation in a variety of tissues, including blood vessels (MCCULLOCH et al., 1973; RAND et al., 1975; STARKE et al., 1975a; STJÄRNE and BRUNDIN, 1975). Ergotamine, dihydroergotamine, dihydroergotoxine, and bromocriptine diminish the increase in heart rate in response to stimulation of the cardiac sympathetic nerves. The effects of the first three compounds can be blocked, at least partially, with phentolamine. That of bromocriptine is inhibited dose-dependently by haloperidol (SCHOLTYSIK, 1976, 1978). It is possible that these drugs may exert a similar inhibitory effect on sympathetic nerve terminals in vascular smooth muscle, and this could contribute to their blood pressure lowering effects.

D-LSD lowers blood pressure in normotensive animals when given intravenously and following intracerebroventricular administration. Since vagotomy or atropine do not markedly alter the hypotensive effect following both routes of administration, it can be assumed that it is due to a centrally mediated diminution of sympathetic vasomotor activity (GINZEL, 1958; CERVONI et al., 1963). Higher centers are not involved. As with the peptide alkaloids (ROSENBLUETH and CANNON, 1933; KONZETT and ROTHLIN, 1953; TADEPALLI et al., 1976), blood pressure still falls in response to *d*-LSD in decerebrate preparations (CERVONI et al., 1963). *D*-LSD has negligible effect on baroreceptor reflex mechanisms, its action on blood pressure control mechanisms being mainly confined to inhibition of chemoreceptor pressor reflexes. GINZEL showed, however, that the hypotensive effect of the drug is clearly distinct from its effect on chemoreceptor reflexes. A small reduction in a reflex response could be associated with a large fall in blood pressure and the reverse was also true. As with ergotamine, there is no direct evidence supporting the hypothesis that *d*-LSD lowers blood pressure by diminishing sympathetic outflow. Electrical activity in postganglionic sympathetic nerves diminishes transiently following intravenous administration but tends to increase as blood pressure falls (BROGHAMMER et al., 1957; TAUBERGER and KLIMMER, 1968).

A purely central action has also been proposed for methysergide. This compound has no α-adrenoceptor blocking activity (FANCHAMPS et al., 1960; DALESSIO, 1963; SAXENA, 1972; ANTONACCIO et al., 1975), neither does it inhibit transmitter release from noradrenergic nerve endings nor impair impulse transmission in sympathetic ganglia (ANTONACCIO and COTÉ, 1976). In dogs with functional sympathectomy due to pretreatment with guanethidine, methysergide causes a fall in blood pressure significantly smaller than that seen in untreated animals. These results are compatible with the suggestion that high doses of the drug induce a central suppression of sympathetic tone. More direct evidence was provided by the demonstration of a hypotensive effect following intracerebroventricular administration of a dose which was inactive by the intravenous route (ANTONACCIO et al., 1975). Intravenous administration has been shown to diminish sympathetic nerve discharge in cats (ANTONACCIO and TAYLOR, 1977).

There is now substantial evidence suggesting that central noradrenergic, adrenergic, and dopaminergic nerves play a significant role in the regulation of arterial blood pressure. The evidence for the participation of serotonergic nerves is still controversial. Nevertheless, it seems that the activity of bulbospinal serotonergic nerves facilitates the maintenance of arterial blood pressure in normal animals and the increase in blood pressure in some models of hypertension (for review, see CHALMERS, 1975). KRSTIĆ and DJURKOVIĆ (1976) have shown that blood pressure and heart rate increase following intracerebroventricular administration of 5-HT in the rat. Both of these responses are abolished by central administration of methysergide. It is tempting to speculate that methysergide may reduce blood pressure and heart rate by interrupting a central serotonergic link in the pathways concerned in the control of blood pressure. Conversely, stimulation of a noradrenergic inhibitory pathway could provide an explanation for the influence which ergotamine exerts on blood pressure control mechanisms. In the light of evidence reviewed by LAUBIE et al. (1976), it seems unlikely that noradrenergic neurons are an integral part of the central baroreceptor reflex pathway. However, there is no justification for the view that maintenance of blood vessel tone or cardiac rate and force is solely dependent upon impulses which arise in the medullary vasomotor center. On the contrary, much evidence indicates an important role for supramedullary structures in tonic discharge to cardiovascular effectors (PEISS, 1965). The possibility cannot be excluded that ergotamine could be acting at supramedullary sites by stimulating neurons which exert an inhibitory influence upon both pressor and depressor areas of the medulla.

Many authors have interpreted an inhibitory effect on the response to carotid occlusion as evidence that a drug lowers blood pressure by interrupting the efferent limb of the baroreceptor reflex pathway. The experiments of TADEPALLI and his colleagues (1976) emphasize that such an interpretation is an oversimplification. They showed that dihydroergotoxine lowered blood pressure when injected into the 4th ventricle in cats with intact brains and after midcollicular decerebration. When the injected drug was confined to the brain rostral to the cerebral aqueduct, blood pressure did not change. Consequently, the blood pressure lowering effect could be attributed solely to an action in the brainstem caudal to the cerebral aqueduct. On the other hand, inhibition of the baroreceptor reflex was only obtained in animals with intact brains. The response was enhanced following administration into the 3rd ventricle and unchanged in decerebrate animals. Similar results were obtained with phentolamine. These latter findings suggest that drugs which block α-adrenoceptors may inhibit baroreceptor reflexes by acting at an interneuronal site within a central efferent pathway to attenuate excitatory impulses descending from the supracollicular level of the brain.

The foregoing discussion has been confined to the relative importance of peripheral and central actions in the capacity of the ergot alkaloids to decrease vasomotor tone; however, it must not be assumed that vasodilation is the only mechanism by which they may lower blood pressure. Consideration must be given to their cardiac effects. The ergot alkaloids, almost without exception, depress heart rate and, therefore, must influence cardiac output unless a compensatory increase in stroke volume occurs. These aspects are discussed in Sections B and E.

6. Mechanisms Involved in the Pressor Action

There is no doubt that the increases in blood pressure evoked by many ergot alkaloids are of a peripheral nature, since they may be obtained in animals after destruction of the whole nervous system (DALE, 1906; BARGER and DALE, 1907; ROSENBLUETH and CANNON, 1933; HEYMANS and BOUCKAERT, 1933; ROTHLIN, 1946, 1949, 1957; SCHLIENZ et al., 1968; CERLETTI and BERDE, 1969; SCHMITT and PETILLOT, 1969), depletion of catecholamine stores with reserpine (SCHMITT and SCHMITT, 1959, 1960; CHU and HOOL-ZULAUF, 1975), or after ganglion blockade (KONZETT and ROTHLIN, 1953; MORPUGO et al., 1975). Elimination of tonic sympathetic nerve activity and reflex autonomic control mechanisms unmasks vasoconstrictor activity in many compounds which exert only depressor effects in intact animals. HOOL-ZULAUF and CHU (unpublished) compared the pressor activities of 20 ergot alkaloids in pithed rats (Fig. 5). Ergotamine emerged as the most potent. The results clearly demonstrate the radical changes that can be obtained by simple chemical modifications in the lysergic acid moiety. Methylation in position 1 of ergotamine and ergostine (22) [1-methyl-ergotamine (34c); 1-methyl-ergostine] has resulted in a marked decrease in pressor activity compared with the parent compound. Pressor activity has been completely eliminated in methysergide (1-methyl-*d*-lysergic acid *L*-2-butanolamide) (34a). This compound should be compared with methylergometrine (*d*-lysergic acid *L*-2-butanolamide) (73a), which has roughly one-sixth of the pressor activity of ergotamine. Pressor activity is also much reduced or may be absent in compounds in which a bromine atom has been introduced in position 2 as in bromocriptine (2-bromo-α-ergokryptine) (38) and brom-LSD (2-bromo-*d*-lysergic acid diethylamide) (37a). Hydrogenation of the double bond at position 9,10 brings about less marked changes. Even so, the hydrogenated derivatives (102) are, without exception, less potent than the parent compounds.

A further structural manipulation which is worthy of note is that in which the *L*-phenylalanine residue of ergotamine is replaced by a 2-methylalanine residue (5′-methylergoalanine) (119a). Uterotonic activity, compared with ergotamine, is decreased by 95%, whereas pressor activity is increased by 55%, conferring upon the drug a remarkable tissue specificity (HOFMANN, 1972).

Nicergoline (104e), an ergoline derivative, is a potent α-adrenoceptor blocking agent but is devoid of pressor activity in the spinal cat or pithed rat in doses up to 2.5 mg/kg (ARCARI et al., 1972).

BLUNTSCHLI (1948) and KONZETT and ROTHLIN (1953) observed that the depressor effect of dihydro ergot alkaloids was reversed to a pressor effect even if only a portion of the sympathetic outflow was eliminated. Spinal section in cats below the level of the 6th thoracic vertebra did not diminish the depressor response, whereas section above this level resulted in an increase in blood pressure. A similar phenomenon can be demonstrated in man. Spinal anesthesia produces regional

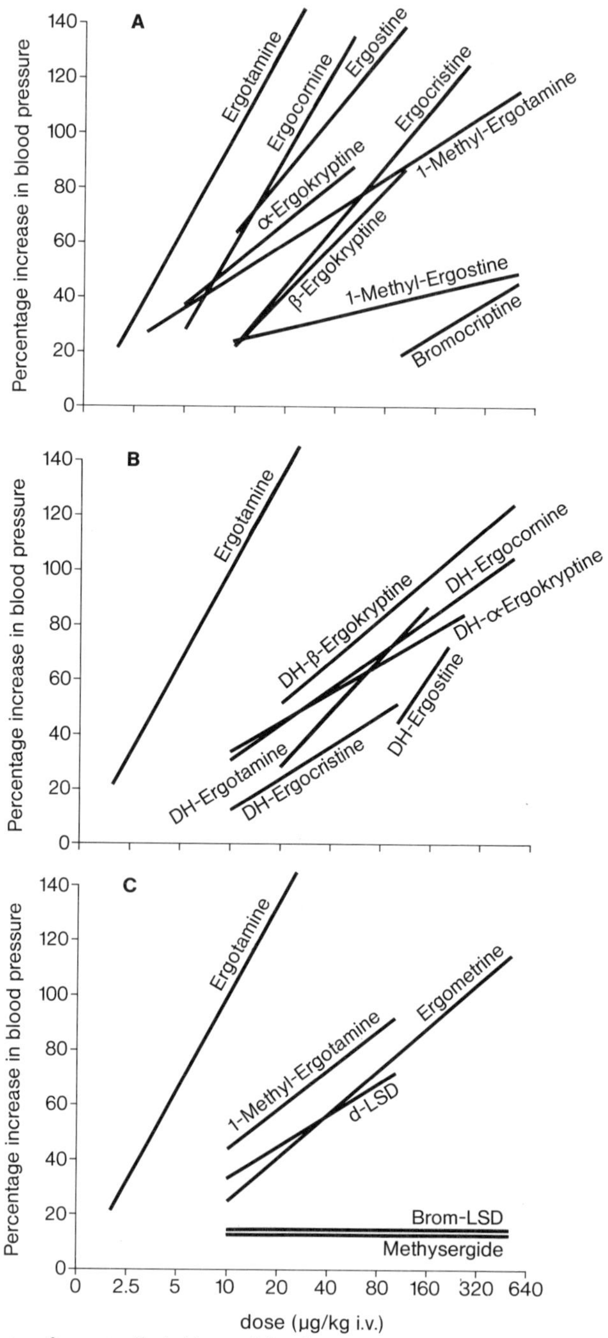

Fig. 5A–C. Effects of ergot alkaloids on blood pressure in pithed rats. Regression lines are derived from responses to 2–3 doses, 3–5 animals tested at each dose level. (A) peptide alkaloids and derivatives substituted in position 1 or 2 of the lysergic acid moiety; (B) hydrogenated derivatives of peptide alkaloids; (C) amide derivatives of lysergic acid. Ergotamine is included in each group for comparison (HOOL-ZULAUF and CHU, unpublished)

sympathetic blockade which results in dilation of resistance and capacitance vessels innervated by sympathetic fibers arising from spinal roots distal to the block. With high spinal anesthesia (to the level of T1–3), blood pressure decreases not only as a result of a decrease in systemic vascular resistance but also as a result of a decrease in cardiac output consequent on peripheral pooling of blood and hence reduced venous return. Both ergotamine (DUNÉR et al., 1960) and dihydroergotamine (BERGENWALD et al., 1972) increase systemic blood pressure to the level preceding anesthesia. Since neither drug increases cardiac output or stroke volume in this situation to levels exceeding pre-anesthetic levels, the restitution of arterial pressure must be due to an effect on resistance vessels. The vasomotor effect of these two compounds in a state of reduced arteriolar tone has provided the basis for its use in clinical practice to stabilize blood pressure during spinal anesthesia.

The hypothesis that the vasoconstrictor actions of ergot alkaloids are at least in part the result of activation of α-adrenoceptors is derived from a number of studies.

Phenoxybenzamine diminishes or abolishes pressor responses to ergotamine, dihydroergotamine, and dihydroergotoxine in the pithed rat (SCHMITT et al., 1971) and to ergotamine in the anesthetized cat (INNES, 1962). Abolition of a pressor response in intact animals, however, does not necessarily imply total elimination of vasoconstrictor effects. Considerable changes in resistance in a given vascular bed can occur without any net change in systemic blood pressure.

Phenoxybenzamine abolishes increases in vascular resistance induced by ergotamine in the perfused spleen of the cat (SALZMANN et al., 1968) and the action of dihydroergotamine in constricting capacitance vessels in muscle (CHU and STÜRMER, 1973) and resistance vessels in skin (CHU and HOOL-ZULAUF, 1975) in the cat hind limb. However, the constrictor action of dihydroergotamine in human hand veins is not always abolished by phentolamine; in some subjects it is only diminished (AELLIG, 1974). Similarly, both phentolamine and dibenzyline induce only a partial inhibition of increases in vascular resistance occurring in response to ergotamine in the dog hind limb (OSSWALD et al., 1970) and carotid vessels (SAXENA and VLAAM-SCHLUTER, 1974). On the other hand, LANDS et al. (1950) were unable to demonstrate any antagonism of the vasoconstrictor effects of ergotoxine by piperoxan in the cat hind limb at a dose which was effective in abolishing pressor responses to adrenaline.

Although, with the exception of the latter, these results suggest that ergot alkaloids interact with α-adrenoceptors, they are not conclusive, since none of the blocking agents used are specific for these receptors. More convincing evidence is provided by studies in isolated tissues. Such experiments show that peptide ergot alkaloids stimulate not only α-adrenoceptors but also 5-HT receptors in vascular smooth muscle (Chapter III). It is likely that 5-HT receptor stimulation contributes to the vasoconstrictor actions of peptide ergot alkaloids in in vivo experiments, especially in the arteries. This might explain the failure of many authors to block the stimulant effects of these drugs with α-adrenoceptor blocking agents.

More emphasis has been placed on demonstrating interaction with 5-HT receptors for non-peptide alkaloids. SHAW and WOOLEY (1956) observed that the initial transient pressor response to *d*-LSD in dogs not only resembled the response to 5-HT, but was abolished by the 5-HT antagonist BAS (1-benzyl-2,5-dimethylserotonin). Similarly, increases in blood pressure in response to *d*-LSD in man can be abolished by the 5-HT antagonist brom-LSD (2-bromo-*d*-lysergic acid diethylamide) (MURPHREE et al., 1958).

B. Hemodynamic Effects

Most of the early studies on the hemodynamic effects of the ergot alkaloids in man were performed using methods based on the WEZLER-BÖGER (1939) technique. Briefly, recordings were made of the pulse waves in the carotid and femoral arteries. From these recordings it was possible to measure directly or derive mathematically a variety of parameters including cardiac output. These techniques are now considered imprecise and unreliable and have given rise to considerable disagreement as to the effects of the alkaloids (STEINMANN et al., 1948; PATTANI, 1949; ZICKGRAF, 1949; DELIUS et al., 1949; KAPPERT, 1949b; STRÖDER and KOPPERMANN, 1952). Since precise measurement of the cardiac output is the pivot of hemodynamic investigations, only those studies in man will be considered in which cardiac output was measured according to the Fick principle or using indicator dilution techniques (Table 3).

No results using the latter methods are available for the effects of ergotamine in man. However, SAXENA and VLAAM-SCHLUTER (1974) have shown that in the dog, dose-dependent reductions in cardiac output are evoked by very small doses (cardiac output was measured as blood flow in the ascending aorta). Despite the reductions in cardiac output, blood pressure is elevated as a result of intense peripheral constriction. Pulmonary pressure was not measured in these experiments, but ROTHLIN (1923) found it to remain constant in the cat and the dog in the presence of considerable increases in systemic pressure. Only when resting pulmonary artery pressure was low at the beginning of an experiment was a rise observed; this latter also applies to patients under spinal anesthesia (DUNÉR et al., 1960). Conversely, LOGARAS (1947) obtained up to threefold increases in pulmonary artery pressure in the cat with a dose of ergotamine which lowered systemic pressure. He attributed the rise to pulmonary vasoconstriction since atrial pressure did not change.

Compounds of the dihydroergotoxine group generally cause decreases in systemic blood pressure and cardiac output in man. It seems that the blood pressure falls can be attributed to reductions in both cardiac output and total peripheral resistance. These compounds do not influence pressure or resistance in the pulmonary vessels if pulmonary arterial pressure is within normal limits (WERKÖ and LAGERLÖF, 1949; FREIS et al., 1949; HALMÁGYI et al., 1953), but pressure may be reduced in patients with pulmonary hypertension (MERIEL et al., 1953).

Results obtained with dihydroergotamine are unpredictable (Table 3). Whereas the effects of ergotamine are mainly pressor and those of dihydroergotoxine mainly depressor, blood pressure may not change in response to dihydroergotamine. When a rise in pressure does occur, it may reflect an increase in total peripheral resistance

(HALMÁGYI et al., 1953; HARRIS, 1963; BEVEGÅRD et al., 1974) or an increase in cardiac output (WERKÖ and LAGERLÖF, 1949; NORDENFELT and MELLANDER, 1972).

NORDENFELT and MELLANDER compared the effects of the drug in the supine and the erect position. In both positions, cardiac output was significantly increased. This reflected an increase in stroke volume, since heart rate was not changed (supine) or only minimally increased (erect). Systolic and mean systemic blood pressures were significantly elevated in the supine but not in the erect position. Dihydroergotamine clearly raised central venous pressure (superior vena cava) in the supine position but did not increase central blood volume. However, changing to the upright position resulted in an increase in the central blood volume without leading to a measurable increase in central venous pressure. The investigation indicated that in both body positions, dihydroergotamine causes such adjustments within the central circulation that diastolic filling of the heart improved.

The differences between these findings and those of HARRIS et al. (1963) (Table 3), who obtained a decrease in cardiac output, may lie in the selection of patients. It is well known that apprehension cannot be entirely avoided in patients exposed to intravascular instrumentation and would tend to increase sympathetic nervous discharge. HARRIS et al. commented that in five of the six patients in their study, heart rate was elevated during the control period, which may have had some bearing on the action of the drug. Bradycardia occurred when dihydroergotamine was given. Cardiac output decreased parallel to the reductions in heart rate, with the result that mean stroke volume did not change.

In accordance with NORDENFELT and MELLANDER's findings, an increase in central venous pressure (right atrium) was obtained by HALMÁGYI et al. (1952), although no significant changes were observed in arterial pressure or cardiac output. In a later study (HALMÁGYI et al., 1953), these investigators found that total peripheral resistance was increased, which accounted for the modest rise in mean blood pressure. The changes which occurred in the pulmonary vessels were far more pronounced.

Pulmonary arterial pressure is generally increased in response to dihydroergotamine, but the contribution made by an increase in tone in the vessels of the pulmonary bed is controversial. WERKÖ and LAGERLÖF (1949) found that the rise in pressure could be attributed almost entirely to an increase in cardiac output. On the other hand, HALMÁGYI and his colleagues (1953) reported that dihydroergotamine caused an elevation of the pulmonary artery pressure without significantly affecting cardiac output or systemic arterial pressure. Whether this effect was due to pulmonary vasoconstriction is in doubt in the absence of a simultaneous estimate of left atrial pressure; several other studies have shown that left atrial pressure is elevated by the drug (HALMÁGYI et al., 1952; NORDENFELT and MELLANDER, 1972; BEVEGÅRD et al., 1974). It would seem that the rise in pulmonary artery pressure is largely due to an increase in pulmonary wedge pressure. HARRIS et al. (1963) showed that the difference between the elevated pulmonary arterial and wedge pressures remained constant in the presence of a fall in pulmonary artery blood flow. This suggested that arterial constriction played a small part. Whether the increase in wedge pressure was simply an expression of an increase in left atrial pressure or whether it was due to constriction of pulmonary veins is not known, but the former seems the more likely. Dihydroergotamine has been

Table 3. Hemodynamic effects of ergot alkaloids. Changes induced in man and anesthetized animals; + = increase, − = decrease. Cardiac output in man measured according to the Fick principle (*) or using indicator dilution techniques (**). Number of patients in parentheses. Cardiac output in dogs (blood flow in ascending aorta) measured with an electromagnetic flow probe

Ergot alkaloid (dose and route of administration)	Species	Mean syst. art. pressure mm Hg	Heart rate beats/min	Stroke volume %	Cardiac output %	Tot. periph. resistance %	Mean pul. art. pressure mm Hg	Pul. art. resistance %	Venous pressure mm Hg	Reference
Ergotamine										
0.1–0.4 mg/kg i.v.	Dog	+	−						+	Guimarães and Osswald (1969)
1–32 μg/kg i.v.	Dog	+4 to +19			−18 to −47	+31 to +163				Saxena and Vlaam-Schluter (1974)
Dihydroergotamine										
10 μg/kg i.v.	Man (4)	+			0**	+			+	Bevegård et al. (1974)
0.5 mg i.v.	Man (4)	+18	− 2		+21*	+ 3	+6 (55%)	+ 6	0	Werkö and Lagerlöf (1949)
1 mg i.v.	Man (28)	0			0*				+7 (80%)	Halmágyi et al. (1952)
1 mg i.v.	Man (8)	+ 4			0*	+11	+9 (38%)	+44		Halmágyi et al. (1953)
1 mg i.pul.art.	Man (6)	+11	−13	+ 2	−12*	+	+3 (16%)	+		Harris et al. (1963)
10–15 μg/kg i.v.	Man (10)	*Supine* + 9	0	+ 8	+ 8**	0			+3 (54%)	Nordenfelt and Mellander (1972)
		Erect. + 5	− 4	+20	+14**	0			0	

Table 3 (continued)

Dihydroergocornine										
0.5 mg i.v.	Man (4)	−15	− 9		− 8*	0	0	0	0	Werkö and Lagerlöf (1949)
0.3–0.4 mg i.v.	Man (4)	−21	− 7		− 9*	−19	0			Freis et al. (1949)
Dihydroergotoxine										
100 μg/kg i.v.	Dog	+25	−19	0	−18	+36	+1 (8%)	+15		Schmitt et al. (1971)
0.3 mg i.m.	Man (6)	−12							+1.5(17%)	Halmágyi et al. (1952)
0.3–0.5 mg i.v.	Man (9)	− 5			− 5	− 5	0	0		Halmágyi et al. (1953)
Methysergide										
20–640 μg/kg i.v.	Dog	+10	+		0					Saxena (1974)
3 mg/kg i.v.	Dog	−40	−34		−10	−25				Antonaccio et al. (1975)
0.5 mg/kg i.v.	Sheep	+13			0*	+13	+3 (20%)	23%		Halmágyi and Colebatch (1961)
Nicergoline										
50–500 μg/kg i.v.	Dog	0		+	+					Arcari et al. (1972)

shown to induce considerable increases in pulmonary artery pressure in patients undergoing spinal anesthesia (BERGENWALD et al., 1972). Both left atrial and pulmonary artery pressures increased to levels significantly above the control values. In spite of the high filling pressure, stroke volume and cardiac output did not increase. A rough estimate of pulmonary vascular resistance from the data reported suggests that a small increase in resistance had occurred. Since the systemic arterial pressure did not increase above the control value and the filling pressure did, there is reason to believe that in this study dihydroergotamine had a more pronounced effect on peripheral capacitance vessels than on resistance vessels, resulting in an increase in the venous return to the heart (see Section C I).

C. Effects on Regional Hemodynamics

The mechanisms considered to be involved in the changes in blood pressure produced by the ergot alkaloids are numerous, and for no drug can a single mechanism be claimed to be wholly responsible. The changes in total peripheral resistance evoked by these drugs probably reflect their composite effects at a number of different sites. The situation is further complicated by the fact that not all vascular beds respond in the same way to a given drug, neither do different compartments of a single vascular bed respond uniformly, with the result that significant redistribution of blood within the organism can occur with no detectable change in blood pressure. This is well illustrated in the experiments of SAXENA and VLAAM-SCHLUTER (1974) and SAXENA (1974) with ergotamine and methysergide in anesthetized dogs (Fig. 6). Ergotamine increased blood pressure dose-dependently, but the changes were not pronounced; methysergide, on the other hand, affected blood pressure only minimally. Ergotamine decreased blood flow (measured with electromagnetic flow probes) and increased vascular resistance in almost all of the regions studied, but at most doses the changes recorded in the carotid and femoral vessels were significantly greater than those in the mesenteric, renal, vertebral, and coronary vascular beds. The selectivity observed with methysergide for the region supplied by the carotid vessels was even more striking. Even here, not all vessels responded uniformly. At some doses, the effects were significantly greater in the internal carotid than in the common carotid bed. This emphasizes the fact that receptors of different types are not uniformly distributed throughout the vasculature. This has been clearly demonstrated in experiments in vitro (Chapter III).

1. Effects on Limb Blood Vessels

The first reported laboratory demonstration of the stimulant effect of ergot alkaloids on peripheral arteries came from KOBERT in 1884 (cited by DALE, 1906). The gangrenous phenomena which he observed in the comb and other peripheral structures of the fowl and pig as a result of administering sphacelinic acid were attributed to "powerful and persistent constriction of the arterioles". DALE (1906) suggested that ergot-induced vasoconstriction could be mediated either directly

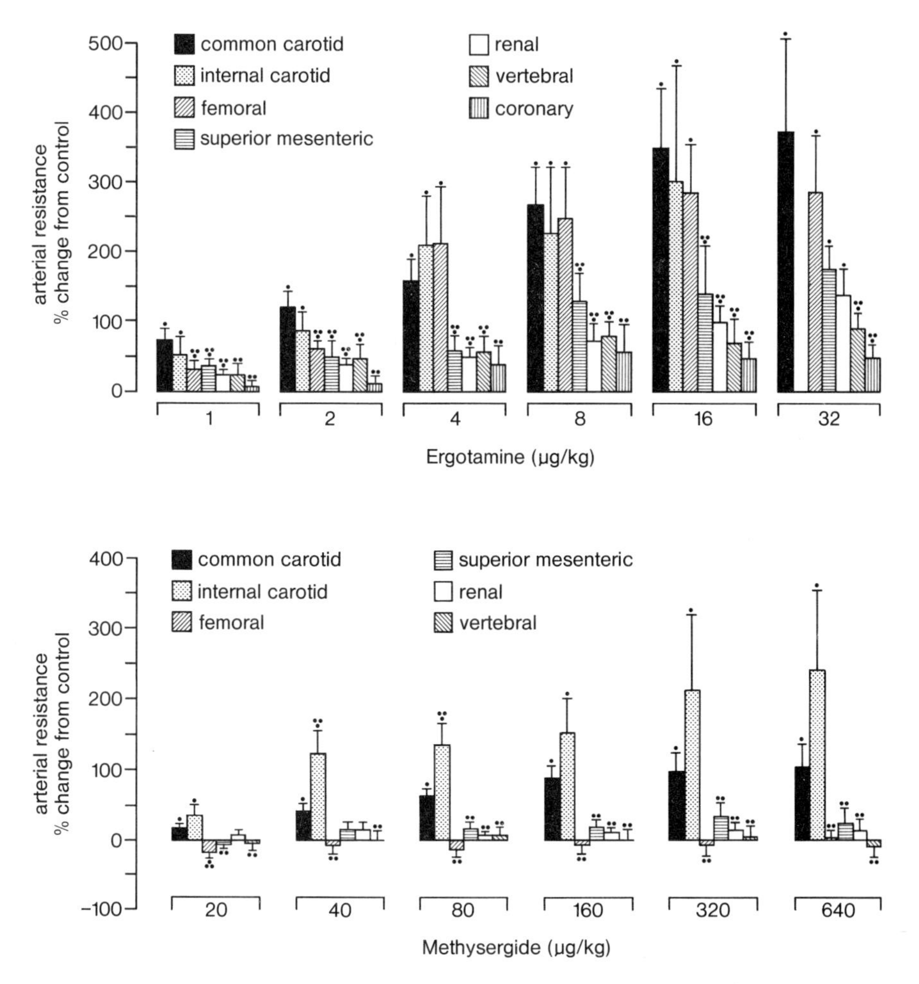

Fig. 6. Effects of ergotamine and methysergide on regional vascular resistance in anesthetized dogs (means ± S.E.M.). • = significantly ($p < 0.05$) different from the control value; •• = significantly ($p < 0.05$) different from the corresponding effect on the common carotid vascular bed (SAXENA, 1974; SAXENA and VLAAM-SCHLUTER, 1974)

by stimulating the arterial smooth muscle or indirectly by stimulation of sympathetic ganglia. Shortly thereafter, BARGER and DALE (1907) showed that ergotoxine administered intravenously in pithed cats, evoked a sharp rise in mean arterial pressure, which was accompanied by a fall in hind limb volume. They argued that since the animal was pithed and the stellate ganglia removed, the action of ergotoxine was mediated through a stimulant effect on vascular smooth muscle. DALE (1906) also correctly deduced that ergot paralyses "the motor elements in the structures associated with sympathetic innervation which adrenaline stimulates". This dual action, which is common to most ergot alkaloids, is to some extent responsible for the seemingly irreconcilable reports as to the action of ergot alkaloids in certain vascular beds.

a) Effects on Blood Flow and Vascular (Arterial) Resistance

Ergotamine, like ergotoxine, exerts mainly vasoconstrictor effects in the extremities both in animals (DALE and SPIRO, 1922; ROTHLIN, 1923; KARR, 1948; FANCHAMPS et al., 1960; WELLENS and WAUTERS, 1968; GUIMARÃES and OSSWALD, 1969; OSSWALD et al., 1970; SAXENA and VLAAM-SCHLUTER, 1974; DE MICHELI and GLÄSSER, 1975) and in man (ABRAMSON and LICHTMAN, 1937; TILLGREN, 1947; BLUNTSCHLI and GOETZ, 1948; GATZEK et al., 1949; LUGARESI and REBUCCI, 1962). Nevertheless, vasodilation has also been reported in the rabbit paw (HEYMANS and REGNIERS, 1927) and in the limbs of human subjects in whom the initial flow rate is low (BLUNTSCHLI and GOETZ, 1948). In perfused hind limbs of cats and dogs, HEYMANS and REGNIERS (1927) observed varying vascular effects, ranging from vasoconstriction to vasodilation. In a subsequent report, HEYMANS et al. (1932a) showed that in intact anesthetized dogs, ergotamine invariably provoked a vasoconstrictor response. However, when the hind limb was perfused with defibrinated blood, which itself increased vascular tone, subsequent administration of ergotamine provoked vasodilation. ROTHLIN and CERLETTI (1949a) showed that ergotamine elicited a marked reduction in flow in both the femoral artery and vein in dogs, but a second dose led to much smaller reductions in flow, implying that ergotamine, a long-acting vasoconstrictor agent, has the capacity to inhibit its own action. In the cat, the response was more variable, and a marked reduction in femoral blood flow after ergotamine such as that observed in the dog could not be demonstrated; the small increases in femoral flow which occurred were considered to be a passive response to the increase in systemic blood pressure. In accordance with ROTHLIN and CERLETTI's findings in the dog, HALEY and MCCORMICK (1956) demonstrated that small doses of ergotamine (0.01–0.1 μg/kg), administered intra-arterially to the autoperfused skeletal muscle of the dog hind limb, decreased muscle blood flow without altering systemic blood pressure. Increasing the dose beyond 2 μg/kg (which induced the greatest increase in resistance) resulted in a progressive diminution of the constrictor effect. Comparable results were obtained in the autoperfused skin vasculature, but in this tissue, the constrictor effect of ergotamine was about 10 times more intense than in muscle. In contrast to these findings, GANTER (1926) and RETTORI and HALEY (1967) found that small doses of ergotamine induced vasodilation in femoral vessels, but at higher doses vasoconstriction was the dominant effect.

Similar contradictory results have been reported for the effects of the dihydro derivatives of the natural alkaloids in experimental animals, which cannot be attributed to differences in species, anesthetic, or route of administration. Several authors have observed only vasoconstrictor effects in innervated preparations (SCHMITT et al., 1971; MANZ and FELIX, 1974; DE MICHELI and GLÄSSER, 1975), whereas others have observed mainly dilator effects (ROTHLIN and CERLETTI, 1949b; HALEY and MCCORMICK, 1956; SCHMITT and SCHMITT, 1960) which are emphasized when femoral blood flow is reduced by hyperventilation (SCHNEIDER and WIEMERS, 1951). The latter authors suggested that the vasodilation might be explained in terms of central parasympathetic nerve stimulation. A small relaxant effect has been demonstrated for dihydroergotoxine in depolarized segments of the central ear artery and saphenous artery of the rabbit, but a dose of 160 μg is required to obtain a measurable effect (VAN NUETEN, 1969).

Responses obtained in man are less variable. Investigations are normally carried out with the patients resting or in the supine position. Anesthetics, which interfere to a greater or lesser extent with normal blood pressure control mechanisms, are not used and there is no surgical intervention (flow changes are measured by plethysmography, rheography, oscillometry, or thermography). Increases in limb (mostly muscle) blood flow usually occur in response to the dihydro derivatives of both ergotamine and alkaloids of the ergotoxine group in patients with normal or low initial flow rates following single parenteral doses (FREIS et al., 1949; BARCROFT et al., 1951; LUGARESI and REBUCCI, 1962; BECATTINI et al., 1964; MELLANDER and NORDENFELT, 1970; ULRICH and SIGGAARD-ANDERSEN, 1971; LÜBKE, 1972; ULRICH et al., 1973; CASTENFORS et al., 1975; BOISMARE et al., 1975a) or after prolonged oral treatment (SIGGAARD-ANDERSEN et al., 1971, 1973). When initial flow to the limb is high as in paraplegic patients subjected to head-up tilt (BIDART and MAURY, 1974) or during spinal anesthesia (CASTENFORS et al., 1975), a decrease in flow occurs. A distinction can be made between dihydroergotamine and dihydroergotoxine and its components with respect to their effects on skin vessels. The latter compounds, whether administered intravenously or intra-arterially, induce up to sixfold increases in blood flow in the hand or foot (BLUNTSCHLI and GOETZ, 1948; BARCROFT et al., 1951; PUGLIONISI and EPPINGER, 1953; GOETZ, 1956; EHRINGER, 1970), whereas dihydroergotamine causes vasoconstriction (BLUNTSCHLI and GOETZ, 1948; MELLANDER and NORDENFELT, 1970; TRONNIER, 1970). In patients with sympathectomized limbs and consequently elevated skin blood flow, dihydroergotoxine and its components induce a further small increase in flow if the compound under test is given intravenously but decrease flow when given by close intra-arterial injection (BLUNTSCHLI and GOETZ, 1948; BARCROFT et al., 1951; PUGLIONISI and EPPINGER, 1953).

The controversy as to the effects of the natural alkaloids and their derivatives on blood flow in the extremities has been largely resolved by the work of AELLIG (1967) in the perfused innervated hind limbs of the dog. One limb was used for measuring the effect of the compounds given intra-arterially. The other served as control, so that spontaneous changes in vascular tone during the experiment could be discounted as a source of error. The effect of ergotamine, dihydroergotamine, and 1-methyl-ergotamine was found to be ambivalent; sometimes there was a vasoconstrictor and sometimes a vasodilator effect. The nature of the response did not depend on the dose, nor was it related to the α-adrenoceptor blocking activity of the substance. It was determined solely by the pre-existing sympathetic tone of the resistance vessels. When control resistance was less than 4 R.U. (resistance units = $mmHg \cdot ml^{-1} \cdot min^{-1}$), ergotamine always induced constriction. Conversely, when vascular resistance was above 4 R.U., the so-called "inversion point" for ergotamine, the drug elicited a dilator response. The inversion points for dihydroergotamine and 1-methyl-ergotamine were 4 R.U. and 2.3 R.U., respectively. In an extension to this work, AELLIG and BERDE (1969) showed that the dual nature of the vascular activity of ergotamine, 1-methyl-ergotamine, and dihydroergotamine was found in at least four other ergot alkaloids. The estimated inversion point for ergostine and dihydroergostine was about 4 R.U., for 1-methyl-ergostine, 2.3 R.U., and dihydroergocristine, 2 R.U. However, 1-methyl-dihydroergocristine consistently elicited vasodilation at initial vascular resistance values down to 1.3 R.U., and 5′-methyl-ergoalanine always caused vasoconstriction at initial values

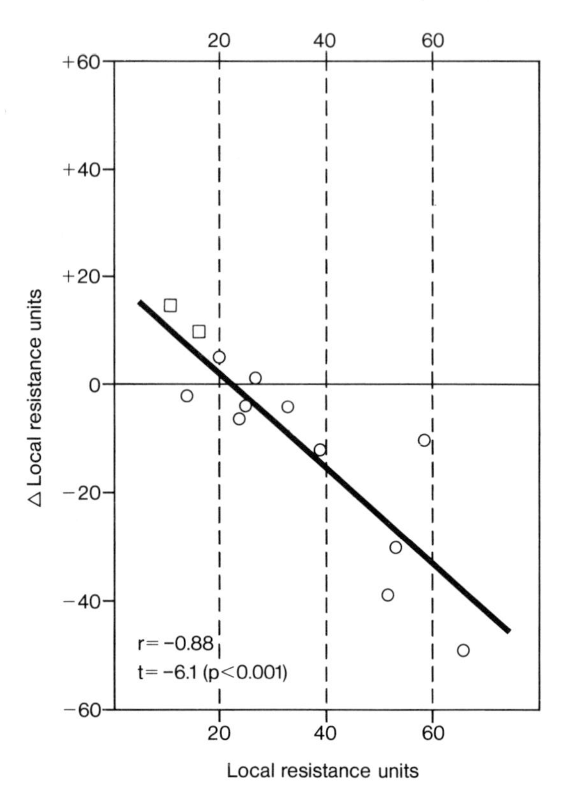

Fig. 7. Correlation between forearm vascular resistance and the change in local resistance induced by dihydroergotamine in man under spinal anesthesia (nerve block to T8) (CASTENFORS et al., 1975)

up to 5.8 R.U. Such a relationship between responses and initial vascular resistance was implied by the results obtained in man and has been substantiated in patients undergoing epidural anesthesia. Nerve block to the level of the 8th thoracic segment results in a decrease in resistance in the lower limbs and a variable increase in the upper limbs. CASTENFORS et al. (1975) observed that dihydroergotamine increased resistance in the nerve-blocked calf but decreased resistance in the forearm of those patients in whom local resistance was above the mean control value. There was a significant correlation between pre-existing local resistance and the change in resistance induced by the drug (Fig. 7).

Nicergoline, like 1-methyl-dihydroergocristine, has only vasodilator effects in the femoral vasculature, which are attributed to blockade of α-adrenoceptors. This compound increases blood flow in dogs over a wide dose range when given either intravenously or by the intra-arterial route (ARCARI et al., 1968, 1972; DE MICHELI and GLÄSSER, 1975), the latter in the absence of changes in systemic blood pressure. Profound reductions in femoral resistance have also been found to occur with methysergide but only when given intravenously in doses (1–3 mg/kg) sufficient to cause a reduction in blood pressure. Intra-arterial administration of similar doses are without effect (ANTONACCIO et al., 1975). Likewise, intravenous doses below 1 mg/kg, although inducing marked increases in resistance in the carotid vascular bed, have negligible effects on femoral arterial resistance (FANCHAMPS et al., 1960; SAXENA, 1974).

b) Effects on Veins

Most of the early workers deduced an increase in vascular resistance from a decrease in limb volume. It was not appreciated at the time that a reduction in the volume of an organ supplied with an intact circulation is no guarantee that the flow rate through the organ has diminished. Changes in volume reflect an action principally on the veins. It is curious that the effects of drugs on the venous system in whole animal preparations is a field which has been, until recently, almost totally neglected by pharmacologists. Not so for the clinician and clinical pharmacologist. The effects of the ergot alkaloids on venous pressure and vein compliance have been dealt with fairly extensively, especially in patients with impaired venomotor regulation (see Section E I). Although an increase in venous tone may give rise to an increase in venous pressure, measurement of central or peripheral venous pressure alone gives no indication of the nature of the changes in venomotor tone and will not be discussed here. In plethysmographic studies, quite dramatic changes in venous tone have been observed, in contrast to the relatively small and variable effects recorded in arterial resistance by other investigators. A single dose of dihydroergotamine (0.5 mg i.v.) has been reported to increase venous tone by 150–250% and to increase central venous (right atrial) pressure by 3 mmHg (LANGE and ECHT, 1972; ECHT and LANGE, 1974). In contrast to the striking effect on venous tone, systolic and diastolic blood pressure rose by less than 10 mmHg. Similarly, the pressure-volume curve (derived from changes in the volume of a limb resulting from changes in the pressure applied with a cuff) was shifted to the left by dihydroergotamine, indicating venoconstriction. The increase in limb volume which occurred on standing was reduced by about one-third (RIECKERT and PAUSCHINGER, 1967; RIECKERT, 1971).

Local venoconstrictor effects have been demonstrated for ergotamine, dihydroergotamine (102b), dihydroergovaline (108b), and dihydroergostine (102g) by infusing the drugs into a superficial hand vein and measuring the change in vein diameter (AELLIG, 1976a,b). A surprising finding was that methysergide, which is devoid of significant effects on flow and resistance in the femoral vascular bed (FANCHAMPS et al., 1960; SAXENA, 1974), was almost as potent as ergotamine and more potent than dihydroergotamine in inducing venoconstriction (Fig. 8). Another unexpected observation, reported by BROOKE and ROBINSON (1970), is that ergometrine, which is considered to have little activity on the cardiovascular system, is also almost as effective as ergotamine in inducing venoconstriction. This drug decreases venous compliance in the forearm by 40% (ergotamine by 50%) and causes a considerable rise in central venous pressure but has no significant effect on forearm blood flow. These findings emphasize the importance of making simultaneous measurements of the effects of a drug on all segments of the vasculature in a single tissue in order to characterize adequately its circulatory actions. It is clear from the foregoing that not only methysergide and ergometrine but other ergot alkaloids have profoundly different actions on the arterial and venous compartments of the circulation.

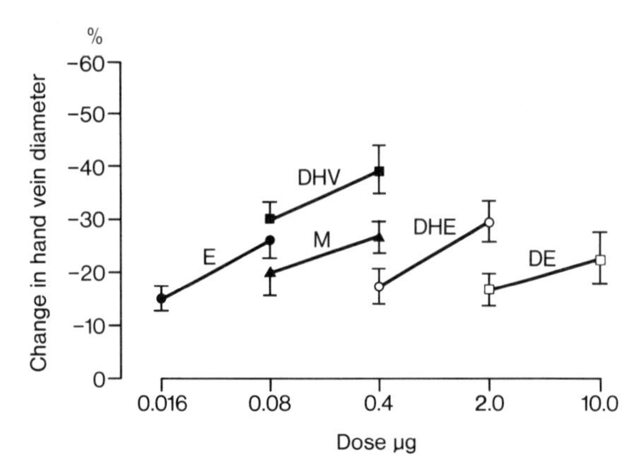

Fig. 8. Venoconstrictor effects of ergot alkaloids in man. Changes in hand vein diameter expressed as percentage of control values after local infusion of ergotamine (E), methysergide (M), dihydroergovaline (DHV), dihydroergotamine (DHE) and dihydroergostine (DE). Mean ±S.E.M., n=5 (AELLIG, 1976b)

Changes in the tone of resistance vessels induced by a vasoactive substance influence regional blood supply. The activity of the precapillary sphincters determines the number of patent capillaries and hence the size of the functional surface available for exchange. Alterations of the pre- to postcapillary resistance ratio affect the hydrostatic capillary pressure, which leads to net transcapillary fluid movements, thus influencing plasma volume. Finally, changes in the tone of the capacitance vessels cause redistribution of blood volume and hence modify venous return and cardiac filling (see MELLANDER and JOHANSSON, 1968).

MELLANDER (1960, 1966) has described an experimental technique which permits simultaneous study of the responses of consecutive vascular segments in a given organ or tissue to physiologic and pharmacologic stimuli. In principle, the tissue is surgically isolated and supplied by one major artery and vein. The inflow blood pressure and the blood flow rate are monitored, and changes in tissue volume are continuously measured by means of a water-filled plethysmograph. From these three parameters, changes in precapillary resistance, precapillary sphincter activity, transcapillary fluid filtration, and capacitance can be derived. Using this technique, MELLANDER and NORDENFELT (1970) studied the vascular effects of dihydroergotamine in the skeletal muscle and skin of cats in the innervated limb and after regional sympathectomy. In innervated muscle, they observed that dihydroergotamine (15 µg/kg) administered intravenously or into the femoral artery caused a slight decrease in arterial resistance with a corresponding constriction of the capacitance vessels; noradrenaline constricted both vascular segments. In acutely denervated muscle, however, constriction was observed in resistance and capacitance segments of the vascular bed. In innervated skin preparations, dihydroergotamine induced constriction in both resistance and capacitance vessels. Denervation enhanced only the resistance response. The compound increased the ratio of pre-/postcapillary resistance but did not significantly influence precapillary sphincter vessels.

A similar study performed in man produced results which corresponded well with those obtained in animals. Hand and calf volumes were measured by plethysmography. Direct recordings of blood pressure and local venous pressures in the hand and calf were taken from cannulated vessels. Data concerning resistance function were obtained from pressure/flow recordings. By continuous measurements of volume changes in the hand or calf, it was possible to follow the shifts in regional blood content, which reflected the reactions of the capacitance vessels (abrupt and fairly rapid changes in tissue volume) as well as the rate of net fluid movement across capillary walls (slower, continuous change in tissue volume). The amount of blood pooled in the hand and calf in response to a given rise of venous outflow pressure (pressure/volume relationship in the capacitance vessels) and the amount of blood (ml/100 g tissue) expelled or mobilized from the region in response to constrictor stimuli were calculated (Fig. 9).

In the hand, the constrictor effects in the resistance vessels were roughly comparable for dihydroergotamine and noradrenaline, but at almost any given level of

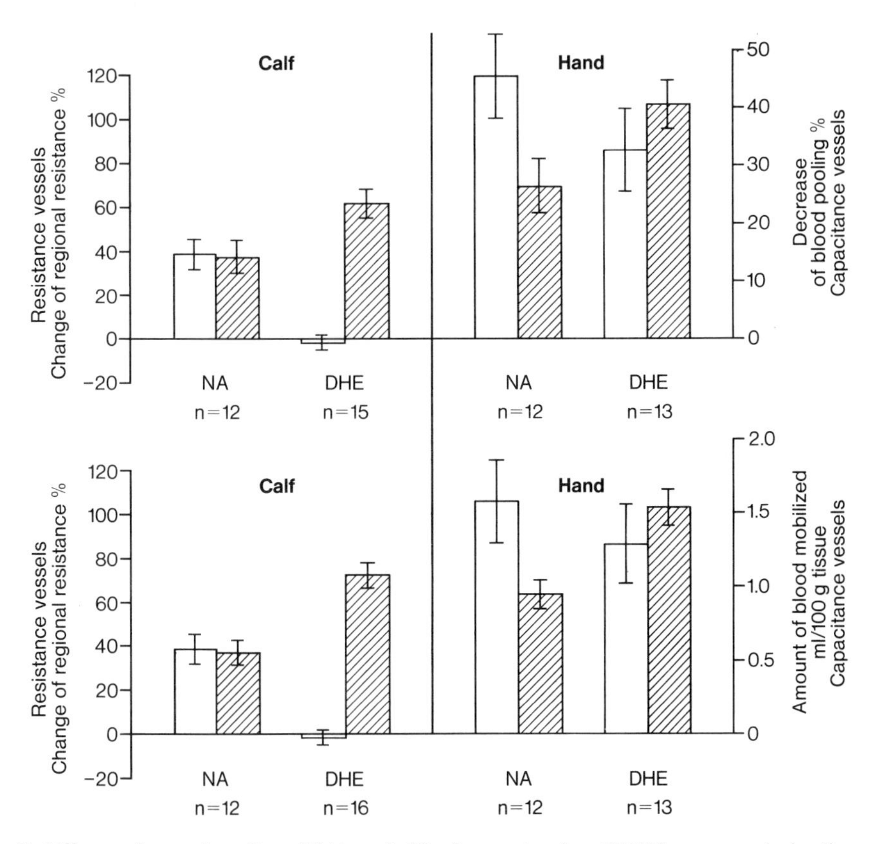

Fig. 9. Effects of noradrenaline (NA) and dihydroergotamine (DHE) on vessels in the calf and hand of healthy male subjects (mean values ± S.E.M.). Open columns indicate resistance response and shaded columns, capacitance response. The capacitance response is expressed in terms of decrease in blood pooling (upper diagram) and blood mobilization (lower diagram) (MELLANDER and NORDENFELT, 1970)

resistance vessel constriction, the concomitant effect in the capacitance vessels was more pronounced for dihydroergotamine than for noradrenaline (Fig. 9). In the calf, noradrenaline always elicited a constriction of the resistance vessels, whereas in two-thirds of the subjects, dihydroergotamine evoked dilator responses in these vessels. Despite these different effects on resistance vessels, dihydroergotamine elicited significantly more pronounced constriction of the capacitance vessels. Assuming the regional blood volume of the leg to be 5.5 ml/100 g tissue, the average capacitance response in terms of blood mobilization produced by dihydroergotamine was calculated to be 20% of regional blood volume in muscle and 29% in skin. These changes were long-lasting; no diminution of the effect occurred within 2 h. There was no net transcapillary fluid movement as evidenced by establishment of isovolumic states of the tissue in the steady-state phase of drug action. The capillary filtration coefficient was largely unaltered. Data obtained in the forearm were similar to the mean values found for the calf. This suggests that changes obtained in calf muscle are representative of the vascular reaction of skeletal muscle in general. The authors concluded that dihydroergotamine is a more efficient constrictor of capacitance vessels than noradrenaline in both skin and muscle, and that in skeletal muscle, dihydroergotamine, in contrast to noradrenaline, can elicit this constrictor response without much affecting resistance vessels.

Comparisons between the constrictor effects of dihydroergotamine and endogenous (OWEN and STÜRMER, 1971) and injected noradrenaline (MANZ and FELIX, 1974) on resistance and capacitance vessels in the cat hind limb have confirmed MELLANDER and NORDENFELT'S findings. OWEN and STÜRMER (1971) showed in acutely denervated calf muscle that the maximum capacitance response to intra-arterial administration of dihydroergotamine is similar in magnitude to that obtained during supramaximal sympathetic nerve stimulation. In the arterial segment, however, the maximum constriction induced by dihydroergotamine is only 9% of the maximum response obtained during nerve stimulation (Fig. 10).

A differential effect on resistance and capacitance vessels has also been demonstrated for ergotamine and dihydroergotoxine in the cat. Ergotamine is a weak constrictor of resistance vessels in denervated calf muscle but is about 10 times more potent than dihydroergotamine in constricting capacitance vessels. It differs from the latter in its effects on skin. Dihydroergotamine was found to constrict mainly capacitance vessels, whereas ergotamine had no such selective effect (OWEN and STÜRMER, 1972a). The results obtained in cats are substantiated by those obtained in man. BROOKE and ROBINSON (1970) reported a 50% reduction in forearm venous compliance following a dose of ergotamine. Venous compliance was calculated as the change in volume/100 ml of forearm for a fall in pressure from 25 mmHg to 5 mmHg. No significant changes in forearm blood flow occurred.

Dihydroergotoxine evokes effects in the cat which are similar to those of dihydroergotamine, but weaker. In contrast to both dihydroergotamine and ergotamine, this compound dilates precapillary sphincter vessels at doses which produce virtually no change in resistance vessels (OWEN and STÜRMER, 1972b). Such an effect would increase the capillary surface area available for filtration and might be expected to result in an increase in lymph flow. This has been borne out in the dog. Femoral lymph flow increases by approximately 55% in response to infusion of

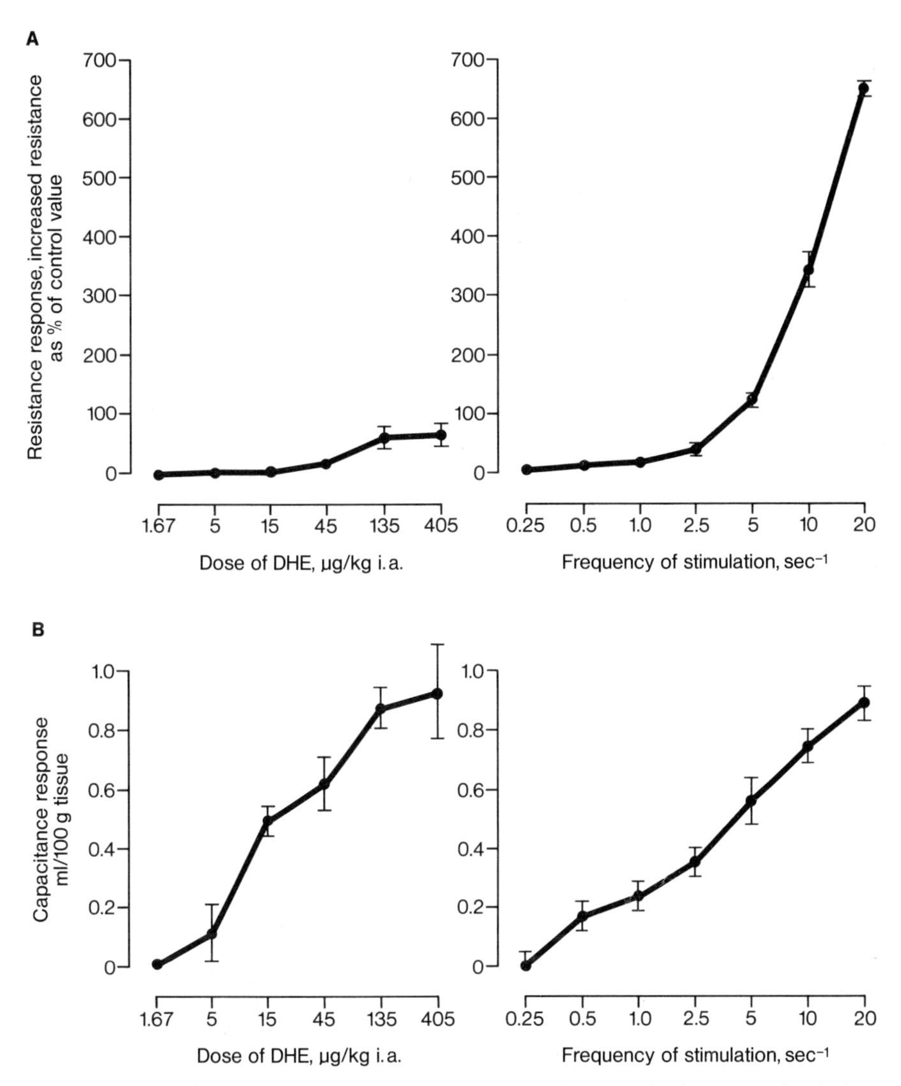

Fig. 10A and B. Effects of dihydroergotamine (DHE) and sympathetic nerve stimulation on resistance (A) and capacitance vessels (B) in denervated skeletal muscle of the cat hind limb (means ± S.E.M., n = 5). Doses are expressed as µg/kg calf muscle tissue (CHU et al., 1976)

150 µg/kg dihydroergotoxine (STÜRMER, 1977).[1] The effects of dihydroergotoxine on precapillary sphincters and vessel tone observed in the cat have not been confirmed in man. ULRICH et al. (1973) found that the compound significantly increased resting blood flow in the calf and decreased the capillary filtration rate, presumably as a result of the decrease in perfusion pressure. No effect was observed

[1] Ergotamine decreases lymph flow in the dog; methysergide and nicergoline have no effect (STÜRMER and CERLETTI, 1966; DE MICHELI and GLÄSSER, 1975).

on the venous side. The reduction in tone in resistance vessels was directly proportional to the pre-existing tone of the vessels. In patients with arterial insufficiency of the lower limbs, similar effects on resistance vessels were observed, but there was no change in capillary filtration rate after dihydroergotoxine (SIGGAARD-ANDERSEN et al., 1971). OWEN and STÜRMER argued that arterial insufficiency would lead to the accumulation of metabolic products which dilate precapillary sphincter vessels (COBBOLD et al., 1963). It is possible that precapillary sphincter tone might have been low in these patients prior to administration of dihydroergotoxine, thereby masking the effects observed in cats with normal vessels. Despite these conflicting findings with dihydroergotoxine, the effects which ULRICH and his colleagues (1973) obtained with dihydroergotamine correspond very closely to those obtained in both animals and man by MELLANDER and NORDENFELT (1970). Limb volume was decreased by 10 ml/l, corresponding to a decrease in venous volume of approximately 20%. No significant changes in blood flow or capillary filtration rate occurred.

Dihydroergostine has effects which are similar to those of dihydroergotoxine in man. Dihydroergostine increases blood flow in the calf in normal subjects but has no effect on capacitance vessels at a dose of 1 mg i.v. (ULRICH and SIGGAARD-ANDERSEN, 1971). Local venoconstriction can be demonstrated but only at doses five times greater than those required to obtain a similar effect with dihydroergotamine (Fig. 8) (AELLIG, 1976a).

These studies raise two interesting questions. Firstly, ergotamine, dihydroergotamine, and dihydroergotoxine are known to interact with α-adrenoceptors. Why, then, do they not affect vessels in the extremities in a manner comparable to noradrenaline; in other words, why should they show a preference for the vein? Even in vitro, the maximum response to ergotamine obtained in canine veins is greater than that in arteries using noradrenaline as the reference compound (MÜLLER-SCHWEINITZER and STÜRMER, 1974; MÜLLER-SCHWEINITZER, 1976). MÜLLER-SCHWEINITZER (1976) produced evidence suggesting that ergotamine exerts its constrictor action in the canine saphenous artery primarily by stimulating 5-HT receptors. In the femoral vein an action on α-adrenoceptors was confirmed in that the stimulant effect of the compound was antagonized competitively by phentolamine ($pA_2 = 6.8$) (MÜLLER-SCHWEINITZER and STÜRMER, 1974). AELLIG (1973) had previously shown that the venoconstrictor effect of dihydroergotamine in superficial hand veins in man was antagonized by phentolamine, but in two of the five subjects investigated, 54% and 38% of the initial response to dihydroergotamine could still be obtained after administration of the blocking drug. It could be that the dose of antagonist was not sufficient to induce blockade in all subjects, but it is of interest that in in vitro experiments, increases in venous tone induced by both ergotamine and dihydroergotamine cannot be completely blocked with phentolamine. The residual increase in tension can be abolished by indomethacin (MÜLLER-SCHWEINITZER, 1974; MÜLLER-SCHWEINITZER and BRUNDELL, 1975a, b). Both ergot alkaloids were found to provoke a significant increase in the level of prostaglandin E-like substance(s) in the bathing fluid. The authors concluded that contraction of vascular smooth muscle by certain ergot alkaloids is associated with increased synthesis of prostaglandin-like substance(s) having, like arachidonic acid, constrictor activity in veins but relaxant effects in arteries. They suggested that this differential effect could be the underlying mechanism for selective venoconstrictor activity.

Nevertheless this phenomenon does not provide an explanation for the second question which is, why do the alkaloids dilate resistance vessels in muscle and not skin and what mechanism underlies the vasodilation? Stimulation of β-adrenoceptors and blockade of α-adrenoceptors were eliminated as possible mechanisms by MELLANDER and NORDENFELT (1970), who showed that propranolol did not alter the response, and the dose of dihydroergotamine used did not significantly affect responses to noradrenaline. These authors were of the opinion that the dilation represented a central inhibitory action on adrenergic vasoconstrictor fiber discharge which was not counterbalanced by any significant direct constrictor effect. The fact that it is absent in the denervated preparation certainly suggests a nervously mediated phenomenon. This was shown to be so by CHU and STÜRMER (1973), who suggested an alternative explanation. Vasodilation was still present in animals pretreated with propranolol, chlorpheniramine, and acetylsalicylic acid, eliminating β-adrenoceptor and histamine receptor stimulation as well as prostaglandin synthesis as contributory factors. Phenoxybenzamine abolished the venoconstrictor response but enhanced the dilator effect in resistance vessels. The latter was abolished by atropine, revealing a constrictor effect similar in magnitude to that observed in the denervated preparation, implying involvement of a cholinergic mechanism. This thesis was strengthened by the finding that the dilator effect was enhanced by eserine. The authors therefore proposed that constriction of the capacitance vessels induced by intravenous administration of dihydroergotamine is mediated peripherally, principally by an action on α-adrenoceptors, whereas the dilator effect in resistance vessels is mediated centrally through the release of acetylcholine.

Whether this latter is a valid explanation for the vasodilator response to dihydroergotamine in resistance vessels in man (MELLANDER and NORDENFELT, 1970) is open to some doubt. Cholinergic vasodilator fibers have been shown to exist in the cat, dog, sheep, goat, and fox but not in the rat, hare, or monkey. A selective and pronounced increase in muscle blood flow has been observed in man during emotional stress, and this can be somewhat reduced by atropine, but as yet, histochemical evidence for the existence of cholinergic nerve terminals in skeletal muscle vessels in man is lacking (UVNÄS, 1971).

2. Effects on Cranial Blood Vessels

Many aspects of the actions of ergot alkaloids on blood vessels supplying the head (cranial vessels) or brain (cerebral vessels) are reviewed elsewhere (Chapters III, VI, and VII). This section will be concerned largely with findings obtained in animal experiments. Observations relevant to their therapeutic action in migraine are discussed in Section E4 of this chapter.

POOL and NASON (1935) made direct observations on the effects of ergotamine and found that it constricted vessels of the dura without significantly influencing pial vessels. Other studies using tissue thermometry (LUBSEN, 1940; SCHMIDT, 1934), perfusion methods (HEYMANS and REGNIERS, 1927), blood flow determinations in the internal carotid artery (SCHNEIDER and SCHNEIDER, 1934; DUMKE and

SCHMIDT, 1943), plethysmography, registration of cerebrospinal fluid pressure (KOOPMANS, 1939; LENNOX et al., 1935), or the nitrous oxide inhalation method (ABREU et al., 1947, 1948) in different animal species have not demonstrated clear-cut vascular activity with ergotamine or ergotoxine. On the one hand, cerebral vasoconstriction has been shown with relatively high doses of ergotamine (DUMKE and SCHMIDT, 1943; SCHNEIDER and SCHNEIDER, 1934; KOOPMANS, 1939; LEY and DE LA FONTAINE-VERWEY, 1929; POOL and NASON, 1935). On the other hand, the drug has also been reported to increase cerebral blood flow (HEYMANS and REGNIERS, 1927; SCHMIDT, 1934; LENNOX et al., 1935; ABREU et al., 1947). According to LENNOX et al. (1935), this could be considered to be a passive response to the blood pressure rise induced by the drug.

Most of the hydrogenated derivatives are effective hypotensive agents (Section A). However, despite a reduction in perfusion pressure, cerebral blood flow remains unimpaired following their administration (HAFKENSCHIEL et al., 1950a, b; ABREU et al., 1948). Since the cerebral vessels are not under any demonstrable neurogenic influence (HARMEL et al., 1949; SCHEINBERG, 1950), it is unlikely that cerebral vasodilation is mediated through a depression of sympathetic tone.

The outstanding impression obtained from an overall view of the effects of drugs on the cerebral circulation is the great resistance of cerebral blood flow to change (SOKOLOFF, 1959). This stability is probably achieved by a combination of two mechanisms. The baroreceptor reflexes, including those activated by receptors in the internal carotid artery, operate to maintain a relatively constant inflow pressure to the cerebral vessels without involving these vessels in the adjustments in tone necessary to accomplish it. In addition, cerebrovascular resistance is altered by the oxygen and carbon dioxide tensions in the blood (GUYTON, 1961) and also by chemical products of metabolism, which are probably the more potent agents affecting the cerebral circulation (SOKOLOFF, 1959). The net result is that blood flow in the brain is less readily changed by drugs than flow in other tissues. Consequently, it is not surprising that early studies in which the effects of ergot alkaloids on cerebral blood flow were measured using relatively insensitive methods, have yielded contradictory results.

Recent investigations, aided by highly sensitive methods, have partially resolved some of the early controversies. SAXENA (1972) determined the effects of ergotamine on the rate of blood flow in the canine external carotid vascular bed using an electromagnetic flow probe. Intravenous administration of the drug (1–32 μg/kg) elicited dose-dependent reductions in blood flow. Since blood pressure was not much changed, the author suggested that vasoconstriction in the external carotid bed induced by ergotamine might be selective. Subsequently, SAXENA and VLAAM-SCHLUTER (1974) studied the regional hemodynamic effects of ergotamine in the anesthetized dog in which the vagosympathetic trunks were divided in the cervical region to achieve dilation of the carotid vessels. Again, the authors showed that ergotamine elicited a constrictor effect in this vascular bed without simultaneously raising the systemic blood pressure. Blood flow in other regions was also decreased by ergotamine but to a smaller extent than in the carotid bed. The capacity of ergotamine to cause peripheral vasoconstriction in the seven vascular beds studied decreased in the following order: common carotid > internal carotid > femoral > superior mesenteric > renal > vertebral > coronary (Fig. 6, p. 353). The results demonstrated the selective action of ergotamine on carotid vessels. The sensitivity of the carotid vasculature to ergotamine has also been shown in canine nasal blood vessels (VARGAFTIG and LEFORT, 1974; SCHÖNBAUM et al., 1975). SPIRA et al. (1976) investigated the effects of ergotamine on the carotid circulation in anesthetized monkeys. Electromagnetic flow probes were placed on both common and external carotid arteries. Internal carotid flow was determined by subtracting the external from the common carotid flow. They found that intravenous administration of 3.6 and 15 μg/kg ergotamine elicited marked increases in resistance in the external carotid bed. Resistance in the internal carotid vessels also rose, but the increase was not statistically significant. Although changes in blood flow in other organ systems were not determined, the absence of any change in systemic blood pressure suggested a selective constrictor effect in the carotid vessels. These results indicate that ergotamine does not significantly influence the cerebral circulation, possibly because of the efficiency of cerebral autoregulatory mechanisms. In contrast, the external carotid vascular bed appears to be the most sensitive of all to the vasoconstrictor action of ergotamine.

Similar techniques have also been applied to studies of the effects of the hydrogenated ergot alkaloids on the cranial circulation. VAN DEN BERGH (1956), using arteriography, could not show an effect with dihydroergotamine on the cerebral circulation of anesthetized dogs. However, when the cerebral vessels were dilated by either nicotinic acid or caffeine, the compound induced marked vasoconstriction. Similarly, BOISMARE et al. (1975b) did not observe changes in cerebral blood flow following dihydroergotamine administration using an electromagnetic flow probe in anesthetized dogs in the supine position. In the erect position however, the drug provoked a slow, but significant increase in vertebral blood flow. Blood pressure was not influenced.

Earlier studies on the effects of dihydroergotoxine on cerebral vessels produced inconsistent and inconclusive results (TAESCHLER et al., 1952; KNAPP et al., 1955; BALDY-MOULINIER, 1968; GOTTSTEIN et al., 1959). In particular, it is difficult to distinguish between direct effects of the drug on vessels and secondary effects related to changes in perfusion pressure or pCO_2 (SZEWCZYKOWSKI et al., 1970). REGLI et al. (1971) examined the effects of dihydroergotoxine on the cerebral vessels of anesthetized cats in which pO_2, pCO_2, pH, and temperature were maintained within physiologic limits. Cortical blood flow was monitored by the external detection of the *beta* activity of ^{85}Kr injected into the bracheocephalic artery. At intravenous doses of 16–52 μg/kg, dihydroergotoxine changed neither blood flow nor blood pressure. The authors concluded that the drug was devoid of significant effects on cerebral blood flow. In view of the enormous capacity of the brain to maintain a constant perfusion, it is not surprising that the hydrogenated ergot alkaloids, which possess weaker vascular activity than their natural counterparts, do not modify the cerebral circulation.

The hallucinogenic property of *d*-LSD has prompted investigations of its effect on cerebral blood flow. In anesthetized and conscious cats, intravenous administration of *d*-LSD 10–100 μg/kg did not alter the rate of venous outflow from the superior sagittal sinus (INGVAR and SÖDERBERG, 1956). However, when the drug was administered via the carotid artery, there was a transient increase in cerebral blood flow which was not associated with any change in blood pressure. GOLDMAN et al. (1975) used an indicator-fractionation technique to determine regional cerebral blood flow changes following the administration of *d*-LSD in conscious rats. They found that the drug induced a significant increase in flow rate only in the cerebellum and frontal and parietal cortex. In contrast, 1-methyl-LSD (34b), 6-nor-LSD (72i) and 8,9-dihydro-LSD (74b) had no effect.

SAXENA (1972) showed that methysergide elicited a significant decrease in the rate of blood flow in the external carotid vascular bed without altering blood pressure in anesthetized dogs. Subsequently, the responses of several vascular beds to methysergide were compared (SAXENA, 1974), and it was found that whereas the common and internal carotid vascular beds constricted, those supplied by the vertebral and femoral arteries dilated (Fig. 6). Similar results have also been reported in monkeys. SPIRA et al. (1976) showed that intravenous administration of methysergide led to increases in resistance in both external and internal carotid beds. Furthermore, the response of the external carotid vascular bed was more profound. Although the authors did not study the regional hemodynamic effects of methysergide, they argued that the absence of any change in systemic blood pressure could be taken as evidence for a selective constrictor effect on cranial vessels.

In general, it can be concluded that the extracranial vessels are most sensitive to the constrictor action of the ergot alkaloids. Although the ergot alkaloids have little influence on total cerebral blood flow, the possibility that they may have significant effects on local flow in specific regions of the brain cannot be excluded.

3. Effects on Renal Blood Vessels

Ergometrine and methysergide have negligible effects on renal vessels (FANCHAMPS et al., 1960; SAXENA, 1974; BELL et al., 1974), whereas bromocriptine induces dilation in the dog (CLARK, 1977). Not unexpectedly, ergotamine constricts these vessels, but the effects in this organ are considerably smaller than those observed in carotid vessels. In the dog, dose-dependent reductions in arterial resistance and renal volume occur from an intravenous dose of 1 μg/kg (CARPI and VIRNO, 1957; SAXENA and VLAAM-SCHLUTER, 1974). Responses to small doses are transient, in contrast to those in cranial vessels which may last for 30 min or more (CARPI and VIRNO, 1957). This probably reflects autoregulation taking place in the kidney. Larger doses (from 50 μg/kg i.v.) in the cat and dog induce marked reductions in renal vein flow or renal volume, which are evident before the onset of the blood pressure rise and which may persist after blood pressure has returned to normal levels (BARRY, 1937; ROTHLIN and CERLETTI, 1949a; WEIDMANN and TAESCHLER, 1966). Ergostine elicits similar effects (WEIDMANN and TAESCHLER, 1966).

The effects of dihydroergotamine in the cat are variable. MELLANDER and NORDENFELT (1970) found that this compound increased renal resistance in some animals but caused a decrease in others. ROTHLIN (1946) detected no significant change in renal volume despite the fact that the drug depressed blood pressure. Effects obtained on renal vessels in man are likewise minimal (REUBI, 1949).

Circulation in the kidney in anesthetized cats is modified to a greater extent by dihydroergotoxine and dihydroergocristine. Reductions occur in renal plasma flow (measured by PAH clearance) or kidney volume but only if blood pressure falls. In contrast to the effects on blood pressure, changes which are observed in the kidney circulation are relatively short-lasting (KONZETT and ROTHLIN, 1953; LOCKETT and WADLEY, 1969). Whether reductions in flow are passive responses to a reduction in perfusion pressure or due to reflex intrarenal vasoconstriction is unclear. In the isolated kidney perfused with blood at constant pressure, concentrations of dihydroergocristine of up to 2.5 μg/ml have no significant effect (LOCKETT and WADLEY, 1969).

Changes in renal plasma flow and glomerular filtration rate induced by dihydroergotoxine in anesthetized dogs are negligible or inconstant, despite the fact that reductions in blood pressure may occur (BLAKE, 1953; HANDLEY and MOYER, 1954; MOYER et al., 1955; LONGO and SANTA, 1968). The disadvantages inherent in renal hemodynamic studies in animals under anesthesia are obvious, particularly those in which the kidney is manipulated. Experiments in conscious animals, on the other hand, provide results which are more comparable to those obtained in man. Renal plasma flow is reduced by dihydroergotoxine. Glomerular filtration rate is either unchanged or decreased, indicating that the filtration fraction is elevated (BLAKE, 1953; OYEN, 1956). Maximal changes in renal plasma flow are obtained at very low doses (12 μg/kg i.v.); in OYEN's study, decreases in renal plasma flow of 25–30% occurred at this dose in both normotensive and hypertensive dogs. The changes observed in the hypertensive animals were associated with falls in blood pressure of up to 40 mmHg, but reductions in flow of a similar magnitude occurred in normotensive animals in the absence of significant blood pressure changes.

Comparable changes have been obtained following acute parenteral administration of dihydroergocornine in normotensive and hypertensive patients (FREIS et al., 1949; CROSLEY et al., 1950), although DEUTSCH and MARKOFF (1953) reported variable effects in response to dihydroergotoxine. The disproportionately greater decrease in renal plasma flow than in blood pressure indicated renal vasoconstriction. CROSLEY and his colleagues suggested that the kidney, in its function as a circulatory regulator, diverts a large fraction of its normal 25% of cardiac output to the more essential brain.

This protective mechanism apparently serves to overcome the effects of the peripheral α-adrenoceptor blocking action of dihydroergocornine which might be expected to cause renal vasodilation. REUBI (1949, 1950) found renal plasma flow decreased by 15–20% following administration of the components of dihydroergotoxine (dihydroergocornine, dihydroergocristine, and dihydroergokryptine). Calculated resistance was increased over a long period, and the filtration fraction was elevated. Resistance in the efferent arterioles was estimated to be increased by 50–60%, whereas afferent arteriolar resistance was not significantly changed. Dihydroergotoxine does not raise the maximum excretory capacity for PAH nor the maximum reabsorptive capacity for glucose, which implies that the drug does not materially affect tubular activity (REUBI, 1952a). REUBI concluded that increases in PAH extraction which occurred in response to dihydroergotoxine in patients in which initial extraction was low may represent a modification of the intrarenal distribution of blood, the blood flow in the medulla, capsule, and cicatricial zones being decreased.

The results of these studies demonstrate clearly that the response to a single parenteral dose of dihydroergotoxine is to cause (indirectly) vasoconstriction in renal vessels. Nevertheless, following prolonged therapy with the drug in both normotensive and hypertensive patients, renal vessels dilate. Renal plasma flow may not change (Reubi, 1952b) or may increase (Deutsch and Markoff, 1953; Lasch, 1954). Blood pressure is usually reduced by the drug in hypertensive patients, but regardless of the effects on blood pressure, renal vascular resistance decreases. These findings underline how misleading an acute experiment can be and emphasize the caution that is necessary in predicting the pharmacologic effects of a drug during long-term therapy from results obtained following a single dose.

4. Effects on Mesenteric Blood Vessels

As in most other vascular beds, ergotamine constricts mesenteric vessels. In the dog, dose-dependent reductions in blood flow, measured by an electromagnetic flow meter, and increases in resistance occur from a dose of 1 μg/kg given intravenously. The changes are, however, much smaller than those obtained in carotid vessels (Saxena and Vlaam-Schluter, 1974). This finding is in agreement with that of Rothlin and Cerletti (1949a) in the cat. Topical application of the natural and hydrogenated alkaloids to the rat mesoappendix causes constriction of the arterioles and precapillary sphincters. Haley et al. (1954) rated them in order of decreasing potency: dihydroergokryptine, ergokryptine, ergotamine, dihydroergocornine, dihydroergotoxine, ergosine, ergocornine, dihydroergocristine, dihydroergotamine, and ergocristine. Ergometrine was ineffective. Apart from finding ergokryptine and dihydroergokryptine slightly more potent than ergotamine, their results correspond fairly well with their relative pressor activities in the pithed rat (Fig. 5). By the intravenous route, ergotamine, dihydroergotamine and dihydroergotoxine all induced dilation. It would seem likely that the dilator effect of the latter two drugs reflected blockade of α-adrenoceptors; closure of precapillary sphincters by adrenaline was inhibited by both alkaloids at the dose effective in causing dilation of these vessels. The dose of ergotamine necessary to demonstrate α-adrenoceptor blockade, however, was 10 times that inducing vasodilation. It is therefore likely that vasodilation was the result of an action on central vasomotor control mechanisms.

A number of other studies have confirmed a vasodilator effect in mesenteric vessels for dihydro ergot alkaloids in cats. Flow was measured either by monitoring venous outflow from a segment of small intestine or recording intestinal volume with a plethysmograph (Rothlin, 1946; Rothlin and Cerletti, 1949b; Konzett and Rothlin, 1953; Biber et al., 1974). Mellander and Nordenfelt (1970) observed variable effects; resistance vessels dilated in some experiments (mean −17%) but constricted in others (mean +14%). After denervation, dihydroergotamine always elicited increases in resistance. The capacitance vessels of the gut showed small constrictor responses both before and after denervation. Capillary filtration coefficient was slightly reduced. The duration of the vascular responses in the intestine was always shorter than that in muscle and skin. The difference between these results and those of other workers may lie in the fact that the dose used by MELLANDER and NORDENFELT did not exert significant blockade of α-adrenoceptors.

Methysergide decreases blood flow slighty in the dog but less so than in the carotid vascular bed. Vascular resistance, however, is not significantly affected (SAXENA, 1974). Neither *d*-LSD, brom-LSD nor nicergoline exert demonstrable effects (ALTURA, 1971; ARCARI et al., 1968). In contrast, the marked dilator effect of bromocriptine in this vascular bed appears to be largely responsible for the hypotensive action of this drug (CLARK, 1977).

5. Effects on Coronary Blood Vessels

Little attention has been paid to the actions of the ergot alkaloids on coronary vessels. The aggravation of angina pectoris that sometimes follows the administration of ergotamine in patients with coronary heart disease has been assumed to result from drug-induced coronary artery spasm. There is little evidence to support this view. Occasionally, ergotamine has been shown to cause powerful constriction of the coronary vessels in the isolated, fibrillating heart of the dog, perfused in situ (KATZ and LINDNER, 1939). According to the authors, this suggested that coronary spasm can and may occur in man. In the isolated, perfused heart of the rabbit, dihydroergotamine and even ergometrine (although at very high doses) decrease coronary artery flow, implying vasoconstriction (SHERIF et al., 1956; KARP et al., 1960).

For practical purposes, the important criterion in determining the deleterious or beneficial effect of a drug on the coronary circulation is not whether it causes dilation or constriction of the coronary vessels but rather whether it changes the ratio between myocardial blood flow and the energy expenditure of the heart. Sympathomimetic amines, for instance, would be expected to induce constriction in coronary vessels as a result of stimulation of α-adrenoceptors. In fact, they induce vasodilation which is largely secondary to the increase in oxygen demand resulting from myocardial stimulation; the contribution made by activation of β-adrenoceptors to vasodilation in the coronary vessels is very small (BERNE, 1958). Conversely, reductions in coronary flow induced by β-adrenoceptor blocking drugs are the consequence of a decrease in cardiac work and/or oxygen demand and not to unmasking of active vasoconstriction (DAVIS et al., 1969; LADDU and SOMANI, 1972). Many ergot compounds, and especially ergotamine, not only alter peripheral resistance and venous return, which would result in reflex changes in cardiac performance, but also directly influence cardiac function by modifying vagal and cardiac sympathetic nerve activity. These effects are likely to bring about changes in myocardial work and oxygen requirements. Little useful information can be provided, therefore, by experiments in isolated (i.e., denervated) hearts perfused under constant pressure or flow conditions.

According to SAXENA and VLAAM-SCHLUTER (1974), significant decreases in blood flow and increases in resistance can occur in most vascular beds without corresponding changes taking place in coronary vessels following i.v. administration of ergotamine in anesthetized dogs with intact cardiac innervation. Coronary vascular resistance is increased only from a dose of 16 μg/kg, i.e., eight times the threshold dose for increasing resistance in the carotid, femoral, superior mesenteric, renal, and vertebral vascular beds. Even a relatively high dose of ergotamine (50 μg/kg) reduces coronary blood flow only slightly, while causing a significant increase in blood pressure and decreases in heart rate and cardiac output. The minimal effects observed on myocardial blood flow and vascular resistance probably reflect the lack of significant alterations in contractility and left ventricular work. Similar effects were obtained with dihydroergotamine and dihydroergotoxine (SCHMITT et al., 1971).

If the findings in anesthetized dogs reflect the situation in patients treated with ergot alkaloids, there is no evidence for the assumption that ergotamine-induced anginal pain is a consequence of a diminution in myocardial perfusion brought about by constriction of the coronary vessels. BROOKE and ROBINSON (1970) have suggested an alternative explanation, namely that it may be due to the venoconstrictor action of the drug. The rise in venous filling pressure that results would tend to increase the metabolic needs of the myocardium. This change would be expected to facilitate the development of angina pectoris in response to exercise or other stress in patients with impaired myocardial perfusion.

6. Effects on Uterine Blood Vessels

In contrast to its potent effects on uterine contractility, methylergometrine has little effect on uterine blood vessels. Slight arteriolar constriction has been observed (by colpomicroscopy) in one of four nonpregnant women following i.v. administration of a high dose (0.6 mg) of the compound, but a lower dose induced no change (KOFLER, 1972). More precise measurements of uterine blood flow, also in nonpregnant women, have been made during surgery using an electromagnetic flowmeter. The dose of methylergometrine usually used therapeutically (0.1 mg) induced no change in flow. In contrast, oxytocin 5 I.U. reduced flow by 26–78%, and calculated uterine vascular resistance increased (KLINGENBERG, 1973). The absence of vasoconstrictor activity observed with ergometrine is in accord with results obtained in post partum cats and sheep (CERLETTI, 1949; ASSALI et al., 1959).

A vasoconstrictor effect for methylergometrine can be shown following topical application to vessels in the uterine omentum of the rat, but a very high concentration (0.2 mg/ml) is necessary to obtain a visible effect. Ergometrine and especially ergotamine are more potent. A vasoconstrictor response to the latter can be obtained at a concentration of 0.5 μg/ml (LANDESMAN and MENDELSOHN, 1956). The potent effect of ergotamine in constricting maternal uterine and placental vessels is considered to be responsible for death in rat fetuses following administration of very high doses (from 10 mg/kg p.o.). Anomalies, typical of those resulting from uterine clamping, are seen on days 13–16 of pregnancy when fetal mortality is maximal (60%). Ergometrine, which has similar uterotonic activity to ergotamine but far less cardiovascular activity, has no such effect. Blood supply to the embryo was determined by measuring transplacental passage of ^{3}H-1-leucine. Three hours after an i.v. dose of ergotamine (2.5 mg/kg) administered on day 14 of pregnancy, blood supply to the fetus was reduced by almost 90%, resulting in 63% embryo mortality. In contrast, fetal blood supply was reduced by only 30% following a dose of ergometrine four times as great and all embryos survived. The authors considered that the action of ergotamine on fetal development and survival was due exclusively to the drug's action on maternal cardiovascular function (LEIST and GRAUWILER, 1974; SCHÖN et al., 1975).

D. Actions on the Heart

1. Effects in Mammals

a) Nature of the Effect

A property which is common to peptide ergot alkaloids and their dihydro derivatives is their ability to reduce heart rate. Bradycardia is almost invariably observed following their administration in conscious and anesthetized animals and in man regardless of the nature of the blood pressure response. This effect of the alkaloids reflects a fundamental difference between these drugs and non-ergot α-adrenoceptor blocking drugs, all of which induce tachycardia, in most cases as a consequence of a blood pressure fall (NICKERSON, 1949). Reflex tachycardia during the depressor phase of the response to dihydro derivatives occurs only in the rabbit, but bradycardia ensues when the blood pressure has returned to control levels (KÜHNS, 1949; ROTHLIN and CERLETTI, 1953). Reductions in heart rate are not necessarily paralleled by reductions in contractility (LANDS et al., 1950; COTTEN et al., 1957; WELLENS and WAUTERS, 1968; OSSWALD et al., 1970; SCHMITT et al., 1971).

In experimental animals, bradycardia is often profound, especially if resting heart rate is very high. Individual responses to a given dose are very variable, however, and no clear relationship can be determined between dose or resting heart rate and the magnitude of the response (Table 4).

Bromination of α-ergokryptine not only alters the receptor stimulating properties of the parent compound but also to a certain extent its action on heart rate. Of 12 dogs under chloralose-urethane anesthesia treated with bromocriptine 12.5 μg/kg i.v., bradycardia occurred in only five. An increase in heart rate occurred in three dogs, but this was of shorter duration and more rapid onset than the accompanying blood pressure reduction. In the remaining four animals there was no significant change in rate, although blood pressure fell by up to 80 mmHg (CLARK et al., 1978).

Bradycardia is not a property confined to the peptide alkaloids; *d*-LSD induces bradycardia in anesthetized cats from a dose of 50 μg/kg i.v. (ROTHLIN, 1957; TAUBERGER and KLIMMER, 1968). Severe conduction disturbances develop at high doses (CERVONI et al., 1963). In man the effects of the compound are reversed. Tachycardia occurs after oral doses of 1–1.5 μg/kg. These doses, although far lower than those effective in inducing cardiovascular changes in animals, are sufficient to induce psychologic changes in normal and psychotic subjects (GRAHAM and KHALIDI, 1954; ISBELL, 1959). The effects on the cardiovascular system can probably be considered as a component of or the response to the motor and behavioural effects observed. *D*-lysergic acid methylcarbinolamide (12) induces only moderate

Table 4. Effect of ergot alkaloids on heart rate

Experimental animal	Compound	Dose	Heart rate (beats/min)		Reference
			Resting level	Decrease	
Conscious cat	Ergotoxine	1 mg/kg	122	43	1
			104	13	
			98	18	
			96	28	
			94	6	
			60	9	
Anesthetized cat	Ergotamine	0.5 mg	180	60	2
			172	16	
Anesthetized dog (vagi divided)	Ergotamine	70 µg/kg	250	83	3
		80 µg/kg	250	63	
		1 mg/kg	244	72	
		160 µg/kg	222	55	
		200 µg/kg	167	52	
		1 mg	136	17	
Anesthetized dog (vagi divided)	Ergotamine	50 µg/kg	192	45	4
			186	78	
			183	54	
			178	30	
			162	36	
			156	54	
			150	30	

References: 1. MOORE and CANNON (1930); 2. ROTHLIN (1925); 3. ANDRUS and MARTIN (1927); 4. WOODS et al. (1932).

decreases in heart rate (GLÄSSER, 1961). Bromination of LSD (brom-LSD) has resulted in a complete loss of cardiovascular activity both in animals (CERLETTI and ROTHLIN, 1955; CERVONI et al., 1963) and in man (MURPHREE et al., 1958). Methysergide has negligible effects on heart rate in cats at doses which abolish pressor responses to 5-HT, i.e., 5–20 µg/kg i.v. (FANCHAMPS et al., 1960), but doses in excess of 1 mg/kg induce pronounced bradycardia in dogs (ANTONACCIO et al., 1975; HELKE et al., 1976) and hypertensive rats (ANTONACCIO and COTÉ, 1976).

Like bromocriptine, 1,1-dimethyl-3-(6-methyl-8β-ergolenyl-methyl)-urea (88 h) (FEHR et al., 1974) has variable effects on heart rate. In anesthetized cats, heart rate usually falls in response to i.v. doses below 40 µg/kg but increases at higher doses (CLARK, unpublished). In the conscious, hypertensive dog (resting heart rate <80 beats/min) the drug induces tachycardia, whereas in the hypertensive rat (resting heart rate >300 beats/min) it causes bradycardia (SALZMANN, unpublished).

b) Effects on Vagosympathetic Control of Heart Rate

When atropine is given to an animal in which heart rate has been depressed by an ergot alkaloid, heart rate may return to normal (ANDRUS and MARTIN,

1927; LOCKETT and WADLEY, 1969). Such experiments have provided the basis for the belief that the alkaloids induce bradycardia solely by stimulating vagal motor nuclei (ROTHLIN, 1946, 1957; NICKERSON, 1949). An alternative explanation is that the alkaloids may act to diminish the accelerating action of the sympathetic, or both mechanisms may be involved.

Numerous studies have shown that if the alkaloids are injected *after* vagotomy or administration of atropine, bradycardia still occurs, although the effect may be slightly attenuated. This has been demonstrated for the natural alkaloids (ROTHLIN, 1923, 1925; ANDRUS and MARTIN, 1927; OTTO, 1928; WOODS et al., 1932; ROSENBLUETH and CANNON, 1933; LANDS et al., 1950; LEVY and AHLQUIST, 1961; SCHMITT et al., 1971), their dihydro derivatives (BAUMANN et al., 1954; ABEL et al., 1963; SCHMITT et al., 1971), *d*-LSD (CERVONI et al., 1963; TAUBERGER and KLIMMER, 1968), and methysergide (ANTONACCIO et al., 1975) in several species using a variety of anesthetics. Although these findings do not provide positive evidence for a reduction in sympathetic nerve activity, they do raise the question as to whether vagal stimulation is a contributory factor at all in ergot-induced bradycardia. That the alkaloids do exert an effect on the vagus under certain conditions is evident from experiments reported by MOORE and CANNON (1930). These authors studied the effects of ergotoxine in resting conscious cats. Ergotoxine induced a decrease in heart rate of 14 beats/min from a mean resting rate of 94 beats/min. After sympathectomy, which depressed heart rate to 76 beats/min, ergotoxine still caused bradycardia. In animals with vagi divided (sympathetic nerves intact), reductions in heart rate occurred in response to ergotoxine in only two of five animals, despite the fact that resting heart rate was much higher in these animals than in sympathectomized animals. These authors also showed that the increase in heart rate which occurred when the animals struggled under restraint was reduced by 50% following ergotoxine administration, implying an inhibitory effect on reflex sympathetic nerve activity. The observation that the ergot alkaloids enhance the effects of vagal stimulation and acetylcholine on the heart (DALE, 1906; ROTHLIN, 1923; OTTO, 1928; DE VLEESCHHOUWER, 1949) has also been explained in terms of a possible removal of reflex accelerator impulses (DALE, 1906).

More direct evidence for an inhibitory action on cardiac sympathetic nerve activity is provided by experiments showing that bradycardia induced by the alkaloids is attenuated by the adrenergic neuron-blocking drug, guanethidine (ANTONACCIO et al., 1975) or by spinal section at the level of the first thoracic vertebra (BLUNTSCHLI, 1948). Although these latter studies suggest that in anesthetized animals, reductions in heart rate are almost entirely due to depression of cardic sympathetic nerve function, they do not provide information on the site of action. Some of the ergot alkaloids have pronounced effects on noradrenaline release from cardiac sympathetic nerve endings, which may well contribute to their cardiac slowing effects. Nevertheless, it would seem that inhibition of sympathetic nerve activity takes place predominantly at some site within the central nervous system. Ergotamine, dihydroergotamine, methysergide, and bromocriptine have all been shown to induce bradycardia when injected directly into the cerebral ventricles (RETTORI and HALEY, 1967; SHARE, 1973; ANTONACCIO et al., 1975; CLARK et al., 1978); the effects of methysergide and bromocriptine occur at doses ineffective by the intravenous route. This action does not require the integrity of higher central nervous structures. Bradycardia is not diminished and may even be augmented in decorticate and decerebrate preparations (ROSENBLUETH and CANNON, 1933; CERVONI et al., 1963).

c) Effects on Prejunctional Receptor Sites

It has been proposed that noradrenergic nerve endings are endowed with sites resembling α-adrenoceptors in effector cells. Activation of these prejunctional α-adrenoceptors by liberated noradrenaline or exogenous agonists depresses the quanta of transmitter released per impulse. Conversely, α-adrenoceptor blocking agents interrupt the negative feedback mechanism and facilitate transmitter release (FARNEBO and HAMBERGER, 1971; KIRPEKAR and PUIG, 1971; LANGER et al., 1971; STARKE, 1971). Evidence in support of this hypothesis has been reviewed by LANGER (1974), STJÄRNE (1975), and STARKE (1977). It might be expected that ergot alkaloids would influence noradrenaline efflux and cardiac stimulant effects in response to sympathetic nerve stimulation according to the relative preponderance of their α-adrenoceptor agonist or antagonist activity (see also Chapter III).

STARKE (1972) has presented evidence that dihydroergotamine augments the overflow of noradrenaline evoked by sympathetic nerve stimulation in the isolated perfused rabbit heart. A significant effect was obtained at a concentration of 0.19 μg/ml without any change occurring in the spontaneous outflow of noradrenaline. No effect on noradrenaline uptake was detected in concentrations up to 6 μg/ml. In this respect, the effect of the compound resembled that of low concentrations of phentolamine (STARKE et al., 1971). Phenoxybenzamine has been reported to induce five- to sixfold increases in noradrenaline overflow, whereas dihydroergotamine (0.19 μg/ml) increases it by a factor of only two or less (LANGER et al., 1972; MCCULLOCH et al., 1972). An increase in noradrenaline overflow would be expected to enhance the motor response to nerve stimulation. In experiments in vivo, however, dihydroergotamine appears to inhibit the release of transmitter, i.e., it diminishes the positive chronotropic response of the heart to nerve stimulation (SCHOLTYSIK, unpublished). Frequency-response curves were obtained in pithed cats for increases in heart rate in response to stimulation of spinal segments C7 and T1. Dihydroergotamine caused a significant displacement of the frequency-response curve to the right at a dose of 15 μg/kg i.v.. Higher doses (up to 155 μg/kg) induced little further change. Dihydroergotoxine (0.1–3.5 μg/kg) and ergotamine (0.5–7.5 μg/kg) exerted similar effects (SCHOLTYSIK, 1975 and unpublished observations). Both compounds induced a parallel displacement of the frequency-response curve for heart rate to the right. The effects were dose-dependent. There was no convincing evidence that the inhibitory effects of the ergot alkaloids on heart rate were mediated entirely by prejunctional α-adrenoceptor stimulation. Phentolamine failed to influence the effect of ergotamine and only partially reversed the effect of dihydroergotoxine.

A preferential interaction with either pre- or postjunctional α-adrenoceptors has been demonstrated with both agonists and antagonists in the rat pulmonary artery. Methoxamine and phenylephrine, for example, have a predominant action on postjunctional receptors, i.e., much higher concentrations are needed to reduce the stimulation-induced overflow of noradrenaline (prejunctional effect) than to elicit smooth muscle contraction (postjunctional effect) (STARKE et al., 1975a). Conversely, yohimbine acts predominantly on prejunctional α-adrenoceptors. A concentration of 3×10^{-8}M significantly enhances stimulation-evoked noradrenaline overflow, whereas contractions of the pulmonary artery induced by phenylephrine are not inhibited at concentrations below 3×10^{-7}M (STARKE et al., 1975b; STARKE and ENDO, 1976). These findings are compatible with the concept that pre- and postjunctional α-adrenoceptors may have different physico-chemical characteristics (DUBOCOVICH and LANGER, 1974).

DREW (1976) has confirmed a preferential stimulant action on postjunctional receptors for methoxamine and phenylephrine in the pithed rat and has shown in addition that α-LSD is more active at prejunctional than postjunctional adrenoceptors. Heart rate was elevated by continous stimulation of the cardiac sympathetic nerves. The doses of the agonists which reduced heart rate by 50 beats/min (prejunctional effect) and raised diastolic blood pressure by 50 mmHg (postjunctional effect) were determined. The mean doses of methoxamine and phenylephrine which reduced heart rate were 23 and >20 times the doses increasing blood pressure respectively. *D*-LSD, on the other hand, did not increase blood pressure at a dose four times that which decreased heart rate by 50 beats/min.

The urea derivative of lysergol (88h) (FEHR et al., 1974), for which there is evidence for postjunctional α-adrenoceptor stimulant activity, inhibits responses to pre- and postganglionic stimulation of the cardiac sympathetic nerves in anesthetized cats. The compound exerts this effect from a dose of 80 μg/kg. A greater inhibitory effect was obtained on responses to low frequency (2–8 Hz) than to high frequency stimulation (>8 Hz). Responses to stimulation frequencies above 16 Hz were potentiated (CLARK, unpublished).

Methysergide does not interact with postjunctional α-adrenoceptors (FANCHAMPS et al., 1960), and there is no evidence to date that 5-HT receptors are involved in the modulation of transmitter release from noradrenergic nerves. Not unexpectedly, methysergide does not affect frequency-response curves for electrically stimulated increases in heart rate in anesthetized dogs (ANTONACCIO et al., 1975).

There is evidence, however, that noradrenergic nerve endings are endowed with dopamine receptors. Dopamine has been found to depress stimulation-induced noradrenaline release in the perfused cat spleen (LANGER, 1973), rabbit ear artery (MCCULLOCH et al., 1973), nictitating membrane (ENERO and LANGER, 1975), and cat and dog heart (LONG et al., 1975). The inhibitory effect of dopamine can be blocked by dopamine receptor antagonists but not by phentolamine (RAND et al., 1975). Bromocriptine, a potent dopamine receptor stimulant in vascular smooth muscle (CLARK, 1977) and the central nervous system (HÖKFELT and FUXE, 1972; CORRODI et al., 1973; JOHNSON et al., 1976) also activates dopamine receptors at the nerve terminal (SCHOLTYSIK, 1978). Significant inhibition of heart rate responses to sympathetic nerve stimulation was obtained in pithed cats at a dose of 10 μg/kg i.v. This dose of bromocriptine is comparable to that which stimulates postjunctional dopamine receptors in the superior mesenteric vascular bed of the dog (CLARK, 1977). The dopamine receptor blocking agent, haloperidol, inhibited the prejunctional effects of infusions of bromocriptine dose-dependently. A small part of the effect of bromocriptine may be mediated by prejunctional α-adrenoceptor stimulation, since phentolamine induced a partial reversal.

d) Interaction with Cardiac β-Adrenoceptors

DALE's early observation that the excitatory effects of adrenaline on the heart were not inhibited by ergotamine (DALE, 1906; BARGER and DALE, 1907) has been substantiated by many authors. OTTO (1928) made the interesting observation that administration of very large doses of ergotamine and ergotoxine in anesthetized dogs and cats cause quite dramatic falls in body temperature. Reductions in the cardiac responses to adrenaline and sympathetic nerve stimulation attributed to the alkaloids were in fact the result of hypothermia. When body temperature was maintained at 30° C, no diminution in responses to adrenergic stimuli appeared, even after a total intravenous dose of 90 mg/kg.

There is no evidence that any of the natural ergot alkaloids interact with β-adrenoceptors in the heart. In anesthetized cats and dogs, intravenous doses between 50 and 200 μg/kg not only do not block but invariably enhance the positive inotropic and positive chronotropic effects of adrenaline, noradrenaline, and isoprenaline, regardless of the type of anesthetic used (WOODS et al., 1932; LANDS et al., 1950; LEVY and AHLQUIST, 1961; WENZEL et al., 1964; WELLENS and WAUTERS, 1968; OSSWALD et al., 1970; MOUILLÉ, 1970; SCHMITT et al., 1971). A similar effect has been obtained with methysergide in dogs treated with atropine. Following a dose of 3 mg/kg i.v., which is 100 times that which abolishes pressor responses to 5-HT (FANCHAMPS et al., 1960), chronotropic responses to isoprenaline and sympathetic nerve stimulation are unaltered, but responses to adrenaline, noradrenaline, tyramine, and the ganglionic stimulant DMPP (1,1-dimethyl-4-phenylpiperazinium iodide) are all significantly increased (ANTONACCIO et al., 1975).

Divergent opinions have been expressed on the interaction between dihydro ergot alkaloids and β-adrenoceptors. According to ROTHLIN (1944), DE VLEESCHHOUWER (1949) and SCHMITT et al. (1971), none of these compounds depress cardiac responses to adrenaline in anesthetized dogs at doses up to 200 μg/kg or in heart-lung preparations. LEVY and AHLQUIST (1961), on the other hand, considered that both dihydroergotamine and dihydroergocornine (500 μg/kg) possess β-adrenoceptor blocking activity on the heart, although their statement was not supported by any experimental data. Apparent antagonism of both chronotropic and inotropic responses to catecholamines has also been reported for dihydroergotoxine in the dog, but whereas α-adrenoceptor blockade was evident following a dose of 40 μg/kg, a dose of 5 mg/kg was required to depress the effects of β-adrenoceptor stimulation by 15–30% (COTTEN et al., 1957).

Results obtained in vitro suggest that the apparent β-adrenoceptor blocking activity observed with the dihydro derivatives is nonspecific. Experiments in isolated tissues have the advantage that extraneous factors can be controlled more effectively. In addition, such preparations allow the use of a wider concentration range of the blocking agents than do studies on the heart in situ. Inhibition of excitatory responses to adrenaline have been demonstrated with dihydroergotamine (20 μg/ml) and dihydroergotoxine (50 μg/ml) in the isolated rabbit heart (MORAN and PERKINS, 1961; NICKERSON and CHAN, 1961). These effects were attributed to deterioration of the preparations, since the positive inotropic and chronotropic responses to calcium chloride were reduced to essentially the same extent. The apparent antagonism occurred at doses far in excess of those required to block excitatory responses of smooth muscle tissue to α-adrenoceptor stimulation. Conversely, the β-adrenoceptor blocking drug dichlorisoprenaline effectively inhibited cardiac responses to adrenaline at concentrations which had little effect on responses to calcium. On the basis of these results, it must be concluded that dihydro ergot alkaloids do not possess β-adrenoceptor blocking activity.

OSSWALD et al. (1970) attributed the potentiating effect of the alkaloids on responses to injected catecholamines to the lower basal values for heart rate and contractile force observed following their administration. Although this may be a contributing factor, it does not fully explain the phenomenon, since a similar effect is obtained in vitro in electrically-driven rat ventricle strips (WENZEL and SU, 1966). Ergotamine (1.5 μg/ml) and ergometrine (0.5 μg/ml) increased the positive inotropic effects of catecholamines by 47–160% (Table 5). The greatest increase occurred with noradrenaline, the least with isoprenaline. The effects on responses to adrenaline was intermediate. Potentiation of responses to catecholamines on the heart is not a property only of ergot alkaloids; an even more marked effect was obtained with phentolamine (1 μg/ml). Slight inhibition of responses to isoprenaline occurred when the dose of ergometrine was increased to 2 μg/ml. Although this latter was interpreted as evidence for β-adrenoceptor blockade, such an assumption is unwise on the basis of results obtained at a single dose. The α-adrenoceptor

Table 5. Interaction of sympathomimetic amines with adrenoceptor blocking agents in electrically driven rat ventricle strips. Maximum mean percentage changes (±S.E.M.) in the amplitude of contraction in response to α- and β-adrenoceptor agonists alone and in the presence of ergometrine and adrenoceptor blocking agents. Number of determinations in parentheses. Responses significantly different from control: *$p<0.005$, **$p<0.025$ (after WENZEL and SU, 1966)

Antagonist	Agonist			
	Noradrenaline (2.5×10^{-7} g/ml)	Adrenaline (2.7×10^{-7} g/ml)	Isoprenaline (5.4×10^{-9} g/ml)	Phenylephrine (1×10^{-5} g/ml)
Control (no antagonist)	46± 3 (5)	48±2 (4)	49± 5 (8)	25±3 (5)
Ergometrine maleate (5×10^{-7} g/ml)	100± 8* (4)	80±7* (6)	77± 4* (4)	
Ergometrine maleate (2×10^{-6} g/ml)	112±11* (4)	44±6 (5)	36± 3** (5)	
Ergotamine tartrate (1.5×10^{-6} g/ml)	121± 4* (5)	92±1* (4)	72± 3* (4)	
Phentolamine (1×10^{-6} g/ml)	173± 6* (5)	157±5* (5)	96±10* (6)	21±4 (4)
Phentolamine (1×10^{-5} g/ml)				2±0.1* (4)
Pronetholol (1×10^{-6} g/ml)	26± 2* (6)	−13±1* +41±5 (4)	(0)* (4)	22±4 (4)

stimulant phenylephrine was shown to increase contractility in this preparation at a concentration of 10 μg/ml, but the response was small. This effect was abolished by phentolamine but not by the β-adrenoceptor blocking agent pronethalol. WENZEL and SU suggested that the rat myocardium contains both α- and β-adrenoceptors, both mediating stimulant effects. Occupation of the less responsive α-adrenoceptors by the antagonists would result in preferential occupation of β-adrenoceptors by catecholamines, resulting in a potentiation of their effects. This explanation is probably oversimplified, since under certain circumstances the ergot alkaloids also enhance the effects of α-adrenoceptor stimulation (see Section A4).

The doses of catecholamines used in WENZEL and SU's experiments were chosen to give a response two-thirds of the maximum. The fact that the response to noradrenaline increased approximately three-fold in the presence of ergotamine suggests receptor sensitization.

e) Effects on the Denervated Heart

Ergotamine slows the rate of transmission of excitatory impulses in the atria of anesthetized dogs even during electrical pacing (ANDRUS and MARTIN, 1927) but does not influence cardiac function in denervated hearts. None of the ergot alkaloids alter the rate of cardiac contraction in the heart-lung preparation in cats and dogs (ROTHLIN, 1945), or in animals in which the medulla oblongata has been destroyed (BARGER and DALE, 1907; ROTHLIN, 1957; MORPUGO et al., 1975). Small, transient alterations in contractility are observed in isolated heart preparations when relatively high concentrations are used, but no changes in the rate of contraction occur (BARGER and DALE, 1907; DE BOER and VAN DONGEN, 1948; SHERIF et al., 1956; KARP et al., 1960; MORAN and PERKINS, 1961; GLÄSSER, 1961). An action exerted on the myocardium itself (as distinct from actions exerted through extrinsic nerves) cannot be considered to contribute to the bradycardia observed in animals and in man, nor to the effects of the alkaloids in reversing or preventing experimental cardiac dysrhythmias.

f) Antiarrhythmic Effects

Ergot alkaloids are effective antiarrhythmic agents, preventing disorders of cardiac rhythm induced by adrenaline (for references see later), toxic doses of digitalis (EBEN-MOUSSI et al., 1966; ACHARI and AHMAD, 1966; SCHLEIMER et al., 1971; HELKE et al., 1976), local application of aconitine (ROTHLIN and CERLETTI, 1949c; ACHARI and AHMAD, 1966; SCHLEIMER et al., 1971), electrical stimulation (ROTHLIN and CERLETTI, 1949a; ACHARI and AHMAD, 1966), and coronary artery ligation (MANNING and CAUDWELL, 1947; HARRIS and BISTENI, 1955; SCHLEIMER et al., 1971). α-Adrenoceptor blockade, reduction in cardiac excitability, and a central action on heart rate control mechanisms have all been invoked as possible explanations for the antiarrhythmic effects, but none of these mechanisms has been substantiated experimentally.

α) Arrhythmias Associated With Myocardial Infarction

Dihydroergotamine is relatively ineffective in controlling ventricular dysrhythmias once they are established. Cumulative doses of up to 5 mg/kg i.v. induce only transient reductions in ectopic activity in conscious dogs when administered on the day following ligation of a coronary artery (HARRIS and BISTENI, 1955). In contrast, when administered before coronary ligation at a dose of only 0.4 mg/kg i.v., dihydroergotamine reduces the incidence of fatal ventricular tachycardia and fibrillation from 50% to 30% during the first 15 min and reduces 24-h mortality from 75% to 30%. Ergotamine (0.25 mg/kg) also has an effect on cardiac irregularities of early onset but does not substantially reduce the 24-h mortality rate (MANNING and CAUDWELL, 1947). The protective effect of these two drugs against early arrhythmias approximates that obtained in animals following sympathetic denervation of the heart (McEACHERN et al., 1940). This prompted MANNING and CAUDWELL to suggest cardiac adrenoceptor blockade as the most likely mechanism for their antiarrhythmic effect. It has already been established that ergot alkaloids have no β-adrenoceptor blocking activity. Nevertheless, there is evidence that they do diminish cardiac sympathetic nerve activity by an action within the central nervous system. This action might be a possible explanation. Whether increases in sympathetic nerve activity or medullary secretion of catecholamines play an essential role in the production of ventricular tachycardia following myocardial infarction is controversial (HARRIS, 1950; HARRIS et al., 1951).

β) Arrhythmias Induced by Adrenaline

It is well known that administration of catecholamines or hydrocarbon anesthetics alone or in combination may induce severe disturbances of cardiac rhythm, mostly tachycardia of ventricular origin, followed not infrequently by fatal ventricular fibrillation.

Ergotamine (ALLEN et al., 1940, 1941; MOE et al., 1948), dihydroergotamine (ORTH and RITCHIE, 1947; DE BOER and VAN DONGEN, 1948; ORTH, 1949; BENNET et al., 1949; MEIRSMAN-ROOBROECK, 1950; WHITE et al., 1951; O'BRIEN et al., 1953), dihydroergocornine (BENNET et al., 1949; ORTH, 1949), and dihydroergotoxine (ROTHLIN and CERLETTI, 1949a; KÜHNS, 1951) all protect the heart against such arrhythmias in the rabbit, dog, and monkey for 30–120 min. Ergotamine is approximately twice as active as dihydro derivatives. The latter are all effective at a dose of 0.4 mg/kg given i.v., but no one compound is superior to the others in terms of degree or duration of protection (CAPPS et al., 1950). SHEN (1938) postulated that the rise of arterial pressure produced by adrenaline was responsible for such arrhythmias on the ground that the α-adrenoceptor blocking agents piperoxan (933F) and yohimbine, which prevented the blood pressure rise, also prevented adrenaline-induced fibrillation.

The question is raised as to the relevance of a rise in blood pressure in the induction of arrhythmias by catecholamines in unprotected animals. NICKERSON and NOMAGUCHI (1949) found that although actual changes in blood pressure appeared to be of very limited importance, there was a significant correlation between the final level of systemic arterial pressure attained and the incidence of arrhythmia. In addition, if pressure is maintained constant during injections of adrenaline by means of a pressure regulator in the abdominal aorta, doses of adrenaline several times that which induces ventricular tachycardia without the pressure regulator are tolerated without ectopic rhythms occurring. In the heart-lung preparation, in which the heart is separated from any possible reflex phenomena, raising pressure mechanically or with adrenaline induces ectopic ventricular activity only when the heart is exposed to cyclopropane. Nevertheless, it seems that an intact reflex pathway is essential for ventricular fibrillation to occur (Moe et al., 1948).

According to Allen et al. (1940) and Stutzman et al. (1947) procedures such as decerebration superior to the pons or cardiac sympathetic denervation, which do not prevent the pressor response to adrenaline, prevent or greatly reduce the duration of ventricular tachycardia induced by adrenaline in the presence of cyclopropane. They considered that the sensitizing action of cyclopropane can be explained by reflex activation of cardiac sympathetic nerves, the afferent limb of the reflex apparently originating in the mesentery or intestine. Evidence to the contrary is provided by the finding that interruption of autonomic pathways by tetraethylammonium does not alter the threshold dose of adrenaline inducing ectopic ventricular activity (Moe et al., 1948). Although the relevance of intact nervous pathways to the heart is controversial, it is conceivable that the ergot alkaloids may exert their antiarrhythmic effect in adrenaline-induced arrhythmias, as in arrhythmias induced by coronary artery ligation, by virtue of their central inhibitory action on cardiac sympathetic nerve activity.

An increase in the afterload on the heart may be considered a contributory factor in the etiology of arrhythmias induced by adrenaline. Nevertheless, it is questionable whether blockade of the pressor effect of the catecholamine by α-adrenoceptor blocking agents is the mechanism for their antiarrhythmic effects. This is underlined by two findings. The first is that the doses of dibenamine and its derivatives necessary to prevent adrenaline-induced arrhythmias are considerably in excess of those required to abolish the pressor response to adrenaline (Nickerson and Nomaguchi, 1949). The second is that ergot alkaloids have been shown to exert antiarrhythmic activity without significantly influencing the pressor responses to adrenaline (Allen et al., 1940; Moe et al., 1948). The alkaloids must, therefore, prevent the development of ventricular tachycardia and fibrillation by some action other than blockade of vascular α-adrenoceptors.

Liberation of potassium in ischemic heart muscle is considered a significant factor in the production of ventricular tachycardia following occlusion of a coronary artery (Harris et al., 1954). The same may also be true in adrenaline-induced dysrhythmias. O'Brien et al. (1953) have shown that injection of a dose of adrenaline sufficient to induce ventricular tachycardia in animals anesthetized with cyclopropane is followed by a sharp rise (85–125%) in the potassium concentration in arterial blood. Ventricular tachycardia consistently appears during the rapid ascent of potassium concentration and extends beyond its summit to the rapidly falling phase. Dihydroergotamine (0.4 mg/kg) and dibenamine (15 mg/kg) each prevented ventricular tachycardia and also inhibited the potassium elevation. The degree of ectopic activity could not be accounted for entirely by the magnitude of potassium rise, however, since Aranthol (2-methylamino-6-hydroxy-6-methylheptane) produced ventricular tachycardia with little or no rise in potassium.

Adrenaline, noradrenaline, and isoprenaline increase heart rate and contractile force, and shorten the A–V refractory period by virtue of their β-adrenoceptor stimulant activity. A third action on the myocardium, which adrenaline and noradrenaline share with phenylephrine and methoxamine (but not isoprenaline), is to shorten intraventricular conduction time, adrenaline being the most active. This action is not affected by the β-adrenoceptor blocking agent dichloroisoprenaline. In the acutely denervated dog heart, dihydroergotoxine (0.4 mg/kg i.v.) almost abolished the positive dromotropic effect of adrenaline. Before the administration of the alkaloids, the mean maximum shortening of the intraventricular conduction time was 9 msec. After dihydroergotoxine, adrenaline caused a shortening of only 1 msec. None of the other stimulant effects of adrenaline were changed, confirming the absence of β-adrenoceptor blocking activity. The alkaloid itself had no effect on any of the parameters measured (ERLIJ and MENDEZ, 1964). Later work by these authors indicated that the effect of adrenaline on intraventricular conduction is the result of an indirect action mediated through the liberation of K^+ ions from the liver (see also D'SILVA, 1949). Although the positive dromotropic action of adrenergic agents seems to be mediated by activation of α-adrenoceptors, the location of these receptors is presumably extracardiac.

The heart is most prone to develop arrhythmias shortly (8–30 sec) after the injected adrenaline first reaches it, rather than at the time of maximum rise in blood pressure (NICKERSON and NOMAGUCHI, 1949). The time of greatest susceptibility to external stimuli coincides with a primary transient decrease in the fibrillation threshold of both atria and ventricles. This initial effect is common to sympathomimetic agents which stimulate β-adrenoceptors and can be prevented by β-adrenoceptor blocking agents. α-Adrenoceptor blocking agents such as phenoxybenzamine (10 mg/kg) and dihydroergotoxine are without effect (PAPP and SZEKERES, 1968). During continuous i.v. infusions of adrenaline and noradrenaline, the initial decrease in the fibrillation threshold is followed by a lasting increase. This is only induced by compounds which stimulate α-adrenoceptors. During the second phase of their action, bursts of ventricular ectopic beats occur. Phenoxybenzamine does not influence the increase in fibrillation threshold but prevents the late arrhythmogenic effect. PAPP and SZEKERES were of the opinion that the late arrhythmogenic effect was mainly secondary to the rise in blood pressure caused by adrenaline and noradrenaline. This hypothesis was supported by the finding that the incidence of late arrhythmias paralleled the elevation of blood pressure, and that these arrhythmias could be eliminated by preventing the blood pressure rise. This may explain the antiarrhythmic effect of phenoxybenzamine but not that of the ergot alkaloids; it has already been stated that the latter display antiarrhythmic activity at doses lower than those required to abolish pressor effects of adrenaline.

Phenylephrine, methoxamine, and synephrine elevate atrial and ventricular fibrillation thresholds, thus showing primarily an antiarrhythmic tendency. These agents act predominantly on α-adrenoceptors and also possess quinidine-like activity. Several authors have described an antiarrhythmic action for methoxamine and synephrine (see PAPP and SZEKERES, 1968). Whether the secondary rise in the fibrillation threshold induced by these compounds can be attributed to stimulation of cardiac α-adrenoceptors or to membrane stabilization remains unanswered. The former mechanism may provide an explanation for the antiarrhythmic actions of the ergot alkaloids, since those compounds found to possess antiarrhythmic activity are partial agonists at the α-adrenoceptor site. It may be of significance that ergotamine is not only a more potent α-adrenoceptor agonist than the dihydro ergot alkaloids but is also more potent in preventing adrenaline-induced arrhythmias. A further possible mechanism for the antiarrhythmic effects of the ergot alkaloids is blockade of 5-HT receptors. The involvement of 5-HT in the induction of arrhythmias is suggested by the fact that the 5-HT antagonist methysergide is effective in the dog against arrhythmias of both atrial and ventricular origin, although the doses required are relatively high (from 2.5 mg/kg i.v.). This compound is somewhat less potent than cyproheptadine against atrial fibrillation and flutter but is 2–3 times more potent than cyproheptadine in protecting against dysrhythmias induced by adrenaline and in reversing arrhythmias resulting from administration of ouabain (ACHARI and AHMAD, 1966). Whether this latter effect is due to antagonism at 5-HT receptor sites within the heart or in the central nervous system is uncertain.

γ) Arrythmias Induced by Digitalis Glycosides

There is evidence that the toxic effects of cardiac glycosides are not due to a direct action on cardiac cell membranes, but that a sympathetic component is involved. Spinal transection, adrenalectomy, and depletion of catecholamines stores by reserpine all enhance tolerance to the toxic actions of the glycosides (MENDÉZ et al., 1961; CAIROLI et al., 1962). Administration of ouabain into the cerebral ventricles induces arrhythmias, which can be abolished by excising the stellate ganglia (SAXENA and BHARGAVA, 1975). High doses of ouabain increase sympathetic nerve activity (GILLIS, 1969); clonidine depresses this effect while simultaneously converting ventricular tachycardia to sinus rhythm (GILLIS et al., 1972). The transmitter mediating the effect of ouabain in the central nervous system is considered to be 5-HT (HELKE et al., 1976). This hypothesis is based on the fact that inhibition of brain tryptophan hydroxylase with *p*-chlorophenylalanine or destruction of central serotonergic nerves with 5,7-dihydroxytryptamine results in a significant increase in the dose of deslanoside necessary to produce ventricular arrhythmias. In animals which had received arrythmogenic doses of deslanoside, i.v. administration of methysergide (3 mg/kg) induced a return to sinus rhythm. HELKE and his colleagues regarded this as additional evidence for the participation of central serotonergic pathways in the genesis of glycoside-induced arrhythmias.

δ) Antiarrhythmic Effects in Man

Despite extensive investigation of the antiarrhythmic properties of ergot alkaloids in experimental animals, their therapeutic potential in man does not seem to have been explored. Negative results have been reported with dihydroergocornine in a small group of patients with atrial fibrillation and flutter (ELEK et al., 1955). Studies with dihydroergotamine and dihydroergocornine in patients undergoing surgery under cyclopropane anesthesia are inconclusive (ORTH, 1949; BENNET et al., 1949). Such results are not adequate to permit an estimate of their possible value in pathologic disorders of cardiac rhythm in man.

2. Effects in Amphibia

The natural alkaloids ergotamine, ergocristine, ergocornine, their dihydro derivatives, and ergometrine do not influence the function of the isolated heart of the frog or toad at concentrations which evoke pharmacologic effects in mammalian smooth muscle. Concentrations in excess of 10^{-6} depress contractility, but the effects are generally irreversible and are probably a reflection of toxicity (AMSLER, 1920; LOEWI and NAVRATIL, 1926; DAVIS et al., 1935; NAVRATIL and WIENINGER, 1948; FREUDIGER and ROTHLIN, 1949; SHERIF et al., 1956).

Both ergotamine (NAVRATIL, 1927) and dihydroergotamine (NAVRATIL and WIENINGER, 1948) depress responses to stimulation of the sympathetic nerves to the heart as a result, according to NAVRATIL (1927), of blockade of receptors in the heart rather than of a decrease in the quantity of transmitter released. A number of investigators have demonstrated dose-dependent inhibition by ergot alkaloids of positive inotropic and positive chronotropic responses to adrenaline in the frog (NAVRATIL, 1927; NAVRATIL and WIENINGER, 1948; FREUDIGER and ROTHLIN, 1949; NICKERSON and NOMAGUCHI, 1950; SHERIF et al., 1956; ERLIJ et al., 1965), whereas others have been unable to obtain such an effect (BARRY, 1937; DE BOER and VAN DONGEN, 1948). Similar conflicting results have been reported for β-haloalkylamines, benzodioxanes, and yohimbine (NICKERSON, 1949).

A systematic attempt to clarify the conditions necessary for blockade was undertaken by NICKERSON and NOMAGUCHI (1950). Positive chronotropic responses to adrenaline, noradrenaline, and isoprenaline were effectively blocked by ergot alkaloids and congeners of dibenamine only during the winter months. The heart rapidly became resistant to blockade during March and sensitivity returned late in August. The seasonal differences in sensitivity showed little direct relationship to environmental temperature or the temperature at which the experiments were conducted, although sensitivity could be increased by exposing the animals to a lower temperature (8° C) for several days.

Compounds which antagonize responses mediated by α-adrenoceptors in a relatively specific manner do not antagonize the inotropic or chronotropic actions of catecholamines in the mammalian heart. These effects can only be blocked by β-adrenoceptor blocking agents (NICKERSON and CHAN, 1961; MORAN and PERKINS, 1961). Accordingly, it has been assumed that the adrenoceptors of the myocardium are entirely of the *beta* type (AHLQUIST, 1948). On the basis of experiments in isolated mammalian tissues there is no evidence that the ergot alkaloids interact with β-adrenoceptors. However, the blocking effects of the ergot alkaloids on the winter frog heart have the characteristics of competitive antagonism, i.e., the positive chronotropic response to adrenaline is blocked over a tenfold concentration range at a constant ratio of blocking to stimulating agent (NICKERSON and NOMAGUCHI, 1950).

In recent years, the question as to whether α-adrenoceptors mediating positive inotropic and chronotropic effects exist in the mammalian myocardium has evoked considerable investigation and discussion (COTTEN and WALTON, 1951; MORAN and PERKINS, 1961; ERLIJ and MENDEZ, 1964; GOVIER et al., 1966; WENZEL and SU, 1966; GOVIER, 1968; KUNOS, 1977). Recent studies in the isolated heart of frogs have shown that the adrenoceptors mediating inotropic and chronotropic responses can be altered qualitatively by ambient temperature in such a way that their characteristics shift from *beta* towards *alpha* when the temperature of the heart is reduced through a critical range of 17–22° C (KUNOS and SZENTIVÁNYI, 1968; BUCKLEY and JORDAN, 1970; KUNOS et al., 1973; HARRI, 1973). At tempera-

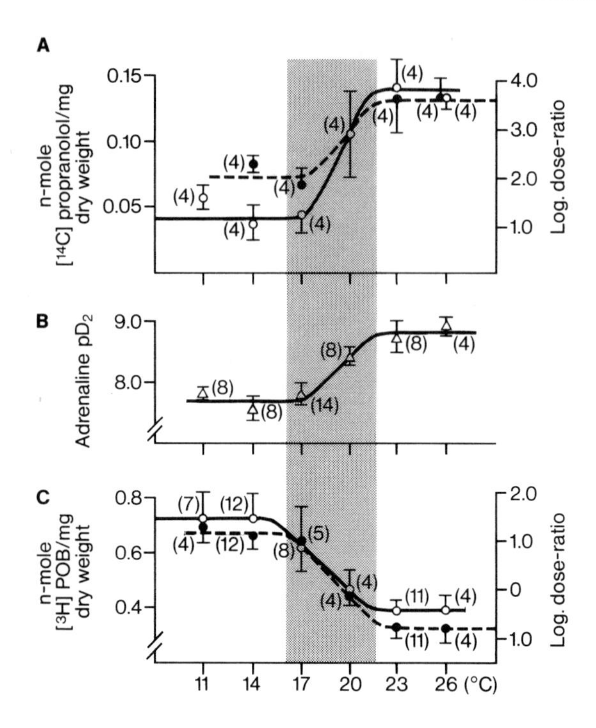

Fig. 11 A–C. Temperature range of receptor interconversion in isolated frog hearts. Block by (●---●) and binding of (○——○) 4 μM [^{14}C]propranolol (A) and 7.3 μM [^{3}H]phenoxybenzamine (C). B shows control sensitivity to adrenaline. Numbers in parentheses show number of experiments and vertical bars the S.E. of means (KUNOS and NICKERSON, 1976)

tures of 23° C and above, inotropic responses to adrenaline are antagonized by propranolol but are unaffected by phentolamine and potentiated by phenoxybenzamine. Below 17° C, the activity of propranolol is reduced at least tenfold, and the α-adrenoceptor antagonists inhibit responses to both adrenaline and isoprenaline but not those to $CaCl_2$ (KUNOS and NICKERSON, 1976). The reciprocal effectiveness of the two types of antagonist suggest either a single type of adrenoceptor whose characteristics are altered by temperature (KUNOS and SZENTIVÁNYI, 1968) or the presence of separate pools of α- and β-adrenoceptors with different sensitivities to or activation by temperature (BUCKLEY and JORDAN, 1970). A number of studies add weight to the former interpretation, namely that the two classes of adrenoceptors may represent allosteric configurations of the same active site (KUNOS et al., 1973; BENFEY et al., 1974; KUNOS and NICKERSON, 1976). KUNOS and NICKERSON showed that significantly more [^{14}C]propranolol is retained by the heart exposed at high temperatures, and significantly more [^{3}H]phenoxybenzamine is bound to the myocardium at low temperatures. The change in binding characteristics with decreasing temperature parallels the change from β- to α-adrenoceptor characteristics and also parallels a decrease in the sensitivity of the heart to adrenaline (Fig. 11).

Based on these considerations, it would seem that the blocking effect of ergot alkaloids on responses to adrenaline in the winter amphibian heart represents interactions of the compounds with α-adrenoceptors.

3. Effects in Molluscs

Electrical stimulation of the visceral ganglion of the lammelibranch mollusc, *Venus mercenaria*, evokes the release of acetylcholine in the heart which, as in the vertebrate heart, induces a decrease in the rate and amplitude of contraction. An opposing excitatory mechanism can be obtained in the presence of an acetylcholine antagonist. This excitatory effect can be mimicked by 5-HT in concentrations as low as 10^{-10} M (WELSH, 1953, 1957). The response of the *Venus* heart to 5-HT is characterized by an increase in amplitude, frequency, and resting tone of the muscle (GREENBERG, 1960b). Adrenaline, noradrenaline, histamine, and dopamine induce qualitatively different effects and are active only in concentrations in excess of 10^{-6} M (WELSH, 1953, 1957; GREENBERG, 1960b). The effect of 5-HT and its presence in large amounts in molluscan nervous systems (WELSH, 1953, 1957; WELSH and MOORHEAD, 1959, 1960) suggest that this indoleamine has a cardioregulatory role in molluscs.

Lysergic acid diethylamide (*d*-LSD) has effects on the heart of *V. mercenaria* which are analogous to those of 5-HT, but it is more potent than the hormone itself (SHAW and WOOLLEY, 1956). *D*-LSD is the most effective known excitor agent for the *Venus* heart (WRIGHT et al., 1962). The heart responds maximally at a concentration of only 10^{-16} M (WELSH and MCCOY, 1957; GREENBERG, 1960a) (Fig. 12). This concentration of *d*-LSD is considerably less than that calculated to be present in human brain tissue to exert psychologic effects in man, i.e., 0.3 ng/kg brain tissue (AXELROD et al., 1956). The excitatory effect of a low concentration of *d*-LSD differs from that of 5-HT in that it takes 1–4 h to reach maximum. High concentrations act more quickly. In contrast to that of 5-HT, the action of *d*-LSD is only slowly reversible on washing (WELSH and MCCOY, 1957; WRIGHT et al., 1962). If left in contact with the tissue without washing, the heart will continue to beat at maximum frequency and amplitude for up to 48 h with little sign of tachyphylaxis (WELSH and MCCOY, 1957; WRIGHT et al., 1962) (Fig. 13).

These latter authors compared the actions of lysergic acid and a number of its derivatives with those of *d*-LSD and 5-HT on the *Venus* heart. Lysergic acid

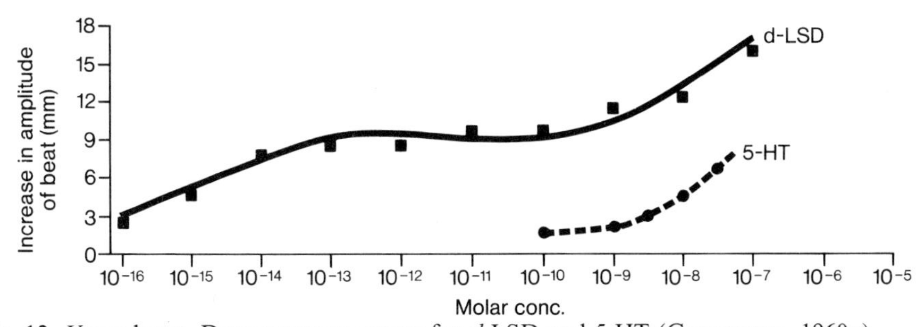

Fig. 12. *Venus* heart. Dose-response curves for *d*-LSD and 5-HT (GREENBERG, 1960a)

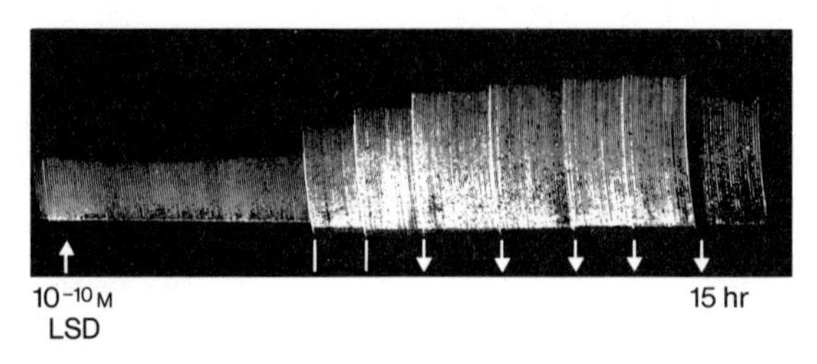

Fig. 13. Effect of *d*-LSD on *Venus* heart. At ↑, 10^{-10}M *d*-LSD; at first four ↓, drum was stopped and bath flushed with sea-water for 10 min. At fifth ↓, sea water was slowly run through the bath for 15 h (WRIGHT et al., 1962)

(8), the monoethylamide (73h), propanolamide (ergometrine, 19), butanolamide (methylergometrine, 73a), and the peptide derivatives dihydroergotamine and ergotoxine all increased the amplitude and the frequency of the heart beat in a manner similar to that of 5-HT. None was more active than *d*-LSD itself. The lowest effective concentration of the most active compounds (dihydroergotamine, ergotoxine, and ergometrine) was 10^{-10} M. Compounds substituted in position 1 or 2 (1-methyl-, 34b, 1-acetyl-, 36a, and 2-bromolysergic acid diethylamide, 37a) had weak excitatory actions, but all induced specific, long-lasting blockade of the actions of 5-HT. Methysergide (1-methyl-lysergic acid butanolamide, 34a) inhibited the action of 5-HT dose-dependently in a molar ratio of about 1:1 (Fig. 14). This compound is the most potent antagonist, not only of the effects of 5-HT but also those of *d*-LSD on this preparation. A concentration of 10^{-5} M blocks effects induced by a very high concentration (10^{-6} M) of *d*-LSD for at least 30 min (WRIGHT et al., 1962).

Brom-LSD also acts on the *Venus* heart as a partial agonist at 5-HT receptor sites. Its stimulant action is much weaker than that of *d*-LSD and is not readily reproducible. At concentrations between 10^{-6} M and 10^{-4} M, the compound inhibits the stimulant effects of *d*-LSD and also those of 5-HT, phenylethylamine and tyramine (WELSH and MCCOY, 1957; GREENBERG, 1960a, b). Blockade of responses to 5-HT can be overcome by increasing the concentration of the agonist indicating competitive antagonism. Specificity for 5-HT receptors is underlined by the fact that brom-LSD does not influence responses to adrenaline, noradrenaline, histamine, or dopamine (GREENBERG, 1960b).

Tapes Watlingi is a member of the same family (Veneridae) as the American clam, *V. mercenaria*. The heart of *T. Watlingi* is very similar in its pharmacologic response to acetylcholine as the *Venus* preparation but is 10–100 times less sensitive to 5-HT. *D*-LSD, ergotamine, ergotoxine, and methylergometrine have powerful, prolonged excitant effects on the *Tapes* heart at concentrations of 10^{-8} M–10^{-7} M when applied for only 1 min. These concentrations are more than 100 times greater than those active on the *Venus* heart. As on the *Venus* heart, methysergide is the least potent excitant and proved to be an effective antagonist of both 5-HT and *d*-LSD at a concentration of 10^{-5} M (CHONG and PHILLIS, 1965).

GADDUM and PAASONEN (1955) studied the actions of ergot alkaloids on the isolated heart of various other molluscs. *D*-LSD, ergometrine, dihydroergotamine, and dihydroergotoxine had excitatory actions on the heart of *Solen siliqua* (razor

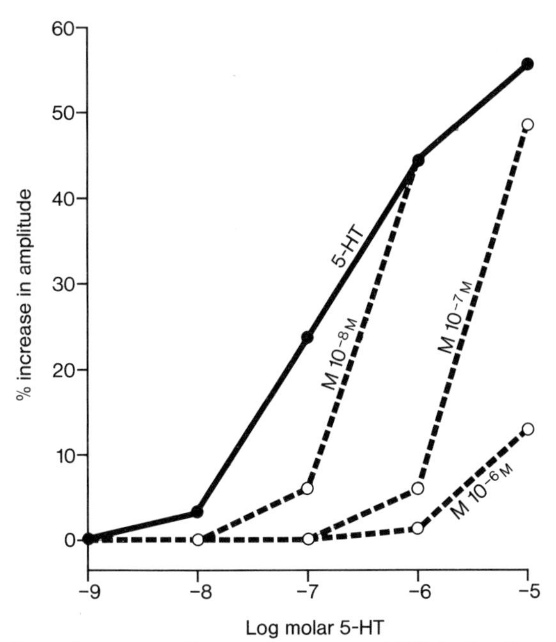

Fig. 14. Inhibitory effect of methysergide on responses to 5-HT in the *Venus* heart. Concentration-response curves for 5-HT alone and in the presence of the indicated concentrations of methysergide (M). Each curve is the average response of three hearts (WRIGHT et al., 1962)

shell), *Cyprina islandica, Mya arenaria, Helix aspersa* (garden snail), and *Spisula* (*Mactra*) *solida*. In contrast to 5-HT, *d*-LSD depressed the heart of *Cardium edule* (cockle). In general the potency of the ergots in these species was 100–1000 times less than that of 5-HT.

E. Pharmacologic Basis for the Clinical Use of Ergot Alkaloids

1. Orthostatic Hypotension

The venous system might be described as the Cinderella of circulatory physiology. It has not been sufficiently appreciated that quite small changes in its capacity produced by venous constriction will have profound effects on the venous return to the heart. FOLKOW (1955) has pointed out that since the veins contain some 60% or more of the total blood volume in a system in which the stroke volume of the pump is only 1–2%, it can be calculated that a 1–2% reduction in venous capacity will double the diastolic inflow to the heart from one beat to the next. A similar constriction of the arterioles would have only a negligible effect on peripheral resistance. The changes in venous tone evoked by activation of sympathetic vasomotor nerves are of great importance in maintaining cardiac output. Their significance lies in the modifications in venous capacity which they induce rather than in changes in resistance to flow to which they give rise.

Large volume shifts occur when changing from the horizontal to the upright position. In normal subjects, the volume of the lower extremities is increased by at least 350 ml (BARBEY and BRECHT, 1965), largely due to increased hydrostatic load. Increased capacity of the venous resevoir decreases the effective blood volume and lowers right atrial filling pressure. The venous return to the heart is compromised, stroke volume is decreased, and consequently blood pressure falls.

Normally, cardiovascular adjustments take place which compensate for these changes. A fall in blood pressure in the sino-aortic reflexogenic zones will activate baroreceptor reflex mechanisms and result in a rapid restoration of blood pressure to normal levels. Although it is true that changes in peripheral resistance caused by arteriolar constriction contribute to the blood pressure rise, according to HEYMANS and NEIL (1958), the most important change is probably that of venoconstriction, i.e., the role of the sino-aortic reflexes is predominantly one of adjusting circulatory capacity (MCDOWELL, 1935). HEYMANS and NEIL have argued that in systemic hypotension (caused, e.g., by hemorrhage), the reflex increase in peripheral resistance in the skin and splanchnic area aids in the distribution of blood to the brain and heart circulations which are themselves relatively independent of the reflex vasoconstriction. However, if arteriolar constriction were the sole result, it is debatable whether any essential benefit would be conferred on the circulation as whole. ALEXANDER (1954) has in fact shown that perfused, innervated segments of the mesenteric veins constrict when carotid sinus pressure is lowered and dilate when intrasinusal pressure is raised. Contraction of the smooth muscle of the capacitance vessels not only mobilizes blood, thereby promoting venous return, but also stiffens the walls of these vessels, enabling them to resist a greater hydrostatic pressure than normal. Accumulation of blood in the dependent regions resulting from increased transmural pressure in the veins is thus reduced.

In some subjects, this compensatory mechanism seems to be impaired, and an abnormal amount of blood is displaced into the dependent regions on changing to the upright position. Such orthostatic intolerance gives rise to an excessive increase in heart rate, a fall in blood pressure, and a decrease in pulse pressure, accompanied by subjective symptoms and sometimes collapse. This circulatory disorder is seen in otherwise healthy people, most commonly in young women. RIECKERT and PAUSCHINGER (1967) suggested that such persons might be relieved of their orthostatic symptoms by a vasoactive drug exerting a powerful constrictor action on the capacitance vessels. MELLANDER and NORDENFELT (1970) showed that dihydroergotamine can elicit such an effect. Both in normal subjects and in patients with impaired regulation of capacitance function (orthostatic hypotension), the drug evoked strong constriction of the capacitance vessels in skeletal muscle and skin but had comparatively small or no constrictor effects on the resistance vessels and precapillary sphincters.

Numerous studies have supported this hypothesis. Dihydroergotamine has been shown to be useful in the treatment of orthostatic disorders, whether idiopathic or functional (ROSMANITZ and BREHM, 1964; BACHMANN et al., 1968; HECK, 1971; ASCHKE et al., 1972; LÜBKE, 1972; BEVEGÅRD et al., 1974; LANG et al., 1975) due to the administration of neuroleptics (BOCCI et al., 1970; RECKEL, 1970; BOISMARE et al., 1974), tricyclic antidepressants (BOCCI et al., 1970; BOJANOVSKY and TOELLE, 1974) or antihypertensives (PARADE et al., 1974), or in paraplegic patients (BIDART and MAURY, 1974).

The results of MELLANDER and NORDENFELT's (1970) study indicated that in the supine subject, dihydroergotamine might cause a mobilization of about 350 ml of blood from the capacitance vessels of all muscle and skin regions. If the amount of blood pooled in the dependent regions of the erect subject decreases by about 25% in response to the drug, the gain for the central circulation would be about 125 ml of blood. It was considered that the gain might be even greater in patients with orthostatic dysregulation, since they have a greater tendency for blood pooling. Such a redistribution of the blood volume would be expected to markedly affect general cardiovascular dynamics. It was predicted that dihydroergotamine would increase central venous pressure and central blood volume and thereby augment stroke volume and cardiac output. The central cardiovascular adjustments evoked by the drug in patients with orthostatic hypotension were found to be those predicted in all essential respects (NORDENFELT and MELLANDER, 1972). In the supine position, cardiac output was significantly increased by nearly half a liter, due solely to an increase in stroke volume, since heart rate did not change. Systolic and mean pressures were also raised significantly by about 10 mmHg, which was caused by the increased cardiac output, since total peripheral resistance was unaltered. Central venous pressure was also increased, but there was no significant change in central blood volume. In the erect position, however, dihydroergotamine caused an increase in central blood volume of 120 ml.

BEVEGÅRD and his colleagues (1974) performed a similar study in which orthostatic stress was applied using a tilt table or simulated by applying lower body negative pressure. In the control phase, central venous and systemic pressures increased after administration of dihydroergotamine, but the effect on cardic output was negligible, and calculated total peripheral resistance increased slightly as a result. During orthostatic stress, blood pressure and cardiac output was maintained at a higher level, and stroke volume decreased much less than before drug administration. Venous tone, which increased in response to dihydroergotamine, was not significantly changed during orthostatic stress. The changes were similar following a single i.v. injection (10 μg/kg) or following long term oral treatment (4–10 mg/day).

It may be concluded that dihydroergotamine improves orthostatic tolerance and the central hemodynamic state in a way which would be expected from a drug exerting a powerful and relatively selective constrictor action on capacitance vessels.

2. Venous Thrombosis

A further clinical application for selective venoconstriction is found in the prevention of postoperative venous thrombosis and pulmonary embolism.

Hemostasis in the deep veins of the lower limbs and changes in blood coagulability are important factors in the pathogenesis of deep vein thrombosis following surgery. It is logical that prophylaxis should be directed towards eliminating both factors. The efficacy of pre- and postoperative administration of low doses of heparin is now established (see SAGAR et al., 1976).

Hemostasis occurs as result of a loss of venous tone induced by inactivity. Physiotherapy may induce up to fourfold increases in the velocity of blood flow in the leg veins, but the effect only lasts for 5–10 min after exercise has ended. Elastic stockings may reduce hemostasis in the limbs but not in the pelvis. The favourable results obtained with intermittent pneumatic compression of the leg and electrical stimulation of the gastrocnemius suggest that sustained venoconstriction induced pharmacologically might also reduce venous stasis and thereby decrease local thrombin generation.

Dihydroergotamine not only increases the tone of capacitance vessels but increases the velocity of blood flow within them. The velocity of venous blood flow can be measured by injecting a radioactive tracer (^{125}I or ^{133}Xe) into a vein on the dorsum of the foot and registering radioactivity over the calf and inguinal region. RIECKERT (1971) showed that dihydroergotamine accelerates venous blood flow in the lower limbs of recumbent healthy subjects from 7.7 cm/sec to 10 cm/sec. The velocity of blood flow in the lower limbs and pelvis in the patients studied by MÜHE and his colleagues (1975) was considerably lower (approximately 3 cm/sec). A single i.v. dose of dihydroergotamine doubled venous flow velocity for at least 8 h.

The therapeutic effect of dihydroergotamine in diminishing the incidence of postoperative deep vein thrombosis has been evaluated in a number of studies comprising large groups of patients. Thrombus formation was detected using the radioactive fibrinogen uptake test. Injected ^{125}I-fibrinogen accumulates in thrombi. The number of thrombi formed is estimated by monitoring radioactivity at several points on each leg. Therapy with dihydroergotamine reduces the incidence of postoperative deep vein thrombosis and pulmonary embolism by 40–60% (FEY et al., 1975; MÜHE et al., 1975; BUTTERMANN et al., 1975). When treatment is combined with low dose heparin, the reduction is at least 75% (SAGAR et al., 1976; BUTTERMANN et al., 1976; HÖR et al., 1977).

3. Shock

The essential features of shock are lowered arterial and venous pressures, diminished venous return, and hence reduced cardiac output. The prime causal factor appears to be loss of circulating fluid, which could be blood from external or internal hemorrhage, plasma as in burns, or effective loss from the circulation due to pooling in capacitance vessels and increased capillary permeability. Increased venous compliance has been reported in patients with cardiogenic shock (WEIL and SHUBIN, 1970). It is possible that a selective venoconstrictor substance might enhance the effects of reflex activation of sympathetic venomotor mechanisms, thereby increasing venous return to the heart without further impairing tissue perfusion. This hypothesis requires investigation.

4. Migraine

a) Clinical Features

The outstanding feature of the migraine syndrome is recurrent, severe headache which is usually unilateral in onset but which may extend to encompass the whole head and even neck and shoulders. The headache is usually accompanied by nausea and vomiting. Photophobia and painful sensations in the skin of the face and scalp are common. Incoming stimuli of any kind will usually accentuate the headache. Frequently, the attacks are ushered in by visual disturbances (scotomata, hemianopia, diplopia) or visual hallucinations. These are thought to be due to functional disturbances in the occipital cortex. Prodromal symptoms arising elsewhere in the cerebral cortex, cerebellum, and brain stem, such as hyperesthesia and paresthesia of the finger tips, lips and tongue, speech disorders, vertigo, ataxia, fainting, and pyschic changes are not uncommon. Although the neurologic symptoms are transient in the majority of patients, recurrent attacks of migraine may be followed by permanent sequelae making their appearance in the function which is predominantly affected (RILEY, 1932).

b) Pathophysiology

Migraine headaches appear to result largely from stretch and dilation of the arteries of the scalp and dura. In 1937, GRAHAM and WOLFF published the first important experimental evidence that distension of vessels in the external carotid vascular bed is involved in the production of pain in migraine. They made quantitative determinations of the magnitude of pulsations in the temporal arteries during a migraine attack by means of tambours placed on the vessels. Manual compression of the common carotid artery on the affected side resulted in a marked diminution in the amplitude of pulsations in the temporal artery (on the same side) and amelioration of the headache, although in some subjects a residuum of deep pain persisted.

Subcutaneous administration of adrenaline was followed by a reduction in the amplitude of arterial pulsations and a temporary reduction in the intensity of the headache. When pulsations returned to the original level, the headache also returned. Similar results were obtained with infusions of noradrenaline (OSTFELD and WOLFF, 1955). In one patient, in whom pressure on the temporal artery abolished the headache in the temporal region, periarterial infiltration of this vessel near its source with procaine hydrochloride was found to have the same effect. Sudden distension of the artery by increasing the intramural hydrostatic pressure experimentally resulted in pain referred to the temporal region. This portion of the artery and the surrounding nerve fibers were ligated and cut. In subsequent headaches, the tempoparietal region was spared (GRAHAM and WOLFF, 1937).

Cutaneous blood flow in the frontotemporal region on the affected side is significantly greater than that on the contralateral side during the headache, although the latter flow is also significantly higher than in headache-free periods (ELKIND et al., 1964). Measurements were made using the radioactive sodium clearance technique. Fundamentally, this technique involves measurement of the rate at which the isotope is removed from the tissue injected, which in turn, is proportional to blood flow through that tissue. Since removal occurs only from blood traversing capillaries, this method provides an index of effective capillary circulation in contrast to flow across arteriovenous communications.

Correlation between headache and locally increased blood flow does not establish the causal nature of the headache. The failure of bradykinin, which enhances blood flow, to produce pain suggests that factors other than increased skin flow contribute to the induction of pain (ELKIND et al., 1964). These findings are difficult to reconcile with the fact that most patients look pale during migraine headache (LANCE, 1973). Thermographic studies have shown that skin temperature is lower on the affected side during the headache phase in the majority of migraine patients (LANCE and ANTHONY, 1971). HEYCK (1956, 1969) suggested that significant blood shunting might take place during the headache and that this may be of importance in the pathophysiology of the migraine attack.

Although emphasis has been placed on the importance of distension of the extracranial arteries in the pain of migraine headache, distension and dilation of intracranial arteries, particularly those supplying the dura and the base of the brain, also results in headache. As in migraine, the pain is associated with nausea (RAY and WOLFF, 1940).

Regional cerebral (intracranial) blood flow is currently estimated by the intracarotid ^{133}Xenon or ^{85}Krypton clearance techniques (LASSEN et al., 1963; OLESEN et al., 1971). Briefly, the method consists in introducing a fine polyethylene catheter into the internal carotid artery and injecting the radioactive material rapidly. The clearance of the isotope from the brain is recorded with multiple external scintillation detectors. The regional cerebral blood flow values are calculated from the initial slope of the clearance curves. During the prodromal phase of a migraine attack, cerebral blood flow is reduced (NORRIS et al., 1975; MATHEW et al., 1976). In some cases, perfusion in the cortex may decline to levels known to be critical for adequate oxygenation (SKINHØJ and PAULSON, 1969; SKINHØJ, 1973). Angiographic studies during the prodromal phase have shown abnormal filling of the internal carotid artery or the basilar artery systems (DUKES and VIETH, 1966; SKINHØJ, 1973; NORRIS et al., 1975). During the headache phase there is cortical hyperperfusion (SKINHØJ and PAULSON, 1969; NORRIS et al., 1975; MATHEW et al., 1976). Intracerebral lactic acidosis has been found during the period of increased flow, indicating that migraine headache is preceded by subclinical cerebral hypoxia (SKINHØJ, 1973).

There is agreement that an attack of migraine starts with a period of cerebral vasoconstriction during which the vessels lack their normal sensitivity to carbon dioxide (INGVAR, 1974). This vasoconstriction, when excessive, is generally considered to be responsible for the (prodromal) symptoms of focal cerebral ischemia. After the vasoconstriction, there is a phase of marked vasodilation as the headache develops. INGVAR (1976) has suggested that the beginning of pain may result in an increase in cerebral metabolism, which in turn would augment the cerebral vasodilation – and the pain – still further, thus setting up a vicious circle which would result in a steady increase in the intensity of the headache.

There is as yet no convincing evidence that the sympathetic nervous system is involved in migraine. It is known that the sympathetic nervous system exerts some control over the cranial vessels, but this effect appears to be weak and inconsistent (LANCE, 1973). Stimulation of the cervical sympathetic trunk decreases blood flow in both internal and external carotid arteries in monkeys, but section of the nerve does not increase cerebral blood flow, suggesting that the sympathetic nervous system is not responsible for maintaining tone in these vessels (MEYER et al., 1967).

Neither cervical sympathectomy nor transection of the greater superficial petrosal nerve provides any lasting benefit in migraine (WHITE and SMITHWICK, 1944; ROWBOTHAM, 1949). The only predictable surgical treatment to ameliorate migraine headache is section of the trigeminal pathways, which relieves pain at the expense of permanent facial analgesia (PENFIELD, 1932; OLIVECRONA, 1947; ROWBOTHAM, 1949).

c) Role of Humoral Mediators in Migraine Headache

Acetylcholine. OSTFELD et al. (1957) showed that the bulbar conjunctival vessels are more sensitive to the dilator effect of acetylcholine during migraine headache, but acetylcholine is not found in the cerebrospinal fluid of migraine patients. Furthermore, i.v. administration of acetylcholine or methacholine does not precipitate headaches in migraine patients (OSTFELD, 1960).

Histamine. Administration of histamine (PICKERING, 1933) or compound 48/80, a histamine liberator (SICUTERI et al., 1957), induces headache. Antihistamines reduce the intensity of histamine headaches but do not influence migraine headaches (OSTFELD et al., 1957). A sharp rise in blood histamine levels can be detected at the conclusion of a migraine headache, but this contrasts with the marked rise in blood histamine levels which follows cluster headaches (LANCE, 1973).

Kinins. Plasmakininogen levels in blood are reduced at the end of a migraine headache (SICUTERI, 1963). Perivascular edematous fluid contains a polypeptide of the plasmakinin type called "neurokinin" by WOLFF (1963). The fall in plasmakininogen levels could indicate an increase in the formation of plasmakinin. KANGASNIEMI et al. (1972) found an increase in activity of proteolytic enzymes in the CSF in some migraine patients during and after a migraine attack. Although injection of bradykinin into arteries produces pain (SICUTERI et al., 1963) and intradermal administration of bradykinin into the temporal area causes transient local pain, no headache ensues (ELKIN et al., 1964; FOX et al., 1961).

Prostaglandins. Infusions of prostaglandin E_1 (PGE_1) in man produce flushing, suggesting vasodilation in the external carotid bed (CARLSON et al., 1968). Although PGE_1 has been shown to dilate internal carotid vessels in baboons (PELOFSKY et al., 1972) and exposed pial arteries of cats (WELCH et al., 1974a), SPIRA et al. (1976) obtained an apparent constrictor effect in the external carotid bed of the monkey.

A role for PGE_1 in the pathogenesis of vascular headaches was originally suggested by the observations of CARLSON et al. (1968) who infused PGE_1 into 11 non-migraine volunteers. All but one developed headache (two with visual disturbances). Recent studies by ANTHONY (1974) have shown, however, that the plasma level of PGE_1 or PGE_2 is not changed during migraine headache (ANTHONY, 1974; OLESEN, 1976; BENNETT et al., 1974). These negative findings do not preclude the involvement of prostaglandins in migraine. They could contribute, for example, to the pain of migraine headache by sensitizing sensory nerve endings to pain-producing stimuli (FERREIRA, 1972).

Noradrenaline. In 1955, OSTFELD and WOLFF reported that the sensitivity of the bulbar conjunctival vessels to the constrictor effect of noradrenaline was increased during the prodromal phase of a migraine attack and decreased during the headache phase. When noradrenaline was infused for up to 3 h in the headache-free period, headache did not occur. SICUTERI (1962) and CURRAN et al. (1965) found that the excretion of VMA (3-methoxy-4-hydroxymandelic acid), the end product of catecholamine metabolism, is increased during attacks of migraine. Their findings have not been confirmed by other investigators (CURZON et al., 1966). According to HINTERBERGER (cited by LANCE, 1973), there is no significant change in the blood and urinary levels of noradrenaline in migraine patients. However, FOG-MØLLER et al. (1976) reported that the plasma level of noradrenaline decreases and reaches a minimum 1.5 h before peak intensity of headache.

5-Hydroxytryptamine. A connection between 5-HT and migraine was first suggested by the finding that during attacks of migraine headache the urinary excretion of 5-hydroxyindoleacetic acid (5-HIAA), the principal degradation product of 5-HT, is often increased (SICUTERI et al., 1961; CURRAN et al., 1965; CURZON et al., 1966). CURRAN et al. (1965) and ANTHONY et al. (1967) found that the 5-HT content of platelets in the serum of migraine patients changed in the course of the migraine attack. Expressing results in terms of $\mu g/10^9$ platelets, ANTHONY et al. found a mean value in 15 patients of 0.72 in headache-free periods, 0.82 in the 24 h preceding the headache, 0.45 during a migraine attack, and 0.71 in the 24 h following the headache. The fall during the attack was statistically highly significant and presumably reflects a fall in total serum 5-HT, since the number of platelets did not change noticeably. These changes were not due to stress, since they could not be reproduced by a stressful procedure such as pneumoencephalography. Very similar changes in the 5-HT level were produced by reserpine, a known depletor of 5-HT, causing migraine-like headache in migraine patients. The mechanism of the fall in platelet 5-HT is not fully understood. Cross-incubation experiments suggested that a 5-HT releasing factor might be involved which appears in the plasma during migraine attacks.

A possible interpretation of these findings is that the maintenance of an adequate 5-HT level provides the tonic vasoconstrictor stimulus required for the prevention of a migraine attack. Conversely, a sudden fall in 5-HT levels may precipitate an attack.

Certain experimental observations in man support the view of a protective role of 5-HT in migraine. KIMBALL et al. (1960) found that i.v. injection of 5-HT or 5-HTP (5-hydroxytryptophan) did not induce attacks in migraine subjects, while both substances relieved migraine headache to some extent. Both substances also relieved the "migraine model" (reserpine-induced) headache. When the amine oxidase inhibitor phenelzine, which would be expected to raise 5-HT levels, was administered to migrainous subjects over a period of 1 week, it reduced the frequency and intensity of headaches in nine out of 10 patients.

It has been remarked that these experiments do not conclusively prove the involvement of 5-HT in migraine. Other humoral mediators may also be involved. Thus, the effects of phenelzine could equally be attributed to interference with catecholamine metabolism.

d) Clinical Use of Ergot Alkaloids in Migraine

One of the earliest reports on the use of ergot alkaloids for the treatment of migraine was published by THOMSON (1894). He recorded the histories of a number of cases of "severe periodic neuralgias" in whom the symptoms were promptly relieved by the use of a fluid extract of ergot. The foundations for the modern use of ergot alkaloids in the treatment of migraine headaches were laid by TZANCK (1928) and TRAUTMANN (1928), who observed that oral administration of ergotamine not only aborted migraine headache and the associated symptoms, but if given daily, also prevented recurrence of migraine attacks. Since the publication of these pioneering studies, the efficacy of ergotamine in the treatment of migraine has been confirmed by numerous investigators, and other ergot alkaloids have been added to the armamentarium of antimigraine agents.

Dihydroergotamine was tried in migraine therapy on the basis of the belief that migraine headache resulted from an increase in sympathetic activity. Accordingly, dihydroergotamine was expected to be more efficacious than ergotamine in treating migraine headache, since it possesses greater α-adrenoceptor blocking activity. However, early clinical experience showed that dihydroergotamine, although effective in aborting migraine headache, must be given in much higher doses than ergotamine (HORTON et al., 1945; FRIEDMAN and FRIEDMAN, 1945; HARTMAN, 1945). Subsequent studies showed that the weaker vasoconstrictor effect of the drug made it suitable for migraine prophylaxis (SPÜHLER, 1946; CHAPUIS, 1948; KRÁL, 1948).

The hypothesis that 5-HT was implicated in migraine headache (OSTFELD et al., 1957) led to the trial of the 5-HT antagonist 2-bromo-LSD in migraine prophylaxis (OSTFELD, 1959). OSTFELD showed that given over a period of 6 weeks, this drug almost completely suppressed headache in subjects in whom i.v. infusions of 5-HT induced migraine-like headache but was only mildly active in preventing migraine headache in patients who did not respond to 5-HT. The modest antimigraine effect of 2-bromo-LSD was confirmed by HEYCK (1960) and KIMBALL et al. (1960). In the meantime, a more potent 5-HT antagonist, methysergide, made its appearance (DOEPFNER and CERLETTI, 1958; FANCHAMPS et al., 1960). The effectiveness of methysergide in migraine prophylaxis and its lack of activity during an attack has been confirmed by many investigators (for review, see CURRAN et al., 1967).

α) Mechanism of Action of Ergotamine

Extracranial Vessels

GRAHAM and WOLFF (1937) studied the effect of i.v. injections of 0.373–0.5 mg ergotamine tartrate in patients during an attack of migraine, recording pulsations of the temporal or occipital branch of the external carotid artery by means of tambours placed on the blood vessels. They carried out the measurements at a stage when the prodromal phenomena, such as scotomata, blurring of vision, and paresthesia, had already passed and headache had commenced. In each case, three control measurements of the amplitude of pulsations were made prior to

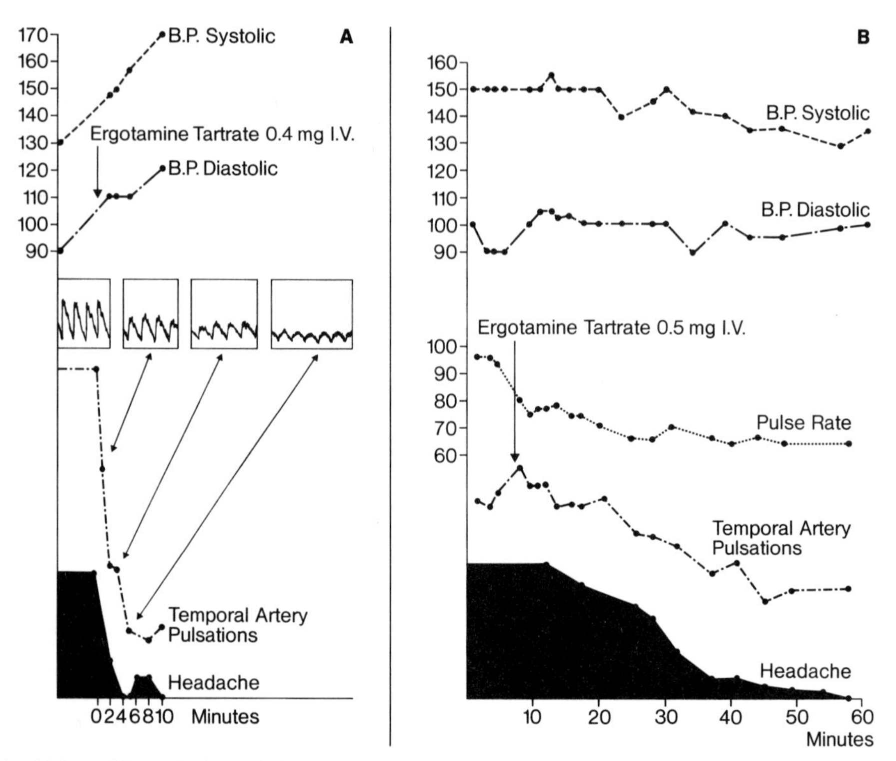

Fig. 15A and B. Relation of the amplitude of pulsation of the temporal artery to the intensity of migraine headache after administration of ergotamine in two patients. The average amplitude of pulsation for any given minute ascertained by measuring the individual pulsations from the photographic record (representative sections of the record are inserted in panel A). Averages are expressed as percentages of the initial amplitude (WOLFF, 1948)

the administration of ergotamine, the patients estimating the subjective intensity of their headache.

Typical results obtained in two out of about 20 experiments are shown in Figure 15. In panel A, ergotamine produced a sharp decrease in the amplitude of pulsation, which was closely paralleled by a rapid decrease in the intensity of the headache. In panel B the amplitude of pulsations decreased slowly after the injection of ergotamine, and headache likewise decreased slowly. Comparable results were obtained in the other experimental subjects, in most of whom a close correlation was obtained between the effect of ergotamine in decreasing pulsations in the external carotid bed and in reducing headache.

As a further test of the assumption that ergotamine relieves migraine headache by virtue of its vasoconstrictor action, OSTFELD and WOLFF (1955) administered noradrenaline as a 0.2% i.v. infusion to patients with migraine. The headache began to diminish in 10–60 min and disappeared within an hour or so. In general, the more intense the headache, the longer the time required for its elimination by noradrenaline. Signs of eye involvement, such as tears or blurred vision, were also eliminated. These findings suggest that vasoconstriction *per se,* by reducing the painful distension of the extracranial arteries, is the cause of relief of migraine headache. This view is supported by the experimental finding (WOLFF, 1963) that subjects suffering from headache experience instant relief if they are placed under increased positive *g* (when acceleration acts in a head-to-foot direction) in a human centrifuge. WOLFF also found that pressure on the common carotid artery or on a particular extracranial artery supplying a painful region diminishes the intensity of headache during a migraine attack. The author's conclusion that pain relief in migraine by ergotamine is due to vasoconstriction in the extracranial arterial bed has since been generally accepted.

Although ergotamine does not alter the pain threshold of normal skin (WOLFF et al., 1941) and lacks significant analgesic activity, it does affect the deep pain threshold of the skin in migraine, but indirectly, as a consequence of its vasoconstrictor action. TUNIS and WOLFF (1952) noticed that many patients exhibited an increased tenderness of the scalp during a migraine attack. Sites of lowered deep-pain threshold occurred particularly around swollen temporal arteries and disappeared after the administration of either ergotamine or noradrenaline (OSTFELD and WOLFF, 1955). The following mechanism was postulated to explain this finding. The increased capillary hydrostatic pressure brought about by arterial vasodilation causes the appearance and accumulation in the tissues of a pain threshold lowering "P" substance (not to be confused with substance P of EULER and GADDUM). During vasoconstriction, the capillary pressure falls but the continued presence of the "P" substance could explain the frequent persistence of local tenderness even after the migraine headache has subsided.

Cerebral Vessels

The intracranial blood supply in man is derived mainly from the internal carotid and vertebral arteries but also partly from the external carotid. The principal dural artery, the middle meningeal, is a branch of the external carotid, while the anterior meningeal artery derives from the internal carotid. With regard to pain sensitivity of intracranial structures, WOLFF (1963) concluded that the great venous sinuses, dural arteries, and cerebral arteries at the base of the brain are pain-sensitive, while the parenchyma of the brain is not sensitive. For a detailed discussion of cranial pain-sensitive structures reference should be made to RAY and WOLFF (1940) and WOLFF (1972).

The role of intracranial vessels in migraine and its relief by ergotamine has not been fully clarified, and information is based on few observations. Direct inspection of the middle meningeal artery during craniotomy revealed a decrease in diameter of the vessel following intravenous injection of 0.5 mg ergotamine (GRAHAM and WOLFF, 1937). Since stimulation of this artery causes pain localized in the temporal region (FAY, 1936; CRAIG, 1933), it seems likely that its constriction by ergotamine will contribute to pain relief. DICKERSON (1933) reported that ligation of this vessel abolished migraine attacks in some subjects. The role of branches of the internal carotid artery was studied by GRAHAM and WOLFF by recording the amplitude of pulsations in the lumbar subarachnoid space through a spinal needle or by inspecting and photographing retinal vessels. Intravenous injections of ergotamine caused a decrease in the amplitude of pulsations of the spinal fluid in some migraine subjects, but no correlation could be established between the amplitude of pulsations and the intensity of the headache. The caliber of retinal vessels was only marginally decreased by ergotamine.

Progress in this field has been impeded by lack of adequate methodology, but it seems likely that a clearer picture of cerebral vascular changes in migraine will emerge from newer methods, such as arteriography and particularly the intracarotid ^{133}Xe injection method. The latter has the advantage over the earlier inhalation method in that the internal carotid blood supply can be sampled without contamination by the external carotid area. Quantitative estimates of regional cerebral blood flow using this method have shown that an attack of migraine starts with a period of cerebral vasoconstriction which characterizes the prodromal stage and is followed by a stage of vasodilatation when the headache develops.

NORRIS et al. (1975) applied the intracarotid ^{133}Xe clearance method to ergotamine studies. They injected 0.25–1 mg ergotamine intramuscularly and carried out the regional cerebral blood flow study 15–30 min afterwards. They investigated 17 patients, three of whom had migraine and were studied during attacks. In none of the patients was regional cerebral blood flow altered by ergotamine. Using this method, SIMARD and PAULSON (1973) investigated a migrainous patient and demonstrated that 1 mg ergotamine given i.v. had no effect on regional cerebral blood flow either in the aura phase of the migraine attack or when repeated 3 months later when the patient was asymptomatic. In conclusion, there is no evidence at present that the therapeutic action of ergotamine is due to an effect on the internal carotid circulation, but obviously more experiments in man with a wider range of doses will be required to establish the point.

β) *Mechanism of Action of Methysergide*

Methysergide is a powerful antagonist of 5-HT on smooth muscle preparations such as the isolated rat uterus and isolated blood vessels (Chapter III). The antagonism between methysergide and 5-HT is of the "noncompetitive" type, i.e., there is a progressive decrease of maxima of the log dose-response curves. In view of the undoubted effectiveness of methysergide in the interval treatment of migraine, it has been difficult to reconcile its antagonistic effect against 5-HT with the apparent protective effect of 5-HT in migraine.

Various attempts have been made to account for the discrepancy. Some workers have considered that the protective action of methysergide is exerted on central serotonergic mechanisms (FANCIULLACCI et al., 1976), but several recent investigations suggest that methysergide may exert, under certain conditions, peripheral effects which are serotonin-like. SAXENA (1974) showed that in the anesthetized dog, methysergide has relatively little effect on general hemodynamics but has a marked effect in the carotid vascular bed, producing dose-dependent vasoconstriction in both internal and external carotid arteries. This effect is similar to that of 5-HT. CARROLL et al. (1974) investigated the effect of methysergide on isolated rabbit ear arteries and human temporal arteries. Methysergide stimulated (contracted) human arteries in relatively high doses, but much lower doses (5×10^{-9}–5×10^{-8}) caused a dose-dependent potentiation of the constrictor response to noradrenaline. The authors conclude that the catecholamine-potentiating effect rather then the direct effect of methysergide represents its most significant action, since it occurs at much lower doses. Other constrictor substances, e.g., histamine, were also potentiated by methysergide and other ergot alkaloids. SCHÖNBAUM et al. (1975) employed a preparation of nasal vessels, studied in the anesthetized dog; 5-HT produced a vasoconstriction which was potentiated by methysergide as well as by the non-ergot 5-HT antagonists cyproheptadine and pizotifen. FANCIULLACCI et al. (1976) investigated the action of methysergide in man by cannulating a hand vein. 5-HT produced venoconstriction which was at first antagonized by methysergide but later potentiated. The effect of a threshold dose of 5-HT was significantly potentiated within 15 min by 10 ng methysergide.

Several drugs which are effective in the prophylaxis of migraine attacks, namely ergotamine, dihydroergotamine, methysergide, and pizotifen, all lead to marked venoconstriction when infused into superficial hand veins in man (AELLIG, 1976b, 1978). During the past years of research into the pathophysiology of migraine and the mechanisms underlying the therapeutic action of drugs effective in preventing or treating the condition, emphasis has been place on changes occurring in cerebral and extracranial arteries. The question as to the involvement of the venous compartment of the cranial circulation in the genesis of migraine headache has received little attention.

F. References

Abel, F.L., Pierce, J.H., Guntheroth, W.G.: Baroreceptor influence on postural changes in blood pressure and carotid blood flow. Amer. J. Physiol. **205**, 360–364 (1963)

Abramson, D.I., Lichtman, S.S.: Influence of ergotamine tartrate upon peripheral blood flow in subjects with liver disease. Proc. Soc. exp. Biol. (N.Y.) **37**, 262–267 (1937)

Abreu, B.E., Liddle, G.W., Handley, C.A., Elliott, H.W.: Preliminary observations on the influence of ergotamine and dihydroergotamine on cerebral blood flow in the dog. Fed. Proc. **6**, 304 (1947)

Abreu, B.E., Liddle, G.W., Burks, A.L., Simon, A., Sutherland, V., Gordan, G.S.: Effects of amphetamine, dihydroergotamine and methadon on human cerebral blood flow and oxygen uptake. Fed. Proc. **7**, 201 (1948)

Achari, G., Ahmad, M.: Antiarrhythmic activity of cyproheptadine and methysergide. Indian Heart J. **18**, 4–16 (1966)

Aellig, W.H.: Periphere Kreislaufwirkungen von Ergotamin, Dihydroergotamin und 1-Methylergotamin an der innervierten, perfundierten Hinterextremität des Hundes. Helv. physiol. pharmacol. Acta **25**, 374–396 (1967)

Aellig, W.H.: Venoconstrictor effect of dihydroergotamine in superficial hand veins. Europ. J. clin. Pharmacol. **7**, 137–139 (1974)

Aellig, W.H.: Venentonisierende Wirkung von Ergotalkaloiden, untersucht an oberflächlichen Handvenen in situ. Cardiology **61** (Suppl.), 302–308 (1976a)

Aellig, W.H.: Influence of ergot compounds on compliance of superficial hand veins in man. Postgrad. med. J. **52** (Suppl. 1), 21–23 (1976b)

Aellig, W.H.: Clinical pharmacological experiments with pizotifen (Sanomigran®) on superficial hand veins in man. In: Current Concepts in Migraine Therapy. Green, R. (ed.), pp. 53–62. New York: Raven Press 1978

Aellig, W.H., Berde, B.: Studies of the effect of natural and synthetic polypeptide type ergot compounds on a peripheral vascular bed. Brit. J. Pharmacol. **36**, 561–570 (1969)

Aellig, W.H., Nüesch, E.: Comparative pharmacokinetic investigations with tritium-labelled ergot alkaloids after oral and intravenous administration in man. Int. J. clin. Pharmac. **15**, 106–112 (1977)

Ahlquist, R.P.: A study of the adrenergic receptors. Amer. J. Physiol. **153**, 586–599 (1948)

Alexander, R.S.: The participation of the venomotor system in pressor reflexes. Circulat. Res. **2**, 405–409 (1954)
Allen, C.R., Stutzman, J.W., Meek, W.J.: The production of ventricular tachycardia by adrenaline in cyclopropane anaesthesia. Anesthesiology **1**, 158–166 (1940)
Allen, C.R., Stutzman, J.W., Slocum, H.C., Orth, O.S.: Protection from cyclopropane-epinephrine tachycardia by various drugs. Anesthesiology **2**, 503–514 (1941)
Altura, B.M.: Chemical and humoral regulation of blood flow through the precapillary sphincter. Microvasc. Res. **3**, 361–384 (1971)
Amsler, C.: Über inverse Adrenalinwirkung. Arch. Physiol. **185**, 86–92 (1920)
Andrus, E.C., Martin, L.E.: The action of the sympathetic upon the excitatory process in the mammalian heart. J. exp. Med. **14**, 1017–1024 (1927)
Anthony, M.: Patterns of plasma free fatty acid and prostaglandin E_1 changes in migraine and stress. Sixth Migraine Symposium. London, England, Sept., p. 4, 1974
Anthony, M., Hinterberger, H., Lance, J.W.: Plasma serotonin in migraine and stress. Arch. Neurol. (Chic.) **16**, 544–552 (1967)
Antonaccio, M.J., Coté, D.: Centrally mediated antihypertensive and bradycardic effects of methysergide in spontaneously hypertensive rats. Europ. J. Pharmacol. **36**, 451–454 (1976)
Antonaccio, M.J., Kelly, E., Halley, J.: Centrally mediated hypotension and bradycardia by methysergide in anaesthetised dogs. Europ. J. Pharmacol. **33**, 107–117 (1975)
Antonaccio, M.J., Taylor, D.G.: Reduction in blood pressure, sympathetic nerve discharge and centrally evoked pressor responses by methysergide in anaesthetized cats. Europ. J. Pharmacol. **42**, 331–338 (1977)
Arcari, G., Dorigotti, L., Fregnan, G.B., Glässer, A.H.: Vasodilating and alpha-receptor blocking activity of a new ergoline derivative. Brit. J. Pharmacol. **34**, 700P (1968)
Arcari, G., Bernardi, L., Bosisio, G., Coda, S., Fregnan, G.B., Glässer, A.H.: 10-Methoxyergoline derivatives as α-adrenergic blocking agents. Experientia (Basel) **28**, 819–820 (1972)
Ariëns, E.J., Simonis, A.M.: Receptors and receptor mechanisms. in: Beta-Adrenoceptor Blocking Agents. Saxena, P.R., Forsyth, R.P. (eds.). Amsterdam: North Holland Publishing Co. 1976
Aschke, J., Trieb, G., Nusser, E.: Die dynamische Labilität der Blutdruckregulation und ihre therapeutische Beeinflussung. Münch. med. Wschr. **114**, 97–102 (1972)
Assali, N.S., Dasgupta, K., Kolin, A.: Measurement of uterine blood flow and uterine metabolism. VI. Effects of oxytocic, vasopressor and vasodepressor drugs on the blood flow to the postpartum uterus in unanaesthetised sheep. Amer. J. Obstet. Gynec. **78**, 313–321 (1959)
Athanasiou, D.J.: Die pharmakologische Beeinflussung des Valsalva-Versuches bei fortlaufender Blutdruckregistrierung. Z. klin. Med. **145**, 340–345 (1949)
Axelrod, J., Brady, R.O., Witkop, B., Evarts, E.V.: Metabolism of lysergic acid diethylamide. Nature (Lond.) **178**, 143–144 (1956)
Bachmann, K., Graf, N., Heynen, H.-P.: Regulationsstörungen des Kreislaufs und ihre Behandlung mit Dihydroergotamin. Fortschr. Med. **86**, 535–537 (1968)
Bacq, Z.M., Brouha, L., Heymans, C.: Recherche sur la physiologie et la pharmacologie du système nerveux autonome. Arch. int. Pharmacodyn. **48**, 429–456 (1934)
Bacq, Z.M., Bremer, F., Brouha, L., Heymans, C.: Reflexes vasomoteurs chez le chat sympathectomisé non anaesthésié. Arch. int. Pharmacodyn. **62**, 460–473 (1939)
Baldy-Moulinier, M.: Influence de l'hydergine sur les variations physiologiques et pathologiques de debit sanguin du cortex cerebral. Path. et Biol. **16**, 759–764 (1968)
Bálint, G.: Effect on blood pressure of drug combinations containing phenothiazine derivatives and hydergine. Acta physiol. Acad. Sci. hung. **26**, 361–368 (1965)
Baráth, E.: Untersuchungen über die Ergotaminwirkung bei Menschen, mit besonderer Rücksicht auf seine klinischen Anwendungsmöglichkeiten bei inneren Erkrankungen. Z. klin. Med. **104**, 712–718 (1926)
Barbey, K., Brecht, K.: Venentonus, Venenkapazität und ihre Messung. Med. Welt **1**, 727–732 (1965)
Barcroft, H., Konzett, H., Swan, H.J.C.: Observations on the action of the hydrogenated alkaloids of the ergotoxine group on the circulation in man. J. Physiol. (Lond.) **112**, 273–291 (1951)

Barger, G., Dale, H.H.: Ergotoxine and some other constituents of ergot. Biochem. J. **2**, 240–299 (1907)
Barry, D.T.: Some features of the pharmacological actions of yohimbine and ergotamine. Arch. int. Pharmacodyn. **55**, 385–401 (1937)
Baumann, D.P., Jerram, D.C., Seager, L.D.: Mechanism of bradycardia induced by hydrogenated ergot alkaloids. Fed. Proc. **13**, 334–335 (1954)
Becattini, U., Cangi, G., Termini, F.: Azione dell'Hydergina sul flusso sanguigno degli arti inferiori. Settim. Med. **52**, 703–707 (1964)
Bell, C., Conway, E.L., Lang, W.J.: Ergometrine and apomorphine as selective antagonists of dopamine in the canine renal vasculature. Brit. J. Pharmacol. **52**, 591–595 (1974)
Bell, C., Conway, E.L., Lang, W.J., Padanyi, R.: Vascular dopamine receptors in the canine hindlimb. Brit. J. Pharmacol. **55**, 167–172 (1975)
Benfey, B.G., Kunos, G., Nickerson, M.: Dissociation of cardiac inotropic and adenylate cyclase activating adrenoceptors. Brit. J. Pharmacol. **51**, 253–257 (1974)
Bennett, W.D., Dhuner, K.-G., Orth, O.S.: A comparison of the effectiveness of dihydroergotamine (DHE-45) and dihydroergocornine (DHO-180) in the prevention of cardiac irregularities during cyclopropane anesthesia. J. Pharmacol. exp. Ther. **95**, 287–292 (1949)
Bennett, A., Magnaes, B., Sandler, M., Sjaastad, O.: Prostaglandins and headache. Sixth Migraine Symposium, London, Sept., p12, 1974
Bergenwald, L., Ecklund, B., Kaijser, L., Klingenström, P.: Haemodynamic effects of dihydroergotamine during spinal anaesthesia in man. Acta anaesthesiol. scand. **16**, 235–239 (1972)
Bergh, R. van den: L'influence de quelques médicaments usuels sur la vasomotricity carotidienne. Acta neurol. belg. **56**, 459–475 (1956)
Berne, R.M.: Effect of epinephrine and norepinephrine on coronary circulation. Circulat. Res. **6**, 644–655 (1958)
Bernsmeier, A.: Die chemische Blockierung des adrenergischen Systems am Menschen. Acta neuroveg., Suppl. 5. Wien: Springer 1954
Bevegård, S., Castenfors, J., Lindblad, L.E.: Haemodynamic effects of dihydroergotamine in patients with postural hypotension. Acta med. scand. **196**, 473–477 (1974)
Bianco, P.L. del, Fanciullacci, M., Franchi, G., Sicuteri, F.: Human 5-hydroxytryptamine venomotor receptors. Pharmacol. Res. Commun. **7**, 395–408 (1975)
Biber, B., Fara, J., Lundgren, O.: A pharmacological study of intestinal vasodilator mechanisms in the cat. Acta physiol. scand. **90**, 673–683 (1974)
Bidart, Y., Maury, M.: Effets de la dihydroergotamine sur l'adaption vaso-motrice à l'orthostatisme chez les paraplégiques. Ann. Méd. phys. **17**, 235–242 (1974)
Bircher, R., Cerletti, A.: Pharmakodynamische Grundlagen der Therapie von Kreislaufstörungen mit den dihydroalkaloiden des Mutterkorns. Helv. med. Acta, Suppl. XXII, 13–26 (1949)
Blake, W.D.: Some effects of dihydrogenated ergot alkaloids on renal haemodynamics, water and electrolyte excretion in the dog. Amer. J. Physiol. **173**, 337–344 (1953)
Bluntschli, H.J.: Über die Wirkung eines Ergot-Derivates (Dihydroergocornin) auf Blutdruck, Respiration und Elektrokardiogramm der Katze nach Querschnittsdurchtrennung des Rückenmarks im Bereich der Thoracal-Segmente. Helv. physiol. pharmacol. Acta **6**, C50–C51 (1948)
Bluntschli, H.J., Goetz, R.H.: The effect of ergot derivatives on the circulation in man with special reference to two new hydrogenated compounds (dihydroergotamine and dihydroergocornine). Amer. Heart J. **35**, 873–894 (1948)
Bluntschli, H.J., Eyband, M., Staub, H.: Über Blutdruckwirkungen von Angiotonin und hydrierten Ergotoxinderivaten (Dihydroergocornin, Hydergin) an der Katze. Helv. physiol. pharmacol. Acta **7**, 406–409 (1949)
Bocci, U., Bignotti, N., Luzi, T.: L'azione normotensiva della diidroergotamina nelle alterazioni pressorie da psicofarmaci. Riv. sper. Freniat. **94**, No. 2 (1970)
Boer, J. de, Van Dongen, K.: Experiments with dihydroergotamine. Arch. int. Pharmacodyn. **77**, 434–441 (1948)
Boismare, F., Derrey, D., Adisio, M., Brocheriou, J.: Hypotension posturale provoquée par les neuroleptiques: étude rhéographique de l'effet de correcteurs (néosynéphrine, dihydroergotamine et chlorhydrate d'heptaminol). Thérapie **29**, 435–446 (1974)

Boismare, F., Hacpille, L., Belliard, J.P.: Etude rhéographique des effets de la dihydroergotamine sur l'hemodynamique encéphalique et périphérique chez les sujets sains. Thérapie **30**, 149–156 (1975a)

Boismare, F., Hacpille, L., Belliard, J., Colin, C.: Effects of dihydroergotamine on postural hypotension induced by levomepromazine. J. Pharmacol. (Paris) **6**, 391–400 (1975b)

Bojanovsky, J., Toelle, R.: Dihydroergotamin gegen die Kreislaufwirkungen der Thymoleptika. Dtsch. med. Wschr. **99**, 1064–1069 (1974)

Bouckaert, J.J., Grimson, K.S., Heymans, C., Samaan, A.: Sur la méchanisme de l'influence de l'hypoxémie sur la respiration et la circulation. Arch. int. Pharmacodyn. **65**, 63–100 (1941)

Broghammer, H., Takagi, K., Schaefer, H.: Die Wirkung von Lysergsäure-Diäthylamid (LSD) und Urethan auf die Tätigkeit eines sympathischen Ganglions. Naunyn-Schmiedebergs Arch. exp. Path. Pharmak. **230**, 358–366 (1957)

Brooke, O.G., Robinson, B.F.: Effect of ergotamine and ergometrine on forearm venous compliance in man. Brit. med. J. **1**, 139–142 (1970)

Buckley, G.A., Jordan, C.C.: Temperature modulation of α- and β-adrenoceptors in the isolated frog heart. Brit. J. Pharmacol. **38**, 394–398 (1970)

Buñag, R.D., Walaszek, E.J.: Blockade of depressor responses to serotonin and tryptamine by lysergic acid derivatives in the chicken. Arch. int. Pharmacodyn. **135**, 142–151 (1962)

Buttermann, G., Hör, G., Pabst, H.W.: Progress in prevention of postoperative thromboembolism – a controlled clinical trial using radio-fibrinogen-uptake-test and lung-perfusion-scan. 4th Mediterranean congress on thromboembolism. Athens, Greece, May 2–6, Abstr. 25 (1976)

Buttermann, G., Theisinger, W., Oechsler, H., Hör, G.: Untersuchungen über die postoperative Thromboembolieprophylaxe nach einem neuen medikamentösen Behandlungsprinzip. Dtsch. med. Wschr. **41**, 2065–2069 (1975)

Cairoli, V., Reilly, J., Ito, R., Roberts, J.: The relation of the digitalis-induced arrhythmia to catecholamine release. Fed. Proc. **21**, 127 (1962)

Capps, R.T., Suckle, H.M., Orth, O.S.: A comparison of protective action of the dihydrogenated ergot alkaloids to cyclopropane-epinephrine ventricular tachycardia. Amer. J. Physiol. **163**, 702–703 (1950)

Carlson, L.A., Ekelund, L.G., Orö, L.: Clinical and metabolic effects of different doses of prostaglandin E in man. Acta med. scand. **183**, 423–430 (1968)

Carpi, A., Virno, M.: The action of ergotamine on the intracranial venous pressure and on the cerebral venous outflow of the dog. Brit. J. Pharmacol. **12**, 232–239 (1957)

Carroll, P.R., Ebeling, P.W., Glover, W.E.: The responses of the human temporal and rabbit ear artery to 5-hydroxytryptamine and some of its antagonists. Aust. J. exp. Biol. med. Sci. **52**, 813–823 (1974)

Castenfors, J., Lindblad, L.E., Mortasawi, A.: Effect of dihydroergotamine on peripheral circulation during epidural anaesthesia in man. Acta anaesth. scand. **19**, 79–84 (1975)

Cerletti, A.: Lysergic acid diethylamide (LSD) and related compounds. Neuropharmacology: Trans. 2nd Conf. Princeton, 1955. Abramson, H.A. (ed.), pp. 9–84. Josiah Macy Jr. Foundation 1956

Cerletti, A.: Gynaecologia (Basel) **128**, 452–453 (1949)

Cerletti, A., Berde, B.: New approaches in the development of compounds from ergot with potential therapeutic use in migraine. In: Background to migraine. 2nd migraine symposium. Smith, R. (ed.), pp. 53–65, London 1969

Cerletti, A., Doepfner, W.: Comparative study on the serotonin antagonism of amide derivatives of lysergic acid and of ergot alkaloids. J. Pharmacol. exp. Ther. **122**, 124–136 (1958)

Cerletti, A., Rothlin, E.: Role of 5-hydroxytryptamine in mental diseases and its antagonism to lysergic acid derivatives. Nature (Lond.) **176**, 785–786 (1955)

Cervoni, P., Bertino, J.R., Geiger, L.E.: Medullary vagal effects of *d*-lysergic acid diethylamide in the decerebrate cat. Nature (Lond.) **199**, 700–701 (1963)

Chalmers, J.P.: Brain amines and models of experimental hypertension. Circulat. Res. **36**, 469–480 (1975)

Chapuis, J.P.: Migraines, céphalées et sympathicolytiques. Schweiz. med. Wschr. **78**, 1125–1126 (1948)

Chong, G.C., Phillis, J.W.: Pharmacological studies on the heart of *Tapes Watlingi*: A mollusc of the family veneridae. Brit. J. Pharmacol. **25**, 481–496 (1965)
Chu, D., Hool-Zulauf, B.: Studies on the reserpine-induced potentiation of the peripheral vascular effect of DHE in cats. Naunyn-Schmiedebergs Arch. exp. Path. Pharmak. **287**, R22 (1975)
Chu, D., Stürmer, E.: Studies on the mechanism of dihydroergotamine (DHE) on the vascular bed of cat skeletal muscle. Brit. J. Pharmacol. **48**, 331P–332P (1973)
Chu, D., Owen, D.A.A., Stürmer, E.: Effects of ergotamine and dihydroergotamine on the resistance and capacitance vessels of skin and skeletal muscle in the cat. Postgrad. med. J. **52** (Suppl. l), 32–36 (1976)
Clark, B.J.: Dopamine receptor stimulants in hypertension. Acta med. scand. Suppl. **606**, 95–99 (1977)
Clark, B.J., Scholtysik, G., Flückiger, E.: Cardiovascular actions of bromocriptine. In: The dopamine agonist, Bromocriptine. Hökfelt, B., Nillius, S.J. (eds.). Acta endocr. (Kbh.) Suppl. (1978) in press
Cobbold, A., Folkow, B., Kjellmer, I., Mellander, S.: Nervous and local chemical control of pre-capillary sphincters in skeletal muscle as measured by changes in filtration coefficient. Acta physiol. scand. **57**, 180–192 (1963)
Corrodi, H., Fuxe, K., Hökfelt, T., Lidbrink, P., Ungerstedt, U.: Effect of ergot drugs on central catecholamine neurons: evidence for a stimulation of central dopamine neurons. J. Pharm. Pharmacol. **25**, 409–412 (1973)
Corsi, V., Dohrn, P.: Ergotamina e attività reflessogena senocarotidea (Nota I: Attività sinusale alla compressione nei normotesi). Boll. Soc. med.-chir. Catania **14**, 245–250 (1946)
Corsi, V.: Contributo di recerche cliniche ed elettrocardiografiche sull' ipertensione da noradrenalina. G. Med. Tisiol. **1**, 21 (1952)
Cotten, M. de V., Walton, R.P.: Dibenamine blockade as a method of distinguishing between inotropic actions of epinephrine and digitalis. Proc. Soc. exp. Biol. (N.Y.) **78**, 810–815 (1951)
Cotten, M. de V., Moran, N.C., Stopp, P.E.: A comparison of the effectiveness of adrenergic blocking drugs in inhibiting the cardiac actions of sympathomimetic amines. J. Pharmacol. exp. Ther. **121**, 183–190 (1957)
Craig, W.M.: Localised headache associated with lesion of meningeal vessels. J. Amer. med. Ass. **100**, 816 (1933)
Crosley, A.P., Cummins, A.J., Barker, H.G., Clark, J.K.: The renal hemodynamic effects of dihydroergocornine (DHO-180) in man. J. Pharmacol. exp. Ther. **98**, 138–143 (1950)
Curran, D.A., Hinterberger, H., Lance, J.W.: Total plasma serotonin, 5-hydroxyindoleacetic acid and p-hydroxy-m-methoxymandelic acid excretion in normal and migrainous subjects. Brain **88**, 997-1010 (1965)
Curran, D.A., Hinterberger, H., Lance, J.W.: Methysergide. Res. Clin. Stud. Headache **1**, 77–122. Basel-New York: Karger 1967
Curzon, G., Theaker, P., Phillips, B.: Excretion of 5-hydroxyindolyl acetic acid (5HIAA) in migraine. J. Neurol. Neurosurg. Psychiat. **29**, 85 (1966)
Dale, H.H.: On some physiological actions of ergot. J. Physiol. (Lond.) **34**, 163–206 (1906)
Dale, H.H., Spiro, K.: Die wirksamen Alkaloide des Mutterkorns. Naunyn-Schmiedebergs Arch. exp. Path. Pharmak. **95**, 337–350 (1922)
Dalessio, D.J.: Recent experimental studies on headache. Neurology (Minneap.) **13**, 7–10 (1963)
Dalessio, D.J., Camp, W.A., Goodell, H., Wolff, H.G.: Studies on headache. Arch. Neurol. (Chic.) **4**, 235–240 (1961)
David, N.A., Kirchof, A.C.: Studies on d-lysergic acid and hydrobutylamide- (2) (methergine). Schweiz. med. Wschr. **77**, 13–17 (1947)
Davis, M.E., Adair, F.L., Chen, K.K., Swanson, E.E.: The pharmacologic action of ergotocin, a new ergot principle. J. Pharmacol. exp. Ther. **54**, 398–407 (1935)
Davis, W.G., McDonald, D.C., Mason, D.F.J.: The effects of pronethalol and propranolol on the coronary circulation of the dog. Brit. J. Pharmacol. **37**, 338–356 (1969)
Delaunois, A.L., Martini, L.: Adrenolytic drugs and action of adrenaline and noradrenaline on carotid sinus wall and blood pressure. Arch. int. Pharmacodyn. **94**, 430–438 (1953)

Delius, L., Hammerschmidt, D., Odenthal, F.: Klinisch-experimentelle Untersuchungen über die kreislaufdynamischen Wirkungen der dihydrierten Mutterkornalkaloide. Klin. Wschr. **27**, 33–34 (1949)
Deutsch, E., Markoff, T.: Mitteilungen zur Nierenclearance. Klin. Med. **8**, 105–115 (1953)
Dickerson, D.G.: The surgical relief of the headache in migraine. J. nerv. ment. Dis. **77**, 42 (1933)
Doepfner, W., Cerletti, A.: Comparison of lysergic acid derivatives and antihistamines as inhibitors of the edema provoked in the rat's paw by serotonin. Int. Arch. Allergy **12**, 89–97 (1958)
Drew, G.M.: Effects of α-adrenoceptor agonists and antagonists on pre- and postsynaptically located α-adrenoceptors. Europ. J. Pharmacol. **36**, 313–320 (1976)
D'Silva, J.L.: Action of adrenaline-like substances on the serum potassium. J. Physiol. (Lond.) **108**, 218–225 (1949)
Dubocovich, M.L., Langer, S.Z.: Negative feedback regulation of noradrenaline release by nerve stimulation in the perfused cat's spleen: differences in potency of phenoxybenzamine in blocking the pre- and post-synaptic adrenergic receptors. J. Physiol. (Lond.) **237**, 505–519 (1974)
Dukes, H.T., Vieth, R.G.: Cerebral arteriography during migraine prodrome and headache. Neurology (Minneap.) **14**, 636–639 (1966)
Dumke, P.R., Schmidt, C.F.: Quantitative measurements of cerebral blood flow in the macaque monkey. Amer. J. Physiol. **138**, 421–431 (1943)
Dunér, H., Granath, A., Klingenström, P.: The effect of ergotamine on blood pressure and cardiac output during spinal anaesthesia in man. Acta anaesthesiol. scand. **4**, 5–11 (1960)
Duret, R.-L.: Action des dérivés d-hydrogénés de l'ergot dans hypertension artérielle. Acta clin. belg. **6**, 85–106 (1951)
Eben-Moussi, E., Allain, P., Van den Driessche, J.: Hydergine et troubles du rythme cardiaque provoqués par la K-strophantine. Thérapie **21**, 375–378 (1966)
Echt, M., Lange, L.: Experimentelle Untersuchungen über die Wirkung venentonisierender Pharmaka auf das Niederdrucksystem des Menschen. In: Das Orthostasesyndrom. 5. Rothenburger Gespräch 25./26.5.73. Dengler, H.J. (ed.), pp. 109–123. Stuttgart-New York: Schattauer 1974
Ehringer, H.: Zur Wirkung von reinem Dihydroergocristin auf Extremitätendurchblutung und periphere Venentonisierung des Menschen. Int. J. clin. Pharmacol. Biopharm. **3**, 81–86 (1970)
Elek, S.R., Hoffman, I., Griffith, G.C., Leik, D.W.: The cardiac effects of dihydroergocornine (DHO-180). Arch. int. Pharmacodyn. **100**, 249–264 (1955)
Eliasson, S., Folkow, B., Lindgren, P., Uvnäs, B.: Activation of sympathetic vasodilator nerves to the skeletal muscles in the cat by hypothalamic stimulation. Acta physiol. scand. **23**, 333–351 (1951)
Eliasson, S., Lindgren, P., Uvnäs, B.,: Representation in the hypothalamus and the motor cortex in the dog of the sympathetic vasodilator outflow to the skeletal muscles. Acta physiol. scand. **27**, 18–37 (1952)
Elkind, A.H., Friedman, A.P., Grossman, I.: Cutaneous blood flow in vascular headaches of the migraine type. Neurology (Minneap.) **14**, 24–30 (1964)
Enero, M.A., Langer, S.Z.: Inhibition by dopamine of ^{3}H-noradrenaline release elicited by nerve stimulation in the isolated cat's nictitating membrane. Naunyn-Schmiedebergs Arch. exp. Path. Pharmak. **289**, 179–203 (1975)
Erlij, D., Mendez, C.: Adrenergic actions on heart rate, atrioventricular refractory period and intraventricular conduction in dogs. Arch. int. Physiol. Biochim. **72**, 44–65 (1964)
Erlij, D., Cefrangolo, R., Valadez, R.: Adrenotropic receptors in the frog. J. Pharmacol. exp. Ther. **149**, 65–70 (1965)
Euler, U.S. v., Hesser, C.M.: Beobachtungen über Hemmungen der Sinusdruckreflexe durch Ergotamin, Dihydroergotamin und Hyperventilation. Schweiz. med. Wschr. **77**, 20–21 (1947)
Euler, U.S. v., Liljestrand, G.: The role of the chemoreceptors of the sinus region for the occlusion test in the cat. Acta physiol. scand. **6**, 319–323 (1943)
Euler, U.S. v., Liljestrand, G.: The regulation of the blood pressure with special reference to muscular work. Acta physiol. scand. **12**, 279–300 (1946)

Euler, U.S. v., Schmiterlöw, C.G.: The action of ergotamine on the chemical and mechanical reflexes from the carotid sinus region. Acta physiol. scand. **8**, 122–133 (1944)
Eyzaguirre, C., Lewin, J.: Chemoreceptor activity of the carotid body of the cat. J. Physiol. (Lond.) **159**, 222–237 (1961)
Fahim, I., Botros, M., Merhom, K., Saad, Y.: The central hypotensive effects of ergotamine and its possible mechanism. Ain Shams Med. **25**, 355–357 (1974)
Fanchamps, A., Doepfner, W., Weidmann, H., Cerletti, A.: Pharmakologische Charakterisierung von Deseril, einem Serotonin-Antagonisten. Schweiz. med. Wschr. **90**, 1040–1046 (1960)
Fanciullacci, M., Granchi, G., Sicuteri, F.: Ergotamine and methysergide as serotonin partial agonists in migraine. Headache **16**, 226–231 (1976)
Farnebo, L.O., Hamberger, B.: Drug-induced changes in the release of (^{3}H)-noradrenaline from field stimulated rat iris. Brit. J. Pharmacol. **43**, 97–106 (1971)
Fay, T.: Mechanism of headache. Trans. Amer. neurol. Ass. **62**, 74–77 (1936)
Fehr, T., Stütz, P., Stadler, P.A., Hummel, R., Salzmann, R.: Antihypertensiv wirksame Harnstoffderivate des 8β-aminomethyl-6-methyl-ergolens. Europ. J. Med. Chem. **9**, 597–601 (1974)
Ferreira, S.H.: Prostaglandins, aspirin-like drugs and analgesia. Nature New Biol. **240**, 200–203 (1972)
Fey, K.H., Herzfeld, U., Saggau, W., Oehlschläger, M.: Postoperative Thromboprophylaxe durch Tonisierung des kaudalen Venensystems. Med. Klin. **70**, 1553–1558 (1975)
Fitzgerald, W.J.: Methergine: a study of its effect on blood pressure. Obstet. and gynec. **8**, 167–169 (1956)
Fog-Møller, F., Kemp-Genefke, I., Bryndum, B.: Changes in concentration of catecholamines in blood during spontaneous migraine attacks and reserpine-induced attacks. The Migraine Trust International Symposium, London, p. 10 (16–17 Sept. 1976)
Folkow, B.: Nervous control of blood vessels. Physiol. Rev. **35**, 629–663 (1955)
Folkow, B., Uvnäs, B.: Do adrenergic vasodilator nerves exist? Acta physiol. scand. **20**, 329–337 (1950)
Fox, R.H., Goldsmith, R., Kidd, D.J., Lewis, G.P.: Bradykinin as a vasodilator in man. J. Physiol. (Lond.) **157**, 589–602 (1961)
Franke, H.: Die pharmakologische Beeinflussung der kardialen Form des hypersensitiven Carotissinus-Syndroms durch hydrierte Mutterkornalkaloide. Z. exp. Med. **116**, 463–477 (1950)
Freis, E.D., Stanton, J.R., Litter, J., Culbertson, J.W., Halperin, M.H., Moister, F.C., Wilkins, R.W.: The hemodynamic effects of hypotensive drugs in man. II. Dihydroergocornine. J. clin. Invest. **28**, 1387–1402 (1949)
Freis, E.D., Stanton, J.R., Finnerty, F.A., Schnaper, H.W., Johnson, R.L., Rath, C.E., Wilkins, R.W.: The collapse produced by venous congestion of the extremities or by venesection following certain hypotensive agents. J. clin. Invest. **30**, 435–444 (1951)
Freudiger, A., Rothlin, E.: Ueber die Wirkung der natürlichen und dihydrierten Mutterkornalkaloide auf das isolierte Froschherz. Arch. int. Pharmacodyn. **78**, 445–455 (1949)
Friedman, M.D., Friedman, D.A.: Dihydroergotamine (DHE-45) in the treatment of migraine: Preliminary clinical observations. Ohio med. J. **41**, 1099–1100 (1945)
Gaddum, J.H., Paasonen, M.K.: The use of some molluscan hearts for the estimation of 5-hydroxytryptamine. Brit. J. Pharmacol. **10**, 474–483 (1955)
Ganter, G.: Ueber die Ausschaltung des vegetativen Nervensystems am Kreislauf. Naunyn-Schmiedebergs Arch. exp. Path. Pharmak. **113**, 129–150 (1926)
Gatzek, H., Matthies, K., Mechelke, K.: Untersuchungen über das Wirkungsbild der Mutterkornalkaloide Ergotamin, Dihydroergotamin und Dihydroergocornin am gesunden Menschen. Naunyn-Schmiedebergs Arch. exp. Path. Pharmak. **207**, 720–730 (1949)
Gernandt, B., Zotterman, Y.: The splanchnic efferent outflow of impulses in the light of ergotamine action. Acta physiol. scand. **11**, 301–317 (1946)
Gernandt, B., Liljestrand, G., Zotterman, Y.: Efferent impulses in the splanchnic nerve. Acta physiol. scand. **11**, 230–247 (1946)
Gillis, R.A.: Cardiac sympathetic nerve activity: changes induced by ouabain and propranolol. Science **166**, 508–510 (1969)

Gillis, R.A., Dionne, R.A., Standaert, F.G.: Suppression by clonidine (St-155) of cardiac arrhythmias induced by digitalis. J. Pharmacol. exp. Ther. **182**, 218–226 (1972)
Ginzel, K.H.: The effect of (+)-lysergic acid diethylamide and other drugs on the carotid sinus reflex. Brit. J. Pharmacol. **13**, 250–259 (1958)
Ginzel, K.H., Kottegoda, S.R.: A study of the vascular actions of 5-hydroxytryptamine, tryptamine, adrenaline and noradrenaline. Quart. J. exp. Physiol. **38**, 225–231 (1953)
Glässer, A.: Some pharmacological actions of d-lysergic acid methyl carbinolamide. Nature (Lond.) **189**, 313–314 (1961)
Goetz, R.H.: The action of dihydroergocornine on the circulation with special reference to hypertension. Lancet **I**, 510–514 (1949)
Goetz, R.H.: The effect of intra-arterial injections of Hydergine and dihydroergocornine on the peripheral circulation in man. Circulation **13**, 63–74 (1956)
Goetz, R.H., Katz, A.: The adrenolytic action of dihydroergocornine in man. Lancet **256**, 560-563 (1949)
Goldberg, L.I.: Cardiovascular and renal actions of dopamine: potential clinical applications. Pharmacol. Rev. **24**, 1–29 (1972)
Goldman, H., Fischer, R., Nicolov, N., Murphy, S.: Lysergic acid diethylamide affects blood flow to specific areas of the conscious rat brain. Experientia (Basel) **31**, 328–330 (1975)
Gottstein, U., Niedermauer, W., Bernsmeier, A.: Die Gehirndurchblutung unter dem Einfluß vasoaktiver Substanzen. Z. ges. exp. Med. **131**, 430–439 (1959)
Govier, W.C.: Myocardial alpha adrenergic receptors and their role in the production of a positive inotropic effect by sympathomimetic agents. J. Pharmacol. exp. Ther. **159**, 82–90 (1968)
Govier, W.C., Mosal, N.C., Whittington, P., Broom, A.H.: Myocardial alpha and beta adrenergic receptors as demonstrated by atrial functional refractory period changes. J. Pharmacol. exp. Ther. **154**, 255–263 (1966)
Graham, J.R., Wolff, H.G.: Mechanism of migraine headache and action of ergotamine tartrate. Proc. Ass. Res. nerv. ment. Dis. **18**, 638–669 (1937)
Graham, J.D.P., Khalidi, A.I.: The actions of d-lysergic acid diethylamide. J. Fac. Med. Baghdad **18**, 1–10 (1954)
Greenacre, J.K., Teychenne, P.F., Petrie, A., Calne, D.B., Leigh, P.N., Reid, J.L.: The cardiovascular effects of bromocriptine in parkinsonism. Brit. J. clin. Pharmacol. **3**, 571–574 (1976)
Greenberg, M.J.: Structure-activity relationship of tryptamine analogues on the heart of *Venus mercenaria*. Brit. J. Pharmacol. **15**, 375–388 (1960a)
Greenberg, M.J.: The response of the *Venus* heart to catecholamines and high concentrations of 5-hydroxytryptamine. Brit. J. Pharmacol. **15**, 365–374 (1960b)
Guimarães, S., Osswald, W.: Adrenergic receptors in the veins of the dog. Europ. J. Pharmacol. **5**, 133–140 (1969)
Guyton, A.C.: Textbook of medical physiology. 2nd ed., pp. 398–400. Philadelphia-London: W.B. Saunders Co. 1961
Gyermek, L., Sztanyik, L., Láng, E.: The adrenolytic and sympathicolytic efficiency of ergot alkaloids. Acta physiol. Acad. Sci. hung. **1**, 65–74 (1950)
Haddy, F.J., Gordon, P., Emanuel, D.A.: The influence of tone upon responses of small and large vessels to serotonin. Circulat. Res. **7**, 123–130 (1959)
Hafkenschiel, J.H., Crumpton, C.W., Moyer, J.H.: The effect of intramuscular dihydroergocornine on the cerebral circulation in normotensive patients. J. Pharmacol. exp. Ther. **98**, 144–146 (1950a)
Hafkenschiel, J.H., Crumpton, C.W., Moyer, J.H., Jeffers, W.A., Hanley, B.F., Harned, S.C.: The effects of dihydroergocornine on the cerebral circulation of patients with essential hypertension. J. clin. Invest. **29**, 408–411 (1950b)
Haley, T.J., McCormick, W.G.: Effect of ergotamine and hydergine on muscle blood flow in the dog. Fed. Proc. **14**, 348–349 (1955)
Haley, T.J., McCormick, W.G.: Comparison of the effect of ergotamine and hydergine on muscle and skin blood flow in the anaesthetised dog. J. Pharmacol. exp. Ther. **117**, 406–413 (1956)
Haley, T.J., Andem, M.R., Liebig, C.: Comparison between capillary effects produced by

topical application and intravenous injection of ergot alkaloids. Arch. int. Pharmacodyn. **98**, 373–378 (1954)
Halmágyi, D.F.J., Colebatch, H.J.H.: Serotonin-like cardiorespiratory effects of a serotonin antagonist. J. Pharmacol. exp. Ther. **134**, 47–52 (1961)
Halmágyi, B., Felkai, J., Iványi, J., Hetényi, J.Jr.: The role of the nervous system in the maintainance of venous hypertension in heart failure. Brit. Heart J. **14**, 101–111 (1952)
Halmágyi, D., Iványi, J., Felkai, B., Zsótér, T. Tényi, M., Szücs, Z.: The effect of dihydroergotamine and Hydergin on pulmonary arterial pressure in man. Scand. J. clin. Lab. Invest. **5**, 85–89 (1953)
Hammerschmidt, D., Odenthal, F.: Ueber die Wirkung der hydrierten Mutterkornalkaloide auf den arteriellen und venösen Blutdruck. Z. Kreisl.-Forsch. **39**, 150–160 (1950)
Handley, C.A., Moyer, J.H.: Changes in sodium and water excretion produced by vaso-active and by ganglionic and adrenergic blocking agents. Amer. J. Physiol. **178**, 309–314 (1954)
Härich, B.K.S., Nissen, H., Stauch, M.: Die Alpha-Sympathikolyse im arteriellen und venösen Kreislaufschenkel nach Hydergin®. Herz/Kreisl. **7**, 194–198 (1975)
Harmel, M.H., Hafkenschiel, J.H., Austin, G.M., Crumpton, C.W., Kety, S.S.: The effect of bilateral stellate ganglion block on the cerebral circulation in normotensive and hypertensive patients. J. clin. Invest. 28, 415–418 (1949)
Harri, M.N.E.: Temperature-dependent sensitivity of adrenoceptors in the toad heart. Acta pharmacol. toxicol. (Kbh.) **33**, 273–279 (1973)
Harris, A.S.: Delayed development of ventricular ectopic rhythms following experimental coronary occlusion. Circulation **1**, 1318–1328 (1950)
Harris, A.S., Bisteni, A.: Effects of sympathetic blockade drugs on ventricular tachycardia resulting from myocardial infarction. Amer. J. Physiol. **181**, 559–566 (1955)
Harris, A.S., Estandia, A., Tillotson, R.F.: Ventricular ectopic rhythms and ventricular fibrillation following cardiac sympathectomy and coronary occlusion. Amer. J. Physiol. **165**, 505–512 (1951)
Harris, A.S., Bisteni, A., Russell, R.A., Brigham, J.C., Firestone, J.E.: Excitatory factors in ventricular tachycardia resulting from myocardial ischaemia. Potassium a major excitant. Science **119**, 200–203 (1954)
Harris, P., Bishop, J.M., Segel, N.: The effects of dihydroergotamine tartrate on the pulmonary and systemic circulations in man. Clin. Sci. molec. Med. **25**, 443–447 (1963)
Hartman, M.M.: Parenteral use of dihydroergotamine in migraine. Ann. Allergy **3**, 440–442 (1945)
Harvey, S.C., Nickerson, M.: Adrenergic inhibitory function in the rabbit: epinephrine reversal and isopropylnorepinephrine vasodepression. J. Pharmacol. exp. Ther. **108**, 281–291 (1953)
Harvey, S.C., Wang, C.Y., Nickerson, M.: Blockade of epinephrine-induced hyperglycemia. J. Pharmacol. exp. Ther. **104**, 363–376 (1952)
Harvey, S.C., Copen, E.G., Eskelson, D.W., Graff, S.R., Poulsen, L.D., Rasmussen, D.L.: Autonomic pharmacology of the chicken with particular reference to adrenergic blockade. J. Pharmacol. exp. Ther. **112**, 8–22 (1954)
Hazard, R., Beauvallet, M., Giudicelli, R., Mouillé, P., Renier-Cornec, A.: Modifications apportées par divers adrénalinotoniques et adrénalinoverseurs aux effect tensionnels de l'isoprénaline (Aleudrine®) chez le chat. Arch. int. Pharmacodyn **143**, 331–336 (1963)
Heck, J.: Dihydroergotamin bei orthostatischer Dysregulation. Med. Klin. **66**, 601–604 (1971)
Heimdal, À., Nordenfelt, O.: The effect of Hydergine on the electrocardiogram. Cardiologia (Basel) **23**, 361–372 (1953)
Heise, A.: Hypotensive action by central α-adrenergic and dopaminergic receptor stimulation. In: New antihypertensive drugs. Scriabine, A., Sweet, C.S. (eds.), New York: Spectrum Publications, Inc. 1976
Helke, C.J., Souza, J.D., Hamilton, B.L., Morgenroth, V.H., Gillis, R.A.: Evidence for a role of central serotonergic neurones in digitalis-induced cardiac arrhythmias. Nature (Lond.) **263**, 246–248 (1976)
Herwick, R.P., Linegar, C.R., Koppanyi, T.: The effect of anaesthesia on the vasomotor reversal. J. Pharmacol. exp. Ther. **65**, 185–190 (1939)
Heyck, H.: Neue Beiträge zur Klinik und Pathogenese der Migräne, pp. 28–37, Stuttgart: Thieme 1956

Heyck, H.: Serotoninantagonisten in der Behandlung der Migräne und der Erythroprosopalgie Bings oder des Horton-Syndroms. Schweiz. med. Wschr. **90**, 203–209 (1960)
Heyck, H.: Pathogenesis of migraine. Res. Clin. Stud. Headache **2**, 1–28, Basel: Karger 1969
Heymans, C., Bouckaert, J.J.: Au sujet de l'action vasomotrice et vasculaire de l'ergotamine. Arch. int. Pharmacodyn **46,** 129–136 (1933)
Heymans, C., Heuvel-Heymans, G. van den: Action of drugs on arterial wall of carotid sinus and blood pressure. Arch. int. Pharmacodyn. **83**, 520–528 (1950)
Heymans, C., Neil, E.: Reflexogenic areas of the cardiovascular system. London: J. and A. Churchill Ltd. 1958
Heymans, C., Regniers, P.: Sur l'action vasculaire et sympathique de l'ergotamine et de l'ergotinine. Arch. int. Pharmacodyn. **33**, 236–249 (1927)
Heymans, C., Regniers, P.: Influence de l'ergotamine sur les réflexes cardio-vasculaires du sinus carotidien. Arch. int. Pharmacodyn. **36**, 116–121 (1929)
Heymans, C., Regniers, P., Bouckaert, J.J.: Ergotamine et réflexes vasomoteurs. La localisation de l'action de l'ergotamine sur les réflexes vasomoteurs du sinus carotidien. Arch. int. Pharmacodyn. **39**, 213–224 (1930)
Heymans, C., Bouckaert, J.J., Dautrebande, L.: Sinus carotidien et refléxes respiratoirs. III Sensibilité des sinus carotidiens aux substances chimiques. Action stimulant respiratoire réflexe du sulfure de sodium, du cyanure de potassium de la nicotine et de la lobéline. Arch. int. Pharmacodyn. **40**, 54–91 (1931)
Heymans, C., Bouckaert, J.J., Moraes, A.: Inversion par l'ergotamine de l'action vasoconstrictice des 'vasotonines' du sang défibriné. Arch. int. Pharmacodyn. **43**, 468–479 (1932a)
Heymans, C., Bouckaert, J.J., Euler, U.S. v., Dautrebande, L.: Sinus carotidiens et réflexes vasomoteurs. Arch. int. Pharmacodyn. **43**, 86–110 (1932b)
Hökfelt, T., Fuxe, K.: On the morphology and the neuroendocrine role of the hypothalamic catecholamine neurons. In: Brain Endocrine Interaction. Knigge, K.M., Scott, D.E., Weindl, A. (eds.), pp. 181–223, Basel: S. Karger 1972
Hör, G., Buttermann, G., Theisinger, W., Pabst, H.W.: Prevention of postoperative thromboembolism by various treatments. Controlled clinical trial in 632 patients using ^{125}I-fibrinogen-uptake-test and lung-perfusion-scans in patients with deep venous thrombosis. Europ. J. nucl. Med. **1**, 197–203 (1976)
Hofmann, A.: Ergot—a rich source of pharmacologically active substances. In: Plants in the development of modern medicine. Swain, T. (ed.), pp. 235–260, Cambridge, Mass.: Harvard University Press 1972
Horton, B.T., Peters, G.A., Blumenthal, L.S.: A new product in the treatment of migraine: a preliminary report. Proc. Mayo Clin. **20**, 241–248 (1945)
Immerwahr, P.: Über die Wirkung des Ergotamin auf Puls, Blutdruck und Blutzucker und ihre Beeinflussung durch Atropin. Med. Klin. **23**, 1–3 (1927)
Ingvar, D.H.: Discussion of Professor Marshall's paper: The regulation of cerebral blood flow; its relationship to migraine. Arch. Neurobiol. **37**, (Extranr.), 21–25 (1974)
Ingvar, D.H.: Pain in the brain and migraine. Hemicrania **7**, 2–6 (1976)
Ingvar, D.H., Söderberg, U.: The effect of LSD-25 upon the cerebral blood flow and EEG in cats. Experientia (Basel) **12**, 427–429 (1956)
Innes, I.R.: Identification of the smooth muscle excitatory receptors for ergot alkaloids. Brit. J. Pharmacol. **19**, 120–128 (1962)
Isbell, H.: Comparison of the reactions induced by psilocybin and LSD-25 in man. Psychopharmacologia **1**, 29–38 (1959)
Johnson, A.M., Loew, D.M., Vigouret, J.M.: Central dopaminergic stimulant properties of bromocriptine in comparison to apomorphine, d-amphetamine and L-DOPA. Brit. J. Pharmacol. **56**, 59–68 (1976)
Kangasniemi, P., Sonninen, V., Rinne, U.K.: Excretion of free and conjugated 5-HIAA and VMA in urine and concentration of 5-HIAA and HVA in CSF during migraine attacks and free intervals. Headache **12**, 62–65 (1972)
Kappert, A.: Untersuchungen über die Wirkungen neuer dihydrierter Mutterkornalkaloide bei peripheren Durchblutungsstörungen und Hypertonie. Helv. med. Acta, Suppl. **22**, 27–64 (1949a)
Kappert, A.: Untersuchungen über die Wirkungen neuer dihydrierter Mutterkornalkaloide

bei peripheren Durchblutungsstörungen und Hypertonie. Helv. med. Acta, Suppl. **22**, 95–126 (1949b)
Kappert, A., Hadorn, W.: Experimental and therapeutic investigations with certain new hydrogenated ergot alkaloids in peripheral vascular disorders. Angiology **1**, 520–529 (1950)
Kappert, A., Sutton, G.C., Reale, A., Skoglund, K.-H.: Untersuchungen über die Wirkung von Hydergin (CCK) auf die durch Noradrenalin ausgelöste Hypertension. Cardiologia (Basel) **16**, 129–144 (1950)
Karlsberg, P., Elliott, H.W., Adams, J.E.: Effect of various pharmacologic agents on cerebral arteries. Neurology (Minneap.) **13**, 772–778 (1963)
Karp, D., Rinzler, S.H., Travell, J.: Effects of ergometrine (ergonovine) on the isolated atherosclerotic heart of the cholesterol-fed rabbit. Brit. J. Pharmacol. **15**, 333–344 (1960)
Karr, N.W.: Circulatory and adrenolytic actions of DHE and DHO. Fed. Proc. **7**, 232 (1948)
Katz, L.N., Lindner, E.: The reaction of the coronary vessels to drugs and other substances. J. Amer. med. Ass. **113**, 2116–2119 (1939)
Kaye, S.B., Shaw, K.M., Ross, E.J.: Bromocriptine and hypertension. Lancet **I**, 1176–1177 (1976)
Kimball, R.W., Friedman, A.P., Vallejo, E.: Effect of serotonin in migraine patients. Neurology (Minneap.) **10**, 107–111 (1960)
Kirpekar, S.M., Puig, N.: Effect of flow-stop on noradrenaline release from normal spleens and spleens treated with cocaine, phentolamine or phenoxybenzamine. Brit. J. Pharmacol. **43**, 359–369 (1971)
Klingenberg, I.: Measurement of uterine blood flow in non-pregnant women by electromagnetic flowmeter. Acta obstet. gynec. scand. **52**, 317–321 (1973)
Knapp, F.M., Hyman, C., Bercel, N.A.: A method for the estimation of regional cerebral blood flow. Yale J. Biol. Med. **28**, 363–371 (1955)
Kofler, E.: Ueber die Mikrozirkulation an der Portio vaginalis uteri. Wien. klin. Wschr. **84**, Suppl. 3, 3–16 (1972)
Kohn, R.: Ueber den Mechanismus der Blutdruckregulation im indifferenten Bade. Z. ges. exp. Med. **85**, 483–494 (1932)
Konzett, H., Rothlin, E.: Investigations on the hypotensive effect of the hydrogenated ergot alkaloids. Brit. J. Pharmacol. **8**, 201–207 (1953)
Koopmans, S.: The function of the blood vessels in the brain. II. The effects of some narcotics, hormones and drugs. Arch. néerl. Physiol. **24**, 250–266 (1939)
Král, U.A.: Neurologische Erfahrungen mit 'Dihydroergotamine'. Schweiz. Arch. Neurol. Psychiat. **62**, 128–150 (1948)
Krause, D.: Die Wirkung von Ergotamin und Hydergin auf die zentrale Kreislaufregulation. Naunyn-Schmiedebergs Arch. exp. Path. Pharmak. **222**, 212–214 (1954)
Krause, D., Schmidtke-Ruhnau, D., Moursi Ali, H.: Zentrale Sympathikusdämpfung und adrenolytische Wirkung genuiner und hydrierter Mutterkornalkaloide. Dtsch. tierärztl. Wschr. **78**, 292–294 (1971)
Krstić, M.K., Djurković, D.: Hypertension mediated by the activation of the rat brain 5-hydroxytryptamine receptor sites. Experientia (Basel) **32**, 1187–1189 (1976)
Kühns, K.: Untersuchungen über die Wirkung eines neuen Sympathicolyticums (Hydergin) und anderer vegetativer Pharmaka auf Elektrokardiogramm und Herzfrequenz des wachen Kaninchens. Helv. med. Acta **16**, 90–109 (1949)
Kühns, K.: Zur Behandlung ventrikulärer Tachykardien. Z. Kreisl.-Forsch. **40**, 415–422 (1951)
Kunos, G.: Thyroid hormone-dependent interconversion of myocardial α- and β-adrenoceptors in the rat. Brit. J. Pharmacol. **59**, 177–189 (1977)
Kunos, G., Nickerson, M.: Temperature-induced interconversion of α- and β-adrenoceptors in the frog heart. J. Physiol. (Lond.) **256**, 23–40 (1976)
Kunos, G., Szentiványi, M.: Evidence favouring the existence of a single adrenergic receptor. Nature (Lond.) **217**, 1077–1078 (1968)
Kunos, G., Yong, M.S., Nickerson, M.: Transformation of adrenergic receptors in the myocardium. Nature New Biol. **241**, 119–120 (1973)
Laddu, A.R., Somani, P.: Direct and beta-adrenoceptor blocking effects of 4-(2-hydroxy-3-isopropylaminopropoxy)-indol (LB46) on myocardial hemodynamics. Arch. int. Pharmacodyn. **196**, 5–15 (1972)

Lake, C.L.: Vasopressor effects of intravenous and intramuscular injections of methergine in the postpartum patient. Obstet. and Gynec. **4**, 308–310 (1954)
Lance, J.W.: Mechanism and management of headache, 2nd ed., pp. 113–133. London: Butterworths 1973
Lance, J.W., Anthony, M.: Thermographic studies in vascular headache. Med. J. Aust. **1**, 240–243 (1971)
Landesman, R., Mendelsohn, B.: The uterine omentum of the rat and its response to vasoconstrictor drugs. Amer. J. Obstet. Gynec. **72**, 84–92 (1956)
Landgren, S., Neil, E.: The contribution of carotid chemoreceptor mechanisms to the rise of blood pressure caused by carotid occlusion. Acta physiol. scand. **23**, 152–157 (1951)
Lands, A.M., Luduena, F.P., Grant, J.I., Ananenko, E., Tainter, M.L.: Reversal of the depressor action of N-isopropylarterenol (isuprel) by ergotamine and ergotoxine. J. Pharmacol. exp. Ther. **100**, 234–297 (1950)
Lang, E., Jansen, W., Pfaff, W.: Orthostatische Hypotonie bei älteren Menschen. Häufigkeit und Therapie. Med. Klin. **70**, 1976–1981 (1975)
Lange, L., Echt, M.: Vergleichende Untersuchungen über venentonisierende Pharmaka. Fortschr. Med. **90**, 1161–1164 (1972)
Langer, S.Z.: Presynaptic regulation of norepinephrine release elicited by nerve stimulation. Life Sci. **13**, xcvii-xcix (1973)
Langer, S.Z.: Presynaptic regulation of catecholamine release. Biochem. Pharmacol. **23**, 1793–1800 (1974)
Langer, S.Z., Adler, E., Enero, M.A., Stefano, F.J.E.: The role of the alpha receptor in regulating noradrenaline overflow by nerve stimulation. Proc. XXVth. Int. Congr. Physiol. Sci., München, p. 335 (1971)
Langer, S.Z., Enero, M.A., Adler-Graschinsky, E., Stefano, F.J.E.: The role of the alpha receptor in the regulation of transmitter overflow elicited by stimulation. V Int. Congr. Pharmacol. San Fransisco, USA, 23/28th July, 1972, Abstr. No. 802
Lasch, F.: Über die Beeinflussung der Nierenclearance durch Hyderginbehandlung. Cardiologia (Basel) **24**, 155–166 (1954)
Lassen, N.A., Høedt-Rasmussen, K., Sørensen, S.C., Skinhøj, E., Cronquist, S., Bodforss, B., Eng, E., Ingvar, D.H.: Regional cerebral blood flow in man determined by krypton^{85}. Neurology (Minneap.) **13**, 719–727 (1963)
Laubie, M., Delbarre, B., Bogaievsky, D., Bogaievsky, Y., Tsoucaris-Kupfer, E., Senon, D., Schmitt, H., Schmitt, H.: Pharmacological evidence for a central α-sympathomimetic mechanism controlling blood pressure and heart rate. Circulat. Res. **38**, Suppl. II, 35–41 (1976)
Leist, K.H., Grauwiler, J.: Ergometrine and uteroplacental blood supply in pregnant rats. Teratology **10**, 316 (1974)
Lennox, W.G.: Ergonovine versus ergotamine as a terminator of migraine headaches. Amer. J. med. Sci. **195**, 458–468 (1938)
Lennox, W.G., Gibbs, E.L., Gibbs, F.A.: Effect of ergotamine tartrate on the cerebral circulation of man. J. Pharmacol. exp. Ther. **53**, 113–119 (1935)
Levy, B., Ahlquist, R.P.: An analysis of adrenergic blocking activity. J. Pharmacol. exp. Ther. **133**, 202–210 (1961)
Ley, J., De La Fontaine-Verwey, B.-C.: A propos de certaines réactions des vaisseaux cerebraux du lapin dans leurs rapports avec les conditions humorales et avec leur innervation sympathique. C.R. Soc. Biol. (Paris) **101**, 478–480 (1929)
Liljestrand, A.: Interaction of ergotamine and carbon dioxide on blood pressure and respiration. Acta physiol. scand. **15**, 198–206 (1948)
Lindgren, P., Uvnäs, B.: Postulated vasodilator centre in the medulla oblongata. Amer. J. Physiol. **176**, 68–76 (1954)
Lindgren, P., Uvnäs, B.: Vasoconstrictor inhibition and vasodilator activation—two functionally separate vasodilator mechanisms in the skeletal muscles. Acta physiol. scand. **33**, 108–119 (1955)
Lipton, B., Gittler, R.D., Slotnik, H.O., Rockaway, F.: Cardiovascular effects of oxytocin injection (USP) synthetic, prepared oxytocin and the ergot alkaloids. N.Y. St. J. Med. **60**, 4006–4015 (1960)

Lockett, M.F., Wadley, R.: Renal actions of dihydroergocristine and of phentolamine in anaesthetised cats. Brit. J. Pharmacol. **37**, 595–608 (1969)
Loewi, O., Navratil, E.: Ueber den Mechanismus der Vaguswirkung von Physostigmin und Ergotamin. Pflügers Arch. ges. Physiol. **214**, 689–696 (1926)
Logaras, G.: Further studies of the pulmonary arterial blood pressure. Acta physiol. scand. **14**, 120–135 (1947)
Lohmann, F.W., Gotzen, R., Ungewiss, U.: Der Einfluss von Dihydroergotamin (Dihydergot) auf die Kreislaufveränderungen und die Funktion des sympathischen Nervensystems in Orthostase. Med. Welt **26**, 1416–1420 (1975)
Long, J.P., Heintz, S., Cannon, J.G., Kim, J.: Inhibition of the sympathetic nervous system by 5,6-dihydroxy-2-dimethylamino-tetralin (M-7), apomorphine and dopamine. J. Pharmacol. exp. Ther. **192**, 336–342 (1975)
Longo, T., Santa, A.: The effects of catecholamines on renal artery flow before and after alpha-receptor blockade. Comparative experimental research on the conscious and anaesthetised dog. J. cardiovasc. Surg. **9**, 195–200 (1968)
Lottenbach, K.: Sympathikolyse und Erregbarkeit der Karotissinusreflexe am Menschen. Z. Kreisl.-Forsch. **42**, 98–103 (1953)
Lübke, K.O.: Der Einfluß von Dihydroergotamin auf Herzfrequenz, Blutdruck und Hautdurchblutung während orthostatischer Belastung. Herz-Kreislauf **4**, 52–55 (1972)
Lubsen, N.: Experimental studies on the cerebral circulation of the unanaesthetised rabbit. III. The action of ergotamine tartrate and of some vasodilator drugs. Arch. néerl. Physiol. **25**, 361–365 (1940)
Lugaresi, E., Rebucci, G.G.: Prime esperienze sull'azione di alcuni farmaci alla luce de registrazioni reografiche contemperanee cerebrali e periferiche. G. Psichiat. Neuropat. **90**, 881–895 (1962)
Manning, G.W., Caudwell, G.C.: The effect of demerol, ergotamine and dihydroergotamine on mortality after coronary occlusion in dogs. Brit. Heart J. **9**, 85–95 (1947)
Manz, M., Felix, W.: Effects of dihydroergotamine (DHE) on the capacitance and resistance vessels of the cat hindleg (chloralose anaesthesia). Naunyn-Schmiedebergs Arch. exp. Path. Pharmak. **282** (Suppl.), R62 (1974)
Marques, M.G., Rato, J.A.: Quelques action des alcaloides hydrogénés de l'ergot de seigle sur l'appareil cardio-vasculaire. Cardiologia (Basel) **24**, 196–206 (1954)
Marsh, D.F., Liere, E.J. van: The effect of adrenergic blocking agents on the vasoconstriction produced by acute oxygen lack. J. Pharmacol. exp. Ther. **44**, 221–224 (1948)
Mathew, N.T., Hrastnik, F., Meyer, J.S.: Regional cerebral blood flow in the diagnosis of vascular headache. Headache **15**, 252–260 (1976)
Mazzella, H.: On the reactivity of the wall of the carotid sinus. Arch. int. Pharmacodyn. **116**, 37–44 (1958)
McCall, M.L., Taylor, H.W., Read, A.W.: The action of hydergine on the circulation and metabolism of the brain in toxemia of pregnancy. Amer. J. med. Sci. **226**, 537–540 (1953)
McCulloch, M.W., Rand, M.J., Story, D.F.: Inhibition of ^{3}H-noradrenaline release from sympathetic nerves of guinea-pig atria by a presynaptic α-adrenoceptor mechanism. Brit. J. Pharmacol. **46**, 523P-524P (1972)
McCulloch, M.W., Rand, M.J., Story, D.F.: Evidence for a dopaminergic mechanism for modulation of adrenergic transmission in the rabbit ear artery. Brit. J. Pharmacol. **49**, 141 P (1973)
McDowell, R.J.S.: Capacity effects from the carotid sinus. J. Physiol. (Lond.) **84**, 24P (1935)
McEachern, G.G., Manning, G.W., Hall, G.E.: Sudden occlusion of coronary arteries following removal of cardiosensory pathways. Arch. int. Med. **65**, 661–670 (1940)
Meirsman-Roobroeck, G.C.: The protective action of parpanit, diparcol and some other drugs against chloroform-adrenaline ventricular fibrillation. Arch. int. Pharmacodyn. **83**, 353–385 (1950)
Mellander, S.: Comparative studies on the adrenergic neuro-hormonal control of resistance and capacitance blood vessels in the cat. Acta physiol. scand. **50**, suppl. 176, 1–86 (1960)
Mellander, S.: Comparative effects of acetylcholine, butyl-norsynephrine (vasculat), noradrenaline and ethyl-adrianol (Effortil) on resistance, capacitance and pre-capillary sphincter vessels and capillary filtration in cat skeletal muscle. Angiology **3**, 77–99 (1966)

Mellander, S., Johansson, B.: Control of resistance, exchange and capacitance functions in the peripheral circulation. Pharmacol. Rev. **20**, 117–196 (1968)

Mellander, S., Nordenfelt, I.: Comparative effects of dihydroergotamine and noradrenaline on resistance, exchange and capacitance functions in the peripheral circulation. Clin. Sci. **39**, 183–201 (1970)

Mendéz, C., Aceves, J., Mendéz, R.: Inhibition of adrenergic cardiac acceleration by cardiac glycosides. J. Pharmacol. exp. Ther. **131**, 191–198 (1961)

Meriel, P., Bollinelli, R., Calazel, P., Cassagneau, J.: Epreuve à l'hydergine et pressions pulmonaires. Arch. Mal. Coeur **46**, 329–340 (1953)

Meyer, J.S., Yoshida, K., Sakamoto, K.: Autonomic control of cerebral blood flow measured by electromagnetic flowmeters. Neurology (Minneap.) **17**, 638–648 (1967)

Micheli, P. de, Glässer, A.H.: The effects of catecholamines and adrenoceptor blocking drugs on the canine peripheral lymph flow. Brit. J. Pharmacol. **53**, 499–504 (1975)

Moe, G.D., Malton, S.D., Rennick, B.R., Freyburger, W.A.: The role of arterial pressure in the induction of idioventricular rhythms under cyclopropane anesthesia. J. Pharmacol. exp. Ther. **94**, 319–327 (1948)

Moore, R.M., Cannon, W.B.: The heart rate of unanaesthetised normal, vagotomised and sympathectomised cats as affected by atropine and ergotoxine. Amer. J. Physiol. **94**, 201–208 (1930)

Moran, N.C., Perkins, M.E.: An evaluation of adrenergic blockade of the mammalian heart. J. Pharmacol. exp. Ther. **133**, 192–201 (1961)

Morpugo, C., Faini, D., Falcone, A.: The effects of phentolamine, dihydroergocristine and isoxsuprine on the blood pressure and heart rate in normotensive, hypotensive and hypertensive rats. Naunyn-Schmiedebergs Arch. exp. Path. Pharmak. **290**, 335–346 (1975)

Mouillé, P.: Interactions entre divers inhibiteurs α et β adrenergiques et l'ergotamine au cours de l'inversion des effets trusionnels de l'isoprenaline chez le chien. C.R. Soc. Biol. (Paris) **164**, 1003–1006 (1970)

Moyer, J.H., Handley, C.A., Seibert, R.A.: Effect of adrenergic blockade on renal hemodynamics and excretion of water and electrolytes. Amer. J. Physiol. **180**, 146–150 (1955)

Mühe, E., Burhardt, K.-H., Kolb, W., Strobel, G.: Eine neue Methode zur Prophylaxie postoperativer Venenthrombosen. Klinikarzt **4**, 88–92 (1975)

Müller-Schweinitzer, E.: Studies on the peripheral mode of action of dihydroergotamine in human and canine veins. Europ. J. Pharmacol. **27**, 231–237 (1974)

Müller-Schweinitzer, E.: Responsiveness of isolated canine cerebral and peripheral arteries to ergotamine. Naunyn-Schmiedebergs Arch. exp. Path. Pharmak. **292**, 113–118 (1976)

Müller-Schweinitzer, E., Brundell, J.: Modification of canine vascular smooth muscle responses to dihydroergotamine by endogenous prostaglandin synthesis. Europ. J. Pharmacol. **34**, 194–206 (1975a)

Müller-Schweinitzer, E., Brundell, J.: Enhanced prostaglandin synthesis contributes to the venoconstrictor activity of ergotamine. Blood Vessels **12**, 193–205 (1975b)

Müller-Schweinitzer, E., Stürmer, E.: Investigations on the mode of action of ergotamine in the isolated femoral vein of the dog. Brit. J. Pharmacol. **51**, 441–446 (1974)

Murphree, H.B., De Maar, E.W.J., Williams, H.L., Bryan, L.L.: Effects of lysergic acid derivatives on man; antagonism between d-lysergic acid diethylamide and its 2-brom congener. J. Pharmacol. exp. Ther. **122**, 55A (1958)

Murray, R., Beck, L., Rondell, P.A., Bohr, D.F.: A study of the central action of ganglionic blocking agents. J. Pharmacol. exp. Ther. **127**, 157–163 (1959)

Navratil, E.: Ueber humorale Uebertragbarkeit der Herznervenwirkung. Pflügers Arch. ges. Physiol. **217**, 610–617 (1927)

Navratil, E., Wieninger, E.: Beitrag zur adrenolytischen Wirkung des Dihydroergotamins am Kaltblüterherz. Klin. Med. **3**, 990–994 (1948)

Nickerson, M.: The pharmacology of adrenergic blockade. Pharmacol. Rev. **1**, 27–101 (1949)

Nickerson, M., Chan, G.C.-M.: Blockade of responses of isolated myocardium to epinephrine. J. Pharmacol. exp. Ther. **133**, 186–191 (1961)

Nickerson, M., Nomaguchi, G.M.: Mechanism of dibenamine protection against cyclopropane-epinephrine cardiac arrhythmias. J. Pharmacol. exp. Ther. **95**, 1–11 (1949)

Nickerson, M., Nomaguchi, G.M.: Blockade of epinephrine-induced cardioacceleration in the frog. Amer. J. Physiol. **163**, 484–504 (1950)
Nickerson, M., Henry, J.W., Nomaguchi, G.M.: Blockade of responses to epinephrine and norepinephrine by dibenamine congeners. J. Pharmacol. exp. Ther. **107**, 300–309 (1953)
Niesel, P., Weigelin, E., Mohr, H.: Untersuchungen über die Wirkung von Hydergin und DHE 45 am intrakraniellen Kreislauf beim "Cold-Pressor-Test". Klin. Wschr. **31**, 948 (1953)
Nilsson, A., Hökfelt, B.: Effect of bromocriptine on blood pressure, plasma and urinary catecholamines and plasma renin activity (PRA) in patients with acromegaly. Acta endocr. (Kbh.) Suppl. **212**, 95 (1977)
Nimmerfall, F., Rosenthaler, J.: Ergot alkaloids: Hepatic distribution and estimation of absorption by measurement of total radioactivity in bile and urine. J. Pharmacokinet. Biopharm. **4**, 57–66 (1976)
Nishi, K.: The action of 5-hydroxytryptamine on chemoreceptor discharges of the cat's carotid body. Brit. J. Pharmacol. **55**, 27–40 (1975)
Nordenfelt, I., Mellander, S.: Central haemodynamic effects of dihydroergotamine in patients with orthostatic hypotension. Acta med. scand. **191**, 115–120 (1972)
Norris, J.W., Hachinski, V.C., Cooper, P.W.: Changes in cerebral blood flow during a migraine attack. Brit. med. J. **3**, 676–677 (1975)
Nueten, J.M. van: Comparative bioassay of vasoactive drugs using isolated perfused rabbit arteries. Europ. J. Pharmacol. **6**, 286–293 (1969)
O'Brien, G.S., Murphy, Q.R., Meek, W.J.: The effect of sympathomimetic amines on arterial plasma potassium and cardiac rhythm in anaesthetised dogs. J. Pharmacol. exp. Ther. **109**, 453–460 (1953)
Olesen, J.: Prostaglandin action on cerebral vessels. Headache 1976. Meeting of Ital. and Scand. Migraine Socs., Florence, June 2–3, 1976, p. 27
Olesen, J., Paulson, O.B., Lassen, N.A.: Regional cerebral blood flow in man determined by the initial slope of the clearance of intra-arterially injected ^{133}Xe. Stroke **2**, 519–539 (1971)
Olivecrona, H.: Notes on the surgical treatment of migraine. Acta med. scand. Suppl. **196**, 229–238 (1947)
Orth, O.S.: The use of dihydroergotamine (DHE 45) and dihydroergocornine (DHO 180) to prevent cardiac irregularities during cycloproprane anaesthesia. Arch. int. Pharmacodyn. **78**, 163–173 (1949)
Orth, S., Ritchie, G.: A pharmacological evaluation of dihydroergotamine methanesulphonate (DHE-45). J. Pharmacol. exp. Ther. **90**, 166–173 (1947)
Osswald, W., Guimarães, S., Garrett, J.: Influence of propranolol and ICI 50,172 on the cardiovascular actions of catecholamines as modified by ergotamine. J. Pharmacol. exp. Ther. **174**, 315–322 (1970)
Ostfeld, A.M.: Some aspects of cardiovascular regulation in man. Angiology **10**, 34–42 (1959)
Ostfeld, A.M.: Migraine headache. Its physiology and biochemistry. J. Amer. med. Ass. **174**, 1188–1190 (1960)
Ostfeld, A.M., Wolff, H.G.: Studies on headache observations on the behaviour of the conjunctival vessels in vascular headache. Trans. Amer. neurol. Ass. **80**, 216–219 (1955)
Ostfeld, A.M., Chapman, L.F., Goodell, H., Wolff, H.G.: Studies in headache: Summary of evidence concerning a noxious agent active locally during migraine headache. Psychosom. Med. **19**, 199–208 (1957)
Otto, H.L.: Upon the action of ergotoxin in the mammalian heart. J. Pharmacol. exp. Ther. **33**, 285–293 (1928)
Owen, D.A.A., Stürmer, E.: Effect of dihydroergotamine (DHE) on the capacitance, resistance and precapillary sphincter vessels of denervated cat skeletal muscle. Brit. J. Pharmacol. **42**, 655P–656P (1971)
Owen, D.A.A., Stürmer, E.: The effects of ergotamine and dihydroergotamine on skin and skeletal muscle vasculature. Experientia (Basel) **28**, 743 (1972a)
Owen, D.A.A., Stürmer, E.: The effects of Hydergine on acutely denervated cat skeletal muscle vasculature. Naunyn-Schmiedeberg's Arch. exp. Path. Pharmak. **272**, 395–401 (1972b)

Oyen, I.H.: Mechanism of early and chronic experimental renal hypertension as tested by CCK-179. Amer. J. Physiol. **186**, 161–166 (1956)
Page, I.H., McCubbin, J.W.: Modification of vascular response to serotonin by drugs. Amer. J. Physiol. **174**, 436–444 (1953)
Papp, J.G., Szekeres, L.: The arrhythmogenic action of sympathomimetic amines. Europ. J. Pharmacol. **3**, 4–14 (1968)
Parade, D., Schwarz, W., Kroenig, B., Brocke, B., Jahnecke, J.: Durch Antihypertensiva hervorgerufener orthostatischer Blutdruckabfall und seine medikamentöse Beeinflussbarkeit. Med. Welt **25**, 179–182 (1974)
Pattani, F.: Die Kreislaufwirkung der Dihydroderivate der genuinen Mutterkornalkaloide am kreislaufgesunden Menschen. Schwarzenburg: Gerber-Buchdruck 1949 (Diss.)
Peiss, C.N.: Concepts of cardiovascular regulation: past, present and future. In: Nervous control of the heart. Randall, W.C. (ed.), pp. 154–197. Baltimore: Williams and Wilkins Co. 1965
Pelofsky, S., Jacobson, E.D., Fischer, R.G.: Effects of prostaglandin E_1 on experimental cerebral vasospasm. J. Neurosurg. **36**, 634–639 (1972)
Penfield, W.: Operative treatment of migraine and observations on the mechanism of vascular pain. Trans. Amer. Acad. Ophthal. Otolaryng. **37**, 50–64 (1932)
Pichler, E., Ostfeld, A.M., Goodell, H., Wolff, H.G.: Central versus peripheral action of ergotamine tartrate and its relevance to the therapy of migraine headache. Arch. Neurol. Psychiat. (Chic.) **76**, 571–577 (1956)
Pickering, G.W.: Observations on the mechanism of headache produced by histamine. Clin. Sci. **1**, 77–101 (1933)
Pool, J.L., Nason, G.J.: Comparative effects of ergotamine tartrate on the arteries of the pia, dura and skin of cats. Arch. Neurol. Psychiat. (Chic.) **33**, 276–282 (1935)
Pool, J.L., Storch, T.J.C., Lennox, W.G.: Effect of ergotamine tartrate on pressure of cerebrospinal fluid and blood during migraine headache. Arch. int. Med. **57**, 32–45 (1936)
Prochnik, G., Maison, G.L., Stutzman, J.W.: Carotid-occlusion-pressor reflex: influence of existing mean arterial pressure, of anaesthetics and of ganglionic- and adrenergic-blocking drugs. Amer. J. Physiol. **162**, 553–559 (1950)
Proosdij-Hartzema, E.G. van, De Jongh, D.K.: Investigations into experimental hypotension. III. Dosage and effect of drugs in experimental renal hypertension in the rat. Acta physiol. pharmacol. néerl. **4**, 160–174 (1955)
Puglionisi, A., Eppinger, S.: L'azione dell'Hydergina sulla circolazione degli arti normali e nelle arteriopatie obliteranti periferiche croniche. Minerva chir. **8**, 61 (1953)
Rand, M.J., Story, D.F., McCulloch, M.W.: Inhibitory feedback modulation of adrenergic transmission. Clin. exp. Pharmacol. physiol., Suppl. **2**, 21–26 (1975)
Ray, B.S., Wolff, H.G.: Experimental studies on headache. Painsensitive structures of the head and their significance in headache. Arch. Surg. **41**, 813–856 (1940)
Reckel, K.: Zur Behandlung pharmakogen bedingter orthostatischer Kreislaufdysregulationen. Ther. d. Gegenw. **109**, 694–704 (1970)
Regli, F., Yamaguchi, T., Waltz, A.G.: Effects of vasodilating drugs on blood flow and the microvasculature of ischaemic and nonischaemic cerebral cortex. Arch. Neurol. (Chic.) **24**, 467–474 (1971)
Rettori, O., Haley, T.J.: Peripheral versus central sites of action of ergotamine on blood flow. Arch. int. Pharmacodyn. **167**, 473–478 (1967)
Reubi, F.: L'action de quelques dérivés de l'ergot de seigle sur la circulation rénale. Experientia (Basel) **5**, 296–297 (1949)
Reubi, F.: Le flux sanguin rénal. Helv. med. Acta **17**, Suppl. XXVI, Fasc. 2 (1950)
Reubi, F.: L'Hydergine modifie-t-elle l'activité tubulaire rénale? Helv. med. Acta **19**, 1–8 (1952a)
Reubi, F.: Les fonctions rénales des hypertendus au cours d'un traitement prolongé par les dérivés dihydrogénés de l'ergot de seigle (Hydergine). Helv. med. Acta **19**, 29–41 (1952b)
Rieckert, H.: Primäre Therapieziele bei der hypotonen Fehlregulation. Fortschr. Med. **89**, 175–176 (1971)
Rieckert, H., Pauschinger, P.: Die Beeinflussung des peripheren Venentonus durch Dihydergot®. Ärztl. Forsch. **21**, 99–101 (1967)

Riley, H.A.: Migraine. Bull. neurol. Inst. N.Y. **2**, 429–544 (1932)
Ripa, R., Frangipane, G., Gilli, P., Tura, S.: Azione della diidroergotamina sulla pressione arteriosa di ratta con ipertensione renale cronica. Boll. Soc. ital. Biol. sper. **43**, 883–887 (1967)
Rosenblueth, A., Cannon, B.: Some circulatory phenomena disclosed by ergotoxine. Amer. J. Physiol. **105**, 373–382 (1933)
Rosmanitz, I.J., Brehm, H.: Klinisch-experimentelle Studie zur Kreislaufwirkung des Dihydergot beim Orthostasesyndrom. Med. Welt **2**, 2618–2625 (1964)
Rothlin, E.: Recherche experimentales sur l'ergotamine, alcaloïde spécifique de l'ergot de seigle. Arch. int. Pharmacodyn. **27**, 459–479 (1923)
Rothlin, E.: Ueber die pharmakologische und therapeutische Wirkung des Ergotamins auf den Sympathikus. Klin. Wschr. **4**, 1437–1443 (1925)
Rothlin, E.: Zur Pharmakologie der hydrierten natürlichen Mutterkornalkaloide Helv. physiol. pharmacol. Acta **2**, C48–C49 (1944)
Rothlin, E.: Ueber die adrenergischen Funktionen am Herz und an Gefässen. Bull. schweiz. Akad. med. Wiss. **1**, 194–207 (1945)
Rothlin, E.: The pharmacology of the natural and dihydrogenated alkaloids of ergot. Bull. schweiz. Akad. med. Wiss. **2**, 249–273 (1946)
Rothlin, E.: Zur Analyse der Blutdruckwirkung der natürlichen und dihydrierten Mutterkornalkaloide. Experientia (Basel) **5**, 78–79 (1949)
Rothlin, E.: Pharmacology of lysergic acid diethylamide and some of its related compounds. J. Pharm. Pharmacol. **9**, 569–587 (1957)
Rothlin, E., Cerletti, A.: Untersuchungen über die Kreislaufwirkung des Ergotamins. Helv. physiol. pharmacol. Acta **7**, 333–370 (1949a)
Rothlin, E., Cerletti, A.: Pharmakologie des Hochdrucks. Verh. dtsch. Ges. Kreisl.-Forsch. **15**, 158–185 (1949b)
Rothlin, E., Cerletti, A.: Ueber die Schutzwirkung von Hydergin gegen heterotope Reizbildungsstörungen. Cardiologia **15**, 184–185 (1949c)
Rothlin, E., Cerletti, A.: Experimentelle Untersuchungen über die cardiale Wirkung hydrierter Mutterkornalkaloide. Z. ges. exp. Med. **122**, 335–345 (1953)
Rothlin, E., Cerletti, A., Emmeneger, H.: Experimental psychoneurogenic hypertension and its treatment with hydrogenated ergot alkaloids (Hydergine). Acta med. scand., Suppl. **312**, 27–35 (1956)
Rothman, S., Drury, D.R.: Role of autonomic nervous system in maintainance of cerebral and renal hypertension. Amer. J. Physiol. **188**, 371–374 (1957)
Rowbotham, G.F.: Long term results of injuries of head (medical, economical and sociological survey). J. ment. Sci. **95**, 336–354 (1949)
Sagar, S., Stamatakis, J.D., Higgins, A.F., Nairn, D., Maffei, F.H., Thomas, D.P., Kakkar, V.V.: Efficacy of low-dose heparin in prevention of extensive deep-vein thrombosis in patients undergoing total-hip replacement. Lancet **I**, 1151–1154 (1976)
Salmoiraghi, G.C., McCubbin, J.W., Page, I.H.: Effects of d-lysergic acid diethylamide and its brom derivative on cardiovascular responses to serotonin and on arterial pressure. J. Pharmacol. exp. Ther. **119**, 240–247 (1957)
Salzmann, R., Pacha, W., Taeschler, M., Weidmann, H.: The effect of ergotamine on humoral and neuronal actions in the nictitating membrane and the spleen of the cat. Naunyn-Schmiedebergs Arch. exp. Path. Pharmak. **261**, 360–378 (1968)
Sankar, D.V. Siva: LSD—a total study. Westbury, N.Y.: PJD Publications Ltd. 1975
Saxena, P.R.: The effects of antimigraine drugs on the vascular responses by 5-hydroxytryptamine and related biogenic substances on the external carotid bed of dogs; possible pharmacological implications to their antimigraine action. Headache **12**, 44–54 (1972)
Saxena, P.R.: Selective vasoconstriction in carotid vascular bed by methysergide: possible relevance to its antimigraine effect. Europ. J. Pharmacol. **27**, 99–105 (1974)
Saxena, P.R., Bhargava, K.P.: The importance of a central adrenergic mechanism in the cardiovascular responses to ouabain. Europ. J. Pharmacol. **31**, 332–346 (1975)
Saxena, P.R., Vlaam-Schluter, G.M. de: Role of some biogenic substances in migraine and relevant mechanisms in antimigraine action of ergotamine—studies in an experimental model for migraine. Headache **13**, 142–163 (1974)

Schade, F.: Methergine: A study of its vasomotor properties. Amer. J. Obstet. Gynec. **61**, 187–192 (1951)
Scheinberg, P.: Cerebral blood flow in vascular disease of the brain, with observations on the effect of stellate ganglion block. Amer. J. Med. **8**, 139–147 (1950)
Schleimer, R., Zitowitz, L., Wohl, A.: The antiarrhythmic activity of dihydroergotamine (DHE). Pharmacologist **13**, (2), 225 (1971)
Schlientz, W., Brunner, R., Rüegger, A., Berde, B., Stürmer, E., Hofmann, A.: β-Ergokryptin, ein neues Alkaloid der Ergotoxingruppe. Pharm. Acta Helv. **43**, 497–509 (1968)
Schmidt, C.F.: The intrinsic regulation of the circulation in the hypothalamus of the cat. Amer. J. Physiol. **110**, 137–152 (1934)
Schmitt, H.: Recherches sur le système nerveux sympathique. III Dissociation des effects des médiateurs chimiques de ceux de l'excitation des nerfs sympathiques. Arch. int. Pharmacodyn. **114**, 381–396 (1958)
Schmitt, H., Fenard, S.: Effets des alcaloïdes de l'ergot de seigle sur les vasomoteurs et leur inhibition par la clonidine. C.R. Soc. Biol. (Paris) **164**, 1006–1009 (1970)
Schmitt, H., Petillot, N.: Potentialisation des effets hypertenseurs de l'angiotensine par les alcaloides de l'ergot de seigle et par la vasopressine. C.R. Soc. Biol. (Paris) **163**, 2551–2553 (1969)
Schmitt, H., Schmitt, H.: Action de l'ergotamine, de la hydroergotamine et de l'hydergine chez le lapin réserpiné. C.R. Soc. Biol. (Paris) **153**, 748–749 (1959)
Schmitt, H., Schmitt, H.: Sur le méchanisme de l'action hypotensive de la dihydroergotamine. J. Physiol. (Paris) **52**, 517–523 (1960)
Schmitt, H., Schmitt, H.:: Modifications de l'excitabilité des centres vasomoteurs par des substances interférant périphériquement avec les effets du systeme sympathique. Arch. int. Pharmacodyn. **150**, 322–335 (1964)
Schmitt, H., Laubie, M., Fenard, S.: Effets hémodynamiques des alcaloides de l'ergot de seigle. J. Pharmacol. (Paris) **2**, 131–140 (1971)
Schneider, M., Schneider, D.: Untersuchungen über die Regulierung der Gehirndurchblutung. II Einwirkung verschiedener Pharmaka auf die Gehirndurchblutung. Naunyn-Schmiedebergs Arch. exp. Path. Pharmak. **175**, 640–664 (1934)
Schneider, M., Wiemers, K.: Ueber die Wirkung der hydrierten Mutterkornalkaloide auf die Gehirndurchblutung. Klin. Wschr. **29**, 580–581 (1951)
Scholtysik, G.: Inhibition of accelerator nerve stimulation in cats by dihydroergotoxine. 6th Int. Congr. Pharmacol. Helsinki, Finland, Abstr. 742 (1975)
Scholtysik, G.: Dopamine receptor mediated inhibition by bromocriptine of accelerator nerve stimulation effects in the pithed cat. Brit. J. Pharmacol. (1978) in press
Schön, H., Leist, K.H., Grauwiler, J.: Single day treatment of pregnant rats with ergotamine. Teratology **11**, 32A (1975)
Schönbaum, E., Vargaftig, B.B., Lefort, J., Lamar, J.C., Haseneck, T.: An unexpected effect of serotonin antagonists on the canine nasal circulation. Headache **15**, 180–187 (1975)
Share, N.N.: "Alpha" and "beta" adrenergic receptors in the medullary vasomotor centre of the cat. Arch. int. Pharmacodyn. **202**, 362–373 (1973)
Shaw, E., Woolley, D.W.: Some serotonin-like activities of lysergic acid diethylamide. Science **124**, 121–122 (1956)
Shen, T.C.R.: The protective action of piperido-methyl-3-benzodioxane (F-933), diethyl-amino-methyl-3-benzodioxane (F-883) and yohimbine upon the chloroform-adrenaline ventricular fibrillation. Arch. int. Pharmacodyn. **59**, 243–251 (1938)
Sherif, M.A.F., Effat, S., Razzak, M.A.: Comparative study of some imidazoline derivatives and dihydrogenated ergot alkaloids on the cardiovascular system. Arch. int. Pharmacodyn. **108**, 5–18 (1956)
Sicuteri, F.: L'acido vanilmandelico (VMA) il maggior metabolita urinario delle catecolamine. Sett. Med. **50**, 227 (1962)
Sicuteri, F.: Mast cells and their active substances. Their role in the pathogenesis of migraine. Headache **3**, 86–92 (1963)
Sicuteri, F., Ricci, M., Monfardini, R., Ficini, M.: Experimental headache with endogenous histamine. Acta allerg. (Kbh.) **11**, 188–192 (1957)

Sicuteri, F., Testi, A., Anselmi, B.: Biochemical investigations in headache: increase in hydroxyindoleacetic acid excretion during migraine attacks. Int. Arch. Allergy **19**, 55–58 (1961)
Sicuteri, F., Fanciullacci, M., Anselmi, B.: Bradykinin release and inactivation in man. Int. Arch. Allergy **22**, 77–84 (1963)
Sicuteri, F., Franchi, G., Fanciullacci, M.: Serotonin potentiation of methysergide, LSD-25 and ergotamine in man: an informal approach to migraine pharmacology. In: Headache, 62 contributions to the present situation of headache research in the international and interdisciplinary view. II. Biochemical bases and drug therapy. Münch. Med. Wschr. (ed.), pp. 101–104. München 1975
Siggaard-Andersen, J., Bonde Petersen, F., Ulrich, J.: Treatment of arterial insufficiency in the lower limbs by Hydergin®. Angiology **22**, 311–319 (1971)
Siggaard-Andersen, J., Petersen, F.B., Ulrich, J.: A double-blind cross-over examination studied by plethysmography. In: Gerontology. Proc. VIth Congr. Clin. Gerontol., Berne, Sept. 8/11th, 1971, pp. 259–261. Bern: H. Huber 1973
Simard, D., Paulson, O.B.: Cerebral vasomotor paralysis during migraine attacks. Arch. Neurol. (Chic.) **29**, 207–209 (1973)
Skinhøj, E.: Hemodynamic studies within the brain during migraine. Arch. Neurol. (Chic.) **29**, 95–98 (1973)
Skinhøj, E., Paulson, O.B.: Regional blood flow in internal carotid distribution during migraine attack. Brit. med. J. **3**, 569–570 (1969)
Sokoloff, L.: The actions of drugs on the cerebral circulation. Pharmacol. Rev. **11**, 2–85 (1959)
Sokoloff, L., Perlin, S., Kornetsky, C., Kety, S.S.: Effects of lysergic acid diethylamide on cerebral circulation and metabolism in man. Fed. Proc. **15**, 174 (1956)
Spira, P.J., Mylecharane, E.J., Lance, J.W.: The effects of humoral agents and antimigraine drugs on the cranial circulation of the monkey. Res. Clin. Stud. Headache **4**, 37–75 (1976)
Spühler, O.: Dihydroergotamin (DHE) als Sympathicolyticum in der inneren Medizin. Schweiz. med. Wschr. **76**, 1259–1263 (1946)
Starke, K.: Influence of α-receptor stimulants on noradrenaline release. Naturwissenschaften **58**, 420 (1971)
Starke, K.: Alpha sympathomimetic inhibition of adrenergic and cholinergic transmission in the rabbit heart. Naunyn-Schmiedebergs Arch. exp. Path. Pharmak. **274**, 18–45 (1972)
Starke, K.: Regulation of noradrenaline release by presynaptic receptor systems. Rev. Physiol. Biochem. Pharmacol. **77**, 1–124 (1977)
Starke, K., Endo, T.: Presynaptic α-adrenoceptors. Gen. Pharmacol. **7**, 307–312 (1976)
Starke, K., Montel, H., Wagner, J.: Effect of phentolamine on noradrenaline uptake and release. Naunyn-Schmiedebergs Arch. Pharmak. **271**, 181–192 (1971)
Starke, K., Endo, T., Taube, H.D.: Relative pre- and postsynaptic potencies of α-adrenoceptor agonists in the rabbit pulmonary artery. Naunyn-Schmiedebergs Arch. exp. Path. Pharmak. **291**, 55–78 (1975a)
Starke, K., Borowski, E., Endo, T.: Preferential blockade of presynaptic α-adrenoceptors by yohimbine. Europ. J. Pharmacol. **34**, 385–388 (1975b)
Steinmann, B., Lüdi, H., Barben, H.P.: Kreislaufuntersuchungen mit vegetativ dämpfenden Pharmaka. Helv. med. Acta **15**, 1–19 (1948)
Stjärne, L.: Basic mechanisms and local feedback control of secretion of adrenergic and cholinergic neurotransmitters. In: Handbook of Psychopharmacology, Vol. 6. Iverson, L.L., Iverson, S.D., Snyder, S.H. (eds.), pp.179–233. New York: Plenum Press 1975
Stjärne, L., Brundin, J.: Dual adrenoceptor-mediated control of noradrenaline secretion from human vasoconstrictor nerves. Facilitation by β-receptors and inhibition by α-receptors. Acta physiol. scand. **94**, 139–141 (1975)
Ströder, U., Koppermann, E.: Der Einfluß hydrierter Mutterkornalkaloide auf das Steh-Ekg unter besonderer Berücksichtigung der Hämodynamik. Z. Kreisl.-Forsch. **41**, 21–31 (1952)
Stumpe, K.O., Kolloch, R., Higuchi, M., Krück, F., Vetter, H.: Hyperprolactinaemia and antihypertensive effect of bromocriptine in essential hypertension. Lancet **2**, 211–214 (1977)
Stürmer, E., Cerletti, A.: The effect of drugs on spontaneous and bradykinin-stimulated lymph flow in dogs. 3rd Int. Congr. Pharmacol. São Paulo, Brazil; Int. Symp. on Vaso-active

polypeptides: Bradykinin and related kinins. Rocha e Silva, M., Rothschild, A. (eds.), pp. 74–80. São Paulo: Edart Livraria Editora Ltda. 1967
Stürmer, E.: The effect of Hydergine® on spontaneous and bradykinin-stimulated lymph flow in dogs. In: Progress in lymphology. Mayall, R.C., Witte, M.H. (eds.), pp. 47–54. Plenum Press 1977
Stutzman, J.W., Murphy, Q., Allen, C.R., Meek, W.J.: Further studies on the production of cyclopropane-epinephrine tachycardia. Anesthesiology **8**, 579–583 (1947)
Sugaar, S., Fried, G.H., Kalberer, J., Antopol, W.: Effect of lysergic acid diethylamide and its brom analogue on arterial hypertension in the rat. Amer. J. Physiol. **201**, 1131–1133 (1961)
Sutton, G.C., Cerletti, A., Taeschler, M.: Comparative analysis of the effect of hydrogenated ergot alkaloids upon presso- and chemoreceptive reflexes in the cat. Arch. int. Pharmacodyn. **84**, 393–400 (1950)
Szewczykowski, J., Meyer, J.S., Kondo, A., Nomura, F., Teraura, T.: Effects of ergot alkaloids (Hydergine) on cerebral hemodynamics and oxygen consumption in monkeys. J. Neurol. Sci. **10**, 25–31 (1970)
Tadepalli, A.S., Mills, E., Schanberg, S.M.: Depression and enhancement of baroreceptor pressor response in cats after intracerebroventricular injection of noradrenergic blocking agents. Circulat. Res. **39**, 724–730 (1976)
Taeschler, M.: Pharmacologie classique de l'Hydergine. Ann. Anesth. Franç. **6**, spécial 2, 97–104 (1965)
Taeschler, M., Cerletti, A., Rothlin, E.: Zur Frage der Hyderginwirkung auf die Gehirnzirkulation. Helv. physiol. pharmacol. Acta **10**, 120–137 (1952)
Tauberger, G. von, Klimmer, O.R.: Die Wirkungen hoher Dosen von d-Lysergsäurediäthylamid auf die Atmung, den Kreislauf und den zentralen Sympathicus-Tonus der Katze. Arzneimittel-Forsch. **18**, 1489–1491 (1968)
Teychenne, P.F., Calne, D.B., Leigh, P.N., Greenacre, J.K., Reid, J.L., Petrie, A., Bamji, A.N.: Idiopathic parkinsonism treated with bromocriptine. Lancet **3**, 473–476 (1975)
Thomson, W.H.: Ergot in the treatment of periodic neuralgias. J. nerv. ment. Dis. **19**, 124–125 (1894)
Thorner, M.O., Chait, A., Aitken, M., Benker, G., Bloom, S.R., Mortimer, C.H., Sanders, P., Mason, A.S., Besser, G.M.: Bromocriptine treatment of acromegaly. Brit. med. J. **1**, 299–303 (1975)
Tillgren, N.: Huvudvärksundersökningar med dihydroergotamintartrat. Huvudvärk och kärlens kontraktionstillständ. (Kopfschmerzuntersuchungen mit DHE. Kopfschmerz- und Kontraktionszustand der Gefäße.) Nord. Med. **33**, 502 (1947)
Trautmann, E.: Die Beeinflussung migräneartiger Zustände durch ein sympathikushemmendes Mittel (Gynergen). Münch. med. Wschr. **75**, 513 (1928)
Tronnier, H.: Gefäßwirksame Kosmetika. J. Soc. Cosmet. Chemists **21**, 299–311 (1970)
Tunis, M.M., Wolff, H.G.: Analysis of cranial artery pulse waves in patients with vascular headache of the migraine type. Amer. J. med. Sci. **224**, 565–568 (1962)
Tzanck, A.: Le traitement des migraines par le tartrate d'ergotamine. Bull. Soc. Méd. Paris **44**, 1057 (1928)
Ulrich, J., Siggaard-Andersen, J.: Vascular effects of dihydrogenated ergot alkaloids. Angiology **22**, 622–628 (1971)
Ulrich, J., Jessen, B., Siggaard-Andersen, J.: Comparative effects of dihydroergotamine and Hydergin® on the blood flow, capillary filtration rate and the capacitance vessels in the human calf studied by plethysmography. Angiology **24**, 657–663 (1973)
Uvnäs, B.: Cholinergic muscle vasodilation. In: Cardiovascular regulation in health and disease. Bartorelli, C., Zanchetti, A. (eds.), pp. 7–32. Milan: Grafiche Elli and Pagani 1971
Vargaftig, B.B., Lefort, J.: Pharmacological evidence for a vasodilator receptor to serotonin in the nasal vessels of the dog. Europ. J. Pharmacol. **25**, 216–225 (1974)
Vleeschhouwer, G.R. de: On the pharmacology of dihydroergotamine. Arch. int. Pharmacodyn. **78**, 461–473 (1949)
Volkman, P.H., Goldberg, L.I.: Lack of correlation between inhibition of prolactin release and stimulation of dopaminergic renal vasodilation. Pharmacologist **18**, 130 (1976)
Walker, R.J., Woodruff, G.N., Glaizner, B., Sedden, C.B., Kerkut, G.A.: The pharmacology

of *Helix* dopamine receptor of specific neurones in the snail, *Helix aspersa*. Comp. Biochem. Physiol. **24**, 455–469 (1968)
Weidmann, H., Cerletti, A.: Weiterer Beitrag zur Pharmakologie von d-Lysergsäure-diäthylamid: Die Wirkung von LSD auf Kreislaufreflexe. Helv. physiol. pharmacol. Acta **16**, C38–C40 (1958)
Weidmann, H., Taeschler, M.: Influence des substances antimigraineuses sur les effets des catecholamines, de la sérotonin et de la stimulation des nerfs sympathiques. Symp. sur les cephaleés vasculaires, 15–16 October, St-Germain-en-Laye. Sandoz éditions, pp. 33–40, 1966
Weil, M.H., Shubin, H.: Changes in venous capacitance during cardiogenic shock—a search for the third dimension. Amer. J. Cardiol. **26**, 613–614 (1970)
Welch, K.M.A., Knowles, L., Spira, P.: Local effect of prostalandins on cat pial arteries. Europ. J. Pharmacol. **25**, 155–158 (1974a)
Welch, K.M.A., Spira, P.J., Knowles, L., Lance, J.W.: Simultaneous measurement of internal and external carotid blood flow in the monkey. An approach to the study of migraine mechanisms. Neurology (Minneap.) **24**, 450–457 (1974b)
Wellens, D., Wauters, E.: Norepinephrine-induced reflex vasodilation and adrenergic beta-receptors. Arch. int. Pharmacodyn. **159**, 401–406 (1966a)
Wellens, D., Wauters, E.: Norepinephrine-induced reflex vasodilation and vascular effects of serotonin. Arch. int. Pharmacodyn. **164**, 140–149 (1966b)
Wellens, D., Wauters, E.: Modification of the haemodynamic effects of isoproterenol by ergotamine. Arch. int. Pharmacodyn. **171**, 246–250 (1968)
Welsh, J.H.: Excitation of the heart of venous mercenaria. Naunyn-Schmiedebergs Arch. exp. Path. Pharmak. **219**, 23–29 (1953)
Welsh, J.H.: Serotonin as a possible neurohumoral agent: evidence obtained in lower animals. Ann. N. Y. Acad. Sci. **66**, 618–630 (1957)
Welsh, J.H., McCoy, A.C.: Actions of d-lysergic acid diethylamide and its 2-bromo derivative on heart of venus mercenaria. Science **125**, 348 (1957)
Welsh, J.H., Moorhead, M.: Identification and assay of 5-hydroxytryptamine in molluscan tissues by fluorescence method. Science **129**, 1491–1492 (1959)
Welsh, J.H., Moorhead, M.: The quantitative distribution of 5-hydroxytryptamine in the invertebrates, especially in their nervous systems. J. Neurochem. **6**, 146–169 (1960)
Wenzel, D.G., Su, J.L.: Interactions between sympathomimetic amines and blocking agents on the rat ventricle strip. Arch. int. Pharmacodyn. **160**, 379–389 (1966)
Wenzel, D.G., Ingianna, J., Grundeman, B.E.: Vascular interaction of ergonovine with nicotine or epinephrine in the rat tail. Arch. int. Pharmacodyn. **150**, 186–190 (1964)
Werkö, L., Lagerlöf, H.: The effect of dihydroergotamine and dihydroergocornine on cardiac output and blood pressure in hypertension. Cardiologia **15**, 120–126 (1949)
Wezler, K., Boeger, A.: Die Dynamik des arteriellen Systems. Ergebn. Physiol. **41**, 292–606 (1939)
White, J.C., Smithwick, R.H.: The autonomic nervous system, p. 255. London: Kimpton 1944
White, J.M. Jr., Noltensmeyer, M.H., Morris, L.E.: The influence of dihydroergotamine methanesulphonate (DHE-45) on epinephrine induced cardiac irregularities in dogs during anaesthesia with several agents. Arch. int. Pharmacodyn. **88**, 361–367 (1951)
Wolff, H.G.: Headache and other head pain. New York: Oxford University Press 1948
Wolff, H.G.: Headache and other head pain, 2nd ed. New York: Oxford University Press 1963
Wolff, H.G.: Headache and other head pain, 3rd ed., rev. by D.J. Dalessio. New York: Oxford University Press 1972
Wolff, H.G., Hardy, J.D., Goodell, H.: Measurement of the effect on the pain threshold of acetylsalicylic acid, acetanilid, acetophenetidin, aminopyrine, ethyl alcohol, trichlorethylene, a barbiturate, quinine, ergotamine tartrate and caffeine: an analysis of their relation to the pain experience. J. clin. Invest. **20**, 63–80 (1941)
Woods, G.G., Nelson, V.E., Nelson, E.E.: The effect of small amounts of ergotamine on the circulatory response to epinephrine. J. Pharmacol. exp. Ther. **45**, 403–418 (1932)
Wright, S.: Studies of reflex activity in involuntary nervous system. II Action of ergotamine on vasomotor reflexes. J. Physiol. (Lond.) **69**, 331–348 (1930)

Wright, A.McC., Moorhead, M., Welsh, J.H.: Actions of derivatives of lysergic acid on the heart of venus mercenaria. Brit. J. Pharmacol. **18**, 440–450 (1962)
Yeh, B.J., McNay, J.L., Goldberg, L.I.: Attenuation of dopamine renal and mesenteric vasodilation by haloperidol: evidence for a specific receptor. J. Pharmacol. exp. Ther. **168**, 303–309 (1969)
Youmans, J.B., Trabue, C., Buvinger, R.S., Frank, H.: Experimental and clinical studies of ergotamine. V. The action of ergotamine on the sympathetic nervous system stimulated by epinephrine. Studies of the metabolic rate, pulse rate, blood pressure, blood sugar and the total leukocyte count. Ann. int. Med. **7**, 653–663 (1933)
Zickgraf, H.: Die Wirkung der dihydrierten Mutterkornalkaloide auf den Kreislauf. Z. klin. Med. **145**, 34–50 (1949)

CHAPTER VI

Effects on the Central Nervous System

D.M. LOEW, E.B. VAN DEUSEN, and W. MEIER-RUGE

A. Introduction

Since the publication of the review by BARGER on "The Alkaloids of Ergot" (1938), the study of the effects of ergot alkaloids on the central nervous system has changed its focus from the mere prediction of undesirable side effects, such as emesis or sedation or convulsive ergotism, to the search for pharmacodynamic effects which are potentially useful in the treatment of nervous and mental disease states.

In his first paper on ergotamine ROTHLIN (1923) reports that central effects of ergotamine in animals occur after administration of high doses only. Assuming that these are toxic dose levels, ROTHLIN concludes that they reflect "les actions collatérales si redoutées de l'ergotisme aigu, à savoir les convulsions et la gangrène." In fact, the first experimental studies on *d*-LSD conducted in 1938 did not reveal particular effects on the central nervous system (ROTHLIN, 1957). It was only after the discovery of the mental effects of *d*-LSD by HOFMANN (STOLL, 1947) that its pharmacologic effects underwent a systematic study. A particular interest was attributed to the peripheral antagonism between *d*-LSD (73b)[1] and serotonin (5-hydroxytryptamine) (GADDUM, 1953). Based on this antagonism, WOOLLEY and SHAW (1954) proposed that serotonin could be involved in *d*-LSD-induced hallucinosis and in schizophrenia. However, subsequent investigations of *d*-LSD and its congeners indicated that hallucinogenic potency does not run parallel to serotonin antagonism in peripheral tissue (CERLETTI and ROTHLIN, 1955a; CERLETTI and DOEPFNER, 1958; ISBELL et al., 1959), but that an excitatory syndrome (ROTHLIN et al., 1956) is observed in the rabbit at a dose level comparable to that which induces hallucinations in man. Thus, CERLETTI (1959) describes a central effect of ergot derivatives which occurs in the animal at low nontoxic dose levels.

The assumption that the central actions of *d*-LSD involve serotonin has provoked extensive research on the effects of ergot derivatives on synaptic function. Early studies on serotonin metabolism (FREEDMAN, 1961; ANDÉN et al., 1968) and subsequent investigations on single serotoninergic neurons (AGHAJANIAN, 1972; HAIGLER and AGHAJANIAN, 1974a) indicate that *d*-LSD, depending on the experimental conditions, mimics or counteracts central effects of serotonin. Recently, these studies have been extended to include other ergot derivatives (HAIGLER and AGHAJANIAN, 1974b; CORRODI et al., 1975; SOFIA and VASSAR, 1975). Furthermore, a number of authors have suggested that ergot derivatives stimulate central dopamine

[1] *D*-lysergic acid diethylamide, LSD-25. This and the subsequent numbers in brackets refer to Chapter II of this volume (RUTSCHMANN and STADLER, 1978).

receptors as well (CORRODI et al., 1973; JOHNSON et al., 1973b; PIJNENBURG et al., 1973). In particular, bromocriptine (38)[2] was shown to imitate the effects of dopamine in the extrapyramidal system, an action which is assumed to be responsible for its therapeutic effects in patients with idiopathic Parkinsonism (CALNE et al., 1974a, b).

Studies of the effects of ergot derivatives on cerebral blood flow and brain metabolism in animals were initiated after the observation of POPKIN (1951) that dihydroergotoxine[3] affected the behavior of geriatric patients suffering from peripheral vascular disease. Based on the pharmacologic data available at that time (ROTHLIN, 1946, 1947; ROTHLIN and FANCHAMPS, 1955), this therapeutic effect was assumed to be related to vasodilation. However, based on a study in an isolated perfused cat head preparation, EMMENEGGER and MEIER-RUGE (1968) proposed that under certain experimental conditions dihydroergotoxine primarily influences brain metabolism, and that changes in cerebral blood flow may depend on these metabolic effects. Subsequently, similar studies were carried out with nicergoline (BENZI et al., 1971), dihydroergonine (CERLETTI et al., 1973), and ergotamine (BOISMARE and STREICHENBERGER, 1973).

The present review intends to cover the time span between the early description of central effects of ergot derivatives as reviewed by BARGER (1938) and the more recent work on the effects of ergot derivatives on central synaptic function and brain metabolism. The material on central cardiovascular control is treated in Chapter V (CLARK et al., 1978) of this volume. The effects of ergot derivatives on the hypothalamo-pituitary axis are reviewed in Chapter IX (FLÜCKIGER and DEL POZO, 1978) of this volume. Experimental work on hallucinogenic ergot derivatives is only included when required to illustrate results reported on other ergot derivatives. For a thorough review of the pharmacologic effects of *d*-LSD the reader is referred to the recent book of SANKAR (1975) and to Chapter VIII of this volume (FANCHAMPS, 1978). Some central effects of ergot derivatives have been covered in recent reviews by HOFMANN (1964) and BRADLEY and BRIGGS (1974a).

B. Early Evidence of Central Effects

Early observation of central nervous system stimulation by ergot alkaloids came from descriptions of ergot poisoning recorded between the end of the 16th and the end of the 19th centuries. During this time and even into this century, central stimulation by ergot compounds was thought to be mainly a sign of its toxicity (BARGER, 1938).

I. Convulsive Ergotism in Man

Two types of ergotism, the convulsive and gangrenous, have been described and are sharply differentiated only in severe cases (BARGER, 1931). The early and mild

[2] 2-Bromo-α-ergokryptine, CB 154, Parlodel.

[3] Dihydroergotoxine consists of one-third of dihydroergocristine (102c), one-third of dihydroergocornine (102d), the rest being a mixture of dihydro-α-ergokryptine (102e) and dihydro-β-ergokryptine (102f) in a proportion of about 2:1. In the form of the methane sulphonate, dihydroergotoxine has the trade name Hydergine.

symptoms in subacute convulsive ergotism are common to both types and include slight giddiness, feeling of frontal pressure in the head, fatigue, depression, nausea with or without vomiting, and pains in the limbs and lumbar region which make walking difficult. Most of these symptoms of ergot poisoning have been observed within 1 h after an i.v. injection of 0.5 mg ergotamine or ergotoxine and in cases of ergot ingestion can last several weeks. A later and more severe symptom of convulsive ergotism after poisoning with larger doses (over 3 mg) is "formication" or tingling of the skin "as if ants crawled under it" and coldness of the extremities. *Sensus formicationis* is most common in the fingers and arms, where it leads to muscle twitching and after a few weeks to clonic muscular twitching and tonic spasms of the limbs. Often the tongue and whole facial muscles (orbicularis oris) are affected. In the most severe cases the onset of convulsions is sudden and, depending on their regularity, they either force the sufferer into a rolled-up position or stretch him out like a statue for several minutes or even hours at a time. Between these painful convulsions patients are usually ravenously hungry. In extreme cases patients lie for 6–8 h as if dead, after which time there follows a pronounced anesthesia of the skin, paralysis of the lower limbs, jerking of the arms and often epileptic convulsions, delirium, and loss of speech. These patients generally become unconscious and die on day 3 after the onset of the first symptoms. In severe, nonfatal cases the disease often lasts for 6–8 weeks and convalescence takes several months. Convalescents remain very sensitive to ergot and relapses are frequent and sometimes regular, accompanied by epilepsy, hemi-, and paraplegia. The most common aftereffects of severe poisoning include general weakness, trembling of the limbs, gastric pains, giddiness, permanent contractures of the hands and feet, anesthesia of the fingers and toes, impairment of hearing and sight, and a variety of mental problems which remain for years.

2. Early Description of Central Effects in Animals

Early quantitative experiments sought to explain the symptoms of convulsive ergotism by studying the effects of sublethal doses of ergot in intact animals. Muscular "fatigue" and lethargy were described by BARGER and DALE (1907) as the most characteristic symptoms in 30 g *frogs* which had received between 0.1 and 1.0 mg of ergotoxine[4]. In contrast, ROTHLIN (1923) observed exophthalmos but not miosis in frogs of a similar size after subcutaneous injections of 0.1–1.0 mg of ergotamine (20).

The effects of ergotamine, ergotoxine, and ergometrine (19) on *cocks* have been reported most extensively by DALE and SPIRO (1922), ROTHLIN (1923), and BROWN and DALE (1935) and are similar to the effects of sensibamine[5] reported by ROESSLER and UNNA (1935). Although the potency of these compounds to produce their effects varied, doses between 0.3 and 1 mg/kg produced poor coordination, general weakness, rapid breathing, staggering gait, drooping wings, salivation, and diarrhea.

Tremors, extreme excitability, and weakness of the hind limbs without permanent injury or lethality were also described by BROWN and DALE (1935) in

[4] Ergotoxine is a mixture of ergocornine (24), ergokryptine (25, 26), and ergocristine (23) in equal parts.

[5] Sensibamine is an equimolar mixture of ergotamine (20) and ergotaminine.

mice which had received 10–150 mg/kg i.v. of ergotoxine ethane sulphonate. The symptoms of ergosine poisoning in mice were similar to those of ergotoxine according to WHITE (quoted by BARGER, 1938); tremor, exophthalmos, piloerection, gasping, and ataxia. The d-isomer, ergosinine, had a similar, but slower effect. KREITMAIR (1934) reported the nonlethal range of intoxication produced by ergotoxine (up to 32 mg/kg i.v.) to be wider than that of ergoclavine[6] (up to 20 mg/kg i.v.). Ergotamine was shown to be lethal at doses above 50 mg/kg (ROTHLIN and HAMET, 1930).

Ergometrine, in contrast, at doses between 10 and 100 mg/kg i.v., produced only slight exophthalmos and piloerection but no other symptoms (BROWN and DALE, 1935). The minimal lethal dose of 250 mg/kg i.v., reported by DAVIS et al. (1935), produced dragging of the hind legs and periodic clonic convulsions prior to death. Sensibamine at 20 mg/kg i.v., or 150 mg/kg s.c., produced tonic and clonic convulsions, sprawling of the hind limbs, and slowing of the respiration. All these symptoms disappeared in a few days. Fifty to 100 mg/kg i.v., however, lead to prolonged intoxication and death of some of the mice (ROESSLER and UNNA, 1935).

In early studies by GITHENS (1917) small doses of ergotoxine (1.0 mg/kg s.c.) produced "dullness," slight ataxia, and hypothermia in *rats*. ROTHLIN (1923) reported that subcutaneous injections of 25–100 mg/kg ergotamine into rats caused dyspnea almost immediately, after 20 min ataxia and after 1 h violent scratching, which was interpreted as a response to itching. Larger doses caused involuntary contractions of the legs.

In *guinea pigs* s.c. injections of ergotamine had an effect similar to that in rats. ROTHLIN (1923) reported that from 4–36 mg/kg i.v. caused immediate excitement, convulsions, and a great acceleration of respiration. After 10–12 h, these animals were normal and suffered no aftereffects. DAVIS et al. (1935) reported that ergometrine at the i.v. lethal dose (80 mg/kg) produced the same symptoms as in mice which had received 250 mg/kg.

Early studies with *rabbits* (GITHENS, 1917) showed that 2.0 mg/kg i.v. of ergotoxine produced maximal pupil dilation after 1 min, after 10 min extreme restlessness which lasted 30 min, and after about 1 h gasping respiratory behavior which was accompanied by piloerection and ataxia in all four limbs. A rapid rise in temperature during the first 2 h was accompanied by "anxiety" and "fear" when the animals were handled. After 3–4 h, when hyperthermia reached a maximum, rapid breathing was the only outstanding symptom. The most important difference between ergotoxine and ergotamine in rabbits was that the latter is only one-third to one-half as potent as ergotoxine in raising the body temperature (ROTHLIN, 1923). ROTHLIN found sensibamine to be about one and one-half times as active as ergotamine but less active than ergotoxine in producing hyperthermia. Otherwise, ROTHLIN reported only slight differences between the minimal lethal i.v. doses of sensibamine (2.5–3 mg/kg) and ergotamine (3 mg/kg). Interestingly, repeated administration of ergotoxine (DALE, 1906), ergotamine (ROTHLIN, 1923), or sensibamine (ROESSLER and UNNA, 1935) did not produce the original symptoms observed after the initial treatment. In rabbits there were striking similarities between the effects of ergotox-

[6] Ergoclavine is an equimolar mixture of ergosine (21) and ergosinine.

ine or ergotamine and ergometrine. BROWN and DALE (1935) reported that 1.8–2.8 mg/kg i.v. ergometrine almost immediately produced wide pupil dilation restlessness, excitability, "sham rage," a crawling gait, acceleration of respiration, and hyperthermia. Smaller doses of ergometrine did not modify the temperature and never lowered it as did small doses of ergotoxine, ergotamine, and ergoclavine. In addition to those symptoms reported by BROWN and DALE, ROTHLIN (1936) observed piloerection, salivation, and convulsions. At the lower end of this dose range he found that as little as 0.1 mg/kg i.v. ergotamine caused hyperthermia.

The effects of ergometrine in *cats* have been reported extensively by BROWN and DALE (1935). In their studies the effect of a 2–2.5 mg/kg i.v. dose was immediately apparent and included rapid mydriasis and piloerection, leading to progressively poor muscle coordination, excitability, and sham rage in response to visual or auditory stimuli of any kind. Within 5 h of ergometrine injection, excitability had subsided and movements became stronger and more coordinated. All of these symptoms resembled those seen in the early excitatory phases of ergotoxine or ergotamine treatment. However, the effects of the latter derivatives were progressively more severe and lead to long-lasting semiconsciousness and incontinence. After oral administration of 5 mg of ergotoxine, BROWN and DALE (1935) observed pupil dilatation, retraction of the nictitating membrane and slight exophthalmos within 5 min but no excitement or sham rage. After subcutaneous injection of 2–2.5 mg/kg, sham rage appeared within 30 min, which was followed by exophthalmos. These effects were perceptible even at doses as low as 0.2 mg/kg s.c. Similar effects were described by GILMAN (1934) after the intracardial injection of 1 mg ergotoxine.

In *dogs* receiving small doses of ergotamine (0.25–0.5 mg/animal) YOUMANS and TRIMBLE (1930) observed mydriasis and often vomiting. FARRAR and DUFF (1928) reported vomiting a few minutes after an i.v. injection of 0.13–0.4 mg/kg ergotamine and later profuse salivation, pupil dilation, tremors, extensive rigidity, and accelerated heartbeat. BROWN and DALE (1935) found that a 0.8 mg/kg i.v. dose of ergotamine produced a short period of excitability after 5 min but otherwise only repeated vomiting and weakness of the hind legs during the subsequent 3 h. Ergotamine induced vomiting in dogs after an initial s.c. dose as low as 0.025 mg/kg (STAHNKE, 1928a, 1928b) but not after repeated higher doses. Similarly, 2 h after an initial i.m. injection of ergotoxine (HATCHER and WEISS, 1923) or after tolerance to ergotamine had developed (STAHNKE, 1928a, 1928b), apomorphine-induced vomiting was also blocked.

It appears that the *monkey* is more sensitive to the central depressant effect of ergot derivatives than other species of laboratory animals. WHITE (1943) studied the symptoms induced by some ergot alkaloids in Silenus Rhesus monkeys weighing between 2 and 4 kg. This author reports that i.m. injection of 4 mg ergosine (21) or intracardial injections of 2 mg ergosinine, 3 mg ergocristine (23), or 12 mg ergometrine induced difficulty of maintaining movement and drowsiness and even sleep. In cats or rabbits WHITE's results were similar to those reported above.

Based on a review of early pharmacologic studies on both peptide derivatives and on ergometrine, WHITE (1944b) concludes that, as opposed to peripheral "sympatholytic" action, nonpeptide and peptide derivatives share a number of central actions, such as temperature changes, somnolence, "sham rage," and polypnoea.

3. The Question of "Toxic" versus "Therapeutic" Dose

The early literature concerning the effects of ergot derivatives is dominated by the assumption that the so-called central effects of ergot alkaloids observed in animals only occur after administration of high, sublethal, i.e., "toxic," doses and reflect the symptoms of ergot poisoning in humans. It is true that rats treated with high doses of ergotamine develop a behavioral pattern reminiscent of formication (ROTHLIN, 1923), and that motor incoordination and convulsions have been reported after administration of sublethal doses of various ergot alkaloids to different species. Thus, some of the symptoms of ergot poisoning reported in humans can be reproduced in animals. On the other hand, other central effects of ergot alkaloids, such as emesis in the dog or hyperthermia in the rabbit, are observed at dose levels far below a maximal tolerated dose.

An experiment in the pigeon, which was carried out by J. GRAUWILER in our laboratories, may serve to illustrate this point. This author investigated ergotamine over a wide dose range in pigeons and determined the dose levels: ED_0 (maximal dose without emesis), LD_0 (maximal dose without lethality), ED_{50} for the induction of emesis, and LD_{50}, using the method of MILLER and TAINTER (1944). After oral administration the following dose levels were calculated: ED_0 1 mg/kg, ED_{50} for emesis 5 mg/kg, LD_0 100 mg/kg, LD_{50} 340 mg/kg. After i.v. administration the respective values were 0.003, 0.07, 0.1, and 0.88 mg/kg. These results indicate that in the pigeon a central effect of ergotamine, i.e., emesis, is observed in doses far below the toxic dose levels, particularly after oral administration. However, the doses used in the pigeon are still considerably higher than the recommended human therapeutic doses, which are in the range of 2 mg p.o. and 0.25–0.5 mg parenterally. The first central effect of an ergot derivative in an animal observed to occur in a dose range similar to an effective dose in humans was the hyperthermic action of *d*-LSD in the rabbit. Hyperthermia induced by *d*-LSD in the rabbit was proposed by CERLETTI (1956) to be predictive of a hallucinogenic effect in humans, which was seen in the microgram dose range as well.

C. Whole-Animal Studies

From the early studies reviewed in the preceding section we see that ergot derivatives exert a variety of pharmacodynamic effects which reflect changes in the function of the central nervous system. Both behavioral excitation and depression are reported, which are frequently accompanied by changes in autonomic regulation, for instance, alterations in rectal temperature or respiration, variations in pupil diameter, or emesis. Some of these central effects have found particular attention, because they have been proposed to be linked to therapeutic or to side effects in humans, e.g., psychomotor depression. Others, such as emesis or alterations of the electroencephalogram, were more thoroughly investigated, because they lend themselves to quantification. The common denominator of the effects which will be reviewed in this section is the fact that they all can be observed in the whole animal.

1. Behavioral Excitation

As described in the previous section, i.v. administration of 2–2.5 mg/kg of ergometrine (19) to cats induced a particular pattern of overresponsiveness to external stimuli. This syndrome was called "sham rage" by BROWN and DALE (1935). Sham rage comprises startling, snarling, spitting, baring of the teeth, and extension of the claws in response to auditory or visual stimulation but no purposeful movements of attack or defense. Similarly, GILMAN (1934) reported excitement and sham rage after intracardiac administration of 1 mg/kg ergotoxine to cats. Following injection of 2 mg ergometrine (19) into the lateral ventricle of conscious cats, GADDUM and VOGT (1956) observed behavioral alterations similar to sham rage. Unfortunately, no detailed further analysis of the mechanism underlying ergot-induced sham rage is available. It was only in 1956 that ROTHLIN et al. studied the effects of *d*-LSD (73b) and related ergot compounds in the rabbit (CERLETTI, 1959) and described a syndrome of "central sympathetic stimulation," consisting of hyperthermia, hyperglycemia, mydriasis, piloerection, electroencephalographic arousal, and an enhanced responsiveness to environmental stimulation. This excitatory syndrome was observed at doses as low as 0.5 µg/kg i.v. of *d*-LSD and was proposed to be predictive of hallucinogenic potency in man (CERLETTI, 1959). As an increase in rectal temperature is the most prominent feature of this syndrome, we will discuss it further in the section on body temperature.

In 1968, DIXON reported that a dose of 5 mg/kg *d*-LSD administered i.p. to rats induced 'aberrant' behavior comprising aimless sniffing, shaking movements of the head, and biting of the mesh floor of the cage. At the same time, locomotor activity was reduced. Later authors described similar stereotyped behavior after the administration of agroclavine (5) (STONE, 1973), ergometrine (PIJNENBURG et al., 1973), bromocriptine (38) (JOHNSON et al., 1973b), or ergocornine (24) (CORRODI et al., 1973) to rats. As it is assumed that stereotyped behavior induced by ergot derivatives relates to stimulation of central dopamine receptors, a detailed review will be found in the section on central synaptic transmission (see Sect: D).

A number of authors have investigated behavioral stimulation after ergot treatment under experimental conditions which produce low rates of baseline responding. GRAEFF and SCHOENFELD (1970) trained pigeons to peck on a key for a food reward in a behavioral program consisting of a fixed interval and of a fixed-ratio-electric-shock-punishment schedule. The rate of key-pecking produced by this multiple schedule in control animals was low in the early part of the fixed interval and under the fixed-ratio-shock schedule. During these parts of the program, treatment with 0.1–3 mg/kg i.m. of methysergide (34a) or with the same doses of 2-Br-LSD (37a)[7] increased rates of responding, whereas 3 mg/kg i.m. of either methysergide or 2-BR-LSD reduced the high rates of responding which occurred at the end of the fixed-interval components of the multiple schedule. WINTER (1972), using a similar procedure in rats, found that methysergide, at doses of 1–10 mg/kg i.p., increased low rates of responding which were produced by concomitant punishment. WINTER (1972) concluded that the behavioral changes observed after methysergide treatment are unrelated to serotonin antagonism, because they were not seen after the nonergot serotonin antagonist cinanserine. In rats trained to

[7] 2-Bromo-d-lysergic acid diethylamide, BOL 148.

work in a Sidman avoidance schedule, low rates of responding were produced by a reduction in the oxygen content of the inspired air to 9% (JÄGGI and LOEW, 1976). Under these conditions, 3 mg/kg i.p. of bromocriptine or dihydroergotoxine enhanced response rate. The same authors reported similar effects of L-DOPA and apomorphine and suggested that increased response rates might be related to central dopaminergic stimulation. In similar experiments in rats, BOISMARE et al. (1978) investigated the acquisition of a conditioned avoidance response which was depressed by hypoxia. Dihydroergocornine (102d), dihydroergokryptine (102e, f), but not dihydroergocristine (102c), when administered during acquisition, counteracted hypoxic depression of acquisition. In addition, the decrease in brain concentrations of dopamine and noradrenaline observed in untreated rats was not seen in animals administered dihydroergocornine or dihydroergokryptine.

Similar to the stimulants of the central nervous system, some ergot derivatives were reported to decrease the time required by experimental animals to meet a certain performance criterion. RAY and WONG (1967) studied the ability of rats to acquire avoidance of a puff of air in a shuttle box. They found that pretreatment with 0.2–0.4 mg/kg s.c. of elymoclavine (6) reduced the number of trials to make five correct responses during six subsequent trials. However, HOOD et al. (1974), when investigating the ability of hamsters to acquire avoidance of an electric shock in a runway, were unable to find a reduction of trials to criterion after 2 mg/kg i.p. of agroclavine. Six or 10 mg/kg i.p. retarded avoidance acquisition. Incidentally, these authors reported dose-dependent gnawing which might have interfered with successful completion of the task, at the higher doses. Indeed, HARSH and WITTERS (1970) report that only low doses of elymoclavine stimulated wheel-turning of mice, whereas high doses impaired it. VILLA and PANCERI (1973) investigated the ability of mice to maintain themselves on a horizontal rod rotating at 16 rpm. under daily treatment with 0.1–10 mg/kg i.p. of nicergoline (104e). The time until the animal fell off the rod increased when the drug was administered 10 min, 1, and 2 h before testing. This effect was observed after the first dose and was maintained over the whole treatment period of 5 days. These authors reported similar effects whether nicergoline was administered by the oral or the intramuscular route.

2. Behavioral Depression

One of the first and most striking experiments to demonstrate behavioral depression induced by an ergot derivative was reported by HESS (1925). HESS administered 1 mg of ergotamine into the lateral or the third brain ventricle of unrestrained cats which were habituated to the laboratory conditions. After a lapse of 50–100 min the cats quieted down and displayed the preparatory activities typical of a cat looking for a quiet place to sleep. After having arranged their bodies to a *regelrechte Schlafstellung*, the cats lowered their heads, shut their eyes, and fell asleep. If disturbed by a visual, acoustic, or tactile stimulus the animals were able to respond and would even catch a mouse which was presented by the observer. This behavioral state lasted for 2–6 h. As emphasized by HESS, intraventricular administration of 1 mg ergotamine induced "readiness for sleep" but not general anesthesia. A similar state of sleep following intraventricular administration of 1 mg ergotamine to dogs also has been mentioned by MARINESCO et al. (1931).

As opposed to intraventricular injection, systemic administration of ergotamine and other ergopeptine derivatives leads to behavioral stimulation in most animal species. However, as summarized in the preceding section, WHITE (1943) noted that the prominent symptoms of systemic administration of ergot derivatives to rhesus monkeys consisted of behavioral depression and even sleep. More recent studies of MELDRUM and NAQUET (1970, 1971) and of VUILLON-CACCIUTTOLO and BALZANO (1972) indicated that in the baboon methysergide, 2-Br-LSD, methergoline (89d), and methylergometrine (73a) all induced drowsiness and muscle atonia, whereas ergotamine, lysergic acid (8), and dihydroergotoxine were without effect. *D*-LSD treatment resulted in stupor, akinesia, or stereotyped movements (WALTER et al., 1971a, b). These results are summarized in Table 1.

In species other than monkeys dihydrogenated ergot alkaloids have been reported to induce less pronounced central nervous system stimulation or even behavioral depression. ROTHLIN (1946, 1947) mentions that in contrast to the genuine nondihydrogenated ergot compounds [ergotamine, ergosine (21), ergocristine (23), ergokryptine (25, 26), and ergocornine (24)], the central stimulant effects of their dihydrogenated derivatives are much less pronounced. ROBERTS et al. (1950), who administered 4 mg/kg i.p. of dihydroergocristine, dihydroergokryptine, or dihydroergocornine to rats, reported that the administration of these dihydrogenated compounds failed to elicit hyperactivity and hyperresponsiveness typical of their parent compounds. At the same time, these authors found their rats to be more docile and less resistant to handling. YUI and TAKEO (1958a) administered fixed doses of various ergot derivatives to rabbits, cats, and dogs (0.2 mg/kg i.v.) or to mice (20 mg/kg i.p.). As opposed to the nondihydrogenated ergots agroclavine, elymoclavine (6), triseclavine, penniclavine, lysergine, lysergene (79f), lysergol (79a), and *d*-LSD, the dihydrogenated derivatives dihydroagroclavine, dihydroelymoclavine, and dihydroergokryptine invariably produced apathy, drowsiness, and sedation and in dogs even sleep.

Studies carried out by BOISSIER et al. (1967a, 1967b, 1968) indicate that 5–40 mg/kg i.p. dihydroergotamine (102b) reduced exploratory activity of mice in a light beam cage by about 40%. However, this effect did not depend on the dose. The same authors found an ED_{50} of 72 mg/kg i.p. for the induction of ptosis in the rat. At a still higher dose, a blockade of apomorphine-induced stereotypies of rats was reported, the ED_{50} being 240 mg/kg i.p. Based on these results, BOISSIER et al. (1968) conclude that dihydroergotamine exerts "psycholeptic effects." In the test procedures employed, the active doses were found to be considerably higher than that of chlorpromazine. *D*-LSD was reported by DHAWAN et al. (1961) to antagonize apomorphine-induced pecking in pigeons with an ED_{50} of 0.052 mg/kg i.m. 2-Br-LSD (0.2–0.4 mg/kg i.m.) only increased the latency of the response, whereas dihydroergotamine or ergotoxine were without effect. In "waltzing mice," ROTHLIN and CERLETTI (1952) and ROTHLIN (1953) reported that 1–2 mg/kg s.c. of dihydroergotoxine reduced the number of turns. At the same doses, dihydroergotamine was inactive in this test.

BALINT and ANOKBONGGO (1968) found that 0.1 mg/kg i.p. dihydroergotoxine slightly increased the latency of rats trained to respond in a conditioned avoidance schedule. In a similar procedure, 0.05–0.5 mg/kg i.p. methysergide did not alter performance, whereas *d*-LSD at doses of 0.05 and 0.1 mg/kg i.p. increased exploration and shuttle-box performance. At 0.5 mg/kg i.p., *d*-LSD inhibited exploration and reduced performance (TORRE and FAGIANI, 1968). Since both drugs decreased brain serotonin levels, TORRE et al. (1975) concluded that their behavioral effects were unrelated to brain serotonin concentrations.

It is questionable whether the "analgesic" effects of ergometrine which were reported by CONTRERAS et al. (1967a, 1967b) reflect central depression. These authors found that 0.5 mg/kg i.p. ergometrine raised the threshold for electrical stimulation of the genital papilla in male rats but not in female rats. Castration abolished the ergometrine effect, which was restored by testosterone administration. Previous administration of α-adrenergic blocking agents or reserpine antagonized ergometrine-induced analgesia, but nalorphine was without an effect.

It is not surprising that ergotamine (GRINKER and SPIVEY, 1945; HEATH and POWDERMAKER, 1944; BAER, 1947) and particularly dihydrogenated ergot derivatives were investigated in mentally ill patients. PRITZKER (1947) administered dihydroergotamine orally at daily doses of 15–30 mg (in some cases up to 200 mg) to agitated patients and reported a beneficial effect in 32 out of 34 patients. SCHNEIDER (1950) and SOLMS (1952) used dihydroergotamine (6–150 mg), dihydroergocornine (6–60 mg), or dihydroergotoxine (6–21 mg) in patients displaying psychomotor excitation. SOLMS (1952) concluded that dihydrogenated ergot derivatives were beneficial to patients suffering from psychomotor excitation as long as there were no concomitant delusions or hallucinations. EY et al. (1968) were able to reduce the doses of neuroleptic drugs without detriment to 43 of 57 mental patients by simultaneous administration of a daily oral dose of 4.5 mg dihydroergotoxine.

3. Interaction With Centrally Depressant Drugs

a) Barbiturates

In 1934, ROTHLIN reported that s.c. administration of 0.25–0.5 mg/kg ergotamine to guinea-pigs or rabbits enhanced the sedation and slight motor incapacitation induced by 20–40 mg/kg s.c. phenobarbital. In cats, the excitatory effects of phenobarbital were inhibited by ergotamine. At the doses of ergotamine investigated by ROTHLIN (1934), no effect of the drug alone was seen. A number of authors report that dihydrogenated ergopeptine derivatives potentiate the effects of subhypnotic doses of barbiturates. ISSEKUTZ and GYERMEK (1949) found that 2 mg/kg s.c. dihydroergocornine potentiated the depressant effect of a subthreshold phenobarbital dose in rats. GRIFFITH et al. (1955) and DAVID et al. (1956) reported a more rapid onset of hypnosis induced in rats by 15–25 mg/kg s.c. of secobarbital or pentobarbital, when dihydroergotoxine at a dose of 0.06 mg/kg s.c. was administered to rats 15 min previously. BALINT (1964) studied sleeping time, i.e., the loss of righting reflex of mice treated with 50 mg/kg i.p. hexobarbital. He found that 0.04 mg/kg i.p. dihydroergotoxine administered i.p. 20 min previously prolonged sleeping time. When in addition to 40 mg/kg i.p. hexobarbital, 2 mg/kg i.p. of various phenothiazines were administered, dihydroergotoxine enhanced the potentiating action of promethazine and methopromazine, whereas the effects of

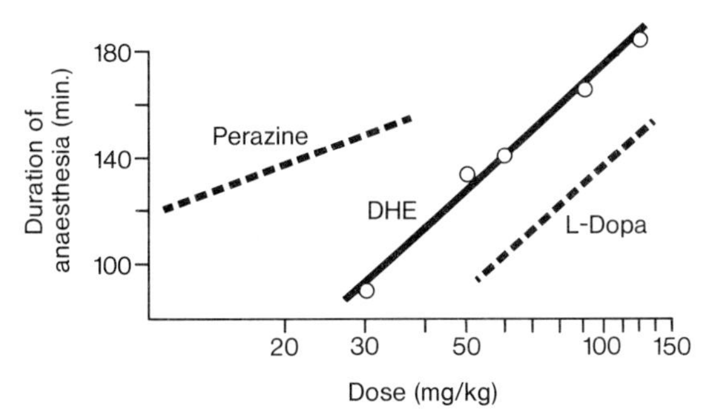

Fig. 1. Dose-dependent prolongation of loss of righting reflex (anesthesia) induced by 10 mg/kg i.p. hexobarbital after i.p. administration of dihydroergotamine (DHE), perazine, and 1-3-(3,4-dihydroxyphenyl)-alanine (L-DOPA) in rats. (From JEND and COPER, 1974)

levopromazine and acepromazine were counteracted by dihydroergotoxine. Similarly, BALINT and ANOKBONGGO (1968) investigated the inhibition of a conditioned avoidance response by phenothiazines in the rat and found that dihydroergotoxine (0.1 mg/kg i.p.) enhanced the effects of 10 mg/kg i.p. promethazine, while counteracting those of 5 mg/kg i.p. levopromazine.

Dihydroergotamine was shown by BOISSIER et al. (1967b) to increase the number of mice losing their righting reflex after a subhypnotic dose (25 or 30 mg/kg i.p.) of pentobarbital. The minimal effective dose was 10 mg/kg i.p. of dihydroergotamine. After 40 mg/kg i.p. of the drug, the effect lasted over 2 h. A careful analysis of the effects of dihydroergotamine in prolonging the hypnosis induced by 100 mg/kg i.p. hexobarbital was carried out in rats by JEND and COPER (1974). In doses of 30–120 mg/kg i.p., dihydroergotamine induced a dose-dependent prolongation of loss of righting reflex (Fig. 1). No effect of dihydroergotamine on the elimination rate of hexobarbital from blood or brain was observed. Based on the investigations of JEND and COPER, the hypothermia induced by dihydroergotamine at an ambient temperature of 22° C did not account for its prolongation of the hexobarbital effect, as similar prolongations were observed at an ambient temperature of 33° C, an ambient temperature at which dihydroergotamine did not lower rectal temperature.

A prolongation of hypnosis induced by 40 mg/kg i.v. thiopental was reported by VOTAVA and LAMPLOVA (1964) after pretreatment with a number of ergolenyl and isoergolenyl derivatives at a dose of 5 mg/kg i.v. At this dose, *d*-LSD also was found to prolong thiopental-induced hypnosis, which contradicts earlier findings of SHORE et al. (1955b) and TAESCHLER and ROTHLIN (1956), who were not able to demonstrate a potentiation of barbiturate effects in mice by *d*-LSD.

b) Reserpine-Induced Behavioral Depression

Early studies on the interaction between ergot derivatives and reserpine were based on the hypothesis that the behavioral depression of reserpine was caused by a release of serotonin (PLETSCHER et al., 1955; BRODIE et al., 1956), and that inhibition of serotonin should antagonize such an effect. Indeed, SHORE et al. (1955 a) reported an antagonism of reserpine-induced barbiturate potentiation by *d*-LSD in mice. At a dose of 10 mg/kg i.p., *d*-LSD shortened the duration of loss of righting reflex induced by 100 or 150 mg/kg i.p. hexobarbital in mice treated with 5 mg/kg i.p. reserpine. TAESCHLER and CERLETTI (1957), using 20 mg/kg i.v. thiopental and 0.5 or 1 mg/kg s.c. reserpine, essentially confirmed these results, and found that the antagonism of 2 mg/kg s.c. *d*-LSD towards reserpine was not shared by the same dose of 2-Br-LSD. These authors suggest that the inhibitory effect of *d*-LSD on reserpine-induced barbiturate hypnosis is not due to its antiserotonin activity but is related to another mechanism, possibly central stimulation. A higher dose of 2-Br-LSD (10 mg/kg i.p.) inhibited reserpine potentiation of hexobarbital hypnosis (SALMOIRAGHI et al., 1956). Inhibition of reserpine-induced hexobarbital potentiation by elymoclavine was reported by YUI and TAKEO (1958a).

BURTON et al. (1957) were the first to show that ergot derivatives counteracted behavioral depression induced in mice by a high dose (>10 mg/kg s.c.) of reserpine. These authors report that *d*-LSD inhibited the reserpine syndrome at doses from 1 to 10 mg/kg i.p., whereas *d*-lysergic acid monoethylamide (LAE 32, 73 h) was only active at a dose above 2.5 mg/kg i.p. 2-Br-LSD or *l*-lysergic acid diethylamide (61) showed virtually no antagonistic effect. Furthermore, BURTON et al. (1957) confirmed the results of TAESCHLER and CERLETTI (1957) by showing that *d*-LSD but not 2-Br-LSD counteracted reserpine-induced barbiturate hypnosis. SAAVEDRA and FISCHER (1970) report that both *d*-LSD (1 mg/kg i.p.) and methysergide (5 mg/kg i.p.) completely counteracted behavioral depression and locomotor inhibition of mice treated 24 h previously with 2 mg/kg i.p. reserpine. Elymoclavine and agroclavine at doses of 1–10 mg/kg i.p. were even more potent antagonists than *d*-LSD in mice which received 2.5 mg/kg i.p. reserpine 15 h previously. Lysergine and lysergene were about as active as *d*-LSD, whereas dihydroergokryptine was virtually inactive (YUI and TAKEO, 1958a). Behavioral depression induced by 5 mg/kg i.m. reserpine was also counteracted in cats by agroclavine or elymoclavine at doses of 0.2–0.5 mg/kg i.v. (YUI and TAKEO, 1958b). In addition, GARCIA LEME and ROCHA E SILVA (1963) reported that "analgesia" induced by 5 mg/kg i.p. reserpine, as measured by the hot-plate (55° C) method, was partially counteracted by 0.5 mg/kg i.p. *d*-LSD.

VOTAVA et al. (1967) investigated the interaction between various doses of *d*-LSD and reserpine (5 mg/kg s.c., 20 h previously). At the same time, brain concentrations of serotonin and catecholamines were measured. *D*-LSD at a dose of 0.1 mg/kg i.p. completely abolished blepharospasm and sedation induced by reserpine, but higher doses from 0.5–2 mg/kg i.p. elicited strong motor excitation and aggressiveness in reserpine-pretreated animals. Methysergide (2 mg/kg i.p.) only counteracted the behavioral depression and blepharospasm but did not produce the motor excitation observed after high doses of *d*-LSD and reserpine. At all doses the administration of *d*-LSD did not influence reserpine-induced depletion of brain serotonin, noradrenaline, or dopamine.

An increased responsiveness of reserpinized animals to *d*-LSD was also found by GRABOWSKA et al. (1974a) when studying locomotor activity of mice treated 20 h previously with 2.5 or 5 mg/kg s.c. reserpine. *D*-LSD at doses of 0.05 or 0.1 mg/kg i.p. did not affect locomotor activity, whereas 0.5 or 1 mg/kg i.p. stimulated locomotor activity. A similar effect was also mentioned by TAESCHLER and

CERLETTI (1957). Methysergide (5.0 mg/kg i.p.) partially suppressed blepharospasm of reserpine-treated animals but did not influence locomotor activity. The administration of haloperidol or pimozide (1.0 mg/kg i.p.) or spiroperidol (1.2 mg/kg i.p.), as opposed to α-adrenoceptor or serotonin receptor blocking agents, completely abolished this locomotor excitation produced by the combination of *d*-LSD and reserpine. Based on their observations, GRABOWSKA et al. (1974a) have suggested that locomotor stimulation induced by *d*-LSD in reserpinized mice might be due to a stimulation of brain dopamine receptors.

Based on the hypothesis that bromocriptine stimulated central dopaminergic receptors (JOHNSON et al., 1974, 1976) VIGOURET et al. (1978) investigated the effects of a number of ergot derivatives on akinesia which was induced by 5 mg/kg i.p. reserpine in mice. When administered 17 h after reserpine, bromocriptine, CF 25-397 (90d)[8] and CM 29-712 (8 epimer of 83b)[9] provided a strong and long-lasting suppression of reserpine akinesia (VIGOURET et al., 1978, Fig. 8). As reported earlier by CARLSSON et al. (1957), L-DOPA counteracted reserpine induced akinesia. In rats, VIGOURET et al. (1977) found a blockade of α-rigidity induced by 10 mg/kg i.v. reserpine when bromocriptine was administered 30 min later, in doses of 0.03 to 1 mg/kg i.v. (for further discussion, see Sec. D).

c) Reserpine-Induced Ponto-Geniculo-Occipital Waves

The occurrence of repetitive electrical potentials in pons, lateral geniculate body, and occipital cortex after reserpine administration to cats provides another model for the study of the interaction of ergot derivatives and reserpine. These so-called PGO waves occur just prior to and during rapid eye movement sleep in normal animals or can be induced independently of the sleep-wakefulness cycle by drugs which deplete the stores of catecholamines and particularly serotonin (DELORME et al., 1965, 1966; BROOKS and GERSHON, 1971). PGO waves seem to be triggered by a noradrenergic "pacemaker" located in the dorsolateral pontine tegmentum, possibly the medial part of the locus coeruleus. This pacemaker, in turn, is under inhibitory serotoninergic control (JOUVET, 1972). PGO waves can be induced outside of rapid eye movement sleep by the administration of reserpine or parachlorophenylalanine (PCPA), which deplete serotonin centrally, by methiothepin, a central 5-HT antagonist (MONACHON et al., 1972), or by the production of raphe lesions (SIMON et al., 1973). Furthermore, drug-induced PGO waves can be suppressed by the administration of 5-hydroxytryptophan (JOUVET, 1972).

As summarized in Table 2, a number of ergot derivatives have been reported to reduce PGO waves elicited by reserpine, PCPA, or the benzoquinolizine derivative Ro 4-1284 (2-hydroxy-2-ethyl-3-isobutyl-9,10-dimethoxy-1,2,3,4,6,7-hexahydro-11bH-benzo(a)quinolizine hydrochloride) (PLETSCHER et al., 1962). The most potent compounds were found to be lysergic acid derivatives, such as PTR 17-402 (88e), *d*-LSD, and CF 25-397 (90d). Higher doses of methysergide or 2-Br-LSD were required to reduce the number of PGO waves elicited by reserpine, PCPA (FROMENT and ESKAZAN, 1971), or Ro 4-1284 (RUCH-MONACHON et al., 1976b).

[8] CF 25-397 is 9,10 didehydro-6-methyl-8β-[2-pyridylthiomethyl] ergoline.

[9] 29-712 is 6-methyl-8α-cyanomethyl-ergoline-I.

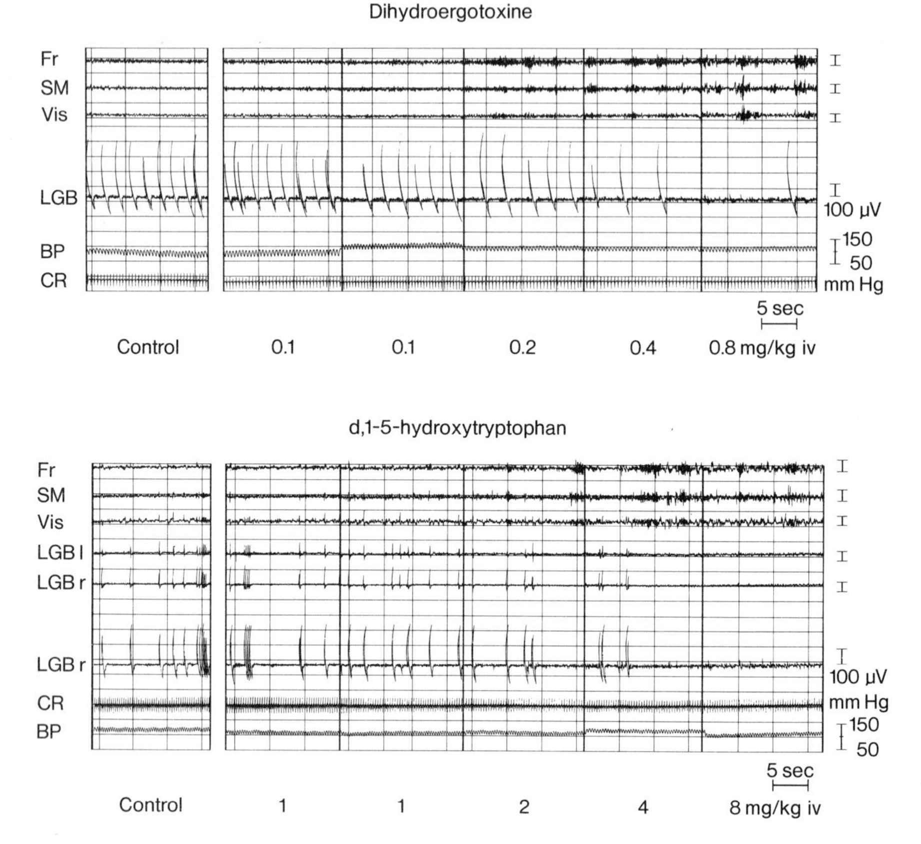

Fr: Frontal cortex
SM: Sensorimotor cortex
Vis: Visual cortex
LGB: Lateral geniculate body
BP: Blood pressure
CR: Cardiac rate
r: right
l: left

Fig. 2. Effects of dihydroergotoxine and of d,1,5-hydroxytryptophan on reserpine-induced ponto-geniculo-occipital waves in the cat. (From DEPOORTERE et al., 1975)

However, FROMENT and ESKAZAN (1971) found that effective doses of methysergide resulted in depression of reserpine-induced PGO waves which lasted longer than similarly effective doses of *d*-LSD. DEPOORTERE (1973) reported that low doses (0.05–0.3 mg/kg i.v.) of 2-Br-LSD increased reserpine-induced PGO waves. After administration of moderate doses of 2-Br-LSD, a short-lasting depression was followed by facilitation. Bromocriptine and a number of dihydrogenated ergopeptine derivatives have also been shown to inhibit reserpine-induced PGO waves (DEPOORTERE and MATEJCEK, 1973; DEPOORTERE et al., 1975; ZÜGER et al., 1978). In addition, RUCH-MONACHON et al. (1976b) reported that dihydroergotamine also reduces PGO density in animals treated with Ro 4-1284 or PCPA. As first shown by FROMENT and ESKAZAN (1971) for *d*-LSD, the reduction of the number of reserpine-induced PGO waves after administration of ergot derivatives was also accompanied by a reversal of the high-frequency, low-amplitude pattern in the electroencephalogram recorded from the cerebral cortex (DEPOORTERE, 1973; DEPOORTERE and MATĚJČEK, 1973; DEPOORTERE et al., 1975; ZÜGER et al., 1978). Figure 2 shows the effects of dihydroergotoxine as compared to those of 5-hydroxytryptophan on reserpine-induced PGO waves of the cat.

The inhibitory effect of ergot derivatives on drug-induced PGO waves can be reduced by methiothepin treatment. MONACHON et al. (1972) reported that 3 mg/kg i.v. methiothepin, besides increasing the frequency of PGO waves in control animals, prevented the inhibitory effect of 0.1 mg/kg i.v. *d*-LSD on PCPA-induced PGO waves. In reserpinized cats, ZÜGER et al. (1978) found that 10 mg/kg i.p. methiothepin reduced the inhibitory effect of dihydroergotoxine and shifted the dose-response curve to the right, in a way similar to the one of 5-hydroxytryptophan (Fig. 3). ZÜGER et al. (1978) were unable to influence the inhibitory effect of dihydroergotoxine by 10 mg/kg i.p. of either phenoxybenzamine or of pimozide. In agreement with earlier authors ZÜGER et al. (1978) point out that the inhibitory effect of ergot derivatives on drug-induced PGO waves may be primarily related to a restoration of the inhibitory serotoninergic control over the pontine pacemaker responsible for controlling the generation of PGO waves.

4. Anticonvulsant Effects

Early reports indicate that ergotamine and ergometrine raise the threshold for electrical convulsions and protect animals from the convulsive effects of seizure-inducing agents. HANZLIK et al. (1948) investigated the convulsive threshold to alternating current applied to the head of rabbits and rats. In the rabbit, s.c. administration of ergotamine (1.25 mg/kg) or ergometrine (0.05–0.1 mg/kg) raised the convulsive threshold by 30–40% and potentiated the effects of 25 mg/kg i.v. diphenylhydantoin. In the rat, i.p. administration of fluid extract of ergot induced a small rise of 12% in threshold. RIECHERT (1951) investigated the protective effects of 5 mg/kg i.m. ergotamine in rats receiving supramaximal doses of various convulsant agents and found that it protected the animals from the seizures induced by cocaine, novocaine, pantocaine, metrazol, nikethamide, and picrotoxine. Dihydroergotamine (1 mg/kg i.m.) also afforded protection against cocaine-induced convulsions. However, in patients, LOSCALZO (1937) was unable to prevent or control the frequency or severity of epileptic convulsions with a daily oral dose of 2–3 mg ergotamine. In cats treated with doses between 0.1 and 0.8 mg/kg s.c. or i.v., dihydroergotoxine afforded a protection from electroconvulsive shocks (JÖTTEN, 1951).

In the brain cortex of untreated animal controls decapitated 10 min after the last electroshock, JÖTTEN (1951) observed microscopic changes indicative of "capillary anemia", whereas animals receiving dihydroergotoxine showed a dilatation of capillary vessels. Ergotamine, at a dose of 0.6 mg/kg s.c., did not provide protection, despite the fact that the capillaries of brain cortex appeared dilated under the microscope.

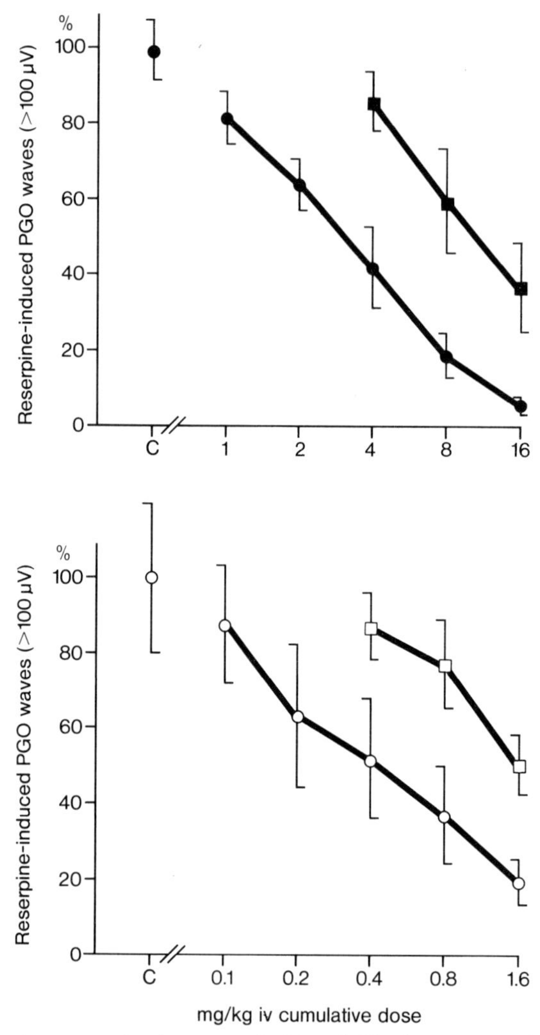

Fig. 3. Effects of dihydroergotoxine (open symbols) and 5-hydroxytryptophan (closed symbols) on ponto-geniculo-occipital waves induced by 0.5 mg/kg i.p. reserpine in the cat. Pretreatment with 10 mg/kg i.p. methiothepin (squares) reduced the inhibitory effects of both compounds. (From ZÜGER et al., 1978)

NAQUET and his collegues have carried out a number of studies on photically induced epilepsy in baboons (*Papio papio*) from the Casamance region of Senegal which, when exposed to intermittent light stimulation of 25 Hz, commonly show myoclonic responses and polyspikes and waves in the electroencephalogram, particularly in that recorded from the fronto-rolandic cortex (KILLAM et al., 1967; BALZANO et al., 1975). *D*-LSD (WALTER et al., 1971a, 1971b), methysergide, 2-Br-LSD and methergoline (MELDRUM and NAQUET, 1970, 1971), and ergotamine and methylergotmetrine (VUILLON-CACCIUTTOLO and BALZANO, 1972) were all found to abolish the clinical and electroencephalographic symptoms of photically induced epilepsy. No anticonvulsant effect was seen after lysergic acid or dihydroergotoxine. The results summarized in Table 1 indicate that the anticonvulsant effects are not necessarily related to behavioral depression or electroencephalographic signs of drowsiness. However, those ergot derivatives which abolished myoclonic and paroxysmal responses to light stimulation also reduced the amplitude of the first wave of the visual evoked response recorded from the occipital cortex or the lateral geniculate body, which would suggest that the reduction of photosensitivity seen after some ergot derivatives could be, at least in part, the result of impaired afferent transmission along the visual pathway (VUILLON-CACCIUTTOLO, 1970; WALTER et al., 1971a, b; MELDRUM and NAQUET, 1970, 1971; VUILLON-CACCIUTTOLO and BALZANO, 1972). In addition, MELDRUM et al. (1972) and WADA et al. (1972) reported that 5-hydroxytryptophan but not l-tryptophan reduced photosensitivity in baboons. On this basis, it was suggested that ergot derivatives block photically induced responses by acting synergistically with serotonin. However, based on the observation that the administration of apomorphine led to a reduction in myoclonic responses to light stimulation, MELDRUM et al. (1975) suggested that central dopamine receptors might be involved as well.

In 1961 KÄRJÄ et al. demonstrated an anticonvulsant effect of methysergide against 5-hydroxytryptophan-induced seizures in mice. Further studies on methysergide were reported by KLAWANS et al. (1973). These authors induced rhythmic myoclonus in guinea-pigs induced by s.c. injection of 300 mg/kg 5-hydroxytryptophan and found that methysergide blocked myoclonus without preventing the rise in whole brain serotonin following 5-hydroxytryptophan treatment. In contrast, after receiving single daily injections of 1 mg/kg s.c. methysergide, the animals' sensitivity to 5-hydroxytryptophan was increased, which was interpreted as "denervation supersensitivity at central serotonin receptors" (KLAWANS et al., 1975). In curarized cats, FANCHAMPS et al. (1960) found 5 mg/kg i.v. methysergide to reduce the convulsant effect of electrical stimulation. No protection from seizures induced by electroshock or metrazol was seen in mice. Only limited therapeutic success has been reported in man with methysergide in temporal lobe and other forms of epilepsy (SICUTERI and COSSIO, 1960; VIPARELLI et al., 1966; ARMBRUST-FIGUEIREDO, 1967).

Anticonvulsant effects of ergocornine (24) were studied by DOW et al. (1974). These authors produced epileptogenic lesions in the frontal motor cortex of rats by the implantation of cobalt pellets and found that ergocornine (2.5–10 mg/kg i.p.) suppressed firing from both primary and secondary foci. This effect could be reduced by prior administration of spiroperidol. ANLEZARK and MELDRUM (1975) administered ergocornine to an inbred DBA/2 strain of mice, which upon exposure to a loud noise showed a sequence of epileptic-like activity. In doses of 2–8 mg/kg i.p. ergocornine delayed the onset and abolished seizures. Protection against audiogenic seizures was also reported after the administration of bromocriptine, ergometrine, *d*-LSD, and methysergide (ANLEZARK et al., 1976) Doses of 1–5 mg/kg i.p. of *d*-LSD reduced audiogenic seizures in mice (LEHMANN, 1964), but only 0.18 mg/kg i.p. were required to facilitate learned inhibition of audiogenic seizure susceptibility (ROUSE and FRANK, 1974). ANLEZARK and MELDRUM (1975) and ANLEZARK et al. (1976) also have presented evidence that the effects of ergot derivatives on audiogenic seizures in mice and on cobalt-induced epilepsy in rats

Table 1. Effects of ergot derivatives on photically induced epilepsy: behavior and background EEG in the baboon

Code No	Compound (Dose mg/kg i.v.)	Myoclonic response	Paroxysmal EEG response	Behavior	Background EEG	Reference
73b	*d*-LSD (0.005–0.4)	Abolished at 0.04 mg/kg i.v.		Stupor, stereotyped behavior, akinesia, reduced aggression, mydriasis, salivation, increased heart rate	Increased frequency, decreased amplitude, spontaneous paroxysms abolished	WALTER et al. (1971a, b)
34a	Methysergide (0.5–5.0)	Abolished at 2–5 mg/kg i.v.		Somnolence and muscular hypotonia, salivation	Slowing, increased Delta waves mixed with fast activity, spikes, and waves	MELDRUM and NAQUET (1971)
37a	2-Br-LSD (1.0–4.0)	Abolished at 4 mg/kg i.v.		Somnolence and muscular hypotonia, salivation	Theta and Delta activity, spikes, and waves	MELDRUM and NAQUET (1970, 1971)
89d	Methergoline (0.5–4.0)	Abolished at 4 mg/kg i.v.		Somnolence and muscular hypotonia, salivation	EEG slowing	MELDRUM and NAQUET (1970, 1971)
8	Lysergic acid (0.1 and 2.0)	No effect		No effect	No effect	VUILLON-CACCIUTTOLO and BALZANO (1972)
—	Dihydroergotoxine (0.1–2.0)	No effect		Decreased heart rate, no change in behavior	No effect, facilitation of spontaneous paroxysms in 2/16 animals	VUILLON-CACCIUTTOLO and BALZANO (1972)
20	Ergotamine (0.1–0.3)	Abolished at 0.15 mg/kg i.v.		Decreased heart rate	Increased amplitude and frequency. Facilitation of spontaneous paroxysms	VUILLON-CACCIUTTOLO and BALZANO (1972)
73a	Methylergometrine (0.2–2.0)	Abolished at 0.4 mg/kg i.v.		Stupor, stereotyped behavior, akinesia, reduced aggression, mydriasis, salivation, decreased heart rate	Increased frequency, decreased amplitude, spontaneous paroxysms abolished	VUILLON-CACCIUTTOLO and BALZANO (1972)

Table 2. Inhibitory effect of ergot derivatives on PGO waves in the cat

Code No	Compound	PGO waves induced by	Approximate E.D.$_{50}$ mg/kg i.v.	References
73b	*d*-LSD	Reserpine	0.03	FROMENT and ESKAZAN (1971) ZÜGER et al. (1978)
		Ro 4-1284	0.05	JALFRE et al. (1970)
		PCPA	<0.1	RUCH-MONACHON et al. (1976a) RUCH-MONACHON et al. (1976b) FROMENT and ESKAZAN (1971)
37a	2-Br-LSD	Reserpine Ro 4-1284	1.5 0.5	DEPOORTERE (1973) RUCH-MONACHON et al. (1976a)
34a	Methysergide	Reserpine	— 0.4	FROMENT and ESKAZAN (1971) ZÜGER et al. (1978)
		Ro 4-1284 PCPA	0.15 —	RUCH-MONACHON et al. (1976a) FROMENT and ESKAZAN (1971)
88c	PTR 17-402	Reserpine	<0.01	ZÜGER et al. (1978)
90d	CF 25-397	Reserpine	0.06	ZÜGER et al. (1978)
8-Epimer of 83b	CM 29-712	Reserpine	0.5	ZÜGER et al. (1978)
38	Bromocriptine	Reserpine	2.0	ZÜGER et al. (1978)
102b	Dihydro-ergotamine	Reserpine	0.2	DEPOORTERE and MATEJCEK (1973) ZÜGER et al. (1978)
109b	Dihydro-β ergosine	Reserpine	0.2	ZÜGER et al. (1978)
102g	Dihydro-ergostine	Reserpine	1.4	ZÜGER et al. (1978)
110b	Dihydro-ergonine	Reserpine	0.6	ZÜGER et al. (1978)
—	Dihydro-ergotoxine	Reserpine	0.4	DEPOORTERE et al. (1975) ZÜGER et al. (1978)

are similar to those of apomorphine and are related to central dopamine receptor activation. DOW et al. (1974) have reported that apomorphine suppressed firing of cobalt-induced foci in the rat, and MCKENZIE and SOROKO (1972) found that apomorphine protected rats against maximal electroshock seizures.

5. Electroencephalogram

Effects of ergot derivatives on the animal electroencephalogram (EEG) have been mentioned previously when discussing ponto-geniculo-occipital waves induced by reserpine-like drugs in the rat and seizure activity in photosensitive baboons. Among the other EEG studies published, the largest number of papers concern *d*-LSD.

This material, recently reviewed by Bradley and Briggs (1974b), Goldstein (1975) and Sankar (1975), aims mostly at elucidating the neurophysiologic basis of hallucinations induced by *d*-LSD and will be discussed further in Chapter VIII of this volume (Fanchamps, 1978). However, a few authors have described such effects of *d*-LSD on the EEG which are shared by other nonhallucinogenic ergot derivatives and therefore will be included in this section. In addition to investigations on the spontaneous EEG and on the sleep-wakefulness cycle of undisturbed animals, a number of studies will be reviewed where the EEG was studied under defined pathologic conditions such as brain ischemia or hypoxemia.

a) Spontaneous Electronencephalogram

In their review of the effects of ergot derivatives on arousal and sleep, Bradley and Briggs (1974b) emphasize that *d*-LSD increases arousal levels and reflex responses to sensory stimuli probably by an action on the reticular formation of the lower brain stem. However, as seen from the electroencephalographic studies with ergot derivatives in the baboon (Table 1), not only *d*-LSD (Walter et al., 1971a, b) but also methylergometrine (Vuillon-Cacciuttolo and Balzano, 1972) elicited a low-voltage, high-frequency pattern typical of behavioral arousal. Brooks (1975), in his discussion of the effects of *d*-LSD on the cat EEG, points out that the low-frequency, high-voltage EEG reported by many authors is not merely a symptom of arousal. This pattern consists of 4–8 Hz activity which is always suppressed by visual stimuli and, in untreated animals, normally reflects a quiet resting behavioral state. Brooks (1975) has compared this pattern to human alpha activity. In the baboon methysergide, 2-Br-LSD and methergoline (Meldrum and Naquet, 1970, 1971) induced slow waves which were accompanied by behavioral depression (Table 1). Drowsiness and an increased amount of 4–6 Hz theta activity were reported by Feldman and Glaser (1963) in patients with vascular headaches of the migraine type upon i.v. administration of 2–4 mg of methysergide. In spite of these changes, therapeutic administration of a maximum daily oral dose of 4–8 mg methysergide over 4–8 months did not produce significant changes in the EEG recordings (Feldman and Glaser, 1963).

In the baboon (Table 1), ergotamine increased both amplitude and frequency, whereas lysergic acid and dihydroergotoxine were without an effect on the EEG (Vuillon-Cacciuttolo and Balzano, 1972).

Comparative studies carried out in the rabbit (Yui and Takeo, 1958b) show that agroclavine (0.05–0.2 mg/kg i.v.) or *d*-LSD (0.01–0.03 mg/kg i.v.) induced a disappearance of slow waves and spindles and elicited fast EEG activity which was not distinguishable from arousal produced by external stimulation. In contrast, dihydroagroclavine or dihydroelymoclavine (0.5–1 mg/kg i.v.) increased the amount of slow waves and spindles. This difference between the EEG effects of two nondihydrogenated ergot alkaloids and their dihydrogenated derivatives is in agreement with the observation that in most animal species, nondihydrogenated ergot derivatives are more likely to elicit behavioral stimulation, whereas dihydrogenated derivatives mostly induce slight depression of behavior.

In two studies carried out in the rat, the distribution of cortical EEG power in the different frequency bands was computed. During slow-wave sleep, DEPOORTERE and MATĚJČEK (1973) reported that 1 mg/kg i.p. dihydroergotamine increased total power and relative power in the delta and theta bands. At similar doses dihydroergotoxine and dihydro-β-ergosine (109b) increased total power in waking rats. In addition, dihydro-β-ergosine increased relative power in the theta and in the fast beta bands of the cortical EEG during wakefulness (CARRUTHERS-JONES et al., 1977). Although behavioral depression was noted after dihydro-β-ergosine, these changes in EEG power distribution were thought to reflect a change in alertness and attention.

In human volunteers, ITIL et al. (1975) found that the isoergolenyl derivative lisuride (96a) at oral doses of 0.025–0.1 mg induced a decrease of power in the low and very high frequency bands and an increase in the range of the 7.5–26.6 Hz bands. This effect was similar to the one observed after 10 mg amphetamine and was interpreted by ITIL et al. (1975) as an index of psychostimulation. In geriatric patients, quantitative EEG studies were carried out by MATĚJČEK and DEVOS (1976) and MATĚJČEK et al. (1976) during treatment with dihydroergonine (DN 16-457, 110b). A single i.v. dose of 0.2 mg increased the amplitude of the dominant frequency and the power in the alpha band of 6.5–12 Hz. At the same time, relative power in the delta band (1–3.5 Hz) was diminished. Treatment with an oral dose of 2.5 mg t.i.d. led to an acceleration of the dominant frequency. Similar changes in the EEG power distribution were reported by MATĚJČEK et al. (1976) after the administration of 1 mg i.v. or 2.5 mg t.i.d. p.o. of dihydroergostine (DE 145, 102 g). These results corroborate earlier conclusions reached by visual inspection of the EEG of geriatric patients treated with dihydroergotoxine (BORENSTEIN et al., 1969; HERZFELD et al., 1972; ROUBICEK et al., 1972; ARRIGO et al., 1973). According to these authors, the shift induced by dihydrogenated ergopeptine derivatives in the power distribution of the EEG was opposed to the EEG changes typical of senescence (MATĚJČEK and DEVOS, 1976) and corresponded to an improvement of symptoms of senile cerebral insufficiency.

b) Sleep-Wakefulness Cycle

In 1924–25, HESS reported that the intraventricular injection of 1 mg ergotamine in cats resulted in behavioral sleep. However, the results of studies published more recently indicate that when administered systemically, most ergot derivatives tend to reduce the amount of time spent in sleep and to prolong the duration of the waking states. LOEW et al. (1970) used behavioral criteria to assess the different stages of the sleep-wakefulness cycle of the rat and found that *d*-LSD (0.1 or 1 mg/kg i.p.) retarded the onset of all the sleep stages studied and enhanced the intensity of body movements during rapid eye movement (REM) sleep. Pretreatment with 2-Br-LSD (1 or 3 mg/kg i.p.) did not delay sleep onset but resulted in blockade of the effects of *d*-LSD on sleep latency. Thus, as opposed to the results of HESS (1925) with intracerebro-ventricular ergotamine, no evidence was found that i.p. *d*-LSD or 2-Br-LSD would prolong the duration of behavioral sleep.

Table 3. Effects of ergot derivatives on the sleep-wakefulness cycle in the rat

Code No	Compound (Dose mg/kg)	Route of adminis-tration	Duration of wakefulness	Duration of NREM sleep	Duration of REM sleep	Reference
73b	*d*-LSD					
	(1.0)	i.p.	+43%	−18%	−51%	Depoortere and Loew (1971)
61	*l*-Lysergic acid diethylamide					
	(1.0, 3.0)	i.p.	no effect	no effect	no effect	Depoortere and Loew (1972)
37a	2-Br-LSD					
	(3.0)	i.p.	no effect	+14%	−27%	Depoortere and Loew (1972)
90d	CF 25-397					
	(10.0)	p.o.	+25%	− 6%	−85%	Vigouret et al. (1977b)
38	Bromocriptine					
	(1.0)	i.p.	−28%	+18%	+46%	Loew and Spiegel (1976)
	(3.0)	i.p.	−10%	+ 6%	+16%	Loew and Spiegel (1976)
102b	Dihydroergotamine					
	(1.0)	i.p.	+54%	−21%	−51%	Depoortere and Matejcek (1972)
109b	Dihydro-β-ergosine					
	(1.0)	i.p.	+45%	−26%	−87%	Loew et al. (1976a)
	(3.0)	i.p.	+57%	−32%	−96%	Loew et al. (1976a)
102g	Dihydroergostine					
	(1.0)	i.p.	+38%	−14%	−29%	Loew et al. (1976a)
	(3.0)	i.p.	+67%	−15%	−81%	Loew et al. (1976a)
110b	Dihydroergonine					
	(1.0)	i.p.	+22%	− 7%	−45%	Loew et al. (1976a)
	(3.0)	i.p.	+31%	− 6%	−59%	Loew et al. (1976a)
—	Dihydroergotoxine					
	(1.0)	i.p.	+23%	−10%	−60%	Loew et al. (1976a, b)
	(3.0)	i.p.	+38%	−12%	−68%	Loew et al. (1976a, b)
	(10.0)	p.o.	+28%	−11%	−54%	Loew et al. (1976a, b)

When studying the effects of ergot derivatives on the sleep-wakefulness cycle of the rat, most authors recorded the EEG by means of chronically implanted cortical electrodes. In the studies contained in Table 3, the recordings were carried out for 6 h during the light part of a controlled light/darkness cycle. The ergot derivatives were administered 15 min before the onset of the recording period, and the effects were compared to solvent control experiments carried out on the preceding day.

The results summarized in Table 3 indicate that in the rat, *d*-LSD 2-Br-LSD, CF 25-397, and a number of dihydrogenated ergot derivatives reduced the amount of time spent in REM and, to some extent, in nonrapid eye movement (NREM) sleep. Concomitantly, the time spent awake was prolonged. After the administration of 1 mg/kg i.p. of dihydroergotamine to rats, DEPOORTERE and MATĚJČEK (1973) reported that the dominant frequency during wakefulness and NREM sleep was increased, whereas total electrical energy was decreased during wakefulness and increased during NREM sleep. An enhancement of the frequency of hippocampal theta activity occurred after s.c. infusions of 0.125 mg/kg *d*-LSD into rats during REM sleep (BILKOVA et al., 1971a, b). Further studies with 2-Br-LSD indicated that the time of administration may be critical for the effects observed. With a pretreatment time of 15 min, 3 mg/kg i.p. 2-Br-LSD slightly, but significantly enhanced the duration of NREM sleep (DEPOORTERE and LOEW, 1972). When 2-Br-LSD was administered once, 3 h before the experiment, or twice, 3 and 27 h before the experiment, the duration of NREM sleep was decreased without any significant effect on REM sleep. As opposed to the other ergot derivatives studied, bromocriptine increased the time spent in NREM and REM sleep (LOEW and SPIEGEL, 1976). Similar experiments were carried out by TABUSHI and HIMWICH (1971) with 1 and 4 mg/kg i.v. methysergide in the rabbit. These authors found that methysergide markedly delayed or abolished REM sleep, increased the duration of wakefulness, and decreased the duration of NREM sleep. As reported in the rat (Table 3) for dihydrogenated ergot derivatives, the effects of methysergide in the rabbit were found to be dose-dependent. In the cat, HOBSON (1964) found that 2 or 20 μg/kg i.p. of *d*-LSD reduced the amount of REM sleep. However, this author did not find a consistent effect on the duration of wakefulness. In the same species FROMENT and ESKAZAN (1971) found that *d*-LSD (10–160 μg/kg i.v.) or methysergide (0.5–10 mg/kg i.v.) induced a dose-dependent suppression of REM sleep. BALDY-MOULINIER et al. (1969) have also reported that dihydroergotoxine enhanced the duration of wakefulness at the expense of NREM sleep in the cat. In patients, methysergide induced insomnia as a side effect (FRIEDMAN and ELKIND, 1963). In human volunteers, a total oral dose of 16 mg, evenly distributed over 48 h, was found to shorten REM time by 36%. This effect was accompanied by a small increase in NREM time. However, no changes in total sleep time or sleep latency were observed (MENDELSON et al., 1975). After a daily oral dose of 4 or 6 mg over 6 or 4 days, respectively, PACK and SCHMIDT (1972) reported an increase in REM latency and a decrease in REM time. In addition, during REM sleep, these authors found a shift to the lighter stages as the deeper stages were suppressed. WYLER et al. (1975) studied five narcoleptic patients with diurnal REM sleep verified by EEG investigations. After treatment with an oral daily dose of 2 or 4 mg methysergide, these patients obtained good control of their sleep attacks. However, MUZIO et al. (1966) report that *d*-LSD at a single oral dose of 0.08–0.73 μg/kg, given to volunteers, increased the duration of the first and the second REM period and induced a reverse rebound effect in the second half of the night. Similar effects were reported by HARTMANN (1967) after the administration of 2.5–10 μg/kg of *d*-LSD to rats. No pronounced effects of 2 mg p.o. bromocriptine were observed by LOEW and SPIEGEL (1976) in a polygraphic sleep study carried out in human volunteers.

The typical response reported after the administration of *d*-LSD, 2-Br-LSD, and a number of dihydrogenated ergot derivatives to rats (Table 3), methysergide to rabbits, cats, and humans (TABUSHI and HIMWICH, 1971; FROMENT and ESKAZAN, 1971; MENDELSON et al., 1975; WYLER et al., 1975), of *d*-LSD or dihydroergotoxine to cats (HOBSON, 1964; BALDY-MOULINIER et al., 1969) consisted of a shortening of the REM stage and a possible shift from the deeper sleep stages to lighter sleep and wakefulness. In discussing such an effect of ergot derivatives (which is particularly well documented for methysergide), TABUSHI and HIMWICH (1971), MENDELSON et al. (1975), and WYLER et al. (1975) suggested that it may be related to an antagonistic action of methysergide at central serotonin receptor sites. However, comparative studies carried out in the rat reveal a striking similarity between the action of 5-hydroxytryptophan and dihydrogenated ergot derivatives on the sleep-wakefulness cycle (LOEW et al., 1976 a, b). These authors, therefore, proposed that this action would be due to a stimulation rather than an antagonism at central serotonin receptor sites.

c) Electroencephalogram Under Defined Pathologic Conditions

Interest in the pharmacologic effects of ergot derivatives on the brain under defined pathologic conditions increased following several reports indicating that some ergot derivatives provided a therapeutic benefit to patients suffering from senile cerebral insufficiency (VENN, 1978, Chapter VII of this volume). In one of the first papers on the effects of dihydroergotoxine in patients suffering from chronic peripheral vascular diseases, POPKIN (1951) found an "improved sense of well being" in about one-quarter of the older age group. As a consequence of this finding and similar studies, animal models of impaired brain function were developed for determining whether ergot derivatives would increase the brain's resistance to noxious conditions, e.g., hypoxia or ischemia (MEIER-RUGE, 1976). In order to indicate changes in overall function of these experimental preparations, metabolic parameters (see Section F of this chapter) or the measurement of spontaneous or evoked electrical activity of the brain were used. In some experiments the concomitant changes in cerebral blood flow were also assessed (see following Section).

The extensive studies carried out in cats treated with dihydrogenated ergot derivatives were recently summarized by MEIER-RUGE et al. (1975). As a model

Fig. 4. Effects of an i.v. infusion of physiologic saline (50–70 min) on cortical blood flow ▷ (CBF) and EEG power under conditions of oligemic hypotension in cats. (From GYGAX et al., 1978)

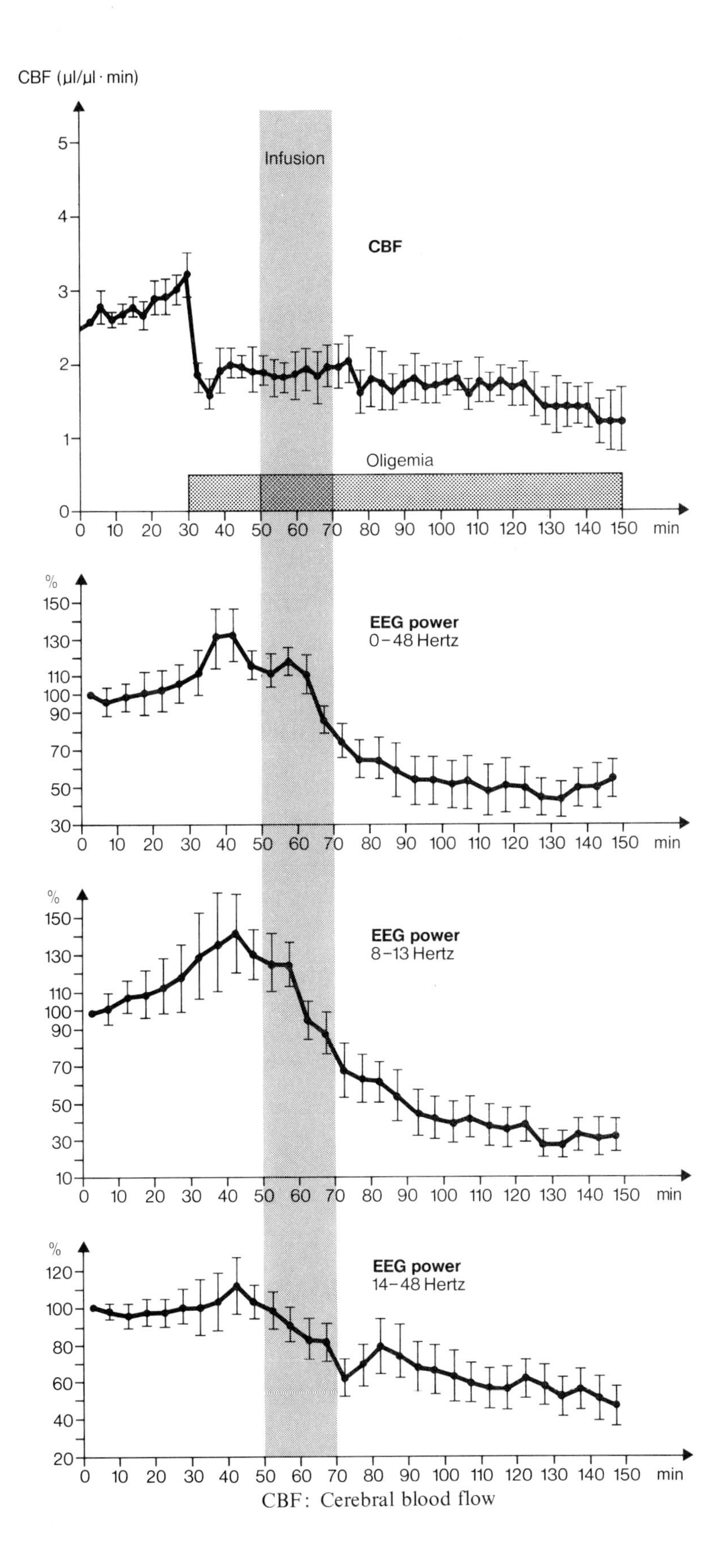

CBF: Cerebral blood flow

of impaired brain function, oligemic hypotension (GYGAX et al., 1973, 1974), temporary ischemia (CERLETTI et al., 1973; EMMENEGGER et al., 1973b), or hypothermia (EMMENEGGER and MEIER-RUGE, 1968; EMMENEGGER et al., 1973a) in cats was used. EEG was recorded from the brain cortex and the power spectra were calculated.

Intravenous infusion of 80 μg/kg dihydroergotoxine administered over 20 min prevented the decline of total power of the EEG recorded from the frontal and the occipital cortex of cats subjected to oligemic hypotension under a light nitrous oxide anesthesia. A significant effect in the same direction was also seen in the alpha (8–13 Hz) and the beta (14–48 Hz) bands (Figs. 4 and 5). In contrast, dihydroergotoxine did not alter the experimentally reduced cortical blood flow in these preparations as measured by the ^{2}H-clearance technique of STOSSECK et al. (1974) (GYGAX et al., 1975, 1976, 1978). In an isolated cat head preparation, the reduction in EEG power brought about by ischemia was counteracted by an i.v. infusion of 80 μg dihydroergotoxine or of 6 μg dihydroergonine (CERLETTI et al., 1973; EMMENEGGER et al., 1973a). Using hypothermia, EMMENEGGER and MEIER-RUGE (1968) reported a partial recovery in electrical activity of the cat EEG after a total i.v. dose of 160 μg dihydroergotoxine. In subsequent experiments EMMENEGGER et al. (1973b) found that a lowering of the body temperature of the cat to 30° C led to a reduction of EEG power in the alpha and beta bands, which could be partially counteracted by dihydroergotoxine.

In an isolated dog brain preparation in situ, BENZI et al. (1971) reported that an infusion of nicergoline (104e) into the superior thyroid artery (5×10^{-5} M, 0.5 ml/min for 30 min) tended to partially reverse the EEG changes caused by halting the respiratory pump. Similar effects of dihydroergotoxine had been reported previously by BALDY-MOULINIER and PASSOUANT (1967).

Drug-induced changes in the amplitude of a cortical potential evoked in the sigmoid gyrus by stimulation of the interdigital space of the forepaw of the cat have been reported during recovery from ischemia (STREICHENBERGER et al., 1970). The drugs were administered into the carotid artery of one side, the other side being treated with solvent. Nicergoline (20–400 μg), ergotamine (2 and 6 μg), dihydroergocornine (0.5 μg), dihydroergokryptine (2–20μg), and dihydroergotoxine (6 and 20 μg) accelerated the recovery of the evoked potential on the treated side, as compared to the untreated side. None of these compounds, when aministered without previous ischemia, changed the amplitude of the potentials (BOISMARE et al., 1970; BOISMARE and STREICHENBERGER, 1973, 1974; BOISMARE and MICHELI, 1974; BOISMARE and LORENZO, 1975). Under the experimental conditions used, these effects of nicergoline increased with the dose over a range of 20–200 μg (BOISMARE and LORENZO, 1975), whereas the other ergot derivatives, at higher doses, tended to prolong recovery time. Dihydroergocristine was inactive at doses from 2 to 100 μg (BOISMARE and MICHELI, 1974). Intracarotid administration of

Fig. 5. Effects of an i.v. dihydroergotoxine infusion (80 μg/kg, 50–70 min) on cerebral blood flow (CBF) and EEG power under condition of oligemic hypotension. (From GYGAX et al., 1978) ▷

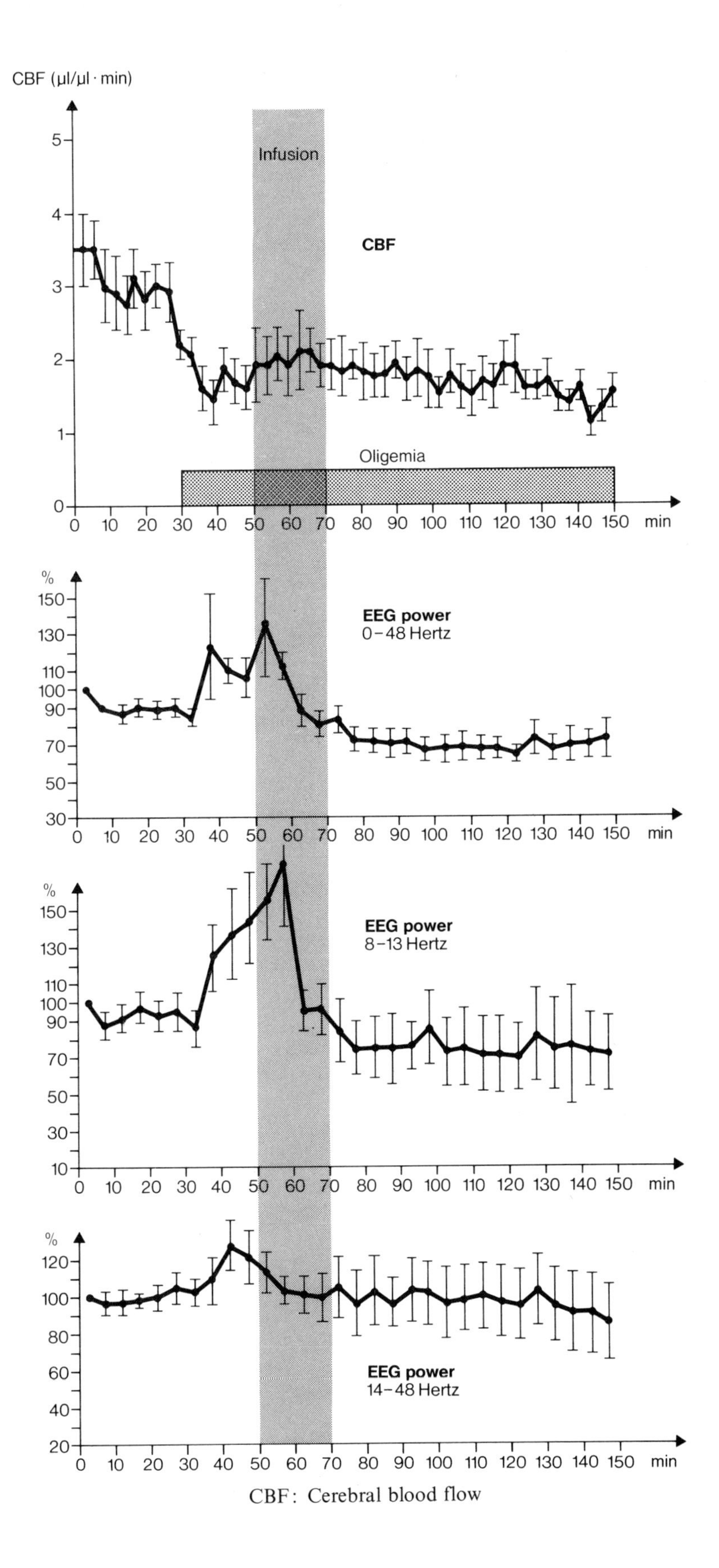

CBF: Cerebral blood flow

sodium malonate but not of trimethadione blocked the effects of nicergoline (BOISMARE and LORENZO, 1975) and of dihydroergotoxine (BOISMARE and MICHELI, 1974). These authors concluded that the acceleration of the recovery from ischemia under treatment with ergot derivatives did not result from an increase in cerebral blood flow, since maximal vasodilatation was already induced by the hypercapnia due to hypoventilation.

Similar studies were carried out by ROSSIGNOL et al. (1972) and by PERRAULT et al. (1976) in cats subjected to ischemia. These authors report that dihydroergotoxine (0.3 and 0.6 mg/kg i.v.) shortened recovery times of evoked potentials in the posteroventral thalamus and of the indirect corticopyramidal response.

6. Cerebral Blood Flow

Studies on the action of ergot derivatives on cerebral blood flow (CBF) have long attracted attention, since it was assumed that ergopeptine derivatives, particularly the dihydrogenated compounds, would cause cerebral vasodilatation by virtue of their α-adrenergic blocking properties (ROTHLIN, 1946/47). Some of their effects on extracranial and intracranial regional blood flow are discussed in Chapter V of this volume (CLARK et al., 1978). In this chapter only those studies of CBF in animals which are pertinent to the interpretation of the therapeutic action of ergot derivatives in patients suffering from senile cerebral insufficiency will be reviewed. For a discussion of clinical studies see VENN (1978), Chapter VII of this volume.

Before reviewing the results of drug studies on CBF, a short comment on the methods for measuring CBF and on its regulation is required. Mean total CBF can be measured based on the Fick principle, by the nitrous oxide technique of KETY and SCHMIDT (1945), or by radioisotope and thermal clearance techniques. Radioisotope clearance is particularly useful in the measurement of regional CBF (INGVAR and LASSEN, 1961). In general, similar techniques are applied for CBF assessment in human and animal studies.

When studying changes in CBF, it should be borne in mind that, despite fluctuations in systemic blood pressure, total blood supply to the brain is maintained within narrow limits by a process called autoregulation. It is thought that autoregulation involves changes in the calibers of both extraparenchymal and intraparenchymal vessels (HARPER, 1966; HARPER et al., 1972; JAMES, 1975). Regional distribution of flow appears to be controlled by changes in the diameter of the arterioles containing muscles which respond to adrenergic nerve impulses and to changes in local concentrations of CO_2. Distribution within the capillary network depends mainly on the metabolic state of the surrounding brain tissue (SEVERINGHAUS et al., 1971/72; RAICHLE et al., 1976). It thus appears that physiologic, pathologic, and pharmacologic stimuli, when provided alone or in combination, will first influence regional CBF before altering total CBF.

In normal anesthetized animals, ergot derivatives have little effect on total CBF. Equivocal results have been reported for the actions of ergotamine (ABREU

Fig. 6. Effects of an i.v. papaverine infusion (1 mg/kg 50–70 min) on cerebral blood flow (CBF) and EEG power under conditions of oligemic hypotension. (From GYGAX et al., 1978) ▷

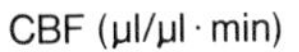

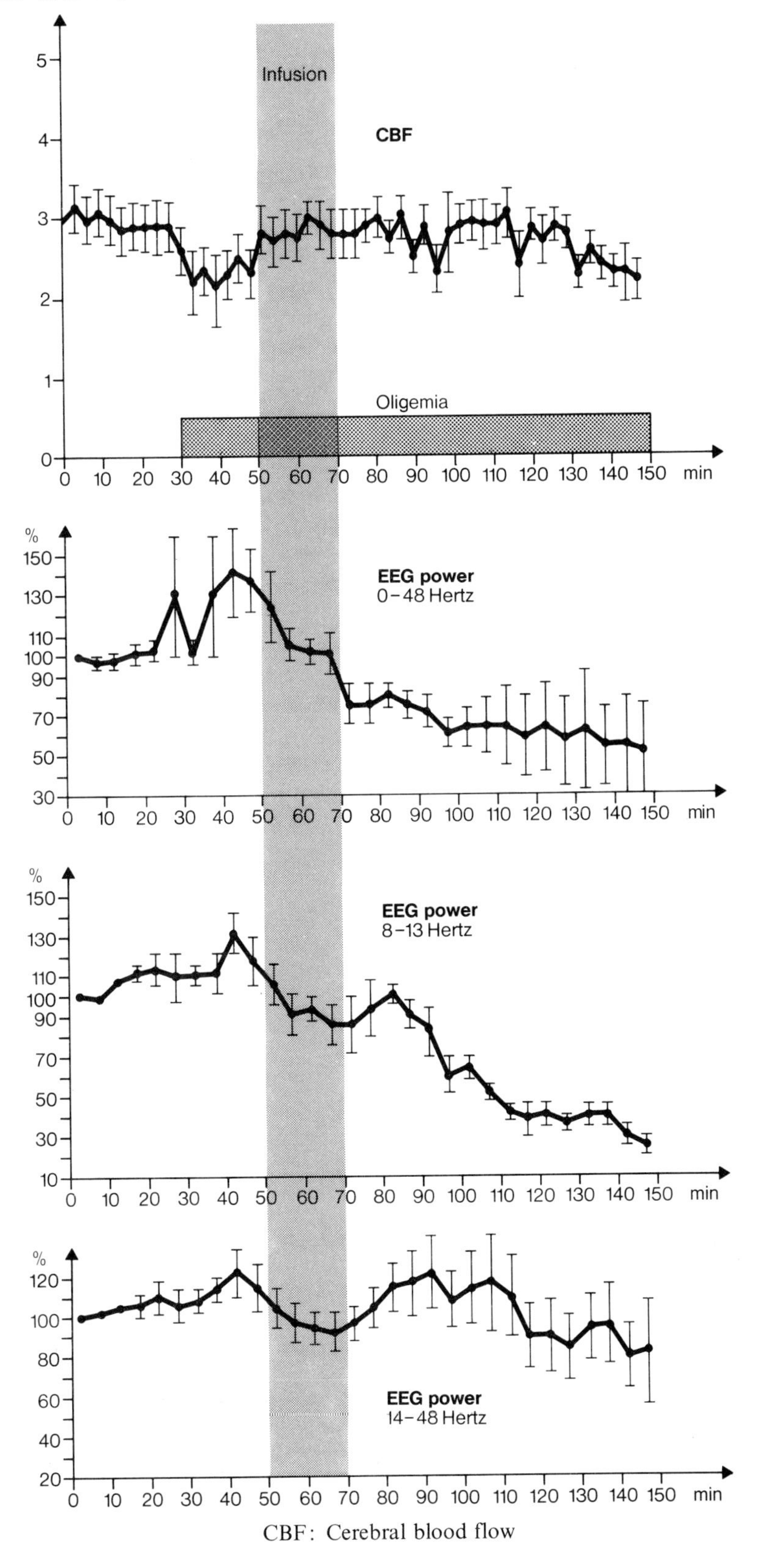

CBF: Cerebral blood flow

et al., 1947; LUBSEN, 1949), dihydroergotamine (ABREU et al., 1947), and dihydroergotoxine (ROTHLIN and TAESCHLER, 1951; SCHNEIDER and WIEMERS, 1951; TAESCHLER et al., 1952; LUDWIGS and SCHNEIDER, 1954; LABORIT et al., 1965; SZEWCZYKOWSKI et al., 1970). Using regional blood flow measurements, KNAPP et al. (1955/56) found that dihydroergotoxine (0.025–0.25 μg/kg into the internal carotid artery of the cat) increased the clearance of ^{131}I or ^{22}Na when injected into the internal capsule. POURRIAS and RAYNAUD (1972) reported an increased cortical blood flow in rabbits, measured by an intracortical thermoelement after the administration of 0.25 mg/kg i.v. dihydroergotoxine. BALDY-MOULINIER and PASSOUANT (1967) and BALDY-MOULINIER (1968), using ^{85}Kr clearance in the cat, were unable to confirm these results. No change was found in microflow within the occipital cortex of the cat after an intracarotid administration of 0.15 or 0.3 mg dihydroergotoxine. However, when cortical microflow was reduced by hyperventilation, ischemia, or cerebral edema, treatment with 0.15 mg dihydroergotoxine counteracted the reduction.

Intravenous ergotamine or dihydroergotoxine did not increase the cerebral blood flow in brains of cats made ischemic by occlusion of one A. cerebri media (REGLI and WALTZ, 1971; REGLI et al., 1971). Similarly, nicergoline was found to have no clear action on cortical or total CBF in normal cats and pigs or in an isolated perfused hypoxic dog brain preparation (BIENMÜLLER and BIETZ, 1972; BENZ et al., 1973).

A series of carefully controlled studies on the effects of dihydroergotoxine on cortical microflow in cats subjected to oligemic hypotension were reported by GYGAX et al. (1975, 1976, 1978). After lowering mean arterial blood pressure to 45 mm Hg, i.e., below the threshold of autoregulation, those authors found cortical microflow as measured by the local ^{2}H microclearance technique of STOSSECK et al. (1974) to be reduced by about 30%. Under a barbiturate anesthesia with 40 mg/kg i.p. pentobarbital sodium, no change in EEG power was observed (GYGAX et al., 1973), whereas under a superficial nitrous oxide anesthesia, the power of the EEG was reduced by oligemic hypotension (Fig. 4) (GYGAX et al., 1974, 1975, 1976, 1978). Under these conditions, an i.v. infusion of 80 μg/kg dihydroergotoxine did not alter the reduced cortical microflow, but EEG power increased (Fig. 5). The administration of papaverine (1 mg/kg) prevented the decline in microflow without significantly changing EEG power (Fig. 6). Under identical conditions WIERNSPERGER et al. (1978) measured cortical tissue pO_2 with a polarographic gold microelectrode technique and reported that oligemia increased the frequency of low pO_2 values at the expense of the higher pO_2 values (Fig. 7). Dihydroergotoxine reduced the frequency of low pO_2 values in the oligemic cat's cortex, whereas after papaverine treatment, the pO_2 histograms were flattened (Fig. 7).

In cats showing similar reductions in cortical microflow during oligemic hypotension, HUNZIKER et al. (1974b) analyzed the shapes of cortical capillary vessels by electronic image processing and found a reduced diameter, an increased surface/volume ratio, and prolongation of capillary length per unit brain volume. After treatment with 80 μg/kg i.v. dihydroergotoxine, a significant increase in diameter and a reduction in capillary length was found. No changes were seen after the administration of 1 mg/kg papaverine (HUNZIKER et al., 1974a; MEIER-RUGE et al., 1975; GYGAX et al., 1975). However, these morphometric studies were carried out under pentobarbitone anesthesia.

When discussing the results of their studies with dihydroergotoxine on the electrical activity and on cerebral microflow in cats subjected to oligemic hypotension, GYGAX et al. (1978) and WIERNSPERGER et al. (1978) concluded that the primary effect of ergot derivatives on impaired brain function does not appear to be related to total or regional blood flow. Similar conclusions have been reached by BENZI et al. (1971, 1972, 1973) and BENZI (1975), who investigated the effects of nicergoline in an hypoxic isolated dog brain preparation. Although the evidence is limited that nicergoline or dihydroergotoxine enhance total or regional CBF under the conditions of acute animal experiments, it will be seen in Section F of this chapter that both compounds have actions on brain metabolism, particularly under conditions of hypoxia or ischemia. Thus, MEIER-RUGE et al. (1975) proposed that the partial protection provided by dihydroergotoxine from some of the consequences of temporary ischemia, as seen in the EEG or in the distribution of local pO_2 concentrations, may result from an "improving" effect of the drug

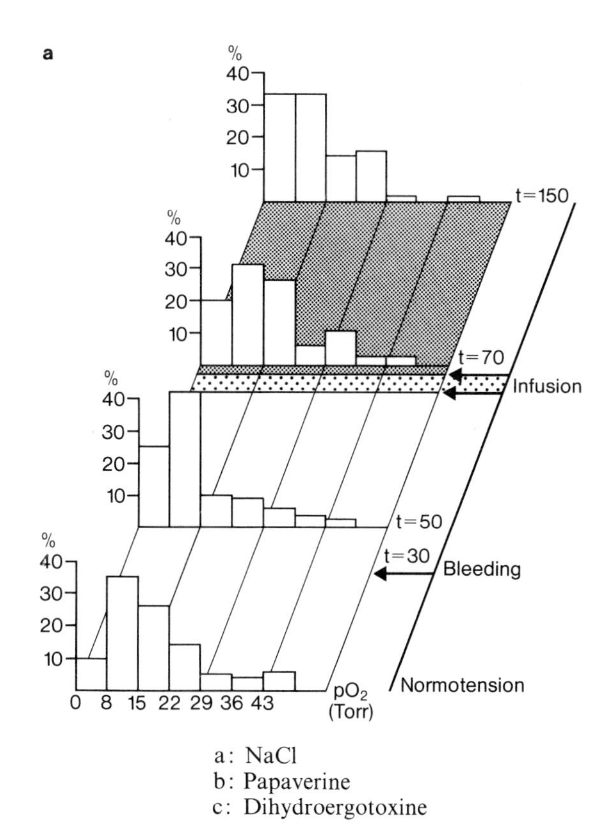

a: NaCl
b: Papaverine
c: Dihydroergotoxine

Fig. 7a–c. Effects of i.v. infusions of physiologic saline (*a*), papaverine (1 mg/kg) (*b*), and dihydroergotoxine (80 μg/kg) (*c*) on cortical O_2 pressure in cats before (normotension) and during oligemic hypotension in cats. (From WIERNSPERGER et al., 1978)

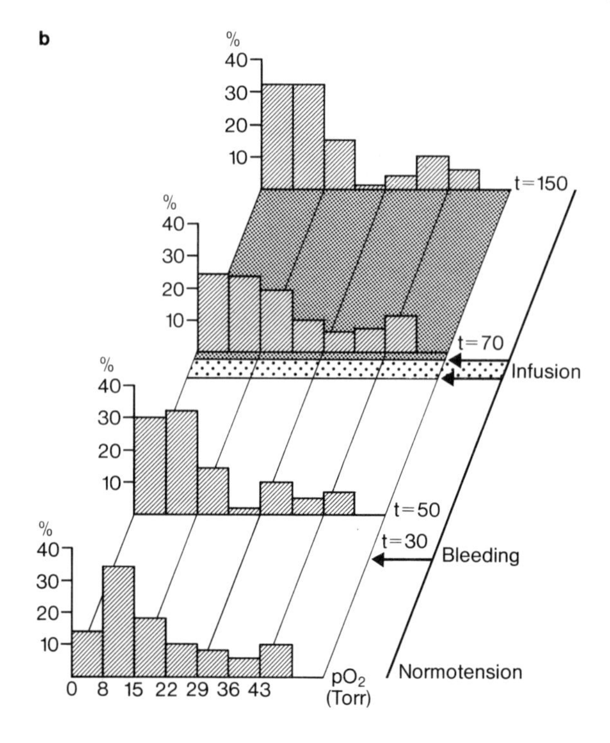

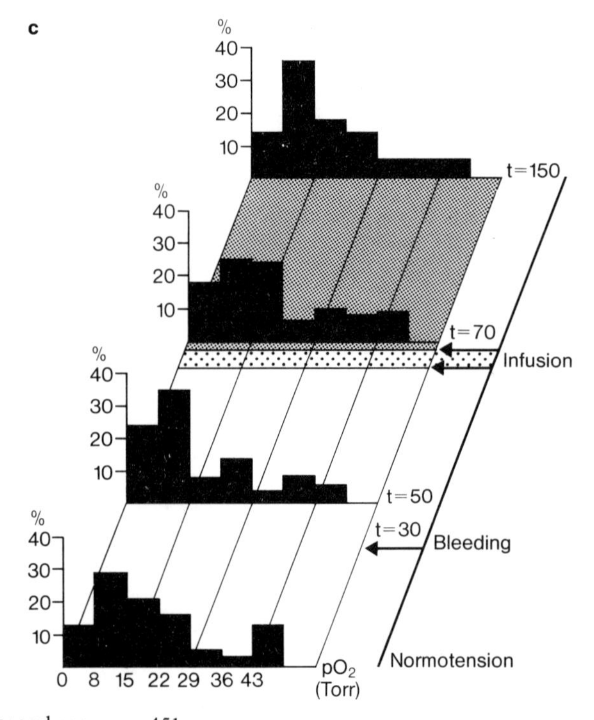

Fig. 7 (cont.). Legend see page 451

on brain metabolism. This may allow the neuronal cell to maintain a functional steady state, even under conditions when its metabolic tolerance is limited. Such a view is also consistent with the observations of HERZFELD et al. (1972) and of MONGEAU (1974) that in patients suffering from senile cerebral insufficiency, dihydroergotoxine increases CBF only when administered over a prolonged period of time.

7. Body Temperature

Effects of ergot preparations on body temperature were already known at the end of the last century. The work of BARGER and DALE (1907), however, for the first time in this century focused attention on rapid ergotoxine-induced hyperthermia in rabbits. Similar observations were reported by MICULICICH (1912) and by CLOETTA and WASER (1915), but the first extensive investigation of this phenomenon was the work of GITHENS (1917) on the effects of s.c. and i.v. injections of ergotoxine phosphate into rabbits, cats, rats, mice, and pigeons. Out of 10 rabbits receiving 2 mg/kg i.v. of ergotoxine, eight survivors showed an average temperature rise of 3.4° to between 42° and 42.5° C; temperature was highest from 2 to 2.5 h after the injection and became normal again in 6–8 h. The other two rabbits showed a more rapid rise to 43.6° and died. Subcutaneous injections produced similar results more slowly. Most of this hyperthermia in the rabbit was considered to be the result of muscle tremor during ergot poisoning, since it could be limited to an average increase of 0.6° C by prior immobilization with curare. However, since sectioning the spinal cord abolished hyperthermia without affecting muscle tremor after 2 mg/kg i.v. of ergotoxine, GITHENS suggested that ergot-induced hyperthermia was caused by a direct action of ergotoxine on a central "heat regulating center." In contrast, ergotoxine produced hypothermia in rats (1–4 mg/kg s.c.), in mice (2 mg/kg s.c.), and in pigeons. Thus, from these early studies it became clear that changes in body temperature induced by ergot are but one symptom of a behavioral syndrome comprising inter alia motor phenomena. In addition, differential responses of various animal species to a given ergot preparation were already noted.

a) Ambient Temperature

Subsequent investigations of the effects of various ergot compounds, including ergotamine and ergometrine, on rabbit temperature made by ROTHLIN (1923), RIGLER and SILBERSTERN (1927), BRINK and RIGLER (1929), SAWYER and SCHLOSSBERG (1933), ROTHLIN (1933, 1935, 1936, 1938), and VARTIAINEN et al. (1937) all suffered from an inadequate control of environmental temperature. WHITE (1944a) found the mouse to be a more suitable species in which ergotoxine, ergosine, ergotamine, ergosinine, and ergometrine lowered rectal temperature, whereas ergotinine, ergotaminine, and lysergic acid were inactive at the doses studied. Based on a survey of the literature, WHITE (1944a) considered the temperature effects of ergot preparations to be a symptom of acute ergot poisoning and proposed the involvement of hypothalamic substrates. Referring to ergometrine he noted that peripheral "sympathetic paralysis is not a necessary component of central effects."

The mechanisms involved in temperature changes have been studied by MARINE et al. (1927), FÖRSTER (1935), DIMITRIJEVIC (1937), BUCHANAN et al. (1948, 1950), and ROBERTS et al. (1949). After treating rats at ambient temperatures above 28° C with 4.5 mg/kg i.p. ergotoxine, ROBERTS et al. (1949) reported a rise in rectal temperature which was accompanied by peripheral vasoconstriction and increased oxygen consumption. They concluded that this temperature rise was caused by a diminution of heat loss and an enhanced heat production and involved central mechanisms. In young rats of 20–28 days of age and in older rats primarily exposed to or transferred to an ambient temperature of 5–8° C, rectal temperature was lowered by treatment with 4.5 mg/kg i.p. of ergotoxine. The effect was accompanied by peripheral vasodilatation and decreased oxygen consumption. These studies indicate that the direction of these temperature changes observed results not only from the particular ergot derivative and the dose administered but also from species, age, and the ambient temperature.

b) Controlled Experiments in the Rabbit

In our laboratories, the effects of a large number of ergot derivatives on rabbit rectal temperature have been investigated under standard conditions, and some of these results are included in this section. The method used for the determination of rabbit body temperature in our laboratories was as follows:

Rabbits (mixed breeds or hare-type or Yellow-Silver) of both sexes were housed in individual cages. Room temperature was kept constant at $25 \pm 3°$ C. During the experiment all food was withheld from the animals, but free access to water was allowed. Syringes, needles, and glassware were rendered free from pyrogens according to USP XVIII. A thermocouple probe was inserted into the rectum of the test animal to a depth of not less than 6 cm, and the body temperature of the animal was recorded. Thirty minutes prior to and immediately before the i.v. injection of the test dose, the control temperature of each animal was determined. The injection volume was kept between 1 and 3 ml/kg. The average number of rabbits used per dosage group was six. Temperature was recorded at 0.5, 1, 1.5, 6, and 8 h following injection. From the individual temperature readings of the animals in each dosage group, an individual temperature curve was drawn, which was superposed on a standard temperature curve which reflected the circadian rhythm of body temperature in 18 control rabbits. Superposition was done in such a way that the control temperatures of both the test curve and the standard curve were as close together as possible. Finally the maximum deviation of each individual temperature curve from the standard curve was read for each animal and the mean was calculated.

Table 4 summarizes the results of these investigations on rabbit rectal temperature. In a separate column i.v. LD_{50}'s are indicated. The method used for the determination of LD_{50}'s is described in Chapter XII of this volume (GRIFFITH, 1978). It can be seen that all but one (nicergoline) simple lysergic acid derivative increased rectal temperature. Whereas most ergopeptine derivatives caused a rise in temperature, all dihydrogenated peptide derivatives investigated lowered rabbit

Table 4. Effect of ergot derivatives on rabbit body temperature

Code No	Compound	Direction of temperature change	Dose (mg/kg i.v.) changing temperature by		LD_{50} mg/kg i.v.
			0.5°C	1.0°C	
Simple lysergic acid derivatives					
5	Agroclavine	↗		<0.3	<1
—	Elymoclavine	↗	0.05		1.2
19	Ergometrine	↗		0.24	3.2
73a	Methylergometrine	↗	0.05	0.22	2
73b	*d*-LSD	↗	0.00033	0.0031	0.31
34a	Methysergide	↗	13.4	19.0	28
104e	Nicergoline	↗	0.4		
		↙	1.5–4.4		28.5
88e	PTR 17-402	↗	0.038	0.078	1.2
Ergopeptine derivatives					
20	Ergotamine	↗	0.68	0.9	3
34c	*l*-Methylergotamine	↗	1.1	2.1	21
21	Ergosine	↗	0.53	0.78	1.23
22	Ergostine	↗		1.0	
		↙	0.03–0.6		1.2
110a	Ergonine	↗	0.14	0.23	1.1
23	Ergocristine				1.9
24	Ergocornine	↗	0.025	0.1	
38	Bromocriptine	↗	0.75	1.2	12
26	β-Ergokryptine	↗		0.22	0.78
108a	Ergovaline	↗	0.26	0.46	1.7
Dihydrogenated ergopeptine derivatives					
102b	Dihydroergotamine	↙	0.7	2.0	37
102a	Dihydroergosine	↙	0.25	1.6	21
102g	Dihydroergostine	↙	0.34		12.5
110b	Dihydroergonine	↙	0.5	3.6	19
102c	Dihydroergocristine	↙	0.25	2.0	33.2
102d	Dihydroergocornine	↙	0.65	1.9	34.5
108b	Dihydroergovaline	↙	0.34	3.4	19
—	Dihydroergotoxine	↙	0.4	3.0	18.5

rectal temperature. Among the *lysergic acid derivatives*, *d*-LSD was found to be the most potent compound. The ratios LD_{50}/dose required to increase rectal temperature by 0.5 or 1.0° C were 1000 and 100, respectively. Such high ratios indicate that a rise of temperature was induced by a dose of *d*-LSD much lower than the lethal dose. Thus, this effect of *d*-LSD appears to be specific. With other lysergic acid derivatives, e.g., elymoclavine, methylergometrine, and PTR 17-402 (88e), smaller ratios were found. In the group of *ergopeptine derivatives* which caused a rise in body temperature, the active doses were closer to the lethal dose range. Thus, our results agree with earlier reports which indicated that hyperthermic effects of ergopeptine derivatives in the rabbit occur at sublethal doses. As reported first by ROTHLIN (1944, 1946/47), *dihydrogenated ergopeptine derivatives* lowered rabbit rectal temperature. From Table 4 it can be seen that, in most instances, a fall in body temperature of 0.5° C was observed at doses 40–100 times lower than the LD_{50}, and a fall of 1° C at doses 5–18 times lower than the LD_{50}.

c) Hyperthermia

From the figures contained in Table 4, it is evident that *d*-LSD is the most specific ergot derivative to cause an elevation of rabbit temperature. Thus, most studies of the mechanisms involved in ergot-induced rabbit hyperthermia were done on this compound. Studies of HORITA and DILLE (1954, 1955) and of NEUHOLD et al. (1957) confirmed WHITE's (1944a) view that central, possibly hypothalamic, substrates are involved in ergot-induced hyperthermia. ROTHLIN et al. (1956) described an excitatory syndrome in the rabbit which included hyperthermia, piloerection, tachycardia, electroencephlographic arousal, mydriasis, and increased excitability, a syndrome which was attributed to "sympathetic excitation." Based on studies of a number of derivatives of *d*-LSD, CERLETTI (1956, 1959) concluded that this excitatory syndrome in the rabbit is predictive of hallucinogenic effects in man. However, HORITA and HAMILTON (1969) have shown that the excitatory effects of *d*-LSD could be dissociated from its hyperthermic action by pretreatment with α-methylparatyrosine, an observation which sheds some doubt on ROTHLIN's earlier interpretation. In fact, hyperthermia without excitation had been reported after administration of 2-Br-LSD by ROTHLIN et al. (1956), CERLETTI (1959), JACOB et al. (1962), and by JACOB and LAFILLE (1963).

Increases in rabbit rectal temperatures after cycloalkylamid derivatives of *d*-lysergic acid have been reported by VOTAVA (1957) and by VOTAVA and PODALOVA (1958).

Hyperthermia induced by *d*-LSD in rabbits has been proposed to depend on serotoninergic mechanisms. HORITA and GOGERTY (1958) have shown that the temperature rise after the administration of 5-hydroxytryptophan was similar to that after *d*-LSD, and that in both cases hyperthermia could be blocked by 2-Br-LSD. However, RUCKEBUSCH et al. (1965) reported that, as opposed to its hyperthermic effects in cats (FELDBERG and MYERS, 1963) and dogs (FELDBERG et al., 1966, 1967), intracerebroventricular serotonin did not enhance rabbit rectal temperature but lowered it. Intracerebroventricular injections of noradrenaline increased rabbit temperature (COOPER et al., 1965). Thus, it was suggested that noradrenergic mechanisms are involved in *d*-LSD-induced hyperthermia. This interpretation is in agreement with the observation that α-adrenergic blockade or pretreatment with chlorpromazine reduced *d*-LSD-induced excitation and hyperthermia (DHAWAN, 1959; GUJRAL and DHAWAN, 1959; ELDER and SHELLENBERGER, 1962; NAKAJIMA et al., 1964). However, more recent work has shown that chlorpromazine-induced blockade could also be due to its dopamine antagonist effect. In the rabbit, neuroleptic agents appear to reduce hyperthermic responses to *d*-amphetamine (HILL and HORITA, 1971; MATSUMOTO and GRIFFIN, 1971), apomorphine (HILL and HORITA, 1972) or intracerebroventricular dopamine (GIRAULT et al., 1975). In several species, including the rabbit, some ergot derivatives have been shown to possess dopamine agonist properties. Thus, the possibility that rabbit hyperthermia could involve a central dopaminergic mechanism is not excluded.

As seen from the results given in Table 4, hyperthermic effects of *ergopeptine derivatives* in the rabbit occur, in general, at doses which are below but close to the lethal range. We, therefore, would caution against extrapolation from the results with *d*-LSD to the ergopeptine derivatives. On the other hand, SELINSKY and BIERMAN (1938) reported that ergotamine tartrate, at a therapeutic dose of 0.5 mg i.v., increased rectal temperature in 15 out of 17 human subjects. In the cock kept at an ambient temperature of 22° C, ergotamine produced a rise in rectal temperature. This effect was abolished by the α-adrenergic blocking agent dibenzyline (KLISSIUNIS et al., 1967/68).

d) Hypothermia

The *dihydrogenated ergot alkaloids* dihydroergotamine, dihydroergosine, dihydroergocristine, dihydroergocryptine, and dihydroergocornine were first reported by ROTHLIN (1944, 1946/47) to lower rabbit temperature. In addition, the dihydrogenated compounds failed to elicit the hyperactivity, emotional lability, and hypersensitivity to environmental stimuli observed after administration of their natural parent compounds (ROBERTS et al., 1950). ROBERTS et al. (1950), CERLETTI and FANCHAMPS (1955), and CERLETTI and ROTHLIN (1955b) reported that hypothermia induced by dihydroergotoxine was observed in the rat at ambient temperatures of 27–28° C. A concomitant small decrease in oxygen consumption and peripheral vasodilatation were also seen. At ambient temperatures of 15–19° C, heat production was decreased. However, SEMLER and DAVID (1954) reported a rise in rabbit rectal temperature after 0.1–0.3 mg/kg i.v. dihydroergotoxine. CAHN et al. (1954/55) and CAHN and CAMPAN (1955) studied the hypothermic effects of dihydroergotoxine within the framework of providing experimental information for the use of adequate combinations of centrally acting drugs for "hibernation artificielle," i.e., controlled hypothermia in human surgery (LABORIT and HUGUÉNARD, 1954). These authors found that dihydroergotoxine, at parenteral doses of 0.1–0.3 mg/kg, lowered temperature in rabbits, rats, and dogs.

Based on the observation that dihydroergotamine at a dose of 10–80 mg/kg i.p., as well as α-adrenergic blocking agents, lowered rectal temperature of mice and rats, BOISSIER et al. (1967a) suggested the possibility that this effect is due to peripheral or central α-adrenergic blockade.

Two nondihydrogenated ergot derivatives, bromocriptine and lisuride, have recently been reported to lower body temperature in mice (FUXE et al., 1975b; HOROWSKI and WACHTEL, 1976). This fall in temperature was counteracted by pimozide and haloperidol, respectively. As these two ergot compounds have been shown to exert central dopamine receptor agonist effects, it has been suggested that their hypothermic effect is mediated by central dopaminergic stimulation. Such a mechanism has also been implicated in the hypothermic effect of apomorphine in the mouse (FUXE and SJÖQVIST, 1972; BARNETT et al., 1972).

8. Emesis

Nausea and vomiting are well-known side effects of ergot compounds in humans (ergotamine: VON STORCH, 1938; FRIEDMAN et al., 1959; ergometrine: LAUERSEN and CONRAD, 1974). However, HATCHER and WEISS (1923) in their "Studies on Vomiting" were unable to show the emetic action of ergot compounds in the dog, but reported that ergotoxine abolished the effects of emetic agents such as apomorphine or pilocarpine. Ergotoxine, even when applied directly to the floor of the fourth ventricle, did not elicit vomiting. These authors have suggested that the emetic action of fluid extract of ergot reported earlier by EGGLESTON and HATCHER (1915) was due to an effect of nonergot contaminants. Subsequent work by KOPPANYI and EVANS (1932) indicated that ergotamine at small doses of 0.02–0.2 mg/kg i.v. elicited retching and vomiting in the dog, but that doses above 0.5 mg/kg i.v. failed to do so. Similarly, in the cat 0.01–0.02 mg/kg i.v. of ergotamine produced emesis, but doses above 0.3 mg/kg i.v. were inactive. Vomiting after ergotamine administration to dogs was also reported by STAHNKE (1928a, 1928b), FARRAR and DUFF (1928), YOUMANS and TRIMBLE (1930), and by BROWN and DALE (1935). However, CHEYMOL and QUINQUAUD (1945, 1948) showed that a high systemic dose of ergotamine (1 mg/kg i.v.) or instillation of ergotamine at a concentration of 2×10^{-3} into the fourth ventricle prevented vomiting usually observed after morphine, emetine, or pilocarpine treatment. In reviewing the literature BORISON and WANG (1953) and WANG (1965) concluded that low doses of ergot compounds elicited emesis in dogs, but that after single administration of a high dose or after repeated treatment (STAHNKE, 1928a, b) antiemetic effects would be observed.

In order to facilitate the discussion of emetic effects of ergot derivatives, we have compiled the results of a number of studies in the dog which were carried out in our own laboratories. The method is as follows: Mongrel dogs of either sex were injected i.v. with the compound dissolved in a volume of 0.2 ml/kg of the appropriate solvent. The injection was slow and lasted 1 min, after which the animals were observed for more than 1 h and the number of retchings was noted. ED_{50}'s were calculated according to the method of MILLER and TAINTER (1944). The ED_{50}'s are given in Table 5. Among the *simple lysergic acid derivatives*, all three compounds investigated failled to induce vomiting. However, JOHNSON et al. (1973a), when testing a number of lysergamides, found the 9,10-dihydrolysergamides of primary amines to be potent emetic compounds. Another lysergic acid derivative, lisuride, has been reported by HOROWSKI and WACHTEL (1976) to induce emesis at 0.01 mg/kg s.c. in the dog. In the group of *ergopeptine derivatives*, it is interesting to note that 1-methylergotamine (34c) did not induce emesis at a dose of 0.3 mg/kg i.v., whereas all other ergopeptine derivatives elicited vomiting at i.v. doses below 0.01 mg/kg. The emetic potency of the *dihydrogenated ergopeptine derivatives* varied considerably. The most potent compounds were dihydroergocornine, dihydroergonine, dihydroergosine (102a), dihydroergovaline (108b), and dihydroergotoxine. As opposed to other central actions, such as hyperthermia in the rabbit (see Table 4) or induction of contralateral turning in the model of UNGERSTEDT in the rat (see Table 6), dihydrogenated ergopeptine derivatives share the emetic action of ergopeptines and of some simple lysergic acid derivatives. Indeed, dihydroergotoxine has become the representative of ergot alkaloids whose emetic action has been studied most extensively.

Systematic studies on emetic responses of dogs to i.v. administration of dihydroergotoxine have been carried out by WANG and GLAVIANO (1954), GLAVIANO

Table 5. Emetic effect of ergot derivatives in the dog

Code No	Compound	ED_{50} µg/kg i.v.	Code No	Compound	ED_{50} µg/kg i.v.
Simple lysergic acid derivatives			*Dihydrogenated ergopeptine derivatives*		
73b	*d*-LSD	> 3000	102b	Dihydroergotamine	36.5
34a	Methysergide	> 3000	102a	Dihydroergosine	3.6
104e	Nicergoline	> 1000	102g	Dihydroergostine	44.0
			110b	Dihydroergonine	3.3
Ergopeptine derivatives			102c	Dihydroergocristine	14.3
			102d	Dihydroergocornine	2.8
20	Ergotamine	3.1	108b	Dihydroergovaline	4.0
34c	*l*-Methylergotamine	> 300	—	Dihydroergotoxine	5.7
22	Ergostine	7.5			
110a	Ergonine	1.75			
24	Ergocornine	3.0			
25	α-Ergokryptine	2.6			
38	Bromocriptine	7.5			
108a	Ergovaline	2.3			
111a	Ergoptine	2.7			

and WANG (1955), BOISSIER and PAGNY (1962), and CERLETTI et al. (1962). WANG and GLAVIANO (1954) reported a minimal emetic dose of 6 µg/kg i.v. and found that 10 µg/kg i.v. induced vomiting in 90% of the dogs. Ninety µg/kg, administered by intragastric route, induced emesis in 50% of the dogs, but a further increase of the intragastric dose failed to enhance the incidence of vomiting. Emesis was observed neither in the cat after i.v. doses of 30–400 µg/kg or an i.m. dose of 100 µg/kg (BRAND et al., 1954) nor in *Macacca mulatta* or *M. cyclopis* (BRIZZEE et al., 1955; PENG and WANG, 1962). Chronic destruction of the chemoceptive trigger zone of the area postrema in the dog abolished the emetic response to i.v. or i.g. dihydroergotoxine (WANG and GLAVIANO, 1954). Vomiting was observed after intracerebroventricular injection of as little as 0.002 µg into the fourth brain ventricle of dogs. By contrast, the ED_{50} was 0.15 µg for the third ventricle and 0.55 µg for the lateral ventricle (PAPP et al., 1966). Emetic responses to intraventricular dihydroergotoxine were blocked by destruction of the chemoceptive trigger zone. Based on these results, PAPP et al. (1966) concluded that the emetic action of dihydroergotoxine in the dog is mediated solely through the chemoceptive trigger zone in the floor of the fourth ventricle in the region of the area postrema. Thus, the mechanism involved in emesis after dihydroergotoxine would be the same as that suggested for apomorphine (SHARE et al., 1965).

The antiemetic action of i.v. ergotoxine or of ergotamine applied topically to the floor of the fourth ventricle (HATCHER and WEISS, 1928; CHEYMOL and QUINQUAUD, 1945, 1948) has been interpreted by PAPP et al. (1966) as central nervous system depression which would include direct depression of the vomiting center situated in the lateral reticular formation (BORISON and WANG, 1953) by high doses of ergot derivatives. However, DHAWAN and GUPTA (1961) reported that *d*-LSD was a potent antiemetic in the dog. It blocked emetic responses to i.m. apomorphine, i.v. morphine, or i.v. dihydroergotoxine at respective ED_{50}'s

Table 6. Induction of contralateral turning in the rat with unilateral degeneration of the nigrostriatal tract by 6-OHDA

Code No	Substance	Dose mg/kg	Route	n	Total number of rotations × 10 ± S.e.m.	Maximal intensity/min	Effect latency (min)	Duration (h)
Simple lysergic acid derivatives								
5	Agroclavine	1	i.p.	3	206 ± 44	10.7	< 10	> 6
—	Elymoclavine	1	s.c.	3	191 ± 18	14.3	< 10	$4^1/_2$
19	Ergometrine	3	s.c.	6	109 ± 16	6.8	30	$4^1/_2$
73a	Methylergometrine	3	s.c.	3	239 ± 66	17.3	30	4
73b	*d*-LSD	1	i.p.	6	106 ± 5	15.2	< 10	$1^1/_2$
34a	Methysergide	30	s.c.	3	∅	∅	∅	∅
39	Lergotrile	1	s.c.	3	199 ± 26	9.2	< 10	7
8-Epimer of 83b	CM 29-712	1	i.p.	6	261 ± 16	14.4	< 10	> 8
96a	Lisuride	0.1	i.p.	3	77 ± 40	17.5	< 10	4
90d	CF 25-397	1	s.c.	6	113 ± 12	12.4	< 10	$1^1/_4$
88e	PTR 17-402	2.5	s.c.	3	184 ± 21	5.3	< 10	> 8
Ergopeptine derivatives								
20	Ergotamine	30	s.c.	∅	∅	∅	∅	∅
21	Ergosine	10	s.c.	3	82 ± 27	6.2	210	> 7
110a	Ergonine	10	s.c.	3	114 ± 35	6.8	70	> 7
23	Ergocristine	1	s.c.	6	75 ± 40	3.1	60	> 7
24	Ergocornine	1	s.c.	6	322 ± 84	11.5	> 10	> 7
25	α-Ergokryptine	1	s.c.	6	394 ± 35	12.3	60	> 7
26	β-Ergokryptine	1	s.c.	6	320 ± 131	12.7	30	> 7
38	Bromocriptine	1	s.c.	6	172 ± 51	8.2	60	> 7
Dihydrogenated ergopeptine derivatives								
102b	Dihydroergotamine	30	s.c.	3	∅	∅	∅	∅
110b	Dihydroergonine	30	s.c.	3	3 ± 0.3	1	< 10	$1^1/_4$
102c	Dihydroergocristine	30	s.c.	3	∅	∅	∅	∅
102d	Dihydroergocornine	30	s.c.	3	9 ± 6	1.3	120	7
102e	Dihydro-α-ergokryptine	30	s.c.	3	100 ± 50	8.8	180	7
102f	Dihydro-β-ergokryptine	30	s.c.	6	15 ± 15	0.9	120	7
—	Dihydroergotoxine	30	s.c.	6	26 ± 11	6.5	60	7
—	Apomorphine	0.25	s.c.	16	56 ± 9	16.5	< 10	$1^1/_2$

of 13, 26, and 39 μg/kg i.v. As *d*-LSD did not prevent emesis induced by protoveratrine, emetine, or ouabain, these authors suggest that it has a direct depressing effect on the chemoceptive trigger zone. The antiemetic action of *d*-LSD was not shared by 2-Br-LSD (DHAWAN and GUPTA, 1961).

The emetic response to i.v. dihydroergotoxine in the dog also could be blocked by metoclopramide (JUSTIN-BESANÇON and LAVILLE, 1964), chlorpromazine (GLAVIANO and WANG, 1955; BRAND et al., 1954), and other phenothiazines, including prochlorperazine, thiethylperazine, and perphenazine (BOISSIER and PAGNY, 1962; CERLETTI et al., 1962). GLAVIANO and WANG (1955) also reported unpublished experiments of WANG showing that emesis induced by i.v. apomorphine or dihydroergotoxine was abolished by placing 0.25 mg of chlorpromazine on the floor of the fourth ventricle. These authors have suggested that chlorpromazine competes with the two emetic agents for receptors at the chemoceptive trigger zone. WANG and GLAVIANO (1954) proposed that this emetic effect of dihydroergotoxine might be related to adrenergic blockade. Indeed, FUXE and OWMAN (1965) pointed out that in the area postrema, which acts as a chemoceptive trigger zone for emesis, monoamines are localized in nerve cells and that monoaminergic mechanisms could be involved in the central emetic reflex chain. As mentioned above, the chlorpromazine-induced blockade of the emetic actions of apomorphine and dihydroergotoxine are strikingly similar. Furthermore, the possibility that phenothiazines prevent emesis induced by either drug through a direct interaction at the chemoceptive trigger zone also suggests that dihydroergotoxine and apomorphine might influence monoaminergic mechanisms in the area postrema. Apomorphine has been shown to stimulate dopaminergic receptors in the central nervous system, particularly those of the extrapyramidal system (ANDÉN et al., 1967), effects which also could be counteracted by dopamine receptor antagonists such as phenothiazines (CORRODI et al., 1967a). It might well be that dopaminergic stimulation is involved in the emetic actions of apomorphine and dihydroergotoxine.

Central dopaminergic effects of various ergot derivatives have been reported and are reviewed in this chapter. It should be noted that no correlations are observed when comparing the emetic potency rank order of ergot derivatives in the dog (Table 5) to their ability to induce contralateral turning in the UNGERSTEDT model in the rat (Table 6). This may be related to the different species and routes of administration used. However, it should be mentioned that the area postrema is notable for a relative deficiency in the blood-brain barrier system (WISLOCKI and PUTNAM, 1920, 1924; WISLOCKI and LEDUC, 1952), which might be responsible for a different accessibility and, therefore, sensitivity of the chemoceptive emetic trigger zone to some ergot derivatives.

D. Synaptic Transmission: Catecholaminergic Mechanisms

1. Criteria of Catecholaminergic Stimulation and Antagonism at the Synaptic Level

In the foregoing sections it has been suggested that some actions of ergot derivatives on central regulation of motor behavior, arousal, sleep, temperature, and emesis involve monoaminergic mechanisms. This section deals with ergot action on neuronal functions known to be served by specific catecholaminergic mechanisms in the brain. In general, the pharmacologic criterion of stimulation or antagonism of a catecholaminergic mechanism used most often here is that an ergot derivative mimics well-established noradrenergic and dopaminergic agonists or antagonists, respectively, at *behavioral*, as well as at *biochemic* and *electrophysiologic* levels of function.

The effect of a drug on catecholamine-dependent behavior of whole animals following pretreatment with agents which inhibit synthesis, deplete stores, block receptors, or destroy specific neuronal pathways can be used to indicate which catecholamine may be involved in drug action and frequently indicates the direction of further biochemic and electrophysiologic studies. It seems to be a general rule that when monoamine receptors are stimulated, the turnover of that transmitter is depressed, but when receptors are blocked the turnover is enhanced (FUXE and HÖKFELT, 1971; CARLSSON, 1974). However, catecholamine turnover reflects overall synaptic function, which includes transmitter synthesis, release, binding to the receptor, reuptake, and degradation and has become a routinely used index of receptor and synaptic function. The most direct experimental evidence that a substance can interact with central catecholaminergic mechanisms has come from studies which permit local, direct drug administration to a relatively small numer of biochemically defined neuronal cell bodies, axons, or synapses and measurement of responsiveness in the treated neurons themselves or in neurons receiving an input from the treated cells. Any study of biologically active compounds in the central nervous system should attempt to apply as many of these functional criteria as possible to the system, but, unfortunately, most of the criteria summarized below are rarely satisfied for any one of the ergot derivatives reviewed.

a) Behavioral Effects

Behavioral studies with intact animals have shown that neostriatal dopaminergic function is essential for the regulation of motor activity. Very small doses of apomorphine administered neostriatally to rats produced stereotyped sniffing, licking, and biting behavior, and, when injected into the nucleus accumbens, produced a long-term increase in locomotor activity (ERNST and SMELIK, 1966; ERNST, 1967). Larger i.p. doses of L-DOPA plus benserazide or apomorphine enhanced locomotor activity in rats and mice (ANDÉN et al., 1973), which could be blocked by either pimozide or haloperidol. Unilateral injection of low doses of L-DOPA, dopamine (DA), or apomorphine into the medial two-thirds of the caudate nucleus of the cat induced turning contralateral to the injected side (COOLS and VAN ROSSUM, 1976). This turning behavior was reversibly counteracted by haloperidol and was blocked after synthesis inhibition by the tyrosine hydroxylase inhibitor, a-methyl-p-tyrosine (aMPT) methyl ester. Similar studies on the caudate nucleus of rhesus monkeys have shown that stimulation of DA-sensitive sites elicited skilled manipulation movements and various dyskinetic activities in the face and extremities. The induction of the first type of movements was blocked by haloperidol (COOLS et al., 1975a).

Relief of reserpine-induced akinesia has been used as an index of dopaminergic stimulation in intact animals, because it has been shown that amphetamine (MORPURGO, 1962) and L-DOPA (CARLSSON et al., 1957) antagonized this effect.

Behavioral studies in lesioned animals also have shown that apomorphine induced turning in rats lesioned unilaterally with 6-hydroxydopamine (6-OHDA) in the substantia nigra (UNGERSTEDT, 1971) or the median forebrain bundle (PIERI et al., 1974, 1975). Since after 6-OHDA treatment, unilateral degeneration of dopaminergic neurones presynaptic to the basal ganglia predisposes these animals to rotate contralaterally to the denervated side, UNGERSTEDT (1971) has suggested that postsynaptic DA receptors on the degenerated side of the striatum exhibit "denervation supersensitivity," and that contralateral turning demonstrates their direct activation by DA agonists. As will be discussed below, these and similar animal models are considered as models of Parkinson's disease and are frequently used as valuable screening tests in the search for new antiparkinsonian agents.

In recent years, a considerable number of ergot derivatives have been investigated in our laboratories using behavioral models. In order to facilitate comparison between individual compounds, some of the results of these investigations are included in this section. The methods have been recently described in detail (JOHNSON et al., 1976; VIGOURET et al., 1978) and can be summarized as follows:

The *induction of contralateral turning* in rats with unilateral degeneration of the nigrostriatal pathway was studied according to the technique of UNGERSTEDT and ARBUTHNOTT (1970). Male OFA rats (140–160 g) were administered a 4 µl solution of 6-hydroxydopamine hydrochloride (2 mg/ml with 0.2 mg/ml ascorbic acid as antioxidant) in the zona reticulata of the right substantia nigra. One week later, the animals were challenged with 0.25 mg/kg s.c. apomorphine, and the number of rotations was counted. To facilitate comparison between different compounds and different groups of animals, the number of rotations in each animal was corrected by a factor derived from the response to 0.25 mg/kg i.p. apomorphine.

Stereotyped behavior was rated in male OFA rats (180–250 g) according to the method of COSTALL et al. (1972) in perspex cylinders of 30-cm diameter with a wire grid floor. The compounds were administered 30 min after placing the animal in the cage, and each dose was administered to at least six rats.

Spontaneous locomotor activity in groups of five male NMRI mice (18–22 g) was measured in a light beam chamber as described by DEWS (1953). Each treatment condition was investigated in six groups to give a total of 30 mice per treatment.

Reserpine-induced akinesia was investigated in male NMRI mice (18–25 g) which had received 5 mg/kg i.p. reserpine 17 h before the test. Antagonism to akinesia was assessed as the ability of the mice to walk off a twine-covered vertical pole in a coordinated manner. Each treatment condition was investigated in at least 10 animals.

The results are contained in Tables 6, 7, and 8 and in Figure 8.

b) Biochemic Effects

Studies of ANDÉN et al. (1967) have shown that apomorphine retarded the depletion of rat brain DA but not noradrenaline (NA) following inhibition of catecholamine synthesis with αMPT. This action of apomorphine was blocked by haloperidol. Similarly, apomorphine enhanced the intensity of DA specific fluorescence in dopa-

Table 7. Induction of stereotyped behavior in the rat

Code No	Substance	Dose mg/kg	Route	Total activity per rat (0–7 h)[a]	Maximal activity per rat ±S.e.m.	Effect		p X^2 test
						Latency (min)	Duration (h)	
Simple lysergic acid derivatives								
5	Agroclavine	30	s.c.	17.9	4±0	<10	7	0.01
19	Ergometrine	30	i.p.	1	0.5±0	<20	1/3	0.01
73a	Methylergometrine	30	i.p.	5.5	1±0	<10	4	0.01
73b	*d*-LSD	30	i.p.	19	4±0	<10	4	0.01
34a	Methysergide	30	i.p.	∅	—	—	—	n.s.
39	Lergotrile	30	i.p.	27	4±0	<10	7	0.01
8-Epimer of 83b	CM 29-712	30	i.p.	14.3	2±0.2	<10	>7	0.01
96a	Lisuride	30	i.p.	12	4±0	<10	5	0.01
90d	CF 25-397	30	s.c.	1.5	0.3±0.2	—	—	n.s.
88e	PTR 17-402	20	i.p.	4	1±0	<10	>7	0.01
Ergopeptine derivatives								
20	Ergotamine	30	i.p.	∅	—	—	—	n.s.
21	Ergosine	30	i.p.	12	3±0	30	3	0.01
22	Ergostine	30	i.p.	∅	—	—	—	n.s.
110a	Ergonine	30	i.p.	14	4±0	<10	2	0.01
23	Ergocristine	20	s.c.	∅	—	—	—	n.s.
25	α-Ergokryptine	20	s.c.	13.1				
26	β-Ergokryptine	5	s.c.	1.8				
38	Bromocriptine	30	i.p.	13	3±0	60	>7	0.01
24	Ergocornine	10	s.c.	16.1	2.3±0.5	<10	>7	0.01
108a	Ergovaline	10	s.c.	∅	—	—	—	n.s.
111a	Ergoptine	30	i.p.	10	3.3±0.2	<10	6	0.01
Dihydrogenated ergopeptine derivatives								
102b	Dihydroergotamine	30	i.p.	0.3	0.3±0.2	—	—	n.s.
102a	Dihydroergosine							
102g	Dihydroergostine	30	i.p.	∅	—	—	—	n.s.
110b	Dihydroergonine	30	i.p.	∅	—	—	—	n.s.
102c	Dihydro-ergocristine	30	i.p.	∅	—	—	—	n.s.
102e	Dihydro-α-ergokryptine	30	i.p.	∅	—	—	—	n.s.
102f	Dihydro-β-ergokryptine	30	i.p.	∅	—	—	—	n.s.
—	Dihydro-ergotoxine	30	i.p.	1.3	0.2±0.1	—	—	n.s.
—	Apomorphine	10	s.c.	12.7	3.3±0.2	<10	1	0.01

[a] Stereotyped behaviour was rated in each rat according to the criteria of COSTALL et al. (1972 which included sniffing, licking and biting.

Table 8. Spontaneous locomotor activity in the mouse ($1^{1}/_{2}$–7 h). Lightbeam chamber: number of light beam interruptions

Code No	Substance	Dose mg/kg s.c.	Total motility × 100 ± S.e.m.	% Change from control	p "t test"
Simple lysergic acid derivatives					
19	Ergometrine[a]	—	43 ± 4.4	—	
		3	41 ± 4.4	− 5	n.s.
		10	56 ± 4.6	+ 30	n.s.
		30	115 ± 6.4	+169	<0.05
73b	*d*-LSD	—	34 ± 6.4	—	—
		2.5	48 ± 6.7	+ 41	0.02
		5	60 ± 9.6	+ 77	0.01
		10	60 ± 7.0	+ 77	0.01
34a	Methysergide[a]	—	36 ± 4.7		
		3	39 ± 3.3	− 9	n.s.
		10	23 ± 2.7	− 37	n.s.
		30	33 ± 8.8	− 9	n.s.
8-Epimer of 83b	CM 29-712	—	40 ± 2.8	—	—
		2.5	63 ± 7.8	+ 58	0.01
		5	62 ± 12.1	+ 56	n.s.
		10	68 ± 9.2	+ 70	0.02
88e	PTR 17-402	—	23 ± 1.9	—	—
		2.5	46 ± 4.9	+ 99	<0.01
90d	CF 25-397	—	30 ± 6.3	—	—
		2.5	29 ± 3.3	− 43	n.s.
		5	24 ± 3.2	− 22	n.s.
		10	23 ± 7.5	− 24	n.s.
Ergopeptine derivatives					
20	Ergotamine	—	40 ± 7.0	—	—
		10	63 ± 11.9	+ 57	<0.05
21	Ergosine	—	39 ± 6.4	—	—
		10	52 ± 7.2	+ 32	n.s.
110a	Ergonine	—	33 ± 0.8	—	—
		10	52 ± 8.3	+ 57	<0.05
23	Ergocristine	—	36 ± 4.0	—	—
		10	94 ± 14.8	+160	<0.01
24	Ergocornine	—	36 ± 4.0	—	—
		2.5	72 ± 12.0	+100	<0.01
		—	36 ± 4.0	—	—
		5	105 ± 14.8	+191	<0.01
		—	36 ± 7.0	—	—
		10	110 ± 7.6	+203	<0.01
25	α-Ergokryptine	—	51 ± 8.2	—	—
		10	206 ± 29.6	+298	<0.01
38	Bromocriptine	—	38 ± 5.5	—	
		2.5	51 ± 6.0	+ 32	<0.1
		5	105 ± 12.2	+178	<0.001
		10	283 ± 19.1	+653	<0.001

[a] 0–3 h.

Table 8 (continued)

Code No	Substance	Dose mg/kg s.c.	Total motility × 100 ± S.e.m.	% Change from control	p "t test"
Ergopeptine derivatives					
26	β-Ergokryptine	—	51 ± 8.2		
		10	120 ± 23.3	+133	<0.01
108a	Ergovaline	—	48 ± 6.6	—	—
		10	83 ± 9.1	+ 76	<0.05
Dihydrogenated ergopeptine derivatives					
102b	Dihydroergotamine	—	31 ± 5.4	—	—
		20	50 ± 3.9	+ 63	<0.05
102g	Dihydroergostine	—	31 ± 5.4	—	—
		20	25 ± 3.2	− 11	n.s.
110b	Dihydroergonine	—	38 ± 4.1	—	
		20	57 ± 4.5	+ 49	n.s.
102d	Dihydroergocornine	—	51 ± 8.2	—	
		20	102 ± 25.9	+ 99	<0.05
102c	Dihydroergocristine	—	35 ± 3.8	—	
		20	45 ± 3.4	+ 29	n.s.
102e	Dihydro-α-ergokryptine	—	35 ± 3.8	—	
		20	38 ± 6.6	+ 9	n.s.
102f	Dihydro-β-ergokryptine	—	35 ± 3.8	—	
		20	54 ± 2.9	+ 53	n.s.
—	Dihydroergotoxine	—	42 ± 4.1	—	—
		100	61 ± 5.9	+ 44	<0.05
—	*d*-Amphetamine	—	74 ± 15.2	—	
		1.25	77 ± 8.9	+ 4	n.s.
		—	41 ± 18.3	—	—
		2.5	84 ± 13.8	+103	
		—	41 ± 18.3	—	<0.05
		5	136 ± 18.2	+202	
—	Apomorphine	—	71 ± 12.6	—	
		5	80 ± 10.0	+ 13	n.s.

mine-containing terminals in the striatum of rats pretreated with αMPT above that of rats pretreated with the tyrosine hydroxylase inhibitor alone.

When impulse flow in the nigrostriatal pathway was blocked by mechanical transection or an electrolytic lesion, a marked increase in neostriatal DA was observed (ANDÉN et al., 1971). This increase could be prevented by systemic administration of apomorphine, which also inhibited DA synthesis in the neostriatum (KEHR et al., 1972; CARLSSON, 1974). This effect of apomorphine, in turn, was effectively blocked by haloperidol (KEHR et al., 1972). Apomorphine was also shown to block the release of DA from neostriatal slices, whereas haloperidol treatment under similar conditions enhanced release (FARNEBO and HAMBERGER, 1971).

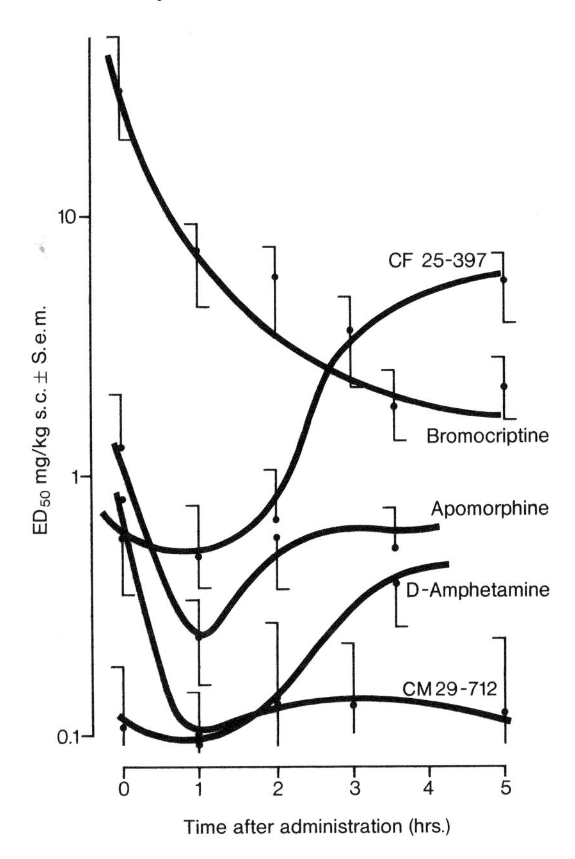

Fig. 8. Antagonism of akinesia induced by 5 mg/kg i.p. reserpine in mice. The antagonists were administered 17 h after reserpine, CF 25-397 (90d), bromocriptine (38), and CM 29-712 (8-epimer of 83b). (From VIGOURET et al., 1978)

Thus biochemic evidence from experiments with intact animals suggests that dopaminergic stimulation by apomorphine and similarly acting substances is accompanied by reduced transmitter synthesis and turnover. This adds support to the conclusion reached from studies in animals with nigrostriatal degeneration that dopamine and apomorphine most probably activate postsynaptic DA receptors in the caudate nucleus. However, a more complex picture of dopaminergic stimulation emerges from these studies. It has been proposed (see AGHAJANIAN and BUNNEY, 1973) that in the absence of impulse flow, DA release is diminished so that DA disappears from its receptors sites on the transected dopaminergic neurons themselves and on neurons receiving these dopaminergic inputs. Transmitter disappearance from receptors on the dopaminergic neurons (presynaptic sites) would especially cause a compensatory increase in DA synthesis, which is actually observed. Reduced synthesis and release of DA observed following systemic administration of apomorphine has been explained by a negative feedback by apomorphine on these presynaptic DA sites as well. Thus, stimulation of DA receptors by apomorphine-like drugs may involve agonist interactions with presynaptic and/

or postsynaptic sites, depending, perhaps, on the prevailing physiologic and pharmacologic conditions.

Since the activation of catecholaminergic receptors in the CNS appears to be coupled to increased cyclic adenosine monophosphate (cAMP) formation, the identification of potential dopaminergic and noradrenergic agonists or antagonists also can be made by measuring their ability to stimulate or depress, respectively, adenylate cyclase activity in biochemically defined neuronal populations (see review of IVERSEN, 1975). The DA receptors of the rat caudate nucleus, which have been well characterized pharmacologically, have been the object of a most intense study of catecholamine-dependent adenylate cyclase by several laboratories. Both DA and, to a lesser extent, NA stimulated adenylate cyclase activity in homogenates of caudate nuclei (KEBABIAN et al., 1972). The effect of apomorphine, like that of DA, on caudate homogenates was to stimulate dopamine-sensitive adenylate cyclase. The effect of either was blocked by low concentrations of haloperidol and of chlorpromazine (GREENGARD, 1974). In addition, GREENGARD (1974) has reported that α-adrenergic antagonists but not β-adrenergic antagonists weakly blocked DA-stimulated adenylate cyclase activity in caudate homogenates, an effect which was qualitatively similar to that reported by ANDÉN et al. (1966a) for α-adrenergic agonists.

Noradrenaline-sensitive adenylate cyclase has been found in various parts of the brain (PALMER et al., 1973). In the cerebellum, unlike the dopamine-sensitive enzyme of the caudate, it was antagonized preferentially by β-adrenoceptor blocking agents (BLOOM et al., 1974; BLOOM, 1975; IVERSEN, 1975). In the rat cortex stimulation of both α- and β-adrenoceptors appeared to elicit increased cAMP production (MARKSTEIN and WAGNER, 1978). Isoprenaline stimulation of adenylate cyclase was antagonized by the β-adrenergic blocking drug pindolol, while NA stimulation of the enzyme could be antagonized only by α-adrenergic blocking drugs such as phentolamine (for further discussion, see Section D IV).

Dopamine might also be able to regulate the level of intracellular cAMP by controlling the activity of the enzyme cAMP-phosphodiesterase which cleaves cAMP to 5′-AMP. MCAFEE and GREENGARD (1972) have shown that phosphodiesterase inhibitors potentiated the hyperpolarization and increased ganglionic cAMP concentrations over the levels induced by stimulation of the preganglionic nerve in the superior cervical ganglion of the rabbit. These inhibitors also potentiated similar responses of the ganglion to exogenous DA.

c) Electrophysiologic Effects

The most commonly observed action of catecholamines on extracellular potentials recorded from single neurons in a variety of brain regions is inhibitory (see review, KRNJEVIC, 1974). BLOOM (1975) has reported evidence for a β-adrenergic inhibitory system in the cerebellar neocortex of rats. Either noradrenaline or cAMP applied iontophoretically to the surface of Purkinje cells caused a hyperpolarization. A similar inhibitory effect also could be produced by electrical stimulation of the noradrenergic pathways originating from the locus coeruleus. In a large proportion of the hyperpolarized cells, this reaction was shown immunologically to be coupled with an increase in their cAMP levels. These inhibitory effects of both NA and cAMP on spontaneous activity in Purkinje cells could be potentiated by cAMP-phosphodiesterase inhibitors (BLOOM, 1975). Cyclic AMP also inhibited the activity of hippocampal pyramidal cells, cerebral pyramidal tract cells and caudate neurons, on which the effects of their natural catecholamines were known to be inhibitory (BLOOM, 1975). In the forebrain, upper brainstem, and cerebellum the action of DA is rather consistently inhibitory, with a potency usually greater than that of NA. In the rat caudate nucleus, dopamine or apomorphine, when applied iontophoretically to single neurons, inhibited firing of the majority of cells. The potency of both agonists on caudate neurons was enhanced in animals in which the striatum had been denervated by 6-hydroxydopamine (6-OHDA) (SIGGINS et al., 1974).

Thus, it appears that DA agonists inhibit caudate neurons regardless of whether their postsynaptic DA receptors are normal or "super-sensitive." However, HULL et al. (1974) have reported that when intracellular potentials were recorded in the cat, the most frequent initial response to DA was excitation.

In both intact and nigrostriatally transected acute preparations (where dopaminergic cells fire at abnormally high rates), apomorphine depressed the firing of dopaminergic neurons when administered systemically (BUNNEY et al., 1973) or directly by microiontophoresis to nigrostriatal neurons (AGHAJANIAN and BUNNEY, 1973). Microiontophoretic applications of DA at low ejection currents had the same depressing effect on these neurons (AGHAHANIAN and BUNNEY, 1973). Systemic administration of haloperidol was able to reverse the apomorpine- and DA-induced depression of firing. Since the nigrostriatal transection blocks all functional communication between dopaminergic neurons and their postsynaptic receptors without blocking the inhibitory action of apomorphine, apomorphine appears to act on presynaptic dopamine sites as well.

2. Agroclavine-Type Ergot Derivatives

a) Behavioral Effects

As seen in Table 6, agroclavine (5), elymoclavine (6), CF 25-397 (90d), CM 29-712 (8 epimer of 83b), lisuride (96a), and lergotrile (39) induced contralateral turning in rats, following unilateral degeneration of the substantia nigra with 6-hydroxydopamine (6-OHDA). FUXE et al. (1978) have also shown that agroclavine (0.025–0.1 mg/kg) and elymoclavine (0.025–0.075 mg/kg) had the same or an even higher potency than the same dose of apomorphine for inducing rotation contralateral to the degenerated side. A possible stimulatory effect of these ergot derivatives on postsynaptic dopamine receptors in the striatum has been postulated, since the classical DA receptor stimulating agent, apomorphine, induced the same rotational behavior (UNGERSTEDT, 1971). The ability of pimozide to block ergot- and apomorphine-induced rotational behavior supports this conclusion.

Agroclavine (0.5–2 mg/kg s.c.) induced sniffing, licking, and biting behavior that was similar to but longer-lasting than that observed following the administration of apomorphine or amphctamine to rats (STONE, 1973; FUXE et al., 1978). Thus, it appears that agroclavine may also produce stereotyped behavior by activating dopaminergic mechanisms in the basal ganglia or in other parts of the brain

(RANDRUP and MUNKVAD, 1967; ERNST, 1967). The same conclusion could be drawn from the action of elymoclavine, CM 29-712, lisuride, and lergotrile (Table 7). Lisuride (ED_{50} between 1.0 and 2.0 mg/kg) also induced a strong stereotypy which was somewhat less pronounced and striking than that seen after either apomorphine and *d*-amphetamine but which could be blocked by haloperidol (HOROWSKI and WACHTEL, 1976). Like apomorphine and amphetamine, lisuride partially antagonized the motor depression produced by reserpine pretreatment. Elymoclavine (0.2 mg/kg i.v.) was shown by YUI and TAKEO (1958b) to be most potent in inducing stereotypies in mice, rabbits, cats, and dogs when compared to the action of other agroclavine-like ergots in order of decreasing potency: agroclavine, triseclavine, penniclavine, LSD-25, lysergene, lysergine, and lysergol. CF 25-397 (Table 7), however, virtually lacked the ability to induce stereotypy.

Subcutaneous injection of agroclavine (0.1–1.0 mg/kg) into normal rats caused dose-dependent effects on locomotor activity (FUXE et al., 1978). All doses in this range inhibited locomotion during the first 10 min and even up to the first hour after injection, whereas only doses above 0.5 mg/kg enhanced the prolonged activity in the period starting 1 h after injection. In contrast, apomorphine (2 mg/kg)-induced activity was maximal only during the first hour after injection. As shown in Table 8, CM 29-712 induced a slight enhancement of locomotion in mice, but CF 25-397 had a tendency to inhibit locomotion. The ability of pimozide to block agroclavine-induced enhancement of locomotor activity in addition to the above effects strengthens the conclusion that most agroclavine-like compounds stimulate catecholaminergic, particularly dopaminergic mechanisms in the brain.

In green monkeys with unilateral lesions in the ventromedial tegmentum, administration of 2.5 and 5 mg/kg i.p. of lergotrile diminished the intensity of tremors and at the higher dose, abolished it for 1–2 h. At the same time, sedation and compulsive contralateral circling was observed (LIEBERMAN et al., 1975).

Both elymoclavine and agroclavine (0.2–0.5 mg/kg i.v.) had a powerful analeptic action on reserpine-induced sedation in mice, rabbits, and cats, which was superior to the arousal effect of equal or even higher doses of *d*-LSD under the same conditions. Thus, the central stimulatory action of these ergot alkaloids can override the monoamine-depleting effects of reserpine (YUI and TAKEO, 1958a), an observation which has been used to suggest that they activate monoaminergic, and especially catecholaminergic, mechanisms. As shown in Figure 8, CF 25-397 and CM 29-712 as well counteracted reserpine-induced akinesia in mice.

b) Biochemic Effects

When catecholamine stores were depleted by αMPT, agroclavine at a dose of 1 mg/kg caused a reduction of DA depletion and a significant acceleration of NA depletion in all the DA-rich regions of the forebrain studied by FUXE et al. (1978). After a dose of 0.3 mg/kg, these authors observed a preferential reduction of turnover only in the diffuse DA terminal systems of the tuberculum olfactorium and the islandic DA system of the nucleus caudatus but not in nucleus accumbens or the dotted tuberculum. Further support for the hypothesis that agroclavine acts as a potent dopaminergic agonist comes from the work of SCHORDERET (1976), who has shown that it (100 μM) stimulated cAMP levels by 74% over control values in the rabbit retina. The concentration of DA required to maximally increase cAMP levels in the retina is also 100 μg. Agroclavine at a concentration of 1 μM continued to induce a significant increase in cAMP accumulation. Thus, it appears to be active in the same concentration range as is DA, which at 1 μM induced half-maximal stimulation of adenylate cyclase. Fluphenazine (5×10^{-4} M) was able to inhibit the maximal adenylate cyclase response to agroclavine.

FUXE et al. (1978) have also observed that CF 25-397, which lacked the ability to induce stereotyped behavior in normal rats (JATON et al., 1976), at doses above 3 mg/kg reduced DA turnover in the subcortical limbic systems and the islandic DA systems of the neostriatum but not in the large diffuse DA systems of the neostriatum. These results underline the view that stereotyped behavior following treatment with DA agonists is related to their action on the large diffuse dopaminergic terminals of the neostriatum. Lergotrile, which produced clearcut stereotyped behavior in doses of 1–10 mg/kg, caused a reduction in DA turnover in all these dopaminergic systems at doses between 3 and 10 mg/kg. Moreover, VIGOURET et al. (1978) have shown that CF 25-397 induced only a weak elevation of the striatal 3,4-dihydroxyphenylacetic acid (DOPAC) concentration in the first hour after administration. On the other hand, CM 29-712 reduced DA turnover and the DOPAC concentration, an observation which has been used by these authors to suggest that this ergot derivative might stimulate postsynaptic DA receptors. The elevation of 3-methoxy-4-hydroxyphenylethanol (MOPEG) after CM 29-712 was similar to that seen after bromocriptine treatment. KEHR (1977) reported that in rats doses of 0.05 to 0.5 mg/kg i.p. lisuride increased DA concentrations, particularly in the striatum and mesolimbic forebrain, retarded the rate of disappearance after synthesis inhibition by αMPT methyl ester, and reduced tyrosine hydroxylation rate in DA-rich areas. These effects were also observed after the interruption of impulse flow in dopaminergic neurons by axotomy. In intact and axotomized rats, the lisuride-induced increase in DOPAC formation was antagonized by haloperidol. Based on these results, KEHR (1977) proposed that lisuride acted directly on the DA-containing neurons of the rat brain. In addition, lisuride slightly enhanced NA concentrations of the rat brain, particularly in the neocortex. After inhibition of NA synthesis, NA disappearance was accelerated (KEHR, 1977).

Agroclavine-type ergot alkaloids have been shown to exert various types of interactions with DA-sensitive adenylate cyclase of the rat striatum and nucleus caudatus (FUXE et al., 1978). At concentrations between 10^{-8} and 10^{-7} M, agroclavine produced a 10–15% increase in striatal cAMP, which was about 25% higher than the increase produced by the addition of either bromocriptine, lergotrile, or CF 25-397. Since agroclavine did not appear to inhibit phosphodiesterase activity at a concentration of 25 μM, the effects of agroclavine on cAMP levels are thought to reflect its effect on the adenylate cyclase itself. Agroclavine also potentiated the activity of adenylate cyclase in the intact and 6-OHDA-denervated caudate nucleus. Unlike agroclavine, CF 25-397 was more effective in stimulating adenylate cyclase activity in the presence of DA (FUXE et al., 1978).

c) Electrophysiologic Effects

Agroclavine applied topically to the somatosensory cortex of the rat had by itself no significant action on the cortical response evoked by stimulation of the contralateral foreleg. If, however, NA was applied to the cortex immediately after the removal of agroclavine (100 μg/ml), the depressant action of NA (50 μg/ml) was almost completely antagonized (DAVIDSON et al., 1969). It was not clear from these results, however, whether or not antagonism of topically applied NA by agroclavine reflected its ability to block a noradrenergic mechanism in the cortex.

Further support for the suggestion that agroclavine activates central dopaminergic receptors has come from the results of in vivo experiments comparing the unit responses of single neurons in the parietal cortex of the rat to microiontophoretically applied agroclavine, DA, NA, and serotonin (5-HT) (STONE, 1974a). When the response to agroclavine was compared with the response of the same cell to either DA, NA, or 5-HT, the percentage of cells responding in the same way were 78%, 48%, and 48%, respectively. In other words, when a cell was depressed, excited, or unaffected by DA, for example, it most frequently showed the same response to agroclavine. Chlorpromazine was able to selectively block the depression of the firing rate induced by either DA or agroclavine but not by 5-HT. Since both DA and agroclavine had similar effects on cortical neurons and were equally susceptible to chlorpromazine antagonism (JARVIK, 1970), it was suggested that agroclavine acted like a dopaminergic agonist in this system as well.

3. Ergometrine

a) Behavioral Efects

BROWN and DALE (1935) were the first to interpret "sham rage" as a central effect of ergometrine (19). A similar effect of ergometrine was reported by GADDUM and VOGT (1956) after the injection of 2 mg of the ergot derivative into the lateral brain ventricle of conscious cats. Several lines of evidence suggested that some of these central effects like "sham rage" could be brought about by the action of ergometrine on central DA receptors.

PIJNENBURG and VAN ROSSUM (1973) and PIJNENBURG et al. (1973) have described strong, long-lasting locomotor stimulation in rats following the injection of small amounts of ergometrine (2–5 μg, bilaterally) into the nucleus accumbens but not into adjacent structures. This stimulation could be prevented or antagonized by low doses (0.1 mg/kg i.p.) of either haloperidol, pimozide, or by inhibition of DA synthesis with αMPT methyl ester. Apomorphine was less effective than ergometrine in producing locomotor stimulation, and, furthermore, these apomorphine-induced effects could not be abolished or antagonized by inhibiting DA synthesis. In contrast, apomorphine and ergometrine both induced stereotyped behavior when administered into the neostriatum (PIJNENBURG et al., 1973; POIGNANT et al., 1974). When injected i.p. or i.v., ergometrine did not have these effects but instead induced a crawling behavior similar to ergometrine-induced behavior in rabbits and cats reported by BROWN and DALE (1935).

The nucleus accumbens contains a high density of DA nerve terminals, which comprise one part of the mesolimbic DA system (ANDÉN et al., 1966b; ARBUTHNOTT et al., 1970; UNGERSTEDT, 1971; FUXE et al., 1969). Axons of DA-rich cell bodies dorsocranial to the interpeduncular nucleus in the ventral mesencephalon (A_{10}-group according to DAHLSTRÖM and FUXE, 1965) ascend together with axons of the nigrostriatal DA system and enter the nucleus accumbens, nucleus interstitialis striae terminalis, and the tuberculum olfactorium. It is difficult to explain why administration of ergometrine in the nucleus accumbens could induce strong locomotor activity, since the nucleus accumbens is not known to control arousal: electrical stimulation of this structure is known to influence only a few brain stem units and to cause hypoactivity instead of arousal. In spite of this uncertainty, ergometrine-induced activity starts abruptly, remains at a constant high level, and stops abruptly as if some DA-sensitive mechanism in the mesolimbic system was being triggered "on and off" by ergometrine. Presently, there is insufficient information concerning the functional significance of the nucleus accumbens or the A_{10}-group of axons or the metabolism of ergometrine in those structures to suggest a mechanism of action.

In Ungerstedt rats, ergometrine (25 mg/kg i.p.) caused turning towards the intact side within 5–12 min, which lasted for about 3 h (WOODRUFF et al., 1974). In our laboratory, ergometrine (3 mg/kg s.c.) also induced turning contralateral to the degenerated nigrostriatal tract, indicating that this ergot derivative probably stimulated DA receptors in the striatum as well. Although it produced a less intense reaction than apomorphine (0.25 mg/kg s.c.), the effect of ergometrine lasted three times as long (Table 6). Haloperidol (1 mg/kg) abolished contralateral turning in rats induced by up to 10 mg/kg of ergometrine but only attenuated responses to higher doses of the ergot derivative (WOODRUFF et al., 1974).

b) Biochemic Effects

Recent biochemic evidence that ergometrine stimulates DA-sensitive adenylate cyclase activity adds further support to the functional evidence for its dopaminergic effects. ELKAWAD et al. (1975) have shown that ergometrine (30 μM) injected into the lateral brain ventricle of rats caused a significant stimulation (160%) of DA-sensitive adenylate cyclase in the striatum, which was about one-half of that (270%) produced by an injection of 30 μM DA injected under the same conditions. This effect of ergometrine appeared to be somewhat specific for dopaminergic neurons, since no adenylate cyclase stimulation at these doses could be observed in the cortex. This probably reflects the relatively low number of dopaminergic neurons in the cortex more than the failure of the ergot derivative to stimulate individual neurons in this area. The concentration of ergometrine required to stimulate adenylate cyclase under these conditions was less than that used by PIJNENBURG et al. (1973) to stimulate locomotor activity.

The accumulation for cAMP induced in the rabbit retina by 1 μM and 100 μM of ergometrine was, respectively, 50% and 44% of that induced by the same concentration of DA, indicating that ergometrine and DA act within the same concentration range (SCHORDERET, 1976). This stimulatory effect on cAMP could also be mimicked by apomorphine (BUCHER and SCHORDERET, 1975) but not by isoproterenol up to concentrations of 100 μM. While stimulation of retinal cAMP does not appear to involve ergot interactions with β-adrenergic receptors, the presence of both α- and β-receptors in the rat striatum indicates that such an interaction cannot be ruled out as one mode of ergot action on dopaminergic mechanisms. The interpretation that ergot derivatives directly activate DA receptors in the brain is also supported by the ability of fluphenazine to block the cAMP-stimulating effects of apomorphine and ergometrine under conditions where the agonist effect of each drug is maximal (IVERSEN, 1975).

c) Electrophysiologic Effects

Preliminary results of studies on both vertebrate and invertebrate neurons have indicated that ergometrine may selectively activate inhibition-mediating DA receptors. Electrophysiologic studies on the caudate nucleus of the cat have shown that this structure may contain two functionally distinct types of DA-sensitive receptors. The rostromedial part of the caput contains the highest density of DA-containing cells which could be excited by nigral stimulation, selectively activated by L-DOPA, DA, apomorphine, and *d*-amphetamine, and selectively inhibited by haloperidol (reviewed by COOLS and VAN ROSSUM, 1976). These authors have termed these cells "excitation-mediating" DA receptors or "DA_e" receptors. In contrast, sites within intracaudate structures surrounding the rostromedial part contain mostly cells which were inhibited either by nigral stimulation or by microiontophoretic application of DA and amphetamine but which were insensitive to apomorphine and haloperidol. Receptors on these intracaudate cells, therefore, have been termed "inhibition-mediating" or "DA_i" receptors by COOLS and VAN ROSSUM (1976).

Furthermore, there is a reasonable correlation between these electrophysiolgic data and other pharmacologic studies which indicates as well that the nucleus caudatus of the cat contains two distinct dopaminergic units with unique topographic and pharmacologic features. Application of low doses of L-DOPA, DA, apomorphine, and amphetamine to the rostromedial part resulted in the so-called contralateral turning syndrome, which could be reversibly counteracted by haloperidol or synthesis inhibition, but not by ergometrine (COOLS and VAN ROSSUM, 1970; COOLS, 1971; COOLS et al., 1975b; also reviewed by COOLS and VAN ROSSUM, 1976). At some intracaudate sites outside the rostromedial area, low doses of L-DOPA, DA, amphetamine, and 3,4-dihydroxy-phenylamino-2-imidazoline (DPI) were able to elicit the so-called ipsilateral turning syndrome. But both haloperidol and apomorphine were ineffective antagonists of this behavior when applied to these sites (COOLS et al., 1975b). Since ergometrine effectively blocked DPI- and DA-induced turning (unpublished results of STRUYKER BOUDIER cited in COOLS and VAN ROSSUM, 1976), it has been suggested for the first time by COOLS and VAN ROSSUM (1976) that only the postulated DA_i receptors in the caudate nucleus are sensitive to ergometrine antagonism. An antagonist effect of ergometrine on DA-induced inhibition of neurons in the rat cerebral cortex (CROSSMANN et al., 1973) may have a similar explanation.

Selective activation of so-called DA_i but not DA_e receptors in the caudate nucleus by ergometrine also has an important parallel in the DA-sensitive neurons of *Helix aspersa,* where ergometrine has been shown to be a potent antagonist of the inhibitory action of DA on neurons in the parietal ganglion (WALKER et al., 1968; WOODRUFF and WALKER, 1969; WOODRUFF et al., 1970) and of the inhibitory action of DPI on DA neurons in the subesophageal ganglion (STRUYKER BOUDIER et al., 1975). STRUYKER BOUDIER and VAN ROSSUM (1974) and STRUYKER BOUDIER et al. (1974) have also postulated the existence of two types of DA receptors in *Helix* on the basis of the differential sensitivity of two groups of dopaminergic neurons towards antagonistic drugs. In both groups the duration of a DA-induced inhibition or excitation and the increase in action potential frequency were always dose related. Out of nine cells located in either the parietal or visceral ganglion, six neurons were consistently (9–21 trials/cell) hyperpolarized and inhibited by DA (thus the term "dopamine-inhibited" or "DI" receptors) and depolarized by acetylcholine. When a variety of ergot derivatives were tested on these DI neurons, ergometrine (0.03–0.08 μM), ergotamine (0.2–0.5 μM), dihydroergotamine (1–5 μM) and dihydroergotoxine (3–10 μM), each blocked DA-induced inhibition of spontaneous activity without affecting the excitation caused by acetylcholine. Neuroleptics such as haloperidol used at concentrations up to 1000 μM were unable to block DA-induced inhibition in these DI neurons and also had no effect on acetylcholine-induced excitation. The remaining three neurons tested were consistently (3–26 trials/cell) depolarized and excited (thus termed "dopamine-excited" or "DE" receptors) by the same concentration of DA which had inhibited the other six but were always inhibited by acetylcholine. These DE neurons were also excited by *d*- or *l*-adrenaline, *l*-isoprenaline, 5-methyldopamine and apomorphine. Haloperidol reversibly antagonized DA-induced excitation as well at 1–10 μM and 5–20 μM, respectively. The effects of ergot derivatives on DA-induced excitation in this system have not yet been reported.

The ability of ergometrine (10 nM) to totally abolish only the inhibitory effects of both DA and DPI (each 1–10 nM) in dopaminergic *Helix* neurons was first used to suggest that DPI is a specific, potent agonist at the DI receptors (STRUYKER BOUDIER et al., 1975). The subsequent finding in the caudate nucleus of the cat that DPI-activation of the putative DA_i receptors could also be blocked by ergometrine (see above) further supports the existence of DA_i as well as DA_e receptors in the mammalian brain and the conclusion that the inhibition-mediating DA receptors are specifically blocked by ergometrine.

The available evidence seems to indicate that actual pharmacologic distinctions between excitation-mediating and inhibition-mediating DA receptors possibly exist in both mammals and in *Helix*. This might explain why ergometrine can under certain conditions act either as a DA agonist or an antagonist.

4. *D*-LSD, 2-Br-LSD, and Methysergide

It is not surprising that recent studies have shown *d*-LSD (73b) to be a stimulator of dopamine receptors in the brain, since other structurally related ergot derivatives, such as ergometrine and the agroclavine-type derivatives, already have been shown to be DA receptor agonists. The nature of this interaction between *d*-LSD and catecholaminergic neurons is just beginning to be investigated.

a) Behavioral Effects

D-LSD induced strong locomotor excitement in rats with accompanying sympathetic stimulation and "aberrant behavior," which has been described by DIXON (1968) as consisting of strong sniffing, licking, chewing, regular side-to-side movements of the head, and biting of the wire mesh floor. Similar "stereotyped behavior" in rats (FOG, 1969) and in several other animal species (RANDRUP and MUNKVAD, 1967) was also described after *d*-amphetamine or apomorphine.

Stereotypies induced by 5 mg/kg s.c. *d*-LSD have been shown by DIXON (1968) to be selectively inhibited by β-adrenoceptor blocking drugs, whereas both locomotor excitation and stereotyped behavior were antagonized by α-adrenergic blocking agents. It appears that 5-HT does not play a major role on this behavior, since parachlorophenylalanine (PCPA) pretreatment had no effect on either *d*-LSD-elicited stereotypies or locomotor excitation. However, a significant inhibition of *d*-LSD action was seen after inhibition of catecholamine synthesis by aMPT. DA appeared to play a more crucial role than NA, since chlorpromazine was more effective in antagonizing *d*-LSD-elicited stereotypies than was disulfiram.

The hypothesis that *d*-LSD may act through dopaminergic mediation also has received support from studies showing that *d*-LSD, like apomorphine, induced rotation in rats lesioned unilaterally in the median forebrain bundle (MFB) (PIERI et al., 1974, 1975). Relatively high i.p. doses (100–200 μg/kg) of *d*-LSD induced turning contralateral to the MFB lesion, an effect which was quantitatively similar to that induced by apomorphine. The probability that *d*-LSD has DA receptor-stimulating properties in this model system is supported further by the observation that both apomorphine- and *d*-LSD-induced rotation were almost completely blocked by haloperidol (1 mg/kg i.p.) but not by αMPT (200 mg/kg i.p.) pretreatment. Methysergide (39a) or 2-Br-LSD (37a) (20 mg/kg i.p.) were unable to induce turning at all (PIERI et al., 1975). Recent results in our laboratories have also shown that *d*-LSD (1 mg/kg i.p.) but not methysergide was able to induce contralateral turning in rats which had been lesioned unilaterally by an injection of 6-hydroxydopamine (6-OHDA) into the nigrostriatal tract. Maximal intensity and duration of rotations towards the intact side were almost identical to that produced by 0.25 mg/kg s.c. apomorphine (Table 6).

b) Biochemic Effects

The cerebral content of DA and NA has been shown to be slightly increased following relatively high doses of *d*-LSD (BARCHAS and FREEDMAN, 1963; DIAZ et al., 1968). Studies of DA PRADA et al. (1975) in the rat have also indicated that the concentration of homovanillic acid (HVA) was diminished to about 70% of control values in the striatum following i.p. administration of 0.2 mg/kg and in the retina by 0.5 mg/kg *d*-LSD. In addition, an i.p. dose of 1 mg/kg *d*-LSD delayed αMPT-induced disappearance of DA in the telencephalon and diencephalon and reduced the output of DA from the perfused caudate nucleus of the cat. In contrast, NA turnover was unaffected by these doses. The suggestion (CARLSSON, 1974) that direct stimulation of DA receptors is responsible for this reduced DA release and turnover is further supported by the fact that *d*-LSD itself activated adenylate cyclase in vivo (UZUNOV and WEISS, 1972; SPANO et al., 1975) and antagonized DA-induced activation of the enzyme (see also VON HUNGEN et al., 1974, 1975a) in striatal homogenates (DA PRADA et al., 1975) but not in brain slices (UZUNOV and WEISS, 1972). Maximal stimulation of adenylate cyclase which was reached with 10^{-5} M *d*-LSD in the striatal homogenates was half the maximal activation induced by 10^{-5} M DA. These results together suggest that by directly stimulating the DA receptors in the brain, *d*-LSD inhibits DA synthesis, release from nerve terminals, and reduces the turnover of DA. Adenylate cyclase systems in cell-free preparations from the cerebral cortex of the adult rat are highly responsible to NA and DA stimulation but are relatively insensitive to 5-HT (VON HUNGEN and ROBERTS, 1973; VON HUNGEN et al., 1974). *D*-LSD and 2-Br-LSD (both at 10 μM) completely abolished the stimulation of cerebral adenylate cyclase activity by NA alone (PALMER and BURKS, 1971) or by 10 μM NA plus 10 μM DA (VON HUNGEN et al., 1974). On the other hand, 5-HT was able to strongly stimulate adenylate cyclase activity in cell-free preparations from the colliculus of neonatal rats (VAN HUNGEN et al., 1975b) and the cockroach ganglion (NATHANSON and GREENGARD, 1974), and *d*-LSD only partially blocked this stimulation. The suggestion that *d*-LSD effects are mediated by central receptors for transmitters other than 5-HT has received further support from studies in which lysergic acid derivatives were tested against equimolar amounts of either DA or NA at concentrations of these catecholamines which alone produced maximal stimulation of the adenylate cyclase activity in particulate fractions from adult rat hippocampus or cerebral cortex (VON HUNGEN et al., 1975a). *D*-LSD, 2-Br-LSD, and methysergide (all 100 μM) abolished or markedly reduced either DA or NA stimulation of cerebral adenylate cyclase activity. *D*-LSD strongly inhibited this enzyme activity in the hippocampal preparation as well.

Furthermore, low concentrations of *d*-LSD, DA, and NA but not 5-HT or high concentrations of *d*-LSD were able to evoke large increases in adenylate cyclase activity in the particulate fraction of the rat corpus striatum. Maximal activation obtained in the striatal preparation with 5 μM *d*-LSD was about half of that produced by 10 μM DA. Since it could be blocked by haloperidol or chlorpromazine but not by propranolol, a *β*-adrenergic blocking agent, this stimulation may be mediated largely by DA receptors. In addition, the well-known response of striatal adenylate cyclase to 10 μM of DA was also eliminated or markedly reduced by 10 μM *d*-LSD or 2-Br-LSD as well as by DA antagonists such as haloperidol. Serotonin itself (10–100 μM) slightly increased the activity of striatal adenylate cyclase, but only very high concentrations (1000 μM) strongly inhibited DA-induced stimulation of the enzyme (VON HUNGEN et al., 1974; 1975a). These results have been confirmed and extended by SPANO et al. (1975), who showed that the in vitro addition of *d*-LSD (2×10^{-5} M) stimulated formation of cAMP in striatum, nucleus accumbens, tuberculum olfactorium, and limbic cortex of rats. At the same concentration, 2-Br-LSD was inactive in these isolated brain tissues. These results have been confirmed in vivo following *d*-LSD (0.25 mg/kg i.p.) administered 15 min before sacrifice.

Thus, *d*-LSD seems to behave as a mixed agonist-antagonist with respect to its ability as an agonist to enhance adenylate cyclase activity and as an antagonist to block DA stimulation of this enzyme. The fact that *d*-LSD can stimulate DA receptors is consistent with the observation that it also produces stereotypy in rats. It has been suggested (COOLS and VAN ROSSUM, 1976) that receptors may not have the unique specificity formerly attributed to them but rather possess a flexibility or "duality," which in this case enables *d*-LSD to act as an agonist or as an antagonist at central receptors, depending on the particular conditions. Such characteristics of *d*-LSD are consistent with a "two-state" model of a neurotransmitter receptor discussed by SNYDER et al. (1975). These authors assume that if ^{3}H-dopamine and ^{3}H-haloperidol label the agonist and antagonist states of the dopamine receptor, respectively, then mixed agonist-antagonist drugs should have similar affinities for the same two sites or states of the receptor. *D*-LSD showed the same high affinity for the ^{3}H-dopamine-labeled binding site as for the ^{3}H-haloperidol-labeled binding site, and these affinities were about 1000 times greater than those of the *l*-isomer for the same sites. However, if two such functional states do in fact exist for the same receptor, not all ergot derivatives may act on both. For example, 2-Br-LSD antagonized the DA-induced stimulation of adenylate cyclase but, in contrast to *d*-LSD, did not itself stimulate adenylate cyclase activity (VON HUNGEN et al., 1975a). Likewise, 2-Br-LSD had about five times more affinity than *d*-LSD for the antagonist state (^{3}H-haloperidol-labeled) of the putative receptor but only half the affinity of *d*-LSD for the agonist state (^{3}H-dopamine-labeled).

5. PRT 17-402

a) Behavioral Effects

PTR 17-402 (88e) induced turning towards the intact side of rats in which the nigrostriatal tract had been unilaterally destroyed by 6-hydroxydopamine (FUXE et al., 1975b; and Table 6). The threshold dose was reported as 0.25–0.5 mg/kg i.p. In the same animals, FUXE et al. (1975b) reported behavioral effects (tremors, flatness, and abduction of the limbs) which they related to an increased 5-HT receptor activity (CORRODI et al., 1975). JOHNSON and GRIFFITH (unpublished, 1972) also reported stereotypies in rats. However, when rating according to the criteria of COSTALL et al. (1972), they observed sniffing (Table 7), which would indicate that in intact animals the stereotypies induced by PTR 17-402 are similar to those observed after 5-HTP but different from those seen after apomorphine. FUXE et al. (1975b) reported that pimozide, even in a high dose of 5 mg/kg i.p., only marginally counteracted contralateral rotations. In mice, PTR 17-402 increased locomotor activity (Table 8).

b) Biochemic Effects

Compared to ergocornine (24) and bromocriptine (38), PTR 17-402 induced only a weak decrease in DA turnover in the whole rat brain (FUXE et al., 1974). However, subsequent studies indicated that this agent preferentially reduced DA turnover in subcortical limbic structures and in the islandic system of the neostriatum (FUXE et al., 1975b). Pretreatment of rats with 0.5–5 mg/kg i.p. PTR 17-402 reduced αMPT methyl ester-induced disappearance of DA from nucleus accumbens, tuberculum olfactorium, and in the islandic system of the neostriatum. In further experiments, adenylate cyclase activity in homogenates of the rat subcortical limbic regions could be stimulated by concentrations of 1–100 μM PTR 17-402. This effect was more pronounced than that observed in the rat caudate nucleus. At a concentration of 50 μM, PTR 17-402 activity approached the activity of DA in subcortical limbic structures (FUXE et al., 1978).

6. Ergocornine

a) Behavioral Effects

Ergocornine (24) induced rapid turning towards the intact side of rats in which unilateral degeneration of the nigrostriatal tract had been caused by 6-hydroxydopamine (FUXE et al., 1974, and Table 6). FUXE et al. (1974) also found that threshold doses of ergocornine (0.25–5.0 mg/kg) as low as those of apomorphine initiated this turning behavior. In our laboratories a small dose of ergocornine (1 mg/kg s.c.) induced both a high maximal frequency and prolonged duration of turning; in addition, 10 mg/kg also induced stereotypy similar to but longer lasting than that seen after apomorphine administration (JOHNSON et al., 1973b; Tables 6 and 7). The lower peak activity induced by ergocornine when compared to that produced by apomorphine in the Ungerstedt model has been attributed to the tendency of this ergot derivative to act also on 5-HT receptors, an effect which would partly counteract the behavior induced simultaneously by DA receptor stimulation (CORRODI et al., 1975). In contrast to apomorphine, however, ergocornine was inactive in rats which had been reserpinized or depleted of their DA stores by inhibition of DA synthesis.

b) Biochemic Effects

Ergocornine (0.5–5 mg/kg i.p.) has been shown to retard DA turnover in the basal ganglia and the limbic forebrain of rats pretreated with a tyrosine hydroxylase inhibitor in a dose-dependent fashion (FUXE et al., 1974). This reduction of turnover is probably related to activation of postsynaptic DA receptors. However, ergocornine alone up to doses of 100 μM was unable to activate striatal adenylate cyclase above control levels, or to inhibit cAMP-phosphodiesterase, or to enhance the stimulatory effects of DA on cAMP levels in vitro (FUXE et al., 1978).

Ergocornine (5 mg/kg) also exerted a releasing effect on NA nerve terminals, leading to a partial depletion of whole brain and hypothalamic NA stores (FUXE et al., 1974). Shortly after tyrosine hydroxylase inhibition, NA turnover was increased in the subcortical brain, and after 2 h in the cortex as well. *D*-amphetamine caused similar changes in NA turnover and release (CORRODI et al., 1973). It appears that the effect of this ergot derivative on noradrenergic neurons is not mediated by NA receptor blockade, since even in the presence of large doses (10 mg/kg), there was no significant reduction of hindlimb flexor reflex intensity observed by FUXE et al. (1974).

Thus, ergocornine appears to act in part by decreasing DA turnover and directly stimulating the supersensitive striatal DA receptors of the Ungerstedt rat. However, in this case behavioral stimulation cannot be explained by the ability of this ergot alkaloid to increase striatal adenylate cyclase activity.

7. Bromocriptine

As a result of the pioneering work on ergotoxine and ergocornine (SHELESNYAK, 1954, 1958), bromocriptine (38) was the first drug selected and developed with the aim to suppress prolactin secretion in man (FLÜCKIGER and WAGNER, 1968;

FLÜCKIGER, 1976). In subsequent studies, FUXE and HÖKFELT (1970) and HÖKFELT and FUXE (1972) found that administration of ergocornine or bromocriptine to lactating rats affected the DA neurons of the tubero-infundibular system of the hypothalamus. Furthermore, since these authors and CORRODI et al. (1973) observed a decrease of DA turnover in the striate nucleus of the rat, they proposed that bromocriptine acts as a central DA agonist. The DA agonist actions of bromocriptine at hypothalamic and pituitary sites are discussed further by FLÜCKIGER and DEL POZO (1978) in Chapter IX of this volume.

The action of bromocriptine on the extrapyramidal motor system (CORRODI et al., 1973) probably accounts for its therapeutic effects in Parkinsonism.

a) Behavioral Effects

In behavioral tests, bromocriptine was reported to exert effects similar to apomorphine. At doses as low as 0.25 mg/kg i.p., it induced rotations towards the intact side of rats with unilateral degeneration of the nigrostriatal tract caused by intranigral 6-hydroxydopamine (CORRODI et al., 1973; JOHNSON et al., 1974, 1976). This effect of bromocriptine was dose-dependent and lasted up to 10 h (Table 6), but unlike apomorphine, ergocornine, and most of the lysergic acid derivatives, this effect appeared after a latency of about 1 h. Because of its long action, even at low doses, bromocriptine was able to induce a total number of turns which was greater than the totals produced by similar doses of apomorphine, or *d*-amphetamine, or L-DOPA in combination with benserazide (JOHNSON et al., 1976). These effects were markedly reduced (CORRODI et al., 1973) or abolished (LOEW et al., 1976b) by pretreatment with pimozide. Previous administration of reserpine or tyrosine hydroxylase inhibition by αMPT reduced the total number of turns elicited by bromocriptine (FUXE et al., 1974; JOHNSON et al., 1976). PIERI et al. (1975) reported that 5 mg/kg i.p. bromocriptine elicited contralateral rotations in rats with a unilateral degeneration of the median forebrain bundle caused by intracerebral 6-hydroxydopamine. Bromocriptine also produced contralateral rotations in mice with unilateral lesions of the nigrostriatal pathway (ANLEZARK et al., 1976) or in rats with 6-OHDA lesions in the lateral hypothalamus (COSTALL et al., 1975). In some of these models, bromocriptine potentiated the effects of *d*-amphetamine or of L-DOPA but inhibited that of apomorphine (DRAY and OAKLEY, 1976; FUXE et al., 1978). Thus, in rats or mice with a unilateral degeneration of the nigrostriatal tract, the induction of contralateral turning would be interpreted as evidence for a direct stimulant action at "super-sensitive" postsynaptic DA receptors in the striate nucleus. In addition, the antagonistic effect on this action brought about by αMPT or reserpine was interpreted to indicate that intact synthesis and presynaptic stores are necessary for its action (JOHNSON et al., 1976; LOEW et al., 1976b).

When administered in doses from 1 to 10 mg/kg s.c. to rats, bromocriptine induced dose-dependent stereotypies (JOHNSON et al., 1973b). The intensity of this behavior was less than that observed after apomorphine or some simple lysergic acid derivatives but lasted well over 7 h (Table 7). Bromocriptine-induced stereotypies were suppressed by previous administration of pimozide, reserpine, αMPT (JOHNSON et al., 1976), or amantadine (SCHNIEDEN and COX, 1976).

Low doses of bromocriptine counteracted akinesia induced in mice by previous administration of 5 mg/kg i.p. reserpine (JOHNSON et al., 1974, 1976; VIGOURET et al., 1978, Fig. 8). In addition, reserpine-induced α-rigidity (JURNA, 1976) in rats was reduced or abolished by bromocriptine (VIGOURET et al., 1977). After 0.03–1 mg/kg i.v. of bromocriptine, administered 30 min after an i.v. dose of 10 mg/kg reserpine, a dose-dependent reduction of rigidity was observed. Under these experimental conditions, bromocriptine was as potent as apomorphine, and its effect was evident within a few minutes after i.v. administration. In contrast, neither apomorphine nor bromocriptine was able to reduce γ-rigidity in the rat decerebrated at the intercollicular level. As reserpine-induced rigidity is assumed to be related to an enhanced discharge rate of α-motoneurons (ROOS and STEG, 1964; JURNA, 1976), VIGOURET et al. (1977) proposed that the observed action of bromocriptine on reserpine rigidity reflects its potential for relieving the symptoms of rigor in human Parkinsonism.

At doses from 1 to 25 mg/kg i.p., bromocriptine decreased audiogenic seizures in mice in the same dose range as apomorphine (ANLEZARK et al., 1976).

The stimulation of locomotor activity of mice treated with 2.5–10 mg/kg s.c. bromocriptine lasted over 6 h but only appeared after a suppression of the initial exploratory phase (JOHNSON et al., 1973b, 1976). A similar biphasic pattern was reported for the action of apomorphine (CARLSSON, 1975), whereas *d*-amphetamine increased locomotor activity also during the exploratory phase (VIGOURET et al., 1978). SNIDER et al. (1976), DI CHIARA et al. (1976) and DI CHIARA et al. (1977), when studying this initial depressant effect of bromocriptine or apomorphine, showed that exploratory activity was depressed at the same time as the content of striatal dihydroxyphenylacetic acid (DOPAC) was reduced, and that these effects could be counteracted by pimozide. These authors have proposed that direct inhibition of (presynaptic) dopamine release by bromocriptine could account for the observed initial depression of motor activity. A biphasic effect on motor activity has also been observed after several other ergot derivatives. The increase in motor activity has been proposed to be related to stimulation of central postsynaptic receptors (JOHNSON et al., 1976) which would be consistent with the observation that, after 10 mg/kg s.c. of bromocriptine, the elevation of striatal DA follows the same time course as stereotypies and locomotor stimulation (VIGOURET et al., 1978).

COSTALL and NAYLOR (1976) have reported that 50 mg/kg i.p. bromocriptine or 0.0625–0.25 mg/kg s.c. apomorphine inhibited hyperactivity induced by a local injection of DA into the nucleus accumbens of rats. These results are consistent with the views of COOLS and VAN ROSSUM (1976) that some ergot derivatives, in particular ergometrine, block DA receptors in the brain. However, PIJNENBURG et al. (1973) found that ergometrine but not bromocriptine or ergocornine induced hyperactivity after their local injection into the nucleus accumbens. Thus, the conclusion reached by COOLS and VAN ROSSUM (1976) that ergometrine is an antagonist at DA_i receptors cannot yet be generalized to include other ergot derivatives such as bromocriptine.

Dopaminergic stimulants have the tendency to reduce the antinociceptive activity of morphine, which has been shown (VIGOURET et al., 1973) to produce an increase in latency of the hindleg flexor reflex elicited by radiant heat stimulation.

This test has been used in an attempt to localize the effect of bromocriptine in the rabbit brain, where the cerebroventricular system was divided into two parts by plugging the aqueduct of Sylvius (DEPOORTERE et al., 1975; LOEW et al., 1976b; VIGOURET et al., 1978). Intravenous injections of bromocriptine (1–5 mg/kg i.v.) reduced the antinociceptive effects of morphine which had been introduced into the rhomboid fossa. This antagonistic effect of bromocriptine could be blocked only if pimozide was introduced into the anterior part, i.e., the third brain ventricle. Apomorphine also antagonized morphine only when it was injected into the anterior part of the divided cerebroventricular system. This action of apomorphine suggested that antagonism of morphine could depend on apomorphine or bromocriptine reaching the striate area.

Bromocriptine, when administered at a dose of 6 mg/kg i.p. provided long-lasting blockade of tremors produced in green monkeys by electrolytically lesioning the ventromedial tegmentum (MIYAMOTO et al., 1974). At the dose investigated, involuntary movements similar to the ones observed after L-DOPA or lergotrile were reported. Unlike lergotrile, no tolerance to the antitremor effects of bromocriptine was observed after repeated administration.

b) Biochemic Effects

HÖKFELT and FUXE (1972) were the first to report that bromocriptine decreased DA turnover in the median eminence of the rat, and to suggest that it might interfere with dopaminergic tubero-infundibular neurons, which presumably control prolactin secretion. Similarly, CORRODI et al. (1973) found that bromocriptine at a dose of 5 mg/kg retarded the disappearance of DA in the whole brain of rats pretreated with a tyrosine hydroxylase inhibitor, αMPT methyl ester. The extent of catecholamine depletion after treatment with bromocriptine and αMPT methyl ester was less than that after the inhibitor alone. In contrast, the level of NA in whole brain after αMPT methyl ester was decreased further after treatment with the inhibitor and bromocriptine. Histochemic examination of the fluorescence intensity of neostriatal and limbic dopamine nerve terminals also revealed a dose-dependent ability of bromocriptine to prevent the loss of DA fluorescence seen after tyrosine hydroxylase inhibition alone. Thus, bromocriptine decreased DA turnover in the neostriatum and limbic system but increased NA turnover in cortical and hypothalamic nerve terminals. In rats treated with 1 or 5 mg/kg i.p. of bromocriptine alone, neither alterations of DA or NA content in various brain areas (FUXE et al., 1974), nor effects on uptake or spontaneous release of NA (FUXE, 1974; personal communication) were observed. However, VIGOURET et al. (1978) have reported a small, but significant increase in the DA content of the rat striate nucleus after the administration of 10 mg/kg s.c. of bromocriptine. At the same dose, DA turnover and DOPAC content were reduced. In addition, these authors reported that NA turnover was accelerated and 4-hydroxy-3-methoxy-phenylethylene glycol sulphate (MOPEG) content enhanced in the rat brain stem.

These neurochemic results in rats indicate that bromocriptine reduced DA turnover in the brain, particularly in the striate nucleus. Thus, they support the hypothesis that bromocriptine is a direct agonist at dopamine receptor sites. SCHORDERET (1976) has reported that bromocriptine (100 μM), like ergometrine and agroclavine, stimulated DA-sensitive adenylate cyclase in the rabbit retina. TRABUCCHI et al. (1976) administered bromocriptine (0.5–4 mg/kg i.p.) to rats and found a dose-dependent increase in cAMP concentration in the striatum. However, this effect was maximal 10–15 min after the injection of the drug and had disappeared after 2 h. In striatal homogenates, bromocriptine at concentrations as high as 10^{-4} M failed to stimulate adenylate cyclase activity. However, at concentrations of 10^{-6} M, bromocriptine noncompetitively inhibited adenylate cyclase stimulation induced by 5×10^{-6} M DA. Similar results were reported by MARKSTEIN et al. (1978), who found no stimulation of DA-sensitive adenylate cyclase activity in rat striatal homogenates or slices incubated between 8 and 60 min with bromocriptine at concentrations of 10^{-10} and 10^{-3} M. However, these authors reported that the presence of bromocriptine (5×10^{-8}–1×10^{-5} M) shifted the dose-response curves of NA and DA (10–1000 μM) to the right. In striatal homogenates the pA_2 values were calculated as 5.6 and 4.9, respectively, and in striatal slices as 7.5 and 6.1, respectively, and indicate a receptor blocking effect particularly on noradrenergic receptors. This latter effect would be consistent with the acceleration of NA disappearance following inhibition of its synthesis (CORRODI et al., 1973) and with the observed increase in the concentration of the NA metabolite, MOPEG sulphate (VIGOURET et al., 1977).

In contrast to the results of TRABUCCHI et al. (1976) and of MARKSTEIN et al. (1978), FUXE et al. (1978) found that bromocriptine (10^{-7}–10^{-5} M) increased adenylate cyclase activity in rat striate homogenates. However, this effect was never more than 110% of the controls. In addition, bromocriptine at concentrations of 10^{-7} or 10^{-8} M also enhanced the effects of 4 μM DA on adenylate cyclase. With greater concentrations of bromocriptine, this effect disappeared.

Most of the results from behavioral studies and from investigations of DA metabolism in the rat striate nucleus favor the hypothesis that bromocriptine in fact stimulates central DA receptors. However, there is at present insufficient evidence that the stimulant effects of bromocriptine at central DA receptor sites are brought about by a stimulation of striatal DA-sensitive adenylate cyclase. These views are also consistent with the therapeutic results of bromocriptine treatment for idiopathic Parkinsonism and with the mechanisms involved in the inhibition of pituitary prolactin secretion (see FLÜCKIGER and DEL POZO, 1978; Chapter IX of this volume). FLÜCKIGER (1976) has reported that chlorpromazine pretreatment protects rats against the consequences of prolactin suppression by bromocriptine, i.e., inhibition of ovum implantation. Evidence that this effect of bromocriptine is probably due to its direct action on the anterior pituitary was first shown in vitro by PASTEELS et al. (1971) and later confirmed by many authors (see TASHJIAN and HOYT, 1972; GAUTVIK et al., 1973; NAGASAWA et al., 1973). Based on an analysis of the mechanisms involved in the actions of DA, apomorphine, and α-ergokryptine on the anterior pituitary MACLEOD and LEHMEYER (1974) concluded that the inhibition of prolactin secretion by these agents is a result of stimulation of DA receptors at the level of the prolactin secreting cells of the anterior pituitary.

The effects of bromocriptine have been ascribed by HÖKFELT and FUXE (1972) to its direct stimulation of hypothalamic DA sites, since they found that bromocriptine specifically reduced DA turnover in the tubero-infundibular dopaminergic neurons of the nucleus arcuatus of rats. Furthermore, FLÜCKIGER (1976) reported that stereotactic placement of 25–50 μg of bromocriptine in the nucleus arcuatus of the rat inhibited ovum implantation. However, since the dopaminergic neurons of the tubero-infundibular system also respond to alterations in circulating prolactin, lowered serum prolactin levels induced by a direct action of bromocriptine on the pituitary could explain the reduced DA turnover in the tuberoinfundibular neurons.

8. Other Ergopeptine Derivatives

Other ergopeptine derivatives besides ergocornine and bromocriptine showed effects typical of an agonist action at central dopaminergic sites. As seen from Tables 6, 7, and 8, a number of genuine ergopeptine derivatives, such as ergosine (21), ergonine (110a), ergocristine (23), α-ergokryptine (25), and β-ergokryptine (26), elicited contralateral turning in rats with a unilateral degeneration of the nigrostriatal pathway and stereotypies in intact rats and increased locomotor activity of mice. Ergotamine was found to be inactive in all three tests. The dihydrogenated ergopeptine derivatives in general were found to be less potent than their nondihydrogenated parent compounds (Tables 6, 7, and 8). However, when administered at a parenteral dose of 30 mg/kg, some of these dihydrogenated derivatives, e.g., dihydro-α-ergokryptine (102e) elicited strong and long-lasting contralateral turning in lesioned rats (Table 6).

Further results with dihydroergotoxine were reported by DEPOORTERE et al. (1975) and by LOEW et al. (1976b). At doses of 2.5–10 mg/kg i.v. this compound reduced the antinociceptive action of morphine in rabbits. However, unlike the antagonism of apomorphine or bromocriptine, it counteracted this reduction of analgesia only when applied intraventricularly to the fourth ventricle, an observation which was interpreted by these authors as indicating a stimulant action on dopaminergic sites in the pontomedullary region of the fourth ventricle. In other studies, LOEW et al. (1976a) and VIGOURET et al. (1977) reported dopaminergic effects of dihydroergotoxine, which at doses of 10 to 100 reduced the concentrations of HVA and DOPAC in the striate nucleus of the rat. In addition, dihydroergotoxine counteracted the elevations of striate homovanillic acid induced by morphine or haloperidol pretreatment (LOEW et al., 1976a). A slight reduction of the NA content in the brain stem as well as an enhancement of MOPEG sulphate content and NA turnover were reported in the same two papers. MARKSTEIN and WAGNER (1978) also found that dihydroergotoxine (5×10^{-9} M) antagonized maximal NA (100 μM) stimulation of cAMP levels in rat cortex slices of homogenates. This blockade was also seen in vivo after 3 or 6 weeks of daily dihydroergotoxine (3 mg/kg) treatment. Based on studies with phentolamine and pindolol, these authors concluded that dihydroergotoxine exerts an α-adrenergic blocking effect at α-receptors of the rat brain cortex (see also MÜLLER-SCHWEINITZER and WEIDMANN, 1978 in Chapter III of this volume and Section F this chapter).

9. Efficacy of Ergot Derivatives as Antiparkinsonian Agents

a) Animal Models of Parkinsonism

Dopamine agonists have proved to be particularly active in alleviating the principal symptoms of Parkinson's disease. The good correspondence between the results from animal and clinical studies using a variety of DA-agonists has confirmed the validity of these animal models of Parkinson's disease in the development of new antiparkinsonian agents, clarified their mechanisms of action, and provided some insight into the etiology of the disease. In these respects the application of ergot pharmacology to the understanding and cure of extrapyramidal disease, namely Parkinson's disease, has been a major development in neuropharmacology during the last 25 years.

The first reports by EHRINGER and HORNYKIEWICZ (1960), BARBEAU (1960), and BARBEAU et al. (1961) of a DA deficiency in the striatum of parkinsonian patients, together with the discovery that DA is a transmitter in the central nervous system (CARLSSON, 1959), led directly to the hypothesis that a loss of transmitter function was either the cause or the consequence of irreversible functional degeneration of the basal ganglia, which is associated with the three characteristic symptoms of Parkinson's disease: rigidity, hypokinesia, and tremor. The striatal deficiency which is due to degeneration of the nigrostriatal system (BERNHEIMER et al., 1973) is also accompanied by decreased levels of 5-HT (BERNHEIMER et al., 1961) and of the GABA-synthesizing enzyme GAD (LLOYD and HORNYKIEWICZ, 1973) in the nigrostriatal-pallidal complex as well as of NA in the nucleus accumbens and other limbic-hypothalamic structures (FARLEY and HORNYKIEWICZ, 1975). Our present understanding of the mechanisms underlying Parkinson's disease and the development of ergot derivatives as new antiparkinson agents have come directly from studies of the anatomic, physiologic, behavioral, and biochemic bases of dopaminergic transmission in animal models and from careful extrapolation of these principles to clinical situations. These studies have led to the general assumption that DA (and perhaps other) receptors on neurons postsynaptic to the degenerated striatal axons would cease to function normally in the parkinsonian patient, thereby producing the symptoms of rigidity, hypokinesia, and tremor. For this reason, tests at the present time are designed to evaluate the ability of prospective antiparkinson drugs to stimulate postsynaptic dopamine receptors.

One of the most satisfactory pharmacologic models of Parkinson's disease has been developed by ANDÉN et al. (1966a) and UNGERSTEDT (1971), who found that unilateral degeneration of the dopaminergic nigrostriatal pathway of the rat led to a characteristic behavior which could be measured and quantified. In these rats a facsimile of the disease was constructed by unilaterally making an electrolytic lesion in the nigrostriatal pathway or injecting 6-hydroxydopamine (6-OHDA) into the substantia nigra. The latter procedure leads to the degeneration of only its DA- and NA-containing neurons that innervate the striatum on the injected side. Although these 6-OHDA-treated rats do not display typical parkinsonian symptoms, the difference in responsiveness of the intact and lesioned sides allows the differentiation between substances which act relatively selectively on the postsynaptic DA striatal receptors of the degenerated side (which have lost their DA inputs) and those which act predominantly (presynaptically) on the striatal DA neurons of the intact side. Thus, activation of the nigrostriatal system in the "Ungerstedt rat" by drugs leads to the production of asymmetric postures and turning behavior toward the side which is activated less. Rotation toward the intact side (contralateral to the lesioned side) implies activation primarily of postsynaptic striatal DA receptors on the degenerated side which develop "denervation supersensitivity" (UNGERSTEDT, 1971). Apomorphine, which mimics the action of

DA, causes turning contralateral to the lesioned side, presumably because it directly stimulates these supersensitive receptors. Presynaptic action on this side is ruled out in the absence of all or most of the dopaminergic inputs to the neostriatum. Consequently, other drugs inducing contralateral turning can be tentatively classified as direct DA receptor agonist. In contrast, drugs like *d*-amphetamine which release dopamine from the nerve terminals induce turning ipsilateral to the lesioned side. Since they act predominantly on the intact side, drugs which induce ipsilateral rotation presumably act presynaptically.

Since antiparkinsonian efficacy is assumed to be related mainly to the ability of a drug to stimulate postsynaptic dopamine receptors in the absence of normal presynaptic function, those drugs which induce turning contralateral to the lesioned side are considered useful antiparkinsonian agents. Drugs like amphetamine which act presynaptically can be considered potential antiparkinsonian agents only if some nigrostriatal dopaminergic neurons remain functional in the parkinsonian patient.

Animal models have been developed to represent the primary symptoms of Parkinson's disease. One of these is the reserpinized rodent, in which reserpine depletes almost all the monoamine stores to produce an akinetic, cataleptic animal whose coordinated motor activity can be restored by apomorphine or L-DOPA plus benserazide (CARLSSON et al., 1957). Although such extreme akinesia is not wholly representative of the comparable parkinsonian symptom and may even reflect the impairment of several transmitter systems within and outside the CNS, its rapid amelioration by dopamine agonists alone has made the reserpine-induced akinesia an invaluable model in the search for new antiparkinsonian agents.

A further effect of reserpine in rodents, i.e., rigidity, provides a model of the rigidity in Parkinson patients. Experimental investigations of reserpine-induced rigidity in animals have indicated that after reserpine the activity of α-motoneurons is enhanced, and that this effect can be reduced by drugs which stimulate central DA receptors (ROOS and STEG, 1964; STEG, 1964; JURNA et al., 1972; JURNA, 1976). The value of the reserpinized rodent model is supported as well by the fact that reserpine increases the intensity of akinesia, tremor, and rigidity in parkinsonian patients (BIRKMAYER and HORNYKIEWICZ, 1964). It also has been demonstrated that L-DOPA treatment can relieve surgically induced tremors in monkeys with a unilateral electrolytic lesion in the ventromedial tegmental region of the brain stem (GOLDSTEIN et al., 1973). Administration of DA agonists also often produces circling towards the denervated side and involuntary movements (MIYAMOTO et al., 1974) which have been used to suggest that degeneration of ascending DA pathways may have produced marked DA receptor sensitivity. Since these results have been interpreted to mean that DA receptor stimulation in the forebrain leads to the relief of tremor, this model also may be relevant to Parkinson's disease.

In another rodent model, DA receptor stimulation, in part, is thought to protect genetically susceptible DBA/2 mice against audiogenic seizures (LEHMANN, 1970; ANLEZARK and MELDRUM, 1975; ANLEZARK et al., 1976). The validity of this model as a possible basis for evaluating antiparkinsonian drugs is based on the observation that apomorphine (1–10 mg/kg) can almost completely block the audiogenic seizure response, and that haloperidol reduces this protective effect of apomorphine. However, serotonin receptor stimulation cannot be ruled out as a component of this protective mechanism, since an increase in cerebral 5-HT also leads to a decrease in seizure susceptibility and vice versa (LEHMANN, 1970).

Stereotypies consisting of compulsive biting, gnawing, and sniffing following the administration of apomorphine to rats were first described by RANDRUP and MUNKVAD (1970). Since then, such drug-elicited stereotypies in rodents are being interpreted as an index of stimulation of central DA receptors. It remains uncertain, however, whether or not the induction of stereotypies by a drug can predict its therapeutic potential for treating the primary symptoms of Parkinsonism such as akinesia or, instead, its propensity to produce side effects such as dyskinesia and involuntary movements which often accompany antiparkinsonian treatment.

Various ergot derivatives studied in our laboratories induced contralateral turning in the Ungerstedt model for a much longer time than doses of apomorphine, which induced a similar or slightly higher rotational frequency (Table 6). Based on the maximal number of rotations per minute achieved at a dose of 1 mg/kg or less, the order of potency was found to be lisuride (0.1 mg/kg) > apomorphine (0.25 mg/kg) > *d*-LSD > elymoclavine = CM 29-712 > CF 25-397 = α-ergokryptine = β-ergokryptine > ergocornine > agroclavine > lergotrile > bromocriptine. The potential usefulness of these ergot derivatives as antiparkinsonian agents is supported as well by observations that doses between 0.5 and 30 mg/kg of agroclavine, *d*-LSD, lisuride, lergotrile, ergosine, ergonine, a-ergokryptine, bromocriptine, and ergocornine could also induce stereotypy in rats (Table 7). Reserpine-induced akinesia in the rat has also been shown in our laboratories and by JOHNSON et al. (1974, 1976) to be inhibited by bromocriptine, CF 25-397 (JATON et al., 1976), and CM 29-712 (VIGOURET et al., 1977) (Figure 8). Recently, lisuride has been shown to be about as effective as apomorphine and *d*-amphetamine in inducing stereotyped behavior in normal as well as reserpinized mice and in antagonizing motor depression induced by reserpine (HOROWSKI and WACHTEL, 1976). In addition, bromocriptine has been shown to reduce reserpine-induced α-rigidity in rats (VIGOURET et al., 1978). Furthermore, lergotrile, bromocriptine, and ergocornine possessed long-lasting antitremor activity in monkeys with brain stem lesions (MIYAMOTO et al., 1974; LIEBERMAN et al., 1975). Ergocornine, bromocriptine, ergometrine, *d*-LSD, and methysergide, in order of decreasing potency, were active in blocking audiogenic seizures in DBA/2 mice as well (ANLEZARK et al., 1976).

b) Therapeutic Advances With Ergot Derivatives in Parkinsonism

Rational steps in the development of new therapeutic agents in the treatment of morbus Parkinson were not taken for 100 years after CHARCOT (cited in ORDENSTEIN, 1867) first advocated the use of atropine and similar synthetic muscarinic blockers in conventional antiparkinsonian therapy. It was only after the discoveries by BLASCHKO (1957) and CARLSSON (1959) of a transmitter role for DA in the central nervous system and by EHRINGER and HORNYKIEWICZ (1960), BARBEAU (1960) and BARBEAU et al. (1961) of a DA deficiency in the brains of parkinsonian patients that the potential efficacy of dopaminergic stimulants underwent systematic study. Therapeutic investigations were subsequently pursued with L-DOPA, which is rapidly converted to DA in the brain. The initial reports of BIRKMAYER and

HORNYKIEWICZ (1961) and of BARBEAU et al. (1961) have since been confirmed and indicate that L-DOPA is an effective treatment for Parkinsonism (COTZIAS et al., 1967; YAHR et al., 1969; CALNE and STERN, 1969; CALNE, 1971). Further progress was made possible by the introduction of extracerebral decarboxylase inhibitors (BARTHOLINI et al., 1967) which allowed a reduction of both the L-DOPA dose and its side effects, particularly of those of peripheral origin (BIRKMAYER and MENTASTI, 1967; SIEGFRIED, 1969; TISSOT, 1969; CHRISTIANI and MÖLLER, 1973; FEISE and PAAL, 1974; BARBEAU and ROY, 1976). In fact, L-DOPA with or without peripheral decarboxylase inhibition provides substantial symptomatic improvement in about two-thirds of the patients. However, L-DOPA does not reverse the disease, and its therapeutic success is often limited by side effects such as nausea, vomiting, and dyskinesias. Less frequently, hallucinations, confusion, and postural hypotension are observed. A therapeutic response to L-DOPA is often slow to appear and, after a few years treatment, response swings ("on-off" phenomena) related to fluctuations in plasma DOPA levels may occur (MARSDEN and PARKES, 1976).

As possible alternatives to L-DOPA therapy, central DA agonist drugs are thought to offer an important advance in the treatment of parkinsonism. In addition to pyrimidyl-piperonyl-piperazine, piribedil (LIEBERMAN et al., 1974), and an apomorphine derivative, norpropyl aporphine (COTZIAS et al., 1976), two ergot derivatives, lergotrile and bromocriptine have been investigated as antiparkinsonian drugs in patients. Lergotrile was found to provide moderate antiparkinson effect when administered at doses up to 20 mg a day (LIEBERMAN et al., 1975). In subsequent studies LIEBERMAN et al. (1976 a) increased the daily oral dose of lergotrile to 60 mg and concomitantly reduced the doses of levodopa. Under these conditions, a significant improvement over the results achieved with the combination of levodopa and benserazide was observed: a diminished frequency of abnormal involuntary movements and of response swings. Delusions and hypotension remained the most commonly observed side effects.

Therapeutic investigations of bromocriptine as an antiparkinson agent have now been reported in over 350 patients. CALNE et al. (1974a), who were the first to add a mean daily oral dose of 19 mg bromocriptine to conventional levodopa therapy, found an improvement which was more pronounced in the more severe cases. When they simultaneously reduced the levodopa dosage during bromocriptine therapy, CALNE et al. (1974b) found that a mean daily dose of 42 mg bromocriptine allowed complete withdrawal of the previous levodopa treatment of 1.6 g/day in six patients, while in 13 patients the levodopa dose was reduced by over 50%. A substitution of placebo for bromocriptine resulted in a pronounced exacerbation of symptoms (CALNE et al., 1974a; LEES et al., 1975).

In another study, KARTZINEL et al. (1976b) reported that a mean daily dose of 80 mg bromocriptine was slightly, but significantly superior to L-DOPA. Optimal benefit was achieved when combining L-DOPA and bromocriptine together in patients who responded to each alone. PARKES et al. (1976a, 1976b) and DEBONO et al. (1976), when scoring total functional disability, found a dose of 2 g of L-DOPA to be slightly more potent than 100 mg bromocriptine. In addition, these authors reported that within a dose range of 12.5–100 mg of bromocriptine, the higher bromocriptine dosages were generally more potent than the lower dosages. These results are in agreement with those obtained by LEES et al. (1975), LIEBERMAN et al. (1976b) and LUDIN et al. (1976).

The side effects reported during bromocriptine therapy were qualitatively rather similar to those observed under L-DOPA, but their relative frequency differed. Nausea and vomiting were rather uncommon, whereas confusion and delusions limited the use of higher doses and even necessitated termination of treatment in one-fifth of the patients. Symptomatic postural hypotension was found to be infrequent, but unvoluntary movements were reported, particularly at higher dose levels (PARKES et al., 1976a, 1976b).

The therapeutic effect of bromocriptine treatment has been maintained over a period of up to 1 year (TEYCHENNE et al., 1976; PARKES et al., 1976a, 1976b). While bromocriptine was not found to be clearly more potent than L-DOPA, its action had an earlier onset and was more sustained. These same authors as well as FRATTOLA et al. (1976) and MCLELLAN (1976) have shown that bromocriptine treatment also led to a reduction of response swings which are characteristic of prolonged L-DOPA treatment.

When studying the cerebrospinal fluid of parkinsonism patients receiving bromocriptine, KARTZINEL et al. (1976a) found that cerebrospinal homovanillic acid concentrations were reduced. Furthermore, PARKES et al. (1976a) reported that the administration of the DA blocking agent metoclopramide (60 mg p.o., 30 min previously) reduced the antiparkinson effects of a single bromocriptine dose. These results indicate that in parkinsonism patients bromocriptine reduces DA turnover and suggest that its therapeutic effects are associated with stimulation of central DA receptors.

E. Synaptic Transmission: Serotoninergic Mechanisms

1. Criteria of Serotoninergic Stimulation and Antagonism at the Synaptic Level

In the preceding section the effects of ergot derivatives on catecholaminergic mechanisms were reviewed using defined criteria applied to pharmacodynamic effects at the behavioral, biochemic, and electrophysiologic levels. In general, similar criteria should be established when discussing serotoninergic mechanisms. For instance, functional criteria of stimulation or antagonism would be that an ergot derivative mimics the effects of well-established serotoninergic agonists or antagonists. There are however, serious drawbacks to such a definition, because no well-established competitive antagonists are available for the study of serotoninergic transmission, and most ergot derivatives which are used as tools in the central nervous system are known to have antagonist effects primarily in peripheral smooth muscle preparations. In addition, in contrast to the study of catecholaminergic transmission, no simple behavioral model similar to the induction of rotations in rats with a unilateral degeneration of the nigrostriatal dopaminergic pathway has found general acceptance.

The biochemic effects on 5-HT turnover have become the most widely used index of central serotoninergic functions. As stated in the discussion of catecholaminergic mechanisms, turnover reflects overall synaptic function, including synthesis, release, binding to receptors, reuptake, and degradation of the transmitter. In spite of the difficulties in differentiating effects on single components of synaptic function, it still is widely accepted that when a serotonin receptor is stimulated, serotonin turnover is depressed, but when a serotonin receptor is blocked, the turnover is enhanced (Andén et al., 1968).

Studies of the turnover of 5-HT in the whole brain do not take into account that 5-HT is unevenly distributed over the brain. Dahlström and Fuxe (1964) and Fuxe (1965a) used a fluorescence technique to demonstrate that 5-HT is primarily contained in neuronal elements, and that the majority of 5-HT-containing neurons are situated in the raphe nuclei of the brain stem and project into the forebrain and other brain regions. Densely packed terminals of serotoninergic raphe neurons have been found in the ventral lateral geniculate body, in the cortical and basal lateral parts of the nucleus amygdalae, in the tectum opticum, and in the subiculum (Aghajanian et al., 1973). However, diffuse 5-HT nerve terminals have also been described in the cortex and in the reticular formation (Fuxe, 1965b). Aghajanian and others have repeatedly emphasized that understanding the effects of putative 5-HT agonists and antagonists, such as *d*-LSD (73b), 2-Br-LSD (37a), or methysergide (34a), on 5-HT turnover or on any other index of serotoninergic function in the brain must be based upon a rigorous description of these effects on defined serotoninergic systems, such as the raphe nucleus or its so-called "postsynaptic" areas which receive a defined, uniform 5-HT input. The possibilities of making electrophysiologic measurements from single cells in the raphe or its projections and of applying drugs iontophoretically to small numbers of these cells have made these the most direct approaches to a well-defined study of 5-HT neurons.

A number of chemically unrelated drugs have been proposed to imitate the effects of 5-HT in the central nervous system. Systemic administration of 5-hydroxytryptophan (5-HTP) increases brain 5-HT, which is in part due to a selective accumulation in neurons (Udenfriend et al., 1957; Fuxe, 1965a; Corrodi et al., 1967b). However, high doses of 5-HTP not only lead to 5-HT accumulation in cells that do not ordinarily contain this amine but also interfere with catecholamines and their precursors for transport, storage, and metabolism (Johnson et al., 1968; Fuxe et al., 1971; Ng et al., 1972). The evidence that quipazine imitates the effects of 5-HT in the central nervous system is mainly based on its effect on 5-HT turnover. This compound was shown by Grabowska et al. (1974b) to reduce brain 5-HT turnover in a similar way to *d*-LSD (Andén et al., 1968). An ever-increasing number of compounds are being described as 5-HT antagonists (Gyermek, 1966). Besides methysergide and *d*-LSD (Cerletti and Doepfner, 1958), methergoline (89d) (Ferrini and Glasser, 1965), cinanserine (Rubin et al., 1964), cyproheptadine (Stone et al., 1961), and mianserine (Vargaftig et al., 1971) are the most frequently cited. Monachon et al. (1972) and Tebecis (1972) have described central 5-HT antagonist effects of methiothepin, which also was reported to block NA and DA receptors.

In addition to investigations of the effects of 5-HT agonists and antagonists and the electrical characteristics of defined 5-HT neurons, a number of studies have been devoted to the search for behavioral models which reflect changes in central serotoninergic transmission. In 1961, HESS and DOEPFNER described that 5-HTP induced head twitches in rats, an effect which was later reported in mice by CORNE et al. (1963). Similar effects of 5-HTP were described by GRAHAME-SMITH (1971 a, 1971 b) and JACOBS (1974 a, 1974 b) in mice, rats, and hamsters. Myoclonus also could be induced by tryptamine in mice (TEDESCHI et al., 1959) and by 5-HTP in guinea-pigs (KLAWANS et al., 1973). In most of these tests the 5-HT antagonists cited above counteracted the behavioral syndromes induced by 5-HTP or tryptamine.

When reviewing the effects of ergot derivatives in the whole animal (Section C of this chapter), reference was made to effects which were attributed to their interaction with central 5-HT receptors. The ability of ergot derivatives to counteract reserpine-induced behavioral depression or reserpine-induced ponto-geniculo-occipital waves was proposed to be related to an imitation of central effects of 5-HT by the ergot derivatives. Furthermore, the results of studies on photogenic seizures, on the sleep-wakefulness cycle, and on body temperature were suggestive of interference with serotoninergic synaptic transmission. Further indirect evidence from behavioral or other intact animal studies which suggest that ergot derivatives affect serotoninergic transmission will not be cited in this section. Instead, emphasis will be given to biochemic and electrophysiologic investigations which provide more direct evidence for an action of ergot derivatives on 5-HT mediated synaptic transmission.

2. *D*-LSD

a) Biochemic Effects

Proposals that the hallucinogenic potency of *d*-LSD (73b) could be explained by the effects of the drug on brain 5-HT were originally based on observations of such an interaction in peripheral organs (GADDUM, 1953; WOOLLEY and SHAW, 1954).

FREEDMAN (1961) was the first to show that *d*-LSD induced a small, but significant increase in the level of 5-HT in the rat brain and thus to infer the existence of central receptors with a similar affinity to both 5-HT and *d*-LSD. Later experimental work by ANDÉN et al. (1968) and by CORRODI et al. (1975) extended this interpretation to suggest that *d*-LSD directly stimulated 5-HT receptors, since the drug reduced the turnover rate of brain and spinal cord 5-HT after inhibition of tryptophan hydroxylase by α-propyldopacetamide (H22/54). Furthermore, in the acutely spinalized rat ANDÉN et al., (1968) showed that nialamide pretreatment followed by either 5-HTP (10–75 mg/kg i.v.) or by *d*-LSD (0.5–2 mg/kg i.p.) caused a dose-dependent increase in the intensity of the hindlimb extensor reflex, tremors in the forelimbs, and involuntary movements of the head. These doses of *d*-LSD were similar to those required to reduce 5-HT turnover. Neither 2-Br-LSD nor methysergide administered instead of *d*-LSD had such effects, nor did they block the action of 5-HTP or *d*-LSD. The action of 5-HTP and *d*-LSD was not even blocked after pretreatment with reserpine plus α-propyldopacetamide or by various catecholamine receptor blockers. The significant feature of these results was that after 5-HT depletion produced by chemical or surgical procedures, sensitivity to the motor excitatory effects of *d*-LSD was maintained. After an electrolytic lesion of the midbrain raphe nucleus, APPEL et al. (1970) even observed an enhanced sensitivity to *d*-LSD. Thus, it was ruled out that *d*-LSD enhanced 5-HT release from raphe terminals. Instead, it was suggested that *d*-LSD might directly stimulate 5-HT receptors postsynaptic to the depleted or degenerated raphe inputs.

An inverse relationship between brain 5-HT levels and the firing rate of raphe neurons has been reported by AGHAJANIAN et al. (1967) and WEISS and AGHAJANIAN (1971), who demonstrated that electrical stimulation of the rat brain raphe decreased 5-HT and increased the 5-hydroxyindoleacetic acid (HIAA) concentrations in the forebrain. Both of these changes could be prevented by *d*-LSD pretreatment, suggesting that *d*-LSD might also have a presynaptic action on raphe neurons, resulting in an increased 5-HT level, inhibition of their firing rate, and reduced 5-HT turnover. In fact, elevation of brain 5-HT levels also resulted in an inhibition of spontaneous activity of raphe neurons (AGHAJANIAN et al., 1970).

The possibility that *d*-LSD inhibits 5-HT release in intact animals cannot be ruled out. Concentrations of *d*-LSD from 2 to 200 μM inhibited selectively the release of 5-HT from field stimulated guinea-pig and rat brain slices in vitro (CHASE et al., 1967, 1969; FARNEBO and HAMBERGER, 1971). Furthermore, i.p. doses of *d*-LSD as low as 75 μg/kg have been shown to decrease the efflux of ^{3}H-5-HT (synthesized in vivo from ^{3}H-tryptophan) into the cerebrospinal fluid (GALLAGER and AGHAJANIAN, 1975). Simultaneous inhibition of raphe cell firing observed at these doses may have accounted for this decrease in 5-HT release. In addition, CARLSSON and LINDQVIST (1972) reported that *d*-LSD decreased the rate of 5-HT synthesis from tryptophan, presumably at the point where tryptophan is converted to 5-HTP by tryptophan hydroxylase.

Vertebrate adenylate cyclase systems which are highly sensitive to 5-HT have been found in the superior and inferior colliculi of 1–3-day-old rats (VON HUNGEN et al., 1975b) and in synaptosomal plasma membranes of adult rats (PAGEL et al., 1976). Half-maximal stimulation of adenylate cyclase in the particulate fraction from collicular cells could be produced by 1 μM 5-HT. In this system, *d*-LSD (100μM) alone was also capable of slightly stimulating enzyme activity, whereas several 5-HT antagonists, including *d*-LSD, 2-Br-LSD, methysergide, and methergoline, produced a significant, but partial blockade of 5-HT-stimulated collicular adenylate cyclase activity. This response to 5-HT declined markedly during early development and was very low at maturity.

b) Electrophysiologic Effects

The most direct approach to testing the original hypothesis of WOOLLEY and SHAW (1954) has been to investigate the effects of *d*-LSD and related compounds when applied microiontophoretically to single brain cells with a clearly identified 5-HT content or input. AGHAJANIAN and coworkers were the first to test *d*-LSD by recording from single cells in the brain stem raphe nucleus. The raphe nucleus is the presumptive source of most 5-HT-containing "presynaptic" neurons, which project to various forebrain "postsynaptic" regions, i.e., the ventral lateral geniculate, amygdala, optic tectum and subiculum (AGHAJANIAN et al., 1973), and hippocampus and superior colliculus (BLOOM et al., 1972, 1973). The apparent histochemic homogeneity of the raphe correlates well with the almost uniform inhibition of its neurons by either systemic or direct iontophoretic application of *d*-LSD (AGHAJANIAN et al., 1968, 1970; HAIGLER and AGHAJANIAN, 1974a). These and subsequent studies have done more than any others to clearly demonstrate the primary action of *d*-LSD and of methysergide (HAIGLER and AGHAJANIAN, 1974b) on 5-HT-containing neurons in the raphe nucleus and their postsynaptic components. In many other iontophoretic studies in which *d*-LSD usually inhibited the unit response to 5-HT (see reviews of BRADLEY, 1972; and BLOOM et al., 1972), it was not clear whether the responding neurons actually received serotoninergic inputs in vivo. In the following discussion we will examine the effects of *d*-LSD mainly on brain structures where 5-HT input and/or content has already been reasonably well established. For a more expanded discussion of *d*-LSD, the reader is referred to Chapter III (MÜLLER-SCHWEINITZER and WEIDMANN, 1978) of this volume.

AGHAJANIAN et al. (1968) have shown that small i.v. doses (10 μg/kg) of *d*-LSD selectively and reversibly inhibited spontaneous unit activity in the nucleus dorsalis raphe and nucleus medianus raphe of the rat. Identical effects of *d*-LSD were reported when it was administered iontophoretically to single raphe neurons (AGHAJANIAN et al., 1972). 5-HT applied directly to these cells inhibited firing as well, and the effects of submaximal doses of both 5-HT and *d*-LSD were additive. Only at i.v. doses between 70 and 300 μg/kg or at very high iontophoretic ejection currents did *d*-LSD inhibit nonraphe units (AGHAJANIAN et al., 1972; BRAMWELL and GÖNYE, 1976). In contrast, iontophoretically applied 2-Br-LSD was unable to inhibit raphe neurons (AGHAJANIAN et al., 1972; AGHAJANIAN and HAIGLER, 1974). Thus, these authors concluded that *d*-LSD imitates the effects of 5-HT on the surface of the raphe cell. Since an elevation of brain 5-HT levels has been observed to inhibit the firing rate of raphe neurons (AGHAJANIAN et al., 1970) and to enhance the availability of 5-HT at postsynaptic sites (AGHAJANIAN, 1972), the reduced turnover of 5-HT as seen in biochemic experiments was thought to be due to a negative feedback mechanism which originates in "postsynaptic" neurons receiving serotoninergic inputs and impinging on the raphe cells.

Further experiments were carried out using iontophoretic or intravenous administration of *d*-LSD or 5-HT to neurons receiving a serotoninergic input. Each of these "postsynaptic" areas mentioned above appears to be uniform in the sense that all of the cells in a given stucture are surrounded by terminals which have been identified histochemically and fluorimetrically as containing 5-HT and which are consistently inhibited by low ejection currents of 5-HT. HAIGLER and AGHAJANIAN (1974a) found that these "postsynaptic" cells also responded to *d*-LSD with a weak inhibition. As compared to the raphe nucleus, cells in these postsynaptic neurons were relatively intensitive to microiontophoretically ejected or systemically administered *d*-LSD. Raphe cells could be totally inhibited at ejection currents too low to have any effect on the postsynaptic neurons. In contrast, 5-HT depressed presynaptic raphe cells and postsynaptic cells at similar concentrations.

Low i.v. doses of *d*-LSD which inhibited raphe neurons accelerated the spontaneous firing rate of postsynaptic neurons of the lateral geniculate nucleus (PHILLIS et al., 1967; TEBECIS and DIMARIA, 1972) and the ventral lateral geniculate, amygdala, optic tectum, and subiculum (HAIGLER and AGHAJANIAN, 1974a) of the rat brain. This acceleration appeared not to be due to blocking of the inhibitory effect of endogenous 5-HT on the postsynaptic neurons, since iontophoretically applied 5-HT was found to be inhibitory to these neurons even after i.v. administration of *d*-LSD. These data have been used to suggest that *d*-LSD, like 5-HT, acts primarily by inhibiting raphe activity, and that this action subsequently releases the postsynaptic cells from their inhibitory raphe influence to produce an acceleration of their firing rate. Other evidence supports this interpretation. For example, electrical stimulation of raphe cells caused inhibition of firing in single cells of the suprachiasmatic nucleus (BLOOM et al., 1972). It is assumed that under most conditions, spontaneous raphe cell activity would exert the same inhibition. Since this strong direct inhibitory effect of *d*-LSD on raphe neurons was produced by i.v. doses (as low as 3 μg/kg) that had little inhibitory effect on the cells receiving 5-HT inputs, an indirect action of *d*-LSD on the raphe via a postsynaptic neuronal feedback loop was excluded. Further support for a direct inhibiting effect of *d*-LSD on raphe cells also has come from evidence that raphe inhibition by i.v. *d*-LSD was neither prevented nor decreased following transection of the 5-HT raphe projections to the forebrain (HAIGLER and AGHAJANIAN, 1974a).

COUCH (1970, 1976a) has recently identified an excitatory serotoninergic synapse originating in the nucleus paragigantocellularis lateralis (NPL) of the medulla oblongata and terminating on pontine and midbrain raphe neurons. Synaptic excitation of these raphe neurons by NPL stimulation could be mimicked by direct iontophoresis of 5-HT on 97 out of 100 raphe neurons ("D" cells) tested. An inhibitory synapse was also postulated in another group of 25 raphe neurons ("I" cells) that were inhibited by NPL stimulation, of which 20 were also inhibited by direct iontophoresis of 5-HT. When COUCH (1976b) tested *d*-LSD as a possible 5-HT blocking agent on these putative raphe synapses, he found that it could block the excitatory 5-HT synapses but not the inhibitory ones. In 17 out of 19 "D" cells, *d*-LSD was shown to simultaneously block synaptic excitation and excitation by iontophoresed 5-HT, results which seem to show that *d*-LSD can specifically block these excitatory central 5-HT synapses. The data on "I" cells which showed that *d*-LSD did not block the inhibitory synapses were consistent with all other studies showing that *d*-LSD consistently mimicked but did not block the inhibitory effects of 5-HT in the dorsal raphe nucleus and its forebrain projections. Thus, the work of COUCH extends our understanding of *d*-LSD action by suggesting that in addition to directly stimulating inhibitory 5-HT receptors on the raphe neurons, *d*-LSD also might play a second role in blocking excitatory serotoninergic synapses to the raphe. The ultimate effect of *d*-LSD on serotoninergic transmission in the above systems is probably the same whether it directly inhibits 5-HT neurons presynaptic to their synapses with other cells, or blocks the postsynaptic effects of 5-HT released from their terminals. In both cases a failure of serotoninergic transmission occurs.

These observations of COUCH (1976) are very similar to those made on the effects of *d*-LSD in the reticular formation (BOAKES et al., 1970; BRADLEY, 1972; GUILBAUD et al., 1973) and in the cortex (ROBERTS and STRAUGHAN, 1967) of the unanesthetized cat, where it also blocked excitatory responses to iontophoretically applied 5-HT. HAIGLER and AGHAJANIAN (1974a) also have found excitatory responses which were blocked by *d*-LSD, but only in the reticular formation of the rat brain where 5-HT terminals are sparse. However, these authors question the importance of this action for the in vivo effects of *d*-LSD, since it remains yet to be determined if the cells excited by 5-HT in fact receive a serotoninergic synaptic input.

3. 2-Br-LSD

Systemically administered 2-Br-LSD is much less potent than *d*-LSD in inhibiting the spontaneous firing rate of midbrain raphe neurons of the rat (AGHAJANIAN et al., 1970; see previous discussion of *d*-LSD). Also, in the forebrain of the rat (HAIGLER and AGHAJANIAN, 1974a) and the cat (HORN and McKAY, 1973) neurons receiving an identified 5-HT input from the midbrain raphe were found to be more sensitive to inhibition by intravenously administered *d*-LSD than to 2-Br-LSD. In neurons with no identified 5-HT inputs such as those in the brain stem (BOAKES et al., 1970) and the cerebral cortex (ROBERTS and STRAUGHAN, 1967) of the cat, excitatory effects of 5-HT were less readily blocked by 2-Br-LSD than by *d*-LSD. *D*-LSD also was more effective in elevating brain 5-HT levels and reducing the rate of 5-HT turnover (see previous discussion of *d*-LSD).

When these two lysergic acid derivatives were compared for their relative abilities to inhibit either the raphe neurons or those in forebrain areas receiving raphe inputs (amygdala and ventral lateral geniculate), AGHAJANIAN (1976) found that 2-Br-LSD was inactive when applied iontophoretically to raphe neurons. In contrast, both ergot derivatives had a 5-HT agonist-like inhibitory action on cells "postsynaptic" to the raphe which was less than that of 5-HT itself. AGHAJANIAN (1976) concluded that the difference between the effects of 2-Br-LSD and *d*-LSD on intact animals probably lies in their relative abilities to mimic inhibitory effects of 5-HT directly on the raphe cell.

4. Methysergide

Methysergide (34a) (5–20 mg/kg i.p.) lowered whole rat brain 5-HT concentrations in a dose-dependent fashion and increased the turnover rate by about 80% (SOFIA and VASSAR, 1975). However, D'AMICO et al. (1976) have reported that lower doses of 1–5 mg/kg methysergide had no effect on 5-HT turnover (also reported by FREEDMAN et al., 1970) but reduced 5-HT concentration in the guinea-pig brain. This discrepancy might be explained by the observation that the 5-HT content is not equally affected by methysergide in all areas of the brain. SOFIA and VASSAR (1975), for example, found that a dose of 20 mg/kg methysergide which had no effect on 5-HT content in the whole brain, cerebral cortex, and hypothalamus plus midbrain did cause a significant increase in cerebellar concentration and a decrease in the medulla oblongata and pons. Since methiothepin, a compound with serotonin antagonist properties, also increased 5-HT turnover (MONACHON et al., 1972), it has been suggested that methysergide, like methiothepin, blocks serotoninergic mechanisms.

Methysergide, like *d*-LSD, was reported to interfere with the specific interaction of 5-HT and adenylate cyclase in the immature rat brain (VON HUNGEN et al., 1975b). PAGEL et al. (1976) have found that 5-HT-sensitive adenylate cyclase activity located in purified adult rat brain synaptosomal membranes was stimulated by 5-HT concentrations between 5×10^{-10} M and 5×10^{-8} M. Methysergide, ergometrine (19), and tryptamine, each at 1×10^{-5} M, decreased the stimulating effect of 1×10^{-8} M 5-HT by 80%, 57%, and 30%, respectively. Fluphenazine, a potent inhibitor of DA-sensitive adenylate cyclase, had no effect in this synaptosomal system. Although the dependence of cAMP production on 5-HT concentration is not yet understood, these results seem to indicate that methysergide acts at central 5-HT receptors.

Recent electrophysiologic experiments of HAIGLER and AGHAJANIAN (1974b) have shown that methysergide blocked the inhibitory action of 5-HT in only some parts of the rat brain, whereas in other parts it mimicked the action of 5-HT. Methysergide applied at low ejection currents was shown to depress the spontaneous firing of neurons in the raphe nucleus and in postsynaptic areas receiving a defined homogeneous serotoninergic input. However, inhibition produced by 5-HT was not blocked in raphe cells, or in forebrain areas receiving a compact serotoninergic input (ventral lateral geniculate body, optic tectum, and amygdala), or in cells in the reticular formation which receive little 5-HT input. These effects were similar to those seen by CURTIS and DAVIS (1962) in the lateral geniculate body and by KRNJEVIC and PHILLIS (1963) in the cortex, where methysergide had no effect on the depressant effect of 5-HT.

Based on their studies with methysergide HAIGLER and AGHAJANIAN (1974b) emphasize that methysergide does not block the inhibitory effects of 5-HT in the central nervous system. These authors have drawn similar conclusions about the action of *d*-LSD, 2-Br-LSD (see above), methergoline (89d), cyproheptadine, cinanserin, and methiothepin.

However, a divergent conclusion was reached when studying the effects of methysergide on 5-HT-mediated inhibition of hippocampal cells by raphe neurons. Stimulation of dorsal or median raphe nuclei has been shown to generate long-latency and long-duration inhibition of spontaneous firing of hippocampal cells, which are known to contain 5-HT themselves and to receive a 5-HT-input from the raphe. SEGAL (1975) has shown that these hippocampal cells were inhibited if, instead of raphe stimulation, 5-HT was applied iontophoretically to them. Furthermore, depletion of 5-HT by high doses of parachlorophenylalanine (PCPA) also prevented these responses of hippocampal cells to raphe stimulation. Systemic administration of methysergide, 2-Br-LSD, and *d*-LSD all blocked the inhibitory response of hippocampal cells to 5-HT applied onto raphe cells. In addition, the late inhibitory hippocampal responses to raphe stimulation were antagonized by iontophoresis of methysergide, but not *d*-LSD, directly into the hippocampus (SEGAL and BLOOM, 1974; SEGAL, 1976).

Another example of antagonism of 5-HT-mediated inhibition by methysergide has been reported by OLPE and KOELLA (1977). These authors reported that iontophoretic application of methysergide to putamen cells (inhibited by dorsal but not median raphe stimulation) antagonized inhibition by dorsal raphe stimulation in nine out of 15 putamen cells recorded.

Thus, the ability of methysergide to universally antagonize 5-HT-mediated inhibition is still controversial. In contrast, there is little disagreement that methysergide blocks the excitatory response to 5-HT in the cerebral cortex or in the reticular formation (ROBERTS and STRAUGHAN, 1967; BOAKES et al., 1970; BRADLEY and BRIGGS, 1974b). This action may also account for the ability of methysergide, *d*-LSD, or 2-Br-LSD to counteract facilitation of monosynaptic spinal reflexes induced in rats or cats by stimulation of the raphe nucleus or by administration of 5-HT precursors (BANNA and ANDERSON, 1968; CLINESCHMIDT and ANDERSON, 1970; ANDERSON, 1972; BARASI and ROBERTS, 1973, 1974).

5. Other Lysergic Acid Derivatives

a) Methergoline

Behavioral and neuropharmacologic evidence indicates that methergoline (89d) may preferentially block postsynaptic 5-HT receptors in the brain and spinal cord. Methergoline blocked head twitches and decreased hindlimb extensor reflex activity induced by 5-HTP in mice (FERRINI and GLASSER, 1965) and rats (CLINESCHMIDT and LOTTI, 1974). Using the spinalized rat to assess the effects of methergoline on 5-HT receptor activity, FUXE et al. (1975a) found that doses between 0.5 and 5 mg/kg caused a dose-dependent reduction of *d*-LSD and 5-HTP-induced increases in extensor reflex activity, whereas the ergot derivative did not increase extensor reflex activity when administered alone.

FUXE et al. (1975a) also reported that methergoline (5–10 mg/kg) reduced 5-HT levels by about 25% and increased α-propyldopacetamide-induced 5-HT depletion in the rat brain. Furthermore, 5 mg/kg methergoline counteracted the reduction of α-propyldopacetamide-induced 5-HT depletion caused by *d*-LSD. In cortical slices methergoline at 10^{-5} M reduced ^{3}H-5-HT content.

Together these results suggest that methergoline blocks postsynaptic 5-HT receptors in the brain and spinal cord. Enhanced depletion of 5-HT has been explained in part by the fact that 5-HT receptor blocking action would probably lead to a compensatory increase in 5-HT release from serotoninergic neurons.

In more direct experiments designed to test this hypothesis in the rat brain, methergoline, like methysergide, applied at low ejection currents slightly depressed the firing rate of raphe cells or their postsynaptic inputs but failed to block the inhibitory action of 5-HT iontophoresed onto the neurons receiving serotoninergic raphe inputs (ventral lateral geniculate, amygdala, and optic tectum) (HAIGLER and AGHAJANIAN, 1974b). Only in the reticular formation where identified serotoninergic inputs are sparse was methergoline shown in 13 out of 14 cells to block excitation produced by 5-HT. In no case did it block inhibition produced by 5-HT. A systemic dose of 3.2 mg/kg methergoline did not antagonize but rather enhanced 5-HT inhibition of amygdala and ventral lateral geniculate cells.

b) PTR 17-402

In rats, PTR 17-402 (88e) markedly reduced α-propyldopacetamide-induced depletion of 5-HT stores and enhanced by about 50% the 5-HT overflow caused by electrical field stimulation (CORRODI et al., 1975; FUXE et al., 1978). At a concentration of 10^{-6} M it stimulated spontaneous release of radioactive ^{3}H-5-HT from cortex slices taken from nialamide-pretreated rats. Since most of the 5-HT present in the cortex of an untreated animal is probably stored in granular sites, it would appear that these pools of 5-HT are unaffected by PTR 17-402. For this reason, CORRODI et al. (1975) have suggested that PRT 17-402 acts primarily to stimulate 5-HT release from a functionally active extragranular pool in serotoninergic nerve terminals.

Uptake and retention of ^{3}H-5-HT by cortex slices from previously untreated rats were markedly reduced as well in a dose dependent fashion by PTR 17-402 ($ED_{50} = 1.6 \times 10^{-6}$ M) (CORRODI et al., 1975).

PTR 17-402 (0.5 to 10 mg/kg) also produced a dose-dependent increase in hind-limb extensor reflex activity of the spinalized rat which lasted for more than 3 h at a dose of 2.5 mg/kg. α-Propyldopacetamide pretreatment significantly reduced this effect of PTR 17-402, but only after combined pretreatment with reserpine was there complete blockade of the extensor reflex in the presence of PTR 17-402. Pretreatment with the MAO inhibitor nialamide markedly potentiated the strength of the extensor reflex after PTR 17-402 (CORRODI et al., 1975). Thus, it appears that this ergot-induced extensor activity is dependent more on the integrity of presynaptic 5-HT stores than on a direct stimulation of postsynaptic 5-HT receptors.

c) CF 25-397, CM 29-712, and Lisuride

VIGOURET et al. (1978) have suggested that the action of CF 25-397 (90d) and of CM 29-712 (8 epimer of 83 d) is to directly stimulate cortical 5-HT receptors. They have found that CF 25-397 and CM 29-712 (1 mg/kg s.c.) slightly reduced the 5-HT content of the whole rat brain, whereas in the cortex, 10 mg/kg slightly increased the 5-HT concentration and significantly increased cortical concentrations of both 5-HT and 5-HIAA. KEHR (1977) has reported that 1 mg/kg i.p. of lisuride (96a) slightly increased the 5-HT content and reduced the 5-HIAA content of the whole rat brain. In the mesolimbic forebrain, striate nucleus, and neocortex, the levels of 5-HTP measured after decarboxylase inhibition were diminished by 0.03–1 mg/kg i.p. lisuride. These effects were interpreted by KEHR (1977) as a possible consequence of 5-HT receptor stimulation.

6. Ergopeptine Derivatives

a) Ergotamine

Ergotamine (20) in a dose range between 5 and 20 mg/kg i.p. exerted a similar but more significant effect than methysergide on 5-HT metabolism in the rat brain. Thirty minutes after the administration of 20 mg/kg i.p. ergotamine, 5-HT content of the whole brain was reduced maximally by 43% of control values (SOFIA and VASSAR, 1975). Most of this reduction seemed to be due to selective reduction of 5-HT levels by 90% in the medulla oblongata and pons and by 83% in the cerebral cortex. In addition, this dose produced a marked increase of 75% in whole brain 5-HT turnover rate. Thus, the effect of ergotamine, like that of methysergide (HAIGLER and AGHAJANIAN, 1974b), appears to be regional. Ergotamine noncompetitively inhibited the uptake of not only 5-HT

($ED_{50} = 10^{-8}$ M), but also NA ($ED_{50} = 10^{-7}$ M) and DA ($ED_{50} = 10^{-7}$ M) by rat hypothalamic synaptosomes. In general, ergotamine was a less potent inhibitor of 5-HT uptake than reserpine but a more potent inhibitor than *d*-LSD, which at 10^{-5} M had no effect on uptake in these experiments (TUOMISTO, 1974).

b) Ergocornine

Ergocornine (24), like *d*-LSD (ANDÉN et al., 1968) was able to induce athetoid movements, hyperextension of the hindleg, forelimb tremors, and involuntary head movements in acutely spinalized rats. Since these effects of ergocornine could be produced even after severe 5-HT depletion, it was suggested that ergocornine may directly stimulate 5-HT receptors (CORRODI et al., 1975).

Intraperitoneal doses of ergocornine between 0.1 and 5 mg/kg did not significantly increase the levels of 5-HT in the brain but produced dose-dependent reduction of α-propyldopacetamide-induced 5-HT depletion. In vitro ergocornine had no effect on ^{3}H-5-HT uptake into cerebral cortical slices, but at 10^{-6} M it caused a 25% reduction in the release of ^{3}H-5-HT from field-stimulated cortex slices (CORRODI et al., 1975). Even larger doses between 0.5 and 20 mg/kg caused a dose-dependent increase in the strength of the hindlimb extensor reflex of the rat. This increase in reflex activity was not reduced by prior treatment with reserpine, α-propyldopacetamide, or a combination of both, indicating that ergocornine can act independently of presynaptic 5-HT stores and probably acts directly on postsynaptic 5-HT receptors (CORRODI et al., 1975).

c) Bromocriptine

Motor behavior of rats treated with 0.5–50 mg/kg i.p. bromocriptine (38) showed a biphasic response in which an initial lag or inhibition was followed by motor excitation (SNIDER et al., 1975, 1976; VIGOURET et al., 1978). The time course of motor activation has been correlated with an elevation of whole brain 5-HT (SNIDER et al., 1975) and with a decrease in catecholamine synthesis and dopamine turnover (SNIDER et al., 1976). Since these changes otherwise could be obscured by normal circadian fluctuations in 5-HT metabolism, SNIDER et al. (1975, 1976) carefully matched the experimental and control animals with regard to litter, diet, housing conditions, and time of sacrifice. At 2 h after a 5 mg/kg i.p. dose of bromocriptine, brain levels of 5-HT increased to 127% of control values and remained elevated 4 h later. The initial inhibition of motor activity observed after 5 mg/kg of bromocriptine and the subsequent time course of excitation could be correlated approximately with increasing accumulation of 5-HT but not 5-HIAA, which was decreased by 30–40%. The observed reduction of 6-HIAA has been used to suggest that this ergot derivative also has a direct inhibitory effect on 5-HT release.

^{3}H-5-HT release from field stimulated rat cortex slices was also reduced by bromocriptine (10^{-6} M) and ergocornine (10^{-7} M) but not by apomorphine (FARNEBO and HAMBERGER, 1971; CORRODI et al., 1975). Although it had no effect alone on the extensor reflex in the rat, bromocriptine antagonized the enhancement of this reflex activity induced by the putative 5-HT receptor stimulating drug, 5-methoxydimethyl-tryptamine (CORRODI et al., 1975).

d) Dihydroergotoxine

Neurochemic studies on rat brain biogenic amines by LOEW et al. (1976a) have indicated that dihydroergotoxine used only at a very high dose (100 mg/kg i.p.) decreased whole brain 5-HIAA concentration, decreased the rate of 5-HT disappearance after *d*-1,6-fluorotryptophan pretreatment, and strongly antagonized 5-HIAA elevation induced by clozapine. Reduction of 5-HIAA content and 5-HT turnover (also VIGOURET et al., 1978) was thought to reflect a possible inhibitory action of dihydroergotoxine on 5-HT release.

F. Brain Metabolism

1. Brain Cyclic Adenosine Monophosphate

In all species tested, cyclic adenosine monophosphate (cAMP) is involved in the mechanism of synaptic transmission (IVERSEN, 1975; BLOOM, 1975). In addition, cAMP is thought to regulate the rate of transmitter biosynthesis, energy production, and axonal transport in neurons (DALY, 1975). In brain tissue, noradrenaline (NA), dopamine (DA), serotonin (5-HT), and histamine induced increased formation of cAMP in vitro and in vivo (BURKHARD, 1972; PALMER et al., 1973). The effects of agroclavine, ergometrine, *d*-LSD, bromocriptine, dihydroergotoxine, and PTR 17-402 on catecholamine-stimulated cAMP levels have already been mentioned in the two preceding sections when reviewing the effects of ergot derivatives on central synaptic transmission. In this section we will examine the way in which some ergot alkaloids may affect the metabolism of cAMP (see review of MEIER-RUGE et al., 1975; CHAPPUIS et al., 1975; ENZ et al., 1975; MEIER-RUGE and IWANGOFF, 1976).

a) Adenylate Cyclase

Evidence that dihydroergotoxine could influence the level of intracellular cAMP came from studies on rats which had been fed the drug (3.1 mg/kg to females and 6.2 mg/kg to males) daily for 2 years (ENZ et al., 1975). In the treated animals the concentration of cAMP in the cortex and cerebellum was significantly lower than that in the same parts of the untreated control brains or in the striatum of either treated or untreated animals.

Recently, MARKSTEIN and WAGNER (1977) carried out similar experiments in vitro in which cAMP levels were measured in rat cortex slices or homogenates. Under these conditions the addition of NA, isoprenaline, or adenosine to the medium produced dose-dependent increases in cAMP production which could be antagonized by specific antagonists, including dihydroergotoxine. Stimulation by isoprenaline was antagonized competitively (parallel shift of log dose-response curves) by the β-adrenergic blocking agent pindolol but was not appreciably affected by dihydroergotoxine or the α-blocker phentolamine. However, maximal stimulation by NA (10^{-4} M) was antagonized by phentolamine (5×10^{-8} M) as well as by dihydroergotoxine (5×10^{-9} M), suggesting that the latter blocks α-adrenoceptors. The antagonism of dihydroergotoxine and phentolamine was of the "noncompetitive" type. In contrast to pindolol and phentolamine, the blockade of the NA effect by dihydroergotoxine could not be surmounted by increasing the agonist concentration (see Figure 16 in Chapter III of this book, MÜLLER-SCHWEINITZER and WEIDMANN, 1978). These experiments suggest that although rat cortex contains both α- and β-adrenoceptors capable of eliciting increased cAMP production, only the α-receptor mediated stimulation is antagonized by dihydroergotoxine.

When the NA-dependent cAMP-generating system was tested in brain slices from rats which had been fed 3 mg/kg dihydroergotoxine daily for 3–6 weeks, NA had a markedly smaller stimulating effect on cAMP formation than it had in untreated controls. From the shift of the NA dose-response curve after feeding dihydroergotoxine for 3–6 weeks, the effective concentration of dihydroergotoxine was calculated to be in the range of 10^{-8} M (MARKSTEIN and WAGNER, 1978).

In these and similar experiments the measured level of intracellular cAMP reflects the relative rates of its synthesis by adenylate cyclase and degradation by cAMP-phosphodiesterase (PEase). Few studies which relate receptor function to cAMP content have shown how a putative receptor agonist or antagonist, such as the ergot alkaloids mentioned in this chapter, effect one or both of these enzyme systems at the same time.

Changes in the level of cAMP which are brought about by effects on the synthesizing enzyme are usually measured as changes in the conversion of radioactive ATP into cAMP either with or without a PEase inhibitor. SCHULTZ and DALY (1973) have shown that NA-stimulated increases in radioactive cAMP levels in guinea-pig cerebral cortex slices are mediated primarily by interaction of NA with what appears to be a classical α-adrenergic receptor. This stimulation could be strongly inhibited by a concentration of 10^{-4} M of dihydroergokryptine (102e, f) or by methysergide (34a).

b) Cyclic AMP-Phosphodiesterase

Dihydroergotoxine has been found to inhibit membrane-bound PEase to a greater extent than soluble PEase in the mammalian brain cortex (IWANGOFF et al. 1975; ENZ et al., 1978).

When PEase activities estimated under different substrate concentrations (2 and 20 μM cAMP) were compared, dihydroergotoxine (10^{-6}–10^{-5} M) showed a stronger inhibitory effect on the low-K_m cAMP-PEase (6–22%, respectively) than on the high-K_m cAMP-PEase (4–11%, respectively) (ENZ et al., 1975). Inhibition of cAMP degradation by dihydroergotoxine or dihydroergotamine (102b) was always found to be greater in the brain than in the liver, heart, or kidney of the cat (IWANGOFF and ENZ, 1973b; IWANGOFF et al., 1975). It has been noted that the concentration range of dihydroergotoxine required to inhibit the low-K_m-PEase activity in vitro may be reached in vivo. Following infusion of 0.6–0.9 mg/kg ^{3}H-dihydroergotoxine into the internal carotid artery, concentrations of about 10^{-6} M were found in the retina and hypophysis and between 10^{-7} and 10^{-6} M in the cortex, cerebellum, and hippocampus (IWANGOFF et al., 1976). These concentrations are one to two orders of magnitude higher than the effective concentrations of dihydroergotoxine calculated by MARKSTEIN and WAGNER (1978) to be 10^{-8} M in rat brain slices following 3–6 weeks of oral administration. An average concentration of 10^{-7} M was calculated by IWANGOFF et al. (1976) after the infusion of 0.6–0.9 mg/kg i.v. ^{3}H-dihydroergotoxine into the internal carotid artery of the cat. These authors also showed that about 60% of this labeled dihydroergotoxine is localized in the synaptosomal fraction of whole brain. The greatest number of counts was found in the pituitary and, to a lesser extent, the cerebellum (MEIER-RUGE et al., 1973; IWANGOFF et al., 1978).

Like the classical PEase inhibitors caffeine and theophylline, a group of nine dihydrogenated ergot alkaloids have been shown by IWANGOFF and ENZ (1972) to inhibit cAMP hydrolysis in the grey matter of the cat brain. The degree of PEase inhibition by these ergot compounds could be correlated roughly with their molecular weights; the compounds with a higher molecular weight averaging 600 were 1.5–2.0 times more powerful inhibitors than those averaging 540. Taking all the data derived from experiments using both concentrations investigated (2.5×10^{-4} M and 2.5×10^{-5} M), it was possible to rank each ergot alkaloid according to its PEase-inhibiting activity: dihydroergostine (102 g) > dihydroergoptine (112b) > dihydroergocristine (102c) > dihydroergocornine (102d) > dihydroergokryptine (102e, f) > dihydroergosine (102a) > dihydroergotamine (102b) > dihydroergonine (110b) > dihydroergovaline (108b). The significance of this correlation does not apply to other lysergic acid derivatives such as 2-Br-LSD (34a) which also inhibit PEase activity (KUKOVETZ and PÖCH, 1969). Neither does this activity ranking reveal the structural requirements of the inhibitory action.

Dihydroergotamine inhibited the activity of PEase in cat grey matter homogenates at concentrations above 2.5×10^{-6} M. Classical PEase inhibitors caffeine and theophylline were slightly less potent when tested at the same concentrations (IWANGOFF and ENZ, 1971). Both dihydroergotamine and dihydroergotoxine seemed to inhibit PEase in an organ-specific fashion at lower concentrations (IWANGOFF and ENZ, 1973b). Only at the highest concentration used (10^{-3} M) do either of these ergot alkaloids produce uniform, significant inhibition of PEase in all organs. Organ-specific inhibition of PEase has been explained, in part, by the presence of brain-specific PEase isozymes which are exclusive to that organ (MONN and CHRISTIANSEN, 1971; CAMPBELL and OLIVER, 1972) and by brain-specific solubility characteristics of brain PEase (CHEUNG, 1970a, 1970b). Whether or not ergot alkaloids actually capitalize on these brain-specific properties of this enzyme system and thus raise the intracellular cAMP levels remains to be substantiated.

Inhibition of PEase probably explains why incubation of rat astrocytoma C6 cells with dihydroergotamine (2×10^{-6}–7.5×10^{-5} M) increased in a dose-dependent fashion the intracellular cAMP concentration up to seven-fold. Preincubation of these confluent cultures with dihydroergotamine also inhibited the usual stimulatory effect of NA on the cAMP levels (MAURER and GRIEDER, 1975).

The adrenergic receptor blocking action of dihydrogenated ergot alkaloids which leads to a diminished adenylate cyclase activity in vitro would be expected to decrease the cAMP content of noradrenergic neurons in vivo. On the other hand IWANGOFF and ENZ (1972, 1973a, 1973b) found that dihydroergotoxine and other dihydrogenated ergot alkaloids given in rather higher concentrations inhibited degradation of cAMP in vitro, which might be expected to increase the intracellular cAMP content of noradrenergic neurons. Thus, the resultant effect of any dihydrogenated ergot alkaloid on brain cAMP levels in the brain in situ would depend on the dynamic equilibrium of these two functions. This functional equilibrium of adenylate cyclase and PEase activity is a consequence of several factors, such as the rates of enzyme synthesis and turnover and the sizes of the active substrate and metal cation pools which are under genetic and other (drug, environmental) controls.

2. Adenosine Triphosphate Metabolism in the Brain

Adenosine triphosphate (ATP) is the predominant intracellular free energy source of the brain and is generated mainly through the complete oxidation of glucose coupled with mitochondrial phosphorylation of ADP. The free phosphate-bond energy of ATP is utilized in the brain for biosynthesis and ion transport, e.g., ion flux leading to synaptic membrane polarization. In addition, ATP is the principal source of cAMP in the cell.

Although the exact components essential to the maintainance of brain metabolism and function have not yet been fully defined, proper levels of ATP are essential to normal function. When oxygen is deficient, normal ATP levels can only be maintained by anaerobic glycolysis (conversion of glucose to lactate) and to a lesser extent by creatine phosphate and myokinase. Therefore, most studies of the effects of ergot derivatives on brain metabolism have focused on the extent to which they can delay the metabolic consequences of severe hypoxia (defined as reduced oxygen consumption): increased intracellular concentrations of creatine, ADP, and P_i, rapid utilization of glucose, and accelerated lactate production, and ATP degradation. Since it is usually extremely difficult to evaluate O_2 consumption directly during hypoxia, analysis of pyruvate conversion to lactate provides one of the best indices of the state of brain energy metabolism. The lactate/pyruvate ratio is meaningful precisely because these substrates are in equilibrium with the cytoplasmic $NADH/NAD^+$ system, so that reoxidation of NADH to NAD^+ which can continue under anaerobic conditions permits continued conversion of pyruvate to lactate. Thus, ergot alkaloids which increase the lactate/pyruvate ratio under hypoxic conditions or during the first phases of recovery probably enhance ATP production by accelerating anaerobic glycolysis. A lower ratio would indicate a shift toward oxidative pathways again.

The early experiments of LEWIS and MCILWAIN (1954) on the effect of ergot derivatives on respiration and glycolysis in guinea-pig cortical slices indicated that effects of these drugs could be observed only after field stimulation of the tissues. When glucose was used as the substrate, the effects of dihydroergotamine, *d*-LSD, and ergotoxine on O_2 utilization and lactic acid formation in nonstimulated tissue were weak; but when electrical pulses were applied, sensitivity to the same drug concentrations increased so that simultaneous inhibition of respiration and glycolysis occurred. Action with and without pulses was so well differentiated with *d*-LSD and ergotoxine that in the presence of electrical stimulation respiration was sensitive to 1/30 of the concentration required to affect unstimulated brain tissue. For example, stimulation of respiration and glycolysis were inhibited in parallel to about 70% by *d*-LSD (3×10^{-6} M and 10^{-4} M, respectively), by ergotoxine (10^{-5} M and 10^{-3} M, respectively), and by dihydroergotamine (above 3×10^{-6} M for both parameters). In none of these experiments was the action of dihydroergotamine antagonized by adrenaline or that of *d*-LSD antagonized by 5-HT.

a) Changes in Glucose Uptake and the Formation of Lactate and Pyruvate Following Hypoxia

Since normal brain energy metabolism clearly provides the operational basis for the electrical function of central neurons, normal electrical (EEG) function or lack of it has been considered a reflection of the metabolic status of the brain. Depression of the spontaneous EEG induced by halting artificial respiration in curarized dogs can be reversed only partially during the 30 min following restoration of normal ventilation. Only under these conditions of partial recovery were BENZI et al. (1971) able to measure the effects of certain ergot derivatives on brain metabolism and EEG. The degree of EEG recovery 30 min after hypoxia was enhanced significantly after perfusion with nicergoline (104e, 5×10^{-5} M). Similar results with dihydroergonine and dihydroergotoxine have been reviewed in the section on "EEG Under Defined Pathologic Conditions" of this chapter.

The effects of ergot derivatives on glucose uptake, lactic acid, and pyruvic acid formation have been studied in the dog brain in situ before and after the induction of a transient hypoxia. Under normal conditions (normoxia), BENZI et al. (1972) found that about 7% and 3% of the glucose taken up by the brain was metabolized to lactate and pyruvate, respectively. At the end of a 15-min period of hypoxia, brain glucose uptake had been reduced by 52% of control values, but lactate and pyruvate formation accounted for about 35% and 40%, respectively, of the glucose which had been taken up. These results suggested that the rate of glycolysis is increased in the hypoxic brain in order to maintain normal levels of ATP and other energy-rich metabolites.

A significant increase in glucose uptake was induced by nicergoline (5×10^{-5} M) infused during the first 30 min after the hypoxemic phase. Lactate formation expressed as a percentage of glucose uptake remained unchanged during recovery, but the percentage of glucose converted to pyruvate enhanced during hypoxia was significantly reduced during recovery. These results have been interpreted to show that nicergoline may reduce the metabolism of glucose via oxidative pathways during hypoxemia.

BENZI et al. (1973) and BENZI (1975) have made more precise evaluations of the energy state of the brain by calculating the "redox potential" of the brain from the lactate/pyruvate ratio, and the "energy charge potential" (ECP) from the relative proportions of individual adenine nucleotides in dog brain tissue. "Redox potential" is a function of the concentrations of lactate and pyruvate determined in small tissue samples removed from the cortex and was calculated according to the following formula (see BENZI, 1975).

$$E_h = E_o - \frac{RT}{nF} \ln \frac{[\text{reduced form}]}{[\text{oxidized form}]} \, .$$

The ECP has been expressed as a function of the relative proportions of the individual adenine nucleotides or

$$\frac{([ATP]+0.5\ [ADP])}{([ATP]+[ADP]+[AMP])}$$

under the assumption that the balance among concentrations of nucleotides responds to the energy state of the cell rather than to the concentration of a single nucleotide. Neither one of these calculations, however, provides an evaluation of the redox potential of the $NADH/NAD^+$ system.

According to these criteria, the energy state of the cortical motor area could be modified with nicergoline only during posthypoxic recovery but never in the control state or during hypoxia. At PaO_2 levels below 20 mm Hg a decrease in ECP and a negativization of the redox potential was observed. After the first three minutes of posthypoxic recovery, infusion of saline produced a recovery of about 50% of the hypoxia-induced drop in ECP, while the redox potential remained unchanged. Perfusion of nicergoline (10^{-4} M), but not that of papaverine and theophylline, raised the ECP even more above the saline control levels without an accompanying recovery of the redox potential from its hypoxic value (BENZI, 1975). Nicergoline was able to induce this increase in the ECP by significantly decreasing the AMP concentration below levels achieved by saline perfusion alone. Thus, it appears that the brain continues to utilize oxidation and glycolysis during recovery, both of which were accelerated by hypoxia. Furthermore, the dependence on oxidation of glucose may be reduced during recovery in the presence of nicergoline.

The action of nicergoline during recovery from hypoxia could be blocked by simultaneous perfusion of Na-malonate (5×10^{-2} M) or cocaine (5×10^{-3} M). Since malonate is a well-known potent inhibitor of the tricarboxylic acid respiratory cycle (TCA) as well, it has been suggested by these authors that nicergoline action also may be associated with the TCA cycle.

Nicergoline at doses which reduce the duration of EEG recovery from acute ischemia (BENZI et al., 1971; BOISMARE and LORENZO, 1975) also reverses certain changes in mitochondrial metabolism induced by ischemia (MORETTI et al., 1974). Complete ischemia of the cat brain in vivo during 3 min had no effect on oxidative phosphorylation but reduced the activity of 2,4-dinitrophenol (DNP)-stimulated and spontaneous ATPases, while increasing the content of free fatty acids (FFA) of mitochondrial preparations from the frontal lobe. Intravenous infusion of nicergoline (150 μg/kg) for 12 min before the onset of ischemia prevented all these alterations. Nicergoline administered to normal animals enhanced both the DNP- and Mg-stimulated ATPases without affecting the FFA content or the activity of spontaneous ATPase.

Since activation of phospholipase A has been shown to be responsible for release of FFA from phospholipids following postdecapitation ischemia (BAZAN et al., 1971), nicergoline may reduce ischemic degradation of lipids in neuronal and other membranes and thereby affect membrane-associated processes such as ATPase activity and cation permeability. It remains to be shown, however, whether or not the EEG pattern induced by acute ischemia is directly related to changes in mitochondrial function.

The effects of nicergoline in models of hypoxia are difficult to interpret, since the "cerebral energy state" is remarkably resistant to these pathophysiologic conditions above a PaO_2 of 20 mm Hg. For example, between 35 and 20 mm Hg, changes of the redox potential are not accompanied by modifications of the ECP, even though the two phenomena are obviously related. This serves to illustrate as well that changes in O_2 consumption cannot be used to define the cerebral energy state, since several conditions such as those above can produce large changes in the rate of cerebral O_2 metabolism without disrupting the energy balance of the brain. At arterial pO_2 below 35 mm Hg, creatine phosphatase also is activated to maintain and protect normal energy levels as long as possible after the onset of hypoxia. Furthermore, since the lactate/pyruvate ratio is influenced by intracellular pH even in the absence of hypoxia, this ratio must be used with caution. These reservations raise substantial questions about the site of nicergoline action in the cell, especially in the above acute models in which the range of drug effect on cerebral bioenergetics is already not very wide and occurs only during the posthypoxic phase. Whether these effects attributed to nicergoline are due to its activation of specific cerebral metabolic pathways or to changes in already low vascular resistance and PaO_2 has not been differentiated. It has been suggested that, since substances such as papaverine with strong vasodilating effects do not change the energy charge before, during, or after hypoxia, nicergoline probably does exert metabolic effects on astrocytes leading to indirect effects on the capillary network (BENZI, 1975).

b) Cyclic AMP-Dependent Protein Kinase

The involvement of cAMP appears to be essential to the mechanism by which some neurotransmitters act postsynaptically in the central nervous system (IVERSEN, 1975). It was first suggested by GREENGARD and his collegues (GREENGARD et al., 1972; DALY, 1975) that transmitter-induced changes in the intracellular cAMP concentration regulate the activity of cAMP-dependent protein kinase and the state of synaptic membrane protein phosphorylation, which in turn leads directly to modification of ion permeability. Protein kinase, which is associated with nerve ending fractions of brain homogenates (MIYAMOTO et al., 1969), rapidly catalyzes the transfer of phosphate from ATP to specific membrane-associated proteins, PI, and PII (UDEA et al., 1973). Although the role of these proteins remains to be determined, PI appears to be unique to the brain, whereas PII may be present in other organs and also can be rapidly dephosphorylated in vitro.

Among their other effects, ergot derivatives may influence phosphorylation of membrane proteins at the level of protein kinase. The effects of dihydroergotoxine, dihydroergotamine, and dihydroergonine on partially purified soluble ox brain or membrane-bound cat brain protein kinase after stimulation in vitro with cAMP have been reported by REICHLMEIER and IWANGOFF (1974) and MEIER-RUGE et al. (1975). Under in vitro conditions where 5×10^{-6} M cAMP maximally stimulated ox brain protein kinase activity (measured as ^{32}P incorporation into histone), the addition of dihydroergotoxine (10^{-5} and 10^{-6} M) virtually abolished this activity. Nonstimulated protein kinase activity was only very weakly reduced by 10^{-4} M dihydroergotoxine. At these concentrations, no significant effects of dihydroergotamine on cAMP-stimulated protein kinase activity were observed. However, 10^{-4} M dihydroergonine, like dihydroergotoxine, reduced cAMP-stimulated (5×10^{-6} M) phosphate incorporation into histone by about 50%, and this inhibition disappeared at 10^{-6} M. Caffeine and papaverine showed no such inhibitory effects on protein kinase activity.

c) Adenosine Triphosphatase

The activation of Na^+/K^+-adenosine triphosphatase (ATPase) by NA is probably involved in catecholamine-induced hyperpolarization of the synaptic membrane. ATPase constitutes one of the most important transport systems for carrying Na^+ out of and K^+ into cells across a concentration gradient and, therefore, for permitting normal synaptic membrane polarization (CHAPPUIS et al., 1975). Although the mechanism of action is controversial (RACKER, 1976), the Na^+/K^+-ATPase presumably acts as a Na^+ carrier when phosphorylated at the expense of ATP hydrolysis or as a K^+ carrier when reversibly dephosphorylated in the presence of K^+-dependent p-nitrophenylphosphatase (K^+-p-NPPase).

The stimulation of Na^+/K^+-ATPase in cat brain homogenates by 10^{-4} and 10^{-3} M NA has been shown by IWANGOFF et al. (1973) to be inhibited by dihydroergotoxine. NA (10^{-4} M) activation of both Na^+/K^+-ATPase and Mg^{++}-ATPase activity in these homogenates was inhibited by 10^{-5} M dihydroergotoxine (MEIER-RUGE et al., 1975). Following ATPase activation by 10^{-3} M NA, this concentration of dihydroergotoxine was able to specifically inhibit the Na^+/K^+-ATPase activity. A concentration of 4.4×10^{-5} M dihydroergotoxine in this system reduced by 55% the level of Na^+/K^+-ATPase activation induced by 10^{-4} M NA. This inhibition was less than that (90%) produced by the same concentration of propranolol but more than that (20%) produced by phentolamine (MEIER-RUGE and IWANGOFF, 1976).

The inhibitory effects of several other dihydrogenated ergot alkaloids on both the Na^+/K^+-ATPase and the Mg^{++}-ATPase following NA stimulation have also been studied by IWANGOFF and ENZ (1973a). After activation with a 10^{-4} M concentration of NA, dihydroergostine and dihydroergotamine at concentrations of 10^{-4} M inhibited Mg^{++}-ATPase, but at 10^{-5} M inhibited the Na^+/K^+-ATPase as well. Dihydroergocristine (102c) at 10^{-6} M inhibited 16% of the NA-stimulated (10^{-3} M) Na^+/K^+-ATPase activity and at 10^{-4} M inhibited about 23% of the NA-stimulated K^+-p-NPPase activity in cat brain homogenate (MEIER-RUGE et al., 1975). Without prior activation by NA, only Mg^{++}-ATPase was inhibited by a variety of dihydrogenated ergot alkaloids (IWANGOFF and ENZ, 1973b), whereas an inhibition of Na^+/K^+-ATPase activity was observed only after the addition of NA. The intensity of this inhibition increased as follows: dihydroergocornine (102d) < dihydroergokryptine (102e,f) < dihydroergotoxine < dihydroergostine (102g) < dihydroergocristine = dihydroergotamine. However, in none of these cases was the degree of inhibition stronger than the degree of activation due to NA.

3. Transformation of Biosubstrates by Demethylation, Acetylation and Glucuronoconjugation

Some aspects of normal brain metabolism have been evaluated in the dog by measuring the transformation of aminopyrine to 4-aminoantipyrine (demethylation) or 4-aminoantipyrine to N-acetyl-4-aminoantipyrine (acetylation) after infusion of aminopyrine into the circle of Willis, and the transformation of oxazepam to glucuronide (glucuronoconjugation) following similar infusion of oxazepam (BENZI et al., 1971). *D*-LSD (5×10^{-7} M) decreased about equally the disappearance of aminopyrine and oxazepam. Nicergoline (5×10^{-5} M) increased the disappearance of these substrates and the appearance of their demethylated and glucoronoconjugated metabolites. Both of these ergot derivatives increased O_2 consumption, which has been related to the biotransformation of these substrates (BENZI et al., 1967, 1969, 1971).

G. References

Abreu, B.E., Liddle, G.W., Handley, C.A., Elliott, H.W.: Preliminary observation on the influence of ergotamine and dihydroergotamine on cerebral blood flow in the dog. Fed. Proc. **6**, 304 (1947)

Aghajanian, G.K.: LSD and CNS transmission. Annu. Rev. Pharmacol. **12**, 157–168 (1972)

Aghajanian, G.K.: LSD and 2-bromo-LSD: comparison of effects on serotonergic neurons and on neurons in two serotonergic projection areas, the ventral lateral geniculate and amygdala. Neuropharmacology **15**, 521–528 (1976)

Aghajanian, G.K., Bunney, B.S.: Central dopaminergic neurons: Neurophysiological identification and responses to drugs. In: Snyder, S.H., Usdin, E. (eds.): Frontiers in Catecholamine Research, pp. 643–648. New York: Pergamon Press 1973

Aghajanian, G.K., Foote, W.E., Sheard, M.H.: Lysergic acid diethylamide: sensitive neuronal units in midbrain raphe. Science **161**, 706–708 (1968)

Aghajanian, G.K., Foote, W.E., Sheard, M.H.: Action of psychotogenic drugs on single midbrain raphe neurons. J. Pharmacol. exp. Ther. **171**, 178–187 (1970)

Aghajanian, G.K., Haigler, H.J.: Mode of action of LSD on serotoninergic neurons. Adv. Biochem. Psychopharmacol. **10**, 167–177 (1974)

Aghajanian, G.K., Haigler, H.J., Bloom, F.E.: Lysergic acid diethylamide and serotonin: direct actions on serotonin-containing neurons. Life Sci. **11**, 615–622 (1972)

Aghajanian, G.K., Kuhar, M.J., Roth, R.H.: Serotonin-containing neuronal perikarya and terminals: differential effects of p-chlorophenylalanine. Brain Res. **53**, 85–101 (1973)

Aghajanian, G.K., Rosecrans, J.A., Sheard, M.H.: Serotonin: release in the forebrain by stimulation of midbrain raphe. Science **156**, 402–403 (1967)

Andén, N.-E., Corrodi, H., Fuxe, K., Hökfelt, T.: Evidence for a central 5-hydroxytryptamine receptor stimulation by lysergic acid diethylamide. Brit. J. Pharmacol. **34**, 1–7 (1968)

Andén, N.-E., Corrodi, H., Fuxe, K., Ungerstedt, U.: Importance of nervous impulse flow for the neuroleptic-induced increase in amine turnover in central dopamine neurons. Europ. J. Pharmacol. **15**, 193–199 (1971)

Andén, N.-E., Dahlström, A., Fuxe, K., Larsson, K.: Functional role of the nigro-neostriatal dopamine neurons. Acta pharmacol. (Kbh.) **24**, 263–274 (1966a)

Andén, N.-E., Dahlström, K., Fuxe, K., Larsson, K., Olsen, L., Ungerstedt, U.: Ascending monoamine neurons to the telencephalon and diencephalon. Acta physiol. scand. **67**, 313–326 (1966b)

Andén, N.-E., Rubenson, A., Fuxe, K., Hökfelt, T.: Evidence for dopamine receptor stimulation by apomorphine. J. Pharm. Pharmacol. **19**, 627–629 (1967)

Andén, N.-E., Strömbom, U., Svensson, T.H.: Dopamine and noradrenaline receptor stimulation: reversal of reserpine-induced suppression of motor activity. Psychopharmacologia (Berl.) **29**, 289–298 (1973)

Anderson, E.G.: Bulbospinal serotonin-containing neurons and motor control. Fed. Proc. **31**, 107–112 (1972)

Anlezark, G.M., Meldrum, B.S.: Effects of apomorphine, ergocornine and piribedil on audiogenic seizures in DBA/2 mice. Brit. J. Pharmacol. **53**, 419–421 (1975)

Anlezark, G.M., Pycock, C., Meldrum, B.: Ergot alkaloids as dopamine agonists: comparison in two rodent models. Europ. J. Pharmacol. **37**, 295–302 (1976)

Appel, J.B., Lovell, R.A., Freedman, D.X.: Alterations in the behavioral effects of LSD by pretreatment with p-chlorophenylalanine and a-methyl-p-tyrosine. Psychopharmacologia (Berl.) **18**, 387–406 (1970)

Arbuthnott, G.W., Crow, T.J., Fuxe, K., Olson, L., Ungerstedt, U.: Depletion of catecholamines in vivo induced by electrical stimulation of central monoamine pathways. Brain Res. **24**, 471–483 (1970)

Armbrust-Figueiredo, J.: A metisergide no tratamento da epilepsia temporal. Arch. Neuropsychiat. (S. Paulo) **25**, 221–226 (1967)

Arrigo, A., Braun, P., Kauchtschischwili, G.M., Moglia, A., Tartara, A.: Influences of treatment on symptomatology and correlated electroencephalographic (EEG) changes in the aged. Curr. Ther. Res. **15**, 417–426 (1973)

Baer, H.: Psychotische Erregungszustände und ihre Bekämpfung durch Schlafmittel. Schweiz. Arch. Neurol. Neurochir. Psychiat. **60**, 1–47 (1947)

Baldy-Moulinier, M.: Influence de l'hydergine sur les variations physiologiques et pathologiques du débit sanguin du cortex cérébral. Path. et Biol. **16**, 759–764 (1968)

Baldy-Moulinier, M., Passouant, P.: Modifications du débit sanguin cortex cérébral par l'hydergine. C.R. Soc. Biol. (Paris) **161**, 2574–2578 (1967)

Baldy-Moulinier, M., Dapres, G., Passouant, P.: Organization of sleeping and waking in the cat during the 24 hours: pharmacological changes. Electroenceph. Clin. Neurophysiol. **24**, 105 (1969)

Bálint, G.: Experimental comparison of the anaesthesia potentiating effect of Hydergin and some phenothiazine derivatives. Acta physiol. scand. **25**, 295–298 (1964)

Bálint, G., Anokbonggo, W.W.: Effect of dihydroergotoxine (Hydergine) and phenothiazines on conditioned avoidance reflexes and body temperature of the rat. Acta physiol. Acad. Sci. hung. **33**, 95–98 (1968)

Balzano, E., Bert, J., Menini, Ch., Naquet, R.: Excessive light sensitivity in papio papio: Its variation with age, sex and geographic origin. Epilepsia **16**, 269–276 (1975)

Banna, N.R., Anderson, E.G.: The effects of 5-hydroxytryptamine antagonists on spinal neuronal activity. J. Pharmacol. exp. Ther. **162**, 319–325 (1968)

Barasi, S., Roberts, M.H.T.: The action of 5-hydroxytryptamine antagonists and precursors on bulbospinal facilitation of spinal reflexes. Brain Res. **52**, 385–388 (1973)

Barasi, S., Roberts, M.H.T.: The modification of lumbar motoneurone excitability by stimulation of a putative 5-hydroxytryptamine pathway. Brit. J. Pharmacol. **52**, 339–348 (1974)

Barbeau, A.: Preliminary observations on abnormal catecholamine metabolism in basal ganglia diseases. Neurology (Minneap.) **10**, 446–451 (1960)

Barbeau, A.: Six years of high-level levodopa therapy in severely akinetic parkinsonian patients. Arch. Neurol. (Chic.) **33**, 333–338 (1976)

Barbeau, A., Murphy, G.F., Sourkes, T.L.: Excretion of dopamine in diseases of basal ganglia. Science **133**, 1706–1707 (1961)

Barbeau, A., Roy, M.: Six-year results of treatment with levodopa plus benzerazide in Parkinson's disease. Neurology (Minneap.) **26**, 399–404 (1976)

Barchas, J.D., Freedman, D.X.: Brain amines: response to physiological stress. Biochem. Pharmacol. **12**, 1232–1235 (1963)

Barger, G.: Ergot and Ergotism, London: Gurney and Jackson 1931.

Barger, G.: The alkaloids of ergot. In: Handb. Exp. Pharm. Ergänzungswerk **6**, 84–222. Berlin: Springer 1938

Barger, G., Dale, H.H.: Ergotoxine and some other constituents of ergot. Biochem. J. **2**, 240–299 (1907)

Barnett, A., Goldstein, J., Taber, R.I.: Apomorphine induced hypothermia in mice: a possible dopaminergic effect. Arch. int. Pharmacodyn. **198**, 242–247 (1972)

Bartholini, G., Burkard, W.P., Pletscher, A., Bates, H.M.: Increase of cerebral catecholamines caused by 3,4-dihydroxyphenylalanine after inhibition of peripheral decarboxylase. Nature (Lond.) **215**, 852–853 (1967)

Bazán, N.G., de Bazán, H.E.P., Kennedy, W.G., Joel, C.D.: Regional distribution and rate of production of free fatty acids in rat brain. J. Neurochem. **18**, 1387–1393 (1971)

Benzi, G.: An analysis of the drugs acting on cerebral energy metabolism. Jap. J. Pharmacol. **25**, 251–261 (1975)
Benzi, G., Arrigoni, E., Manzo, L., de Bernardi, M., Ferrara, A., Panceri, P., Berte, F.: Estimation of changes induced by drugs in cerebral energy-coupling processes in situ in the dog. J. pharm. Sci. **62**, 758–764 (1973)
Benzi, G., Berte, F., Arrigoni, E., Manzo, L.: Study of the cerebral metabolizing activity in the newborn dog utilizing the isolated perfused brain in situ technique. J. pharm. Sci. **58**, 885–887 (1969)
Benzi, G., Berte, F., Crema, A., Frigo, G.M.: Cerebral drug metabolism investigated by isolated perfused brain in situ. J. pharm. Sci. **56**, 1349–1351 (1967)
Benzi, G., de Bernardi, M., Manzo, L., Ferrara, A., Panceri, P., Arrigoni, E., Berte, F.: Effect of lysergide and nimergoline on glucose metabolism investigated on the dog brain isolated in situ. J. pharm. Sci. **61**, 348–352 (1972)
Benzi, G., Manzo, L., de Bernardi, M., Ferrara, A., Sanguinetti, L., Arrigoni, E., Berte, F.: Action of lysergide, ephedrine, and nimergoline on brain metabolizing activity. J. pharm. Sci. **60**, 1320–1324 (1971)
Bernheimer, H., Birkmeyer, W., Hornykiewicz, O.: Verteilung des 5-Hydroxytryptamin (Serotonin) im Gehirn des Menschen und sein Verhalten bei Patienten mit Parkinson-Syndrom. Klin. Wschr. **39**, 1056–1059 (1961)
Bernheimer, H., Birkmayer, W., Hornykiewicz, O., Jellinger, K., Seitelberger, F.: Brain dopamine and the syndromes of Parkinson and Huntington. J. neurol. Sci. **20**, 415–455 (1973)
Bienmüller, H., Betz, E.: Wirkung von Nicergolin auf die Hirndurchblutung. Arzneimittel-Forsch. **22**, 1367–1372 (1972)
Bílková, J., Radil-Weiss, T., Bohdanecký, Z.: The influence of LSD on sleep cycles in rats. Act. Nerv. Super. (Praha) **13**, 100–101 (1971a)
Bílková, J., Radil-Weiss, T., Bohdanecký, Z.: The influence of low LSD dose administration during sleep in rats. Psychopharmacologia (Berl.) **20**, 395–399 (1971b)
Birkmayer, W., Hornykiewicz, O.: Der L-3,4-dihydroxyphenylalanin-(=DOPA) Effekt bei der Parkinson-Akinese. Wien. klin. Wschr. **73**, 787–788 (1961)
Birkmayer, W., Hornykiewicz, O.: Weitere experimentelle Untersuchungen über L-DOPA beim Parkinson-Syndrom und Reserpin-Parkinsonismus. Arch. Psychiat. Z. ges. Neurol. **206**, 367–381 (1964)
Birkmayer, W., Mentasti, M.: Weitere experimentelle Untersuchungen über den Catecholaminstoffwechsel bei extrapyramidalen Erkrankungen. Arch. Psychol. (Frankf.) **210**, 29–35 (1967)
Blaschko, H.: Metabolism and storage of biogenic amines. Experientia (Basel) **13**, 9–12 (1957)
Bloom, F.E.: The role of cyclic nucleotides in central synaptic function. Rev. Physiol. Biochem. Pharmacol. **74**, 1–103 (1975)
Bloom, F.E., Hoffer, B.J., Nelson, C., Sheu, Y., Siggins, G.R.: The physiology and pharmacology of serotonin-mediated synapses. In: Barchas, J., Usdin, E. (eds.), Serotonin and Behavior, pp. 249–261. New York: Academic Press 1973
Bloom, F.E., Hoffer, B.J., Siggins, G.R., Barker, J.L., Nicoll, R.A.: Effects of serotonin on central neurons: microiontophoretic administration. Fed. Proc. **31**, 97–106 (1972)
Bloom, F.E., Siggins, G.R., Hoffer, B.J.: Interpreting the failure to confirm the depression of cerebellar Purkinje cells by cyclic AMP. Science **185**, 627–629 (1974)
Boakes, R.J., Bradley, P.B., Briggs, I., Dray, A.: Antagonism of 5-hydroxytryptamine by LSD 25 in the central nervous system: a possible neuronal basis for the actions of LSD 25. Brit. J. Pharmacol. **40**, 202–218 (1970)
Boismare, F., Lorenzo, J.: Study of the protection afforded by nicergoline against the effects of cerebral ischemia in the cat. Arzneimittel-Forsch. **25**, 410–413 (1975)
Boismare, F., Micheli, L.: Etude de la protection assurée par la dihydroergotoxine et chacun de ses composants contre les effets de l'ischémie cérébrale chez le chat. J. Pharmacol. (Paris) **5**, 221–230 (1974)
Boismare, F., Streichenberger, G.: Influence de l'ergotamine et de la dihydroergotoxine sur la récupération post-ischémique du potentiel évoqué cortical chez le chat. In: Géraud, J., Lazorthes, G., Bès, A. (eds.), L'ischémie cérébrale dans le territoire carotidien. Journées internationales de circulation cérébrale, Avril 1972., pp. 501–504 Suppl., Toulouse 1973
Boismare, F., Streichenberger, G.: The action of ergot alkaloids (ergotamine and dihydroergo-

toxine) on the functional effects of cerebral ischemia in the cat. Pharmacology **12**, 152–159 (1974)
Boismare, F., LePoncin, M., Lefrancois, J.: Biochemical and behavioural effects of hypoxic hypoxia in rats: Study of the protection afforded by ergot alkaloids. Gerontology **24** (Suppl. 1), 6–13 (1978)
Boismare, F., Streichenberger, G., Schrub, J.C.: Modifications, par l'ergotamine, des effets d'une anoxie ischémique encéphalique chez le chat. In: Migraines et céphalées. Colloque de Lille, 14. 11. 1970, Sandoz Edition, pp. 142–148, 1970
Boissier, J.R., Pagny, J.: Etude pharmacologique d'un phénothiazine neuroleptique, la thiéthylpérazine ou GS 95 (Torecan). Med. exp. **6**, 320–326 (1962)
Boissier, J.R., Simon, P., Giudicelli, J.F.: Effets centraux de quelques substances adréno-et/ou sympatholytiques. I. -Action sur la température rectale. Arch. int. Pharmacodyn. **168**, 180–187 (1967a)
Boissier, J.R., Simon, P., Giudicelli, J.F.: Effets centraux de quelques substances adréno-et/ou sympatholytiques. II. -Action sur la motilité spontanée et potentialisation du Pentobarbital. Arch. int. Pharmacodyn. **169**, 312–319 (1967b)
Boissier, J.R., Simon, P., Giudicelli, J.F.: Effets centraux de quelques substances adréno-et/ou sympatholythiques. III. -Ptosis, catalepsie, antagonisme vis-à-vis de l'apomorphine et de l'amphétamine. Arch. int. Pharmacodyn. **171**, 68–80 (1968)
Borenstein, P., Cujo, P., Bahon, L.: Contribution à l'étude électro-encéphalographique et clinique de l'action des dérivés hydrogénés de l'Ergotoxine. Ann. méd.-psychol. **127**, 410–424 (1969)
Borison, H.L., Wang, S.C.: Physiology and pharmacology of vomiting. Pharmacol. Rev. **5**, 193–230 (1953)
Bradley, P.B.: The actions of drugs on single neurons in the brain. Progr. Brain Res. **36**, 183–187 (1972)
Bradley, P.B., Briggs, I.: Ergot alkaloids and related compounds. In: Simpson, L.L., Curtis, D.R. (eds.), Neuropoisons—Their Pathophysiological Actions, pp. 249–269. New York: Plenum Press 1974a
Bradley, P.B., Briggs, I.: Further studies on the mode of action of psychotomimetic drugs: Antagonism of the excitatory actions of serotonin by methylated derivatives of tryptamine. Brit. J. Pharmacol. **50**, 345–354 (1974b)
Bramwell, G.J., Gönye, T.: Responses of midbrain neurons to microiontophoretically applied 5-hydroxytryptamine: Comparison with the response to intravenously administered lysergic acid diethylamide. Neuropharmacology **15**, 457–461 (1976)
Brand, E.D., Harris, T.D., Borison, H.L., Goodman, L.S.: The antiemetic activity of 10-(γ-dimethylaminopropyl)-2-chlorphenothiazine (chlorpromazine) in dog and cat. J. Pharmacol. exp. Ther. **110**, 86–92 (1954)
Brink, C.D., Rigler, R.: Ueber einen scheinbaren Unterschied in der Wirkung von Ergotamin und Ergotoxin auf die Körpertemperatur. Naunyn-Schmiedebergs Arch. exp. Path. Pharmak. **145**, 321–330 (1929)
Brizzee, K.R., Neal, L.M., Williams, P.M.: The chemoreceptive trigger zone for emesis in the monkey. Amer. J. Physiol. **180**, 659–662 (1955)
Brodie, B.A., Shore, P.A., Pletscher, A.: Serotonin-releasing activity limited to Rauwolfia alkaloids with tranquillizing action. Science **123**, 992–993 (1956)
Brooks, D.C.: The effect of LSD upon spontaneous PGO wave activity and REM sleep in the cat. Neuropharmacology **14**, 847–857 (1975)
Brooks, D.C., Gershon, M.D.: Eye movement potentiates the oculomotor and visual systems of the cat: a comparison of reserpine induced waves with those present during wakefulness and rapid eye movement sleep. Brain Res. **27**, 223–239 (1971)
Brown, G.L., Dale, H.: The pharmacology of ergometrine. Proc. roy. Soc. B **118**, 446–477 (1935)
Buchanan, A.R., Roberts, J.E., Robinson, B.E.: Ergotamine hyper- and hypothermia in albino rats. Proc. Soc. exp. Biol. (N.Y.) **68**, 143–150 (1948)
Buchanan, A.R., Witt, J.A., Roberts, J.E., Massopust, C.C.: Peripheral circulatory and metabolic reactions associated with ergotoxine hyper- and hypothermia in adult albino rats. Amer. J. Physiol. **163**, 62–69 (1950)

Bucher, M.B., Schorderet, M.: Dopamine- and apomorphine-sensitive adenylate cyclase in homogenates of rabbit retina. Naunyn-Schmiedebergs Arch. Pharmacol. **288**, 103–107 (1975)

Bunney, B.S., Aghajanian, G.K., Roth, R.H.: Comparison of effects of L-DOPA, amphetamine and apomorphine on firing rate of rat dopaminergic neurons. Nature (Lond.) New Biol. **245**, 123–125 (1973)

Burkhard, W.P.: Catecholamine-induced increase of cyclic adenosine 3′,5′-monophosphate in rat brain in vivo. J. Neurochem. **19**, 2615–2619 (1972)

Burton, R.M., Sodd, M.A., Goldin, A.: The analeptic action of lysergic acid diethylamide and d-amphetamine on reserpine-sedated mice. Arch. int. Pharmacodyn. **112**, 188–198 (1957)

Cahn, J., Campan, L.: Künstlicher Winterschlaf ohne Chlorpromazin (Megaphen); Anwendung von Hydergin in der Neurochirurgie. Anaesthesist **3**, 155–156 (1954–55)

Cahn, J., Dubrasquet, M., Bodiou, J., Melon, J.M.: Méthodes d'hibernation artificielle. Etude expérimentale comparée. Anesth. et Analg. **11**, 141–146 (1954)

Cahn, J., Melon, J.M., Dubrasquet, M., Bodiou, J.: Die neurovegetative Dämpfung im sogenannten „künstlichen Winterschlaf" mit hydrierten Mutterkornalkaloiden. Physiologische Studie. Anaesthesist **4**, 82–88 (1955)

Calne, D.B.: Parkinsonism-physiology and pharmacology. Brit. med. J. **3**, 693–697 (1971)

Calne, D.B., Stern, G.M.: L-DOPA in idiopathic parkinsonism. Lancet **1969 II**, 973

Calne, D.B., Teychenne, P.F., Claveria, L.E., Eastman, R., Greenacre, J.K., Petrie, A.: Bromocriptine in Parkinsonism. Brit. med. J. **4**, 442–444 (1974a)

Calne, D.B., Teychenne, P.F., Leigh, P.N., Bamji, A.N., Greenacre, J.K.: Treatment of Parkinsonism with bromocriptine. Lancet **1974 II**, 1355–1356

Campbell, M.T., Oliver, I.T.: 3′:5′-Cyclic nucleotide phosphodiesterases in rat tissues. Europ. J. Biochem. **28**, 30–37 (1972)

Carlsson, A.: The occurrence, distribution and physiological role of catecholamines in the nervous system. Pharmacol. Rev. **11**, 490–493 (1959)

Carlsson, A.: Some aspects of dopamine in the central nervous system. In: McDowell, F.H., Barbeau, A. (eds.), Advances in Neurology, Vol. 5, pp. 59–68. New York: Raven Press 1974

Carlsson, A.: Dopamine Autoreceptors. In: Almgren, O., Carlsson, A., Engel, J. (eds.), Chemical Tools in Catecholamine Research, Vol. 2, pp. 219–225. Amsterdam: North Holland Publ. Co. 1975

Carlsson, A., Lindqvist, M.: The effect of l-tryptophan and some psychotropic drugs on the formation of 6-hydroxytryptophan in the mouse brain in vivo. J. Neural. Transm. **33**, 23–43 (1972)

Carlsson, A., Lindqvist, M., Magnusson, T.: 3,4-dihydroxyphenylalanine and 5-hydroxytryptophan as reserpine antagonists. Nature (Lond.) **180**, 1200 (1957)

Carruthers-Jones, D.I., Depoortere, H., Loew, D.M.: Changes in the rat electrocorticogram following administration of two dihydrogenated ergot derivatives. Gerontology **24** (Suppl. 1), 23–33 (1978)

Cerletti, A.: Lysergic acid diethylamide (LSD) and related compounds. In: Abramson, H.A. (ed.), Neuropharmacology, pp. 9–84. New York: Josiah Macy, Jr. Foundation 1956

Cerletti, A.: Comparison of abnormal behavioural states induced by psychotropic drugs in animals and man (Discussion Third Symposium). In: Bradley, P.B., Deniker, P., Radouco-Thomas, C., (eds.), Neuropsychopharmacology, Proceedings of the First International Congress of Neuropsychopharmacology, pp. 117–123. Amsterdam: Elsevier Press 1959

Cerletti, A.: Ergostin – Neue Perspektiven der Chemie und Pharmakologie des Mutterkorns. Med. exp. **8**, 278–286 (1963)

Cerletti, A., Doepfner, W.: Comparative study on the serotonin antagonism of amide dervatives of lysergic acid and of ergot alkaloids. J. Pharmacol. exp. Ther. **122**, 124–136 (1958)

Cerletti, A., Fanchamps, A.: Neuroplegie und kontrollierte Hypothermie. Schweiz. med. Wschr. **85**, 141–145 (1955)

Cerletti, A., Rothlin, E.: Role of 5-hydroxytryptamine in mental diseases and its antagonism to lysergic acid derivatives. Nature (Lond.) **176**, 785–786 (1955a)

Cerletti, A., Rothlin, E.: Untersuchungen zur Frage der pharmakodynamisch induzierten Hypothermie. Acta neuroveg. (Wien) **11**, 260–274 (1955b)
Cerletti, A., Emmenegger, H., Enz, A., Iwangoff, P., Meier-Ruge, W., Musil, J.: Effects of ergot DH-alkaloids on the metabolism and function of the brain. An approach based on studies with DH-ergonine. In: Genazzani, E., Herken, H. (eds.), Central Nervous System. Studies on Metabolic Regulation and Function, pp. 201–212. Berlin-Heidelberg-New York: Springer 1973
Cerletti, A., Streit, M., Taeschler, M.: Thiethylperazin (Torecan) ein spezifisches Antiemeticum. Arzneimittel-Forsch. **12**, 964–968 (1962)
Chappuis, A., Enz, A., Iwangoff, P.: The influence of adrenergic effectors on the cationic pump of brain cell. Triangle **14**, 93–98 (1975)
Chase, T.N., Breese, G.R., Kopin, I.J.: Serotonin release from brain slices by electrical stimulation: regional differences and effect of LSD. Science **157**, 1461–1463 (1967)
Chase, T.N., Katz, R.I., Kopin, I.J.: Release of (^{3}H) serotonin from brain slices. J. Neurochem. **16**, 607–615 (1969)
Cheung, W.Y.: Properties of cyclic 3′,5′-nucleotide phosphodiesterase from rat brain. Biochemistry **6**, 1079–1087 (1970a)
Cheung, W.Y.: Cyclic 3′,5′-nucleotide phosphodiesterase. Biochem. biophys. Res. Commun. **38**, 533–538 (1970b)
Cheymol, J., Quinquaud, A.: Les poisons émétisants devant l'ergotamine. C.R. Soc. Biol. (Paris) **139**, 548–549 (1945)
Cheymol, J., Quinquaud, A.: Application d'ergotamine sur le bulbe émétisant. Arch. int. Pharmacodyn. **77**, 509–512 (1948)
Christiani, K., Möller, W.D.: Die medikamentöse Therapie des Parkinson-Syndroms. Eine klinische Langzeitstudie mit L-Dopa und dem Kombinationspräparat L-Dopa-Decarboxylasehemmer. Münch. med. Wschr. **115**, 711–713 (1973)
Clark, B.J., Aellig, W., Chu, D.: Action on the Circulation. In: Berde, B., Schild, H.O. (eds.), Ergot Alkaloids and Related Compounds. Handbuch der experimentellen Pharmakologie, Ch. V. Berlin-Heidelberg-New York: Springer 1978
Clineschmidt, B.V., Andersson, E.G.: The blockade of bulbospinal inhibition by 5-hydroxytryptamine antagonists. Exp. Brain Res. **11**, 175–186 (1970)
Clineschmidt, B.V., Lotti, V.J.: Indoleamine antagonists: relative potencies as inhibitors of tryptamine- and 5-hydroxytryptophan-evoked responses. Brit. J. Pharmacol. **50**, 311–313 (1974)
Cloetta, M., Waser, E.: Zur Kenntnis des Fieberanstieges, über das Adrenalinfieber. Naunyn-Schmiedebergs Arch. exp. Path. Pharmak. **79**, 30–41 (1915)
Contreras, E., Quijada, L., Tamayo, L.: Influence of nalorphine upon the synergistic effect of methyldopa and ergonovine on morphine analgesia. Med. Pharmacol. exp. **16**, 371–376 (1967a)
Contreras, E., Tamayo, L., Quijada, L.: Analgesic effect of ergonovine in male and female rats. Med. Pharmacol. exp. **16**, 159–164 (1967b)
Cools, A.R.: The function of dopamine and its antagonism in the caudate nucleus of cats in relation to the stereotyped behaviour. Arch. int. Pharmacodyn. **194**, 259–269 (1971)
Cools, A.R., van Rossum, J.M.: Caudate dopamine and stereotyped behaviour of cats. Arch. int. Pharmacodyn. **187**, 163–173 (1970)
Cools, A.R., van Rossum, J.M.: Excitation-mediating and inhibition-mediating dopamine-receptors: a new concept towards a better understanding of electrophysiological, biochemical, pharmacological, functional and clinical data. Psychopharmacologia (Berl.) **45**, 243–254 (1976)
Cools, A.R., Hendriks, G., Korten, J.: The acetylcholine-dopamine balance in the basal ganglia of rhesus monkeys and its role in dynamic, dystonic, dyskinetic and epileptoid motor activities. J. Neurotransmission **36**, 91–105 (1975a)
Cools, A.R., Janssen, H.J., Struyker Boudier, H.A.J., van Rossum, J.M.: Interaction between antipsychotic drugs and catecholamine receptors. In: Wenner-Grenn Center International Symposium Scrics. New York: Pergamon Press 1975b
Cooper, K.E., Cranston, W.I., Honour, A.J.: Effects of intraventricular and intrahypothalamic injection of noradrenalin and 5-HT on body temperature in conscious rabbits. J. Physiol. (Lond.) **181**, 852–864 (1965)

Corne, S.J., Pickering, R.W., Warner, B.T.: A method for assessing the effects of drugs on the central actions of 5-hydroxytryptamine. Brit. J. Pharmacol. **20**, 106–120 (1963)
Corrodi, H., Farnebo, L.-O., Fuxe, K., Hamberger, B.: Effect of ergot drugs on central 5-hydroxytryptamine neurons: evidence for 5-hydroxytryptamine release or 5-hydroxytryptamine receptor stimulation. Europ. J. Pharmacol. **30**, 172–181 (1975)
Corrodi, H., Fuxe, K., Hökfelt, T.: The effects of neuroleptics on the activity of central catecholamine neurons. Life Sci. **6**, 767–774 (1967a)
Corrodi, H., Fuxe, K., Hökfelt, T.: Replenishment by 5-hydroxytryptophan of the amine stores in the central 5-hydroxytryptamine neurons after depletion induced by reserpine or by an inhibitor of monoamine synthesis. J. Pharm. Pharmacol. **19**, 433–438 (1967b)
Corrodi, H., Fuxe, K., Hökfelt, T., Lidbrink, P., Ungerstedt, U.: Effect of ergot drugs on central catecholamine neurons: evidence for a stimulation of central dopamine neurons. J. Pharm. Pharmacol. **25**, 409–412 (1973)
Costall, B., Naylor, R.J.: Apomorphine as an antagonist of the dopamine response from the nucleus accumbens. J. Pharm. Pharmacol. **28**, 592–595 (1976)
Costall, B., Naylor, R.J., Olley, J.E.: Stereotypic and anticataleptic activities of amphetamine after intracerebral injection. Europ. J. Pharmacol. **18**, 83–88 (1972)
Costall, B., Naylor, R.J., Pycock, C.: The 6-hydroxydopamine rotational model for the detection of dopamine agonist activity: reliability of effect from different locations of 6-hydroxydopamine. J. Pharm. Pharmacol. **27**, 943 (1975)
Cotzias, G.C., Papavasiliou, P.S., Tolasa, E.S., Mendez, J.S., Bell-Midura, M.: Treatment of Parkinson's disease with aporphines. Possible role of growth hormone. New Engl. J. Med. **294**, 567–572 (1976)
Cotzias, G.C., van Woert, M.H., Schiffer, L.M.: Aromatic aminoacids and modification of parkinsonism. New Engl. J. Med. **276**, 374–379 (1967)
Couch, J.R.: Responses of neurons in the raphe nuclei to serotonin, norepinephrine, and acetylcholine and their correlation with an excitatory synaptic output. Brain Res. **19**, 137–150 (1970)
Couch, J.R.: Further evidence for a possible excitatory synapse on raphe neurons of pons and lower midbrain. Life Sci. **19**, 761–768 (1976a)
Couch, J.R.: Action of LSD on raphe neurons and effect of presumed serotonergic raphe synapses. Brain Res. **110**, 417–424 (1976b)
Crossman, A.R., El-Khawad, A.O.A., Walker, R.J., Woodruff, G.N.: Effects of ergometrine on dopamine receptors. J. Physiol. (Lond.) **232**, 59P (1973)
Curtis, D.R., Davis, R.: Pharmacological studies on neurons of the lateral geniculate nucleus of the cat. Brit. J. Pharmacol. **18**, 217–246 (1962)
Dahlström, A., Fuxe, K.: Evidence for the existence of monoamine-containing neurons in the central nervous system. I. Demonstration of monoamines in the cell bodies of brainstem neurons. Acta physiol. scand. **62**, Suppl. 232, 1–55 (1964)
Dahlström, A., Fuxe, K.: Evidence for the existence of monoamine neurons in the central nervous system. Acta physiol. scand. **64**, Suppl. 247 1–36 (1965)
Dale, H.H.: On some physiological actions of ergot. J. Physiol. (Lond.) **34**, 163–206 (1906)
Dale, H.H., Spiro, K.: Die wirksamen Alkaloide des Mutterkorns. Naunyn-Schmiedebergs Arch. exp. Path. Pharmak. **95**, 337–350 (1922)
Daly, J.W.: The role of cyclic nucleotides in the nervous system. In: Iversen, L.L., Iversen, S.D., Snyder, S.H. (eds.): Handbook of Psychopharmacology, pp. 47–130. New York: Plenum Press 1975
D'Amico, D.J., Patel, B.C., Klawans, H.L.: The effect of methysergide on 5-hydroxytryptamine turnover in whole brain. J. Pharm. Pharmacol. **28**, 454–455 (1976)
Da Prada, M., Saner, A., Burkard, W.P., Bartholini, G., Pletscher, A.: Lysergic acid diethylamide: evidence for stimulation of cerebral dopamine receptors. Brain Res. **94**, 67–73 (1975)
David, N.A., Griffith, W.B., Porter, G.A., Misko, J.: Hydergine potentiation and antagonism of some effects of secobarbital and pentobarbital in the rat. Curr. Res. Anesth. **35**, 468–475 (1956)
Davidson, N., Edwardson, J.A., Schwab, D.I.: Agroclavine antagonizes depression induced by noradrenaline in the cerebral cortex of the rat. Nature (Lond.) **223**, 1166–1168 (1969)
Davis, M.E., Adair, F.L., Chen, K.K., Swanson, E.E.: Pharmacologic action of ergotocin, new ergot principle. J. Pharmacol. exp. Ther. **54**, 398–407 (1935)

Debono, G., Marsden, C.D., Asselman, P., Parkes, D.J.: Bromocriptine and dopamine receptor stimulation. Brit. J. clin. Pharmacol. **3**, 977–982 (1976)
Delorme, F., Froment, J.L., Jouvet, M.: Suppression du sommeil par la p-chlorométhamphétamine et la p-chlorophénylalanine. C.R. Soc. Biol. (Paris) **160**, 2347–2351 (1966)
Delorme, F., Jeannerod, M., Jouvet, M.: Effets remarquables de la réserpine sur l'activité EEG phasique ponto-géniculo-occipitale. C.R. Soc. Biol. (Paris) **159**, 900–904 (1965)
Depoortere, H.: Effects of BOL-148 on the sleep-wakefulness cycle. In: Koella, W.P., Levin, P. (eds.), Sleep, pp. 360–364. Basel: S. Karger 1973
Depoortere, H., Loew, D.M.: Alterations in sleep/wakefulness cycle in rats following treatment with (+)-lysergic acid diethylamide (LSD-25). Brit. J. Pharmacol. **41**, 402P-403P (1971)
Depoortere, H., Loew, D.M.: Alterations in the sleep/wakefulness cycle in rats after administration of (−)-LSD or BOL-148: a comparison with (+)-LSD. Brit. J. Pharmacol. **44**, 354P-355P (1972)
Depoortere, H., Loew, D.M., Vigouret, J.M.: Neuropharmacological studies on Hydergine®. Triangle **14**, 73–79 (1975)
Depoortere, H., Matějček, M.: Action de la dihydroergotamine sur le système nerveux central. In: Symposium sur la dysrégulation vasculaire. pp. 65–74, Edit. Sandoz Sci. Serv., 1973
Dews, P.B.: The measurement of the influence of drugs on voluntary activity in mice. Brit. J. Pharmacol. **8**, 46–48 (1953)
Dhawan, B.N.: Effect of drugs on LSD-25 induced pyrexia in rabbits. Arch. int. Pharmacodyn. **123**, 186–194 (1959)
Dhawan, B.N., Gupta, G.P.: Antiemetic activity of d-lysergic acid diethylamide. J. Pharmacol. exp. Ther. **133**, 137–139 (1961)
Dhawan, B.N., Saxena, P.N., Gupta, G.P.: Antagonism of apomorphine-induced pecking in pigeons. Brit. J. Pharmacol. **16**, 137–145 (1961)
Diaz, P.M., Ngai, S.H., Costa, E.: Factors modulating brain serotonin turnover. In: Garattini, S., Shore, P.A. (eds.), Advances in Pharmacology, Vol. 6, Part B, pp. 75–92. New York: Academic Press 1968
Di Chiara, G., Porceddu, M.L., Vargiu, L., Argiolas, A., Gessa, G.L.: Evidence for dopamine receptors mediating sedation in the mouse brain. Nature (Lond.) **264**, 564–566 (1976)
Di Chiara, G., Porceddu, M.L., Vargiu, L., Gessa, G.L.: Evidence for Selective and Long-Lasting Stimulation of "Regulatory" Dopamine-Receptors by Bromocriptine (CB 154). Naunyn-Schmiedebergs Arch. Pharmacol. **300**, 239–245 (1977)
Dimitrijevic, I.-N.: Influence de l'ergotamine sur la thermogenèse et la thermo-régulation chez le rat. C.R. Soc. Biol. (Paris) **124**, 474–476 (1937)
Dixon, A.K.: Evidence of catecholamine mediation in the "aberrant" behaviour induced by lysergic acid diethylamide (LSD) in the rat. Experientia (Basel) **24**, 743–747 (1968)
Dow, R.C., Hill, A.G., McQueen, J.K.: Effects of some dopaminergic receptor stimulants on cobalt induced epilepsy in the rat. Brit. J. Pharmacol. **52**, 135P (1974)
Dray, A., Oakley, N.R.: Bromocriptine and dopamine-receptor stimulation. J. Pharm. Pharmacol. **28**, 586–588 (1976)
Eggleston, C., Hatcher, R.A.: The seat of the emetic action of various drugs. J. Pharm. exp. Ther. **7**, 225–253 (1915)
Ehringer, H., Hornykiewicz, O.: Verteilung von Noradrenalin und Dopamin (3-Hydroxytyramin) im Gehirn des Menschen und ihr Verhalten bei Erkrankungen des Extrapyramidalen Systems. Klin. Wschr. 1236–1239 (1960)
Elder. J.T., Shellenberger, M.K.: Antagonism of LSD-induced hyperthermia. J. Pharmacol. exp. Ther. **136**, 293–297 (1962)
Elkawad, A.O., Munday, K.A., Poat, J.A., Woodruff, G.N.: The effect of dopamine receptor stimulants on locomotor activity and cyclic AMP levels in the rat striatum. Brit. J. Pharmacol. **53**, 456P–457P (1975)
Emmenegger, H., Meier-Ruge, W.: The actions of hydergine on the brain. Pharmacology (Basel) **1**, 65–78 (1968)
Emmenegger, H., Gygax, P., Musil, J., Walliser, C.: Hydergine-effects on the ischaemically disturbed EEG in the isolated cat head. Int. Res. Comm. System, Pharmacol. II, 7-10-4 (1973a)
Emmenegger, H., Gygax, P., Walliser, C.: Hydergine effects on the EEG of the hypothermic cat. Int. Res. Comm. System, Pharmacol. II, 7-10-2 (1973b)

Enz, A., Iwangoff, P., Chappuis, A.: The influence of dihydroergotoxine mesylate on the Low-K_M-cAMP-phosphodiesterase of cat and rat brains in vitro. Gerontology (Basel) **24** (Suppl. 1), 115–125 (1978)

Enz, A., Iwangoff, P., Markstein, R., Wagner, H.: The effect of Hydergine® on the enzymes involved in cAMP turnover in the brain. Triangle **14**, 90–92 (1975)

Ernst, A.M.: Mode of action of apomorphine and d-amphetamine on gnaw-compulsion in rats. Psychopharmacologia (Berl.) **10**, 316–323 (1967)

Ernst, A.M., Smelik, P.G.: Site of action of dopamine and apomorphine on compulsive gnawing behaviour in rats. Experientia (Basel) **22**, 837–838 (1966).

Ey, H., Le Borgne, Y.R., Guennoc, A.: Etude de l'action "paraneuroleptique" de l'Hydergine chez les malades mentaux. In: Lopez Ibor, J.J. (ed.), Proceedings of the 4th World Congress of Psychiatry, Madrid, 5–11 Sept., 1966. Part 3, pp. 2225–2226. Amsterdam: Excerpta Medica Found. 1968

Fanchamps, A.: Some compounds with hallucinogenic activity. In: Berde, B., Schild, H.O. (eds.), Ergot Alkaloids and Related Compounds. Handbuch der experimentellen Pharmakologie, Ch. VIII. Berlin-Heidelberg-New York: Springer 1978

Fanchamps, A., Doepfner, W., Weidmann, H., Cerletti, A.: Pharmakologische Charakterisierung von Deseril®, einem Serotonin-Antagonisten. Schweiz. med. Wschr. **90**, 1040–1046 (1960)

Farley, I.J., Hornykiewicz, O.: Noradrenaline in subcortical brain regions of patients with Parkinson's disease and control subjects. In: Birkmayer, W., Hornykiewicz, O. (eds.), Recent Advances in the Research of Parkinsonism. Basel: Editiones Roche 1975

Farnebo, L.O., Hamberger, B.: Drug-induced changes in the release of ^{3}H-monoamines from field-stimulated rat brain slices. Acta physiol. scand., Suppl. **371**, 35–44 (1971)

Farrar, G.E., Duff, A.M.: Ergotamine tartrate; its direct hyperglycemic action and its influence on hyperglycemia produced by epinephrine in normal unanesthetized dogs. J. Pharmacol. exp. Ther. **34**, 197–202 (1928)

Feise, G., Paal, G.: Zur Therapie des Parkinson-Syndroms mit L-Dopa allein und in Kombination mit einem Decarboxylasehemmer – ein Vergleich. Nervenarzt **45**, 126–132 (1974)

Feldberg, W., Hellon, R.F., Lotti, V.J.: Temperature effects produced in dogs and monkeys by injections of monoamines and related substances into the third ventricle. J. Physiol. (Lond.) **191**, 501–515 (1967)

Feldberg, W., Hellon, R.F., Myers, R.D.: Effects on temperature of monoamines injected into the cerebral ventricles of anaesthetized dogs. J. Physiol. (Lond.) **186**, 416–423 (1966)

Feldberg, W., Myers, R.D.: A new concept of temperature regulation by amines in the hypothalamus. Nature (Lond.) **200**, 1325 (1963)

Feldman, R.G., Glaser, G.H.: EEG study of methysergide in migraine. Electroenceph. clin. Neurophysiol. **15**, 699–702 (1963)

Ferrini, R., Glasser, A.: Antagonism of central effects of tryptamine and 5-hydroxytryptophan by 1,6-dimethyl-8β-carbobenzyloxyaminomethyl-10α-ergoline. Psychopharmacologia (Basel) **8**, 271–276 (1965)

Flückiger, E.: The pharmacology of bromocriptine. In: Bayliss, R.I.S., Turner, P., Maclay, W.P. (eds.), Pharmacological and Clinical Aspects of Bromocriptine (Parlodel), pp. 12–26. Turnbridge Wells, G.B.: MCS Consultants 1976

Flückiger, E., Del Pozo, E.: Influence on the endocrine system. In: Berde, B., Schild, H.O. (eds.), Ergot Alkaloids and Related Compounds. Handbuch der experimentellen Pharmakologie, Ch. IX. Berlin-Heidelberg-New York: Springer 1978

Flückiger, E., Wagner, H.R.: 2-Br-α-Ergokryptin: Beeinflussung von Fertilität und Laktation bei der Ratte. Experientia (Basel) **24**, 1130–1131 (1968)

Förster, S.: Über den Einfluß des Gynergens auf den Wärmehaushalt des Organismus. Med. doświadcz. i społ. **19**, 152–175 (1935)

Fog, R.: Stereotyped and non-stereotyped behaviour in rats induced by various stimulant drugs. Psychopharmacologia (Basel) **14**, 299–304 (1969)

Frattola, L., Albizzatti, M.G., Spano, P.F., Trabucchi, M.: Effet de la bromocriptine sur les fluctuations thérapeutiques secondaires à la dopa thérapie. Phénomène "on-off" chez les parkinsoniens. Nouv. Presse Méd. **5**, 1761 (1976)

Freedman, D.X.: Effects of LSD-25 on brain serotonin. J. Pharmacol. exp. Ther. **134**, 160–166 (1961)
Freedman, D.X., Gottlieb, R., Lovell, R.A.: Psychotomimetic drugs and brain 5-hydroxytryptamine metabolism. Biochem. Pharmacol. **19**, 1181–1188 (1970)
Friedman, A.P., Elkind, A.H.: Appraisal of methysergide in treatment of vascular headaches of migraine type. J. Amer. med. Ass. **184**, 125–128 (1963)
Friedman, A.P., von Storch, T.J.C., Araki, S.: Ergotamine tartrate: its history, action and proper use in the treatment of migraine. N. Y. St. J. Med. 59 (12), 2359–2366 (1959)
Froment, J.L., Eskazan, E.: Effets du LSD et du méthysergide sur les pointes ponto-géniculo-occipitales. C.R. Soc. Biol. (Paris) **165**, 2153–2157 (1971)
Fuxe, K.: Evidence for the existence of monoamine-containing neurons in the central nervous system. III. Demonstration of monoamine-containing nerve terminals in the brain. Z. Zellforsch. **65**, 572–596 (1965a)
Fuxe, K.: Evidence for the existence of monoamine neurons in the brainstem. IV. Distribution of monoamine nerve terminals in the central nervous system. Acta physiol. scand. **64**, Suppl. 247, 37–85 (1965b)
Fuxe, K., Hökfelt, T.: Participation of central monoamine neurons in the regulation of anterior pituitary function with special regard to the neuroendocrine role of tubero-infundibular dopamine neurons. In: Bargmann, W., Scharrer, B. (eds.), Aspects of Neuroendocrinology. Berlin-Heidelberg-New York: Springer 1970
Fuxe, K., Hökfelt, T.: Histochemical fluorescence detection of changes in central monoamine neurones provoked by drugs acting on the CNS. Triangle **10**, 73–84 (1971)
Fuxe, K., Owman, C.: Cellular localization of monoamines in the area postrema of certain mammals. J. comp. Neurol. **125**, 337–354 (1965)
Fuxe, K., Sjöqvist, F.: Hypothermic effect of apomorphine in the mouse. J. Pharm. Pharmacol. **24**, 702–705 (1972)
Fuxe, K., Agnati, L., Everitt, B.J.: Effects of methergoline on central monoamine neurons. Evidence for a selective blockade of central 5-HT receptors. Neurosci. Letters **1**, 283–290 (1975a)
Fuxe, K., Agnati, L., Hökfelt, T., Jonsson, G., Lidbrink, P., Ljungdahl, A., Lofstrom, A., Ungerstedt, U.: The effect of dopamine receptor stimulating and blocking agents on the activity of supersensitive dopamine receptors and on the amine turnover in various dopamine nerve terminal systems in the rat brain. J. Pharmacol. **6**, 117–129 (1975b)
Fuxe, K., Butcher, L.L., Engel, J.: DL-5-hydroxytryptophan-induced changes in central monoamine neurons after peripheral decarboxylase inhibition. J. Pharm. Pharmacol. **23**, 420–424 (1971)
Fuxe, K., Corrodi, H., Hökfelt, T., Lidbrink, P., Ungerstedt, U.: Ergocornine and 2-Br-α-ergocryptine. Evidence for prolonged dopamine receptor stimulation. Med. Biol. **52**, 121–132 (1974)
Fuxe, K., Fredholm, B.B., Agnati, L., Ögren, S.-O., Everitt, B.J., Jonsson, G., Gustafsson, J.Å.: Interaction of ergot drugs with central monoamine systems. Evidence for a high potential in the treatment of mental and neurological disorders. Pharmacology (Basel) **16** (Suppl. I), 99–134 (1978)
Fuxe, K., Hökfelt, T., Ungerstedt, U.: Distribution of monoamines in the mamalian central nervous system by histochemical studies. In: Hooper, C. (ed.), Metabolism of Amines in the Brain, pp. 10–32. London: Mac Millan 1969
Gaddum, J.H.: Antagonism between lysergic acid diethylamide and 5-hydroxytryptamine. J. Physiol. (Lond.) **121**, 15P (1953)
Gaddum, J.H., Vogt, M.: Some central actions of 5-hydroxytryptamine and various antagonists. Brit. J. Pharmacol. **11**, 175–179 (1956)
Gallager, D.W., Aghajanian, G.K.: Effects of chlorimipramine and lysergic acid diethylamide on efflux of precursor-formed ^{3}H-serotonin: correlation with serotoninergic impulse flow. J. Pharmacol. exp. Ther. **193**, 785–795 (1975)
Garcia-Leme, J., Rocha e Silva, M.: Effect upon the analgesic action of reserpine of central nervous stimulants and drugs affecting the metabolism of catechol- and indole-amines. J. Pharm. Pharmacol. **15**, 454–460 (1963)
Gautvik, K.M., Hoyt, R.F., Tashjian, A.H.: Effects of colchizine and 2-Br-α-ergocryptine-

methane sulfonate (CB 154) on the release of prolactin and growth hormone by functional tumor cells in culture. J. Cell Physiol. **82**, 401–410 (1973)
Gilman, A.: Ergotoxine excitement. Proc. Soc. Exp. Biol. (N.Y.) **31**, 468–470 (1934)
Girault, J.-M., Kandasamy, B., Jacob, J.: Actions de divers neuroleptiques sur les hyperthermies centrales induites par la dopamine, la noradrénaline et la 5-hydroxytryptamine chez le lapin éveillé. J. Pharmacol. (Paris) **6**, 341–350 (1975)
Githens, T.S.: The influence of ergotoxine on body temperature. J. Pharmacol. exp. Ther. **10**, 327–340 (1917)
Glaviano, V., Wang, S.C.: Dual mechanism of anti-emetic action of 10-(γ-dimethylamino propyl)-2-chlorophenothiazine hydrochloride (chlorpromazine) in dogs. J. Pharmacol. exp. Ther. **114**, 358–366 (1955)
Goldstein, L.: The effect of LSD and other hallucinogens on the electrical activity of brain during wakefulness and sleep. In: Sankar, D.V.S. (ed.), LSD- A Total Study, pp. 395–435. Westbury, New York: P.J.D. Publications 1975
Goldstein, M., Battista, A., Ohmoto, T., Anagnoste, B., Fuxe, F.: Tremor and involuntary movements in monkeys: effect of L-Dopa and of a dopamine receptor stimulating agent. Science **179**, 816–817 (1973)
Grabowska, M., Antkiewicz, L., Michaluk, J.: The influence of LSD on locomotor activity in reserpinized mice. Pol. J. Pharmacol. Pharm. **26**, 499–594 (1974a)
Grabowska, M., Antkiewicz, L., Michaluk, J.: The influence of quipazine on the turnover rate of serotonin. Biochem. Pharmacol. **23**, 3211–3212 (1974b)
Graeff, F.O., Schoenfeld, R.I.: Tryptaminergic mechanisms in punished and unpunished behavior. J. Pharmacol. exp. Ther. **173**, 277–283 (1970)
Grahame-Smith, D.G.: Inhibitory effect of chlorpromazine on the syndrome of hyperactivity produced by L-tryptophan or 5-methoxy-N,N-dimethyltryptamine in rats treated with a monoamine oxidase inhibitor. Brit. J. Pharmacol. **43**, 856–864 (1971a)
Grahame-Smith, D.G.: Studies "in vivo" on the relationship between brain tryptophan, brain 5-HT synthesis and hyperactivity in rats treated with a monoamine oxidase inhibitor and L-tryptophan. J. Neurochem. **18**, 1053–1066 (1971b)
Greengard, P.: Molecular studies on the nature of the dopamine receptor in the caudate nucleus of the mammalian brain. In: Seeman, P., Brown, G.M. (eds.), Frontiers in Neurology and Neuroscience Research, pp. 12–15. Toronto: N. Toronto Press 1974
Greengard, P., McAfee, D.A., Kebabian, J.W.: On the mechanism of action of cyclic AMP and its role in synaptic transmission. In: Greengard, P., Robison, G.A. (eds.), Advances in Cyclic Nucleotide Research, Vol. 1, pp. 337–355. New York: Raven Press 1972
Griffith, R.: Toxicological considerations. In: Berde, B., Schild, H.O. (eds.), Ergot Alkaloids and Related Compounds., Handbuch der experimentellen Pharmakologie, Ch. XII. Berlin-Heidelberg-New York: Springer 1978
Griffith, W.B., Porter, G.A., David, N.A.: Hydergine potentiation of barbiturate depressant effects in the rat. Fed. Proc. **14**, 346–347 (1955)
Grinker, R.R., Spivey, R.J.: Ergotamine tartrate in the treatment of war neuroses. J. Amer. med. Ass. **127**, 158 (1945)
Guilbaud, G., Besson, J.M., Oliveras, J.L., Liebeskind, J.C.: Suppression by LSD of the inhibitory effect exerted by dorsal raphe stimulation on certain spinal cord interneurons in the rat. Brain Res. **61**, 417–422 (1973)
Gujral, M.L., Dhawan, B.N.: Effects of drugs on LSD-25 induced pyrexia in rabbits. Indian J. Physiol. Pharmacol. **3**, 79 (1959)
Gyermek, L.: Drugs which antagonize 5-hydroxytryptamine and related indolealkylamines. In: Eichler, O., Farah. A. (eds.), 5-Hydroxytryptamine and Related Indolealkylamines. Handbuch der experimentellen Pharmakologie, pp. 471–528. Berlin-Heidelberg-New York: Springer 1966
Gygax, P., Emmenegger, H., Dixon, R.: Cortical microflow and electrical brain activity (EEG) of the cat in a state of hypovolaemic shock (Wigger's Model). Int. Res. Comm. System 11-16-1 (1973)
Gygax, P., Emmenegger, H., Dixon, R., Peier, A.: The effect of hypovolaemic oligemia on the cerebral microcirculation and EEG in the cat (Wigger's Model), pp. 386–394. In: Cervos-Navarro, J. (ed.), Pathology of Cerebral Microcirculation. Berlin: Walter de Gruyter 1974

Gygax, P., Hunziker, O., Schultz, U., Schweizer, A.: Experimental studies on the action of metabolic and vasoactive substances in the brain. Triangle **14**, 80–89 (1975)
Gygax, P., Meier-Ruge, W., Schulz, U., Enz, A.: Experimental studies on the action of metabolic and vasoactive substances in the oligemically disturbed brain. Arzneimittel-Forsch. **26**, 1245–1246 (1976)
Gygax, P., Wiernsperger, N., Meier-Ruge, W., Baumann, T.: Effect of papaverine and dihydroergotoxine mesylate on cerebral microflow, EEG and PO_2 in oligemic hypotension. Gerontology (Basel) **24** (Suppl. 1), 14–22 (1978)
Haigler, H.J., Aghajanian, G.K.: Lysergic acid diethylamide and serotonin: A comparison of effects on serotoninergic neurons and neurons receiving a serotoninergic input. J. Pharmacol. exp. Ther. **188**, 688–693 (1974a)
Haigler, H.J., Aghajanian, G.K.: Peripheral serotonin antagonists: Failure to antagonize serotonin in brain areas receiving a prominent serotonergic input. J. Neural Transm. **35**, 257–273 (1974b)
Hanzlik, P.J., Cutting, W.C., Hoskins, D., Hanzlik, H., Barnes, E.W., Doherty, E.W.: Vasomotor drugs on the convulsant threshold in rodent with and without diphenylhydantoin. Stanford med. Bull. **6**, 47–53 (1948)
Harper, A.M.: Autoregulation of cerebral blood flow: Influence of the arterial blood pressure on the blood flow through the cerebral cortex. J. Neurol. Neurosurg. Psychiat. **29**, 398–403 (1966)
Harper, A.M., Deshmukh, V.D., Rowan, J.O., Jennett, W.B.: The influence of sympathetic nervous activity on cerebral blood flow. Arch. Neurol. (Chic.) **27**, 1–6 (1972)
Harsh, J., Witters, W.L.: The effects of elymoclavine on wheel turning activity in mice. Psychonomic Sci. **18**, 301–302 (1970)
Hartmann, E.L.: The sleep-dream cycle and brain serotonin. Psychonom. Sci. **8**, 295–296 (1967)
Hatcher, R.-A., Weiss, S.: Studies on vomiting. J. Pharmacol. exp. Ther. **22**, 139–193 (1923)
Heath, R.G., Powdermaker, F.: The use of ergotamine tartrate as a remedy for "battle reaction". J. Amer. med. Ass. **125**, 111–113 (1944)
Herzfeld, U., Christian, W., Oswald, W.D., Ronge, J., Wittgen, M.: Zur Wirkungsanalyse von Hydergin im Langzeitversuch. Med. Klin. **67**, 1118–1125 (1972)
Hess, S.M., Doepfner, W.: Behavioral effects and brain amine content in rats. Arch. int. Pharmacodyn. **134**, 89–99 (1961)
Hess, W.R.: Über die Wechselbeziehungen zwischen psychischen und vegetativen Funktionen. Schweiz. Arch. Neurol. Neurochir. Psychiat. **15**, 260–277 (1924); **16**, 36–55, 285–306 (1925)
Hill, H.F., Horita, A.: Inhibition of (+)-amphetamine hyperthermia by blockade of dopamine receptors in rabbits. J. Pharm. Pharmacol. **23**, 715–717 (1971)
Hill, H.F., Horita, A.: A pimozide-sensitive effect of apomorphine on body temperature of the rabbit. J. Pharm. Pharmacol. **24**, 490–491 (1972)
Hobson, J.A.: The effect of LSD on the sleep cycle of the cat. Electroenceph. clin. Neurophysiol. **17**, 52–56 (1964)
Hökfelt, T., Fuxe, K.: On the morphology and the neuroendocrine role of the hypothalamic catecholamine neurons. In: Knigge, K.M., Scott, D.E., Weindl, A. (eds.), Brain-Endocrine Interactions, pp. 181–223. Basel: Karger 1972
Hofmann, A.: Die Mutterkorn-Alkaloide. Stuttgart: Ferdinand Enke 1964
Hood, R.D., Melvin, K.B., Starling, P.B.: Effects of agroclavine on avoidance behavior in the hamster. Bull. Psychon. Soc. **3**, 71–72 (1974)
Horita, A., Dille, J.M.: Pyretogenic effect of lysergic acid diethylamide. Science **120**, 1100–1101 (1954)
Horita, A., Dille, J.M.: The pyretogenic effect of lysergic acid diethylamide. J. Pharmacol. exp. Ther. **113**, 29 (1955)
Horita, A., Gogerty, J.H.: The pyretogenic effect of 5-hydroxytryptophan and its comparison with that of LSD. J. Pharmacol. exp. Ther. **122**, 196–200 (1958)
Horita, A., Hamilton, A.E.: Lysergic acid diethylamide: Dissociation of its behavioral and hyperthermic actions by DL-a-methyl-p-tyrosine. Science **164**, 78–79 (1969)
Horn, G., McKay, J.M.: Effects of lysergic acid diethylamide on the spontaneous activity and visual receptive fields of cells in the lateral geniculate nucleus of the cat. Exp. Brain Res. **17**, 271–284 (1973)

Horowski, R., Wachtel, H.: Direct dopaminergic action of lisuride hydrogen maleate, an ergot derivative, in mice. Europ. J. Pharmacol. **36**, 373–383 (1976)
Hull, C.D., Levine, M.S., Buchwald, N.A., Heller, A., Browning, R.A.: The spontaneous firing pattern of forebrain neurons. I. The effects of dopamine and non-dopamine depleting lesions as caudate unit firing patterns. Brain Res. **73**, 241–262 (1974)
Hungen, K. von, Roberts, S.: Adenylate-cyclase receptors for adrenergic neurotransmitters in rat cerebral cortex. Europ. J. Biochem. **36**, 391–401 (1973)
Hungen, K. von, Roberts, S., Hill, D.F.: LSD as an agonist and antagonist at central dopamine receptors. Nature (Lond.) **252**, 588–589 (1974)
Hungen, K. von, Roberts, S., Hill, D.F.: Interactions between lysergic acid diethylamide and dopamine-sensitive adenylate cyclase systems in rat brain. Brain Res. **94**, 57–66 (1975a)
Hungen, K. von, Roberts, S., Hill, D.F.: Serotonin-sensitive adenylate cyclase activity in immature rat brain. Brain Res. **84**, 257–267 (1975b)
Hunziker, O., Emmenegger, H., Frey, H., Schulz, U., Meier-Ruge, W.: Morphometric characterization of the capillary network in the cat's brain cortex. A comparison of the physiological state and hypovolemic conditions. Acta neuropath. (Wien) **29**, 57–63 (1974a)
Hunziker, O., Emmenegger, H., Meier-Ruge, W., Schulz, U.: The behaviour of morphometric parameters of cortical capillaries in the cats brain influenced by DH-ergotoxine and papaverine. Int. Res. Comm. System, Pharmacology II, 1481 (1974b)
Ingvar, D.H., Lassen, N.A.: Quantitative determination of regional cerebral blood flow in man. Lancet **1961 II**, 806–807
Isbell, H., Miner, E.J., Logan, C.R.: Relationship of psychotomimetic to antiserotonin potencies of congeners of lysergic acid diethylamide (LSD-25). Psychopharmacologia (Berl.) **1**, 20–28 (1959)
Issekutz, B., Gyermek, L.: Die Wirkung von Dihydroergotamin und Dihydroergocornin auf den Gaswechsel. Arch. int. Pharmacodyn. **78**, 174–196 (1949)
Itil, T.M., Herrmann, W.M., Akpinar, S.: Prediction of psychotropic properties of lisuride hydrogen maleate by quantitative pharmaco-electroencephalogram. Int. J. clin. Pharmacol. **12**, 221–233 (1975)
Iversen, L.L.: Dopamine receptors in the brain. Science **188**, 1084–1089 (1975)
Iwangoff, P., Enz, A.: The effect of dihydroergotamine on the phosphodiesterase activity of cat grey matter. Experientia (Basel) **27**, 1258–1259 (1971)
Iwangoff, P., Enz, A.: The influence of various dihydroergotamine analogues on cyclic adenosine-3′,5′-monophosphate phosphodiesterase in the grey matter of cat brain in vitro. Agents and Actions **2**, 223–230 (1972)
Iwangoff, P., Enz, A.: The brain-specific inhibition of the cAMP-phosphodiesterase (PEase) of the cat by dihydroergotalkaloids in vitro. Int. Res. Comm. System, Med. Sci., 3-10-9 (1973a)
Iwangoff, P., Enz, A.: Inhibition of phosphodiesterase by dihydroergotamine and hydergine in various organs of the cat in vitro. Experientia (Basel) **29**, 1067–1069 (1973b)
Iwangoff, P., Chappuis, A., Enz, A.: The effect of different dihydroergot alkaloids on the noradrenaline activated ATP-ase of the cat brain. Int. Res. Comm. System, Med. Sci., 3–10–20 (1973)
Iwangoff, P., Enz, A., Chappuis, A.: Inhibition of cAMP-phosphodiesterase of different cat organs by DH-ergotoxine in the micromolar substrate range. Int. Res. Comm. System, Med. Sci. **3**, 403 (1975)
Iwangoff, P., Enz, A., Meier-Ruge, W.: Incorporation, after single and repeated application of radioactively labelled DH-ergot alkaloids in different organs of the cat, with special reference to the brain. Gerontology (Basel) **24** (Suppl. 1), 126–138 (1978)
Iwangoff, P., Meier-Ruge, W., Schieweck, Ch., Enz, A.: The uptake of DH-ergotoxine by different parts of the cat brain. Pharmacology (Basel) **16**, 27–38 (1976)
Jacob, J., Lafille, C.: Caractérisation et détection pharmacologiques des substances hallucinogènes. – I. Activités hyperthermisantes chez le lapin. Arch. int. Pharmacodyn. **145**, 528–545 (1963)
Jacob, J., Lafille, C., Loiseau, G., Echinard-Garin, P., Barthélémy, C.: Recherche d'équivalents expérimentaux au pouvoir hallucinogène. Action des hallucinogènes sur la température rectale du lapin et sur les effets de la morphine chez la souris. Med. exp. (Basel) **7**, 296–304 (1962)

Jacobs, B.L.: Evidence for the functional interaction of two central neurotransmitters. Psychopharmacologia (Berl.) **39**, 81–86 (1974a)
Jacobs, B.L.: Effect of two dopamine receptor blockers on a serotonin-mediated behavioral syndrome in rats. Europ. J. Pharmacol. **27**, 363–366 (1974b)
Jacobs, B.L.: An animal behavior model for studying central serotonergic synapses. Life Sci. **19**, 777–786 (1976)
Jäggi, U.H., Loew, D.M.: Central dopaminergic stimulation and avoidance performance under hypoxia in rats. Experientia (Basel) **32**, 229 (1976)
Jalfre, M., Monachon, M.A., Haefely, W.: Pharmacological modifications of benzoquinolizine induced geniculate spikes. Experientia (Basel) **26**, 691 (1970)
James, I.M.: Autonomic control of cerebral circulation. In: Meldrum, B.S., Marsden, C.D. (eds.), Advances in Neurology, Vol. 10, pp. 167–180. New York: Raven Press 1975
Jarvik, M.E.: Drugs used in the treatment of psychiatric disorders. In: Goodman, L.S., Gilman, A. (eds.), The Pharmacological Basis of Therapeutics., pp. 151–203. London: MacMillan (1970)
Jaton, A.L., Loew, D.M., Vigouret, J.M.: CF 25–397 (9,10-didehydro-6methyl-8β-[-2-pyridyl-thiomethyl]ergoline), a new central dopamine receptor agonist. Brit. J. Pharmacol. **56**, 371P (1976)
Jend, J.-H., Coper, H.: On the mechanism of the synergistic effect of perazine and hexobarbital. Naunyn-Schmiedebergs Arch. Pharmacol. **281**, 219–232 (1974)
Jötten, J.: Die Beeinflussung der paroxysmaler Durchblutungsstörungen und des Auftretens provozierter Krämpfe durch sympathikolytische Stoffe. Arch. Psychiat. Z. Neurol. **187**, 153–164 (1951)
Johnson, F.N., Ary, I.E., Teiger, D.G., Kassel, R.J.: Emetic activity of reduced lysergamides. J. med. Chem. **16**, 532–537 (1973a)
Johnson, A.M., Griffith, R.W.: Exposé: Toxicological and Pharmacological Investigations with PTR 17–402. Basle: Sandoz Ltd., 1972
Johnson, A.M., Loew, D.M., Vigouret, J.M.: Stimulant properties of bromocriptine on central dopamine receptors in comparison to apomorphine, (+)-amphetamine and l-DOPA. Brit. J. Pharmacol. **56**, 59–68 (1976)
Johnson, A.M., Vigouret, J.M., Loew, D.M.: Central dopaminergic actions of ergotoxine alkaloids and some derivatives. Experientia (Basel) **29**, 763 (1973b)
Johnson, A.M., Vigouret, J.M., Loew, D.M.: CB-154 (2-bromo-α-ergocriptine), bromocriptine, a potential antiparkinson agent. Naunyn-Schmiedebergs Arch. exp. Path. Pharmacol. **282**, Suppl. R 40 (1974)
Johnson, G.A., Kim, E.G., Boukma, S.J.: Mechanism of norepinephrine depletion by 5-hydroxytryptophan. Proc. Soc. exp. Biol. (N.Y.) **128**, 509–512 (1968)
Jouvet, M.: Biogenic amines and the state of sleep. Science **163**, 32–41 (1969)
Jouvet, M.: The role of monoamines and acetylcholine-containing neurons in the regulation of the sleep-waking cycle. Ergebn. Physiol. **64**, 166–307 (1972)
Jurna, I.: Striatal monoamines and reserpine and chlorpromazine rigidity. Pharmacol. Ther. B. **2**, 113–128 (1976)
Jurna, I., Theres, C., Bachmann, T.: The effect of physostigmine and tetrabenazine on spinal motor control and its inhibition by drugs which influence reserpine rigidity. Naunyn-Schmiedebergs Arch. Pharmak. exp. Path. **263**, 427–438 (1972)
Justin-Besançon, L., Laville, C.: Action antiémétique du métoclopramide vis-à-vis de l'apomorphine et de l'hydergine. C.R. Soc. Biol. (Paris) **158**, 723–727 (1964)
Kärjä, J., Kärki, N.T., Tala, E.: Inhibition of methysergide of 5-hydroxytryptophan toxicity to mice. Acta pharmacol. (Kbh.) **18**, 255–262 (1961)
Kartzinel, R., Perlow, M., Carter, A.C., Chase, T.N., Calne, D.B.: Metabolic studies with bromocriptine in patients with idiopathic Parkinsonism and Huntington's chorea. Arch. Neurol. (Chic.) **33**, 384 (1976a)
Kartzinel, R., Perlow, M., Teychenne, P., Gielen, A.C., Gillespie, M.M., Calne, B.: Bromocriptine and levodopa (with or without carbidopa) in Parkinsonism. Lancet **1976b II**, 272–275
Kebabian, J.S., Petzold, G.L., Greengard, P.: Dopamine-sensitive adenylate cyclase in caudate nucleus of rat brain, and its similarity to the "dopamine receptor." Proc. nat. Acad. Sci. (Wash.) **69**, 2145–2149 (1972)
Kehr, W.: Effect of lisuride and other ergot derivatives on monoaminergic mechanisms in rat brain. Europ. J. Pharmacol. **41**, 261–273 (1977)

Kehr, W., Carlsson, A., Lindqvist, M., Magnusson, T., Atack, C.V.: Evidence for a receptor-mediated feedback control of striatal tyrosine hydroxylase activity. J. Pharm. Pharmacol. **24**, 744–747 (1972)

Kety, S.S., Schmidt, C.F.: Determination of cerebral blood flow in man by use of nitrous oxide in low concentration. Amer. J. Physiol. **143**, 53–66 (1945)

Killam, K.F., Killam, E.K., Naquet, R.: An animal model of light sensitive epilepsy. Electroenceph. clin. Neurophysiol. **22**, 497–513 (1967)

Klawans, H.L., D'Amico, D.J., Patel, B.C.: Behavioral supersensitivity to 5-hydroxytryptophan induced by chronic methysergide pretreatment. Psychopharmacologia (Berl.) **44**, 297–300 (1975)

Klawans, H.L., Goetz, C., Weiner, W.J.: 5-Hydroxytryptophan-induced myoclonus in guinea pigs and the possible role of serotonin in infantile myoclonus. Neurology (Minneap.) **23**, 1234–1240 (1973)

Klissiunis, N., Kanakis, K., Dosi, I.: Die Wirkung von Ergotamin auf die Körpertemperatur verschiedener Tiere. Naunyn-Schmiedebergs Arch. Pharmak. exp. Path. **259**, 212–213 (1967/68)

Knapp, F.M., Hyman, C., Bercel, N.A.: A method for the estimation of regional blood flow. Yale J. Biol. Med. **28**, 363–371 (1955/56)

Koppanyi, T., Evans, E.I.: Studies on the emetic and antiemetic actions of ergotamine. Proc. Soc. exp. Biol. (N.Y.) **29**, 1181–1182 (1932)

Kreitmair, H.: Über Ergoclavin, ein neu entdecktes Mutterkornalkaloid. Naunyn-Schmiedebergs Arch. exp. Path. Pharmak. **176**, 171–180 (1934)

Krnjević, K.: Chemical nature of synaptic transmission in vertebrates. Physiol. Rev. **54**, 418–540 (1974)

Krnjević, K., Phillis, J.W.: Actions of certain amines on cerebral cortical neurones. Brit. J. Pharmacol. **20**, 471–490 (1963)

Kukovetz, W., Pöch, G.: The action of theophylline, 2-bromo-LSD and imidazole on phosphodiesterase activity in the perfused guinea-pig heart. Fed. Proc. **28**, 741 (1969)

Laborit, H., Huguenard, P.: Pratique de l'hibernothérapie en chirurgie et en médecine. Paris: Masson 1954

Laborit, G., Baron, C., Laborit, H.: Etude expérimentale de la circulation cérébrale et ses rapports avec l'activité des différentes structures métaboliques cérébrales. Aggressologie (Paris) **6**, 721–737 (1965)

Lauersen, N.H., Conrad, P.: Effect of oxytoxic agents on blood loss during first trimester suction curettage. Obstet. Gynec. (N.Y.) **44**, 428–433 (1974)

Lees, A.J., Shaw, K.M., Stern, G.M.: Bromocriptine in parkinsonism. Lancet **1975 II**, 709–710

Lehmann, A.: Contribution à l'étude psychophysiologique et neuropharmacologique de l'épilepsie acoustique de la souris et du rat. II. Etude expérimentale. Aggressologie (Paris) **5**, 311–344 (1964)

Lehmann, A.: Psychopharmacology of the response to noise with special reference to audiogenic seizures in mice. In: Welch, B.L., Welch, A.S. (eds.), Physiological Effects of Noise, p. 227. New York: Plenum Press 1970

Lewis, J.L., Mc Ilwain, H.: The action of some ergot derivatives, mescaline and dibenamine on the metabolism of separated mammalian cerebral tissues. Biochem. J. **57**, 680–684 (1954)

Lieberman, A., LeBrun, Y., Boal, D.: The use of a dopaminergic receptor stimulating agent (Pribedil, ET 495) in Parkinson's disease. Adv. Biochem. Psychopharmacol. **12**, 415–425 (1974)

Lieberman, A., Kupersmith, M., Estey, E., Goldstein, M.: Lergotrile in Parkinson's disease. Lancet **1976a I**, 515–516

Lieberman, A., Kupersmith, M., Estey, E., Goldstein, M.: Treatment of Parkinson's disease with bromocriptine. New Engl. J. Med. **295**, 1400–1404 (1976b)

Lieberman, A., Miyamoto, T., Battista, A.: Studies on the antiparkinsonian efficacy of lergotrile. Neurology (Minneap.) **25**, 459–462 (1975)

Lloyd, K.G., Hornykiewicz, O.: L-glutamic acid decarboxylase in Parkinson's disease: effect of L-dopa therapy. Nature (Lond.) **243**, 521–523 (1973)

Loew, D.M., Spiegel, R.: Polygraphic sleep studies in rats and in humans. Their use in psychopharmacological research. Arzneimittel-Forsch. **26**, 1032–1035 (1976)

Loew, D.M., Depoortere, H., Bürki, H.R.: Effects of dihydrogenated ergot alkaloids on the sleep-wakefulness cycle and on brain biogenic amines in the rat. Arzneimittel-Forsch. **26**, 1080–1083 (1976a)
Loew, D.M., Depoortere, H., Vigouret, J.M.: Effects of d-lysergic diethylamide (LSD-25) and 2-bromo-d-lysergic acid diethylamide (BOL-148) upon behavioral sleep in rats. Naunyn-Schmiedebergs Arch. Pharmak. **266**, 394–395 (1970)
Loew, D.M, Vigouret, J.M., Jaton, A.L.: Neuropharmacological investigations with two ergot alkaloids, Hydergine and bromocriptine, Postgrad. med. J. **52**, Suppl. 1, 40–46 (1976b)
Loscalzo, A.E.: The effect of ergotamine tartrate in idiopathic epilepsy. J. nerv. ment. Dis. **86**, 559–566 (1937)
Lubsen, N.: Experimental studies on the cerebral circulation of the unanaesthetized rabbit. III. The action of ergotamine tartrate and of some vasodilator drugs. Arch. néerl. Physiol. **25**, 361–365 (1949)
Ludin, H.P., Kunz, F., Lörincz, P., Ringwald, E.: Klinische Erfahrungen mit Bromocriptin, einen zentralen dopaminergen Stimulator. Nervenarzt **47**, 651–655 (1976)
Ludwigs, N., Schneider, M.: Über den Einfluß des Halssympathicus auf die Gehirndurchblutung. Pflügers Arch. ges. Physiol. **259**, 43–55 (1954)
McAfee, D.A., Greengard, P.: Adenosine 3′,5′-monophosphate: electrophysiological evidence for a role in synaptic transmission. Science **178**, 310–312 (1972)
McLellan, D.L.: Comparison of reflex effects of levodopa and bromocriptine in parkinsonism. Brit. med. J. **2**, 235–236 (1976)
MacLeod, R.M., Lehmeyer, J.E.: Studies of the mechanism of the dopamine-mediated inhibition of prolactin secretion. Endocrinology **94**, 1077–1085 (1974)
McKenzie, G.M., Soroko, F.E.: The effects of apomorphine (+)-amphetamine and 1-dopa on maximal electroshock convulsions – a comparative study in the rat and mouse. J. Pharm. Pharmacol. **24**, 696–701 (1972)
Marine, D., Deutch, M., Cipra, A.: Effect of ergotamine tartrate on the heat production of normal and thyroidectomized rabbits. Proc. Soc. exp. Biol. (N.Y.) **24**, 662–664 (1927)
Marinesco, G., Sager, O., Kreindler, A.: Action centrale de l'ergotamine sur la tension artérielle. C.R. soc. Biol. (Paris) **107**, 191–192 (1931)
Markstein, R., Wagner, H.R.: Effects of dihydroergotoxine on cyclic-AMP-generating systems in rat cerebral cortex slices. Gerontology (Basel) **24** (Suppl. 1), 94–105, (1978)
Markstein, R., Herrling, P.L., Bürki, H.R., Asper, H., Ruch, W.: The effect of CB-154 (2-Br-α-ergocryptine) on adenylate cyclase and catecholamine metabolism of the rat striatum. (In Preparation 1978)
Marsden, C.D., Parkes, J.D.: On-off effects in patients with Parkinson's disease on chronic levodopa therapy. Lancet **1976 I**, 292–296
Matějček, M., Devos, J.E.: Selected methods of quantitative EEG analysis and their applications in psychotropic drug research. In: Kellaway, P., Petersén, I. (eds.), Quantitative Analytic Studies in Epilepsy, pp. 183–205. New York: Raven Press 1976
Matějček, M., Arrigo, A., Knor, K.: Quantitative EEG in geriatric drug research. Description of a working hypothesis, first results and their relation to clinical symptomatology. In: Matějček, M., Schenk, G.K. (eds.), Quantitative Analysis of the EEG, pp. 127–147. Konstanz: AEG Telefunken 1976
Matsumoto, C., Griffin, W.: Antagonism of (+)-amphetamine-induced hyperthermia in rats by pimozide. J. Pharm. Pharmacol. **23**, 710 (1971)
Maurer, R., Grieder, A.: Effects of dihydroergotamine on cAMP content in cultured glial cells. Experientia (Basel) **31**, 730–731 (1975)
Meier-Ruge, W.: Experimental pathology and pharmacology in brain research and aging. Life Sci. **17**, 1627–1636 (1976)
Meier-Ruge, W., Iwangoff, P.: Biochemical effects of ergot alkaloids with special reference to the brain. Postgrad. med. J. **52**, 47–54 (1976)
Meier-Ruge, W., Enz, A., Gygax, P., Hunziker, O., Iwangoff, P., Reichlmeier, K.: Experimental pathology in basic research of the aging brain. In: Gershon, S., Raskin, A. (eds.), Genesis and Treatment of Psychologic Disorders in the Elderly, pp. 55–126. New York: Raven Press 1975

Meier-Ruge, W., Schieweck, Ch., Iwangoff, P.: The distribution of (^{3}H) Hydergine in the cat brain. Int. Res. Comm. Service., Med. Sci., 7-10-3 (1973)
Meldrum, B.S., Naquet, R.: Effects of psilocybine, dimethyltryptamine and various lysergic acid derivatives on photically-induced epilepsy in the baboon (Papio papio). Brit. J. Pharmacol. **40**, 144P–145P (1970)
Meldrum, B.S., Naquet, R.: Effects of psilocybine, dimethyltryptamine, mescaline and various lysergic acid derivatives on the EEG and on photically induced epilepsy in the baboon (Papio papio). Electroenceph. clin. Neurophysiol. **31**, 563–572 (1971)
Meldrum, B., Anlezark, G., Trimble, M.: Drugs modifying dopaminergic activity and behaviour, the EEG and epilepsy in *Papio papio*. Europ. J. Pharmacol. **32**, 203–213 (1975)
Meldrum, B.S., Balzano, E., Wada, J.A., Vuillon-Cacciuttolo, G.: Effects of l-tryptophan, L-3,4 dihydroxyphenylalanine and tranylcypromine on the electroencephalogram and on photically-induced epilepsy in the baboon, Papio papio. Physiol. Behav. **9**, 615–621 (1972)
Mendelson, W.B., Reichman, J., Othmer, E.: Serotonin inhibition and sleep. Biol. Psychiat. **10**, 459–464 (1975)
Miculicich, M.: Über den Einfluß von Ergotoxin auf die Adrenalin- und Diuretinglykosurie. Naunyn-Schmiedebergs Arch. exp. Path. Pharmak. **69**, 133–148 (1912)
Miller, L.C., Tainter, M.L.: Estimation of ED_{50} and its error by means of logarithmic-probit graph paper. Proc. Soc. exp. Biol. (N.Y.) **57**, 261–264 (1944)
Miyamoto, T., Battista, A., Goldstein, M.: Long-lasting antitremor activity induced by 2-Br-α-ergocriptine in monkeys. J. Pharm. Pharmacol. **26**, 452–454 (1974)
Miyamoto, E., Kuo, J.F., Greengard, P.: Cyclic nucleotide-dependent protein kinases. III. Purification and properties of adenosine 3′,5′-monophosphate dependent protein kinase from bovine brain. J. biol. Chem. **244**, 6395–6402 (1969)
Monachon, M.-A., Burkard, W.P., Jalfre, M., Haefely, W.: Blockade of central 5-hydroxytryptamine receptors by methiothepin. Naunyn-Schmiedebergs Arch. Pharmacol. **274**, 192–197 (1972)
Mongeau, B.: The effect of Hydergine on the transit time of cerebral circulation in diffuse cerebral insufficiency. Europ. J. clin. Pharmacol. **7**, 169–175 (1974)
Monn, E., Christiansen, R.D.: Adenosine 3′,5′-monophosphate phosphodiesterase: multiple molecular forms. Science **173**, 540–542 (1971)
Moretti, A., Pegrassi, L., Suchowsky, G.K.: Effect of nicergoline on some ischemia-induced metabolic changes in the brain of cat. In: Genazzani, E., Herken, H, (eds.), Central Nervous System; Studies on Metabolic Regulation and Function, pp. 213–216. Berlin-Heidelberg-New York: Springer 1974
Morpurgo, C.: Effects of antiparkinson drugs on a phenothiazine-induced catatonic reaction. Arch. int. Pharmacodyn. **137**, 84–90 (1962)
Müller-Schweinitzer, F., Weidmann, H.: Basic pharmacological properties of ergot alkaloids and related compounds. In: Berde, B., Schild, H.O. (eds.), Ergot Alkaloids and Related Compounds., Handbuch der experimentellen Pharmakologie, Ch. III. Berlin-Heidelberg-New York: Springer 1978
Muzio, J.N., Roffwarg, H.P., Kaufman, E.: Alterations in the nocturnal sleep cycle resulting from LSD. Electroenceph. clin. Neurophysiol. **21**, 313–324 (1966)
Nagasawa, H., Yanai, R., Flückiger, E.: Counteraction by 2-Br-α-ergokryptine of pituitary prolactin release provoked by dibutyril-adenosine-3′,5′-monophosphate in rats. In: Pasteels, J.L., Robyn, C. (eds.), Human Prolactin, pp. 313–315. Amsterdam: Excerpta Medica 1973
Nakajima, H., Grandjean, J.L., L'Huillier, J., Thuillier, J.: Neuro-stimulants hallucinogènes et non hallucinogènes: Confrontation expérimentale de leurs effets sur la température centrale et périphérique. In: Proc. 2nd Int. Pharmacol. Meeting, Vol. 2, pp. 263–278. Prag: Czechoslovak Med. Press 1964
Nathanson, J.A., Greengard, P.: Serotonin-sensitive adenylate cyclase in neural tissue and its similarity to the serotonin receptor: a possible site of action of lysergic acid diethylamide. Proc. nat. Acad. Sci. (Wash.) **71**, 797–801 (1974)
Neuhold, K., Taeschler, M., Cerletti, A.: Beitrag zur zentralen Wirkung von LSD: Versuche über die Lokalisation von LSD-Effekten. Helv. physiol. pharmacol. Acta **15**, 1–7 (1957)
Ng, L.K.Y., Chase, T.N., Colborn, R.W., Kopin, I.J.: Release of (3-H) dopamine by L-5-hydroxytryptophan. Brain Res. **45**, 499–505 (1972)

Olpe, H.-R., Koella, W.P.: The response of striatal cells upon stimulation of the dorsal and median raphe nuclei. Brain Res. **122**, 357–360 (1977)
Ordenstein, L.: Sur la Paralysie Agitante, et al Sclérose en plaques généralisées. M.D. Thesis, Paris: Martinet 1867
Pack, A.T., Schmidt, H.S.: Methysergide and sleep in human subjects. Psychophysiology **9**, 88 (1972)
Pagel, J., Christian, S.T., Quayle, E.S., Monti, J.A.: A serotonin sensitive adenylate cyclase in mature rat brain synaptic membranes. Life Sci. **19**, 819–824 (1976)
Palmer, G.C., Burks, T.F.: Central and peripheral adrenergic blocking actions of LSD and BOL. Europ. J. Pharmacol. **16**, 113–116 (1971)
Palmer, G.C., Sulser, F., Robison, G.A.: The effects of neurohumoral and adrenergic agents on cyclic AMP levels in various areas of the rat brain *in vitro*. Neuropharmacol. **12**, 327–337 (1973)
Papp, R.H., Hawkins, H.B., Share, N.N., Wang, S.C.: Emesis induced by the intracerebroventricular administration of hydergine and mechlorethamine hydrochloride. J. Pharmacol. exp. Ther. **154**, 333–338 (1966)
Parkes, J.D., Debono, A.G., Marsden, C.D.: Bromocriptine in Parkinsonism: Long-term treatment, dose-response and comparison with levodopa. J. Neurol. Neurosurg. Psychiat. **39**, 1101–1108 (1976a)
Parkes, J.D., Debono, A.G., Marsden, C.D., Asselman, P.: Clinical pharmacology of bromocriptine in Parkinsonism. In: Bayliss, R.I.S., Turner, P., MacLay, W.P. (eds.), Pharmacological and Clinical Aspects of Bromocriptine (Parlodel), pp. 27–33. Turnbridge Wells, G.B.: MCS Consultants 1976b
Pasteels, J.L., Danguy, A., Frerotte, M., Ectors, F.: Inhibition de la sécrétion de prolactine par l'ergocornine et la 2-Br-α-ergokryptine: action directe sur l'hypophyse en culture. Ann. Endocr. (Paris) **32**, 188–192 (1971)
Peng, M.T., Wang, S.C.: Emetic responses of monkeys to apomorphine, hydergine, deslanoside and protoveratrine. Proc. Soc. exp. Biol. (N.Y.) **110**, 211–215 (1962)
Perrault, G., Liutkus, M., Boulu, R., Rossignol, P.: Modification par l'hypoxie ischémique aiguë de la résponse cortico-pyramidale chez le chat. Application à l'étude des médicaments de l'insuffisance vasculaire cérébrale. J. Pharmacol. (Paris) **7**, 27–38 (1976)
Phillis, J.W., Tebecis, A.K., York, D.H.: The inhibitory action of monoamines on lateral geniculate neurones. J. Physiol. (Lond.) **190**, 563–581 (1967)
Pieri, L., Pieri, M., Haefely, W.: LSD as an agonist of dopamine receptors in the striatum. Nature (Lond.) **252**, 586–588 (1974)
Pieri, M., Pieri, L., Saner, A., da Prada, M., Haefely, W.: A comparison of drug-induced rotation in rats lesioned in the medial forebrain bundle with 5,6-dihydroxytryptamine or 6-hydroxydopamine. Arch. int. Pharmacodyn. **217**, 118–130 (1975)
Pijnenburg, A.J.J., van Rossum, J.M.: Stimulation of locomotor activity following injection of dopamine into the nucleus accumbens. J. Pharm. Pharmacol. **25**, 1003–1004 (1973)
Pijnenburg, A.J.J., Woodruff, G.N., van Rossum, J.M.: Ergometrine-induced locomotor activity following intracerebral injection into the nucleus accumbens. Brain Res. **59**, 289–302 (1973)
Pletscher, A., Brossi, A., Gey, K.F.: Benzoquinolizine derivatives: a new class of monoamine decreasing drugs with psychotropic actions. Int. Rev. Neurobiol. **4**, 275–306 (1962)
Pletscher, A., Shore, P.A., Brodie, B.B.: Serotonin release as a possible mechanism of reserpine action. Science **122**, 374–375 (1955)
Pletscher, A., Shore, P.A., Brodie, B.B.: Serotonin as mediator of reserpine action in brain. J. Pharmacol. exp. Ther. **116**, 89 (1956)
Poignant, J.C., Lejeune, F., Malecot, E., Petitjean, M., Regnier, G., Canevari, R.: Effets comparés du piribédil et de trois de les métabolites sur le système extrapyramidal du rat. Experientia (Basel) **30**, 70–71 (1974)
Popkin, R.J.: An evaluation of some dihydrogenated alkaloids of ergot in the management of chronic peripheral vascular diseases. Angiology **2**, 114–124 (1951)
Pourrias, B., Raynaud, G.: Action de quelques agents vaso-actif sur l'irrigation sous-corticale du lapin et du chien. Therapie **27**, 849–860 (1972)
Pritzker, B.: Die Beeinflussung der psychomotorischen Erregung durch Dihydroergotamin (DHE 45). Schweiz. med. Wschr. **77**, 985–987 (1947)

Racker, E.: Structure and function of ATP-driven ion pumps. Trends in Biochem. Sci. **1**, 244–247 (1976)
Raichle, M.E., Grubb, R.L., Jr., Mokhtar, H.G., Eichling, J.O., Ter-Pogossian, M.M.: Correlation between regional cerebral blood flow and oxidative metabolism. Arch. Neurol. (Chic.) **33**, 523–526 (1976)
Randrup, A., Munkvad, I.: Stereotyped activities produced by amphetamine in several animal species and man. Psychopharmacologia (Berl.) **11**, 300–310 (1967)
Randrup, A., Munkvad, I.: Behavioural stereotypies induced by pharmacological agents. Pharmakopsychiatrie (Stuttg.) **1**, 18–26 (1968)
Randrup, A., Munkvad, I.: Biochemical, anatomical and psychological investigations of stereotyped behavior produced by amphetamines. In: Costa, E., Garattini, S. (eds.), Amphetamines and Related Compounds, pp. 695–715. New York: Raven Press 1970
Ray, A.J., Wong, S.: Effect of elymoclavine on conditioned avoidance. Arch. int. Pharmacodyn. **166**, 253–257 (1967)
Regli, F., Waltz, A.G.: Cerebral circulation. Effects of vasodilating drugs on blood flow and the microvasculature of ischemic and non-ischemic cerebral cortex. Arch. Neurol. (Chic.) **24**, 467–474 (1971)
Regli, F., Yamaguchi, T., Waltz, A.G.: Responses of surface arteries and blood flow of ischemic and nonischemic cerebral cortex to aminophylline, ergotamine tartrate, and acetazolamide. Stroke **2**, 461–470 (1971)
Riechert, W.: Über die antikonvulsive Wirkung des Gynergens. Naunyn-Schmiedebergs Arch. exp. Path. Pharmak. **213**, 82–87 (1951)
Reichlmeier, K., Iwangoff, P.: Influence of phosphodiesterase inhibitors on brain protein kinases in vitro. Experientia (Basel) **30**, 691 (1974)
Rigler, R., Silberstern, E.: Zur Physiologie der Wärmeregulierung. Der Einfluß sympathikushemmender Mittel auf die Körpertemperatur. Naunyn-Schmiedebergs Arch. exp. Path. Pharmak. **121**, 1–22 (1927)
Roberts, J.E., Massopust, L.L., Buchanan, A.R.: Effects in albino rats of dihydrogenated derivatives of the dimethylpyruvic acid group of ergot alkaloids as manifested by thermal reactions and oxygen utilization. J. Pharmacol. exp. Ther. **100**, 51–58 (1950)
Roberts, J.E., Robinson, B.E., Buchanan, A.R.: Oxygen consumption correlated with the thermal reactions of young rats to ergotamine. Amer. J. Physiol. **156**, 170–176 (1949)
Roberts, M.H.T., Straughan, D.W.: Excitation and depression of cortical neurones by 5-hydroxytryptamine. J. Physiol. (Lond.) **193**, 269–294 (1967)
Roessler, R., Unna, K.: Zur Pharmakologie des neuen Mutterkornalkaloides Sensibamin. Naunyn-Schmiedebergs Arch. exp. Path. Pharmak. **179**, 115–126 (1935)
Roos, B.E., Steg, G.: The effect of L-3,4-dihydroxyphenylalanine and DL-5-hydroxytryptophan on rigidity and tremor induced by reserpine, chlorpromazine and phenoxybenzamine. Life Sci. **3**, 351–360 (1964)
Rossignol, P., Boulu, R., Ribart, M., Paultre, C., Bache, S., Truelle, B.: Action de quelques médicaments de l'insuffissance vasculaire cérébrale sur les potentiels primaires somesthétiques evoqués au niveau du cortex et du thalamus chez le rat en état d'ischémie cérébrale aigue. C.R. Acad. Sci. (Paris) Sér. D **274**, 3027–3029 (1972)
Rothlin, E.: Recherches expérimentales sur l'ergotamine, alcaloide spécifique de l'ergot de seigle. Arch. int. Pharmacodyn. **27**, 459–479 (1923)
Rothlin, E.: Zur Frage der pharmakologischen Identität der beiden Mutterkornalkaloide Ergotamin und Ergotoxin. Klin. Wschr. **12**, 25–26 (1933)
Rothlin, E.: Über Wechselbeziehungen in der Wirkung neurovegetativer Pharmaka. Schweiz. med. Wschr. **64**, 188–191 (1934)
Rothlin, E.: Über ein neues Mutterkornalkaloid. Schweiz. med. Wschr. **65**, 947–949 (1935)
Rothlin, E.: Neues zum Mutterkornproblem. Naunyn-Schmiedebergs Arch. exp. Path. Pharmak. **181**, 154–155 (1936)
Rothlin, E.: Beitrag zur differenzierenden Analyse der Mutterkornalkaloide. Schweiz. med. Wschr. **33**, 971–975 (1938)
Rothlin, E.: Zur Pharmakologie der hydrierten natürlichen Mutterkornalkaloide. Helv. physiol. pharmacol. Acta **2**, 48–49 (1944)
Rothlin, E.: The pharmacology of the natural and dihydrogenated alkaloids of ergot. Schweiz. Akad. med. Wiss. **2**, 249–272 (1946/47)

Rothlin, E.: Structure fonctionelle du système neurovégétatif et points d'attaque des alcaloides de l'ergot de seigle. In: Hazard, R. (eds.), Actualités Pharmacologiques, 6 ième Sér., pp. 197–219. Paris: Masson & Cie. 1953
Rothlin, E.: Pharmacology of lysergic acid diethylamide and some of its related compounds. J. Pharm. Pharmacol. **9**, 569–587 (1957)
Rothlin, E., Cerletti, A.: Über einige pharmakologische Untersuchungen an Mäusen mit congenitaler Drehsucht. Helv. physiol. pharmacol. Acta **10**, 319–327 (1952)
Rothlin, E., Fanchamps, A.: Quelques développements récents de la pharmacologie de l'ergot de seigle. Rev. Path. gén. comp. **55**, 1427–1443 (1955)
Rothlin, E., Hamet, R.: Sur l'action utérine de l'Uzara. Rév. Pharmacol. exp. Ther. **2**, 29–47 (1930)
Rothlin, E., Taeschler, M.: Zur Wirkung von Adrenalin und Hydergin auf die Hirndurchblutung. Helv. physiol. pharmacol. Acta **9**, C37–C39 (1951)
Rothlin, E., Cerletti, A., Konzett, H., Schalch, W.R., Taeschler, M.: Zentrale vegetative LSD-Effekte. Experientia (Basel) **12**, 154–155 (1956)
Roubicek, J., Geiger, C., Abt, K.: An ergot alkaloid preparation (hydergine) in geriatric therapy. J. Amer. geriat. Soc. **20**, 222–229 (1972)
Rouse, L.O., Frank, D.L.: Facilitation of learned resistance to audiogenic seizures in Balb/cCrgl mice by d-LSD-25. Nature (Lond.) **248**, 78–81 (1974)
Rubin, B., Piala, J.J., Burke, J.C., Craver, B.N.: A new, potent and specific serotonin inhibitor, (SQ 10,643) 2′-(3-dimethylamino-propylthio) cinnamanilide hydrochloride: Antiserotonin activity on uterus and on gastrointestinal, vascular and respiratory systems of animals. Arch. int. Pharmacodyn. **152**, 132–143 (1964)
Ruch-Monachon, M.A., Jalfre, M., Haefely, W.: Drugs and PGO waves in the lateral geniculate body of the curarized cat. II. PGO wave activity and brain 5-hydroxytryptamine. Arch. int. Pharmacodyn. **219**, 269–286 (1976a)
Ruch-Monachon, M.A., Jalfre, M., Haefely, W.: Drugs and PGO waves in the lateral geniculate. V. Miscellaneous compounds. Synopsis of the role of central neurotransmitters on PGO wave activity. Arch. int. Pharmacodyn. **219**, 326–346 (1976b)
Ruckebusch, Y., Grivel, M.L., Laplace, J.P.: Variations interspécifiques des modifications de la température centrale liées à l'injection cérébroventriculaire de catécholamines et de 5-hydroxytryptamine. C.R. Soc. Biol. (Paris) **159**, 1748–1750 (1965)
Rutschmann, J., Stadler, P.A.: Chemical Background. In: Berde, B., Schild, H.O. (eds.), Ergot Alkaloids and Related Compounds., Handbuch der experimentellen Pharmakologie, Ch. II. Berlin-Heidelberg-New York: Springer 1978
Saavedra, J.M., Fischer, E.: Antagonism of β-phenylethylamine derivatives and serotonin blocking drugs upon serotonin, tryptamine and reserpine induced behavioral depression in mice. Arzneimittel-Forsch. **20**, 952–957 (1970)
Salmoiraghi, G.C., Sollero, L., Page, I.H.: Blockade by Bromlysergic-acid-diethylamide (BOL) of the potentiating action of serotonin and reserpine on hexobarbital hypnosis. J. Pharmacol. exp. Ther. **117**, 166–168 (1956)
Sankar, D.V.S.: Effect of LSD, BOL, and chlorpromazine on "Neurohormone" metabolism. Ann. N.Y., Acad. Sci. **96**, 93–97 (1962)
Sankar, D.V.S.: Effects of LSD on sleep-dream cycles and rhythm. In: Sankar, D.V.S. (ed.), LSD- A Total Study, pp. 464–469. Westbury, N.Y.: P.J.D. Publications 1975
Sawyer, M.E.M., Schlossberg, T.: Studies of homeostasis in normal, sympathectomized and ergotaminized animals; effect of high and low temperatures. Amer. J. Physiol. **104**, 172–183 (1933)
Schneider, M., Wiemers, K.: Über die Wirkung der hydrierten Mutterkornalkaloide auf die Gehirndurchblutung. Klin. Wschr. **29**, 580–581 (1951)
Schneider, P.B.: Recherches expérimentales et cliniques avec les alcaloides dihydrogénés de l'ergot de seigle. Schweiz. Arch. Neurol. Psychiat. **65**, 283–310 (1950)
Schnieden, H., Cox, B.: A comparison between amantadine and bromocriptine using the stereotyped behaviour test (SBR) in the rat. Europ. J. Pharmacol. **39**, 133–141 (1976)
Schorderet, M.: Direct evidence for the stimulation of rabbit retina dopamine receptors by ergot alkaloids. Neurosci. Letters **2**, 87–91 (1976)
Schultz, J., Daly, J.W.: Adenosine 3′,5′monophosphate in guinea pig cerebral cortical slices:

effects of α- and β-adrenergic agents, histamine, serotonin and adenosine. J. Neurochem. **21**, 573–579 (1973)
Segal, M.: Physiological and pharmacological evidence for a serotonergic projection to the hippocampus. Brain Res. **94**, 115–131 (1975)
Segal, M.: 5-HT antagonists in rat hippocampus. Brain Res. **103**, 161–166 (1976)
Segal, M., Bloom, F.E.: The projection of midline raphe nuclei to the hippocampus of the rat. Fed. Proc. **331**, Abstract 538 (1974)
Selinsky, H., Bierman, W.: The effect of ergotamine tartrate on body temperatures. J. Mt Sinai Hosp. **5**, 545–550 (1938)
Semler, H.J., David, N.A.: Potentiation of morphine and 1-isomethadone analgesia by dihydrogenated ergot alkaloids. Amer. J. Med. **13**, 99–100 (1952)
Semler, H.J., David, N.A.: Effects of Hydergine (CCK-179)-1-isomethadone combinations on respiration and temperature in the rabbit. J. Pharmacol. exp. Ther. **110**, 46 (1954)
Severinghaus, J.W., Nemoto, E., Hoff, J.: The CO_2 shuttle in cerebral arteriolar ECF H^3 control. Europ. Neurol. **6**, 56–59 (1971/72)
Share, N.N., Chai, C.Y., Wang, S.C.: Emesis induced by intracerebroventricular injection of apomorphine and deslanoside in normal and C T zone ablated dogs. J. Pharmacol. exp. Ther. **147**, 416–421 (1965)
Shelesnyak, M.C.: Ergotoxine inhibition of deciduoma formation and its reversal by progesterone. Amer. J. Physiol. **179**, 301–304 (1954)
Shelesnyak, M.C.: Action de différents alcaloides de l'ergot sur la formation du déciduome chez les rats en pseudogestation. C.R. Acad. Sci. (Paris) **246**, 2525–2528 (1958)
Shore, P.A., Silver, S.L., Brodie, B.B.: Interaction of reserpine, serotonin and lysergic acid diethylamide in the brain. Science **122**, 284–285 (1955a)
Shore, P.A., Silver, S.L., Brodie, B.B.: Interaction of serotonin and lysergic acid diethylamide (LSD) in the central nervous system. Experientia (Basel) **11**, 272–273 (1955b)
Sicuteri, F., Cossio, M.: Studio clinico sulle proprietà antiepilettiche di un neovo derivato lisergico ad azione antiserotoninica. Minerva med. **51**, 1591–1595 (1960)
Siegfried, J.: Traitement du parkinsonism avec la L-DOPA associée à un inhibiteur de la décarboxylase. Méd. et. Hyg. (Genéve) **27**, 543–545 (1969)
Siggins, G.R., Hoffer, B.J., Ungerstedt, U.: Electrophysiological evidence for involvement of cyclic adenosine monophosphate in dopamine responses of caudate neurons. Life Sci. **15**, 779–792 (1974)
Simon, R.P., Gershon, M.D., Brooks, D.C.: The role of the raphe nuclei in the regulation of ponto-geniculo-occipital wave activity. Brain Res. **58**, 313–330 (1973)
Snider, S.R., Hutt, C., Stein, B., Fahn, S.: Increase in brain serotonin produced by bromocriptine. Neurosci. Letters **1**, 237–241 (1975)
Snider, S.R., Hutt, C., Stein, B., Prasad, A.L.N., Fahn, S.: Correlation of behavioural inhibition or excitation produced by bromocriptine with changes in brain catecholamine turnover. J. Pharm. Pharmacol. **28**, 563–566 (1976)
Snyder, S.H., Burt, D.R., Creese, I.: The dopamine receptor of mammalian brain: direct demonstration of binding to agonist and antagonist states. In: Ferrendelli, J.A., McEwen, B.S., Snyder, S.H. (eds.), Soc. for Neuroscience, Symposia, Vol. I., pp. 28–49. Bethesda 1975
Sofia, R.D., Vassar, H.B.: The effect of ergotamine and methysergide on serotonin metabolism in the rat brain. Arch. int. Pharmacodyn. **216**, 40–50 (1975)
Solms, H.: Psychosedativer Effekt der Sekale-Alkaloide (DHE 45, DHO 180 und Hydergin) auf psychomotorisch Erregte. Schweiz. Arch. Neurol. Psychiat. **68**, 64–84 (1952)
Spano, P.F., Kumakura, K., Tonon, G.C., Govoni, S., Trabucchi, H.: LSD and dopamine-sensitive adenylate cyclase in various rat brain areas. Brain Res. **93**, 164–167 (1975)
Stahnke, E.: Studien zur Wirkung des Ergotamins. Klin. Wschr. **7**, 23–25 (1928a)
Stahnke, E.: Zur Pharmakologie des Ergotamins. Naunyn-Schmiedebergs Arch. exp. Path. Pharmak. **128**, 132–133 (1928b)
Steg, G.: Efferent muscle innervation and rigidity. Acta physiol. scand. 61. Suppl. 225, 1–53 (1964)
Stoll, W.A.: Lysergsäure-diäthylamid, ein Phantastikum aus der Mutterkorngruppe. Schweiz. Arch. Neurol. Psychiat. **60**, 279–323 (1947)

Stone, C.A., Wenger, H.C., Ludden, C.T., Stavorski, J.M., Ross, C.A.: Antiserotonine-antihistamine properties of cyproheptadine. J. Pharmacol. exp. Ther. **131**, 73–84 (1961)
Stone, T.W.: Studies on the central nervous system effects of agroclavine, an ergot alkaloid. Arch. int. Pharmacodyn. **202**, 62–65 (1973)
Stone, T.W.: Further evidence for a dopamine receptor stimulating action of an ergot alkaloid. Brain Res. **72**, 177–180 (1974a)
Stone, T.W.: On the antagonism of ergot alkaloids and dopamine by phenothiazines. Experientia (Basel) **30**, 827–829 (1974b)
Storch, T.J.C. von: Complications following the use of ergotamine tartrate. J. Amer. med. Ass. **111**, 293–300 (1938)
Stosseck, K., Lübbers, D.W., Cottin, N.: Determination of local blood flow (microflow) by electrochemically generated hydrogen. Pflügers Arch. ges. Physiol. **348**, 225–238 (1974)
Streichenberger, G., Boismare, F., Lauressergues, H., Lechat, P.: Modification, par certains médicaments doués d'action vasculaire, des effets d'une anoxie ischémique encéphalique chez le chat. Thérapie **25**, 1003–1016 (1970)
Struyker Boudier, H.A.J., van Rossum, J.M.: Dopamine-induced inhibition and excitation of neurones of the snail, *Helix Aspersa*. Arch. int. Pharmacodyn. **209**, 314–323 (1974)
Struyker Boudier, H.A.J., Gielen, W., Cools, A.R., van Rossum, J.M.: Pharmacological analysis of dopamine-induced inhibition and excitation of neurones of the snail, *Helix Aspersa*. Arch. int. Pharmacodyn. **209**, 324–331 (1974)
Struyker Boudier, H.A.J., Teppema, L., Cools, A.R., van Rossum, J.M.: (3,4-dihydroxyphenylamino)-2-imidazoline (DPI), a new potent agonist at dopamine receptors mediating neuronal inhibition. J. Pharm. Pharmacol. **27**, 882–883 (1975)
Szewczykowski, J., Meyer, J.S., Kondo, A., Nomura, F., Teraura, T.: Effects of ergot alkaloids (Hydergine) on cerebral hemodynamics and oxygen consumption in monkeys. J. neurol. Sci. **10**, 25–31 (1970)
Tabushi, K., Himwich, H.E.: Electroencephalographic study of the effects of methysergide on sleep in the rabbit. Electroenceph. clin. Neurophysiol. **31**, 491–497 (1971)
Taeschler, M., Cerletti, A.: Some observations on the interaction of reserpine and LSD. J. Pharmacol. exp. Ther. **120**, 179–183 (1957)
Taeschler, M., Rothlin, E.: Zur Charakterizierung der zentralen Wirkung von Phenothiazinderivaten. Naunyn-Schmiedebergs Arch. exp. Path. Pharmak. **228**, 184–186 (1956)
Taeschler, M., Cerletti, A., Rothlin, E.: Zur Frage der Hyderginwirkung auf die Gehirnzirkulation. Helv. physiol. pharmacol. Acta **10**, 120–137 (1952)
Tashjian, A.H., Hoyt, R.F.: Transient control of organ specific functions in pituitary cells in culture. In: Sussman, M. (ed.), Molecular Genetics and Developmental Biology, pp. 353–387. Englewood Cliffs, N.J.: Prentice Hall 1972
Tebècis, A.K.: Antagonism of 5-hydroxytryptamine by methiothepin shown in microelectrophoretic studies of neurones in the lateral geniculate nucleus. Nature (Lond.) New Biol. **238**, 63–64 (1972)
Tebècis, A.K., Di Maria, A.: A re-evaluation of the mode of action of 5-hydroxytryptamine on lateral geniculate neurones: comparison with catecholamines and LSD. Exp. Brain Res. **14**, 480–493 (1972)
Tedeschi, D.H., Tedeschi, R.E., Fellows, E.J.: The effects of tyramine on the central nervous system, including a pharmacological procedure for the evaluation of iproniazide-like drugs. J. Pharmacol. exp. Ther. **165**, 251–257 (1959)
Teychenne, P.F., Kartzinel, R., Calne, D.B., Pfeiffer, R.: Longterm experience with bromocriptine in parkinsonism. In: Bayliss, R.I.S., Turner, P., Maclay, W.P. (eds.), Pharmacological and Clinical Aspects of Bromocriptine (Parlodel), pp. 34–38. Turnbridge Wells, G.B.: MCS Consultants 1976.
Tissot, R.: Perturbations du métabolisme des catécholamines (notamment la dopamine) d'un syndrome parkinsonien. Presse méd. **77**, 617–618 (1969)
Torre, M., Fagiani, M.B.: Effects of LSD-25 and dimethysergide bimaleate on a conditioned reflex in the rat. J. Neurol. Sci. **7**, 571–579 (1968)
Torre, M., Torre, E., Bogetto, F.: The relation between cerebral serotonin levels and conditioned behaviour in the rat following the administration of LSD-25 and UML. Psychopharmacologia (Berl.) **41**, 245–247 (1975)

Trabucchi, M., Spano, P.F., Tonon, G.C., Frattola, L.: Effects of bromocriptine on cerebral dopaminergic receptors. Life Sci. **19**, 225–232 (1976)
Tuomisto, J.: Inhibition of noradrenaline (NA), dopamine (DA) and 5HT uptake in synaptosomes by reserpine, 6-hydroxy-1,2,3,4-tetrahydroharmane (6HTH), LSD and ergotamine. J. Pharmacol. (Paris) **5**, Suppl. 2, 100 (1974)
Udea, T., Maeno, H., Greengard, P.: Regulation of endogenous phosphorylation of specific proteins in synaptic membrane fractions from rat brain by adenosine 3′,5′-monophosphate. J. biol. Chem. **248**, 8295–8305 (1973)
Udenfriend, S., Weissbach, H., Bogdanski, D.F.: Increase in tissue serotonin following administration of its precursor 5-hydroxytryptophan. Ann. N.Y. Acad. Sci. **66**, 602–608 (1957)
Ungerstedt, U.: Postsynaptic supersensitivity after 6-hydroxydopamine induced degeneration of the nigro-neostriatal dopamine system. Acta physiol. scand., Suppl. **367**, 69–73 (1971)
Ungerstedt, U., Arbuthnott, G.W.: Quantitative recording of rotational behaviour in rats after 6-OH dopamine lesions of the nigrostriatal dopamine system. Brain Res. **24**, 485–493 (1970)
Uzunov, P., Weiss, B.: Psychopharmacological agents and the cAMP system of rat brain. In: Greengard, P., Robinson, G.A. (eds.), Advances in Cyclic Nucleotide Research, Vol. 1., pp. 435–453. New York: Raven Press 1972
Vargaftig, B.B., Coignet, J.L., de Vos, C.J., Grijsen, H., Bonta, I.L.: Mianserin hydrochloride: Peripheral and central effects in relation to antagonism against 5-hydroxytryptamine and tryptamine. Europ. J. Pharmacol. **16**, 336–346 (1971)
Vartiainen, A., Lassas, B., Paetiaelae, R.: The effects of ergot alkaloids on body temperature of rabbit. Acta Soc. med. ferm. Durdicum, Ser. A., fasc. 3, Art. 12, **19**, 1–21 (1937)
Venn, R.D.: Clinical pharmacology of ergot alkaloids in senile cerebral insufficiency. In: Berde, B., Schild, H.O. (eds.), Ergot Alkaloids and Related Compounds. Handbuch der experimentellen Pharmakologie, Ch. VII. Berlin-Heidelberg-New York: Springer 1978
Vigouret, J.M., Bürki, H.R., Jaton, A.-L., Züger, P.E., Loew, D.M.: Neurochemical and neuropharmacological investigations with four ergot derivatives: Bromocriptine, dihydroergotoxine, CF 25-397, and CM 29-712. Pharmacology (Basel) **16** (Suppl. 1), 156–173 (1978)
Vigouret, J.M., Loew, D.M., Jaton, A.-L.: Effects of bromocriptine on α- and γ-rigidity in rats in comparison to apomorphine and d-amphetamine. Naunyn-Schmiedebergs Arch. Pharmacol. **297**, Suppl. 2, R 54 (1977)
Vigouret, J.M., Teschemacher, H.J., Albus, K., Herz, A.: Differentiation between spinal and supraspinal sites of action of morphine when inhibiting the hindleg flexor reflex in rabbits. Neuropharmacol. **12**, 111–121 (1973)
Villa, R.F., Panceri, P.: Action of some drugs on performance time in mice. Farmaco **28**, 43–48 (1973)
Viparelli, U., Crispi, G., Di Lorenzo, R.: La serotonina nell' epilessia: un dilemma terapeutico. Ann. Neuropsichiat. Psicoanal. **13**, 254–265 (1966)
Votava, Z.: Pharmacologie des cycloalkylamides de l'acide d-lysergique. J. Physiol. (Paris) **49**, 417–419 (1957)
Votava, Z., Lamplova, I.: Action anti-serotonine et autres effets pharmacologiques de quelques analoques des alcaloides naturels de l'ergot. Therapie **19**, 733–742 (1964)
Votava, Z., Podalova, I.: Farmakologické vlastnosti cyckloalkylamidů kyseliny d-lysergové. Čas. Lék. čes. **97**, 1062–1064 (1958)
Votava, Z., Glisson, S.N., Himwich, H.E.: Behavioural reaction of rats pretreated with reserpine to LSD-25. Int. J. Neuropharmacol. **6**, 543–547 (1967)
Vuillon-Cacciuttolo, G.: Etude de la photosensibilité et des réponses évoquées le long de la voie visuelle chez le singe papio papio. Thèse de 3e cycle. Marseille 1970
Vuillon-Cacciuttolo, G., Balzano, E.: Action de quatre dérivés de l'ergot sur la photosensibilité et l'E.E.G. du papio papio. J. Pharmacol. (Paris) **3**, 31–45 (1972)
Wada, J.-A., Balzano, E., Meldrum, B.S., Naquet, R.: Behavioural and electrographic effects of β-5-hydroxytryptophan and D,L$\pm$parachlorophenylalanine on epileptic Senegalese baboon (papio papio) Electroenceph. clin. Neurophysiol. **33**, 520–526 (1972)
Walker, R.J., Woodruff, G.N., Glaizner, B., Sedden, C.B., Kerkut, G.A.: The pharmacology of *Helix* dopamine receptor of specific neurons in the snail, *Helix aspersa*. Comp. Biochem. Physiol. **24**, 455–469 (1968)

Walter, S., Balzano, E., Vuillon, Cacciuttolo, G., Naquet, R.: Changes in visual evoked potentials and in photosensitivity produced by LSD in Papio papio. Electroenceph. clin. Neurophysiol. **30**, 253 (1971a)
Walter, S., Balzano, E., Vuillon-Cacciuttolo, G., Naquet, R.: Effets comportementaux et électrographiques du diéthylamide de l'acide d-lysergique (LSD 25) sur le Papio papio photosensible. Electroenceph. clin. Neurophysiol. **30**, 294–305 (1971b)
Wang, S.C.: Emetic and antiemetic drugs. In: Root, W.S., Hofmann, F.G. (eds.), Physiological Pharmacology, Vol. II, pp. 255–328. New York: Academic Press 1965
Wang, S.C., Glaviano, V.V.: Locus of emetic action of morphine and hydergine in dogs. J. Pharmacol. exp. Ther. **111**, 329–334 (1954)
Weiss, B.L., Aghajanian, G.K.: Activation of brain serotonin by heat: Role of midbrain raphe neurons. Brain Res. **26**, 37–48 (1971)
White, A.C.: A comparison of some of the ergot alkaloids. Part I. General toxicology. Quart. J. Pharm. Pharmacol. **16**, 344–352 (1943)
White, A.C.: A comparison of some of the ergot alkaloids. Part II. Action on temperature regulation in the mouse and the rabbit. Quart. J. Pharm. Pharmacol. **17**, 1–7 (1944a)
White, A.C.: A comparison of some of the ergot alkaloids. Part III. General pharmacology. Quart. J. Pharm. Pharmacol. **17**, 95–102 (1944b)
Wiernsperger, N., Gygax, P., Danzeisen, M.: Cortical PO_2-distribution during oligemic hypotension and its pharmacological modifications. Arzneimittel-Forsch., in press (1978)
Winter, J.C.: Comparison of chlordiazepoxide, methysergide, and cinanserin as modifiers of punished behavior and as antagonists of N,N-dimethyltryptamine. Arch. int. Pharmacodyn. **197**, 147–159 (1972)
Wislocki, G.B., Leduc, E.H.: Vital staining of the hematoencephalic barrier by silver nitrate and trypan blue, and cytological comparison of the neurohypophysis, pineal body, area postrema, intercolumnar tubercle and subraoptic crest. J. comp. Neurol. **96**, 371–413 (1952)
Wislocki, G.B., Putnam, T.J.: Note on the anatomy of the area postrema. Anat. Rec. **19**, 281–287 (1920)
Wislocki, G.B., Putnam, T.J.: Further observations on the anatomy and physiology of the areae postremae. Anat. Rec. **27**, 151–156 (1924)
Woodruff, G.N., Walker, R.J.: The effect of dopamine and other compounds on the activity of neurons of *Helix aspersa*; structure activity relationships. Int. J. Neuropharmacol. **8**, 279–289 (1969)
Woodruff, G.N., Elkhawad, A.O., Crossmann, A.R.: Further evidence for the stimulation of rat brain dopamine receptors by ergometrine. J. Pharm. Pharmacol. **26**, 455–456 (1974)
Woodruff, G.N., Walker, R.J., Kerkut, G.A.: Actions of ergometrine on catecholamine receptors in the guinea-pig vas deferens and in the snail brain. Comp. gen. Pharmacol. **1**, 54–60 (1970)
Woolley, D.W., Shaw, E.: A biochemical and pharmacological suggestion about certain mental disorders. Science **119**, 587–588 (1954)
Wyler, A.R., Wilkus, R.J., Troupin, A.S.: Methysergide in the treatment of narcolepsy. Arch. Neurol. (Chic.), **32**, 265–268 (1975)
Yahr, M.D., Duvoisin, R.C., Schear, M.J., Barret, R.E.: Treatment of parkinsonism with levo-DOPA. Arch. Neurol. (Chic.) **21**, 343–354 (1969)
Youmans, J.B., Trimble, W.H.: Experimental and clinical studies of ergotamine; effect of ergotamine on blood sugar and epinephrine hyperglycemia in trained unanesthetized dogs. J. Pharmacol. exp. Ther. **38**, 121–132 (1930)
Yui, T., Takeo, Y.: Neuropharmacological studies on a new series of ergot alkaloids. Elymoclavine as a potent analeptic on reserpine-sedation. Jap. J. Pharmacol. **7**, 157–161 (1958a)
Yui, T., Takeo, Y.: Neuropharmacological studies on a new series of ergot alkaloids. The effects on electrocorticogram of rabbits. Jap. J. Pharmacol. **7**, 162–168 (1958b)
Züger, P.E., Vigouret, J.M., Loew, D.M.: Effect of ergot derivatives on reserpine induced PGO waves in the cat. Experientia (Basel), in press (1978)

CHAPTER VII

Clinical Pharmacology of Ergot Alkaloids in Senile Cerebral Insufficiency

R.D. VENN

"Age carries all things,
even the mind, away."

VIRGIL

A. Introduction

Aging is one of the biologic processes shared by all living things. Perhaps the inexorable nature of aging and its inevitability have been responsible for its hitherto almost unquestioned acceptance as a normal phenomenon of life and, until recent years, for the relatively low interest in this field of biologic and clinical research, particularly the latter.

The remarkable progress of medical science during the past 40 years has increased the average human life expectancy, so that the shift in the age distribution of the population at large has been towards the older end of the spectrum. The significant increase in the numbers of individuals who now reach geriatric status has demanded a new look at the aging process and its attendant problems and has stimulated a new interest at the biologic, clinical and socioeconomic levels.

There is a trend in gerontologic research away from simple descriptions of changes in the physical and mental characteristics of the aged to the elucidation of the causes of aging at the cellular and molecular level. However, the ultimate goal of geriatric research at all levels is not only to identify the mechanisms of aging and to increase life span but more importantly to preserve mental and physical function, so that the elderly are self-sufficient and productive in their later years and do not become a misery to themselves and a burden to those responsible for their care.

B. Terminology, Etiology, and Pathology of the Aging Process of the Brain

1. Terminology

A review of the relevant gerontologic literature reveals that although there is some agreement on the broad clinical profile of aging, there is still a lack of unanimity as to what constitutes a well-defined valid symptom complex which can reasonably be called the syndrome of mental and behavioral deterioration in the aging person. Furthermore, although considerable advances toward a better understanding of aging have been made in recent years, the exact mechanisms of the aging process at the cellular and molecular levels are still largely unknown. It is not surprising, therefore, that there is also no concordance of opinion as to the nomenclature and definition of these involutional changes.

On the one hand, a terminology has emerged which takes its origin from presumed underlying pathologic changes responsible for the aging process in the brain. Cerebral arteriosclerosis and cerebrovascular insufficiency, for example, are terms still used, based on the popular misconception that the clinical manifestations of the condition are exclusively due to stenotic cerebral vascular disease. On the other hand, in order to avoid nomenclature which specifically involves unproven causative mechanisms, terms such as senile dementia and chronic organic brain syndrome have been applied to the clinical manifestations of the condition. These, too, are not entirely satisfactory, as not all senile persons are demented in the strict sense of the word, and chronic organic brain syndrome might be applied to any organic brain disease regardless of age.

At the present time, senile dementia appears to be the term most often used in context with the aging process in the brain. However, until more is known of the mechanisms underlying this process, the term senile cerebral insufficiency, though not widely used, is probably the most appropriate, as it indicates the general nature of the condition and the age group in which it occurs without suggesting any specific clinical characteristics or possible etiologic or pathologic background.

2. Definition

Senile cerebral insufficiency is a descriptive diagnostic term (synonymous with senile dementia and chronic organic brain syndrome) applied to a clinical symptom complex or syndrome which develops sooner or later in the aging process and which is characterized by: Impairment of cognitive function; changes in affect and behavior; lessened ability to cope with the ordinary tasks of everyday living; and the appearance of certain symptoms not related to concomitant disease processes.

3. Etiology and Pathology

The mechanisms at the morphologic, biochemic, and electrophysiologic levels which determine the deterioration of mental function associated with aging are largely unknown at the present time, and their elucidation presents a formidable challenge to those engaged in gerontologic research.

A number of different theories as to the nature of the aging process in the brain, based mostly on animal experimentation, have been propounded by various investigators in this field of research, but a unifying hypothesis to explain the pathophysiology of aging has yet to be developed.

Consideration of the etiology and pathogenesis of the aging process is of importance, because their investigation—particularly in animal studies—has provided the basis for some of the clinical pharmacologic methods used to measure drug effect on senile cerebral insufficiency. However, many experimental methods used in animals cannot be applied to man.

Progress in this direction has been further hindered by the persistence of a number of conventional conceptions of the etiology of age-related brain dysfunction. Foremost among these conceptions is the commonly held idea that the mental, emotional, and behavioral changes of senescence are the exclusive results of impaired cerebral blood flow secondary to arteriosclerotic changes in the cerebral vasculature.

In a comprehensive review, LASSEN (1959) was among the first who questioned in a broad sense the relationship of psychic disturbance to arteriosclerotic changes in the brain. OBRIST (1972) also questioned whether mental decline in aging is related primarily to arteriosclerosis of the brain vessels.

Comparison of clinical symptomatology and autopsy findings has demonstrated that psychic changes in aging individuals are associated with the stenotic process of cerebral arteriosclerosis in less than 30% of patients. Indeed, it is now established that most patients showing signs of senile mental decline have normal brain vessels on autopsy (TOMLINSON et al., 1968, 1970).

On the other hand, elderly persons with specific neurologic deficits due to cerebrovascular accident, such as hemiplegia and multiple small strokes, are often found to have arteriosclerotic lesions (GELLERSTEDT, 1933; BAKER et al., 1960; HASSLER, 1965; PERESS et al., 1973).

Atherosclerosis of the extracerebral arteries is relatively common with advancing age, and gradual narrowing of the external carotid and vertebral arteries has been held responsible for a state of chronic cerebral ischemia and mental deterioration.

According to CORSELLIS and EVANS (1965), however, when the entire vascular tree from the heart to the brain is examined in mentally deteriorated and nondeteriorated patients of comparable age, both the cerebral and extracerebral vessels are found to be affected to approximately the same extent in the two groups.

JORGENSEN and TORVIK (1969) and BLACKWOOD et al. (1969) have shown that most cerebral infarcts are due to thromboembolism from extracranial arteries and the heart. In only a small minority of cases are cerebral softenings caused by in situ thrombosis of cerebral vessels.

Other studies have shown that cerebral blood flow does not change significantly following carotid endarterectomy, suggesting that arteriosclerotic stenoses of major extracranial arteries are seldom important hemodynamically. The cessation of cerebrovascular occlusive attacks after operation is probably due to removal of an arteriosclerotic focus which was the source of recurrent emboli (ENGELL et al., 1972; BOYSEN, 1972).

A number of investigators have attempted to identify histopathologic changes in the central nervous system which correlate with the process of deterioration of mental function in the aged person. The literature, however, is replete with contradictory findings. TOMLINSON and his co-workers (1970) found no differences in brain weight and ventricular size in old people with and without evidence of senile cerebral insufficiency. On the other hand, the observations of ROESSLE and ROULET (1932), VOGT and VOGT (1954), BURGER (1957), HEMPEL (1968), and PERESS et al. (1973) indicate significant loss of brain weight with aging. Until recently, this was considered to be evidence of age-dependent loss of neuronal cells (BRODY, 1955; WRIGHT and SPINK, 1959). Precise morphometric measurements now possible with the use of electronic image analysis techniques have shown that the stock of neuronal cells is probably not appreciably depleted during aging (TREFF, 1974).

The latter findings are of significance from the therapeutic aspect of senile cerebral insufficiency, because if the mental deterioration in this condition were due to irrevocable neuronal loss, then all forms of drug therapy would be futile.

Histologically, neurofibrillary tangles and senile plaques similar to those found in Alzheimer's disease (ALZHEIMER, 1907) have been observed in elderly persons with and without senile cerebral insufficiency (ROTHSCHILD, 1941; ROTHSCHILD and SHARP, 1941; DAYAN, 1970; TOMLINSON, 1970, 1972; MORIMATSU, et al., 1975). These histologic findings along with others, such as lipofuscin deposits in the brain cells and Hirano bodies and fibres in the astrocytes, have been described by others (BAKER et al., 1960; BONDAREFF, 1964; SEITELBERGER, 1968, 1969; BRODY, 1970; TERRY and WISNIEWSKI, 1970; TERRY, 1971; IGBAL et al., 1974). It is not known, however, whether any one or more of these changes are age-related phenomena fundamental to the aging process.

Apart from well-defined pathologic entities, such as classical Alzheimer's disease, Pick's disease, and Jacob-Creutzfeld's syndrome, it would appear that at the clinicopathologic level there are three pricipal age-dependent disorders which may result in the mental decline so often present in the elderly:

1. Most often encountered (approximately 75% of cases) is senile *cerebral* insufficiency without cerebrovascular arteriosclerosis (simple senile dementia) which OBRIST (1972) terms "psycho-organic defect."

2. Much less frequently present (approximately 15% of cases) is *cerebrovascular* insufficiency due to arteriosclerotic changes in the cerebral or extracerebral vessels, the so-called arteriosclerotic senile dementia.

3. In about 10% of cases of combination of the two disorders may occur. The coincidental development of cerebrovascular disease, however, would merely serve to accelerate deterioration of brain-cell function at the metabolic level rather than be the prime factor in the etiology of the condition.

The working premise, therefore, is that the pathology of the aging brain is often related to a nonvascular metabolic disturbance of brain-cell function and less often related to cerebrovascular insufficiency or a combination of these disorders. The underlying cause of these changes at the molecular, biochemical, and electrophysiologic level, however, still remains to be demonstrated.

C. Research Techniques Used in Clinical Pharmacologic Studies of Ergot Alkaloids in Senile Cerebral Insufficiency

Certain alkaloids of ergot, notably dihydroergotoxine mesylate (Hydergine), dihydroergonine (DN 16-457), an investigational new drug of promise, and nicergoline (Sermion), have been found to be of therapeutic value in senile cerebral insuffiency.

Experimental studies of the effects of dihydroergotoxine and dihydroergonine on the brain at the morphologic, metabolic, and electrophysiologic levels have been carried out on laboratory animals by EMMENEGGER and MEIER-RUGE (1968), MEIER-RUGE et al. (1973a, b, 1974a, b); CERLETTI et al. (1973), GYGAX et al. (1973a, b, 1974), IWANGOFF and ENZ (1972), IWANGOFF et al. (1973a, b, 1974), and STREICHENBERGER et al. (1970).

Many of the laboratory research methods used to study the effects of drugs, however, cannot be applied to man because of the relative inaccessibility of the human brain to biochemical, physiologic, and morphologic techniques, and because ethical considerations preclude the use of the invasive techniques often necessary to study brain function at these levels.

The research techniques currently available for human pharmacology studies in senile cerebral insufficiency have thus been limited to:

1. Measurement of cerebral bloodflow and certain basic biochemical determinations related to cerebral metabolism.
2. Clinical assessment of brain function by means of symptom rating scales and psychometric tests.
3. Electroencephalography (EEG)

As cerebral bloodflow measurements and metabolic determinations are currently of limited pharmacologic applicability, this chapter will deal mainly with clinical assessment and EEG methodology. In reviewing each method, the pertinent findings in untreated geriatric individuals with and without evidence of senile cerebral insufficiency will be presented in order to provide baseline information on the measurable parameters of the aging brain function. The results of treatment of mentally deteriorated elderly patients with ergot alkaloids of therapeutic value for this condition will then be presented in order to define the applicability and usefulness of each method as an adjunct to clinical pharmacology research.

1. Methods for Measuring Cerebral Bloodflow and Metabolism

Quantitative circulatory and metabolic studies on the human brain were first made possible by the pioneer work of KETY and SCHMIDT (1945). The Kety-Schmidt method is based on the Fick principle and requires measurement of the differences in concentration of nitrous oxide in the arterial blood arriving at the brain and the venous blood leaving the brain. The nitrous oxide method measures the total mean cerebral bloodflow and is therefore of limited clinical value, as alterations in cerebral bloodflow are most often regional in nature. Nevertheless, these early studies indicated that the normal aging process of the brain and senile deterioration of brain function are correlated with diminution of total cerebral bloodflow.

When isotope-clearance techniques using Krypton-85 and Xenon-133 were later developed, more informative regional cerebral bloodflow determinations became available (INGVAR and LASSEN, 1961; INGVAR et al., 1965). The further development of noninvasive techniques for the determination of cerebral bloodflow has given further impetus to the study of cerebral hemodynamics and oxygen uptake both in normal young and old human subjects and in patients suffering from a variety of clinical conditions, including senile cerebral insufficiency (HEYMAN et al., 1953; LINDEN, 1955; AIZAWA et al., 1961; GOTTSTEIN, 1963; MCHENRY, 1966; INGVAR and

RISBERG, 1967; MEYER et al., 1967, 1968; INGVAR et al., 1968; INGVAR and LASSEN, 1970; OBRIST et al., 1970).

These studies have revealed that subtle regional circulatory changes occur during normal psychic activity, and that elderly patients with senile cerebral insufficiency may show focal cerebral bloodflow abnormalities, especially in the grey matter of the brain.

It has also been shown that the severity of mental impairment in patients suffering from senile cerebral insufficiency is related to impairment of cerebral bloodflow (OBRIST et al., 1970; HERZFELD et al., 1972; MONGEAU, 1974). Furthermore, LASSEN and his co-workers (1960) have shown cerebral oxygen uptake in elderly subjects with symptoms of senile cerebral insufficiency to be 20–40% below the level of uptake in normal young subjects.

Emerging from these investigations is the important viewpoint that the fundamental cause of changes in cerebral bloodflow is not usually the organic stenotic process of cerebrovascular arteriosclerosis but the direct result of alterations in cerebral cell metabolism (INGVAR and LASSEN, 1970; OBRIST et al., 1970).

Apart from oxygen uptake by the brain, there are other indices of brain metabolism which are of interest in human pharmacologic studies on the aging brain. Among these are the cerebral arteriovenous differences in pCO_2 and changes in pyruvate-lactate ratios. As these measurements require repeated carotid artery and jugular bulb puncture, their applicability to the average clinical situation from an ethical standpoint is severely limited.

Following the demonstration of 5-hydroxyindolacetic acid-5-HIAA (the metabolite of serotonin) and homovanillic acid-HVA (the metabolite of dopamine) in the cerebrospinal fluid (CSF) by ASHCROFT and SHARMAN (1960) and ANDEN et al. (1963), respectively, the CSF has proved to be a relatively accessible source of useful information related to brain catecholamine metabolism in elderly persons with and without senile cerebral insufficiency.

In an investigation of HVA and 5-HIAA levels in the cerebrospinal fluid of normal geriatric volunteers, patients with presenile dementia of the Alzheimer type and patients with senile dementia (senile cerebral insufficiency), GOTTFRIES and his associates (1970) have shown that patients suffering from senile cerebral insufficiency have lower CSF levels of HVA and 6-HIAA than normal geriatric volunteers. Also, patients with presenile dementia have lower values of HVA and 5-HIAA than patients with senile cerebral insufficiency. Furthermore, there is a significant negative correlation between degreee of intellectual and emotional deterioration and the levels of HVA in the CSF, which may reflect a disturbance of dopamine metabolism in the functionally impaired brain. The 5-HIAA levels, though also reduced, were not significantly correlated to mental and emotional deterioration. The effects of ergot alkaloids on HVA and 5-HIAA in the CSF of patients with senile cerebral insufficiency have not been studied.

A further likely metabolic correlate of the aging process of the brain is the blood concentration of dopamine-B-hydroxylase (DBH), the enzyme which converts dopamine to norepinephrine. Humphrey et al. (publication in preparation, 1976) have demonstrated that in an aged population the percentage of subjects with serum DBH levels above upper limits of normal is higher than in nongeriatric adults.

As a sequel to these findings, FRIEDEL (1976, unpublished data) made serum DBH determinations in geriatric patients with mild-to-moderate senile cerebral insufficiency who were participating in a 26-week double-blind, placebo-controlled clinical study of dihydroergotoxine. The patients received 3 mg dihydroergotoxine or matching placebo daily by mouth for the duration of the study, and serum DBH determinations were made predrug and again at week 3, week 15, and week 27. However, no definite correlation between symptomatic improvement and serum DBH was shown. It is possible that, although serum DBH levels change with age, they are not a sufficiently sensitive metabolic correlate of brain function in the aged to be a useful measure in clinical pharmacology.

2. Methods for the Clinical Assessment of Brain Function

The essentially subjective nature of clinical assessment of changes in cognitive function, emotional patterns, and behavior of the aging individual leaves a lot to be desired. In recent years, therefore, the attention of researchers in this field has been directed towards those neurophysiological correlates of symptom change which lend themselves to more objective measurement.

Useful as these more objective parameters are, in the final analysis it is the degree of symptomatic change which determines whether or not the quality of life of the deteriorated geriatric patients has been influenced by treatment, irrespective of changes that may have occured in the correlative measurements. The clinical rating scale, therefore, remains an essential item in the armamentarium of the clinical pharmacologist.

a) Clinical Rating Scales

The methods available at present for the clinical measurement of drug effect on the symptom profile of senile cerebral insufficiency are clinical rating scales and certain psychometric tests. While clinical rating scales have been longest and most often used and are still the mainstay of geriatric psychopharmacologic research, they are, because of the subjective nature of the assessment of change, the least precise of the few research tools available in this field. Also, owing to the lack of rating scales specifically designed for geriatric use, until recently assessment of drug effect in the mentally deteriorated geriatric patient has been made with rating systems created primarily for younger people.

In a comprehensive review of the psychopharmacology literature, SALZMAN et al. (1972a, b, c) found only a few rating instruments specific for research in the elderly. They also noted that rating scales not created specifically for geriatric populations or which do not reflect the wide variability within aged persons have limited usefulness in geriatric clinical pharmacology research.

In 1968, at the start of an extensive clinical research program to evaluate the efficacy of dihydroergotoxine for the treatment of senile cerebral insufficiency, the lack of a symptom rating scale specifically for this purpose was even more evident and prompted the development of the Sandoz Clinical Assessment Geriatric (SCAG) Scale (Table 1).

Table 1. Sandoz clinical assessment-geriatric scale

Assessment of clinical status

Rating key: 1 = Not Present, 2 = Very Mild, 3 = Mild, 4 = Mild to Moderate, 5 = Moderate, 6 = Moderately Severe, 7 = Severe

Patient No.		*Rating Period*	
		Date	
1. Confusion	Lack of proper association for surroundings, persons and time-not with it. Slowing of thought processess and impaired comprehension, recognition and performance; disorganization. Rate on patient response and on reported episodes since last interview.		
2. Mental alertness	Reduction of attentiveness, concentration, responsiveness, alacrity and clarity of thought, impairment of judgment and ability to make decisions. Rate on structured questions and response at interview.		
3. Impairment of recent memory	Reduction in ability to recall recent events and actions of importance to the patient, e.g., visits by members of family, content of meals, notable environmental changes, personal activities. Rate on structured pertinent questions and not on reported performance.		
4. Disorientation	Reduced awareness of place and time, identification of persons including self. Rate on response to questions at interview only.		
5. Mood depression	Dejected, despondent, helpless, hopeless, preoccupation with defeat or neglect by family or friends, hypochondriacal concern, functional somatic complaints, early waking. Rate on patient's statements, attitude and behavior.		
6. Emotional lability	Instability and inappropriateness of emotional response, e.g., laughing or crying or other undue positive or negative response to non-provoking situations as the interviewer sees them.		
7. Self-care	Impairment of ability to attend to personal hygiene, dressing, grooming, eating and getting about. Rate on observation of patient at and outside interview situation and not on statements of patient.		
8. Anxiety	Worry, apprehension, overconcern for present or future, fears, complaints of functional somatic symptoms, e.g., headache, dry mouth, etc. Rate on patient's own subjective experience and on physical signs, e.g., trembling, sighing, sweating, etc., if present.		
9. Motivation initiative	Lack of spontaneous interest in initiating or completing tasks, routine duties and even attending to individual needs. Rate on observed behavior rather than patient's statements.		
10. Irritability (Cantankerousness)	Edgy, testy, easily frustrated, low tolerance threshold to aggravation and stress or challenging situations. Rate on patient's statements and general attitude at interview.		

le 1 (continuation)

ssment of clinical status

ng key: 1 = Not Present 5 = Moderate
2 = Very Mild 6 = Moderately Severe
3 = Mild 7 = Severe
4 = Mild to Moderate

tient No.		*Rating period*	
		Date	
Hostility	Verbal aggressiveness, animosity, contempt, quarrelsome, assaultive. Rate on impression at interview and patient's observed attitude and behavior towards others.		
Bothersome	Frequent unnecessary requests for advice or assistance, interference with others, restlessness. Rate on behavior at and outside the interview situations.		
Indifference to surroundings	Lack of interest in everyday events, pastimes and environment where interest previously existed, e.g., news, TV, heat, cold, noise. Rate on patient's statements and observed behavior at an outside interview.		
Unsociability	Poor relationships with others, unfriendly, negative reaction to social and communal recreational activities, aloof. Rate on observed behavior and not on patient's own impression.		
Uncooperativeness	Poor compliance with instructions or requests for participation. Performance with ill grace, resentment or lack of consideration for others. Rate on attitude and responses at interview and observed behavior out side interview situation.		
Fatigue	Sluggish, listless, tired, weary, worn out, bushed. Rate on patient's statements and observed response to normal daily activities outside interview situation.		
Appetite (Anorexia)	Disinclination for food, inadequate intake, necessity for dietary supplements, loss of weight. Rate on observed attitude towards eating, food intake encouragement required and loss of weight.		
Dizziness	In addition to true vertigo, dizziness in this context includes spells of uncertainty of movement and balance, subjective sensations in the head apart from pain, e.g., lightheadedness. Rate on physical examination as well as patient's subjective experience.		
Overall impression of patient	Considering your total clinical experience and knowledge of the patient, indicate the patient's status at this time, taking into account physical, psychic and mental functioning.		
itials of rater			

Fundamental to the development of a valid and reliable rating instrument for the evaluation of senile cerebral insufficiency is an inventory of symptoms which are consistently present in patients suffering from the condition. Review of the literature available in 1968 revealed a general agreement that the clinical manifestations of senile cerebral insufficiency fall into three main categories: Impairment of cognitive function; dysphoric mood states; and impairment of behavioral functioning. On the other hand, there was no consensus as to the symptoms comprising each of these categories, the sum total of which could justifiably be called the syndrome of senile cerebral insufficiency.

In order to determine which of the many possible symptoms occur with sufficient frequency and consistency in senescent patients to constitute a valid symptom complex or syndrome of senile cerebral insufficiency, a pilot rating scale was constructed which inclued all symptoms most commonly reported in the relevant publications available at that time. This amounted to a formidable list of 38 different symptoms—obviously and excessive number for a meaningful syndrome or for inclusion in a workable general-purpose clinical pharmacologic rating instrument.

The pilot scale was then used in studies involving approximately 150 moderately deteriorated patients over 65 years of age with diagnoses compatible with senile cerebral insufficiency.

In the analysis of the relative frequency with which each of the 38 symptoms presented in the patients participating in the studies, only those symptoms which occurred in 60% or more of the patients were considered to qualify for inclusion in the final symptom profile. Only 18 of the original 38 symptoms met this criterion.

In order to substantiate these early findings and to determine whether or not some symptoms had been included by chance occurrence at the 60% level because of the relatively few patients involved, a running check on the incidence of symptoms was kept in 16 subsequent studies, involving approximately 800 patients. Again, none of the original 18 symptoms were found to occur in less than 60% of the patients (VENN et al., 1975).

The SCAG scale, therefore, embodies an inventory of 18 symptoms which constitute what is considered to be an acceptable syndrome of senile cerebral insufficiency (Table 1). Following the general format of the widely used Brief Psychiatric Rating scale (OVERALL and GORHAM, 1962), each symptom on the SCAG scale has a short descriptor indicating the manner in which the symptom should be rated. A seven-point rating system is used for evaluation of the degrees of severity of each symptom (VENN and HAMOT, 1971).

The reliability and validity of the scale, which became evident from factorial analyses made during its earlier clinical use, was subsequently tested and confirmed in a special study conducted by SHADER et al. (1974).

The SCAG scale has been used in a considerable number of studies for the assessment of the efficacy of dihydroergotoxine and to a lesser extent of dihydroergonine for the treatment of geriatric patients with senile cerebral insufficiency (JENNINGS, 1972; RAO and NORRIS, 1972; SHORT and BENWAY, 1972; ROSEN, 1975; ARRIGO et al., 1973; BAZO, 1973; MATEJCEK et al., 1975; NELSON, 1974, 1975; EINSPRUCH, 1976; WINSLOW, 1974a, b; HOLLINGSWORTH, 1976; GAITZ and VARNER, 1974). It has proved to be sensitive to the often subtle changes that occur as a result of drug therapy and may, therefore, be a useful tool for this aspect of clinical pharmacologic research.

Another general-purpose rating scale which has been used in a clinical pharmacologic trial with dihydroergotoxine (REHMAN, 1973) is the Crichton Royal Behavioral Rating Scale (ROBINSON, 1961). This is a 10-factor scale using a 5-point rating system and, in spite of the title of this scale, is indeed a general-purpose scale.

Other rating scales specific for geriatric populations are available for clinical pharmacologic use. Most of these, however, are designed for the assessment of but one aspect of the complex clinical picture of the aging process of the brain and have not been used in clinical pharmacologic studies with ergot alkaloids. The Geriatric Rating Scale of PLUTCHIK et al. (1970), the Rating Scale for Behavior on a Geriatric Ward (BURDOCK et al., 1960), and the Behavior Rating Scale of LAWTON (1965) and LAWTON and BRODY (1969), for example, rate patient behavior only, while others are confined to the evaluation of social functioning and more specific activities of everyday living. Few geriatric scales cover all the common clinical manifestations.

b) Psychometric Tests

The shortcomings of essentially subjective clinical rating methods have been mentioned. In order to provide more objective measurements of brain function, a variety of psychometric tests have been devised over the years. Among the many tests available are stimulus-response measurements, such as reaction time and flicker fusion tests, and tests of intelligence, of which the Binet Test, the Wechsler Intelligence Scales, the Rorschach Performance Test, Raven's Progressive Matrices, and the Benton Test are examples.

Each one of these tests provides useful information relating to levels of response and intellectual function of both young and old, but for the most part these tests applied singly are not sufficiently sensitive to detect the often subtle changes in response and intellectual function resulting from pharmacotherapy of senile cerebral insufficiency.

On the other hand, it has been found that a properly selected combination of these tests does provide a method for objective evaluation of drug effect, which is of sufficient sensitivity to be of interest to the clinical pharmacologist.

The Nuremberg Geriatric Inventory (NGI) is a battery of suitably modified standard psychometric tests which has been shown to be sensitive to drug effect in senile cerebral insufficiency and which has been successfully used as an adjunct to the SCAG scale for this purpose. The NGI scale (applied in the order presented) comprises:

1. Digit Span Test (after WECHSLER, modified)
2. Labyrinth Test (after CHAPUIS)
3. Benton Test
4. Block Design Test (after WECHSLER mosaic)
5. Dirgit Symbol Test (after WECHSLER, modified).

There can be no doubt that, if the more general subjective clinical impressions recorded by means of a rating scale correlate well with the more precise objective psychometric test scores, confidence in the clinical pharmacologic evaluation of

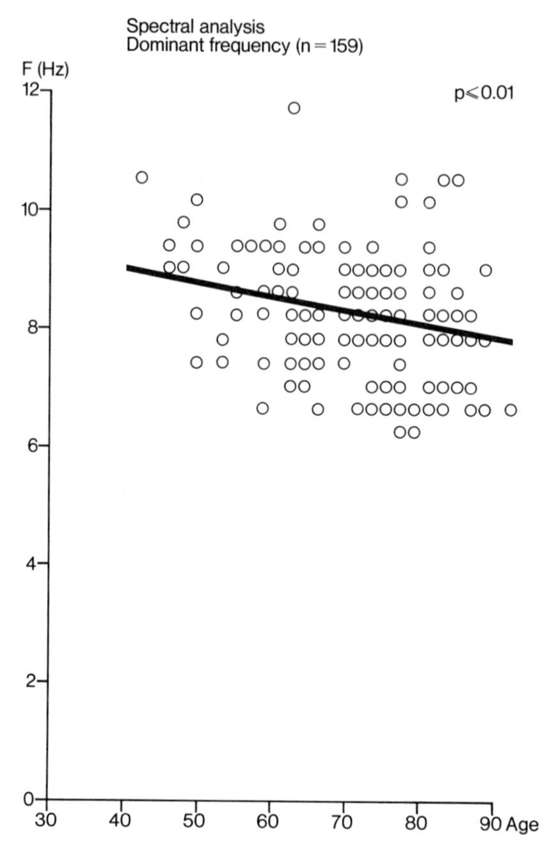

Fig. 1. Slowing of the dominant frequency as a function of age derived by spectral analysis of a 3-minute recording of the resting EEG's (lead O_2–C_z) of 159 persons (MATEJCEK and DEVOS, 1976)

therapeutic response is greatly increased. Every geriatric rating scale should, therefore, be supported by appropriate psychometric tests wherever possible.

3. Electroencephalography

The advent of newer and more sophisticated computer techniques for quantification of the EEG (FINK, 1963; BURCH et al., 1964) has opened a new field of research of brain activity. Using these more precise quantitative analyses, ITIL et al. (1968) have developed methods for differentiation and prediction of activity of psychotropic drugs, based on the hypothesis that psychotropic drugs producing similar EEG changes will display similar clinical activity.

Even prior to the routine use of computer techniques for analysis of EEG recordings, a correlation between frequency-distribution changes in the EEG spectrum and advancing age had been observed (GIBBS and GIBBS, 1950; MUNDY-CASTLE et al., 1954; MAGGS and TURTON, 1956; OBRIST and BISSELL, 1955; OBRIST et al., 1962, 1963; OBRIST and BUSSE, 1965; MATOUSEK et al., 1967; GSCHWEND and KAR-

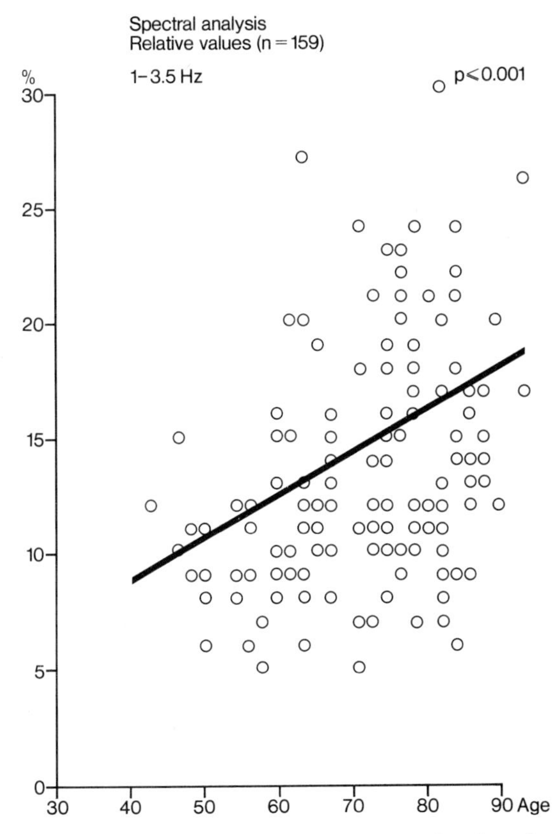

Fig. 2. a Characteristic changes in the various EEG frequency bands as functions of age derived by spectral analysis of the same EEG recordings as in Figure 1 (MATEJCEK and DEVOS, 1976)

BOWSKI, 1970). These investigators have shown that there is a progressive slowing of the alpha frequency with advancing age, and that fast (beta) frequencies are not a constant feature of the senescent EEG but vary with age and mental status. There is some evidence that increase in fast frequencies is most prevalent among intellectually well-preserved subjects during early senescence. Its presence in an elderly person's EEG can probably be regarded as a favorable sign.

The more recent work of ROUBICEK (1975) and MATEJCEK and DEVOS (1976), using spectral and iterative analyses of the EEG, has confirmed the earlier findings.

In an EEG study of 159 subjects ranging in age from 18 to 92 years, these investigators have produced further evidence of a slowing of the dominant occipital alpha frequency with advancing age (Fig. 1).

Spectral analysis of the EEG recordings provided the percentage distribution of energy in the various frequency bands relative to the spectrum as a whole (Fig. 2a, b, c, d).

In the 1–3.5-Hz (delta) range (Fig. 2a) as well as in 3.5–6.5-Hz (theta) range (Fig. 2b), a significant relative increase in percentage activity occurred with advancing age. On the other hand, there was a significant decrease in the percentage

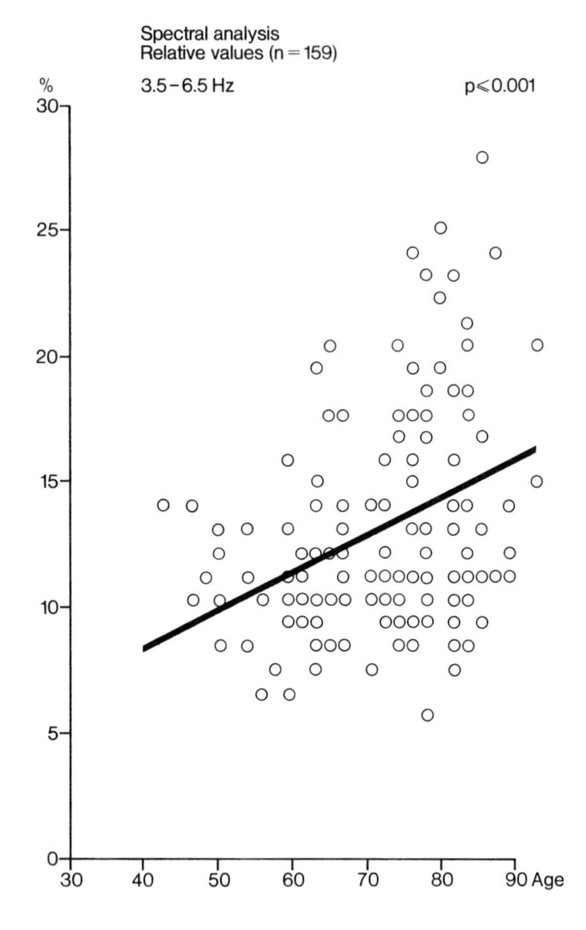

Fig. 2b

activity in both the 6.5–12-Hz (alpha) range (Fig. 2c) and in the 12–30-Hz range (Fig. 2d).

Analysis of segments of the fast-activity 12–40-Hz range demonstrates an interesting age-related decrease in percentage activity in the 12–16-Hz, 16–20-Hz, and 20–25-Hz segments, no change in percentage activity in the 25–30-Hz segment, and an increase in percentage activity in both the 30–35-Hz and 35–40-Hz segments. The mean for the entire 12–40-Hz range shows a slight but insignificant decrease in percentage fast activity. These findings indicate the importance of segmental analysis of fast activity. Figure 3 illustrates how these age-related changes may be represented diagrammatically in the EEG power spectrum.

A study by GERSON and JOHN (1975) provides further evidence that EEG changes occur in geriatric individuals, and that the nature and degree of change are correlated with impairment of cognitive function, affect, and behavior so often afflicting the elderly. Furthermore, this study indicates that the use of evoked potential techniques and correlation of interhemispheric EEG activity are methodologic advances in this type of investigation.

Two groups of individuals over 60 years of age were selected. Each group was as homogeneous as possible in respect to age, socioeconomic status, education,

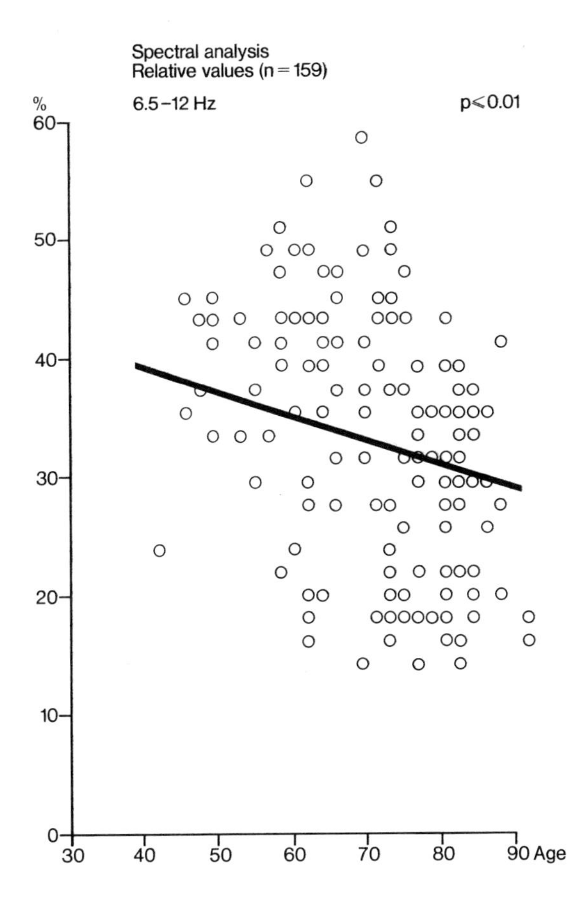

Fig. 2c

and ethnic origin. Based on neurologic, psychiatric, psychologic, and psychometric evaluations, one group comprised normal individuals gainfully employed, and the other group were abnormal in that they exhibited cognitive, emotional, behavioral, and somatic symptoms associated with senile cerebral insufficiency.

Spontaneous EEG and evoked-potential data were available for 107 patients (56 normals and 51 abnormal seniles).

Spectral analysis revealed that the abnormal senile group had a greater percentage of energy in the low frequency 1.5–3.5-Hz (delta 2) frequency band and a smaller percentage of energy in the 7–13-Hz (alpha) band than did the normal group. These differences were highly significant.

Also using evoked potential techniques, the electrical activity in the two hemispheres was significantly less well coordinated or synchronized in the senile group than in the normals. Furthermore, a significant relationship between interhemispheric coordination and psychometric scores was shown (Fig. 4).

The data falls clearly into two separate clusters – one with high (good) interhemispheric coordination and low (good) psychometric impairment scores (57 normals and 9 seniles) and the other with low (poor) interhemispheric coordination and high (poor) psychometric impairment scores (37 seniles and 7 normals) (Fig. 4).

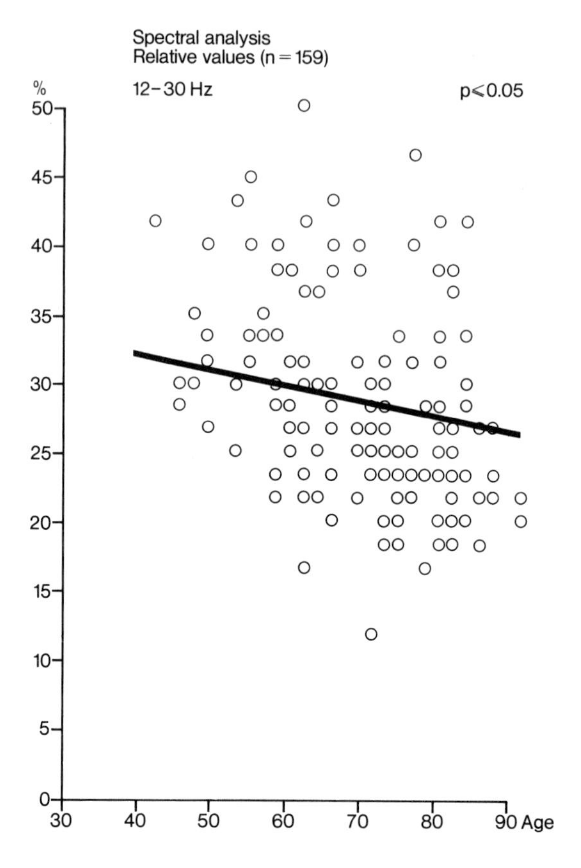

Fig. 2d

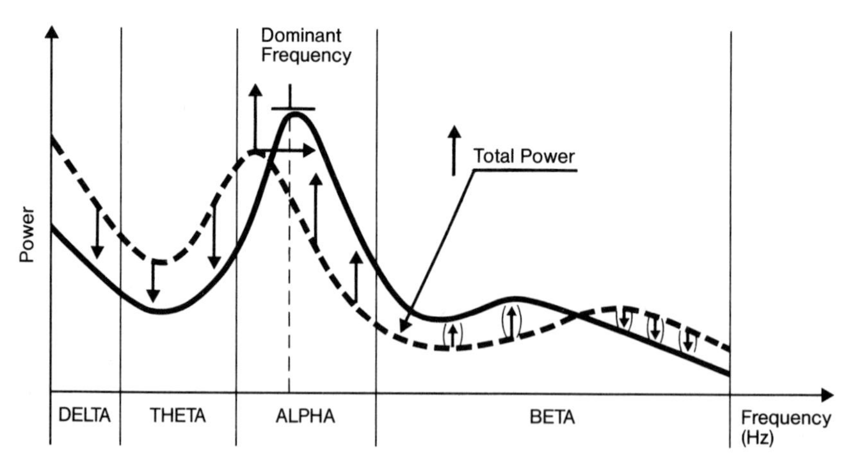

Fig. 3. Median shape of the resting EEG power spectrum in adults below (—) and above (---) the age of 60 years. Arrows indicate the direction of change in the EEG power spectrum theoretically expected to be produced by compounds which are effective in senile cerebral insufficiency (MATEJCEK and DEVOS, 1976)

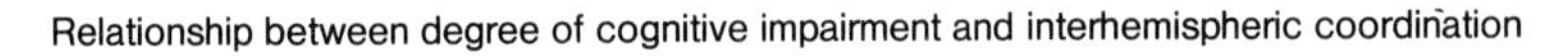

Relationship between degree of cognitive impairment and interhemispheric coordination

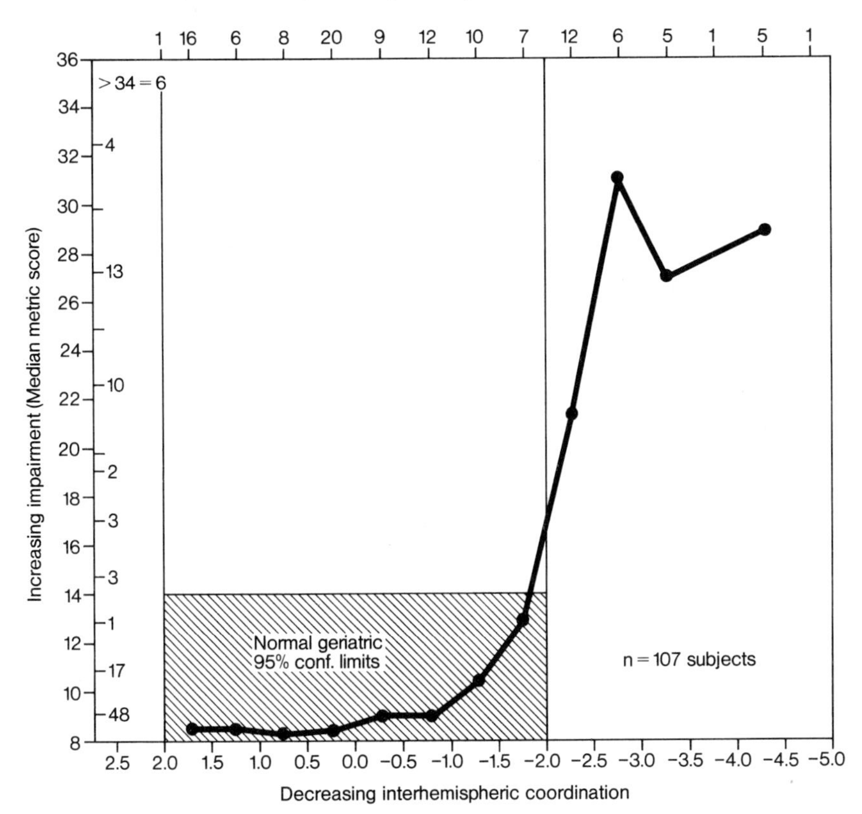

Fig. 4. Scores of increasing mental impairment and the number of geriatric persons with those scores showing significant correlation with scores of decreasing interhemispheric coordination and the number of geriatric persons with those scores. Scores of less than 14 for mental impairment and scores of 2.0 to −2.0 for interhemispheric coordination are normal limits for the geriatric sample under consideration (GERSON and JOHN, 1975)

These results show that the two cerebral hemispheres of the mentally deteriorated senile individual are significantly less well coordinated than those of the normal aged person, and that the degree of incoordination is proportional to the degree of mental impairment. Also, evoked-potential techniques indicate that these incoordinations are further accentuated by imposing an informational burden on the system.

The conclusions that can be drawn from this study are that the pattern of EEG changes occurring with advancing age shown in other studies has been confirmed and that there is a correlation between these EEG changes and mental deterioration in the elderly.

Based on these findings, one might surmise that, since the EEG has been shown to be correlate of age-dependent changes in brain function, the EEG may be an index of therapeutic effect of psychoactive drugs as well as a possible predictor of psychoactivity of drugs whose therapeutic effects on the human brain are not known.

The results of clinical pharmacologic studies with dihydroergotoxine (Hydergine), dihydroergonine (DN 16-457), and nicergoline (Sermion) support these hypotheses.

D. Results of Clinical Pharmacology Studies With Ergot Alkaloids

Although a number of ergot alkaloids have central nervous system effects, the clinical pharmacology of the ergot alkaloids in senile cerebral insufficiency is mainly concerned with three interesting ergot derivatives of known efficacy in the pharmacotherapy of senile cerebral insufficiency. These are:

1. Dihydroergotoxine mesylate (Hydergine)
2. Dihydroergonine (DN 16-457), a new synthetic hydrogenated ergot alkaloid currently under clinical investigation
3. Nicergoline (Sermion), a synthetic derivative of ergoline into which a nicotinic acid radical has been incorporated.

The present knowledge of the clinical pharmacology of these three ergot alkaloids has been determined by studies in which the relatively limited tools available for geriatric pharmacologic research have been used.

As more clinical investigations have been done with dihydroergotoxine than with dihydroergonine or nicergoline, the results presented are mainly those relating to the clinical pharmacology of dihydroergotoxine.

1. Cerebral Bloodflow and Metabolic Studies

The effects of 0.6 mg dihydroergotoxine given i.v. and those of certain vasodilator drugs, including papaverine, were studied by GOTTSTEIN (1965) in senile patients with reduced cerebral bloodflow and oxygen uptake. GOTTSTEIN was unable to demonstrate any significant improvement in cerebral bloodflow or oxygen uptake with any of the drugs used.

MCHENRY et al. (1971) measured regional bloodflow in acute-stroke patients with the 133-Xenon method in association with cerebral angiography. They found that dihydroergotoxine administered in doses of 0.6–1.2 mg i.m. did not change cerebral bloodflow in these stroke patients during the short period of time in which the measurements were made.

On the other hand, in a clinical study conducted by HEYCK (1961), dihydroergotoxine was administered in doses of 0.3 mg i.m. daily for 5–40 days to 13 geriatric patients with diagnoses compatible with senile cerebral insufficiency. Cerebral bloodflow measured by the Kety-Schmidt technique increased by 61%; oxygen uptake increased by 44%; and vascular resistance was reduced by 39% as a result of therapy, with dihydroergotoxine.

GERAUD et al. (1963), using Krypton 85 methodology, obtained similar results in a study of the effects of 0.9 mg dihydroergotoxine infused slowly i.v. on cerebral bloodflow, oxygen uptake, and vascular reistance in 18 elderly patients with diagnoses in keeping with senile cerebral insufficiency. Cerebral bloodflow increased by 33%; oxygen uptake was increased by 24%; and vascular resistance decreased by 33%.

In another study in which the Krypton 85 method for measuring cerebral bloodflow was used, DEPLA (1963) administered 0.9 mg dihydroergotoxine by slow infusion to 18 patients with a variety of what were termed vascular disorders of the brain but which by today's concepts were no doubt in keeping with a diagnosis of senile cerebral insufficiency. In these patients an overall increase in cerebral bloodflow of 23.7% was demonstrated along with a 23.7% increase in oxygen consumption and a decrease in vascular resistance of 56%.

HERZFELD et al. (1972) employed radiocirculographic techniques in a double-blind placebo controlled study of dihydroergotoxine to evaluate the effects of the drug on the cerebral circulation time of geriatric patients with evidence of senile cerebral insufficiency. They found that dihydroergotoxine decreased cerebral circulation time, thus increasing cerebral bloodflow, and that this correlated well with improvement in concurrently measured EEG activity and symptomatic status of the patients.

In a more recent study, also using a radiocirculographic technique and using the SCAG scale, MONGEAU (1974) investigated the cerebral perfusion rates and the clinical responses of 35 elderly patients with senile cerebral insufficiency before and after treatment with dihydroergotoxine by mouth in dosages of 1.0 mg four times daily for 4 weeks followed by 1 mg three times daily for 8 weeks. A good correlation between cerebral perfusion rate and symptom improvement was demonstrated. In patients with normal perfusion, dihydroergotoxine ameliorated clinical symptomatology, while perfusion did not change; in patients with borderline perfusion, the rates returned to normal along with improvement in symptoms; and in patients with poor perfusion, the rates noticeably improved, as did the clinical symptoms. The authors ascribed the improved perfusion to increased neuronal metabolic activity.

In none of these studies was an age-matched control group without cerebral insufficiency included, so there is currently no evidence whether improvement in cerebral bloodflow following therapy with dihydroergotoxine is confined to patients exhibiting this syndrome.

2. Clinical Pharmacologic Studies With Ergot Alkaloids in Senile Cerebral Insufficiency

a) Clinical Rating Scales for Quantitative Assessment of Response

A relatively large number of clinical pharmacologic studies of ergot alkaloids in patients with senile cerebral insufficiency have been conducted over the past 8 years. As dihydroergotoxine has been available for pharmacologic investigation in man for a considerably longer time than dihydroergonine or nicergoline, the majority of studies conducted to date have involved dihydroergotoxine (GERIN, 1969; GRILL and BROICHER, 1969; BANEN, 1972; TRIBOLETTI and FERRI, 1969; JENNINGS, 1972; DITCH et al., 1971; RAO and NORRIS, 1972; SHORT and BENWAY, 1972; BAZO, 1973; RODRIGUEZ, 1973; ROSEN, 1975; RAO, 1973; MCCONNACHIE,

Table 2. Summary of dihydroergotoxine clinical pharmacologic studies in which the SCAG scale or a close modification was used

Investigator	Type of study		Control medication	Dihydro-ergotoxine	Study duration	Patients completing study	Number of symptoms with greater response to dihydroergotoxine than to control		
	In-pat.	Out-pat.	Dosage	Dosage	Weeks		Trends favoring dihydro-ergotoxine	Significant[a] differences at 0.05 level	Global ratings significant at 0.05 level
JENNINGS	×		Placebo	1 mg t.i.d.	12	50	17/17	8/17	S
RAO and NORRIS	×		Placebo	1 mg t.i.d.	12	59	14/16	12/18	S
WINSLOW (1)	×		Placebo	1 mg t.i.d.	12	50	19/19	15/19	S
ARRIGO et al.	×		Placebo	1 mg t.i.d.	12	20	17/18	5/18	S
GAITZ and VARNER	×		Placebo	1 mg t.i.d.	24	47	17/18	9/18	Borderline
BAZO	×		Papaverine HCl 100 mg t.i.d.	1 mg t.i.d.	12	36	13/17	4/17	NS
ROSEN		×	Papaverine HCl 100 mg t.i.d.	1 mg t.i.d.	12	53	15/15	13/15	S
NELSON	(30)	(15)	Papaverine HCl 100 mg t.i.d.	1 mg t.i.d.	12	45	15/15	14/15	S
EINSPRUCH	×		Pavabid 150 mg b.i.d.	1 mg t.i.d.	12	39	17/18	6/18	NS
WINSLOW (2)	×		Pavabid 150 mg b.i.d.	1 mg t.i.d.	12	53	18/18	17/18	S

[a] In none of the studies was there a significant difference in favor of the control.

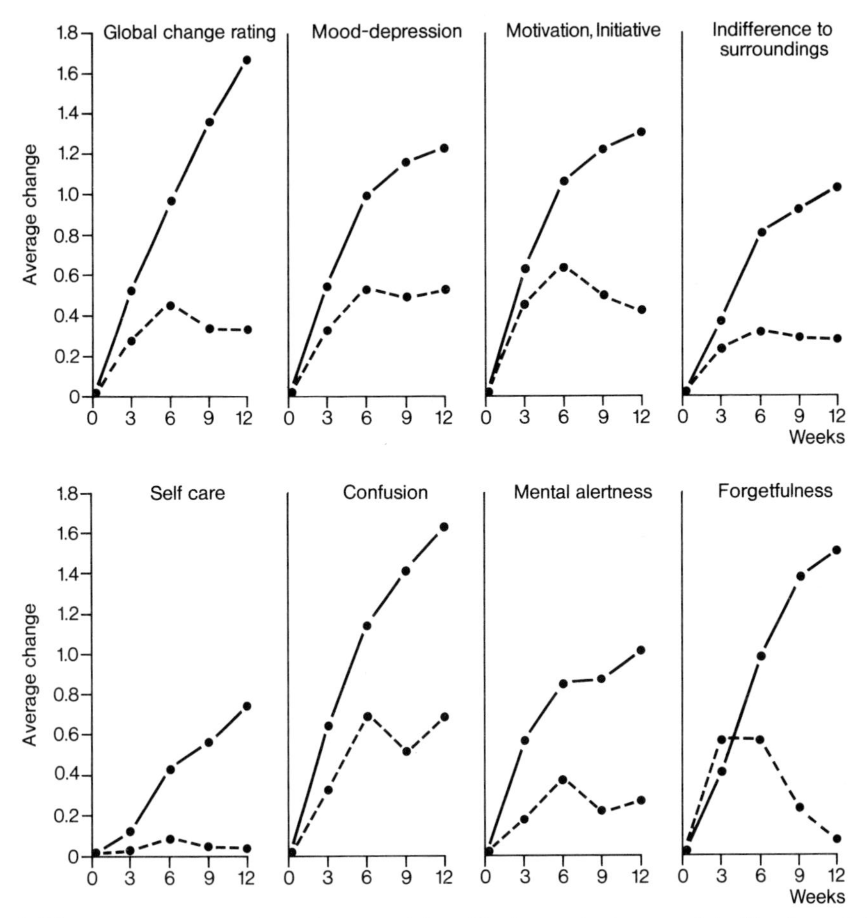

Fig. 5. Time-response curves in patients receiving dihydroergotoxine mesylate (3 × 1 mg daily) n=29 (—) and placebo n=28 (---). Double-blind design using a 7-point rating scale related to SCAG. Average change in rating. Mean age 78 years. (After RAO and NORRIS, 1972)

1973; REHMAN, 1973; BARGHEON, 1973; EINSPRUCH, 1976; WINSLOW, 1974; LINDEN, 1975; HOLLINGSWORTH, 1976; GAITZ and VARNER, 1974; NELSON, 1975).

Furthermore, in most of the dihydroergotoxine studies a double-blind, controlled, parallel treatment-group design was used, and the principal instrument employed for measurement of pharmacotherapeutic response was the SCAG scale.

A summary of double-blind controlled dihydroergotoxine studies in which the SCAG scale was the principal rating instrument is provided in tabular form (Table 2).

The consistent trends of greater symptomatic response in the dihydroergotoxine-treated patient groups as opposed to the control patient groups are evident in this series of investigations as were the very low incidence of adverse reactions.

In a further series of studies involving dihydroergotoxine, different rating scales, based on the Crighton scale, were employed (BARGHEON, 1973; GERIN, 1969; GRILL and BROICHER, 1969; HEISS et al., 1971; MCCONNACHIE, 1973; PAUX et al., 1975;

REHMAN, 1973; ROUBICZEK et al., 1972; THIBAULT, 1974). Groups of geriatric patients—average age 65–82 years—received daily doses of 4.5 mg dihydroergotoxine or placebo, as a rule over a 12-week period in double-blind studies. Symptom ratings improved significantly or highly significantly in the drug groups as compared to placebo. Thus, there is substantial evidence that dihydroergotoxine produces symptomatic improvement of a range of complaints presented by geriatric patients. They become less confused, irritable, and forgetful, their mood improves, and they show greater emotional stability. However the underlying mechanism of the mental effects of this and related ergot alkaloids remains unexplained.

As an example of the type of effect produced in geriatric patients, the study by RAO and NORRIS (1972), who carried out a double-blind investigation of dihydroergotoxine in the treatment of senile cerebral insufficiency, may be quoted Dihydroergotoxine mesylate 1 mg t.i.d. or placebo was administered orally to 59 patients (mean age 77 and 79 years) exhibiting at least two of the following symptoms: Confusion, emotional lability, impairment of recent memory, or decreased mental alertness. Using a rating scale similar to SCAG, they concluded that patients treated with dihydroergotoxine experienced greater symptomatic improvement than those treated with placebo. The differences were significant ($p < 0.05$) in 12 of 17 symptoms, the improvement generally increasing throughout the study (Fig. 5).

b) Clinical Rating Scales Combined With EEG for Quantitative Assessment of Response

While those studies in which the SCAG scale was the principal rating instrument have contributed to the methodology of geriatric research and to the understanding of the clinical pharmacology of dihydroergotoxine, they do lack the desirable more-objective corroborative evidence of response to drug therapy provided by such measures as the EEG and appropriate psychometric tests.

When it was established that the aging brain is associated with a characteristic pattern of EEG changes, the next step was to investigate the possible usefulness of the EEG as an objective correlate of clinically rated response to drug therapy of senile cerebral insufficiency. Furthermore, the availability of new computerized techniques for the more precise multidimensional analysis of the EEG now provides the clinician with far more information on the nature and changes of electrical activity of the brain than can be obtained from the standard visual evaluation techniques.

Clinical pharmacology of the ergot alkaloids is now better understood as a result of a number of controlled double-blind studies of dihydroergotoxine and dihydroergonine in particular in which effects of these drugs on the EEG and symptomatic response have been evaluated concurrently (ROUBICEK et al., 1972; HERZFELD et al., 1972; ARRIGO et al., 1973; WILDER and GONYEA, 1973; MATEJCEK et al., 1975; MATEJCEK and DEVOS, 1976).

In a study already mentioned, where the effects of dihydroergotoxine on cerebral circulation time were studied using a radiocirculographic technique, HERZFELD et al. (1972) also investigated under double-blind, placebo-controlled conditions the effects of dihydroergotoxine on the EEG and on the cognitive performance, mood, and behavior of 44 geriatric patients with clinical and EEG evidence of senile cerebral insufficiency. Compared with placebo, significant increases in the dominant alpha frequency, the alpha index, and reduction in the number of slow waves in the theta and delta bands were demonstrated after 6 weeks of treatment with dihydroergotoxine. Concomitant improvement in mental performance and behavior, assessed by means of psychometric tests and a behavior rating scale, occurred to a greater extent in the dihydroergotoxine-treated patients than in those who received placebo.

The results of the study by HERZFELD et al. (1972) are in agreement with a study carried out by ROUBICEK et al. (1972), in which the effects of dihydroergotoxine on symptoms and EEG patterns were assessed in nonpsychotic mentally deteriorated geriatric patients. Twenty-two pairs of patients (average age, 78.7 years), matched in sex, age, and previous occupation, received orally 4.5 mg of dihydroergotoxine or placebo daily for 3 months, according to a randomization schedule under double-blind conditions. Of 21 clinical variables rated, 13 showed a significant improvement with dihydroergotoxine and 2 with placebo. With regard to the EEG, the dihydroergotoxine-treated group had a significantly greater number of patients with a shift in dominant frequency to the fast part of the spectrum than the placebo group.

In a double-blind study conducted by ARRIGO et al. (1973), dihydroergotoxine or placebo was given orally in daily dosages of 4.5 mg to a total of 20 deteriorated geriatric patients 55–79 years of age, in two randomly constituted groups of 10 patients each. The treatment period was 12 weeks, and evaluations of symptom response and EEG of each patient were made at weeks 0, 4, 8, and 12. Comparison of the two treatment groups after 12 weeks of treatment showed a good correlation between an increased abundance of faster frequencies in the alpha band of the EEG and symptom improvement (Table 3).

In a placebo-controlled, double-blind study (GIOVE and SILVA, 1973) of geriatric patients receiving 4.5 mg dihydroergotoxine daily, correlation was highly significant between clinical improvement (18 parameters) and EEG changes (acceleration and increased amplitude of dominant frequency). Changes were more marked after 4 and 6 months of treatment than after 2 months.

WILDER and GONYEA (1973) carried out a double-blind, placebo-controlled combined EEG and clinical pharmacologic study with dihydroergotoxine. In this study, the relative effects of 1.0 mg of dihydroergotoxine or placebo taken sublin-

Table 3. Relation between improvement (+) and no improvement (0) in clinical symptoms and EEG in the same patient after 12 weeks of treatment with 4.5 mg dihydroergotoxine daily or placebo (see text). (ARRIGO et al., 1973)

	D-H Ergotoxine	Placebo
Clinical status+ and EEG+	6	1
Clinical status+ and EEG0	3	0
Clinical status0 and EEG0	1	9
Clinical status0 and EEG+	0	0
Total	10	10

gually t.i.d. on the EEG and clinical parameters were assessed in 28 hospitalized poststroke male patients, 55–79 years of age (average 68 years), over a 6-week treatment period. All patients had symptoms and signs of cognitive, emotional, and behavioral deterioration attributable to the aging process and were stable insofar as their neurologic deficits were concerned. There were 16 patients in the dihydroergotoxine group and 12 patients in the placebo group.

Symptomatic response was evaluated pretrial and at weeks 3 and 6 by means of the SCAG Scale, by a global assessment, and a neurologic rating scale. EEG recordings were made at the same evaluation periods and interpreted visually according to standard criteria.

The results of the EEG responses revealed a significantly greater increase in abundance of faster frequencies in the alpha band and a greater tendency to normalization of the EEG patterns of those patients on dihydroergotoxine than in those on placebo. Likewise, the symptomatic responses revealed that a significantly greater percentage of patients improved in the dihydroergotoxine treatment group than in the placebo group. Furthermore, the incidence of concomitantly occurring positive EEG changes and symptomatic improvement was shown to be consistently greater in the dihydroergotoxine-treated patients than in those patients who received placebo.

MATEJCEK proposed as a working hypothesis that drugs active in senile cerebral insufficiency normalize age-related EEG changes with associated clinical improvement. (The expected changes in the EEG power spectrum in geriatric patients are shown by arrows in Fig. 3.) According to this hypothesis, useful drugs of this type would be expected to produce the following changes in the EEG power spectrum:

1. An acceleration of the dominant frequency
2. Reduction in percentage delta and theta activities
3. Augmentation of the energy content of the dominant alpha frequency
4. A percentage increase in activity in frequency band 12–25 Hz and a percentage decrease in frequency band 25–40 Hz.

In a test of the hypothesis, dihydroergonine (DN 16-457) was administered to geriatric patients both by single injection and by chronic administration (MATEJCEK et al., 1975). The effects of dihydroergonine on the EEG and symptoms of patients with senile cerebral insufficiency were found to be similar to those of dihydroergotoxine, but the duration of effect following both intravenous and oral administration of dihydroergonine was considerably longer (more than 8 h) than that of dihydroergotoxine (4–6 h).

The EEG responses to a single 0.2 mg intravenous dose of dihydroergonine in geriatric patients with senile cerebral insufficiency of moderate severity and a slow basic EEG have been evaluated in three placebo-controlled studies (MATEJCEK and DEVOS, 1976). EEG recordings were made at 0-, $^1/_2$-, 2-, and 4-hour intervals in study 1; at hour 0, 3, 5, and 8 in study 2; and at hour 0, 1, 2, 4, and 8 in study 3.

The results of the spectral analysis of the EEG's in all three studies show that, compared with baseline, there was a decrease of activity in the 1–3.5-Hz range with dihydroergonine, as opposed to an increase with placebo (Fig. 6).

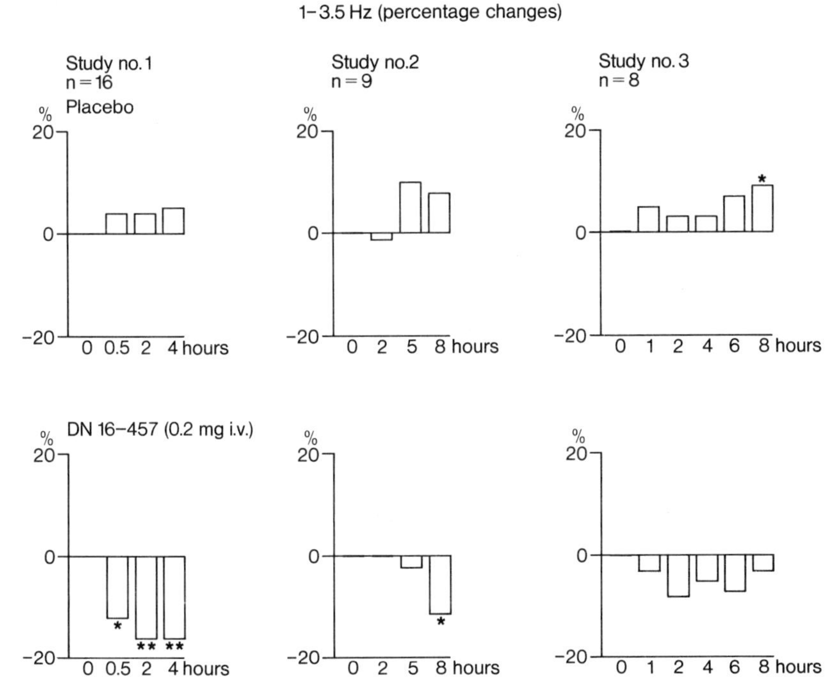

Fig. 6. The effects of a single dose of 0.2 mg dihydroergonine i.v. on slow EEG activity expressed as percentage change from base-line in three studies. Histograms in the upper half of the figure refer to placebo, in the lower half of the figure to DN 16-457 (MATEJCEK et al., 1975)

In the 6.5–12-Hz range, an increase of activity of the dominant frequency occurred in dihydroergonine-treated patients in all three studies; conversely, the placebo patients showed a decrease of activity in this frequency range in all three studies.

In the 12–40-Hz range, the results with dihydroergonine suggest a decrease in relative amount of energy as opposed to an increase with placebo, especially in the higher (30–40 Hz) bands.

In a chronic study (MATEJCEK et al., 1975), 11 geriatric patients suffering from symptoms and signs attributable to senile cognitive, emotional, and behavioral changes were treated with dihydroergonine in dosages of 2.5 mg t.i.d. for a period of 12 weeks. Clinical and EEG assessments were made at weeks 0, 2, 4, 8, and 12.

While in the above-mentioned acute studies with dihydroergonine no significant acceleration of the dominant frequency was noted despite the increase in amplitude, the chronic study revealed a significant acceleration of the dominant frequency starting at week 4.

Furthermore there was good concordance between the EEG frequency shift to the faster end of the alpha band and clinical improvement as assessed by both the global evaluations and the total scores obtained from a symptom rating scale (Fig. 7).

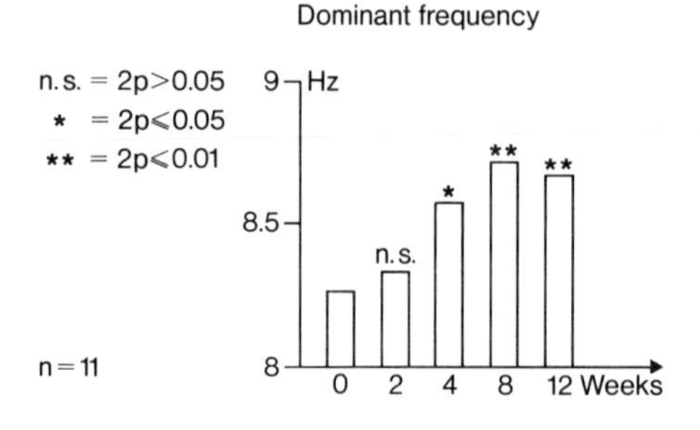

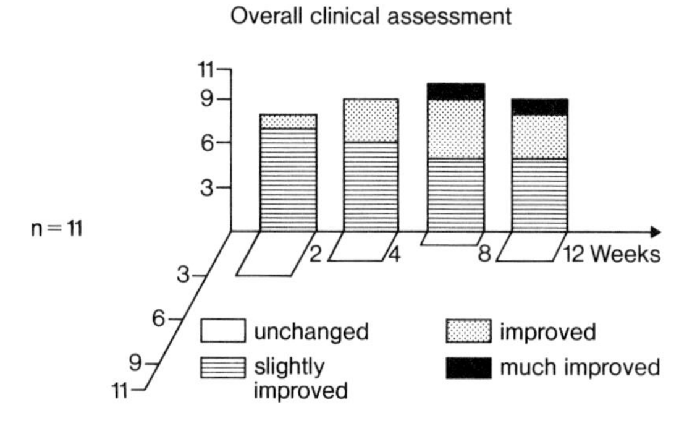

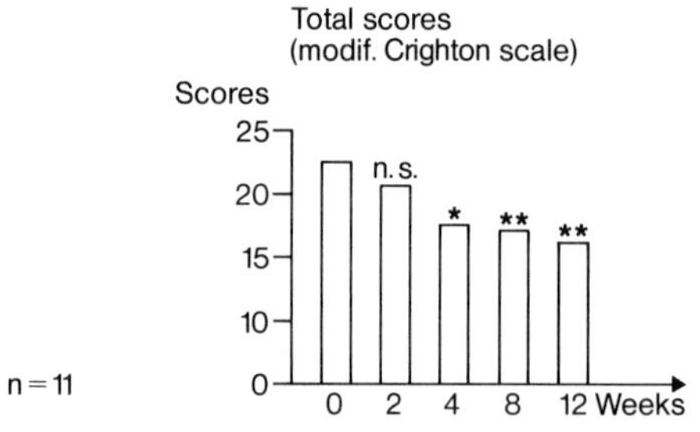

Fig. 7. Concordance of acceleration of the dominant EEG frequency with clinical improvement assessed on a global and symptom basis over the course of 12-weeks treatment with dihydroergonine, 2.5 mg orally, three times daily. Lower total score signifies improvement. (After MATEJCEK et al., 1975)

Clinically, nicergoline (Sermion) has been used as an antihypertensive agent, a peripheral vasodilator, and as a cerebrovascular vasodilator. A number of open uncontrolled clinical studies in geriatric patients suffering from psychic symptoms attributable to cerebrovascular insufficiency have indicated that nicergoline may have a beneficial effect on related symptoms (NEBULONI, 1972; PAZZAGLIA, 1972; GUARDAMAGNA and NEGRI, 1972; ALLORO and TERENZIANI, 1973).

In double-blind, placebo-controlled studies conducted by BOUDOURESQUES et al. (1974), MICHELANGELI et al. (1975), MEMIN and NAJEAN HEUBER (1973), and MOREAU et al. (in press), the trends of improvement favored nicergoline over placebo for a number of symptoms evaluated. In three further unpublished studies conducted by Schott, Moinade and Terrasse, and by Rouzaud in patients suffering from cerebrovascular accidents, the trends of improvement mostly favored nicergoline.

In a study conducted by Montanini et al. (1973), EEG recordings were made on 25 patients suffering from cerebrovascular insufficiency. Visual evaluation of the tracings indicated reduction in slow waves and regularization of irregularities of alpha rhythm in 40% of cases, along with improvement in some of the symptoms of the condition. As this study was uncontrolled, the significance of these findings is difficult to assess.

As clinical studies with dihydroergotoxine, dihydroergonine, and a number of other drugs with central nervous system effects have shown a correlation between clinical findings and EEG changes, the EEG may be regarded as a useful objective tool in geriatric clinical pharmacology. It may provide early essential information on the profile of a psychoactive investigational new drug, including the onset and duration of action, the pattern of action possibly indicating its field of therapeutic usefulness, the optimum dose (oral and parenteral), and comparative activity with standard reference drugs.

E. Summary

There is no generally accepted single term for the symptom profile of the mental, emotional, and behavioral changes which characterize normal biologic aging. Senile cerebral insufficiency is a satisfactory term which provides a diagnostic label without suggesting the possible etiology or underlying pathology and is offered as an acceptable compromise to those who find the existing nomenclature to be unsatisfactory.

The individual symptoms which characterize the mental deterioration, the changes on affect and behavior, the inability to cope with the ordinary tasks of everyday living, and certain autonomic manifestations of senile cerebral insufficiency, have been well defined during the development of a sensitive, valid, and reliable general-purpose clinical rating scale. These symptoms have been shown to be present with sufficient frequency and consistency in deteriorated geriatric patients to warrant this symptom complex being designated the senile cerebral insufficiency syndrome.

Although a number of different hypotheses as to the nature of the aging process, based largely on animal experiments, have been presented by almost as many different investigators, the etiology of the aging process and of senile cerebral insufficiency remains essentially unknown.

With regard to the pathology of the condition, one observation of fundamental importance has emerged from histopathologic studies of the brains of patients with senile cerebral insufficiency. The conventional widely held opinion that senile *cerebral* insufficiency and *cerebrovascular* insufficiency due to cerebral arteriosclerosis are synonymous has been shown to be erroneous. In fact, autopsy studies have demonstrated that less than 30% of the brains of patients who had well-defined senile *cerebral* insufficiency during life showed any evidence of cerebrovascular arteriosclerosis. The weight of evidence favors the concept that the aging processes in the brain are not vascular in origin.

The clinical pharmacology of senile cerebral insufficiency is not well understood, as research has been considerably restricted by the inaccessibility of the human brain for this type of investigation both from the biologic and the ethical points of view.

Three main avenues of human research into the nature and pharmacotherapy of the aging process are available at present:

1. Symptomatic and psychometric clinical evaluations
2. EEG analysis
3. Limited biochemical studies

Studies with dihydroergotoxine, dihydroergonine, and nicergoline have shown that these ergot alkaloids have a beneficial effect on patients with symptoms of senile cerebral insufficiency, and that improvement in the EEG patterns in these patients correlate well with the clinical improvement. There is also evidence that dihydroergotoxine improves the metabolic processes of the aging brain, in that cerebral blood flow and oxygen uptake are augmented by its use.

Although such information on the clinical pharmacology of dihydroergotoxine and dihydroergonine in senile cerebral insufficiency as is available at this time correlates well with the results obtained from morphologic, biochemic, and electrophysiologic experiments in laboratory animals, the precise pharmacologic action of these two psychoactive ergot alkaloids at the metabolic level in the human brain has yet to be determined.

F. References

Aizawa, T., Tazaki, Y., Gotoh, F.: Cerebral circulation in cerebrovascular disease. Wld Neurol. **2**, 635–648 (1961)

Alloro, L., Terenziani, S.: Esperienza clinica con un nuovo farmaco vasoattivo, la nicergolina, nelle vasculopatie cerebrali. Gazz. med. ital. **132**, 81–90 (1973)

Alzheimer, A.: Allg. Z. Psychiat. **64**, 146 (1907)

Anden, M.E., Roos, B.F., Werdinius, B.: On the occurrence of homovanillic acid in brain and cerebrospinal fluid and its determination by a fluorimetric method. Life Sci. **2**, 448–458 (1963)

Arrigo, A., Braun, P., Kautchtschischwilli, G., Moglia, A., Tartara, A., Pavia, L.T.: Influence of treatment of symptomatology and correlated electroencephalographic (EEG) changes in the aged. Curr. ther. Res. **15**(7), 417–426 (1973)

Ashcroft, G.W., Sharman, D.F.: 5-hydroxyindoles in human cerebrospinal fluids. Nature (Lond.) **186**, 1050–1051 (1960)

Baker, A.B., Refsum, S., Dahl, E.: Cerebrovascular disease. IV A study of Norwegian population. Neurology (Minneap.) **10**, 525–529 (1960)

Banen, D.M.: An ergot preparation (Hydergine) for relief of symptoms of cerebrovascular insufficiency. J. Amer. Geriat. Soc. **20**, 22–24 (1972)

Bargheon, J.: Double-blind study of hydergine in geriatric patients. Nouv. Presse Med. **2**, 2053–2055 (1973)

Bazo, A.J.: An ergot alkaloid preparation (Hydergine) versus papaverine in treating common complaints of the aged: double-blind study. J. Amer. Geriat. Soc. **21**, 63–71 (1973)

Blackwood, W., Hallpike, J.F., Kocen, R.S., Mair, W.G.P.: Atheromatous disease of the carotid arterial system and embolism from the heart in cerebral infarction; a morbid anatomical study. Brain **92**, 897–910 (1969)

Bondareff, W.: Histophysiology of the aging nervous system. Adv. Gerontol. Res. **1**, 1–22 (1964)
Boudouresques, J., Vigourous, R.A., Boudouresques, G., Monnier, M.C.: Étude de la nicergoline dans l'insuffisance vasculaire cérébrale. Lyon Mediter. Med. **10**, 989–991 (1974)
Boysen, G.: Acta neurol. scand. (Suppl.) **51**, 421–422 (1972)
Brody, H.: Organization of the cerebral cortex. III. A study of aging in the human cerebral cortex. J. comp. Neurol. **102**, 511–516 (1955)
Brody, H.: Structural changes in the aging nervous system. Interdisc. Top. Geront. **7**, 9–21 (1970)
Burch, N.R., Nettleton, W.J., Sweeney, J., Edwards, R.J.: Period analysis of the electroencephalogram on a general-purpose digital computer. Ann. N.Y. Acad. Sci. **115**, 827–843 (1964)
Burdock, E.I., Hardesty, A.S., Hakerem, G., Zubin, J.: A ward behavior rating scale for mental hospital patients. J. clin. Psychol. **16**, 246–247 (1960)
Burger, M.: Altern und Krankheit. Leipzig: Georg Thieme 1957
Cerletti, A., Emmenegger, H., Enz, A., Iwangoff, P., Meier-Ruge, W., Musil, J.: Effects of ergot DH-alkaloids on the metabolism and function of the brain. An approach based on studies with DH-ergonine. In: Central Nervous System: Studies on Metabolic Regulation and Function. Genazzani, E., Herken, H. (eds.), pp. 201–212. Berlin-Heidelberg-New York: Springer 1973
Corsellis, J.A.N., Evans, P.H.: Proc. V Int. Congr. Neuropathol. 546 (1965)
Dayan, A.D.: Quantitative histological studies on the aged human brain: senile plaques and neurofibrillary tangles in "normal" patients. Acta neuropath. (Berl.) **16**, 85–94 (1970)
Depla, M.: Contribution à l'etude du débit sanguin cérébral mesuré par le Crypton 85; quelques applicationes chiruriques et pharma-dynamiques. Thèse; Toulouse, 1963
Ditch, M., Kelly, F.J., Resnick, O.: An ergot preparation (Hydergine) in the treatment of cerebrovascular disorders in the geriatric patient: a double-blind study. J. Amer. Geriatr. Soc. **19**, 208–217 (1971)
Einspruch, B.C.: Helping to make the final years meaningful for the elderly residents of nursing homes. Dis. nerv. Syst. **37**, 439–442 (1976)
Emmenegger, H., Meier-Ruge, W.: The actions of Hydergine on the brain. A histological, circulatory and neurophysiological study. Pharmacology **1**, 65–78 (1968)
Engell, H.C., Boysen, G., Ladegaard-Pedersen, H.J., Henriksen, H.: Cerebral blood flow before and after carotid endarterectomy. Vasc. Surg. **6**, 14–19 (1972)
Fink, M.: Quantitative electroencephalography in human psychopharmacology II: Drug patterns. In: EEG and Behavior. Glaser, G. (ed.). New York: Basic Books 1963
Friedel, R.O.: Division of psychopharmacology. University of Washington, Seattle (Unpublished data – 1976)
Gaitz, C.M., Varner, R.V.: Pharmacotherapy of late life organic brain syndromes; evaluation of Hydergine (an ergot derivative) versus placebo using double-blind technique. Gerontologist **14** (5/II), 44 (1974)
Gellerstedt, N.: Zur Kenntnis der Hirnveränderungen bei der normalen Altersinvolution. Upsala Läk.-Fören. Förh. **38**, 193–408 (1933)
Geraud, J., Bes, A., Rascol, A., Delpha, M., Marc-Vergnes, J.P.: Measurement of cerebral blood flow using Krypton 85. Some physiopathological and clinical applications. Rev. Neurol. **108**, 542–557 (1963)
Gerin, J.: Symptomatic treatment of cerebrovascular insufficiency with Hydergine. Curr. ther. Res. **11**, 539–546 (1969)
Gerson, I.M., John, R.: Average evoked response (AER) in the electroencephalographic diagnosis of the normally and abnormally aged brain. Presented at Annual AMEEG Meeting, April 12–16, 1975, Scottsdale, Arizona
Gibbs, F.A., Gibbs, E.L.: Electroencephalographic changes with age in adolescent and adult control subjects. Trans. Amer. neurol. Ass. **70**, 154–157 (1950)
Giove, C., Silva, N.: Influence du traitement sur l'EEG et la symptomatologie clinique des sujets âgés. Communication Xe Congrès Internat. Neurologie, Barcelona, 1973
Gottfries, C.G., Gottfries, I., Roos, B.E.: Homovanillic acid and 5-hydroxyindoleacetic acid in cerebrospinal fluid related to rated mental and motor impairment in senile and presenile dementia. Acta psychiat. scand. **46**, 99–105 (1970)

Gottstein, U.: Cerebral blood flow disorders. Therapiewoche **13**, 922–928 (1963)
Gottstein, U.: Pharmacological studies of total cerebral blood flow in man with comments of the possibility of improving regional cerebral blood flow by drugs. Acta neurol. scand. **41** (Suppl. 14), 136–141 (1965)
Grill, P., Broicher, H.: Zur Therapie der zerebralen Insuffizienz Dtsch. med. Wschr. **94**, 2429–2435 (1969)
Gschwend, J., Karbowski, K.: Der Normbereich des Alters-Electroenzephalogramms. Schweiz. Arch. Neurol. Neurochir. Psychiat **106**, 209–281 (1970)
Guardamagna, C., Negri, S.: Efficacia clinica della nicergolina nelle vasculopatie cerebrali. Minerva cardioangiol. 636–641 (1972). English title: Statistical assessment of the clinical effectiveness of Nicergoline in 39 cases of cerebrovascular disease. (Italien)
Gygax, P., Emmenegger, H., Stossek, K.: Quantitative determination of cortical microflow and EEG in graded hypercapnia. Stroke **4**, 360–361 (1973a)
Gygax, P., Emmenegger, H., Dixon, R.: Cortical microflow and electrical brain activity (EEG) of the cat in a state of hypovolemic shock. IRSC Med. Sci. **73-4**, 11–16 (1973b)
Gygax, P., Emmenegger, H., Dixon, R., Peier, A.: The effect of hypovolemic oligemia on the cerebral microcirculation and EEG in the cat In: Pathology of Cerebral Microcirculation. Cervox-Navarro, J. (ed.). Walter de Gruyter 1974
Hassler, O.: Vascular changes in senile brain, a micro-angiographic study. Acta neuropath. (Berl.) **5**, 40–53 (1965)
Heiss, R., Seus, R., Fahrenberg, J.: Eine Studie zur Prüfung der psychodynamischen Wirkung von Dihydroergotoxin. Arzneimittel-Forsch. **21**, 797–800 (1971)
Hempel, K.J.: Quantitative und topische Probleme der Altersvorgänge im Gehirn. Verh. dtsch. Ges. Path. **52**, 179–202 (1968)
Herzfeld, U., Christian, W., Ronge, J., Wittgen, M.: Determinants estimating cerebral functions after long term therapy with Hydergine. Ärztl. Forsch. **26**, 215–228 (1972)
Heyck, H.: The influence of initial values upon sympatholytic effects on brain circulation in cerebral vascular disorders. Arzneimittel-Forsch. **15**, 243–251 (1961)
Heyman, A., Patterson, Jr., J.L., Duke, T.W., Battey, L.L.: The cerebral circulation and metabolism in arteriosclerotis and hypertensive cerebrovascular disease. New Engl. J. Med. **249**, 223–229 (1953)
Hollingsworth, S.W.: Data on file at Sandoz, Inc., U.S.A. (1976)
Humphrey, J.: 1976 (28th Convention, Portland, Oregon, Nov. 30–Dec. 3C, 1974)
Igbal, K., Wisniewski, H.M., Shelanski, M.L., Brostoff, S., Liwnicz, B.H., Terry, R.D.: Protein changes in senile dementia. Brain Res. **77**, 337–343 (1974)
Ingvar, D.H., Lassen, N.A.: Quantitative determination of regional cerebral bloodflow in man. Lancet **1961/II**, 806–807
Ingvar, D.H., Lassen, N.A.: Cerebral blood flow and cerebral metabolism. Triangle **9**, 234–243 (1970)
Ingvar, D.H., Risberg, J.: Increase of regional cerebral bloodflow during mental effort in normals and in patients with focal brain disorders. Exp. Brain Res. **3**, 195–211 (1967)
Ingvar, D.H., Cronqvist, S., Ekberg, R., Risberg, J., Hedt-Rasmussen, K.: Normal values of regional cerebral blood flow in man, including flow and weight estimates of grey and white matter. Acta neurol. scand. **41** (Suppl. 14), 72–78 (1965)
Ingvar, D.H., Obrist, W., Chivian, E., Cronqvist, S., Risberg, J., Gustafson, L., Hägerdal, M., Wittbom-Cigén, G.: General and regional abnormalities of cerebral blood flow in senile and "presenile" dementia. Scand. J. clin. Lab. Invest. 22: (Suppl. 102): XII:B (1968)
Itil, T., Shapiro, D.M., Fink, M.: Differentiation of psychotropic drugs by quantitative EEG analysis. Agressologie **9**, 267–280 (1968)
Iwangoff, P., Enz, A.: The influence of various dihydroergotamine-analogues on cyclic adenosine-3′,5′-monophosphate phosphodiesterase in the grey matter of cat brain in vitro. Agents Actions **2**, 223–230 (1972)
Iwangoff, P., Chappuis, A., Enz, A.: The effect of different dihydroergot alkaloids on the noradrenaline activated ATPase of the cat brain. IRCS Med. Sci. **73**, 8, 3–10–20 (1973a)
Iwangoff, P., Chappuis, A., Enz, A.: The influence of catecholamines on the ATPase in the cat's brain cortex. IRCS Med. Sci. **73**, 8, 3–10–19 (1973b)

Iwangoff, P., Chappuis, A., Enz, A.: Dependence of noradrenaline activated ATPase activity on monovalent and bivalent ions in the brain cortex of the cat. IRCS Med. Sci. **2**, 1182–1186 (1974)

Jennings, W.C.: An ergot alkaloid preparation (Hydergine) versus placebo for treatment of symptoms of cerebrovascular insufficiency: double-blind study. J. Amer. Geriat. Soc. **20**, 407–412 (1972)

Jorgensen, L., Torvik, A.: 1) Ischemic cerebrovascular diseases in an autopsy series. 2) Prevalence location pathogenesis and clinical course of cerebral infarcts. J. neurol. Sci. **9**, 285–320 (1969)

Kety, S.S., Schmidt, C.F.: Determination of cerebral bloodflow in man by use of nitrous oxide in low concentrations. Amer. J. Physiol. **143**, 53–66 (1945)

Lassen, N.A.: Cerebral bloodflow and oxygen consumption in man. Physiol. Rev. **39**, 183–238 (1959)

Lassen, N.A., Feinberg, I., Lane, M.H.: Bilateral studies of cerebral oxygen uptake in young and aged normal subjects and in patients with organic dementia. J. clin. Invest. **39**, 491–500 (1960)

Lawton, M.P.: Geriatric behavior rating scale. Philadelphia, Geriatric Center (unpublished) (1965)

Lawton, M.P., Brody, E.M.: Assessment of older people: self-maintaining and instrumental activities of daily living. Gerontologist **9**, 179–186 (1969)

Linden, L.: The Effect of Stellate Ganglion Block on Cerebral Circulation in Cerebrovascular Accidents. Acta med. scand. (Suppl. 151) **301**, 1–110 (1955)

Linden, M.E.: Scientific exhibit. Amer. Geriat. Soc. 124th Annual Meeting (1975)

McConnachie, R.W.: A clinical trial comparing Hydergine with placebo in the treatment of cerebrovascular insufficiency in elderly patients. Curr. Med. Res. Opin. **1**, 463–468 (1973)

McHenry, Jr., L.C.: Medical progress. Cerebral bloodflow. New Engl. J. Med. **274**, 82–91 (1966)

McHenry, Jr., L.C., Jaffe, M.E., Kawamura, J., Goldberg, H.I.: Hydergine effect on cerebral circulation in cerebrovascular disease. J. neurol. Sci. **13**, 475–481 (1971)

Maggs, R., Turton, E.C.: Some EEG findings in old age and their relationship of affective disorder. J. ment. Sci. **102**, 812–818 (1956)

Matejcek, M., Devos, J.E.: Selected methods of quantitative EEG analysis and their applications in psychotropic drug research. In: Quantitative Analytic Studies in Epilepsy. Kellaway, P., Petersén, I. (eds.), pp. 183–205. New York: Raven Press

Matejcek, J., Arrigo, A., Knor, K.: Quantitative EEG in geriatric drug research: description of a working hypothesis. In: Quantitative Analysis of the EEG. Matejcek, M., Schenk, G.K. (eds.). Proceedings of the 2nd Symposium EEG-Methodology, Jongny sur Vevey pp. 127–147. Konstanz: AEG-Telefunken 1975

Matousek, M., Volavka, J., Roubicek, J., Roth, Z.: EEG frequency analysis related to age in normal adults. Electroenceph. clin. Neurophysiol. **23**, 162–167 (1967)

Meier-Ruge, W., Emmenegger, H., Tobler, H.J., Cerletti, A.: Dihydrogenated alkaloids of ergocornine, ergocritine, ergocryptine effects on the cat EEG after temporary ischemia. Fed. Proc. **32**, 728–2904 (1973a)

Meier-Ruge, W., Schieweck, Chr., Iwangoff, P.: The distribution of (^{3}H-)-Hydergine in the cat brain. IRSC Med. Sci. **73-4**, 7–10–3 (1973b)

Meier-Ruge, W., Emmenegger, H., Gygax, P., Iwangoff, P., Walliser, Ch., Cerletti, A.: About the pathophysiology and therapy of cerebral insufficiency. A contribution to the experimental gerontology of the brain. In: Altern. Platt, D. (ed.), pp. 153–167. Stuttgart-New York: Schattauer 1974a

Meier-Ruge, W., Gygax, P., Iwangoff, P., Schieweck, Chr., Wolff, J.R.: The significance of pericapillary astroglia for cerebral cortical blood flow and EEG activity. In: Pathology of Cerebral Microcirculation. Cervos-Navarro, J. (ed.), pp. 235–243. Berlin: Walter de Gruyter 1974b

Memin, Y., Najean Heuber, E.: Etude à double insu selon une échelle d'appréciation quantitative d'un traitement des troubles vasculaires cérébraux chroniques. Sem. Hôp. Paris **49**, 605–608 (1973)

Meyer, J.S., Gotch, F., Akiyama, M., Yoshitake, S.: Monitoring cerebral blood flow, oxygen and glucose metabolism. Analysis of cerebral metabolic disorder in stroke and some therapeutic trials in human volunteers. Circulation **36**, 197–211 (1967)

Meyer, J.S., Sawado, T., Kitamura, A., Toyoda, M.: Cerebral oxygen, glucose, lactate and pyruvate metabolism in stroke. Therapeutic considerations. Circulation **37**, 1036–1048 (1968)

Michelangeli, J., Sevilla, M., Lavagna, J., Darcourt, G.: Étude de l'action de la nicergoline (Sermion) dans la pathologie vasculaire chronique du 3e âge. Ann. Méd.-psychol. **I, 4**, 499–510 (1975)

Moinade, S., Terrasse, J.: Dossier d'expertise clinique du Sermion.

Mongeau, B.: The effect of Hydergine on cerebral blood perfusion in diffuse cerebral insufficiency. Eur. J. clin. Pharmacol. **7**, 169–175 (1974)

Montanini, R., Gasco, P., Manfredini, G.: Observazioni cliniche ed elettroencefalografiche sull'azione della nicergolina in vasculopatici cerebrali. Acta neurol. (Napoli) **28**, 133–149 (1973)

Moreau, Ph., Beletre, J., Bruneau, M.: Insuffisance circulatoire cerebrale chronique. Etude des effets de la nicergoline. Vie Medicale (a paraitre)

Morimatsu, M., Hirai, H., Martimatsu, A., Yochikawa, M.: Senile degenerative brain lesions and dementia. J. Amer. Geriat. Soc. **23**, 390–405 (1975)

Mundy-Castle, A.C., Hurst, L.A., Beerstecher, D.M., Prinsloo, T.: The electroencephalogram in senile psychoses. EEG Clin. Neurophysiol. **6**, 235–244 (1954)

Nebuloni, G.: Sindromi amnesiche nell'età avanzata e loro possibilità di trattamento. G. Geront. **20**, 451–458 (1972)

Nelson, J.J.: Effects of the dihydrogenated ergot alkaloids on selected symptoms in elderly patients. A 5-year review presented as a scientific exhibit at the annual meeting of the American Geriatrics Society, Toronto, Canada, April 17–18, 1974

Nelson, J.J.: Relieving selected symptoms of the elderly. Geriatrics **30(3)**, 133–142 (1975)

Obrist, W.D.: Cerebral physiology of the aged: influence of circulatory disorders. In: Aging and the Brain. Gaitz, Ch.M. (ed.), pp. 117–133. New York-London: Plenum Press 1972

Obrist, W.D., Bissell, L.F.: The electroencephalogram of aged patients with cardiac and cerebral vascular disease. J. Geront. **10**, 315–330 (1955)

Obrist, W.D., Busse, E.W.: The electroencephalogram in old age. In: Applications of Electroencephalography in Psychiatry. Wilson, W.P. (ed.). Durham: Duke U. Pr. 1965

Obrist, W.D., Busse, E.W., Eisdorfer, C., Kleemeier: Relation of the electroencephalogram to intellectual function in senescence. J. Geront. **17**, 197–206 (1962)

Obrist, W.D., Sokoloff, L., Lassen, N.A., Lane, M.H., Butler, R.N., Feinberg, I.: Relation of EEG to cerebral bloodflow and metabolism in old age. Electroenceph. Clin. Neurophysiol. **15**, 610–619 (1963)

Obrist, W.D., Chivian, E., Cronqvist, S., Ingvar, D.H.: Regional cerebral blood flow in senile and presenile dementia. Neurology **20**, 315–322 (1970)

Overall, J.E., Gorham, D.R.: The brief psychiatric rating scale. Psychol. Rep. Amer. Psychiat. Ass. **10**, 799–812 (1962)

Paux, G., Boismare, F., Delaunay, P.: Étude en double aveugle de l'hydergine chez le sujet âgé. Nouv. Presse méd. **4**, 2529 (1975)

Pazzaglia, P.: Effetti clinici e poligrafici di un nuovo derivato ergolinico, la nicergolina, nei disturbi del circolo cerebrale. Riv. sper. Freniat. **96**, 348–363 (1972)

Peress, N.S., Kane, W.C., Aronson, S.M.: Central nervous system findings in a tenth decade autopsy population. Progr. Brain Res. **40**, 473–483 (1973)

Plutchik, R., Conte, H., Bakur, M., Grossman, J., Lehman, N.: Reliability and validity of a scale for assessing the functioning of geriatric patients. J. Amer. Geriat. Soc. **18**, 491–500 (1970)

Rao, D.B.: Double-blind study of hydergine vs. Papaverine in the treatment of cerebrovascular insufficiency in the elderly. Data on file at Sandoz, E. Hanover, NJ U.S.A. 1973

Rao, D.B., Norris, J.R.: A double-blind investigation of hydergine in the treatment of cerebrovascular insufficiency in the elderly. Johns Hopk. med. J. **130**, 317–324 (1972)

Rehman, S.A.: Two trials comparing Hydergine with placebo in the treatment of patients suffering from cerebrovascular insufficiency. Curr. Med. Res. Opin. **1**, 456–462 (1973)

Robinson, R.A.: Some problems of clinical trials in elderly people. Geront. clin. (Basel) **3**, 247–257 (1961)
Rodriguez, J.M.: A double-blind placebo controlled study of Hydergine in the treatment of cerebrovascular insufficiency in the elderly. Data on file at Sandoz, U.S.A. 1973
Roessle, R., Roulet, F.: Mass und Zahl in der Pathologie. Berlin-Wien: Springer 1932
Rorschach, H.: Psychodiagnostics. New York: Grune and Stratton 1942
Rosen, H.J.: Mental decline in the elderly: pharmacotherapy (ergot alkaloids vs. Papaverine). J. Amer. Geriat. Soc. **23**, 169–174 (1975)
Rothschild, D.: The clinical differentiation of senile and arteriosclerotic psychoses. Amer. J. Psychiat. **98**, 324–333 (1941)
Rothschild, D., Sharp, M.L.: The origin of senile psychoses. Neuropathologic factors and factors of a more personal nature. Dis. nerv. Syst. **2**, 49–54 (1941)
Roubicek, J.: Actividad eléctrica del cerebro en adultos y ancianos. Invest. Méd. Intern. **2**, (Suppl. (1)), 35–44 (1975)
Roubicek, J., Geiger, C., Abt, K.: An ergot alkaloid preparation (Hydergine) in geriatric therapy. J. Amer. Geriat. Soc. **20**, 5, 222–229 (1972)
Rouzaud, M.: Dossier d'expertise clinique du Sermion.
Salzmann, C., Kochansky, G.E., Shader, R.I.: Rating scales for geriatric psychopharmacology: a review. Psychopharmacol. Bull. **8**, 3–50 (1972a)
Salzman, C., Shader, R.I., Kochansky, G.E.: Rating scales for psychotropic drug research with geriatric patients. I. Behaviour ratings. J. Amer. Geriat. Soc. **20**, 209–214 (1972b)
Salzman, C., Kochansky, G.E., Shader, R.I.: Rating scales for psychotropic drug research with geriatric patients. II. Mood ratings. J. Amer. Geriat. Soc. **20**, 215–221 (1972c)
Schott, B.: Dossier d'expertise clinique du Sermion
Seitelberger, F.: Allgemeine Neuropathologie der Alterns- und Aufbrauchkrankheiten des Gehirns. Verh. dtsch. Ges. Path. **52**, 32–64 (1968)
Seitelberger, F.: Neurologie und Pathologie der nicht gefäßbedingten Altersprozesse des Gehirns. Wien. klin. Wschr. **81**, 309–516 (1969)
Shader, R.I., Harmatz, J.S., Salzman, C.: A new scale for clinical assessment (SCAG). J. Amer. Geriat. Soc. **22**, 107–113 (1974)
Short, M.J., Benway, M.: Delivery of mental health services to the elderly: the state hospital and the community. Scientific exhibit. Am. Psychiatr. Assoc. Meeting, Dallas, May 1–5, 1972
Streichenberger, G., Boismare, F., Lauressergues, H., Lechat, P.: Modification of anoxic ischemic encephalopathy in the cat by selected vasoactive drugs. (French) Therapie **25**, 1003–16 (1970)
Terry, R.D.: Presidential address: neuronal fibrous protein in human pathology. J. Neuropath. exp. Neurol. **30**, 8–19 (1971)
Terry, R.D., Wisniewski, H.: The Ultrastructure of the Neurofibrillary Tangle and the Senile Plaque in Alzheimer's Disease. Wolstenholme, G.E.W., O'Connor, M. (eds.). London: Churchill 1970
Thibault, A.: A double-blind evaluation of Hydergine and placebo in the treatment of patients with organic brain syndrome and cerebral arteriosclerosis in a nursing home. Curr. med. Res. Opin. **2**, 482–487 (1974)
Tomlinson, B.E.: Morphological brain changes in non-demented old people. In: Ageing of the Central Nervous System. VanPraag, H.M., Kalverboer, A.F. (eds.). Haarlem: DeErven F. Bohn 1972
Tomlinson, B.E., Blessed, G., Roth, M.: J. neurol. Sci. **7**, 331–356 (1968)
Tomlinson, B.E., Blessed, G., Roth, M.: Observations on brains of demented old people. J. neurol. Sci. **11**, 205–242 (1970)
Treff, W.M.: Das Involutionsmuster des Nucleus dentatus cerebelli. In: Altern. Platt, D. (ed.), pp. 37–54. Stuttgart-New York: F.K. Schattauer 1974
Triboletti, F., Ferri, H.: Hydergine for treatment of symptoms of cerebrovascular insufficiency. Curr. ther. Res. **11**, 609–620 (1969)
Venn, R.D., Hamot, H.: Methodological considerations of the clinical evaluation of drug

effect on chronic cerebrovascular insufficiency of the aged. In: 6. Europäischer Kongreß für Klinische Gerontologie, Bern, Sept. 8–11, Abstr. No. 88, 1971

Venn, R.D., Armellino, J., Hamot, H., Pagano, D.M.: The degenerative symptoms of aging. The symptom profile and a method for assessment of symptom severity and pharmacologic management. Presented at Meeting of New York Academy of Science, Oct., 1975. (To be published)

Vogt, C., Vogt, O.: Gestaltung der topistischen Hirnforschung und ihre Förderung durch den Hirnbau und seine Anomalien. J. Hirnforsch. **1**, 1–46 (1954)

Wechsler, D.: Manual for the Wechsler Adult Intelligence Scale. New York: Psychological Corporation 1955

Wilder, B.J., Gonyea, E.F.: The effects of dehydrogenated ergot alkaloids on syrup forms of aging. A controlled pilot study of clinical, neurologic and EEG changes. Scientific exhibit: Am. Med. Assoc. Ann. Conv., New York, June 23–27, 1973

Winslow, I.E.: The hospitalized geriatric patient. Scientific exhibit: American Med. Assoc. Meeting, Oregon, Nov. 30–Dec. 3, 1974b (to be published)

Winslow, I.E.: Mental decline in the aged: aspects of etiology and therapy. Scientific Exhibit: am. Geriat. Soc. Annual Meeting, Toronto, Canada, April 17–18, 1974a (to be published)

Wright, E.A., Spink, J.M.: A study of the loss of nerve cells in the central nervous system in relation to age. Gerontologia **3**, 277–287 (1959)

CHAPTER VIII

Some Compounds With Hallucinogenic Activity

A. FANCHAMPS

A. Introduction

Although "delusional insanity" has been reported among the manifestations of convulsive ergotism (BARGER, 1931), none of the naturally occurring ergot alkaloids have typical hallucinogenic properties; such properties are confined to a number of semisynthetic derivatives of lysergic acid, the prototype of which is LSD. This substance is the most potent and, by far, the most extensively tested hallucinogen derived from ergot.

This chapter will consequently be centered on LSD. Unlike all other modern drugs, this compound has been assayed in man before an extended pharmacologic testing was performed in animals. Furthermore, its most specific and only interesting activity, the psychotomimetic one, cannot be studied directly in laboratory animals. This is one reason why this chapter is dealing only with human pharmacology. The other reason stems from the fact that all relevant data on animal pharmacology are included anyhow in other parts of this book.

B. Discovery of LSD

LSD[1] was prepared for the first time in 1938 by ALBERT HOFMANN as part of a systematic chemical and pharmacologic investigation of partially synthetic amides of lysergic acid in the Sandoz Research Laboratories (STOLL and HOFMANN, 1943). The diethylamide was synthesized in the hope of obtaining an analeptic, in view of a structural relationship with nikethamide (Fig. 1).

A pharmacologic screening performed by ROTHLIN (quoted by STOLL and HOFMANN, 1943) revealed a marked uterotonic effect on the rabbit uterus in vitro and in situ as well as an excitatory action in these animals; in dogs and cats the substance produced cataleptic phenomena, reminiscent of the action of bulbocapnin (ROTHLIN, quoted by STOLL, 1947; ROTHLIN, 1957). Work on LSD then fell in abeyance for a number of years.

The discovery of its psychotropic effect was partly due to chance, when 5 years later, in April 1943, HOFMANN decided to prepare a fresh quantity of LSD. In the course of this work, he experienced a remarkable state of intoxication, which he described as follows (HOFMANN, quoted by STOLL, 1947; HOFMANN, 1970a):

---

[1] *d*-Lysergic acid diethylamide. Lysergide (INN rec.), Delysid, LSD25, d-LSD, (No. 73b in Chapter II, "Chemical Background").

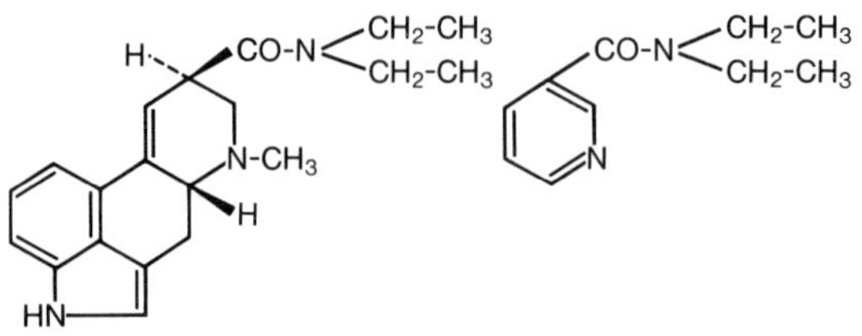

LSD Nikethamide

Fig. 1. Structural relationship between LSD and nikethamide

"Last Friday, April 16, 1943, I was forced to stop my work in the laboratory in the middle of the afternoon and to go home, as I was seized by a peculiar restlessness associated with a sensation of mild dizziness. On arriving home, I lay down and sank into a kind of drunkenness which was not unpleasant and which was characterized by extreme activity of imagination. As I lay in a dazed condition with my eyes closed (I experienced daylight as disagreeably bright) there surged upon me an uninterrupted stream of fantastic images of extraordinary plasticity and vividness and accompanied by an intense, kaleidoscope-like play of colours. This condition gradually passed off after about two hours."

The nature and course of this extraordinary disturbance led him to suspect that he had been intoxicated by the substance with which he had been working that afternoon: He had separated the two isomers formed by this synthesis, the diethylamides of the lysergic and isolysergic acids, and prepared the crystalline water-soluble salt of lysergic acid diethylamide with tartaric acid.

Chance made then way to a planned investigation, which led to the actual discovery. In order to clarify the question, HOFMANN decided to perform some self-experiments, starting with what he thought to be a subthreshold oral dose: 0.25 mg. Forty minutes after having ingested the substance, he noted in his laboratory journal (HOFMANN, 1970b):

"17.00, onset of dizziness, anxiety, visual disturbances, paralysis, urge to laugh."

At this point, the laboratory notes were discontinued; the last words had been written only with great difficulty. A supplementary note was entered 2 days later:

"Went home by bicycle. From 18.00 to 20.00, very severe crisis (see special report)."

From this special report, extracts of which have been published in various scientific papers (STOLL, 1947; HOFMANN 1970a), we learn that while cycling home with his laboratory assistant, HOFMANN realized that the symptoms were much stronger than the first time.

"I had great difficulty in speaking coherently, my field of vision swayed before me, and objects appeared distorted like images in curved mirrors. I had the impression of being unable to move from the spot, although my assistant told me afterwards that we had cycled at a good pace ... Once I was at home a physician was called.

By the time the doctor arrived, the peak of the crisis had already passed. As far as I remember, the following were the most outstanding symptoms: vertigo, visual disturbances; the faces of those around me appeared as grotesque, coloured masks; marked motoric unrest, alternating with paralysis; an intermittent heavy feeling in the head, limbs and the entire body, as if they were filled with lead; dry, constricted sensation in the throat; feeling of choking; clear recognition of my condition, in which state I sometimes observed, in the manner of an independent, neutral observer, that I shouted half insanely or babbled incoherent words. Occasionally I felt as if I were out of my body.

The doctor found a rather weak pulse but an otherwise normal circulation ... Six hours after ingestion of the LSD my condition had already improved considerably. Only the visual disturbances were still pronounced. Everything seemed to sway and the proportions were distorted like the reflections in the surface of moving water. Moreover, all objects appeared in unpleasant, constantly changing colours, the predominant shades being sickly green and blue. When I closed my eyes, an unending series of colourful, very realistic and fantastic images surged in upon me. A remarkable feature was the manner in which all acoustic perceptions (e.g. the noise of a passing car) were transformed into optical effects, every sound evoking a corresponding coloured hallucination constantly changing in shape and colour like pictures in a kaleidoscope. At about one o'clock I fell asleep and awoke next morning feeling perfectly well."

This was the first planned human experiment with LSD. Subsequent, more prudent trials have revealed that the dose chosen by HOFMANN was about five times the average effective amount.

C. Effects of LSD in Man

Effective doses range from 0.5 to 2.0 μg per kg of body weight, either given orally or intravenously. Enteral absorption is fairly complete. Effects usually set in 30–40 min after ingestion and reach a maximum within 90 min. The intensity of the reaction may then show wave-like variations for a further 2–3 h and then begin to decline progressively; most subjects have largely recovered 8–12 h after the start of the experiment. Certain individuals may experience bouts of after-effects, such as strange feelings, mood disturbances, or hallucination, days or even weeks after the drug intake (ROSENTHAL, 1964; HOROWITZ, 1969).

1. Somatic Actions

Autonomic and neurologic disturbances usually become manifest before the effects on mind and perception. In the majority of cases, they are of a mild nature. *Autonomic changes* reflect a stimulation of both branches of the autonomic nervous system. Sympathetic stimulation is evidenced in most subjects by a pupillary dilatation and moderate increases in heart rate and blood pressure; other, inconstant signs are piloerection, a slight blood-sugar elevation, and, rarely, some increase in body temperature. Respiration is generally unchanged. Other symptoms point to a parasympathetic stimulation: Sweating and salivation are frequent; nausea may occur; vomiting is exceptional; an increase in diuresis is occasionally noted; flushing of the face is more frequent than paleness. Sympathicotonia usually predominates, but there are great individual variations and a marked parasympathicotonia with bradycardia and hypotension may be observed in some subjects. Headache and dizziness have sometimes been reported.

The most consistent *neurologic effect* is an exaggeration of the patellar (ISBELL et al., 1956) and other tendon reflexes. Other, less constant signs are a slight unsteadiness of gait, ataxia, a positive Romberg's sign, and mild tremor.

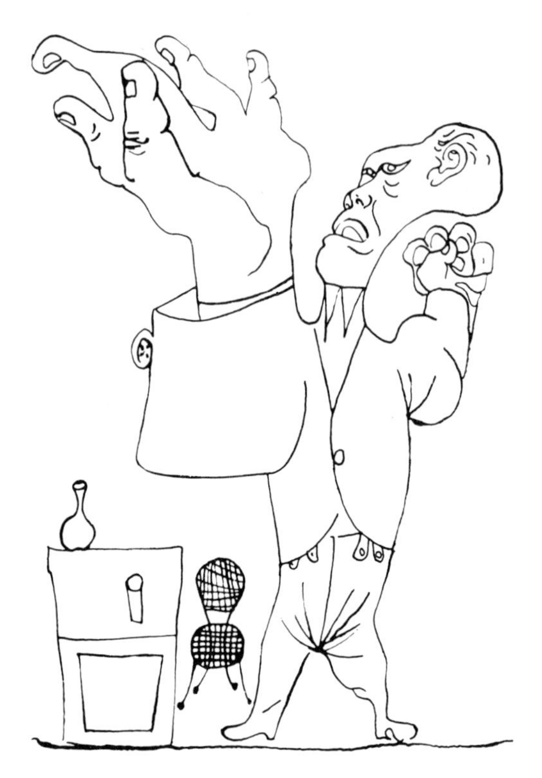

Figs. 2 and 3. Drawings executed during an LSD session (100 µg orally) by painter O. JANECEK. The artist represented hallucinations he was experiencing. In Figure 2, "A politician", the disproportionate right hand and the hollow head are remarkable. The face in Figure 3 has an additional eye and is surrounded by two oversized left hands. (Reproduced with permission of J. ROUBICEK, 1961)

2. Psychic Actions

The characteristic psychic and perceptual effects of LSD have been excellently described by W.A. STOLL (1947) in the very first clinical paper on the new drug, so that later investigators, such as BECKER (1949), CONDRAU (1949), RINKEL et al. (1952), LIDDELL and WEIL-MALHERBE (1953), ABRAMSON et al. (1955d), BERCEL et al. (1956a), and many others could do little more than confirm these observations (while often completing the investigational method with psychologic or psychometric tests, performing laboratory tests, EEG's etc., and expanding the material to various categories of mentally ill subjects).

a) Psychologic Effects in Mentally Normal Subjects

In mentally normal subjects, the most important changes concern perception, mood, relationship to the environment, and ego integrity.

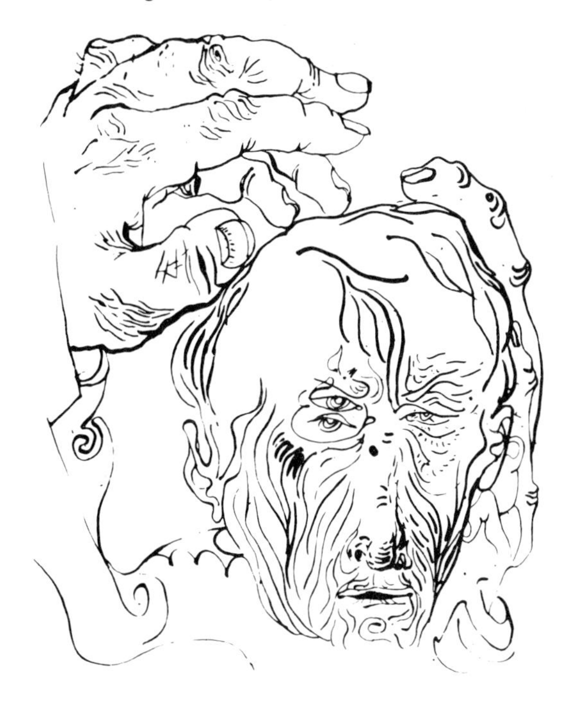

Fig. 3

α) Perception

Most prominent are *visual* phenomena. They usually start as prolonged after-images, then rapidly proceed to illusions and, especially in a dark room, to elementary hallucinations. Finally, formed hallucinations occur in many subjects. Objects, including faces, appear distorted; sizes and distances are misjudged; objects seem to approach or to recede. Perception of colors is altered, yellow and red appearing with particular frequency; in general, colors are perceived brighter than normal, but they may also appear drab and greyish during depressed phases. Elementary hallucinations may start with flickering, glittering points, flashes of light, colored waves, strips, spots, circles, spirals, whirls, and may gradually turn into well-defined objects, animals, human beings (Figs. 2 and 3), or whole sceneries.

Optic sensations may be triggered or modified by auditory stimuli (HOFMANN, quoted by STOLL, 1947; BERCEL et al., 1956a) or by pressure on the eye balls. LSD may also induce visual experiences in blind subjects (KRILL et al., 1963), even after enucleation of both eyeballs (ALEMA, 1952), provided there is a history of previous visual activity.

Acoustic phenomena often consist in hyperacousis; slight noises are perceived very loud, reverberating, filling the space. Acoustic illusions are frequently mentioned, but true acoustic and especially verbal hallucinations are rare (BENEDETTI, 1951; SAVAGE, 1952).

Olfactory and *gustatory* distortions or illusions are less prominent.

Tactile illusions are relatively frequent. On touch, objects including the own body may feel different (harder, or softer, rougher, smoother etc.) from usual. DE SHON et al. (1952) describe "a rather vivid experience in a subject of his trousers being wet from urine."

β) Alterations of Body Image

Alterations of body image form an important part of the LSD syndrome (ARNOLD and HOFF, 1953b). The whole body or part of it is felt to be altered in size, shape, consistency, or to be strange in some way. A limb may be said to be "like detached" from the rest of the body or completely missing (BERCEL et al., 1956a). The body may be perceived either as increased (LIEBERT et al., 1958) or, more often, as reduced in size. The subject feels as if he were transformed into a child; SANDISON et al. (1954) mention a woman 29 years old who became a girl of 5 or 6; she felt that her clothes were huge and hanging loosely about her, and her hand appeared small compared to the doctor's hand grasping hers. Door handles may appear out of reach as they would be to a small child. Such experiences are especially conspicuous in neurotic individuals, where they are usually associated with the reliving of repressed personal memories of childhood.

γ) Time Sense

Time sense is frequently impaired, aberrations occurring both in the direction of acceleration or slowing down even to a feeling of complete arrest of time passage (BECKER, 1949; ARONSON and KLEE, 1960).

δ) Mood Changes

Mood changes are prominent during the LSD experience; there is usually an alternation between euphoric and depressive episodes, with a certain prevalence of the former. The subject may be delighted by the beauty of his hallucinatory experiences. Euphoria may also take the form of a shallow elation with silly smiling and giggling, or unmotivated, uncontrolled laughter. Certain individuals become disinhibited or frankly hypomanic, with an increased urge for action. This, coupled with the mental aberrations, may make the subject dangerous to himself or to others. A man, for instance, jumped out of a window, having complete faith that he could fly (COHEN, 1967), while another tried to walk on the sea (COHEN, 1966). On the other hand, cases of homicide have also been reported (KNUDSEN, 1964). In spite of the disinhibition, sexual stimulation rarely occurs (ANDERSON and RAWNSLEY, 1954).

Emotional indifference is sometimes reported, but dysphoria is more frequent. The experience may be felt as unbearingly flat and dull; depression may take the form of a quiet sadness or be of a more agitated nature. Suicide is a potential danger (COHEN and DITMAN, 1962) and a further reason for the unadvisability of LSD experiments outside strict medical and psychologic supervision.

Tension, anxiety, or a frank panic may develop at the height of the reaction. The hallucinatory experience can be extremely frightening. The feeling of becoming insane is very anguishing to some subjects, especially if they have doubts about the reversibility of their abnormal condition (FROSCH et al., 1965; COHEN, 1966).

ε) Consciousness

Consciousness is maintained, orientation usually remains intact, and the vast majority of subjects remain aware that their uncommon experience is caused by the drug; however, this insight may be lost, especially after high doses. Memory is not impaired, the individual is usually able to remember every detail.

ζ) Ego Integrity

Ego integrity is often disturbed by feelings of depersonalization and derealization—often related to distortions of the body image—or of division of the personality, which may closely mimic schizophrenic symptoms (DE SHON et al., 1952; LANGS and BARR, 1968; YOUNG, 1974). On the whole, however, most experts feel that there are more differences than similarities between the clinical pictures of most types of schizophrenia and the LSD intoxication (ROUBICEK, 1958a, b; LANGS and BARR, 1968).

η) Psychologic and Psychometric Tests

In order to explore more in depth the effects of the LSD intoxication on mental functioning, thought patterns, mood, personality, and psychomotor performance, a large array of psychological and psychometric tests have been applied. Discussion of the results is not possible in the frame of this chapter, but Table 1 will facilitate reference to the original papers. In this connection, it must be pointed out that filling out questionnaires, concentrating on a mental or physical task, or submitting to other test procedures may considerably weaken the LSD experience (the most vivid effects are usually obtained in a dark and quiet surrounding).

b) Psychologic Effects in Mental Patients

Psychotic patients, especially schizophrenics, are more resistant to the psychologic and hallucinogenic (though not necessarily to the somatic) effects of LSD than mentally normal or neurotic individuals (STOLL, 1947, 1952; CONDRAU, 1949; BECKER, 1949; BUSCH and JOHNSON, 1950; FORRER and GOLDNER, 1951; RINKEL et al., 1952; HOCH et al., 1952; ARNOLD and HOFF, 1953a, and many others). With sufficiently high doses, however, an increase in psychomotor activity and verbal exteriorization may be obtained even in stuporous schizophrenics, and patients with mania may become greatly excited. LSD often accentuates the preexisting emotional state, so that melancholic patients become still more depressed and manic patients still more euphoric (CONDRAU, 1949; SLOANE and LOVETT DOUST, 1954). Psychiatric patients are usually able to distinguish between the drug-induced and their usual hallucinations.

In *neurotic patients*, especially when applied in connection with analytic psychotherapy, LSD may produce very conspicuous disinhibiting effects, and thus greatly

Table 1. Psychologic and psychometric tests under LSD

Test	In normal subjects	In mental patients[a]
Mental state, mood		
Questionnaires	ABRAMSON et al. (1955d, e) ABRAMSON (1960a) JARVIK et al. (1955a) KORNETSKY et al. (1957) BRENGELMANN (1958) LEBOVITS et al. (1960a) LINTON and LANGS (1962)	ISBELL et al. (1956) PAUK and SHAGASS (1961)
Clyde mood scale	LEBOVITS et al. (1960b, 1962)	
Powick rating scale	SANDISON (1959b)	SANDISON (1959b)
Anxiety tests	MCGLOTHLIN et al. (1967)	
Personality		
MMPI	KORNETSKY and HUMPHRIES (1957) KLEE and WEINTRAUB (1959) LEBOVITS et al. (1960a, 1962)	BELLEVILLE (1956) UNGERLEIDER et al. (1968a)
Perceptual reaction	BRENGELMANN (1958)	
Personality, attitude, and value test battery	MCGLOTHLIN et al. (1967)	
Aesthetic sensitivity test battery	MCGLOTHLIN et al. (1967)	
Thinking process		
Thematic aperception (TAT)	LEBOVITS et al. (1962)	SANGUINETI et al. (1956)
Projective test battery	MCGLOTHLIN et al. (1967)	
Concrete-abstract thinking, proverb interpretation	DESHON et al. (1952) COHEN et al. (1962)	
Rorschach	DESHON et al. (1952) RINKEL et al. (1952) STOLL (1952) GASTAUT et al. (1953) DELAY et al. (1954) SLOANE and LOVETT DOUST (1954) LEVINE et al. (1955b) BERCEL et al. (1956b) HURST et al. (1956) TALLAFERRO (1956) VON FELSINGER et al. (1956) LEBOVITS et al. (1960b, 1962) PIERCE (1961) AXELROD and KESSEL (1972)	BENEDETTI (1951) SMORTO et al. (1955) ISBELL et al. (1956) SANGUINETI et al. (1956) TALLAFERRO (1956) ZIOLKO (1959)
Goldstein-Scheerer sorting		ISBELL et al. (1956)
Raven progressive matrices	KRUS et al. (1961)	
Color pyramid	LIENERT (1961)	
Four pictures	VAN LENNEP (1960)	VAN LENNEP (1960)
Thurstone hand test	ABRAMSON et al. (1955c)	

Table 1 (continued)

Test	In normal subjects	In mental patients[a]
Zucker		SMORTO et al. (1955)
Word association	WEINTRAUB et al. (1959, 1960)	
Associational fluency (Guilford)	McGLOTHLIN et al. (1969)	McGLOTHLIN et al. (1969)
Creativity test battery	McGLOTHLIN et al. (1967)	
Porteus maze	ARONSON and KLEE (1960) McGLOTHLIN et al. (1969)	McGLOTHLIN et al. (1969)
Spatial orientation map test	McGLOTHLIN et al. (1969)	McGLOTHLIN et al. (1969)
Intelligence		
IQ (Shipley-Hartford)	COHEN et al. (1958) McGLOTHLIN et al. (1969)	McGLOTHLIN et al. (1969)
Wechsler-Bellevue	LEVINE et al. (1955a)	ISBELL et al. (1956)
Digit symbol	KORNETSKY et al. (1957)	
Cattell	GASTAUT et al. (1953)	
IST-Amthauer	LIENERT (1956, 1959)	
Memory and learning		
Memory	BERCEL et al. (1956a) SILVERSTEIN and KLEE (1958a, 1960a)	
Recall and recognition test battery	JARVIK et al. (1955c) ARONSON et al. (1962)	
Picture recognition	BARENDREGT (1960)	BARENDREGT (1960)
Figure reconstruction	BRENGELMANN (1958) BRENGELMANN et al. (1958a) BARENDREGT (1960)	BARENDREGT (1960)
Learning	ARONSON et al. (1962)	
Drawing task		
Bender-Gestalt	ABRAMSON et al. (1955f) BERLIN et al. (1955) TALLAFERRO (1956) BAMBAREN VIGIL (1957)	TALLAFERRO (1956) BAMBAREN VIGIL (1957) PAUK and SHAGASS (1961)
Draw a tree, draw a person	BERLIN et al. (1955) SILVERSTEIN and KLEE (1958b) PIERCE (1961) McGLOTHLIN et al. (1967)	GOMIRATO et al. (1958)
Three tree	VAN LENNEP (1960)	VAN LENNEP (1960)
Mirror-image drawing	ORSINI and BENDA (1960)	
Minnesota percepto-diagnostic (MPDT)	McGLOTHLIN et al. (1969)	McGLOTHLIN et al. (1969)
Spontaneous drawing and painting	MATEFI (1952) BERLIN et al. (1955) RINKEL (1956) ROUBICEK (1956, 1958a, b, 1961)	SAURI and DE ONORATO (1955) ROUBICEK (1958a, b, 1961) MACHOVER and LIEBERT (1960) LEUNER (1962, 1963a)

Table 1 (continued)

Test	In normal subjects	In mental patients[a]
	Tonini and Montanari (1955a) Von Mering et al. (1957) Machover and Liebert (1960)	Maccagnani et al. (1964)
Attention		
Attention and concentration test battery	Jarvik et al. (1955b)	
Düker calculation	Lienert (1956, 1958, 1959)	Wapner and Krus (1960)
Counting backwards	Cohen et al. (1962)	
Adding (Kraepelin, Birren, Pauli)	Hurst et al. (1956) Kornetsky et al. (1957) Krus et al. (1961) Pierce (1961)	
Arithmetic problems	Jarvik et al. (1955d)	
Number square	Horackova et al. (1958)	
Lahy	Gastaut et al. (1953)	
Stroop color-word	Wapner and Krus (1960) Krus et al. (1961)	
Trail making	McGlothlin et al. (1969)	McGlothlin et al. (1969)
Estimation of quantities	Brengelmann (1958)	
Psychomotor functions		
Tapping	Landis and Clausen (1954) Sloane and Lovett Doust (1954) Bercel et al. (1956a) Hurst et al. (1956) Barendregt (1960) Krus et al. (1961)	Barendregt (1960)
Reaction time	Abramson et al. (1955b) Orsini and Benda (1959) Rosenbaum et al. (1959) Edwards and Cohen (1961)	Wikler et al. (1965a)
Purdue pegboard	Landis and Clausen (1954)	
Rotatory pursuit	Abramson et al. (1955a) Kornetsky et al. (1957) Rosenbaum et al. (1959)	
Dual pursuit	Silverstein and Klee (1960b)	
Steadiness	Abramson et al. (1955a) Krus et al. (1961)	
Speed of copying	Kornetsky et al. (1957)	
Handwriting	Stoll (1947) Bercel et al. (1956a) Hirsch et al. (1956) Hurst et al. (1956) Krus et al. (1961)	Thuring (1960)
Language		Priori (1957) Fink et al. (1960)

Table 1 (continued)

Test	In normal subjects	In mental patients[a]
Visual functions		
Flicker fusion	Landis and Clausen (1954) Hurst et al. (1956) Takashina (1960)	
Visual threshold	Carlson (1958) Takashina (1960)	
Retinal function, ERG	Krill et al. (1960)	
Color detection	Edwards and Cohen (1961)	
Tachistoscopic discrimination	Kornetsky et al. (1957)	
Figural after-effects	Smith (1960)	
Embedded figures (Witkin)	McGlothlin et al. (1969)	McGlothlin et al. (1969)
Part-whole relationship	Krus and Wapner (1959)	
Size constancy	Edwards and Cohen (1961)	
After-image duration	Brengelmann (1958)	
Apparent horizontal	Wapner and Krus (1959)	
Apparent eye level	Krus et al. (1966)	
Various physiologic functions		
Patellar reflex	Wikler et al. (1965b)	Isbell et al. (1956) Wikler et al. (1965b)
Galvanic skin response	Fisher and Cleveland (1959) McGlothlin et al. (1967)	
Warmth detection	Edwards and Cohen (1961)	
Tactual threshold	Kornetsky et al. (1957)	
Two-point discrimination	Edwards and Cohen (1961)	
Weight discrimination	Rosenbaum et al. (1959)	
Audiometric threshold	Henkin et al. (1967)	
Subjective time	Boardman et al. (1957) Aronson et al. (1959) Benda and Orsini (1959) Orsini and Benda (1959)	

[a] Including psychotics, psychoneurotics, and former drug addicts.

facilitate release and abreaction of repressed material, while enhancing contact and transference. These properties of LSD have been widely exploited as an adjunct to psychotherapy and psychoanalysis (see D, 1).

Reliving of traumatic childhood experiences is usually accompanied by a regression of the body image to a size corresponding to the relived age. Certain authors even claim that patients under LSD have been able to relive their own birth (Lewis and Sloane, 1958; Sandison, 1960).

The psychologic effects of LSD in neurotic subjects have been analyzed in depth by Leuner in his book *Die experimentelle Psychose* (1962).

3. Effects of LSD on the Human EEG

The first investigators found no LSD-induced changes in the electroencephalogram (FORRER and GOLDNER, 1951). With refined evaluation methods, however, the following effects were observed rather consistently:

1. An accelerated and decreased amplitude of the alpha-rhythm (RINKEL et al., 1952; GASTAUT et al., 1953; ROUBICEK, 1958a; BENTE et al., 1958).
2. An increase in β-activity (GASTAUT et al., 1953), which may become dominant (ROUBICEK, 1958a).
3. In patients with drug-induced slow background rhythm, e.g., during a combined treatment with chlorpromazine and reserpine, LSD increases the frequency and decreases the amplitude (BENTE et al., 1958).
4. In epileptics, slow rhythms are accelerated, but spike activity may be increased (BENTE et al., 1958).
5. Blocking of the α-activity by a visual stimulus is preserved (ROUBICEK, 1958a) and may be prolonged (BERCEL et al., 1956a), which might correlate with the frequently observed persistence of after-images.
6. Evoked potentials due to flicker light are increased (GASTAUT et al., 1953).
7. In the quantified EEG, one observes a decrease in electrical energy with an associated reduction in variability; the tracings becoming strikingly similar to those of chronic schizophrenic patients (PFEIFFER et al., 1965).

On the whole, the effects of LSD on the EEG appear to result from an increased neuronal activity.

The effect of LSD on the depth EEG of patients with convulsive and/or psychotic disorders has been investigated by SCHWARZ et al. (1956); in epileptics, they observed a pronounced quieting effect on the spike and sharp-wave foci, whereas chronic schizophrenics responded with an increase in paroxysmal activity. MONROE et al. (1957) attempted to correlate, in schizophrenic patients with implanted electrodes, the behavioral effects of LSD with EEG modification; paroxysmal activity in the hippocampal, amygdaloid, and septal regions seemed to be associated with overt expressions of disturbed psychotic behavior.
In patients with exposed cerebral cortex, PURPURA et al. (1957) observed that, if perfused locally into a small cortical artery, LSD inhibits the dendritic activity evoked by electrical stimulation of the cortical surface.

4. Clinical Laboratory Investigations

a) Liver Function Tests

Liver function tests, which may be pathologic in schizophrenia, revealed only a mild and transient disturbance under LSD. Quick's hippuric acid excretion test as well as the Hijmans van den Berg and Takata-Ara reactions remain negative (FISCHER et al., 1951; BELSANTI, 1955), whereas the more sensitive cinnamonic acid test of Snapper and Saltzmann revealed a slight dysfunction (FISCHER et al., 1951). After i.v. LSD in schizophrenic patients, SANGUINETI et al. (1956) found no change in bilirubinemia but an increase of the albumin-globulin quotient and some disturbances in tests for serum lability. Curiously enough, liver functions have hardly been tested in more recent studies. According to BROWN (1972), SGOT is unchanged and liver functions unaffected by LSD.

b) Carbohydrate Metabolism

Besides an occasional slight elevation of blood sugar (LIDDELL and WEIL-MALHERBE, 1953), LSD may produce an increase in the plasma concentration of hexosemonophosphate (MAYER-GROSS et al., 1952, 1953); the authors conclude that LSD impairs glycogen mobilization by blocking its metabolism at the level of hexosemonophosphate, but their corroborating in vitro findings were not confirmed by others (BAIN, 1957).

ARNOLD (1955) observed that high oral or intravenous doses of glutamic acid or succinic acid may interrupt or retard the LSD reaction 3–5 h; from this he inferred that the effect of LSD on brain function might be connected to a derangement in the citric acid cycle.

c) Adrenaline Metabolism

The fact that signs of adrenergic stimulation usually precede the mental symptoms points to a possible involvement of the adrenaline system in the mechanism of LSD psychosis (RINKEL et al., 1955). LIDDELL and WEIL-MALHERBE (1953) reported that following LSD, plasma adrenaline first rises, then drops below the starting level, then rises again, but such changes could not be confirmed by MANGER et al. (1956). An increased urinary excretion of adrenaline and noradrenaline was found after LSD in manic-depressive but not in schizophrenic patients (ELMADJIAN et al., 1957).

HOFFER and his group, who from 1954 on investigated this problem in a number of studies (quoted by HOFFER, 1965), thought to have identified adrenochrome and adrenolutin as probable mediators of certain mental effects of LSD as well as possible pathogenic factors in schizophrenia. The main evidence on which they base their theory is as follows: Adrenaline is metabolized into adrenochrome, which in turn is converted into (1) dihydroxyindole or (2) trihydroxyindole, pathway 1 being preferred. LSD (but not the nonpsychomimetic BOL 148, No. 37a in Chapter II) increases the in vitro conversion of adrenaline into adrenolutin as well as the blood levels of adrenochrome and adrenolutin. When adrenochrome is injected into a schizophrenic patient or to an LSD pretreated subject, the adrenochrome blood level remains elevated much longer than in controls (or after treatment with BOL 148). This could be interpreted as resulting from a block of the main metabolic pathway, leading to an accumulation of adrenochrome and to an increased formation of adrenolutin (pathway 2). According to these authors, adrenochrome and adrenolutin induce psychologic changes and hallucinations (HOFFER et al., 1954; OSMOND, 1956), a finding which could not be confirmed, however, by RINKEL et al. (1955), using a stabilized form of adrenochrome nor by the surgical experience with adrenochrome used as an hemostatic; since native adrenochrome is unstable, the psychotic effects observed by HOFFER were possibly caused by a degradation product.

d) Phosphate Excretion

In schizophrenic patients, urinary phosphate excretion is low compared to normal controls but increases after ACTH. LSD produces identical phenomena in normal subjects: Low urinary output of phosphate and increase after ACTH (HOAGLAND et al., 1955); the authors suggest that LSD acts on enzyme systems to facilitate the binding of phosphate, which is reversible by adrenocorticoids; in schizophrenic patients, an endogenous derivative of adrenaline metabolism would have a similar phosphorylation facilitating effect.

e) Enzymatic Systems

Studies on the effect of LSD in various enzymes in man, in animal models, or in vitro have been unrewarding, as far as the psychotomimetic mechanism is concerned. CLARK et al. (1954, 1956) found a slight inhibition of the succinic dehydrogenase system in rat brain homogenates, no effect on lactic dehydrogenase, and a slight activation of malic dehydrogenase as well as a stimulation of cytochrome C oxidase and of alkaline phosphatase. However, the centrally inactive levorotatory isomer 1-LSD (No. 61) has identical effects on malic dehydrogenase and alkaline phosphatase. Among the brain cholinesterases, only pseudocholinesterase is consistently inhibited by LSD (THOMPSON et al., 1955); the same authors found no effect on true cholinesterase and tributyrinase, whereas FOLDES et al. (1959) observed a definite inhibition. Inhibition of human serum cholinesterase (FRIED and ANTOPOL, 1956; ZSIGMOND et al., 1959; EVANS, 1960) and pseudocholinesterase (THOMPSON et al., 1955; ZEHNDER and CERLETTI, 1956) has been regularly demonstrated with LSD concentrations of the order of magnitude of 10^{-6} M but with lower concentrations such as 6×10^{-9} M FRIED and ANTOPOL (1957) found a potentiation of serum pseudocholinesterase. The relevance of these alterations in cholinesterase activity for the psychotomimetic effect is doubtful, since similar inhibitions were demonstrated with the nonpsychotomimetic compounds BOL 148 (No. 37a) (ZEHNDER and CERLETTI, 1956; FOLDES et al., 1959; ZSIGMOND et al., 1959; EVANS, 1960), l-LSD and d-iso-LSD (No. 93c) (ZSIGMOND et al., 1960).

Mono-amino-oxidase is not affected by LSD (CERLETTI, 1956), and the same applies to 5-hydroxytryptophane decarboxylase, dopa decarboxylase, glutamic acid decarboxylase, and amino acid oxidase (CERLETTI, 1958). On the other hand, LSD was found to inhibit glutamic dehydrogenase (SIVA SANKAR et al., 1961).

More recently, an increase of serum creatine phosphokinase (CPK) activity has been observed following ingestion of LSD or of street drugs believed to be LSD (HARDING, 1974; MELTZER, 1975); this was possibly an indirect effect of the psychotic reaction rather than a direct effect of LSD, since experiments in rats failed to show any alteration in CPK activity after i.p. or i.m. injection of LSD (MELTZER, 1975). Increased CPK has also been found in some individuals with spontaneous psychoses (MELTZER, 1968, 1975).

f) Cerebral Circulation and Metabolism

Cerebral circulation and metabolism have been investigated in normal subjects and schizophrenics at the height of the effect of i.v. LSD by SOKOLOFF et al.

(1957). Cerebral blood flow (nitrous oxide method), cerebral vascular resistance, cerebral oxygen consumption, and glucose utilization remained practically unchanged.

5. Tolerance to LSD Effect

If LSD is given daily, tolerance develops very quickly but disappears after a few days off the drug. ABRAMSON et al. (1956) used their questionnaire method to demonstrate such tolerance in normal volunteers receiving fixed or increasing oral doses for 3–6 days. The same was observed by ISBELL et al. (1956, 1961) in former morphine addicts. CHOLDEN et al. (1955) gave daily intramuscular injections to schizophrenics; tolerance was already evident on day 2 and complete on day 3 of drug administration, and a period of 4 to 6 days free of LSD was necessary to reinstate the original reaction.

6. Inhibitors of LSD Reaction

The acute LSD reaction can be aborted by sedatives and tranquilizers. By far the most widely applied antidote is intramuscular or intravenous chlorpromazine. Within a few minutes of an injection of 25–100 mg, most autonomic and psychic disturbances are completely abolished (SCHWARZ et al., 1955; HOCH, 1956a, b; ISBELL and LOGAN, 1957; LESSE, 1958; SANDISON, 1968); the same applies to the EEG alterations (SCHWARZ et al., 1956; MONROE et al., 1957). Oral chlorpromazine is much less effective (ISBELL, 1959; ABRAMSON et al., 1960b); nevertheless, in connection with the therapeutic use of LSD in psychoneurotic patients, MARTIN (1957) terminated the experience by giving one to three oral doses of 50 mg chlorpromazine. A preventive effect on the LSD psychosis may be observed if chlorpromazine is applied orally before the hallucinogen, either in a single dose of 50–100 mg 30 min prior to LSD (ISBELL and LOGAN, 1957) or in repeated daily doses of 200–600 mg (GIBERTI and GREGORETTI, 1955).

Reserpine applied parenterally is definitely less effective than chlorpromazine as an antagonist (HOCH, 1956b; MONROE et al., 1957), and pretreatment may even potentiate the LSD-reaction (ISBELL and LOGAN, 1957; ISBELL, 1959).

On the other hand, strong sedation by intravenous amobarbital (500 mg or more) is a very efficient method to stop the LSD reaction and put the subject eventually to sleep (HOCH, 1956a; HOFFER, 1965).

Among the minor tranquilizers, azacyclonol attracted much interest following reports by FABING (1955) that a pretreatment with oral daily doses of 10–30 mg given for 2–7 days was able to almost block completely the psychic reaction to 100 μg LSD. According to BROWN et al. (1956), 100 mg of i.v. azacyclonol injected at the height of the LSD reaction promptly relieves the symptoms. However, this striking antagonistic effect of azacyclonol could not be confirmed by CLARK (1956), HOCH (1956b), ISBELL and LOGAN (1957); MONROE et al. (1957) observed no effect on the behavioral changes and only a doubtful effect on the LSD-induced alterations of the EEG.

Hydroxyzine, another minor tranquilizer, was tested as a pretreatment by LOEB and GIBERTI (1959) as well as by PIERCE (1961) in a self-experiment; the subsequent LSD experience was attenuated, especially regarding the mood disturbances, but the perceptive alterations were not suppressed; the LSD-induced EEG changes were not modified.

More recently, diazepam, 5–15 mg i.v., 10 mg i.m., 10–50 mg orally, has been described as a very potent antidote of the acute LSD experience (Editorial, 1971); even after oral application, hallucinations, euphoria, panic, and terror disappear in about half an hour (Levy, 1971).

In cases of prolonged psychotic reactions following abuse of LSD, lithium therapy (achieving blood levels ranging from 0.5 to 1.2 mEq/l) proved more effective than phenothiazines in normalizing the psychic state (Horowitz, 1975); the author concludes that, at least in certain individuals, the LSD-induced psychotic reaction is closer to manic-depressive illness than to schizophrenia.

Other attempts at counteracting the effects of LSD were connected with theories on the biochemical mechanism of action. Arnold (1955), suspecting a derangement in the carbohydrate metabolism, observed that glutamic acid, 20 g i.v. or 100 g orally, or succinic acid, 10 g i.v., interrupted or retarded the LSD reaction for several hours. In the hands of Hoch (1956b), however, these two substances didn't prove very effective.

Nicotinic acid has been tested by Agnew and Hofer (1955); they found that in subjects pretreated with 3 g nicotinic acid per day for 3 days, the LSD reaction was modified, exhibiting less visual disturbances but more feeling of unreality and confusion about self-identity. When 200 mg nicotinic acid were injected i.v. at the height of the LSD experience, all the disturbances except affect were markedly reduced within a few minutes. Hoffer (1965) as well as O'Reilly and Reich (1962) used nicotinic acid routinely during LSD therapy to mitigate or terminate the reaction. In a double-blind study by Miller et al. (1957), nicotinic acid did not alter the pattern of the response to LSD, except for a reduced anxiety.

Also steroid hormones have been used in conjunction with LSD. Abramson and Sklarofsky (1960) pretreated normal subjects with 40–165 mg of prednisone per day for 3–7 days; anxiety was reduced, but the other LSD effects were not modified. According to Clark and Clark (1956), premedication of schizophrenic patients with cortisone had no observable effect upon their sensitivity to LSD. Krus et al. (1961), using a battery of tests in a double-blind study in normal subjects, observed that 600 mg progesterone given 1 h before LSD decreased the sensory-motor, perceptual, and conceptual disturbances.

A clear attenuation or even suppression of the LSD reaction was observed by Grof and Dytrych (1965) in patients pretreated for several weeks with the MAO-inhibitor nialamide, 150–500 mg per day parenterally and orally; the protective effect lasted as long as 2 weeks after cessation of the drug. This action might be related to an interference with the metabolism of brain serotonin.

Serotonin itself was also tried (Poloni, 1955), but since it does not cross the blood-brain barrier, it is not surprising that no clear-cut modificaton of the LSD experience could be observed. The precursor 5-hydroxytryptophan (25 mg i.v.), which increases the concentration of serotonin in the brain, did not markedly alter the reaction to i.v. LSD, although the psychologic tests suggest a slight alleviation (Brengelmann et al., 1958b).

Finally, small daily doses of propranolol, a beta-adrenoceptor blocking agent, have been found effective in relieving delayed anxiety reactions after high doses of LSD in subjects who had responded poorly to chlorpromazine and diazepam (LINKEN, 1971).

7. Side-Effects and Complications

As long as LSD is administered under professional supervision, the incidence of side-effects and complications seems to be relatively low. In 1960, COHEN reported the results of an inquiry among 44 LSD researchers covering 5000 individuals who had undergone one or more LSD sessions for experimental or therapeutic purposes and combined these data with a survey of the literature. He estimated the rate of major complications per thousand patients undergoing therapy as follows: 1.2 attempted suicide; 0.4 completed suicide; 1.8 experienced a psychotic reaction over 48 h. The corresponding figures per thousand normal experimental subjects were: O attempted or completed suicide and 0.8 psychotic reactions persisting longer than 2 days. COHEN concluded that LSD induced only very few toxic or psychologic complications.

This reassuring picture changed dramatically with the advent of illicit and unsupervised use, as noted by the same author 2 years later (COHEN and DITMAN, 1962). The complications most frequently encountered are:

1. Acute panic reactions (FROSCH et al., 1965; COHEN, 1966)
2. Acute paranoid state with acting-out behavior (COHEN, 1966)
3. Confusion state with disorganized behavior (COHEN, 1971)
4. Depression, which may lead to suicide attempts (COHEN, 1966; UNGERLEIDER et al., 1966)
5. Late recurrence of symptoms such as depersonalization and perceptual distortions, which may occur intermittently for weeks or months (FROSCH et al., 1965)
6. Chronic anxiety reactions (COHEN, 1966; UNGERLEIDER et al., 1966)
7. Prolonged psychotic episodes (COHEN and DITMAN, 1962), not only after repeated intake, but also after a single ingestion, chiefly in individuals with underlying schizophrenia (FROSCH et al., 1965).

Since the total number of illicit LSD intakes cannot be determined, the proportion of them leading to complications is unknown, but the magnitude of the problem is illustrated by a survey performed in 1966–1967 in Los Angeles County by UNGERLEIDER et al. (1968b): On the basis of a questionnaire filled out by 1584 professionals (psychiatrists, psychiatric residents, internists, general practitioners, psychologists), the total number of adverse reactions to LSD occuring in this area during an 18-month period was estimated at 4100.

Dealing with illicit use, however, the causal relationship between LSD and the reported reactions is obscured by the fact that black market LSD is of questionable purity and very often contains unknown contaminants, and even more because most subjects have been taking other drugs as well, ranging from barbiturates to amphetamine, marijuana, mescaline, or heroin (COHEN and DITMAN, 1962).

On the other hand, the relative safety of LSD when used therapeutically under adequate supervision in a hospital setting was again stressed in 1969 by DENSON: Among 411 LSD sessions in 237 patients, 87% were entirely uncomplicated, and only 4% led to major complications, such as confusion, violence, or depression, scores which compare favorably with those of many widely used medicaments.

Whereas the LSD-induced complications encompass a large array of mental and psychologic disorders, somatic side-effects are rather exceptional. In a review covering the LSD complications published up to 1967, SCHWARZ (1968) found only slight indices of suspicion regarding definite physical effects from LSD. Convulsions have been produced in rare instances (COHEN, 1966, 1971). Slight alterations of the electrocardiogram with T-wave flattening and depression of the S-T segment have been observed by TENENBAUM (1961). Acute overdosage leads to a complex toxic symptomatology, which may include extreme hyperthermia (FRIEDMAN and HIRSCH, 1971), emesis, collapse, coma, respiratory arrest, platelet dysfunction, and mild generalized bleeding (KLOCK et al., 1974).

LSD intoxication in children has occured following accidental intake, which is favored by the fact that black market LSD is often deposited on sugar cubes (COHEN, 1966). Transient or prolonged psychotic reactions resembling those of adults usually ensue, but notable differences may also be observed. MILMAN (1967) describes the case of 5-year-old girl who ingested 100 µg LSD and developed, besides a prolonged psychotic reaction, signs of organic brain dysfunction which persisted for several months, with impaired visual-motor function and EEG abnormalities (diffuse high voltage, slowing, dysrhythmia) opposite to those produced by LSD in adults; a similar discrepancy betwenn LSD-induced EEG changes in children and adults was reported by SCHIEFER et al. (1972). A striking case of intoxication in a 2-year-old boy who ingested the huge amount of 180 µg/kg LSD has been described by SAMUELSSON (1974): After an initial phase of extreme excitability with ataxia and mydriasis, the child, without loosing consciousness, went into a state of total catatonia which lasted for about 4 h. Laboratory investigations as well as ECG and EEG remained normal; recovery was uneventful and there were no lasting sequelae.

The possible genetic effects of LSD including chromosomal anomalies are dicussed in detail by GRIFFITH et al. in Chapter XII.

8. Illicit Use and Addiction

Whereas for nearly 15 years, LSD had been used exclusively for scientific or therapeutic purposes by and under the supervision of responsible researchers and clinicians, unsupervised use and abuse of LSD and other hallucinogens quickly developed in the early 1960's, first in the United States and then spreading to Europe and the rest of the world. LUDWIG and LEVINE (1965a) refer to "abuse" when hallucinogens are taken by individuals who have procured them through illicit channels and/or taken them in medically unsupervised or socially unsanctioned settings.

This unfortunate development started with enthusiastic reports of novelists such as Aldous HUXLEY (1954, 1956) on mescaline and of some psychologists of Harvard Universtity (LEARY and ALPERT, 1963; LEARY, 1964) ascribing to LSD mind expanding, creativity-enhancing properties and describing it, as COHEN puts it in a critical review article (1971), "as a solution to all of one's personal problems and a solution the world's woes if it were universally utilized". A sensational, wide-spread publicity disseminated by the mass media ensued, which triggered the formation of subcultural groups of LSD devotees, some led by psychologists (e.g., the IFIF or International Foundation for Internal Freedom), others formed among students, intellectuals, beatniks, or hippies, many involving a mystique or religious component. Simultaneously, individual use burgeoned among the same categories of people, also including many unstable, emotionally disturbed, unadapted, frustrated persons, neurotics, psychopaths, drug addicts (LUDWIG and LEVINE, 1965a) and permanent dropouts from society (LOURIA, 1968). In 1971, COHEN estimated that 5–10% of all college students in the United States had tried LSD at least once, and that perhaps 1% were regular users. A detailed analysis of the psychologic background of this "epidemy" and of the motives for using LSD has been published by FREEDMAN (1968).

LSD is not physically addicting, and an abstinence syndrome is not identifiable (COHEN, 1971; BROWN, 1972), but a psychologic dependence may be encountered (LUDWIG and LEVINE, 1965a). In a series of LSD users mentioned by SANDISON (1968), nearly three-fourths of all persons who had had LSD expressed an interest in taking it again, and more than half of the regular users showed signs of habituation. Mentions of individuals having taken LSD several hundreds of times are not exceptional in the literature (FROSCH et al., 1965; SANDISON, 1968; MCGLOTHLIN and ARNOLD, 1971). Furthermore, the dose of LSD taken under illicit conditions is often much higher than the 0.5–2.0 or 3.0 µg/kg of body weight, which are regarded as reasonable by responsible researchers and therapists; COHEN (1966) mentions a man who repeatedly took up to 4000 µg at a time, and in his 1971 article, the same author cites one instance where 10 mg was swallowed without a fatal result. The deleterious effects of such chronic use and overdosage may further be aggravated by the fact that many of these individuals are taking not only LSD but indulge in multiple drugs, including other hallucinogens, stimulants, sedatives, and narcotics (COHEN and DITMAN,, 1962; LUDWIG and LEVINE, 1965a; LEUNER, 1971a; TRUBE-BECKER, 1975). Fortunately, according to a follow-up survey of 247 LSD takers, the drug seems to become less attractive with continuous use, so that its abuse becomes self-limiting (MCGLOTHLIN and ARNOLD, 1971).

Up to the early 1960's, Sandoz Ltd. was the sole producer of LSD; it did not introduce the drug commercially and restricted its free-of-charge distribution to carefully selected investigators and experienced therapists. When abuse became evident, in 1965, Sandoz further drastically strengthened its distribution policy for LSD and the related hallucinogen psilocybin; from then on, shipments were made to investigators only if they could produce an official authorization from the health authority of their own country. In the United States, selection of and distribution to the investigators were entirely farmed out to the National Institute of Mental Health. Following these measures, the output of LSD from Sandoz dropped to negligible amounts. Thus, the huge quantities of LSD appearing in illicit trade and use do not originate from a diversion of "legal" LSD but are prepared illegally from lysergic acid (which is now freely available on the fine chemical market), a procedure which does not require particular skill, especially if is not attempted to obtain a completely pure substance. Combined with the above-mentioned lay-press publicity, this easy access to LSD paved the way to the development of abuse. In turn, abuse and misuse imposed severe legal and administrative restrictions which greatly impeded or even sterilized further research with hallucinogenic drugs, since, as LOURIA (1968) puts it, "it is now far easier to obtain LSD for illicit use than for legitimate and important medical experiments."

D. Clinical Applications of LSD

In addition to its use as an experimental tool to produce transient "model psychoses" – in the hope of reproducing at will and studying the psychodynamic, physical, and biochemical anomalies which characterize and perhaps cause spontaneous psychoses – LSD has been widely used for therapeutic purposes. In the frame of this review, only a short account of the main fields of application can be given.

1. Adjuvant to Psychotherapy

The first attempt to use LSD during sessions of psychotherapy in order to reduce repression and permit recall of traumatic experiences was made as early as 1950 by BUSCH and JOHNSON, but 4 years elapsed before the next reports appeared in the literature (FREDERKING, 1953/54; SANDISON, 1954; SANDISON et al., 1954). From then on, the method has been applied by an increasing number of psychotherapists, until the advent of illicit use and the ensuing legal restrictions drastically limited the access of serious clinicians to this drug. Among the people who have gathered the largest experience with LSD as an aid to psychotherapy, one may cite SANDISON and his co-workers (SANDISON 1954, 1959a, 1960; SANDISON and WHITELAW, 1957; SANDISON et al., 1954), MARTIN (1957, 1962), LING and BUCKMAN (1960, 1963), BIERER and BROWNE (1960) in England; ABRAMSON (1955, 1956a, b, 1957, 1960b), SAVAGE (1957, 1961), EISNER and COHEN (1958), COHEN and EISNER (1959), CHANDLER and HARTMAN (1960) in the United States; LEWIS and SLOANE (1958), BAKER (1964) in Canada; WHITAKER (1964) in Australia; LEUNER and HOLFELD (1962), LEUNER (1963a, b, 1971b) in Germany; BAROLIN (1961) in Austria; VAN RHIJN (1960), ARENDSEN HEIN (1963) in Holland; GEERT-JÖRGENSEN et al. (1964) in Denmark,; STEVENIN and BENOIT (1962) in France; ALHADEFF (1963) in Switzerland; GIBERTI et al. (1956) in Italy; ROJO SIERRA (1959) in Spain; FONTANA (1961) and PÉREZ MORALES (1963a, b) in Argentina.

Besides individual psychotherapy, LSD has also been used to facilitate group therapy, e.g., by FONTANA and ALVAREZ DE TOLEDO (1960), ROJO SIERRA (1960), TENENBAUM (1961), SPENCER (1963), PÉREZ MORALES (1963c), EISNER (1964), and HOFFER (1965).

This combined use of psychotherapy and hallucinogens is sometimes referred to as "psycholytic therapy," according to LEUNER's proposal (LEUNER and HOLFELD, 1962). Obsessive-compulsive neuroses, anxiety neuroses, sexual neuroses and deviations, character disorders, and psychopathy are considered the best subjects. LSD is usually applied in small or medium doses for a series of psychotherapeutic or psychoanalytic sessions. It acts by removing the blocks to insight, relieving emotionally charged memories, intensifying affectual responses, and increasing the transference relationship to the therapist; the latter lends support and later interprets. Abreactions may occur and ego defenses may be reduced. According to most authors, the psychotherapeutic process may thus be considerably shortened, and cases resistant to conventional methods can be made amenable to therapy.

The true value of LSD in facilitating psychotherapy, however, has been questioned by some investigators. In a controlled study, ROBINSON et al. (1963) found no difference in the outcome of treatment of neurotic patients undergoing either plain or drug-assisted psychotherapy (with oral LSD or i.v. methamphetamine/hexobarbital being applied to induce abreaction). More recently, SOSKIN (1973) compared LSD and a placebo in two parallel series of patients undergoing psychotherapy; as measured by a battery of rating scales, both groups improved moderately, but the LSD patients didn't do better than the placebo patients, neither after five drug-assisted sessions, nor after a 18-month followup. The author hypothesizes that the impressive improvement rates reported by earlier investigators were due to the heightened therapist motivation and involvement, to the unusual amount of time and attention provided to the patient, and to the tacit permission given to the patient to express otherwise unacceptable thoughts and feelings.

2. Psychedelic Therapy

The term "psychedelic"—which means mind-manifesting—has been proposed by OSMOND (1958) for substances such as LSD which, besides mimicking mental illness, are supposed to "enrich the mind and enlarge the vision." It has subsequently been used to designate a therapeutic method developed in Canada and the USA; after a period of psychologic preparation, a high dose of LSD is given for one single session (or at the utmost for a limited number of sessions), the effect often being reinforced by the therapist's attitude, a religious atmosphere, an esthetic surrounding, music (BONNY and PAHNKE, 1972), or even hypnosis (LUDWIG and LEVINE, 1965b), etc. The aim is to produce an overwhelming, "transcendental" experience with ego-dissolving, expansion of consciousness, sense of harmony, or, according to COHEN's formulation (1971), "a psychological death-rebirth experience with the opportunity for a new beginning."

a) Alcoholism

This method has been applied primarily in the treatment of alcoholism. At first, enthusiastic reports were published by SMITH (1958), CHWELOS et al. (1959), SAVAGE (1962), JENSEN and RAMSAY (1963), KURLAND et al. (1967, 1968, 1971), and others. However, on the basis of their literature review, ABUZZAHAB and ANDERSON (1971) concluded that the overall effectiveness remains disappointing. As a matter of fact, none of the controlled studies in which psychedelic therapy has been compared to a no-drug treatment performed under similar circumstances was able to show a significant superiority in the LSD-treated patients (e.g., SMART et al., 1966; VAN DUSEN et al., 1967; JOHNSON, 1969; LUDWIG et al., 1969; DENSON and SYDIAHA, 1970; BOWEN et al., 1970). In their book devoted to a fair appraisal of the therapeutic efficacy of LSD in alcoholism, LUDWIG et al. (1970) conclude that "the various LSD procedures used do not offer any more for the treatment of alcoholism than an intensive milieu therapy program, and the latter, at best, is quite ineffective in deterring drinking."

b) Narcotic Addicts

The psychedelic method has also been applied on a more limited scale to the treatment of narcotic addicts. Two controlled studies (Ludwig and Levine, 1965b; Savage and McCabe, 1973) have been performed; they are in favor of the LSD-treated groups.

3. Use in Psychoses

The activating effect of LSD on psychotic symptomatology has been used by some psychiatrists for a therapeutic purpose. Basing on the usual observation that acute schizophrenic phases with abundant productive symptoms show a high tendency to spontaneous remission, Jost (1957) performed a series of LSD sessions in patients with slowly developing, nonproductive forms of the illness; in a number of cases, symptoms were markedly enhanced, and Jost claims that the evolution towards remission was accelerated. Sandison and Whitelaw (1957) followed an analogous reasoning, but they aborted the acute LSD reaction by a chlorpromazine injection; they report encouraging results in seven out of 14 psychotic patients resistant to orthodox therapy. Perillo and Garcia de la Villa (1963) succeeded in activating, by means of LSD, cases of schizophrenic dementia and treated them subsequently with thioridazine.

Somewhat similar experiences were made by Itil et al. (1969) in therapy-resistant chronic schizophrenics, characterized by a hypersynchronous EEG with predominant alpha activity, who were given a series of i.v. LSD injections; as soon as an acceleration and desynchronization of the EEG, accompanied by an activation of the psychotic symptomatology, became apparent, the hallucinogenic drug was stopped; conventional psychotropic drugs were then reinstated, and proved more effective than before the LSD course.

Abramson et al. (1958a) followed a different approach. They used LSD to enhance communication between a schizophrenic patient and a nonpsychotic "stablemate" during group therapy.

Other investigators, such as Lesse (1959), Wijsenbeek and Landau (1960), had negative results, and most experts consider that LSD is contraindicated in compensated schizophrenics or patients with schizoid personality because of the possibility of precipitation into a psychosis (Cohen, 1960; Barolin, 1961).

4. Therapeutic Use in Children

LSD has been used in conjunction with psychoanalysis in psychotic children by Rojas Bermudez (1960); communication with the therapist was facilitated, and in spite of the high dosage (50–300 μg), no side effects were encountered. Fontana (1961) notes a progress when associating LSD to psychotherapy in children with character disorder.

BENDER et al. (1962, 1963) and BENDER (1968) applied a different concept in treating schizophrenic children, 6–12 years old, with LSD; the drug was given daily for 2 months or longer in progressively increasing doses of 25–150 µg; no psychotherapy was attempted. Autistic children became less introverted and plastic, more aware and responsive, contact improved, and there was some increase in verbal communication. Intelligent, verbal schizophrenics in the same age group showed an improved behavior, changes in fantasy and bizarre ideation to more insightful and reality-oriented, though often anxious and depressive attitudes, improved maturity and organization. The improvement was confirmed by Rorschach, Bender-Gestalt, and Human Figure Drawing tests. When taken off medication the patients deteriorated and responded again when LSD was resumed. There were no serious side effects. Since BENDER obtained nearly identical results with methysergide, the beneficial effect she observed with LSD was probably not connected to the hallucinogenic action of the latter.

FREEDMAN et al. (1962) also tried LSD in autistic schizophrenic children, not in daily doses like the above authors, but on one single or, at the most, on two occasions, the dose ranging from 50–200 µg. Some reaction was observed, but the hoped-for change from muteness to speech did not occur.

5. Use in Terminal Cancer Patients

KAST (1963) included LSD in his investigations on the analgesic properties of some narcotic compounds in patients suffering from intolerable pain, mostly due to terminal cancer. After a single dose of 100 µg LSD, pain and distress were often relieved for 18 h or longer, and appeared to be reduced for 2 or 3 weeks, the patient becoming indifferent to the pain experience. In addition, depression and apprehension concerning approaching death were lessened. In more recent publications, this author analyzed the psychologic mechanism of the LSD analgesia (KAST and COLLINS, 1964; KAST, 1966) and reported the incidence of adverse reactions in his series of 128 cases: panic episode in 5.5%, mild anxiety in 33%, no adverse somatic effects (KAST, 1967).

A useful pain-relieving and psychologic action in a few patients was also reported by COHEN (1965), who concludes that LSD "may one day provide a technique for altering the meaning—and lessening the dread—of dying"; he doesn't seem, however, to have pursued this line, since no mention is made of this potential use of LSD in his more recent reviews (e.g., COHEN, 1971).

The approach of KURLAND and his group was somewhat different. These investigators (KURLAND et al., 1968, 1973; PAHNKE et al., 1969; GROF et al., 1973) didn't look primarily for an analgesic effect but applied LSD in the frame of a psychedelic therapy, with the aim of alleviating the psychologic stress of the dying patient. After intense preparatory psychotherapy, one session with a high dose of 200–500 µg LSD was conducted and possibly repeated after some time if need arose. For the following days or weeks, the patients exhibited a decrease of their emotional distress, depression, anxiety, insomnia, and psychologic isolation, coupled with a better acceptance and less fear of death; emerging mystical or religious feelings reoriented their philosophy of life, they felt detached from the wordly values. Though analgesia was not the main goal, previously excruciating pain completely disappeared for days or weeks in several patients, even those in whom the organic lesion seemed to make pain inevitable. In most cases, a certain amount of pain persisted but was no longer the primary focus of the patient's attention.

The latest statistics of these authors include 60 cases, of which 29% improved dramatically and 42% moderately, whereas 23% remained unchanged and 6% became worse (GROF et al., 1973). The LSD session appeared to be rather fatiguing for these debilitated patients. Recently, the KURLAND group tended to replace LSD by i.m. dipropyltryptamine or DPT, a shorter acting and therefore less stressful hallucinogen, which has the added advantage of being uncontaminated by adverse lay publicity.

E. LSD Analogues Tested in Man

A large series of chemical analogues of LSD, some natural but most of them semisynthetic, were prepared in the Sandoz Research Laboratories (HOFMANN, 1958, 1964) and tested systematically in vitro, in laboratory animals, and in man. The purpose was twofold:

1. To try and establish a structure-activity relationship
2. To correlate the hallucinogenic effect in man with biochemical and/or pharmacologic activities, in order to gain some clues regarding the mechanism of the model psychosis.

1. LSD Isomers

The levorotatory isomer l-LSD (No. 61[2]) is completely devoid of psychotomimetic activity (GERONIMUS et al., 1956; HOFMANN, 1958; MURPHREE et al., 1958; ISBELL et al., 1959a) and modifies neither the cortical nor subcortical EEG in man (MONROE et al., 1957). Also devoid of psychotomimetic activity are the two derivatives of isolysergic acid, d-iso-LSD (No. 93c) (HOFMANN, 1958; ISBELL et al., 1959a) and l-iso-LSD (No. 62) (HOFMANN, 1958). Compared to LSD, these three inactive isomers are extremely weak serotonin antagonists (CERLETTI and DOEPFNER, 1958a) and are not pyretogenic in the rabbit (Sandoz Research Laboratories, 1958, 1959) (Table 2). On the other hand, l-LSD and d-iso-LSD do not differ from LSD regarding cholinesterase inhibition (ZSIGMOND et al., 1960); rat brain alkaline phosphatase and malic dehydrogenase are activated to the same extent by LSD and l-LSD; the only difference was found with respect to lactic dehydrogenase, which is not affected by LSD but slightly inhibited by l-LSD (CLARK et al., 1956).

2. Hydrogenated Derivatives

Dihydrolysergic acid diethylamide (Dihydro-LSD, No. 74b) is hydrogenated in positions C_9 and C_{10}. In oral doses of 100–200 μg, it produces strong autonomic disturbances (nausea, emesis, tachycardia, shiver, polyuria, headache, and paraesthesias) but no psychic alterations (CERLETTI, 1956). Its antiserotonin effect is about 50% of that of LSD (CERLETTI and DOEPFNER, 1958a). It produces a decrease

[2] Numbers refer to structural formulas in Chapter II.

of the body temperature of the rat in all doses up to 10 mg/kg, whereas LSD produces a decrease only in doses lower than 1 mg/kg but an increase in high doses (Sandoz Res. Lab., 1959).

2,3-Dihydrolysergic acid diethylamide (see general formula in the chapter "Chemical Background," Fig. 15) induces LSD-like autonomic and mental changes; its potency is estimated by GORODETZKY and ISBELL (1964) at about 15% of that of LSD. Its activity in inducing hyperthermia in rabbits is only 4% of the LSD activity (Sandoz Res. Lab., 1959).

3. Unsubstituted and Monosubstituted Amide Derivatives

d-lysergic acid amide (LA 111, ergine, No. 18) is not hallucinogenic; in doses up to 1 mg i.v., it produces – besides autonomic disturbances such as hypersalivation, emesis, dizziness and diarrhea – sedation, clouding of consciousness, and finally sleep (SOLMS, 1956a, 1956b; ISBELL, 1962). Its antiserotonin potency on the isolated rat uterus is 4% of that of LSD (CERLETTI and DOEPFNER, 1958a).

d-lysergic acid ethylamide (LAE 32, No. 73h), the first analogue tested in man, exerts LSD-like hallucinogenic effects, but these are definitely weaker than after LSD and require higher doses – such as 0.25–2.0 mg by injection – in order to become manifest; on the other hand, indifference, apathy, confusion, even lethargy are prevalent (SOLMS, 1953, 1956a, 1956b; JARVIK et al., 1955a). Perceptual alterations, depersonalization, anxiety, and paranoid reactions are less frequent than after LSD (VON FELSINGER et al., 1956; GIBERTI and GREGORETTI, 1958). According to TONINI and MONTANARI (1955b), the LSD-like response lasts only for 2–3 h. In schizophrenic and oligophrenic patients, SOLMS (1953) observed a sedation and sleep-inducing effect after parenteral or oral doses of 0.25–1.5 mg one to three times daily. ABRAMSON (1959) and ISBELL et al. (1959a) took into account not only the intensity of the LSD-like action – as established by their questionnaire method and by rating of the clinical grade – but also the dose relation to assess the comparative potencies of LSD and a series of analogues (Table 2); using this technique, they estimate the psychotomimetic potency of LAE 32 compared to LSD at 3% and 5%, respectively.

As far as the antiserotonin activity is concerned, LAE 32 exhibits 12% of the antagonistic effectiveness of LSD on the isolated rat uterus (CERLETTI and DOEPFNER, 1958a) and 20% on the rat paw edema (DOEPFNER and CERLETTI, 1958). The effect on the various enzymes parallels that of LSD, with the exception of lactic dehydrogenase, which is not affected by LSD but stimulated by LAE 32 (CLARK et al., 1954, 1956; ZSIGMOND et al., 1960). The conversion of adrenaline to adrenolutin is increased to a greater extent than by LSD (HOFFER et al., 1959). On the body temperature of the rat, the effect of LAE 32 exactly mimics the dual action of LSD: Decrease with doses below 1 mg/kg, increase above this dosage (CERLETTI, 1956); in the rabbit its pyretogenic effect amounts to 17% of that of LSD (Sandoz Res. Lab., 1958).

4. Disubstituted Amide Derivatives

Lysergic acid dimethylamide (DAM 57, No. 73c) is about 10 times less active than LSD as a psychotomimetic agent. Using the already-mentioned quantitative methods, ABRAMSON (1959) estimates its potency at 11% and ISBELL et al. (1959a) at 10% of that of LSD. On the other hand, it exhibits 20% of the serotonin antagonism of LSD on the rat uterus (CERLETTI and DOEPFNER, 1958a) and 13% on the rat paw edema (DOEPFNER and CERLETTI, 1958). When applied by intracerebral injection to conscious mice, it does not antagonize the stupor-inducing effect of intracerebral serotonin (HALEY, 1957). In the rabbit, it shows about 40% of the pyretogenic effect of LSD (Sandoz Res. Lab., 1958).

Lysergic acid dibutylamide (LBB66, No. 73e) is devoid of LSD-like mental effects (Sandoz Res. Lab., 1959). Its antiserotonin effect is 30% of that of LSD (CERLETTI and DOEPFNER, 1958a).

5. Cyclic Amide Derivatives

Lysergic acid pyrrolidide (LPD824, No. 73f) exhibits a modest LSD-like psychic effect (MURPHREE et al., 1958), which ABRAMSON (1959) quantifies at 5% and ISBELL et al. (1959a) at 10% of the LSD-activity.

As a serotonin-inhibitor, it shows 5% of the LSD-potency (CERLETTI and DOEPFNER, 1958a). Its dual action on the body temperature of the rat is identical to that of LSD (CERLETTI, 1956); as a pyretogenic in the rabbit, it exhibits 10% of the LSD potency (Sandoz Res. Lab., 1958).

Lysergic acid morpholidide (LSM775, No. 73g) produces LSD-like mental changes of short duration (GOGERTY and DILLE, 1957); both ABRAMSON (1959) and ISBELL et al. (1959a) estimate its potency at 11% of the LSD one. Its serotonin antagonism is only 2% of that of LSD (CERLETTI and DOEPFNER, 1958a), its pyretogenic effect in rabbits 10% (GOGERTY and DILLE, 1957; Sandoz Res. Lab., 1958). Behavior modifications in mice, rabbits, cats, and dogs are similar to those produced by LSD (GOGERTY and DILLE, 1957). LSM775 does not differ from LSD regarding cholinesterase inhibition (ZSIGMOND et al., 1960) but, contrary to LSD, does not increase adrenochrome plasma levels (HOFFER et al., 1959).

6. Ring-Substituted Derivatives

Substitutions in position 1 of the ring complex of lysergic acid do not suppress the psychotomimetic property, whereas the antiserotonin activity may even be increased.

1-Methyl-LSD (MLD41, No. 34b), if given in 1.5–3 times higher doses than LSD to normal or psychotic subjects, produces qualitatively similar mental effects of a somewhat lesser intensity (MALITZ et al., 1960, 1962). ABRAMSON (1959) quantifies the LSD-like potency of MLD41 at 36%, ISBELL et al. (1959a) at 33%. As an antiserotonin, it is 3.7 times more active than LSD on the isolated rat uterus (CERLETTI and DOEPFNER, 1958a) and exhibits 90% of the LSD activity on the rat paw edema (DOEPFNER and CERLETTI, 1958). When given by intracerebral injection to mice, it produces the same hyperexcitability syndrome as LSD and blocks the stuporous effect of intracerebral serotonin (HALEY, 1957). On the body temperature of the rat, it produces a decrease at all doses, and its pyretogenic effect on the rabbit is 5% of that of LSD (Sandoz Res. Lab., 1958, 1959).

1-Acetyl-LSD (ALD 52, No. 36f) is as effective as LSD as a psychotomimetic. MALITZ et al. (1960, 1962) compared the effects of LSD (0.1–2.8 μg/kg) and ALD52

(0.6–3.3 μg/kg) in a large series of subjects and psychotic patients; they found very similar action profiles, but ALD52 produced somewhat more distortions of the body image and thinking disturbances. ABRAMSON (1959) rates its relative effectiveness at 91%, ISBELL et al. (1959a) at 100% of LSD.

As a serotonin antagonist, it is 2.1 times more active than LSD on the isolated rat uterus (CERLETTI and DOEPFNER, 1958a), and upon intracerebral injection in mice, it produces the same excitatory syndrome and serotonin inhibition as LSD and MLD41 (HALEY, 1957). On the other hand, it has only a modest pyretogenic effect in the rabbit, amounting to 13% of the LSD activity (Sandoz Res. Lab., 1958).

1-Hydroxymethyl-LSD (OML632, No. 36h) retains 66% of the mental activity of LSD (ABRAMSON, 1959) and 60% of its antiserotonin potency on the isolated rat uterus (CERLETTI and DOEPFNER, 1958a).

If, however, the 1-substitution is performed on side-chain modifications of LSD, the psychotomimetic effect remains as modest as with the parent compounds, whereas the antiserotonin potency may be dramatically enhanced.

1-Methyl-lysergic acid ethylamide (MLA74, No. 34e) is the methylated analogue of LAE32. According to ISBELL et al. (1959a), its LSD-like activity is 4% of that of LSD (LAE32:5%). Contrasting with this, as a serotonin antagonist on the isolated rat uterus, it is 8.3 times stronger than LSD and 70 times stronger than LAE32 (CERLETTI and DOEPFNER, 1958b), whereas on the rat paw edema, it produces only 60% of the LSD effect (DOEPFNER and CERLETTI, 1958). Unlike LAE32, MLA74 is practically devoid of pyretogenic effect in rabbits (Sandoz Res. Lab., 1958).

1-Methyl-lysergic acid pyrrolidide (MPD75, No. 34d) is the methylated analogue of LPD824. It has only a partial, short-lasting LSD-like psychic action, which ISBELL et al. (1959a) rate at less than 5% of the effect of LSD (LPD824:10%). As a serotonin antagonist on the isolated rat uterus, it is 28 times stronger than LPD824 and 1.3 times stronger than LSD (CERLETTI and DOEPFNER, 1958b). It is not pyretogenic in the rabbit (Sandoz Res. Lab., 1958).

1-Acetyl-lysergic acid ethylamide (ALA10, No. 36g), the acetylated analogue of LAE32, exhibits 7% of the psychotomimetic effect of LSD (ISBELL et al., 1959a). Its antiserotonin potency on the isolated rat uterus is 40% of that of LSD (thus three times stronger than LAE32), whereas its pyretogenic effect in rabbits is only 1% of the LSD action (Sandoz Res. Lab., 1958).

With a substitution in position 2 of the lysergic acid molecule, the psychotomimetic effect is practically cancelled, though the antiserotonin effect is retained or even reinforced.

2-Bromo-lysergic acid diethylamide (2-bromo-LSD, BOL148, No. 37a) has been one of the first and most widely investigated analogues of LSD. The first tests in normal volunteers and carcinoid patients failed to demonstrate any LSD-like action up to doses of 2 mg i.v. or 7.5 mg orally (CERLETTI and ROTHLIN, 1955; SNOW et al., 1955; ROTHLIN, 1957; HOFFER et al., 1959; SCHERBEL and HARRISON, 1959) but only some sedation. In a more sophisticated, cross-over study with placebos, LSD, and other drugs, JARVIK et al. (1955a) found after BOL148 a psychotomimetic effect which was very modest indeed but clearly stronger than after a tap-water placebo. ABRAMSON (1959) ascribes 7% of the LSD activity to BOL 148 but ISBELL et al. (1959a), using a similar method, find only a partial LSD-like effect, smaller than 2%. When administering BOL 148 in very high doses by intravenous infusion (0.5–5.0 mg/min., total doses of 15–160 mg) in normal subjects or carcinoid patients, SCHNECKLOTH et al. (1957) observed psychic changes, such as drowsiness, anxiety, restlessness, feelings of unreality and depersonalization, but there were no hallucinations; oral daily doses up to 20 mg had no psychic effects. Individual hypersensitivity may occur, however, as exemplified by the case, reported by RICHARDS et al. (1958), of a laboratory technician who ingested 0.5 mg BOL 148 during a vascular headache and experienced a clear-cut, LSD-like reaction with distortion of body image, perceptual changes, and a wave-like alternation of euphoria and anxiety.

The antiserotonin effect of BOL 148 is about 100% of that of LSD on the isolated rat uterus (CERLETTI and DOEPFNER, 1958a) and 30% on the rat paw edema (DOEPFNER and CERLETTI, 1958). Regarding cholinesterase inhibition, it does not differ from LSD (ZSIGMOND et al., 1960). Contrary to LSD, BOL 148 does not increase plasma adrenochrome or the conversion of adrenaline to adrenolutin (HOFFER et al., 1959). It decreases the body temperature of the rat at all doses (ROTHLIN, 1957) and exhibits only 5% of the pyretogenic effect of LSD in the rabbit (Sandoz Res. Lab., 1958).

1-Methyl-2-bromo-LSD (MBL 61, No. 37b) was expected to combine the effects of the two ring substitutions. Actually, the psychotomimetic property seems to be completely lost (ISBELL et al., 1959a), whereas the antiserotonin activity on the isolated rat uterus surpasses that of the 1-methyl (370%) and of the 2-bromo (100%) derivatives and amounts to 530% of the LSD effect (CERLETTI and DOEPFNER, 1958a); on the rat paw edema, however, it is only 26% as active as LSD (DOEPFNER and CERLETTI, 1958). It is not pyretogenic in the rabbit (Sandoz Res. Lab., 1958).

7. Ololiuqui

Ololiuqui, one of the three "magic" plants of the Aztecs, has been identified as corresponding to two varieties of morning glory, *Rivea corymbosa* and *Ipomea violacea,* the seeds of which are still being ingested by some Mexican Indians in religious or therapeutic rituals. In a series of self-experiments, OSMOND (1955) developed apathy and hypnagogic phenomena after the ingestion of seeds of *Rivea corymbosa.*

Having succeeded in identifying the active principles of Ololiuqui, HOFMANN and his colleagues (HOFMANN and TSCHERTER, 1960; HOFMANN and CERLETTI, 1961; HOFMANN, 1961, 1963) were surprised to find out that they consisted of six already-known alkaloids of the ergot group, which had all been either prepared synthetically or extracted from various varieties of *Claviceps* but never from higher plants.

One of them was *d-lysergic acid amide* or LA 111 (No. 18), the autonomic and weak psychotomimetic effects of which—chiefly sedation and reduced consciousness—had already been described (page 591).

The second main component was *d-isolysergic acid amide,* or Iso-LA 819 (No. 18a). After its identification in ololiuqui, trials were performed in man with oral doses up to 5 mg; they revealed central effects which were not LSD-like (ISBELL, 1962) but chiefly consisted in relaxation, synesthesias, and altered time experience (HEIMANN, 1965; HEIM et al., 1968).

Elymoclavine (No. 6) produces mainly sedation (ISBELL and GORODETZKY, 1966).

Lysergol (No. 79a) has no effect up to 6 mg, but 8 mg produce a slight sedation (HEIM et al., 1968).

Ergometrine (No. 19) is a specific uterotonic and has very little central effects (JARVIK et al., 1955a).

The last component, *Chanoclavine,* is a tricyclic alkaloid, which is devoid of ergot-like activities.

In a cross-over study on six former opiate addicts, ISBELL and GORODETZKY (1966) compared the effects of a crude extract containing the total alkaloids of *Ipomea violacea* (5 mg) to the effects of 5 mg of a synthetic mixture of the six components (LA 111 45%, Iso-LA 819 25%, elymoclavine 5%, lysergol 5%, ergometrine 10%, and chanoclavine 10%), of 1.5 μg/kg LSD and of a placebo. This study confirmed that the crude extract and the synthetic mixture had practically identical, predominantly sedative properties and produced only slight autonomic changes; this contrasted sharply with the spectacular psychotomimetic and autonomic actions of LSD in the same subjects. In another group of addicts, 6 g of ground seeds of *Ipomea violacea* produced only very little effects.

A similar study was performed by HEIMANN and his colleagues (HEIMANN, 1965; HEIM et al., 1968), comparing the artificial mixture of the six alkaloids with LA 111, Iso-LA 819, and lysergol. They found that low doses of the mixture (2–3 mg) produced a relaxation resembling the effect of Iso-LA 819, whereas high doses (6–7 mg) elicited unpleasant autonomic changes and a reduced consciousness, such as observed after LA 111. They concluded that the central action of ololiuqui was primarily due to its content in these two main alkaloids.

8. Discussion

Table 2 provides a synoptic view of the LSD-like activity of the various analogues and helps to analyze the *structure-activity relationship.*

The three stereoisomers of LSD are devoid of psychotomimetic properties. The same applies to 9,10-dihydro-LSD, whereas the 2,3-dihydro analogue exhibits an appreciable potency.

After substitutions in position 1 of the lysergic acid moiety, the psychotomimetic effect is only slightly reduced, the less so with acetyl (ALD 52) and somewhat more with hydroxymethyl (OML 632) or methyl (MLD 41) substitution. Also if applied to the less potent lysergic acid ethylamide or pyrrolidide, the 1-substitution (ALA 10, MLA 74, MPD 75) only slightly affects the psychotomimetic activity of the parent compounds LAE 32 and LPD 824. In this connection, it is interesting that methysergide (UML 491, No. 34a), which is the 1-methyl analogue of the purely uterotonic methylergometrine (d-lysergic acid L-2-butanolamide, No. 73a), may produce in some migraine patients mental changes reminiscent of a slight LSD reaction, such as unworldly feelings, dreamy state (GRAHAM, 1964), or even

Table 2. Psychotomimetic activity and some pharmacodynamic effects of structural analogues of LSD

LSD-like activity in man				Pharmacological properties		
	①	②	③	5-HT inhibition isol. rat uterus[i,j]	Body temp. rat[a,b,d]	Pyretogenic effect rabbit[d,k,l]
	LSD=100			LSD=100	LSD ↗	LSD=100
High						
1-Acetyl-LSD (ALD 52)	91	100		210		13
1-Hydroxymethyl-LSD (OML632)	66			60		
1-Methyl-LSD (MLD41)	36	33		370	↘	5
Medium						
LA Ethylamide (LAE 32)	3	5		12	↗	17
1-Acetyl-LA ethylamide (ALA 10)		7		40		1
1-Methyl-LA ethylamide (MLA 74)		4		830		0
LA dimethylamide (DAM 57)	11	10		20		40
LA pyrrolidide (LPD824)	5	10		5	↗	10
LA morpholidide (LSM 775)	11	11		2		10
2,3-Dihydro-LSD			15[f]			4
Partial						
2-Bromo-LSD (BOL148)	7	<2	0[b]	100	↘	5
1-Methyl-LA pyrrolidide (MPD75)		<5		130		0
Absent						
LA amide (LA 111)			sed[e,g]	4		
Iso-LA amide (Iso-LA 819)			sed[h]			
l-LSD		0	0[c]	0.05		0
d-Iso-LSD		0	0[c]	0.1		0
l-Iso-LSD			0[c]	0.1		0
9,10-Dihydro-LSD (DH-LSD)			0[a]	50	↘	
1-Methyl-2-bromo-LSD (MBL61)		<1		530		0
LA dibutylamide (LBB66)			0[d]	30		
Lysergol			0[h]			
Elymoclavine			0[g]			1.4

LA stands for d-lysergic acid; sed=sedation

①ABRAMSON (1959). ②ISBELL et al. (1959a). ③[a] CERLETTI, (1956); [b] ROTHLIN (1957); [c] HOFMANN (1958); [d]Sandoz Res. Lab. (1959); [e] SOLMS (1956a, b); [f] GORODETZKY and ISBELL (1964); [g] ISBELL and GORODETZKY (1966); [h] HEIM et al. (1968); [i] CERLETTI and DOEPFNER (1958a); [j] CERLETTI and DOEPFNER (1958b); [k] Sandoz Res. Lab. (1958); [l] Chapter VI hallucinations (HALE and REED, 1962). According to ABRAMSON (1959), this action amounts to 1% of the effect of LSD.

By substitution in position 2 with a bromine atom, on the other hand, the psychotomimetic effect is nearly (BOL 148) or completely (MBL 61) suppressed.

Alterations of the diethylamide side chain have a profound influence on the central activity. The nonsubstituted amides LA 111 and Iso-LA 819 have sedative properties. The monosubstituted ethyl-analogues LAE 32, ALA 10, MLA 74 are psychotomimetic, but about 10–20 times weaker than the corresponding diethylamides LSD, ALD 52, and MLD 41. Regarding disubstituted amides, the psychotomimetic activity is reduced by shortening of the chains (DAM 57) and by ring closure (LPD 824 and LSM 775) and suppressed by lengthening (LBB 66).

In the ergolene derivatives, lysergol and elymoclavine are devoid of psychotomimetic properties.

Table 2 also enables one to examine the *correlation of the psychotomimetic activity with some pharmacological properties.*

The hypothesis that brain serotonin plays a role in maintaining normal mental processes, and that the hallucinogenic effect of LSD and of other psychotomimetic compounds might be connected with their serotonin antagonism has been proposed by various authors, especially by WOOLLEY (WOOLLEY and SHAW, 1954; WOOLLEY, 1958). However, CERLETTI and ROTHLIN (1955) concluded from the lack of LSD-like activity of BOL 148 that such a correlation is not very likely; according to these authors, it cannot be argued that BOL 148 does not penetrate into the brain, since it produces sedation, which is a central effect, and has been detected in the brain in the same amounts as LSD after intravenous injection to mice. Their conclusion is further supported by the complete absence of parallelism between the psychotomimetic activity and the antiserotonin potency, as evidenced by Table 2; very weak as well as very strong serotonin antagonists may be found side by side in the group of compounds with medium as well as in the group with no LSD-like properties.

No correlation exists with the pattern of body temperature reaction in the rat, since the relatively strong hallucinogenic MLD 41 produces a decrease at all dose levels, contrary to LSD and the moderately active hallucinogens LAE 32 and LPD 824, which produce an increase in high doses.

A weak correlation seems to exist with the pyretogenic effect in the rabbit, although there is no parallelism; none of the mentally active analogues possess a pyretogenic potency comparable to that of LSD, and some (ALA 10, MLA 74) have practically no such effect. The nonpsychotomimetic elymoclavine, on the other hand, has a certain hyperthermic effect.

As far as the enzymatic effects are concerned, no correlation emerges from the few results available; cholinesterase inhibition was found in the active compounds LSD, LAE 32, and LSM 775 as well as in inactive ones such as BOL 148, l-LSD, and d-iso-LSD (ZSIGMOND et al., 1960); also regarding dehydrogenases and alkaline phosphatase, there were no striking differences between LSD, LAE 32, and l-LSD (CLARK et al., 1954, 1956).

A further search for such correlations, especially if taking into account more recent findings concerning the biochemistry of brain functions, might have led to a better understanding of the mechanism involved in psychotomimetic reactions.

This was prevented, however, by the decision of Sandoz Ltd. to stop all supply of, and experimentation with, LSD analogues following the surge of hallucinogen abuse in the early 1960's.

F. Cross-Tolerance

Since tolerance to the autonomic and mental effects of LSD rapidly develops upon daily administration, cross-tolerance with closely related hallucinogenic analogues was to be expected (Table 3).

Actually, subjects receiving MLD41 in increasing doses (100–360 μg) for 5–6 days proved totally resistant to the effects of 80–100 μg LSD (ABRAMSON et al., 1958b). Similarly, a partial resistance to LSD was elicited in former narcotic addicts by a 1-week treatment with 0.5–1 mg per day of the weaker hallucinogen LAE32 (ISBELL et al., 1959b), and schizophrenics who had become resistant to LSD following daily i.m. injections of increasing LSD doses (100–400 μg) were also resistant to LAE32 (CHOLDEN et al., 1955).

Cross-tolerance has also been investigated between LSD and hallucinogens unrelated to ergot; here, the results were more variable.

Resistance to *psilocybin* was observed by ISBELL et al. (1961) in subjects who had become resistant to LSD following daily intake for 6–12 days and by ABRAMSON et al. (1960a) after a 5–12 day pretreatment with MLD41; conversely, a few days pretreatment with psilocybin nearly suppressed the autonomic and psychic reactions to LSD (ABRAMSON et al., 1960a; ISBELL et al., 1961); BALESTRIERI (1960), however, did not observe the development of tolerance with psilocybin and cross-tolerance between psilocybin and LSD.

The results are not quite consistent with *mescaline* either. BALESTRIERI and FONTANARI (1959) observed a total resistance to i.v. mescaline after a few days pretreatment with oral LSD and a reduced LSD response in subjects who had become resistant to mescaline following daily i.v. injections. Similarly, WOLBACH et al. (1962) found that subjects receiving 1.5 μg/kg LSD i.m. daily for 14 days became resistant not only to LSD but also to 5 mg/kg mescaline i.m., and conversely, that a 14 days' pretreatment with mescaline produces a tolerance to mescaline and LSD. CHOLDEN et al. (1955), however, did not find a cross-tolerance to mescaline after the development of tolerance to LSD.

N,N-dimethyltryptamine (DMT) produces psychic disturbances resembling the effects of LSD, except for a shorter onset and duration of action. According to ROSENBERG et al. (1964), subjects rendered tolerant to LSD by daily i.m. injections of 1.5 μg/kg for 13 days exhibited no tolerance to 1 mg/kg DMT i.m.; even a LSD tolerance produced by 3 μg/kg i.m. twice daily for 20 days did not suppress, but only attenuated, the response to a small dose of DMT (0.5 mg/kg).

Although *d-amphetamine* is not hallucinogenic, it has certain effects in common with LSD, such as euphoria, anxiety, elevation of body temperature, and blood pressure increase; as with LSD, direct tolerance develops after daily administration. However, subjects tolerant to d-amphetamine are not cross-tolerant to LSD, and subjects tolerant to LSD are not cross-tolerant to d-amphetamine (ROSENBERG et al., 1963).

Table 3. Cross tolerance between LSD, structural analogues, and other hallucinogens in man

Tolerance produced by	Test for cross tolerance with	Cross tolerance present	Remarks
[a] MLD 41	[a] LSD	yes	
[a] LAE 32	[a] LSD	yes	partial tolerance
[a] LSD	[a] LAE 32	yes	
[a] Psilocybin	[a] LSD	yes	BALESTRIERI: no tolerance
[a] LSD	[a] Psilocybin	yes	
[a] MLD 41	[a] Psilocybin	yes	
Mescaline	[a] LSD	yes	
[a] LSD	Mescaline	yes	CHOLDEN: no tolerance
[a] LSD	[a] Dimethyltryptamine	(yes)	slight reduction of response
d-amphetamine	[a] LSD	no	
[a] LSD	d-amphetamine	no	
[a] LSD	JB 336	no	
[a] LSD	Tetrahydrocannabinol	no	
[a] BOL 148	[a] LSD	yes	BALESTRIERI: no tolerance
[a] Methysergide	[a] LSD	yes	

[a] Substances with indole structure

Finally, subjects who had developed tolerance to LSD did not show cross-tolerance to *JB336* (N-methyl-3-piperidyl benzilate) (BALESTRIERI, 1960) or to *tetrahydrocannabinol* or THC, an active principle of marijuana (ISBELL and JASINSKI, 1969); the latter substance causes mental disturbances very similar to the LSD reaction but does not produce the autonomic changes characteristic of LSD, such as elevation in blood pressure and body temperature, pupillary dilatation, and increased knee jerk. The lack of cross-tolerance between LSD and certain other hallucinogens indicates that different mechanisms of action must be involved.

The matter is further complicated by the fact that a certain, albeit inconstant, resistance to LSD may be obtained by a pretreatment with ergot derivatives which are usually devoid of hallucinogenic properties, such as BOL 148 and methysergide. After *BOL 148* given in daily doses of 2–30 mg for periods ranging from 2 days to 5 weeks, the response to LSD was completely abolished (GINZEL and MAYER-GROSS, 1956; TURNER et al., 1959) or attenuated (ABRAMSON et al., 1958b; ISBELL et al., 1959b); only BALESTRIERI and FONTANARI (1959) failed to observe a resistance to LSD after BOL 148 pretreatment. Even more surprising is the finding by BERTINO et al. (1959) that a single oral dose of 32–64 μg/kg BOL 148 applied 1 h before LSD is able to considerably reduce the LSD response; no antagonism was found if BOL 148 was given simultaneously with LSD (ISBELL et al., 1959b) or at the height of the LSD reaction (GINZEL and MAYER-GROSS, 1956). It is interesting to note that in the rabbit a premedication with BOL 148 blocks the pyretogenic effect of LSD given 30 min later (HORITA and GOGERTY, 1958).

With *methysergide,* according to BALESTRIERI (1960), a 5–6 days' oral treatment with 2–4 mg per day markedly reduced the reaction to LSD, but a single dose given 1 h before LSD was without effect.

When considering Table 3, it becomes evident that—with the one exception of mescaline—cross-tolerance with LSD is confined to molecules, hallucinogenic or not, which comprise an indole structure. This suggests the involvement of brain receptors with a particular affinity for the indole nucleus.

G. References

Abramson, H.A.: Lysergic acid diethylamide (LSD-25): III. As an adjunct to psychotherapy with elimination of fear of homosexuality. J. Psychol. **39**, 127–155 (1955)
Abramson, H.A.: Lysergic acid diethylamide (LSD-25): XIX. As an adjunct to brief psychotherapy, with special reference to ego enhancement. J. Psychol. **41**, 199–229 (1956a)
Abramson, H.A.: Lysergic acid diethylamide (LSD-25): XXII. Effect on transference. J. Psychol. **42**, 51–98 (1956b)
Abramson, H.A.: Verbatim recording and transference studies with lysergic acid diethylamide (LSD-25). J. nerv. ment. Dis. **125**, 444–450 (1957)
Abramson, H.A.: Lysergic acid diethylamide (LSD-25): XXIX. The response index as a measure of threshold activity of psychotropic drugs in man. J. Psychol. **48**, 65–78 (1959)
Abramson, H.A.: Lysergic acid diethylamide (LSD-25): XXX. The questionnaire technique with notes on its use. J. Psychol. **49**, 57–65 (1960a)
Abramson, H.A.: Psychoanalytic psychotherapy with LSD. In: The Use of LSD in Psychotherapy. Transactions of a Conference on d-Lysergic Acid Diethylamide (LSD-25). April 22–24, 1959. Abramson, H.A. (ed.), pp. 25–80. New York: Josiah Macy, Jr., Foundation 1960b
Abramson, H.A., Sklarofsky, B.: Lysergic acid diethylamide (LSD-25) antagonists. III. Modifications of syndrome by prior administration of prednisone. Arch. gen. Psychiat. **2**, 89–93 (1960)
Abramson, H.A., Jarvik, M.E., Hirsch, M.W.: Lysergic acid diethylamide (LSD-25): VII. Effect upon two measures of motor performance. J. Psychol. **39**, 455–464 (1955a)
Abramson, H.A., Jarvik, M.E., Hirsch, M.W.: Lysergic acid diethylamide (LSD-25): X. Effect on reaction time to auditory and visual stimuli. J. Psychol. **40**, 39–52 (1955b)
Abramson, H.A., Jarvik, M.E., Hirsch, M.W., Ewald, A.T.: Lysergic acid diethylamide (LSD-25): V. Effect on spatial relations abilities. J. Psychol. **39**, 435–442 (1955c)
Abramson, H.A., Jarvik, M.E., Kaufman, M.R., Kornetsky, C., Levine, A., Wagner, M.: Lysergic acid diethylamide (LSD-25): I. Physiological and preceptual responses. J. Psychol. **39**, 3–60 (1955d)
Abramson, H.A., Jarvik, M.E., Levine, A., Kaufman, M.R., Hirsch, M.W.: Lysergic acid diethylamide (LSD-25): XV. The effects produced by substitution of a tap water placebo. J. Psychol. **40**, 367–383 (1955e)
Abramson, H.A., Waxenberg, S.E., Levine, A., Kaufman, M.R., Kornetsky, C.: Lysergic acid diethylamide (LSD-25): XIII. Effect on Bender-Gestalt test performance. J. Psychol. **40**, 341–349 (1955f)
Abramson, H.A., Jarvik, M.E., Gorin, M.H., Hirsch, M.W.: Lysergic acid diethylamide (LSD-25): XVII. Tolerance development and its relationship to a theory of psychosis. J. Psychol. **41**, 81–105 (1956)
Abramson, H.A., Hewitt, M.P., Lennard, H., Turner, W.J., O'Neill, F.J., Merlis, S.: The stablemate concept of therapy as affected by LSD in schizophrenia. J. Psychol. **45**, 75–84 (1958a)
Abramson, H.A., Sklarosfky, B., Baron, M.O., Fremont-Smith, N.: Lysergic acid diethylamide (LSD-25) antagonists. II. Development of tolerance in man to LSD-25 by prior administration of MLD-41 (l-methyl-d-lysergic acid diethylamide). Arch. Neurol. Psychiat. (Chic.) **79**, 201–207 (1958b)

Abramson, H.A., Rolo, A., Sklarofsky, B., Stache, J.: Production of cross-tolerance to psychosis-producing doses of lysergic acid diethylamide and psilocybin. J. Psychol. **49**, 151–154 (1960a)
Abramson, H.A., Rolo, A., Stache, J.: Lysergic acid diethylamide (LSD-25) antagonists: chlorpromazine. J. Neuropsychiat. **1**, 307–310 (1960b)
Abuzzahab, F.S., Anderson, B.J.: A review of LSD treatment in alcoholism. Int. Pharmacopsychiat. **6**, 223–235 (1971)
Agnew, N., Hoffer, A.: Nicotinic acid modified lysergic acid diethylamide psychosis. J. ment. Sci. **101**, 12–27 (1955)
Alema, G.: Allucinazioni da acido lisergico in cieco senza bulbi oculari. Riv. Neurol. **22**, 720–733 (1952)
Alhadeff, B.W.: Les effets psychotomimétiques du LSD et de la psilocybine dans l'exploration clinique de la personnalité. Schweiz. Arch. Neurol. Neurochir. Psychiat. **92**, 238–242 (1963)
Anderson, E.W., Rawnsley, K.: Clinical studies of lysergic acid diethylamide. Mschr. Psychiat. Neurol. **128**, 38–55 (1954)
Arendsen Hein, G.W.: Treatment of the neurotic patient, resistant to the usual techniques of psychotherapy, with special reference to LSD. Top. Probl. Psychother. **4**, 50–57 (1963)
Arnold, O.H.: Untersuchungen zur Frage des Zusammenhangs zwischen Erlebnisvollzug und Kohlehydratstoffwechsel. Wien. Z. Nervenheilk. **10**, 85–120 (1955)
Arnold, O.H., Hoff, H.: Untersuchungen über die Wirkungsweise von Lysersäurediäthylamid. Wien. Z. Nervenheilk. **6**, 129–150 (1953a)
Arnold, O.H., Hoff, H.: Körperschemastörungen bei LSD 25. Wien Z. Nervenheilk. **6**, 259–274 (1953b)
Aronson, H., Klee, G.D.: Effect of lysergic acid diethylamide (LSD-25) on impulse control. J. nerv. ment. Dis. **131**, 536–539 (1960)
Aronson, H., Silverstein, A.B., Klee, G.D.: Influence of lysergic acid diethylamide (LSD-25) on subjective time. Arch. gen. Psychiat. **1**, 469–472 (1959)
Aronson, H., Watermann, C.E., Klee, G.D.: The effect of D-lysergic acid diethylamide (LSD-25) on learning and retention. J. clin. exp. Psychopath. **23**, 17–23 (1962)
Axelrod, P., Kessel, P.: Residual effects of LSD on ego functioning: an exploratory study with the Rorschach test. Psychol. Rep. **31**, 547–550 (1972)
Bain, J.A.: A review of the biochemical effects in vitro of certain psychotomimetic agents. Ann. N.Y. Acad. Sci. **66**, 459–467 (1957)
Baker, E.F.W.: The use of lysergic acid diethylamide (LSD) in psychotherapy. Canad. med. Ass. J. **91**, 1200–1202 (1964)
Balestrieri, A.: Studies on cross tolerance with LSD-25, UML-491 and JB-336. Psychopharmacol. **1**, 257–259 (1960)
Balestrieri, A., Fontanari, D.: Acquired and crossed tolerance to mescaline, LSD-25, and BOL-148. Arch. gen. Psychiat. **1**, 279–282 (1959)
Bambaren Vigil, C.: La prueba de Bender en la intoxicatión experimental con la LSD 25. Rev. Neuropsiquiat. **20**, 588–607 (1957)
Barendregt, J.T.: Performance on some objective tests under LSD-25. Advanc. psychosom. Med. (Basel) **1**, 217–219 (1960)
Barger, G.: Ergot and Ergotism. London: Gurney and Jackson 1931
Barolin, G.S.: Erstes Europäisches Symposium für Psychotherapie unter LSD-25. Göttingen, November 1960. Wien. med. Wschr. **111**, 466–468 (1961)
Becker, A.M.: Zur Psychopathologie der Lysergsäurediäthylamidwirkung. Wien. Z. Nervenheilk. **2**, 402–440 (1949)
Belleville, R.E.: MMPI score changes induced by lysergic acid diethylamide (LSD-25). J. clin. Psychol. **12**, 279–282 (1956)
Belsanti, R.: Nuove ricerche in psichiatria sperimentale con la dietilamide dell'acido lisergico. Acta neurol. (Napoli) **10**, 460–466 (1955)
Benda, P., Orsini, F.: Etude expérimentale de l'estimation du temps sous LSD-25. Ann. méd.-psychol. **117**, 550–557 (1959)
Bender, L.: Theory and treatment of childhood schizophrenia. Acta paedopsychiat. **34**, 298–307 (1968)

Bender, L., Goldschmidt, L., Siva Sankar, D.V.: Treatment of autistic schizophrenic children with LSD-25 and UML-491. Recent Advanc. Biol. Psychiat. **4**, 170–177 (1962)
Bender, L., Faretra, G., Cobrinik, L.: LSD and UML treatment of hospitalized disturbed children. Recent Advanc. Biol. Psychiat. **5**, 84–92 (1963)
Benedetti, G.: Beispiel einer strukturanalytischen und pharmakodynamischen Untersuchung an einem Fall von Alkoholhalluzinose, Charakterneurose and psychoreaktiver Halluzinose. Z. Psychother. med. Psychol. **1**, 177–192 (1951)
Bente, D., Itil, T., Schmid, E.E.: Elektroencephalographische Studien zur Wirkungsweise des LSD 25. Psychiat. et Neurol. (Basel) **135**, 273–284 (1958)
Bercel, N.A., Travis, L.E., Olinger, L.B., Dreikurs, E.: Model psychoses induced by LSD-25 in normals. I. Psychophysiological investigations, with special reference to the mechanism of the paranoid reaction. Arch. Neurol. Psychiat. (Chic.) **75**, 588–611 (1956a)
Bercel, N.A., Travis, L.E., Olinger, L.B., Dreikurs, E.: Model psychoses induced by LSD-25 in normals. II. Rorschach test findings. Arch. Neurol. Psychiat. (Chic.) **75**, 612–618 (1956b)
Berlin, L., Guthrie, T., Weider, A., Goodell, D., Wolff, H.G.: Studies in human cerebral function: the effects of mescaline and lysergic acid on cerebral processes pertinent to creative activity. J. nerv. ment. Dis. **122**, 487–491 (1955)
Bertino, J.R., Klee, G.D., Weintraub, W.: Cholinesterase, d-lysergic acid diethylamide, and 2-bromolysergic acid diethylamide. J. clin. exp. Psychopath. **20**, 218–222 (1959)
Bierer, J., Browne, I.W.: An experiment with a psychiatric night hospital. Proc. roy. Soc. Med. **53**, 930–932 (1960)
Boardman, W.K., Goldstone, S., Lhamon, W.T.: Effects of lysergic acid diethylamide (LSD) on the time sense of normals. Arch. Neurol. Psychiat. **78**, 321–324 (1957)
Bonny, H.L., Pahnke, W.N.: The use of music in psychedelic (LSD) psychotherapy. J. Music Ther. **9**, 64–87 (1972)
Bowen, W.T., Soskin, R.A., Chotlos, J.W.: Lysergic acid diethylamide as a variable in the hospital treatment of alcoholism. A follow-up study. J. nerv. ment. Dis. **150**, 111–118 (1970)
Brengelmann, J.C.: Effects of LSD-25 on test of personality. J. ment. Sci. **104**, 1226–1236 (1958)
Brengelmann, J.C., Laverty, S.G., Lewis, D.J.: Differential effects of lysergic acid and sodium amytal on immediate memory and expressive movement. J. ment. Sci. **104**, 144–152 (1958a)
Brengelmann, J.C., Pare, C.M.B., Sandler, M.: Alleviation of the psychological effects of LSD in man by 5-hydroxytryptophan. J. ment. Sci. **104**, 1237–1244 (1958b)
Brown, F.C.: Hallucinogenic Drugs. Springfield, Illinois: Charles C. Thomas 1972
Brown, B.B., Braun, D.L., Feldman, R.G.: The pharmacologic activity of (4-piperidyl) benzhydrol hydrochloride (azacyclonol hydrochloride) an ataraxic agent. J. Pharmacol. exp. Ther. **118**, 153–161 (1956)
Busch, A.K., Johnson, W.C.: L.S.D. 25 as an aid in psychotherapy. (Preliminary report of a new drug). Dis. nerv. Syst. **11**, 241–243 (1950)
Carlson, V.R.: Effect of lysergic acid diethylamide (LSD-25) on the absolute visual threshold. J. comp. Physiol. Psychol. **51**, 528–531 (1958)
Cerletti, A.: Lysergic acid diethylamide (LSD) and related compounds. In: Neuropharmacology. Transactions of the second conference, May 25–27, 1955, Princeton, N.J., Abramson, H.A. (ed.), pp. 9–84. New York: Josiah Macy, Jr., Foundation 1956
Cerletti, A.: The LSD psychosis. I. Pharmacological aspects of the LSD psychosis. In: Chemical Concepts of Psychosis. Rinkel, M., Denber, H. (eds.), pp. 63–74. New York: McDowell Obolensky 1958
Cerletti, A., Doepfner, W.: Comparative study on the serotonin antagonism of amide derivatives of lysergic acid and of ergot alkaloids. J. Pharmacol. exp. Ther. **122**, 124–136 (1958a)
Cerletti, A., Doepfner, W.: Spezifische Steigerung der serotonin-antagonistischen Wirkung von Lysergsäurederivaten durch Methylierung des Indolstickstoffes der Lysergsäure. Helv. physiol. pharmacol. Acta **16**, C55–C57 (1958b)
Cerletti, A., Rothlin, E.: Role of 5-hydroxytryptamine in mental diseases and its antagonism to lysergic acid derivatives. Nature (Lond.) **176**, 785–786 (1955)
Chandler, A.L., Hartman, M.A.: Lysergic acid diethylamide (LSD-25) as a facilitating agent in psychotherapy. Arch. gen. Psychiat. **2**, 286–299 (1960)

Cholden, L.S., Kurland, A., Savage, C.: Clinical reactions and tolerance to LSD in chronic schizophrenia. J. nerv. ment. Dis. **122**, 211–221 (1955)
Chwelos, N., Blewett, D.B., Smith, C.M., Hoffer, A.: Use of d-lysergic acid diethylamide in the treatment of alcoholism. Quart. J. Stud. Alcohol. **20**, 577–590 (1959)
Clark, L.D.: Further studies of the psychological effects of Frenquel and a critical review of previous reports. J. nerv. ment. Dis. **123**, 557–560 (1956)
Clark, L.D., Clark, L.S.: The effects of cortisone on LSD-25 intoxication in schizophrenic patients. J. nerv. ment. Dis. **123**, 561–562 (1956)
Clark, L.C., Fox, R.P., Benington, F., Morin, R.: Effect of mescaline, lysergic acid diethylamide, and related compounds on respiratory enzyme activity of brain homogenates. Fed. Proc. **13**, 27 (1954)
Clark, L.C., Fox, R.P., Morin, R., Benington, F.: Effects of psychotomimetic compounds on certain oxidative and hydrolytic enzymes in mammalian brain. J. nerv. ment. Dis. **124**, 466–472 (1956)
Cohen, S.: Lysergic acid diethylamide: side effects and complications. J. nerv. ment. Dis. **130**, 30–40 (1960)
Cohen, S.: LSD and the anguish of dying. Harpers Magazine **231**, 69–72, 77–78 (1965)
Cohen, S.: A classification of LSD complications. Psychosomatics **7**, 182–186 (1966)
Cohen, S.: Suicide or accident? Amer. J. Psychiat. **124**, 111 (1967)
Cohen, S.: The psychotomimetic agents. In: Progress in Drug Research. Jucker, E. (ed.), Vol. XV. pp. 68–102, Basel-Stuttgart: Birkhäuser 1971
Cohen, S., Ditman, K.S.: Complications associated with lysergic acid diethylamide (LSD-25). J. Am. med. Ass. **181**, 161–162 (1962)
Cohen, S., Eisner, B.G.: Use of lysergic acid diethylamide in a psychotherapeutic setting. Arch. Neurol. Psychiat. (Chic.) **81**, 615–619 (1959)
Cohen, S., Fichman, L., Eisner, B.G.: Subjective reports of lysergic acid experiences in a context of psychological test performance. Amer. J. Psychiat. **115**, 30–35 (1958)
Cohen, B.D., Rosenbaum, G., Luby, E.D. Gottlieb, J.S.: Comparison of phencyclidine hydrochloride (sernyl) with other drugs. Arch. gen. Psychiat. **6**, 395–401 (1962)
Condrau, G.: Klinische Erfahrungen an Geisteskranken mit Lysergsäure-diäthylamid. Acta psychiat. neurol. scand. **24**, 9–32 (1949)
Delay, J., Pichot, P., Lainé, B., Perse, J.: Les modifications de la personnalité produites par la diéthylamide de l'acide lysergique (LSD-25). Ann. méd.-psychol. **112** (II), 1–13 (1954)
Denson, R.: Complications of therapy with lysergide. Canad. med. Ass. J. **101**, 659–663 (1969)
Denson, R., Sydiaha, D.: A controlled study of LSD treatment in alcoholism and neurosis. Brit. J. Psychiat. **116**, 443–445 (1970)
De Shon, H.J., Rinkel, M., Solomon, H.C.: Mental changes experimentally produced by L.S.D. (d-lysergic acid diethylamide tartrate). Psychiat. Quart. **26**, 33–53 (1952)
Doepfner, W., Cerletti, A.: Comparison of lysergic acid derivatives and anti-histamines as inhibitors of the edema provoked in the rat's paw by serotonin. Int. Arch. Allergy **12**, 89–97 (1958)
Editorial: Diazepam for LSD intoxication. Int. Drug Ther. Newslett. **6**, 31 (1971)
Edwards, A.E., Cohen, S.: Visual illusion, tactile sensibility and reaction time under LSD-25. Psychopharmacologia (Berl.) **2**, 297–303 (1961)
Eisner, B.G.: Notes on the use of drugs to facilitate group psychotherapy. Psychiat. Quart. **38**, 310–328 (1964)
Eisner, B.G., Cohen, S.: Psychotherapy with lysergic acid diethylamide. J. nerv. ment. Dis. **127**, 528–539 (1958)
Elmadjian, F., Hope, J.M., Lamson, E.T.: Excretion of epinephrine and norepinephrine in various emotional states. J. clin. Endocr. **17**, 608–620 (1957)
Evans, F.T.: The effect of several psychotomimetic drugs on human serum cholinesterase. Psychopharmacologia (Berl.) **1**, 231–240 (1960)
Fabing, H.D.: Frenquel, a blocking agent against experimental LSD-25 and mescaline psychosis. Neurology (Minneap.) **5**, 319–328 (1955)
Fink, M., Jaffe, J. Kahn, R.L.: Drug induced changes in interview patterns: linguistic and

neurophysiologic indices. In: The Dynamics of Psychiatric Drug Therapy. Sarwer-Foner, G.J. (ed.), pp. 29–44. Springfield, Illinois: Charles C. Thomas 1960

Fischer, R. Georgi, F., Weber, R.: Psychophysische Korrelationen. Modellversuche zum Schizophrenieproblem. Lysergsäurediäthylamid und Mezcalin. Schweiz. med. Wschr. **81**, 817–838 (1951)

Fisher, S., Cleveland, S.E.: Right-left body reactivity patterns in disorganized states. J. nerv. ment. Dis. **128**, 396–400 (1959)

Foldes, V., Zsigmond, E.K., Erdos, E.G., Foldes, F.F.: Histochemical demonstration of the inhibitory effect of d-lysergic acid diethylamide (LSD) and its congeners on brain cholinesterases. Fed. Proc. **18**, 389 (1959)

Fontana, A.E.: El uso clínico de las drogas alucinógenas. Acta neuropsiquiat. argent. **7**, 94–98 (1961)

Fontana, A.E., Alvarez de Toledo, L.G.: Psicoterapia de grupo y dietilamida del ácido lisérgico. Nuevas aportaciones. Acta neuropsiquiat. argent. **6**, 68–71 (1960)

Forrer, G.R., Goldner, R.D.: Experimental physiological studies with lysergic acid diethylamide (LSD-25). Arch. Neurol. Psychiat. (Chic.) **65**, 581–588 (1951)

Frederking, W.: Über die Verwendung von Rauschdrogen (Meskalin und Lysergsäurediaethylamid) in der Psychotherapie. Psyche **7**, 342–364 (1953/54)

Freedman, A.M., Ebin, E.V., Wilson, E.A.: Autistic schizophrenic children. An experiment in the use of d-lysergic acid diethylamide (LSD-25). Arch. gen. Psychiat. **6**, 203–213 (1962)

Freedman, D.X.: On the use and abuse of LSD. Arch. gen. Psychiat. **18**, 330–347 (1968)

Fried, G.H., Antopol, W.: The effects of psychotomimetic compounds on human cholinesterase. Anat. Rec. **125**, 610 (1956)

Fried, G.H., Antopol, W.: Effects of psychotomimetic compounds on human pseudocholinesterase. J. appl. Physiol. **11**, 25–28 (1957)

Friedman, S.A., Hirsch, S.E.: Extreme hyperthermia after LSD ingestion. J. Amer. med. Ass. **217**, 1549–1550 (1971)

Frosch, W.A., Robbins, E.S., Stern, M.: Untoward reactions to lysergic acid diethylamide (LSD) resulting in hospitalization. New Engl. J. Med. **273**, 1235–1239 (1965)

Gastaut, H., Ferrer, S., Castells, C., Lesevre, N., Luschnat, K.: Action de la diéthylamide de l'acide d-lysergique (LSD-25) sur les fonctions psychiques et l'électroencéphalogramme. Confin. neurol. (Basel) **13**, 102–120 (1953)

Geert-Jörgensen, E., Hertz, M., Knudsen, K., Kristensen, K.: LSD-treatment. Experience gained within a three-year-period. Acta psychiat. scand. **40** (Suppl. 180), 373–382 (1964)

Geronimus, L.H., Abramson, H.A., Ingraham, L.J.: Lysergic acid diethylamide (LSD-25): XXIII. Comparative effects of LSD-25 and related ergot drugs on brain tissue respiration and on human behavior. J. Psychol. **42**, 157–168 (1956)

Giberti, F., Gregoretti, L.: Prime esperienze di antagonismo psicofarmacologico. Psicosi sperimentale da LSD e trattamento con cloropromazina e reserpina. Sist. nerv. **7**, 301–310 (1955)

Giberti, F., Gregoretti, L.: Studio comparativo degli effetti psicopatologici della monoetilamide dell'acido lisergico (L.A.E.32) e della dietilamide dell'acido lisergico (L.S.D.25) in soggetti neurotici. Sist. nerv. **10**, 97–110 (1958)

Giberti, F., Gregoretti, L. Boeri, G.: L'impiego della dietilamide dell'acido lisergico nelle psiconevrosi. Considerazioni e principii preliminari di valutazione diagnostico-terapeutica. Sist. nerv. **8**, 191–208 (1956)

Ginzel, K.H., Mayer-Gross, W.: Prevention of psychological effects of d-lysergic acid diethylamide (LSD-25) by its 2-brom derivative (BOL 148). Nature (Lond.) **178**, 210 (1956)

Gogerty, J.H., Dille, J.M.: Pharmacology of d-lysergic acid morpholide (LSM). J. Pharmacol. exp. Ther. **120**, 340–348 (1957)

Gomirato, G., Gamna, G., Pascal, E.: Il disegno dell'albero applicato allo studio delle modificazioni pricopatologiche indotte dalla dietilamide dell'acido d-lisergico in schizofrenici. G. Psichiat. Neuropat. **86**, 433–483 (1958)

Gorodetzky, C.W., Isbell, H.: A comparison of 2,3-dihydrolysergic acid diethylamide with LSD-25. Psychopharmacologia (Berl.) **6**, 229–233 (1964)

Graham, J.R.: Methysergide for prevention of headache. Experience in five hundred patients over three years. New Engl. J. Med. **270**, 67–72 (1964)

Grof, S., Dytrych, Z.: Blocking of LSD reaction by premedication with niamid. Activ. nerv. sup. (Praha) **7**, 306 (1965)
Grof, S., Goodman, L.E., Richards, W.A., Kurland, A.A.: LSD-assisted psychotherapy in patients with terminal cancer. Int. Pharmacopsychiat. **8**, 129–144 (1973)
Hale, A.R., Reed, A.F.: Prophylaxis of frequent vascular headache with methysergide. Amer. J. med. Sci. **243**, 92–98 (1962)
Haley, T.J.: 5-hydroxytryptamine antagonism by lysergic acid diethylamide after intracerebral injection in conscious mice. J. Am. pharm. Ass. **46**, 428–430 (1957)
Harding, T.: The effect of lysergic acid diethylamide on serum creatine kinase levels. Psychopharmacologia (Berl.) **40**, 177–184 (1974)
Heim, E., Heimann, H., Lukacs, G.: Die psychische Wirkung der mexikanischen Droge „Ololiuqui" am Menschen. Psychopharmacologia (Berl.) **13**, 35–48 (1968)
Heimann, H.: Die Wirkung von Ololiuqui im Unterschied zu Psilocybin. Neuropsychopharm. **4**, 474–477 (1965)
Henkin, R., Buchsbaum, M., Welpton, D., Zahn, T., Scott, W., Wynne, L., Silverman, J.: Physiological and psychological effects of LSD in chronic users. Clin. Res. **15**, 484 (1967)
Hirsch, M.W., Jarvik, M.E., Abramson, H.A.: Lysergic acid diethylamide (LSD-25): XVIII. Effects of LSD-25 and six related drugs upon handwriting. J. Psychol. **41**, 11–22 (1956)
Hoagland, H., Rinkel, M. Hyde, R.W.: Adrenocortical function and urinary phosphate excretion. Comparison in schizophrenia and in lysergic acid diethylamide-induced psychotic episodes in normal persons. Arch. Neurol. Psychiat. **73**, 100–109 (1955)
Hoch, P.: Studies in routes of administration and counteracting drugs. In: Lysergic Acid Diethylamide and Mescaline in Experimental Psychiatry. Cholden, L. (ed.), pp. 8–12. New York–London: Grune and Stratton 1956a
Hoch, P.H.: The production and alleviation of mental abnormalities by drugs. XXth International Physiological Congress, Brussels, July 30th-August 4th, 1956b. Abstracts of Reviews, pp. 429–442
Hoch, P.H., Cattell, J.P., Pennes, H.H.: Effects of mescaline and lysergic acid (d-LSD-25). Amer. J. Psychiat. **108**, 579–584 (1952)
Hoffer, A.: D-lysergic acid diethylamide (LSD): a review of its present status. Clin. Pharmacol. Ther. **2**, 183–255 (1965)
Hoffer, A., Osmond, H., Smythies, J.: Schizophrenia: a new approach. II. Result of a year's research. J. ment. Sci. **100**, 29–45 (1954)
Hoffer, A., Smith, C., Chwelos, N., Callbeck, M.J., Mahon, M.: Psychological response to d-lysergic acid diethylamide and its relationship to adrenochrome levels. J. clin. exp. Psychopath. **20**, 125–134 (1959)
Hofmann, A.: Relationship between spatial arrangement and mental effects. In: Chemical Concepts of Psychosis. Rinkel, M., Denber, H.C.B. (eds.), pp. 85–90. New York: McDowell-Obolensky 1958
Hofmann, A.: Die Wirkstoffe der mexikanischen Zauberdroge „Ololiuqui". Planta med. (Stuttg.) **9**, 354–367 (1961)
Hofmann, A.: The active principles of the seeds of rivea corymbosa and ipomoea violacea. Botanical Museum Leaflets Harvard University **20**, 194–212 (1963)
Hofmann, A.: Die Mutterkornalkaloide. Stuttgart: Ferdinand Enke Verlag 1964
Hofmann, A.: The discovery of LSD and subsequent investigations on naturally occurring hallucinogens. In: Discoveries in Biological Psychiatry. Ayd, F.J., Blackwell, B. (eds.), pp. 91–106. Philadelphia–Toronto: J.B. Lippincott 1970a
Hofmann, A.: Notes and documents concerning the discovery of LSD. Agents Actions **1**, 148–150 (1970b)
Hofmann, A., Cerletti, A.: Die Wirkstoffe der dritten aztekischen Zauberdroge. Die Lösung des „Ololiuqui"-Rätsels. Dtsch. med. Wschr. **86**, 885–888 (1961)
Hofmann, A., Tscherter, H.: Isolierung von Lysergsäure-Alkaloiden aus der mexikanischen Zauberdroge Ololiuqui. Experientia (Basel) **16**, 414 (1960)
Horackova, E., Mosinger, B., Vojtechovsky, M.: Square test for investigating the concentration of attention in experimental psychosis evoked by diethylamide lysergic acid (LSD-25). Čs. Psychiat. **54**, 236–243 (1958)

Horita, A., Gogerty, J.H.: The pyretogenic effect of 5-hydroxytryptophan and its comparison with that of LSD. J. Pharmacol. exp. Ther. **122**, 195–200 (1958)
Horowitz, H.A.: The use of lithium in the treatment of the drug-induced psychotic reaction. Dis. nerv. Syst. **36**, 159–163 (1975)
Horowitz, M.J.: Flashbacks: recurrent intrusive images after the use of LSD. Amer. J. Psychiat. **126**, 565–569 (1969)
Hurst, L.A., Reuning, H., van Wyk, A.J., Crouse, H.S., Booysen, P.J., Nelson, G.: Experiences with d-lysergic acid diethylamide (LSD). A symposium. S.A.J. Lab. clin. Med. **2**, 289–310 (1956)
Huxley, A.: The Doors of Perception. New York: Harper and Brothers 1954
Huxley, A.: Heaven and Hell. London: Chatto and Windus 1956
Isbell, H.: Effects of various drugs on the LSD reaction. In: Psychopharmacology Frontiers. Kline, N.S. (ed.), pp. 361–364. Boston-Toronto: Little, Brown 1959
Isbell, H.: Personal communication 1962
Isbell, H., Gorodetzky, C.W.: Effect of alkaloids of Ololiuqui in man. Psychopharmacologia (Berl.) **8**, 331–339 (1966)
Isbell, H., Jasinski, D.R.: A comparison of LSD-25 with (-)-Δ^9-Trans-Tetrahydrocannabinol (THC) and attempted cross tolerance between LSD and THC. Psychopharmacologia (Berl.) **14**, 115–123 (1969)
Isbell, H., Logan, C.R.: Studies on the diethylamide of lysergic acid (LSD-25). II. Effects of chlorpromazine, azacyclonol, and reserpine on the intensity of the LSD-reaction. Arch. Neurol. Psychiat. **77**, 350–358 (1957)
Isbell, H., Belleville, R.E., Fraser, H.F., Wikler, A., Logan, C.R.: Studies on lysergic acid diethylamide (LSD-25). I. Effects in former morphine addicts and development of tolerance during chronic intoxication. Arch. Neurol. Psychiat. **76**, 468–478 (1956)
Isbell, H., Miner, E.J., Logan, C.R.: Relationships of psychotomimetic to anti-serotonin potencies of congeners of lysergic acid diethylamide (LSD-25). Psychopharmacologia (Berl.) **1**, 20–28 (1959a)
Isbell, H., Miner, E.J., Logan, C.R.: Cross tolerance between d-2-brom-lysergic acid diethylamide (BOL-148) and the d-diethylamide of lysergic acid (LSD-25). Psychopharmacologia (Berl.) **1**, 109–116 (1959b)
Isbell, H., Wolbach, A.B., Wikler, A., Miner, E.J.: Cross tolerance between LSD and Psilocybin. Psychopharmacologia (Berl.) **2**, 147–159 (1961)
Itil, T.M., Keskiner, A., Holden, J.M.C.: The use of LSD and ditran in the treatment of therapy resistant schizophrenics. Dis. nerv. Syst. **30** (Suppl. 2), 93–103 (1969)
Jarvik, M.E., Abramson, H.A., Hirsch, M.W.: Comparative subjective effects of seven drugs including lysergic acid diethylamide (LSD-25). J. abnorm. soc. Psychol. **51**, 657–662 (1955a)
Jarvik, M.E., Abramson, H.A., Hirsch, M.W.: Lysergic acid diethylamide (LSD-25): IV. Effect on attention and concentration. J. Psychol. **39**, 373–383 (1955b)
Jarvik, M.E., Abramson, H.A., Hirsch, M.W.: Lysergic acid diethylamide (LSD-25): VI. Effect upon recall and recognition of various stimuli. J. Psychol. **39**, 443–454 (1955c)
Jarvik, M.E., Abramson, H.A., Hirsch, M.W., Ewald, A.T.: Lysergic acid diethylamide (LSD-25): VIII. Effect on arithmetic test performance. J. Psychol. **39**, 465–473 (1955d)
Jensen, S.E., Ramsay, R.: Treatment of chronic alcoholism with lysergic acid diethylamide. Canad. psychiat. Ass. J. **8**, 182–188 (1963)
Johnson, F.G.: LSD in the treatment of alcoholism. Amer. J. Psychiat. **126**, 481–487 (1969)
Jost, F.: Zur therapeutischen Verwendung des LSD XXV in der klinischen Praxis der Psychiatrie. Wien. klin. Wschr. **69**, 647–651 (1957)
Kast, E.C.: The analgesic action of lysergic acid compared with dihydromorphinone and meperidine. Bull. Drug Addict. Narcot. Appendix **27**, 3517–3529 (1963)
Kast, E.: LSD and the dying patient. Chicago Med. School Quart. **26**, 80–87 (1966)
Kast, E.: Attenuation of anticipation: a therapeutic use of lysergic acid diethylamide. Psychiat. Quart. **41**, 646–657 (1967)
Kast, E.C., Collins, V.J.: A study of lysergic acid diethylamide as an analgesic agent. Anaesth. Analg. Curr. Res. **43**, 285–291 (1964)
Klee, G.D., Weintraub, W.: Paranoid reactions following lysergic acid diethylamide (LSD-25). In: Neuro-Psychopharmacology. Proc. 1st Int. Congr. Neuro-Psychopharmacology, Rome,

Sept. 1958. Bradley, P.B., Deniker, P., Radouco-Thomas, C. (eds.), pp. 457–460. Amsterdam-London-New York-Princeton: Elsevier 1959
Klock, J.C., Boerner, U., Becker, C.E.: Coma, hyperthermia and bleeding associated with massive LSD overdose: a report of eight cases. West. J. Med. **120** (3), 183–188 (1974)
Knudsen, K.: Homicide after treatment with lysergic acid diethylamide. Acta psychiat. scand. **40** (Suppl. 180), 389–395 (1964)
Kornetsky, C., Humphries, O.: Relationship between effects of a number of centrally acting drugs and personality. Arch. Neurol. Psychiat. (Chic.) **77**, 325–327 (1957)
Kornetzsky, C., Humphries, O., Evarts, E.V.: Comparison of psychological effects of certain centrally acting drugs in man. Arch. Neurol. Psychiat. (Chic.) **77**, 318–324 (1957)
Krill, A.E., Wieland, A.M., Ostfeld, A.M.: The effect of two hallucinogenic agents on human retinal function. Arch. Ophthal. **64**, 724–733 (1960)
Krill, A.E., Alpert, H.J., Ostfeld, A.M.: Effects of a hallucinogenic agent in totally blind subjects. Arch. Ophthal. **69**, 180–185 (1963)
Krus, D.M., Wapner, S.: Effect of lysergic acid diethylamide (LSD-25) on perception of part-whole relationships. J. Psychol. **48**, 87–95 (1959)
Krus, D.M., Wapner, S., Bergen, J., Freeman, H.: The influence of progesterone on behavioral changes induced by lysergic acid diethylamide (LSD-25) in normal males. Psychopharmacologia (Berl.) **2**, 177–184 (1961)
Krus, D.M., Resnick, O., Raskin, M.: Apparent eye level test. Its background and use in psychopharmacology. Arch. gen. Psychiat. **14**, 419–427 (1966)
Kurland, A.A., Unger, S., Shaffer, J.W., Savage, C.: Psychedelic therapy utilizing LSD in the treatment of the alcoholic patient: a preliminary report. Amer. J. Psychiat. **123**, 1202–1209 (1967)
Kurland, A.A., Savage, C., Unger, S.: LSD in psychiatric treatment. Clin. Psychopharmacol. Mod. Probl. Pharmacopsychiat. **1**, 273–284 (1968)
Kurland, A.A., Savage, C., Pahnke, W.N., Grof, S., Olsson, J.E.: LSD in the treatment of alcoholics. Pharmakopsychiatr. Neuropsychopharmakol. **4**, 83–94 (1971)
Kurland, A.A., Grof, S., Pahnke, W.N., Goodman, L.E.: Psychedelic drug assisted psychotherapy in patients with terminal cancer. In: Psychopharmacological Agents for the Terminally Ill and Bereaved. Goldberg, I.K., Malitz, S., Kutscher, A.H. (eds.), pp. 86–133. New York-London: Columbia Univ. Press 1973
Landis, C., Clausen, J.: Certain effects of mescaline and lysergic acid on psychological functions. J. Psychol. **38**, 211–221 (1954)
Langs, R.J., Barr, H.L.: Lysergic acid diethylamide (LSD-25) and schizophrenic reactions. J. nerv. ment. Dis. **147**, 163–172 (1968)
Leary, T.: The religious experience: its production and interpretation. Psychedelic Rev. **1**, 324–346 (1964)
Leary, T., Alpert, R.: The politics of consciousness expansion. Harvard Rev. **1**, 33–37 (1963)
Lebovits, B.Z., Visotsky, H.M., Ostfeld, A.M.: LSD and JB 318: a comparison of two hallucinogens. I. An exploratory study. Arch. gen. Psychiat. **2**, 390–407 (1960a)
Lebovits, B.Z., Visotsky, H.M., Ostfeld, A.M.: Lysergic acid diethylamide (LSD) and JB 318: a comparison of two hallucinogens. II. An exploratory study. Arch. gen. Psychiat. **3**, 176–187 (1960b)
Lebovits, B.Z., Visotsky, H.M., Ostfeld, A.M.: LSD and JB 318: a comparison of two hallucinogens. III. Qualitative analysis and summary of findings. Arch. gen. Psychiat. **7**, 39–45 (1962)
Lesse, S.: Psychodynamic relationships between the degree of anxiety and other clinical symptoms. J. nerv. ment. Dis. **127**, 124–130 (1958)
Lesse, S.: Discussion on drug research. In: IInd International Congress for Psychiatry. Congress Report: Vol. II, pp. 324–325. Zürich: Orell Füssli 1959
Leuner, H.: Die experimentelle Psychose. Berlin-Göttingen-Heidelberg: Springer 1962
Leuner, H.: Die Psycholytische Therapie: klinische Psychotherapie mit Hilfe von LSD-25 und verwandten Substanzen. Z. Psychother. med. Psychol. **13**, 57–64 (1963a)
Leuner, H.: Psychotherapy with hallucinogens. A clinical report with special reference to the revival of emotional phases of childhood. In: Proc. Quart. Meet. Royal Med. Psychol. Assoc., London, February 1961, pp. 67–73. London: H.K. Lewis 1963b

Leuner, H.: Über den Rauschmittelmißbrauch Jugendlicher. Nervenarzt **42**, 281–291 (1971a)
Leuner, H.: Halluzinogene in der Psychotherapie. Pharmakopsychiatr. Neuropsychopharmakol. **4**, 333–351 (1971b)
Leuner, H., Holfeld, H.: Ergebnisse und Probleme der Psychotherapie mit Hilfe von LSD-25 und verwandten Substanzen. Psychiat. et Neurol. (Basel) **143**, 379–391 (1962)
Levine, A., Abramson, H.A., Kaufman, M.R., Markham, S.: Lysergic acid diethylamide (LSD-25): XVI. The effect on intellectual functioning as measured by the Wechsler-Bellevue intelligence scale. J. Psychol. **40**, 385–395 (1955a)
Levine, A., Abramson, H.A., Kaufman, M.R., Markham, S., Kornetsky, C.: Lysergic acid diethylamide (LSD-25): XIV. Effect on personality as observed in psychological tests. J. Psychol. **40**, 351–366 (1955b)
Levy, R.M.: Diazepam for LSD intoxication. Lancet **1971 I,** 1297
Lewis, D.J., Sloane, R.B.: Therapy with lysergic acid diethylamide. J. clin. exp. Psychopath. **19**, 19–31 (1958)
Liddell, D.W., Weil-Malherbe, H.: The effects of methedrine and of lysergic acid diethylamide on mental processes and on the blood adrenaline level. J. Neurol. Neurosurg. Psychiat. **16**, 7–13 (1953)
Liebert, R.S., Werner, H., Wapner, S.: Studies in the effect of lysergic acid diethylamide (LSD-25). Self- and object-size perception in schizophrenics and normal adults. Arch. Neurol. Psychiat. (Chic.) **79**, 580–584 (1958)
Lienert, G.A.: Pharmakopsychologische Untersuchungen über den Abbau der geistigen Leistungsfähigkeit. Bericht über den 20. Kongreß der Deutschen Gesellschaft für Psychologie, Berlin, 1955, pp. 144–147. Göttingen: Verlag für Psychologie (Dr. C.J. Hogrefe) 1956
Lienert, G.A.: Über eigenartige Motivationsvorgänge unter Wirkung von Lysergsäure-Diäthylamid. Bericht über den 21. Kongreß der Deutschen Gesellschaft für Psychologie, Bonn, 1957, pp. 202–205. Göttingen: Verlag für Psychologie (Dr. C.J. Hogrefe) 1958
Lienert, G.A.: Changes in the factor structure of intelligence tests produced by d-lysergic acid diethylamide (LSD). In: Neuro-Psychopharmacology. Proc. 1st Int. Congr. Neuro-Psychopharmacology, Rome, Sept. 1958. Bradley, P.B., Deniker, P., Radouco-Thomas, C. (eds.), pp. 461–465. Amsterdam-London-New York-Princeton: Elsevier 1959
Lienert, G.A.: Die Farbwahl im Farbpyramidentest unter Lysergsäurediätylamid (LSD). Versuch einer experimentellen Prüfung klinischer Gültigkeitshypothesen. Z. exp. angew. Psychol. **8**, 110–121 (1961)
Ling, T.M., Buckman, J.: The use of lysergic acid in individual psychotherapy. Proc. roy. Soc. Med. **53**, 927–929 (1960)
Ling, T.M., Buckman, J.: Lysergic acid (LSD 25) and Ritalin in the treatment of neurosis. London: The Lambarde Press 1963
Linken, A.: Propranolol for LSD-induced anxiety states. Lancet **1971 II**, 1039–1040
Linton, H.B., Langs, R.J.: Subjective reactions to lysergic acid diethylamide (LSD-25). Measured by a questionnaire. Arch. gen. Psychiat. **6**, 352–368 (1962)
Loeb, C., Giberti, F.: Lysergic acid diethylamide effects modified by hydroxyzine hydrochloride. Confin. neurol. (Basel) **19**, 40–51 (1959)
Louria, D.B.: Lysergic acid diethylamide. New Engl. J. Med. **278**, 435–438 (1968)
Ludwig, A.M., Levine, J.: Patterns of hallucinogenic drug abuse. J. Amer. med. Ass. **191**, 92–96 (1965a)
Ludwig, A.M., Levine, J.: A controlled comparison of five brief treatment techniques employing LSD, hypnosis and psychotherapy. Amer. J. Psychother. **19**, 417–435 (1965b)
Ludwig, A., Levine, J., Stark, L., Lazar, R.: A clinical study of LSD treatment in alcoholism. Amer. J. Psychiat. **126**, 59–69 (1969)
Ludwig, A.M., Levine, J., Stark, L.H.: LSD and Alcoholism. A clinical study of treatment efficacy. Springfield, Illinois: Charles C. Thomas 1970
Maccagnani, G., Bobon, J., Goffioul, F.: Exploration sous psychodysleptiques du contenu latent de dessins schizophréniques stéréotypés. Encéphale **53**, 543–552 (1964)
McGlothlin, W., Cohen, S., McGlothlin, M.S.: Long lasting effects of LSD on normals. Arch. gen. Psychiat. **17**, 521–532 (1967)
McGlothlin, W.H., Arnold, D.O., Freedman, D.X.: Organicity measures following repeated LSD ingestion. Arch. gen. Psychiat. **21**, 704–709 (1969)

McGlothlin, W.H., Arnold, D.O.: LSD revisited. A ten-year follow-up of medical LSD use. Arch. gen. Psychiat. **24**, 35–49 (1971)
Machover, K., Liebert, R.: Human figure drawings of schizophrenic and normal adults. Changes following administration of lysergic acid. Arch. gen. Psychiat. **3**, 139–152 (1960)
Malitz, S., Wilkens, B., Roehrig, W.C., Hoch, P.H.: A clinical comparison of three related hallucinogens. Psychiat. Quart. **34**, 333–345 (1960)
Malitz, S., Wilkens, B., Esecover, H.: A comparison of drug-induced hallucinations with those seen in spontaneously occurring psychoses. In: Hallucinations. West, C.J. (ed.), pp. 50–63. New York-London: Grune and Stratton 1962
Manger, W.M., Schwarz, B.E., Baars, C.W., Wakim, K.G., Boliman, J.L., Petersen, M.C., Berkson, J.: Plasma and cerebrospinal fluid concentrations of epinephrine and norepinephrine in certain psychiatric conditons. XXth International Physiological Congress, Brussels 1956. Abstracts of Communications, p. 610
Martin, A.J.: L.S.D. (Lysergic acid diethylamide) treatment of chronic psychoneurotic patients under day-hospital conditions. Int. J. soc. Psychiat. **3**, 188–195 (1957)
Martin, A.J.: The treatment of twelve male homosexuals with L.S.D. (followed by a detailed account of one of them who was a psychopathic personality). Acta psychother. **10**, 394–402 (1962)
Matefi, L.: Mezcalin- und Lysergsäurediäthylamid-Rausch. Selbstversuche mit besonderer Berücksichtigung eines Zeichentests. Confin. neurol. (Basel) **12**, 146–177 (1952)
Mayer-Gross, W., McAdam, W., Walker, J.: Lysergsäure-Diäthylamid und Kohlenhydratstoffwechsel. Vorläufige Mitteilung. Nervenarzt **23**, 30–31 (1952)
Mayer-Gross, W., McAdam, W., Walker, J.W.: Further observations on the effects of lysergic acid diethylamide. J. ment. Sci. **99**, 804–808 (1953)
Meltzer, H.: Creatine kinase and aldolase in serum; abnormality common to acute psychoses. Science **159**, 1368–1370 (1968)
Meltzer, H.Y.: Plasma creatine phosphokinase levels in rats following lysergic acid diethylamide. Psychopharmacologia (Berl.) **44**, 91–93 (1975)
Miller, A.I., Williams, H.L., Murphree, H.P.: Niacin, niacinamide, or atropine versus LSD-25 model psychoses in human volunteers. J. Pharmacol. exp. Ther. **119**, 169 (1957)
Milman, D.H.: An untoward reaction to accidental ingestion of LSD in a 5-year-old girl. J. Am. med. Ass. **201**, 821–824 (1967)
Monroe, R.R., Heath, R.G., Mickle, W.A., Llewellyn, R.C.: Correlation of rhinencephalic electrograms with behavior. A study on humans under the influence of LSD and mescaline. EEG Clin. Neurophysiol. **9**, 623–642 (1957)
Murphree, H.B., de Maar, E.W.J., Williams, H.L., Bryan, L.L.: Effects of lysergic acid derivatives on man; antagonism between d-lysergic acid diethylamide and its 2-brom congener. J. Pharmacol. exp. Ther. **122**, 55A (1958)
O'Reilly, P.O., Reich, G.: Lysergic acid and the alcoholic. Dis. nerv. Syst. **23**, 331–334 (1962)
Orsini, F., Benda, P.: Etude expérimentale du ralentissement de la performance sous LSD-25. Ann. méd.-psychol. **117**, 519–525 (1959)
Orsini, F., Benda, P.: L'épreuve du dessin en miroir sous LSD-25. Ann. méd.-psychol. **118**, 809–816 (1960)
Osmond, H.: Ololiuqui: the ancient aztec narcotic. Remarks on the effects of rivea corymbosa (Ololiuqui). J. ment. Sci. **101**, 526–537 (1955)
Osmond, H.: Research on schizophrenia. In: Neuropharmacology. Transactions of the second conference, Princeton, N.J., May 25–27, 1955. Abramson, H.A. (ed.), pp. 183–233. New York: Josiah Macy, Jr., Foundation 1956
Osmond, H.: A review of the clinical effects of psychotomimetic agents. Ann. N.Y. Acad. Sci. **66**, 418–434 (1958)
Pahnke, W.H., Kurland, A.A., Goodman, L.E., Richards, W.A.: LSD-assisted psychotherapy with terminal cancer patients. In: Psychedelic Drugs. Proceedings of a Hahnemann Medical College and Hospital Symposium, Philadelphia, Nov. 22–24, 1968. Hicks, R.E., Fink, P.J. (eds.), pp. 33–42. New York-London: Grune and Stratton 1969
Pauk, Z.D., Shagass, C.: Some test findings associated with susceptibility to psychosis induced by lysergic acid diethylamide. Comprehens. Psychiat. **2**, 188–195 (1961)

Pérez Morales, F.: El LSD 25 en psicoterapia. Su fundamentación histórica y metodológica. Acta psiquiát. psicol. argent. **9**, 33–39 (1963a)
Pérez Morales, F.: El LSD 25 en la psicoterapia. Psicoterapia individual. Acta psiquiát. psicol. argent. **9**, 136–143 (1963b)
Pérez Morales, F.: Psicoterapia y LSD 25 (III). Acta psiquiát. psicol. argent. **9**, 226–232 (1963c)
Perillo, A.E., Garcia de la Villa, A.: Experiencia farmacológica en el discutido terreno de la demencia esquizofrénica. Acta psiquiát. psicol. argent. **9**, 49–52 (1963)
Pfeiffer, C.C., Goldstein, L., Murphree, H.B., Sugerman, A.: Time-series, frequency analysis, and electrogenesis of the EEGs of normals and psychotics before and after drugs. Amer. J. Psychiat. **121**, 1147–1155 (1965)
Pierce, J.: Zur Wirkung von Atarax auf die LSD-Modellpsychose. Praxis **50**, 486–491 (1961)
Poloni, A.: Serotonina e schizofrenia. Osservazioni sulle interferenze fra l'azione della serotonina (S.) e della dietilamide dell'acido lisergico (LSD-25), mescalina (M.) e bulbocapnina (B.) nell'uomo e nell'animale. Cervello **31**, 271–294 (1955)
Priori, R.: Esperienza interiore e linguaggio nella "model psychosis" indotta da LSD-25. Lav. neuropsichiat. **21**, 209–224 (1957)
Purpura, D.P., Pool, J.L., Ransohoff, J., Frumin, M.J., Housepian, E.M.: Observations on evoked dentritic potentials of human cortex. EEG Clin. Neurophysiol. **9**, 453–459 (1957)
Richards, N., Chapman, L.F., Goodell, H., Wolff, H.G.: LSD-like delirium following ingestion of a small amount of its brom analog (BOL-148). Ann. intern. Med. **48**, 1078–1083 (1958)
Rinkel, M.: Experimentally induced psychoses in man. In: Neuropharmacology. Transactions of the second conference, Princeton, N.J., May 25–27, 1955. Abramson, H.A. (ed.), pp. 235–258. New York: Josiah Macy, Jr., Foundation 1956
Rinkel, M., De Shon, H.J., Hyde, R.W., Solomon, H.C.: Experimental schizophrenia-like symptoms. Amer. J. Psychiat. **108**, 572–578 (1952)
Rinkel, M., Hyde, R.W., Solomon, H.C., Hoagland, H.: Experimental psychiatry II. Clinical and physio-chemical observations in experimental psychosis. Amer. J. Psychiat. **111**, 881–895 (1955)
Robinson, J.T., Davies, L.S., Sack, E.L.N.S., Morrissey, J.D.: A controlled trial of abreaction with lysergic acid diethylamide (LSD 25). Brit. J. Psychiat. **109**, 46–53 (1963)
Rojas Bermudez, J.G.: Tratamiento combinado de psicoanálisis y LSD 25 en niños psicóticos. Acta neuropsiquiát. argent. **6**, 497–500 (1960)
Rojo Sierra, M.: Terapéutica lisérgica en ciertos síndromes obsesivos y neurosis sexuales. Act. luso-esp. Neurol. **18**, 108–113 (1959)
Rojo Sierra, M.: El LSD 25 y la psicoterapia en grupo. Rev. Psiquiat. Psicol. méd. **4**, 419–422 (1960)
Rosenbaum, G., Cohen, B.D., Luby, E.D., Gottlieb, J.S., Yelen, D.: Comparison of sernyl with other drugs. Simulation of schizophrenic performance with sernyl, LSD-25, and amobarbital (amytal) sodium; I. Attention, motor function, and proprioception. Arch. gen. Psychiat. **1**, 651–656 (1959)
Rosenberg, D.E., Wolbach, A.B., Miner, E.J., Isbell, H.: Observations on direct and cross tolerance with LSD and d-amphetamine in man. Psychopharmacologia (Berl.) **5**, 1–15 (1963)
Rosenberg, D.E., Isbell, H., Miner, E.J., Logan, C.R.: The effect of N,N-dimethyltryptamine in human subjects tolerant to lysergic acid diethylamide. Psychopharmacologia (Berl.) **5**, 217–227 (1964)
Rosenthal, S.H.: Persistent hallucinosis following repeated administration of hallucinogenic drugs. Amer. J. Psychiat. **121**, 238–244 (1964)
Rothlin, E.: Pharmacology of lysergic acid diethylamide and some of its related compounds. J. Pharm. Pharmacol. **9**, 569–587 (1957)
Roubicek, J.: Experimentelle psychische Störungen. Vesmir **35**, 291–294 (1956)
Roubicek, J.: Similarities and differences between schizophrenia and experimental psychoses. Rev. Czechoslov. Med. **4**, 125–134 (1958a)
Roubicek, J.: Similarities and dissimilarities between experimental psychoses and schizophrenia. Čsl. Psychiat. **54**, 108–115 (1958b)
Roubicek, J.: Experimentální Psychosy. Praha: Státní Zdravotnické Nakladatelství 1961

Samuelsson, B.O.: LSD intoxication in a two-year-old child. Acta paediat. scand. **63**, 797–798 (1974)
Sandison, R.A.: Psychological aspects of the LSD treatment of the neuroses. J. ment. Sci. **100**, 508–515 (1954)
Sandison, R.A.: The role of psychotropic drugs in individual therapy. Bull. Wld. Hlth. Org. **21**, 495–503 (1959a)
Sandison, R.A.: Discussion fourth symposium: comparison of drug-induced and endogenous psychoses in man. In: Neuro-Psychopharmacology. Proc. 1st Int. Congr. Neuro-Psychopharmacology, Rome, Sept. 1958. Bradley, P.B., Deniker, P., Radouco-Thomas, C. (eds.), pp. 176–182. Amsterdam-London-New York-Princeton: Elsevier 1959b
Sandison, R.A.: The nature of the psychological response to LSD. In: The Use of LSD in Psychotherapy. Transactions of a Conference on D-Lysergic Acid Diethylamide (LSD-25). April 22–24, 1959. Abramson, H.A. (ed.), pp. 81–149. New York: Josiah Macy, Jr., Foundation 1960
Sandison, R.A.: The hallucinogenic drugs. Practitioner **200**, 244–250 (1968)
Sandison, R.A., Spencer, A.M., Whitelaw, J.D.A.: The therapeutic value of lysergic acid diethylamide in mental illness. J. ment. Sci. **100**, 491–507 (1954)
Sandison, R.A., Whitelaw, J.D.A.: Further studies in the therapeutic value of lysergic acid diethylamide in mental illness. J. ment. Sci. **103**, 332–343 (1957)
Sandoz Research Laboratories: Pharmacologic properties and psychotogenic effects of some lysergic acid derivatives. Comparison with Delysid (LSD 25). Scientific Exhibit, Fed. Proc. **17**, 682 (1958)
Sandoz Research Laboratories: Unpublished data, 1959
Sanguineti, I., Zapparoli, G.C., Laricchia, R.: Studio clinico-biologico delle reazioni indotte dal solfato di mescalina e dall'acido lisergico (LSD 25) in malati di mente. Riv. sper. Freniat. **80**, 887–918 (1956)
Sauri, J.J., De Onorato, A.C.: Las esquizofrenias y la dietilamida del acido d-lisergico (LSD-25). I. Variaciones del estado de animo. Acta neuropsiquiát. argent. **1**, 469–476 (1955)
Savage, C.: Lysergic acid diethylamide (LSD-25). A clinical psychological study. Amer. J. Psychiat. **108**, 896–900 (1952)
Savage, C.: The resolution and subsequent remobilization of resistance by LSD in psychotherapy. J. nerv. ment. Dis. **125**, 434–437 (1957)
Savage, C.: The uses and abuses of LSD in psychotherapy. In: Third World Congress of Psychiatry, Montreal 4.–10. 6., 1961, Part II, p. 466
Savage, C.: LSD, alcoholism and transcendence. J. nerv. ment. Dis. **135**, 429–435 (1962)
Savage, C., McCabe, O.L.: Residential psychedelic (LSD) therapy for the narcotic addict. Arch. gen. Psychiatry **28**, 808–814 (1973)
Scherbel, A.L., Harrison, J.W.: Response to serotonin and its antagonists in patients with rheumatoid arthritis and related diseases. Angiology **10**, 29–33 (1959)
Schiefer, I., Bähr, G., Boiselle, I., Kiefer, B.: EEG-Veränderungen von 9 Kindern mit einer LSD-Vergiftung. Klin. Pädiat. **184**, 307–311 (1972)
Schneckloth, R., Page, I.H., Del Greco, F., Corcoran, A.C.: Effects of serotonin antagonists in normal subjects and patients with carcinoid tumors. Circulation **16**, 523–532 (1957)
Schwarz, B.E., Bickford, R.G., Rome, H.P.: Reversibility of induced psychosis with chlorpromazine. Proc. Mayo Clin. **30**, 407–417 (1955)
Schwarz, B.E., Sem-Jacobsen, C.W., Petersen, M.C.: Effects of mescaline, LSD-25, and adrenochrome on depth electrograms in man. Arch. Neurol. Psychiat. (Chic.) **75**, 579–587 (1956)
Schwarz, C.J.: The complications of LSD: a review of the literature. J. nerv. ment. Dis. **146**, 174–186 (1968)
Silverstein, A.B., Klee, G.D.: Effects of lysergic acid diethylamide (LSD-25) on intellectual functions. Arch. Neurol. Psychiat. (Chic.) **80**, 477–480 (1958a)
Silverstein, A.B., Klee, G.D.: A psychopharmacological test of the "body image" hypothesis. J. nerv. ment. Dis. **121**, 323–329 (1958b)
Silverstein, A.B., Klee, G.D.: The effect of lysergic acid diethylamide on digit span. J. clin. exp. Psychopath. **21**, 11–14 (1960a)

Silverstein, A.B., Klee, G.D.: The effect of lysergic acid diethylamide on dual pursuit performance. J. clin. exp. Psychopath. **21**, 300–303 (1960b)

Siva Sankar, D.V., Gold, E., Sankar, B., McRorie, N.: Effect of psychopharmacological agents on DPN-dependent enzymes. Fed. Proc. **20**, 394 (1961)

Sloane, B., Lovett Doust, J.W.: Psychophysiological investigations in experimental psychoses: results of the exhibition of d-lysergic acid diethylamide to psychiatric patients. J. ment. Sci. **100**, 129–144 (1954)

Smart, R.G., Storm, T., Baker, E.F.W., Solursh, L.: A controlled study of lysergide in the treatment of alcoholism. I. The effects on drinking behavior. Quart. J. Stud. Alcohol. **27**, 469–482 (1966)

Smith, C.M.: A new adjunct to the treatment of alcoholism: the hallucinogenic drugs. Quart. J. Stud. Alcohol. **19**, 406–417 (1958)

Smith, R.P.: The effect of LSD-25 and atropine upon figural after-effects. Pharmacologist **2**, 72 (1960)

Smorto, G., Corrao, F., Pagano, M.: Sulle modificazioni psicopatologiche indotte dall'acido lisergico (dietilamide). Pisani **69**, 39 (1955)

Snow, P.J.D., Lennard-Jones, J.E., Curzon, G., Stacey, R.S.: Humoral effects of metastasising carcinoid tumours. Lancet **1955 II**, 1004–1009

Sokoloff, L., Perlin, S., Kornetsky, C., Kety, S.S.: The effects of d-lysergic acid diethylamide on cerebral circulation and over-all metabolism. Ann. N.Y. Acad. Sci. **66**, 468–477 (1957)

Solms, H.: Lysergsäure-äthylamid (LAE), ein neues, stark sedativ wirkendes Psychoticum aus dem Mutterkorn. Schweiz. med. Wschr. **83**, 356–361 (1953)

Solms, H.: Relationships between chemical structure and psychoses with the use of psychotoxic substances. "Comparative pharmacopsychiatric analysis": A new research method. J. clin. exp. Psychopath. **17**, 429–433 (1956a)

Solms, H.: Chemische Struktur und Psychose bei Lysergsäure-Derivaten. Praxis **45**, 746–749 (1956b)

Soskin, R.A.: The use of LSD in time-limited psychotherapy. J. nerv. ment. Dis. **157**, 410–419 (1973)

Spencer, A.M.: Permissive group therapy with lysergic acid diethylamide. Brit. J. Psychiat. **109**, 37–45 (1963)

Stévenin, L., Benoit, J.C.: L'utilisation des médicaments psychotropes en psychothérapie. Encéphale **51**, 420–459 (1962)

Stoll, W.A.: Lysergsäure-diäthylamid, ein Phantastikum aus der Mutterkorngruppe. Schweiz. Arch. Neurol. Psychiat. **60**, 279–323 (1947)

Stoll, W.A.: Rorschach-Versuche unter Lysergsäure-Diäthylamid-Wirkung. Rorschachiana **1**, 249–270 (1952)

Stoll, A., Hofmann, A.: Partialsynthese von Alkaloiden vom Typus des Ergobasins. Helv. chim. Acta **26**, 944–965 (1943)

Takashina, K.: Physiological studies of visual symptoms due to the effects of hallucinogenic agent LSD 25 on the critical fusion frequency of flicker, the electric flicker threshold, and the intensity threshold for light. Psychiat. Neurol. jap. **62**, 1745–1757, 109–110 (1960)

Tallaferro, A.: Mescalina y L.S.D. 25. Experiencias, valor terapéutico en psiquiatría. Buenos Aires: Libreria juridica de Valerio Abeledo 1956

Tenenbaum, B.: Group therapy with LSD-25. A preliminary report. Dis. nerv. Syst. **22**, 459–462 (1961)

Thompson, R.H.S., Tickner, A., Webster, G.R.: The action of lysergic acid diethylamide on mammalian cholinesterases. Brit. J. Pharmacol. **10**, 61–65 (1955)

Thuring, J.P.: The influence of LSD on the handwriting pressure curve. Advanc. psychosom. Med. (Basel) **1**, 212–216 (1960)

Tonini, G., Montanari, C.: Effects of experimentally induced psychoses on artistic expression. Confin. neurol. (Basel) **15**, 225–239 (1955a)

Tonini, G., Montanari, C.: Effetti psichici della monoetilamide dell'acido lisergico (Lae 32). G. Psichiat. Neuropat. **83**, 355–357 (1955b)

Trube-Becker, E.: Drogenabusus mit Todesfolge. Med. Klin. **70**, 133–140 (1975)

Turner, W.J., Almudevar, M., Merlis, S.: Chemotherapeutic trials in psychosis: III. Addendum. 2-Brom-d-lysergic acid diethylamide (BOL). Amer. J. Psychiat. **116**, 261–262 (1959)

Ungerleider, J.T., Fisher, D.D., Fuller, M.: The dangers of LSD. Analysis of seven months' experience in a university hospital's psychiatric service. J. Amer. med. Ass. **197**, 389–392 (1966)
Ungerleider, J.T., Fisher, D.D., Fuller, M., Caldwell, A.: The "bad trip"—The etiology of the adverse LSD reaction. Amer. J. Psychiat. **124**, 1483–1490 (1968a)
Ungerleider, J.T., Fisher, D.D., Goldsmith, S.R., Fuller, M., Forgy, E.: A statistical survey of adverse reactions to LSD in Los Angeles County. Amer. J. Psychiat. **125**, 352–357 (1968b)
Van Dusen, W., Wilson, W., Miners, W., Hook, H.: Treatment of alcoholism with lysergide. Quart. J. Stud. Alcohol. **28**, 295–304 (1967)
Van Lennep, J.E.: Performance on some projective tests under LSD-25. Advanc. psychosom. Med. **1**, 219–222 (1960)
Van Rhijn, C.H.: Symbolysis: Psychotherapy by symbolic presentation. In: The Use of LSD in Psychotherapy. Transactions of a Conference on D-Lysergic Acid Diethylamide (LSD-25). April 22–24, 1959. Abramson, H.A. (ed.), pp. 151–197. New York: Josiah Macy, Jr., Foundation 1960
Von Felsinger, J.M., Lasagna, L., Beecher, H.K.: The response of normal men to lysergic acid derivatives (di-and mono-ethyl amides). Correlation of personality and drug reactions. J. clin. exp. Psychopathol. **17**, 414–428 (1956)
Von Mering, O., Morimoto, K., Hyde, R.W., Rinkel, M.: Experimentally induced depersonalization. In: Experimental Psychopathology. Hoch, P.H., Zubin, J. (eds.), pp. 66–77. New York-London: Grune and Stratton 1957
Wapner, S., Krus, D.M.: Behavioral effects of lysergic acid diethylamide (LSD-25). Space localization in normal adults as measured by the apparent horizon. Arch. gen. Psychiat. **1**, 417–419 (1959)
Wapner, S., Krus, D.M.: Effects of lysergic acid diethylamide, and differences between normals and schizophrenics on the Stroop color-word test. J. Neuropsychiat. **2**, 76–81 (1960)
Weintraub, W., Silverstein, A.B., Klee, G.D.: The effect of LSD on the associative processes. J. nerv. ment. Dis. **128**, 409–414 (1959)
Weintraub, W., Silverstein, A.B., Klee, G.D.: The "correction" of deviant responses on a word association test. A measure of the defensive functions of the ego. Arch. gen. Psychiat. **3**, 17–20 (1960)
Whitaker, L.H.: Lysergic acid diethylamide in psychotherapy. Med. J. Aust. **51** (I), 5–8, 36–41 (1964)
Wijsenbeek, H., Landau, R.: A review on the use of lysergic acid diethylamide (LSD-25) in psychiatry. Harefuah **58**, 281–286 (1960)
Wikler, A., Haertzen, C.A., Chessick, R.D., Hill, H.E., Pescor, F.T.: Reaction time ("mental set") in control and chronic schizophrenic subjects and in postaddicts under placebo, LSD-25, morphine, pentobarbital and amphetamine. Psychopharmacologia (Berl.) **7**, 423–443 (1965a)
Wikler, A., Rosenberg, D.E., Hawthorne, J.D., Cassidy, T.M.: Age and effect of LSD-25 on pupil size and kneejerk threshold. Studies in chronic schizophrenic and nonpsychotic subjects. Psychopharmacologia (Berl.) **7**, 44–56 (1965b)
Wolbach, A.B., Isbell, H., Miner, E.J.: Cross tolerance between mescaline and LSD-25 with a comparison of the mescaline and LSD reactions. Psychopharmacologia (Berl.) **3**, 1–14 (1962)
Woolley, D.W.: Serotonin in mental disorders. Res. Publ. Ass. nerv. ment. Dis. **36**, 381–400 (1958)
Woolley, D.W., Shaw, E.: A biochemical and pharmacological suggestion about certain mental disorders. Proc. nat. Acad. Sci. (Wash.) **40**, 228–231 (1954)
Young, B.: A phenomenological comparison of LSD and schizophrenic states. Brit. J. Psychiat. **124**, 64–74 (1974)
Zehnder, K., Cerletti, A.: Hemmung der Menschenserum-Pseudocholinesterase durch Lysergsäurediäthylamid und 2-Brom-Lysergsäurediäthylamid. Helv. physiol. pharmacol. Acta **14**, 264–268 (1956)
Ziolko, H.U.: Psychotrope Drogenwirkung und psychische Ausgangslage (Neurose). In: Neuro-Psychopharmacology. Proc. 1st Int. Congr. Neuro-Psychopharmacology, Rome, Sept. 1958.

Bradley, P.B., Deniker, P., Radouco-Thomas, C. (eds.), pp. 711–713. Amsterdam-London-New York-Princeton: Elsevier 1959

Zsigmond, E.K., Foldes, F.F., Foldes, V., Erdos, E.G.: The in vitro inhibitory effect of d-lysergic acid (LSD) and its congeners on human cholinesterases. Fed. Proc. **18**, 463 (1959)

Zsigmond, E.K., Foldes, F.F., Foldes, V.: The lack of correlation between the psychopharmacologic and anticholinesterase effect of LSD and its congeners. Fed. Proc. **19**, 266 (1960)

CHAPTER IX

Influence on the Endocrine System

E. FLÜCKIGER and E. DEL POZO. With a Contribution by B.P. RICHARDSON

A. Animal Data

1. Actions on Pituitary Hormones

Ergot alkaloids became known to influence pituitary hormone secretion by the work of the reproduction physiologist SHELESNYAK of the Weizmann Institute of Science, Rehovot, Israel. In the early 1950's, in search of a pharmacologic tool which would interfere with the process of the uterine deciduoma reaction connected with ovum implantation, he applied the ocytocic ergometrine and ergotoxine to rats. Ergotoxine (SHELESNYAK, 1954a) but not ergometrine (SHELESNYAK, 1954b) inhibited the deciduoma reaction of the pseudopregnant rat, and SHELESNYAK (1954a) concluded from his observations and a critical appraisal of the scanty information in the literature, that ergotoxine acts via the hypothalamus and pituitary to inhibit mammotrophin-luteotrophin (=prolactin) secretion. Thus, an entirely new field opened to ergot pharmacology at the time when the concept of hypothalamo-hypophyseal interplay just became generally accepted (HARRIS, 1955). It was not until 17 years later that the first clinical results indicating the suppression of prolactin secretion in man by an ergot alkaloid (CB154, bromocriptine) were published (LUTTERBECK et al., 1971).

Ten years after SHELESNYAK's fundamental paper, ZEILMAKER in his doctoral thesis (Amsterdam, 1964) observed that ergocornine, one of the ergot alkaloids contained in ergotoxine, also inhibits ovulation when administered to proestrus rats. Thus, ergot alkaloids may also influence the control of pituitary gonadotropin secretion—LH in particular. This finding has had little echo outside the field of rodent endocrinology. The secretion of other anterior pituitary hormones may also be influenced by ergot alkaloids as has only very recently been observed. Especially the inhibition by bromocriptine of GH secretion in acromegalic patients (LIUZZI et al., 1974) and of ACTH in Cushing's disease (BENKER et al., 1976) have further stimulated the interest in the endocrine pharmacology of ergot alkaloids.

a) Prolactin

Introduction. In the reviewers' opinion, prolactin is the most interesting pituitary hormone of today. First recognized in 1928 as an extractable hypophyseal factor inducing lactation in rabbits (STRICKER and GRÜTER, 1928) prolactin has only recently been recognized to also exist in man.

We are used to attribute to a hormone of the pituitary one specific action, but prolactin has brought the classical concept of "one hormone–one action" ad absurdum: NICOLL (1974) now counts more than 80 different physiologic actions. The multipurpose hormone prolactin only rarely acts as the "trophic" hormone for a particular peripheral endocrine organ, and it is unknown how the different target systems feed back to control prolactin secretion. But the multiplicity of actions that prolactin exerts among the vertebrates indicates that during evolution of the phylum, the stimuli to enhance or suppress prolactin secretion (i.e., the input of the control system) must have changed several times. The integrative neuronal system which has only been studied in mammals comprises catecholaminergic, serotoninergic, cholinergic, and gabaergic elements. The output of this prolactin regulating system is considered to consist of two hypothalamo-hypophyseotropic messengers, a prolactin-secretion-inhibiting factor (PIF) and a releasing factor (PRF). Both factors still await isolation and chemical identification. At the time of this writing, many researchers favor the idea that PIF may be identical with dopamine. TRH is also a potent prolactin releasing factor of hypothalamic origin, but it is not at all clear whether it functions under physiologic conditions, as such.

In mammals, the prolactin secreting cells of the pituitary are known to be under a predominantly inhibitory hypothalamic influence. The mammalian pituitary, if disconnected from the hypothalamus, secretes prolactin spontaneously. In reptiles and in birds, prolactin secretion from the pituitary is under stimulatory influence of the hypothalamus. With the exception of very few papers, the literature reporting on pharmacologic studies of prolactin secretion is concerned with the situation in mammals, including man and quite especially with the situation in rats. In mammals, the acknowledged major function of prolactin is in female reproduction, classically as the mammotropic hormone and in some species as a luteotropic hormone. More recently, it was recognized as being involved either at the periphery or through hypothalamic mechanisms with reproductive functions also in the male as well as participating in the regulation of many other physiologic systems (COWIE and FORSYTH, 1975).

A number of recent reviews exist which the reader may consult for basic information on various prolactin aspects: COWIE and FORSYTH (1975) on the whole prolactin field; NICOLL (1974) on the physiologic actions of prolactin; MEITES and CLEMENS (1972), MEITES (1973), and TINDAL (1974) on the regulation of its secretion; FLOSS et al., (1973), FLÜCKIGER (1972), MACLEOD (1976), and SULMAN (1970) on aspects of the pharmacologic control of prolactin secretion.

To cope with the information explosion about prolactin to which we are witnesses, HORROBIN admirably reviews the field at yearly intervals (HORROBIN, 1973, 1974, 1975, 1976).

Methodologic Remarks. All important steps in introducing the ergot alkaloids to the field of prolactin (experimental and clinic) were made without the benefit of direct and quantitative hormone measurements (FLÜCKIGER, 1975). Assessment of endocrine effects of the compounds was based on functional changes of target organs. Thus, inhibition in rodents of (1) the deciduoma reaction in the uterus of pseudopregnant animals (SHELESNYAK, 1954a), of (2) ovum implantation (CARLSEN et al., 1961), and of (3) lactation were used and are still being used as indicative of drug-induced prolactin deficiency. The basis of functional tests (1) and (2) is the fact that prolactin appears to provide the critical luteotropic stimulus for progesterone secretion from day 2 to about day 7 of pregnancy and pseudopregnancy (SMITH et al., 1975; DÖHLER and WUTTKE, 1974) and to stimulate the formation of LH-receptors on luteal cells (HOLT et al., 1976). When using test (3), lactation inhibition in the rat, one should be aware that the action of prolactin at the mammary gland involves an important latency of 8–16 h (GROSVENOR and MENA, 1973). It is thus theoretically impossible to reach by prolactin secretion inhibition alone a full inhibition of pups' weight gain when using a 24 h observation period as done by FLÜCKIGER and WAGNER (1968). Full inhibition of pups' weight gain in such a short time may be brought about easily by drugs which, e.g., inhibit milk ejection, as pointed out by NICOLL et al., (1970). Ergot alkaloids, with an important adrenergic α-receptor stimulating activity (e.g., ergotamine, cpd 20), would be likely candidates for showing such an effect. To study the lactation inhibitory activity of ergot compounds, the method described by AUŠKOVÁ et al. (1974a) with a 4-day observation period is very suitable. If used judiciously and with the appropriate control experiments, they make useful quantitative pharmacologic tests (FLÜCKIGER et al., 1976) and can serve for screening purposes (ZIKAN et al., 1972; BERAN et al., 1975). In reverse, induction of pseudopregnancy in cyclic rats (ASTWOOD, 1941, 1953) or induction of lactation, e.g., in rabbits (AUDIBERT et al., 1956) or rats (SULMAN, 1970) by a drug may be used as indication of stimulated prolactin secretion. In contrast to inhibition of pseudopregnancy or ovum implantation (CASTRO-VASQUEZ et al., 1975), induction of pseudopregnancy is easily accomplished in rodents by various sensory stimuli (SALZMANN, 1963; NEILL, 1974) which emphasizes the need of appropriate control experiments.

These tests may be used pharmacologically to determine the dose of a drug which brings about a certain functional change in a prolactin target system. These tests do not tell how much the initial prolactin secretion has been changed and for how long. A drug may fail in such tests to induce a functional change, because its duration of action is too short. A nice example is provided by the early work of SHELESNYAK (1954a, b); he observed that a single injection of the ocytocic ergonovine (=ergometrine, cpd 19) to pseudopregnant rats does not inhibit deciduoma formation, while a similar dose of ergotoxine is active. In the face of similar ocytocic activities of both drugs, he luckily concluded that inhibition of deciduoma formation is not produced by an ocytocic (ergometrine-like) action. Today we know that ergometrine also inhibits prolactin secretion but with a rather short duration of action. Had SHELESNYAK injected ergonovine twice daily, his results could have been positive. It cannot be known for certain what the consequences of such a finding at that time would have been for this particular field of ergot pharmacology. In the case of bromocriptine, some information is available to illustrate the case further. WUTTKE and DÖHLER (1973), treating inseminated female rats with 2 × 50 μg at 8 a.m. and 7 p.m., observed that this treatment was sufficient to inhibit prolactin secretion during the day and first half of the following night but was insufficient to suppress prolactin in the following late night-early morning period. These animals showed ovum implantation. When injecting the animals thrice daily with 70 μg at 8 a.m. and 4 p.m. and 100 μg at midnight, a round-the-clock suppression of prolactin was obtained together with implantation inhibition. To be effective in the implantation inhibition test, the duration of prolactin suppression by a drug must thus also cover the late night and early morning hours of the following day. ED_{50} for implantation inhibition by bromocriptine is 0.75 mg/kg s.c. (single dose on day 5 of pregnancy), which is similar in magnitude to the dose needed to suppress the serum prolactin values 24 hours later by 50% ($ID_{50,24\,h}=1$ mg/kg s.c.) in male adult rats (FLÜCKIGER et al., 1976). Thus, functional tests not only give limited information to the physiologist (NEILL, 1974), but they also have important limitations in pharmacologic work.

Of the more specific tests, bioassay of prolactin (FORSYTH and PARKE, 1973) has found little use in studies with ergot alkaloids (PASTEELS et al., 1971; BESSER et al., 1972) for obvious reasons (NEILL, 1974). An alternative physical method, but also in restricted use, is the polyacrylamid disc gel electrophoresis, with subsequent photometric evaluation (NICOLL et al., 1969; YANAI and NAGASAWA, 1969; CHEEVER et al., 1969). Only the advent of radioimmunoassays (RIA) for prolactin (e.g., rat, KWA and VORHOFSTAD, 1967; cattle, SCHAMS and KARG, 1970; sheep and goats, BRYANT and GREENWOOD, 1968; man, HWANG et al., 1971), and the availability of rat prolactin RIA kits generously distributed worldwide by the US National Institute of Arthritis and Metabolic Diseases (NIAMD) enabled numerous investigators to develop the field so dynamically, as we have witnessed in the past few years. RIA-assisted screening methods for prolactin-secretion inhibitory ergot alkaloids and their selection for potency have been described (CLEMENS et al., 1974; FLOSS et al., 1973).

α) Drug Actions

In Table 1 are assembled, according to the rules laid down in Chapter II of this book, chemically identified compounds together with experimental data relevant for their qualitative and quantitative characterization as inhibitors of prolactin secretion. A number of inactive compounds as well as some active compounds have been omitted from the table, because they are considered to be of lesser importance, but these compounds are mentioned briefly in the text.

General Remarks. The first impression to be gained from Table 1 is that of great diversity of structures compatible with prolactin secretion inhibitory activity. Five classes of 6-methylergoline derivatives contribute to the list: The four main classes of ergot alkaloids, i.e., the clavine alkaloids, the lysergic acids, the simple lysergic acid amides, and the peptide alkaloids, and the fifth class, 8α-aminoergolines of which no natural cogeners are known.

The pharmacologic information published on the different compounds is very heterogeneous, and the greater part of the published material consists unfortunately of one-dose pharmacology only. This allows only for a superficial discussion of structural requirements for activity, although a number of experimental studies on certain structural aspects have been published since 1972 (BERAN et al., 1974; CASSADY et al., 1974; CLEMENS et al., 1974; FLOSS et al., 1973; FLÜCKIGER et al., 1976; LI et al., 1975; SWEENEY et al., 1975; ZIKAN et al., 1972, 1974). The majority of compounds discussed are only of short-term effects (1 h and/or 2 h) on serum prolactin levels. Thus, the important aspect of the duration of drug action cannot be satisfied.

Of most of the compounds mentioned in the table, no information is available about other activities besides that of prolactin secretion. It is, therefore, also not possible to discuss structural aspects relevant for selectivity of prolactin secretion inhibiting action. It seems important in this context to point out that the active minimal structure mentioned in Table 1, 6-methyl-9-ergolene (cpd[1] 79h) also exerts other activities typical for the profile of ergot compounds, i.e., vasoconstrictor uterotonic, serotonin antagonistic, and blood pressure lowering actions (BACH et al., 1974).

Commentary on Individual Compounds or Groups of Compounds in Table 1. The two most simple ergot alkaloids in the list, *agroclavine* (cpd 5) and its oxydation product *elymoclavine* (cpd 6) are both active as inhibitors of prolactin secretion. From the published data given in the table, it is not possible to decide which one is the more active. In the reserpinized rat at 1 h, agroclavine induced a smaller reduction of circulating prolactin than elymoclavine, but at 2 h both were found only marginally effective after 50 μg/kg i.p. Injections of 3 mg/kg s.c. of elymoclavine once daily over 13 days into rat, with 7,12-dimethyl-benz(a)anthrazene (DMBA)-induced mammary tumors and produced a reduction in tumor mass, whereas the same treatment schedule with agroclavine did not arrest tumor growth. It may be assumed that agroclavine has a shorter duration of action than elymoclavine. Substitution of the alcohol group of cpd 6 to produce elymoclavine-0-acetate did not clearly alter the activity of 50 μg/kg i.p. at 1 h (CASSADY et al., 1974), but at 2 h the activity continued (FLOSS et al., 1973). A similar increase in activity was also observed with elymoclavine-β-D-fructoside. Substitutions by carbamate or benzoate at C17 of elymoclavine (FLOSS et al., 1973) did not seem to change the activity. Further derivation (cpds 6a–6i) produced one compound (cpd 6f) with an activity equal to that of ergocornine at 1 h after 50 μg/kg i.p. (LI et al., 1975).

Lysergic acid (cpd 8) has been found inactive in vivo by three laboratories. In contrast to this lysergic acid methylcarbinolamide (cpd 12), a natural derivative of cpd 8 is very active and seems to have a prolonged duration of action. Of a series of synthetic lysergic acid amines studied by SWEENEY et al., (1975) for inhibition of DMBA-induced mammary tumors in rats, only two compounds induced tumor regression: N-lysergyl-2-hydroxy-cyclopentylamine and N-lysergyl-3-hydroxy-n-butylamine.

Ergometrine (cpd 19) is a drug with clinical relevance for its uterotonic activity. SHELESNYAK (1954b, 1958), who injected up to 50 mg/kg s.c., could not inhibit the deciduoma reaction in pseudopregnant rats. This inactivity contrasts with the positive results of SHAAR and CLEMENS (1972), who observed a 73% reduction of serum prolactin levels in lactating rats at about 6 h after the fifth of daily injections of ~20 mg/kg s.c. Ergometrine at ~1 mg/kg d.i.p. inhibited the growth of prolactin-secreting pituitary tumor transplants in rats (QUADRI et al., 1972) but at 3 mg/kg s.c. was unable to inhibit the growth of DMBA-induced mammary tumors (SWEENEY et al., 1975). The difference of these results cannot be explained on the basis of the published material.

[1] cpd = compound

Table 1. Actions of ergot compounds on prolactin (explanation to abbreviated notations)

Notation	*Explanation*	*Notation*	*Explanation*
AMT	α-Methyl-p-tyrosine	DMBA; 3 mg/kg s.c./d, 13 d	7,12-Dimethyl-benz(a)anthrazene was used for induction of mammary tumors; tumor bearing animals were treated with 3 mg/kg s.c. of the test substance for 13 days
ECO	Ergocornine (cpd 24)		
Prl	Use of the word prolactin (Prl) under results implies actual measurement of the peptide by radioimmunoassay or other physical means		
Prl − 52% = 81% ECO	The circulating prolactin concentration was found reduced by 52%, this being 81% of the effect of ergocornine at the same dose, in the same study.	pit. tumor impl.	Animals were implanted s.c. with fragments of a prolactin secreting rat pituitary tumor
		hypex + ect. pit.	Animals were hypophysectomized, then implanted with a pituitary at an ectopic site
implant. inhib.	Inhibition of ovum implantation (pregnancy)		
reserp.; 50 µg/kg i.p., 2 h	Pretreated with reserpine; of the test substance 50 µg/kg was given i.p., 2 h before blood collection	rat, pseudopr.; decid. inhib.	Pseudopregnant rats were induced to produce a deciduoma reaction of the uterine mucosa; inhibition of this reaction by pretreating the rats with the test substance was sought for
ovex + EB	Animals were prepared by ovariectomy and then substituted with estradiol-benzoate		

Cpd[a] number	Name	Experimental condition	Results	Authors
5	Agroclavine	Rat, implant. inhib., oral	Active at ca. 2 mg·d	EDWARDSON (1968)
		Rat, lactation inhib., oral	Active at ca. 2 mg·d	
		Mouse, pregnant, 5 or 7 mg% in feed	Inhibits development of mammary glands and lactation	MANTLE (1968)
		Rat, reserp.; 50 µg/kg i.p., 2 h	Prl marg. reduced	FLOSS et al. (1973)
		Rat, reserp.; 50 µg/kg i.p., 1 h	Prl −46%	CASSADY et al. (1974)
		Rat, ovex + EB; 1 mg s.c., 1 h	Prl reduced signif.	NASR and PEARSON (1975)
		Rat, DMBA; 3 mg/kg s.c./d, 13 d	Tumor growth not stopped	SWEENEY et al. (1975)
6	Elymoclavine	Rat, reserp.; 50 µg/kg i.p., 2 h	Prl marg. reduced	FLOSS et al. (1973)
		Rat, reserp.; 50 µg/kg i.p., 1 h	Prl −71%	CLEMENS et al. (1974)
		Rat, reserp.; 50 µg/kg i.p., 1 h	Prl −71% = 98% of ECO	[illegible]

		Rat, implant. inhib. oral d_6+d_7 Rat, DMBA; 3 mg/kg s.c./d, 13 d	5 mg/kg complete inhib. Tumor growth −41%	Řežábek et al. (1975) Sweeney et al. (1975)
6a	Elymoclavine-pyridinum tosylate	Rat, reserp.; 50 μg/kg i.p., 1 h	Prl −40% = ca. 100% of ECO	Cassady et al. (1974)
6b	6-Methyl-8-piperidino-methyl-8-ergolene	Rat, reserp.; 50 μg/kg i.p., 1 h	Prl −34% = 83% of ECO	Clemens et al. (1974)
6c	6-Methyl-8-diethylamino-methyl-8-ergolene	Rat, reserp.; 50 μg/kg i.p., 1 h	Prl −52% = 81% of ECO	Li et al. (1975)
6d	6-Methyl-8-chloro-methyl-8-ergolene	Rat, reserp.; 50 μg/kg i.p., 1 h	Prl −17% = 40% of ECO	Li et al. (1975)
6e	6-Methyl-8-cyanomethyl-8-ergolene	Rat, reserp.; 50 μg/kg i.p.,1 h	Prl −49% = 85% of ECO	Li et al. (1975)
6f	6-Methyl-8-carboxamidomethyl-8-ergolene	Rat, reserp.; 50 μg/kg i.p.,1 h	Prl −83% = 101% of ECO	Li et al. (1975)
6g	6-Methyl-8-pyrrolidino-methyl-8-ergolene	Rat, reserp.; 50 μg/kg i.p., 1 h	Prl −43% = 60% of ECO	Li et al. (1975)
6h	6-Methyl-8-anilinomethyl-8-ergolene	Rat, reserp.; 50 μg/kg i.p., 1 h	Prl −43% = 64% of ECO	Li et al. (1975)
6i	6-Methyl-8-acetylanilino-8-ergolene	Rat, reserp.; 50 μg/kg i.p., 1 h	Prl −59% = 83% of ECO	Li et al. (1975)
8	Lysergic acid	Rat, pseudopr.; decid. inhib. Rat, reserp.; 50 μg/kg i.p., 1 h Rat, ovex + EB; 1 mg/kg s.c., 1 h	~2.5 mg/kg s.c. no effect No effect No effect	Shelesnyak (1958) Clemens et al. (1974) Nasr and Pearson (1975)
12	d-Lysergic acid-methyl-carbinolamide	Mouse, implant. inhib.; 250 μg d_3–d_5 Rat, reserp.; 50 μg/kg i.p., 2 h Rat, reserp.; 50 μg/kg i.p., 1 h	Full inhibition Prl −74% (ECO = 100%) Prl −53% = 67% of ECO	Mantle (1969) Floss et al. (1973) Cassady et al. (1974)

[a] cdp numbers referring to Chapter II.

Table 1 (continued)

Cpd number	Name	Experimental condition	Results	Authors
19	Ergonovine, ergometrine	Rat, reserp.; decid. inhib.	~5 mg/kg s.c. no effect	SHELESNYAK (1958)
		Rat, pit. tumor impl.; 0.2 mg/d i.p., 21 d	Tumor inhibition	QUADRI et al. (1972)
		Rat, lact. inhib.; 4 mg s.c., d_4–d_8	Prl −73%; pups' weight gain −58%	SHAAR and CLEMENS (1972)
		Rat, DMBA; 3 mg/kg s.c., 13 d	Tumor growth not stopped	SWEENEY et al. (1975)
20	Ergotamine	Rat, pregn.; 2×5 mg/d i.p., 2×1 mg/d, d_{12}–d_{25}	Pups' retarded growth; reduced mammary secretion	SOMMER and BUCHANAN (1955)
		Rat, pseudopr.; decid. inhib.	~5 mg/kg s.c. no effect	SHELESNYAK (1958)
		Rat, 1 mg i.p.; pit. ex vivo pit. in vitro, 2.5–20 µg/ml	Prl secr. reduced	NICOLL et al. (1970)
		Rat, lact. inhib.; 4 mg s.c., d_4–d_8	Prl −50%; pups' weight gain −109%	SHAAR and CLEMENS (1972)
		Rat, 0.2 mg/d s.c., 7 d; pit. ex vivo	Prl not influenced	MACLEOD and LEHMEYER (1973)
		Rat, pit. in vitro, 4 µM	Prl secretion suppressed	
		Rat, pit. tumor impl.; 50 µg s.c., 13 d	Prl suppressed, tumor arrest.	
		Rat, reserp.; 50 µg/kg i.p.; 1 h	Prl −46%	CLEMENS et al. (1974)
		Rat, DMBA; 13 d, 3 mg/kg s.c.	Tumor growth not stopped	SWEENEY et al. (1975)
		Rat, implant. inhib., d_5	ED_{50} = 14 mg/kg s.c.	FLÜCKIGER et al. (1976)
		Rat, females; 0.2 mg/d, 7 d	Prl not reduced	MACLEOD and KRIEGER (1976)
		Rat, pit. tumor impl.; 0.2 mg/d, 7 d	Prl suppressed	
21	Ergosine	Rat, implant. inhib., d_5	ED_{50} = 505 µg s.c./rat (≈3.3 mg/kg s.c.)	KRAICER and SHELESNYAK (1965)
		Rat, implant. inhib., d_5	ED_{50} = 5.7 mg/kg s.c.	FLÜCKIGER et al. (1976)
22	Ergostine	Rat, implant. inhib., d_5	ED_{50} > 20 mg/kg s.c.	FLÜCKIGER et al. (1976)
23	Ergocristine	Rat, pseudopr.; deciduoma inhib.	~5 mg/kg s.c. no effect	SHELESNYAK (1958)
		Rat, reserp.; 50 µg/kg i.p., 1 h	Prl −78%	CLEMENS et al. (1974)

		s.c.		
		Rat, implant. inhib., d_5	$ED_{50}=4.2$ mg/kg s.c.	Flückiger et al. (1976)
24	Ergocornine = ECO 580	Rat, pseudopr., deciduoma inhib.	~5 mg/kg s.c. part. eff.	Shelesnyak (1958)
		Rat, hypex + ect. pit.; funct. c.l.	1 mg inhibits c.l.	Zeilmaker and Carlsen (1962)
		Rat, + ect. pit.; vag. smears	1 mg induces estrus	Zeilmaker and Carlsen (1962)
		Rat, implant. inhib., d_5	$ED_{50}=335$ µg s.c./rat (≈2.1 mg/kg)	Kraicer and Shelesnyak (1965)
		Mouse, + ect. trophoblasts, pseudopr.	0.4 mg without effect	Zeilmaker (1968)
		Rat, proestr. Prl surge, 50 µg/kg s.c.	Prl suppressed	Wuttke et al. (1971)
		Rat, pit. tumor impl.; 0.1 mg or 0.2 mg i.p./d, 21 d	Tumor inhib. −15 and −30%	Quadri et al. (1972)
		Rat, lact. inhib.; 0.5 mg/s.c. d_4–d_8	Prl −78%; pups' weight gain −104%	Shaar and Clemens (1972)
		Rat, lact. inhib.; 1 mg s.c. d_4–d_8	Prl −78%; pups' weight gain −118%	
		Rat, hypex + 2 ect. pit.; 2 mg/d	Prl secr. fully inhibited	
		Rat, reserp.; 50 µg/kg i.p., 2 h	Prl −58% to −75%	Floss et al. (1973)
		Rat, reserp.; 50 µg/kg i.p., 1 h	Prl −83%	Clemens et al. (1974)
		Rat, DMBA; 3 mg/kg s.c., 13 d	Tumor growth −31%	Sweeney et al. (1975)
		Rat, DMBA; 2 mg/animal, 20 d	Tumor area −58%	Nasr and Pearson (1975)
		Rat, proestrus Prl surge; 1 mg	Prl fully inhib., duration 24 h	Nasr and Pearson (1975)
		Rat, reserp.; dose resp. curve 1 h	ID_{50} ~10 µg/kg i.p.	Clemens et al. (1974)
		Rat, implant. inhib.; d_5	$ED_{50}=2.7$ mg/kg s.c.	Flückiger et al. (1976)
25	α-Ergokryptine	Rat, implant. inhib.; d_5	$ED_{50}=1.15$ mg/kg s.c.	Flückiger and Wagner (1968)
		Rat, lact. inhib.: acute pups' weight gain	$ID_{50}=8.7$ mg/kg s.c.	
		Rat, lact. inhib.; 0.5 mg s.c. d_4–d_8	Prl −76%; pups' weight gain −122%	Shaar and Clemens (1972)
		Rat, pit. tumor impl.; 0.3 mg i.p., 21 d	Tumor marg. inhibited	Quadri et al. (1972)

Table 1 (continued)

Cpd number	Name	Experimental condition	Results	Authors
26	β-Ergokryptine	Rat, implant. inhib.; d_5	$ED_{50} = 2.8$ mg/kg s.c.	FLÜCKIGER et al. (1976)
34a	Methysergide	Rat, lact., suckling-induced Prl release	25 mg/kg i.p. full inhib.	RABII and GALLO (1975)
		Rat, ovex, anaesth., 3 and 25 mg/kg	Short-lived Prl increase	GALLO et al. (1975)
		Rat, pit. in vitro; 12.5 and 125 µg/ml	Prl inhib. marginally	GALLO et al. (1975)
		Rat, ether and bleeding stress, 5 mg/kg i.p.	Inhib. Prl stimulation, no effect on resting Prl level	MARCHLEWSKA-KOJ and KRULICH (1975)
37c	2-Bromo-ergocornine	Rat, implant. inhib.; d_5	$ED_{50} = > 5$mg/kg s.c.	FLÜCKIGER et al. (1976)
38	Bromocriptine = CB 154	Rat, implant. inhib.	$ED_{50} = 0.75$ mg/kg s.c.	FLÜCKIGER and WAGNER (1968)
		Rat, implant. inhib.	$ED_{100} = 1.5$ mg/kg s.c. = 6 mg/kg orally	CORBIN (1974)
		Rabbit, implant. inhib. d_5	No effect up to 5 mg/kg s.c.	FLÜCKIGER (1972)
		Pig, lact. inhib.	ID_{50} milk yield < 0.27 mg/kg i.m.	FLÜCKIGER (1972)
		Dog, lact. inhib.	ID_{50} milk yield = 6 µg/kg	MAYER and SCHÜTZE (1973)
		Rabbit, lact. inhib.	1 mg s.c.	TAYLOR and PEAKER (1975)
		Rat, DMBA; d_{1-80}	6 mg/kg·d i.p. but not 1 mg/kg fully suppress tumor development	STÄHELIN et al. (1971)
		Mouse, 0.2 mg/d, 3 weeks	Reduced pit. Prl content, GH unchanged	YANAI and NAGASAWA (1970b)
		Rat, cycling; 3 doses (70–100 µg) daily	Block. of cyclic Prl fluctuations	WUTTKE and DÖHLER (1973)
		Rat, lact.; suckling-induced Prl release	10 mg/kg s.c. or 3 mg/kg s.c. suppress Prl release	FLÜCKIGER and KOVACS (1974), FLÜCKIGER et al. (1976)
		Sheep, cycling; 2×1 mg i.m./d	Prl reduced below 0.5 ng/ml, no effect on cycle	NISWENDER (1974)

		after parturition	attenuates lactogenesis	
		Dog, male 2 mg i.m. daily for 7 d	Prl suppressed from 77 ng/ml to unmeasurable level from 2nd day onward	JONES et al. (1976)
		Macaca fascic. intact and ovex; 0.2 or 2 mg/kg i.v.	Antagonizes TRH-induced Prl release	GALA and SANFORD (1975)
		Rat and human foetal pit. in vitro	Reversible reduction of Prl release	PASTEELS et al. (1971)
		Rat pit. tumor cell cultures	Dose-dependent Prl release inhibition	TASHJIAN and HOYT (1972)
		Rat, pit. tumor cell cultures, depolarized by high [K^+]	Prl release inhibition	GAUTVIK et al. (1973)
39	Lergotrile = Lilly 83636	Rat, reserp.; 50 µg/kg i.p., 1 h	Prl −63%	CLEMENS et al. (1974)
		Rat, reserp.; dose resp., 1 h	ID_{50} ~20 µg/kg i.p.	
		Rat, lact.; 0.6 and 1.25 mg, d_4–d_8	Pups' weight gain −35%, −64%	CLEMENS et al. (1975)
		Rat, DMBA; 3 mg/kg s.c., 13 d	Tumor growth −30%	SWEENEY et al. (1975)
39a	2-Br-6-methyl-8β-cyano-methylergoline	Rat, reserp.; 50 µg/kg i.p., 1 h	Prl −53%	CLEMENS et al. (1974)
		Rat, DMBA; 3 mg/kg s.c., 13 d	Tumor growth −29%	SWEENEY et al. (1975)
39b	2-Iodo-6-methyl-8β-cyano-methylergoline	Rat, reserp.; 50 µg/kg i.p., 1 h	Prl −44%	CLEMENS et al. (1974)
39c	2-Cl-1,6-dimethyl-8β-methyl-ergoline	Rat, reserp.; 50 µg/kg i.p., 1 h	Prl −47%	CLEMENS et al. (1974)
73a	Methylergometrine	Rat, pseudopreg., decid. inhib.	~5 mg/kg s.c. no effect	SOMMER and BUCHANAN (1955)
		Rat, pregnancy; 2×0.5 mg/kg/d i.p., d_{12}–d_{21}	Fetuses marg. retarded	
		Rat, reserp.; 50 µg/kg i.p., 1 h	Prl −47%	CLEMENS et al. (1974)
73b	Lysergidum = LSD 25	Rat, proestrus surge, 0.2, 0.5, 1 mg/kg i.p.	Prl surge fully inhib.	QUADRI and MEITES (1971)
		Rat, DMBA; 5–20 µg/kg s.c., 21 d	Tumor growth inhibited by 20 µg/kg·d	QUADRI et al. (1973)
		Rat, ovex + EB; 1 mg s.c., 1 h	No effect on serum Prl	NASR and PEARSON (1973)
74e	Dihydrolysergic acid-azide	Rat, reserp.; 50 µg/kg i.p., 2 h	Prl ∅	FLOSS et al. (1973)
		Rat, reserp.; 50 µg/kg i.p., 1 h	Prl ∅	CASSADY et al. (1974)

Table 1 (continued)

Cpd number	Name	Experimental condition	Results	Authors
79a	Lysergol = 6-methyl-8β-hydroxymethyl-9-ergolene	Rat, reserp.; 50 μg/kg i.p., 1 h Rat, DMBA; 3 mg/kg s.c., 13 d	Prl −56% Tumor growth −29%	CLEMENS et al. (1974) SWEENEY et al. (1973)
79c	Lysergin = 6,8β-dimethyl-9-ergolene	Rat, reserp.; 50 μg/kg i.p., 2 h Rat, reserp.; 50 μg/kg i.p., 1 h	Prl ∅ Prl ∅	FLOSS et al. (1973) CASSADY et al. (1974)
79d	Isolysergin = 6,8α-dimethyl-9-ergolene	Rat, reserp.; 50 μg/kg i.p., 2 h Rat, reserp.; 50 μg/kg i.p., 1 h	Prl ∅ Prl ∅	FLOSS et al. (1973) CASSADY et al. (1974)
79e	Isolysergol = 6-methyl-8α-hydroxymethyl-9-ergolene	Rat, reserp.; 50 μg/kg i.p., 2 h Rat, reserp.; 50 μg/kg i.p., 1 h	Prl −52% (ECO = 100%) Prl −37%	FLOSS et al. (1973) CASSADY et al. (1974)
79f	Lysergen = 6 methyl-8-methylen-9-ergolene	Rat, reserp.; 50 μg/kg i.p., 2 h Rat, reserp.; 50 μg/kg i.p., 1 h	Prl ∅ Prl ∅	FLOSS et al. (1973) CASSADY et al. (1974)
79g	6-Methyl-8-acetoxymethylen-9-ergolene	Rat, reserp.; 50 μg/kg i.p., 2 h Rat, reserp.; 50 μg/kg i.p., 1 h	Prl −48% (ECO = 100%) Prl −28%	FLOSS et al. (1973) CASSADY et al. (1974)
79h	6-Methyl-9-ergolene	Rat, reserp.; 0.5 mg/kg i.p., 1 h	Prl −45% (<10% of ECO effect)	BACH et al. (1974)
81a	Dihydrolysergol	Rat, reserp.; 50 μg/kg, 2 h Rat, DMBA; 3 mg/kg s.c., 13 d	Prl −82% (ECO = 100%) Tumor growth no effect	FLOSS et al. (1973) SWEENEY et al. (1975)
82b	6-Methyl-8β-chloromethyl-ergoline	Rat, DMBA; 3 mg/kg s.c., 13 d	Tumor growth no effect	SWEENEY et al. (1975)
83a	Homolysergic acid nitrile	Rat, reserp.; 50 μg/kg, 1 h	Prl −61%	CLEMENS et al. (1974)
83b	Dihydrohomolysergic acid nitrile = VUFB6605	Rat, implant. inhib.; ca. 10 mg/kg orally, d_0, d_1... or d_7; 1 mg/kg d_1 or d_3 or d_5 Mouse, implant. inhib.; 250 μg/animal per os, d_1–d_3	Full inhibition Partial inhibition Inhibition	REZABEK et al. (1969) MANTLE and FINN (1971)

		Rat, reserp.; 50 µg/kg, 1 h	Prl −85%	Clemens et al. (1974)
		Mouse, 0.1 mg/d s.c. over 14 months	Mammary hyperpl. alveolar nodules and tumors supressed	Welsch et al. (1974)
		Rat, DMBA; 3 mg/kg s.c., 13 d	Tumor growth −38%	Sweeney et al. (1974)
83c	1-Methyl-dihydrohomolysergic acid nitrile	Rat, reserp.; 50 µg/kg, 1 h	Prl −38%	Clemens et al. (1974)
83d	1-Formyl-dihydro-homolysergic acid nitrile	Rat, reserp.; 50 µg/kg, 1 h	Prl −74%	Clemens et al. (1974)
86b	Dihydrohomolysergic acid amide=VUFB6683	Rat, implant. inhib.; ca. 0.4 mg/kg orally	Implant. inhibited	Semonský et al. (1971)
		Rat, lact. inhib.; 4 d orally		Aušková et al. (1973)
		1) pups' weight gain inhib.:	ID_{50}=0.22 mg/kg·d	
		2) pups' milk spot inhib.:	ID_{50}=0.15 mg/kg·d	
		Rat, lact. inhib.; 1, 4 or 10 mg/kg·d orally, 4 d	Lactation inhibited; Prl content of pit. reduced (=inhib. of Prl synthesis)	Krejčí et al. (1973)
94c	6-Methyl-8β-amino-ergoline	Rat, reserp.; 50 µg/kg i.p., 1 h	Prl −57%=81% of ECO	Cassady et al. (1974)
96a	Lysuride=N-[6-methyl-8α-(9-ergolenyl)]-N′,N-diethyl-urea	Rat, lact. inhib.; orally, 4 d	Pups' weight gain inhib. ID_{50}=0.050 mg/kg·d	Aušková et al. (1974a)
		Rat, reserp.; 0.1, 0.5 mg/kg, 1 h	Prl −76%, −77%	Horowski et al. (1975)
		Rat, reserp.; s.c. minimum effect. dose for Prl inhib.	0.025 mg/kg	
		Rat, reserp.; 0.1 mg/kg s.c. 1 h	Prl −90%	Horowski and Gräf (1975)
		Rat, reserp.+AMT; 0.1 mg/kg s.c. 1 h	Prl −90%	
		Rat, ovex+EB±res., duration of action after 0.1 mg/kg	Prl inhib. 12 h	Gräf et al. (1976)
96c	N-(6-Methyl-8α-ergolinyl)-N′,N′-diethylurea hydrogen-maleinate=VUFB6638	Rat, lact. inhib.; 0.1, 1, 2 mg/kg·d orally, 4 d	Prl content of pit. reduced =inhib. of Prl synthesis	Krejčí et al. (1973)
		Rat, lact. inhib.; orally, 4 d		Aušková et al. (1974b)
		pups' weight gain inhib.,	ID_{50}=0.112 mg/kg·d	
		pups' milk spots inhib.:	ID_{50}=0.084 mg/kg·d	

Table 1 (continued)

Cpd number	Name	Experimental condition	Results	Authors
102a	Dihydroergosine	Rat, implant. inhib., d_5	$ED_{50} = 20$ mg/kg s.c.	FLÜCKIGER et al. (1976)
102b	Dihydroergotamine = DHE	Rat, pseudopr., decid. inhib. Rat, ovex + EB; 1.5 to 3 mg s.c., 1 h Rat, implant. inhib., d_5	~5 mg/kg s.c., no effect Increased Prl serum level signif. $ED_{50} = > 20$ mg/kg s.c.	SHELESNYAK (1958) NASR and PEARSON (1975) FLÜCKIGER et al. (1976)
102c	Dihydroergocristine	Rat, pseudopr.; decid. inhib. Rat, ovex + EB; 1 mg s.c., 1 h Rat, implant. inhib., d_5	~5 mg/kg s.c. no effect Increased Prl serum level signif. $ED_{50} = > 3$ mg/kg s.c.	SHELESNYAK (1958) NASR and PEARSON (1975) FLÜCKIGER et al. (1976)
102d	Dihydroergocornine	Rat, pseudopreg.; decid. inhib. Rat, lact. inhib.; 1 mg·d s.c., d_4–d_8 Rat, reserp.; dose resp. curve, 1 h Rat, ovex + EB; 2 mg s.c., 1 h Rat, DMBA; 3 mg/kg s.c./d, 13 d Rat, implant. inhib.; d_5	~5 mg/kg s.c. no effect Pups' weight gain fully inhibited ID_{50} ca. 12 µg/kg i.p. Lowered Prl serum level signif. Tumor growth +3% (c = +98%) $ED_{50} = > 3$ mg/kg s.c.	SHELESNYAK (1958) SHAAR and CLEMENS (1972) CLEMENS et al. (1974) NASR and PEARSON (1975) SWEENEY et al. (1975) FLÜCKIGER et al. (1976)
102e	Dihydro-α-ergokryptine	Rat, reserp.; 50 µg/kg i.p., 1 h Rat, implant. inhib.; d_5	Prl −82% $ED_{50} = 4.8$ mg/kg s.c.	CLEMENS et al. (1974) FLÜCKIGER et al. (1976)
102g	Dihydroergostine	Rat, implant. inhib.; d_5	$ED_{50} = > 3$ mg/kg s.c.	FLÜCKIGER et al. (1976)
108a	Ergovaline	Rat, implant. inhib.; d_5 Rat, implant. inhib.; d_5	$ED_{50} = 945$ µg s.c./rat (≈6.1 mg/kg s.c.) $ED_{50} = 9$ mg/kg s.c.	KRAICER and SHELESNYAK (1965) FLÜCKIGER et al. (1976)
108b	Dihydroergovaline	Rat, implant. inhib.; d_5	$ED_{50} = > 20$ mg/kg s.c.	FLÜCKIGER et al. (1976)
110a	Ergonine	Rat, implant. inhib.: d_5	$ED_{50} = 4.6$ mg/kg s.c.	FLÜCKIGER et al. (1976)
110b	Dihydroergonine	Rat, implant. inhib.; d_5	$ED_{50} = > 3$ mg/kg s.c.	FLÜCKIGER et al. (1976)
111a	Ergoptine	Rat, implant. inhib.; d_5	$ED_{50} = 4$ mg/kg s.c.	FLÜCKIGER et al. (1976)
111b	Dihydroergoptine	Rat, implant. inhib.; d	ED ... > 3 mg/kg s.c.	FLÜCKIGER et al. (1976)

Ergotamine (cpd 20), of clinical importance for its vascular effects, produces conflicting results in respect to its effects on prolactin secretion: Clear inhibitory effects are found in in vitro experiments (NICOLL et al., 1970; MACLEOD and LEHMEYER, 1973) and in short term in vivo studies (CLEMENS et al., 1974). In functional tests, where only a prolonged inhibition of prolactin secretion produces positive results, ergotamine showed little activity. Thus, SHELESNYAK (1958) could not inhibit the deciduoma reaction in pseudopregnant rats by 5 mg/kg s.c., and we obtained an ED_{50} for implantation inhibition of 14 mg/kg s.c. (FLÜCKIGER et al., 1976). Ergotamine was very effective in reducing weight gain of the young of treated nursing rats (SHAAR and CLEMENS, 1972), although prolactin levels were only partially suppressed. Also, in rats with ectopic pituitary tumors, ergotamine proved very effective in suppressing prolactin secretion and tumor growth (MACLEOD and LEHMEYER, 1973), although the same dose given to normal rats did not influence prolactin levels. It must be assumed that α-receptor stimulation by ergotamine contributes to the overall effect; GROSVENOR (1956) reported that 3 mg/kg s.c., of ergotamine acutely interfered with milk ejection, and GROSVENOR and TURNER (1956) showed that this effect could be overcome by injecting ocytocin. Also, MACLEOD and KRIEGER (1976) pointed out that (peripheral) α-receptor stimulation is probably a determinant in the endocrine of actions of ergotamine.

Ergocornine (cpd 24), first used by SHELESNYAK (1958), is one component of the ergotoxine mixture previously used in his studies on deciduoma formation in pseudopregnant rats. With this compound a number of observations have been made: ZEILMAKER and CARLSEN (1962) provided the first experimental proof that in ergocornine treated pseudopregnant rats inhibition of the deciduoma reaction and interruption of leucocytic vaginal smears by estrus, "are the results of a temporary inhibition of the secretion of luteotropic hormone by the pituitary". These authors also provided experimental proof that ergocornine acts at the pituitary level to inhibit prolactin secretion. ZEILMAKER (1968), using mice, and KISCH and SHELESNYAK (1968), using rats, showed that this action is specific for pituitary prolactin, in that the drug did not inhibit pseudopregnancy nor pregnancy in the presence of the throphoblasts or placentae. This fact explains why ergocornine and similar drugs act as antifertility drug in rodents only in the preimplantation period, i.e., before the luteotrophic complex secreted by the throphoblasts is effective.

α-ergokryptine (cpd 25) is the most active member of the ergotoxine group of alkaloids in inhibiting ovum implantation in rats (FLÜCKIGER and WAGNER, 1968; FLÜCKIGER et al., 1976). MACLEOD and LEHMEYER (1972) reported that daily s.c., injections of 0.2 mg into female rats significantly inhibits prolactin secretion from their pituitaries when incubated in vitro and increases the amount of prolactin retained in the tissue. When added to the incubation medium, 3×10^{-9} α-ergokryptine inhibited prolactin secretion from rat pituitary halves by 95% and reduced prolactin synthesis by 75% (Fig. 3) (MACLEOD and LEHMEYER, 1974a). This inhibitory action of α-ergokryptine could be fully antagonized by perphenazine or haloperidol. In a later study, it was observed that 2×10^{-10}M α-ergokryptine inhibited the release of prolactin from rat pituitaries by 50%, and 4×10^{-10}M reduced prolactin release by 75% (HILL-SAMLI and MACLEOD, 1975). Adding TRH to the incubation medium reduced the effect of the ergot alkaloid. In rats inoculated with the prolactin secreting MtTW5 pituitary tumor, daily s.c. injections of 0.2 mg α-ergokryptine suppressed tumor growth and reduced the high serum prolactin levels (MACLEOD and LEHMEYER, 1973).

Methysergide (cpd 34a), pharmacologically relevant as a serotonin antagonist (see Chapter III), is primarily used by researchers in the prolactin field for this property to analyze the central control of prolactin secretion. It has a doubtful inhibitory effect on in vitro pituitary prolactin release (GALLO et al., 1975).

Bromocriptine (cpd 38), the 2-Bromo derivative of α-ergokryptine (cpd 25), is the first drug selected and developed for the purpose of suppressing prolactin secretion in man. The compound inhibits prolactin secretion in all animal species so far studied, from fish to man (Table 2) under various conditions of in vivo or in vitro experimentation. The experimental data leading to the selection of bromocriptine (FLÜCKIGER et al., 1976) as well as endocrine and nonendocrine pharmacology have recently been presented (FLÜCKIGER, 1975, 1976). In the first publication on bromocriptine (FLÜCKIGER and WAGNER, 1968), we were puzzled over the discrepancy we found when comparing the dose-response curve for implantation inhibition with that for lactation inhibition (Fig. 1). The latter curve is very flat for bromocriptine (Fig. 1 B), while with ergocornine and α-ergokryptine it is steep (Fig. 1 A), and with increasing doses it converges with the dose-response curve for implantation inhibition, so that for the two tests maximal effects are reached with a similar dose. We naively assumed in 1968 that what we observed with the natural compounds α-ergokryptine and ergocornine was "standard," and we therefore sought to explain the divergent behavior of the two slopes obtained with bromocriptine. We put forward the idea of a differential action of bromocrip-

Table 2. First publications on inhibition of prolactin secretion by bromocriptine in different species

Species	Reference
Fishes	
Anguilla anguilla	OLIVEREAU and LEMOINE (1973)[a]
Xiphophorus helleri	MCKEOWN (1972)[a]
Poecilia latipinna	
Mammals	
Mesocricetus auratus	FORD and YOSHINAGA (1975)
Laboratory mouse	YANAI and NAGASAWA (1970a)
Laboratory rat	FLÜCKIGER and WAGNER (1968)[a]
	WUTTKE and DÖHLER (1973)
Rabbit	TAYLOR and PEAKER (1975)[a]
Sheep	NISWENDER (1974)
Goat	HART (1973)
Pig	FLÜCKIGER (1972)[a]
Dairy cow	KARG et al. (1972)
Dog	MAYER and SCHÜTZE (1973)[a]
	JONES et al. (1976)
Macaca fascicularis	GALA and SANFORD (1975)
M. mulata	BUTLER et al. (1975)
Man	LUTTERBECK et al. (1971)[a]
	BESSER et al. (1972)

[a] Statements based on indirect evidence (physiologic or morphologic).

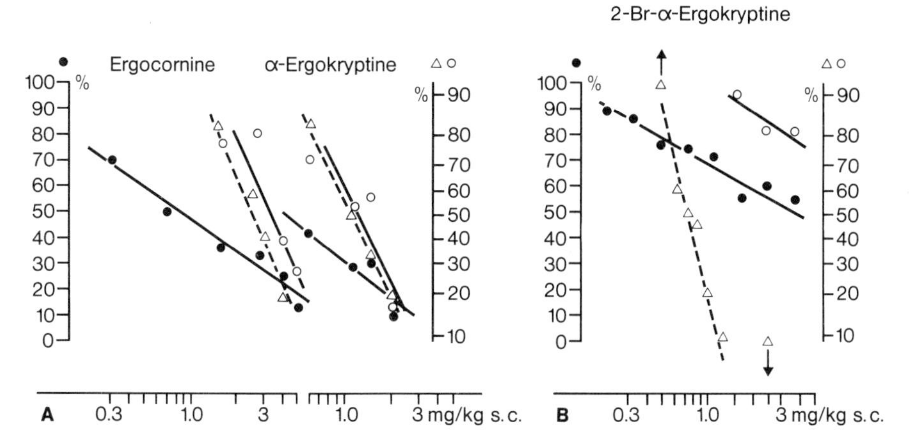

Fig. 1A and B. Dose-response curves for ergocornine (cpd 24), α-ergokryptine (cpd 25), and α-Br-α-ergokryptine (cpd 38) in rats on ovum implantation (△) and on lactation (○●). Number of pregnancies in percent of number of treated females (△) are read on the (right) probit scale. Lactation was assessed in two ways: Weight gain of the pups in percent of controls (●) is read on the (left) linear scale; milk spot occurrence in the pups in percent (○) is read on the (right) probit scale (FLÜCKIGER and WAGNER, 1968). (With permission from Alpha Omega Alpha Publishing for the reproduction of the graphs from FLÜCKIGER, 1972)

tine on the two types of prolactin secretion in early gestation and in lactation. This hypothesis was soon refuted in a discusssion by NICOLL et al. (1970) and by all subsequent experience (see "Methodological Remarks," above). It may be possible, as NICOLL et al. (1970) suggested, that the natural ergot alkaloids, in contrast to bromocriptine, also inhibit the milk ejection reflex as had been shown for several compounds (GROSVENOR and TURNER, 1956, 1957). This suggested difference in the profile of actions has not yet been experimentally tested, but employing the method described by AUSKOVA et al. (1974a) an ID_{50} for pups' weight gain inhibition of 1 mg/kg s.c. was found for bromocriptine. This value agrees well with the ED_{50} for implantation inhibition (0.7 mg/kg s.c.) and with the ID_{50} for serum prolactin suppression in male rats, measured 24 h after drug application (see below). Bromocriptine inhibits the depletion of prolactin from the pituitary in lactating rats stimulated by suckling pups (FLÜCKIGER and KOVACS, 1974) as well as the surge of serum prolactin levels (FLÜCKIGER et al., 1976). For bromocriptine, the dose-response effects on prolactin secretion as a function of pretreatment time has been studied in rats (FLÜCKIGER et al., 1976). At 2, 4, 8, and 24 h a single subcutaneous injection of bromocriptine was determined, which lowers the serum prolactin level of male rats by 50% (ID_{50}). The results are as follows: ID_{50} at 2 h=0.009 mg/kg s.c.; at 4 h=0.006; at 8 h=0.08, at 24 h=1.0 mg/kg s.c.

Lergotrile (cpd 39), the 2-chloro derivative of dihydrohomolysergic acid nitrile (cpd 83b), is a clinical research compound for the suppression of prolactin secretion in man. It is active in vivo and in vitro and is said to be equally potent as its mother compound but less toxic (CLEMENS et al., 1975). Replacement in position 2 of chloro by bromo (cpd 39a) gave a compound of slightly less activity, but the 2-iodo derivative (cpd 39b) seems to be clearly less active than lergotrile. Methylation of N_1 in lergotrile (cpd 39c) did not appreciably change the activity.

Methylergometrine (cpd 73a), a derivative of the natural product ergometrine (cpd 19), and clinically relevant for its uterotonic activity, is also quite active as a suppressor of prolactin secretion in an acute rat test at 50 μg/kg i.p. (CLEMENS et al., 1974) but only marginally active at 0.5 mg i.p. as an inhibitor of mammary development in late pregnancy when injected twice daily (SOMMER and BUCHANAN, 1955) and inactive at 5 mg/kg s.c. in inhibiting the deciduoma reaction in pseudopregnant rats (SHELESNYAK, 1958).

LSD 25 (lysergidum, cpd 73b) also seems to be a potent inhibitor of prolactin secretion and has a prolonged duration of action as judged from the fact of mammary tumor inhibition.

Lysergol (cpd 79a), 6-methyl-8β-hydroxymethyl-9-ergolene, inhibits prolactin secretion in acute tests and mammary tumor growth, both to an extent similar to the results with lergotrile. Isolysergol (cpd 79e), 6-methyl-8α-hydroxymethyl-9-ergolene, seems to be only slightly less active. The analogous 8α- and 8β-methyl compounds (cpd 79c, cpd 79d) seem both to be inactive at 50 μg/kg i.p. Lysergen, the 8-methylene analogue (cpd 79f) is also inactive, but the 8-acetoxymethylene derivative (cpd 79g) produced an effect at 2 h after 50 μg/kg i.p. of 48% of ergocornine (FLOSS et al., 1973). The smallest molecule of the whole list, 6-methyl-9-ergolene (cpd 79h), is said to also be active but to have less than 10% of the ergocornine activity (BACH et al., 1974).

Dihydrolysergol (cpd 81a) was very potent in an acute prolactin secretion suppression test (FLOSS et al., 1973) but did not suppress the growth of DMBA-induced mammary tumors (SWEENEY et al., 1975). This discrepancy could indicate that the drug has only a short duration of action.

Homolysergol (cpd 87a) and *dihydrohomolysergol* (cpd 87b) derivatives have been studied by BERAN et al. (1974) for implantation inhibitory activity at 5 mg/kg·d given orally for 5 days. The dihydro-series proved active.

Homolysergic acid has attracted much attention. *Homolysergic acid nitrile* (cpd 83a) inhibits prolactin secretion quite actively in acute tests, but *dihydrohomolysergic acid nitrile* (cpd 83b) is the more active of the two (CLEMENS et al., 1974). This compound is of particular interest, because it was the first nonpeptide ergot alkaloid derivative reported to inhibit prolactin secretion (ŘEŽÁBEK et al., 1969), and because lergotrile (cpd 39) is its 2-chloroderivative. Methylation of cpd 83b in position N_1 (cpd 83c) reduces the activity considerably, while introducing formyl in position N_1 (cpd 83d) is of little influence on the activity, as assessed in an acute test (CLEMENS et al., 1974).

Dihydrohomolysergic acid amide (cpd 86b) is a very potent and long-acting inhibitor of prolactin secretion. A single dose of ca. ~0.4 mg/kg orally prevents ovum implantation in rats (SEMONSKY et al., 1971). It inhibits weight gain in suckling rats with an ED_{50} of 0.22 mg/kg given orally over 4 days to the nursing rat (AUŠKOVÁ et al., 1973). Unfortunately, similar data to compare with other homolysergic acid derivatives are not available. From the fact that 1 mg/kg of cpd 83b given once orally to rats only partially inhibited implantation (ŘEŽÁBEK et al., 1969), it would seem that cpd 86b is more active than cpd 83b and possibly cpd 39. Substitution of the amide of cpd 86b by diethyl or cyclopentyl gave active compounds, but published results (SEMONSKY et al., 1971) do not permit a comparison with the mother compound.

A series of ergolenes and ergolines in which position 8 is substituted with an amino function is of particular interest: Results with *6-methyl-8β-amino-ergoline* (cpd 94c) in an acute test show a good prolactin secretion inhibitory activity (CASSADY et al., 1974). Unfortunately, no results with the 8α-amino isomer (cpd 94d) have been published nor with the 8α- or 8β-amino-ergolenes (cpd 94a 94b). SWEENEY et al. (1975) reported results from experiments on the inhibition of mammary tumor growth by 3 mg/kg s.c. of formylamino derivatives given for 13 days: 6-methyl-8α-formylamino-9-ergolene produced strong inhibition; 6-methyl-8α-formylamino-10β-ergoline gave medium inhibition; while 6-methyl-8α-formylamino-2,3-dihydro-9-ergolene, 6-methyl-8α-acetylamino-9-ergolene, and N(6-methyl-8α-ergolinyl)-N′-(3-pyrrolyl)-urea were found inactive.

Lysuride (cpd 96a), a 8α-urea derivative, is a clinically interesting compound for its central actions (ITIL et al., 1975). It is also a highly potent inhibitor of prolactin secretion in vivo and in vitro. In inhibits weight gain in suckling rats with an ED_{50} of 0.050 mg/kg given orally over 4 days to the nursing rat (AUŠKOVÁ et al., 1974a). It is, therefore, about four times more active than cpd 86b. Saturation of the double bond in position 9, 10 of cpd 96a produces N-(6-methyl-8α-ergolinyl)-N′N′-diethylurea (cpd 96c). This compound is about two times more potent as an inhibitor of prolactin secretion (as evidenced by the lactation inhibition test) than 86b and just about half as active than the unsaturated lysuride (cpd 96a) (AUŠKOVÁ et al., 1974b).

The 9,10-dihydrogenated series of the natural ergot peptide alkaloids and their analoga are not of great interest as inhibitors of prolactin secretion (cpds 102a–102e, 102 g; 108a/b; 110a/b). Only four of the compounds have been tested in more than one test, and of these the results with *dihydroergocornine* (cpd 102d) are of some heuristic value. CLEMENS et al. (1974) published results of dose-response studies comparing the lowering of serum prolactin levels in reserpine pretreated rats at 1 h after i-p. injection of either ergocornine (cpd 24) or dihydroergocornine (cpd 102d). The results showed both compounds to be equipotent ($ED_{50,1\,h}=10$ and 12 μg/kg i-p., respectively). The authors concluded that dihydrogenated derivatives are as active as their parent molecules. The results of other studies do not agree with this generalized view. SHELESNYAK (1958) found that 5 mg/kg s.c. dihydroergocornine did not inhibit the deciduoma reaction in pseudopregnant rats, in contrast to ergocornine; SWEENEY et al. (1975) observed less mammary tumor growth inhibition with dihydroergocornine than with ergocornine; FLÜCKIGER et al. (1976), using implantation inhibition as the criterion, reported the ED_{50} for dihydroergocornine to be greater than 3 mg/kg s.c., while the ED_{50} for ergocornine is 2.7 mg/kg s.c. Thus, in experiments where a prolonged suppression of prolactin is necessary to produce a functional effect, dihydroergocornine proves less active than ergocornine. The discrepancy between the results of CLEMENS et al. (1974) and those of the other investigators can best be explained by assuming that the duration of prolactin secretion inhibition by dihydroergocornine is shorter than that obtained with the same dose of ergocornine. This has not been tested. If this interpretation is true, then it would seem that using a test system with a prolonged observation period to screen for pharmacologically interesting com-

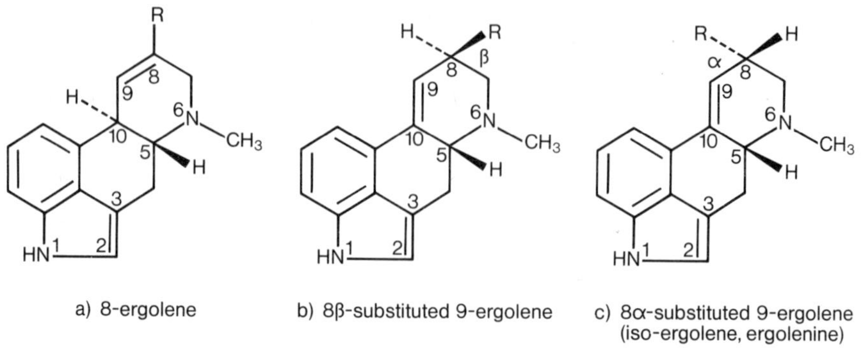

a) 8-ergolene b) 8β-substituted 9-ergolene c) 8α-substituted 9-ergolene (iso-ergolene, ergolenine)

Fig. 2a–c. General structural formulas of ergot derivatives. a) 8-ergolene; b) 8β-substituted 9-ergolene; c) 8α-substituted 9-ergolene (iso-ergolene, ergolenine)

pounds is more informative than using a test with only a short observation period.

Structure-Activity Relationships. It is evident from the foregoing that in this class of compounds greatly divergent derivations of the 6-methylergoline nucleus are compatible with prolactin secretion inhibitory activity. Due to this and due to the nature of the published results (e.g., mostly only one dose employed), the possibility for looking at structure-activity relationships is limited. To facilitate orientation in the following, Figure 2 reproduces the general structural formulas of ergot derivatives.

Substitutions in position 1. Methylation of position 1 of the ergolene nucleus is known to alter the profile of actions of ergot alkaloids profoundly. Considering only prolactin secretion inhibitory activity, the published material shows mostly quantitative changes. Lergotrile (cpd 39) is more active than its 1-methyl-derivative (cpd 39c) (CLEMENS et al., 1974). Methysergide (cpd 34a), which is the 1-methyl derivative of methylergometrine (cpd 73a), is probably less active than the latter, but the published data do not permit a more precise statement. Substitution of dihydrohomolysergic acid nitrile (cpd 83b) by 1-methyl (cpd 83c) reduces the activity considerably, but substitution by 1-formyl (cpd 83d) produces a smaller loss of activity (CLEMENS et al., 1974). Substituting agroclavine (cpd 5) by 1-cyano-methyl gives an inactive compound (CLEMENS et al., 1974).

Substitution in position 2. Introduction of halogen in position 2 is also known to alter the characeristics of ergot alkaloids profoundly. Looking at the prolactin secretion inhibitory activity only, the effects do not seem to be so dramatic as with other aspects of ergot pharmacology: 2-Br-ergocornine (cpd 37c) is several times less potent as an inhibitor of implantation than ergocornine (cpd 24), but bromocriptine (cpd 38) was found to be significantly more potent than α-ergokryptine (cpd 25) (FLÜCKIGER et al., 1976). Dihydrohomolysergic acid nitrile (cpd 83b) is said to be equally potent with its 2-chloro-derivative lergotrile (cpd 39) (CLEMENS et al., 1975). Using bromo instead of chloro substitution (cpd 39a) produced only a slight loss, while the 2-iodo derivative (cpd 39b) seems to have clearly less activity than lergotrile (CLEMENS et al., 1974). Saturation of the double bond between positions 2 and 3 gave only inactive products in the few cases published (CASSADY et al., 1974; SWEENEY et al., 1975).

Substitution at position 8. As previously mentioned five classes of 6-methylergoline derivatives contribute to the list of prolactin secretion inhibiting compounds, and these classes differ in the substituents at position 8: The clavine alkaloids, the lysergic acids, the simple lysergic acid amides, the peptide alkaloids, and the 8-amino-ergolines. Generally speaking, these different types of substituents tend to increase the biologic activity of 6-methyl-9-ergolene (cpd 79h), which itself inhibits prolactin secretion (BACH et al., 1974). Except for the 8-ergolenes (e.g., agroclavine), substitution at position 8 is possible in α or β. Traditionally, the α-isomer is often distinguished from the β-isomer by the prefix iso- or by the suffix -inine. With the lysergic acid derivatives, it is generally held that only the 8β-configuration is biologically active. In agreement with this, ergocorninine, the 8α-stereomer of ergocornine, was reported inactive by MEITES and CLEMENS (1972). With simpler derivatives of the 6-methyl-9-ergolene moiety, both diastereomers of the 8 position seem compatible with biologic activity; Isolysergol (cpd 79e) is probably not less active as a prolactin release inhibitor than lysergol (cpd 79a). In the 8-amino series, both diastereomers seem to allow for biologic activity: 6-methyl-8β-aminoergoline (cpd 94c) inhibits prolactin secretion (CASSADY et al., 1974). No results with the 8α-stereomer are available, but the two most active derivatives of this class of compounds show the 8α-configuration, cpd 96a (AUŠKOVÁ et al., 1974a) and cpd 96c (AUŠKOVÁ et al., 1974b). ZIKAN et al. (1974) reported 1,1-diethyl-4-(6-methyl-8β-ergolinyl)-semicarbazide to inhibit implantation but found the 8α-stereomer inactive.

Saturation of double-bonds Δ8 or Δ9. 6-methyl-8-cyanomethyl-8-ergolene (cpd 6e) (LI et al., 1975) seems to be less active than the saturated compound (cpd 83b), dihydrohomolysergic acid nitrile (β-isomer) (CLEMENS et al., 1974). 6-Methyl-8-carboxamidomethyl-8-ergolene (cpd 6f) was found equally active with ergocornine at 1 h after injection (LI et al., 1975). Its saturated congener (β-isomer) is dihydrohomolysergic acid amide (cpd 86b), a highly potent compound in several functional tests (SEMONSKY et al., 1971; AUŠKOVÁ et al., 1973). Thus, saturation of the double-bond Δ8 does not seem to diminish prolactin secretion inhibitory activity. Lysergol (cpd 79a), a Δ9 unsaturated compound, and dihydrolysergol (cpd 81a) are both quite active in short-term tests, but 3 mg/kg·d s.c. of lysergol was found inactive (SWEENEY et al., 1975). This could mean that saturation of Δ9 induces a shortening of the duration of action. Homolysergic acid nitrile (cpd 83a) at 1 h after injection seems to be less active than dihydrohomolysergic acid nitrile (cpd 83b) (CLEMENS et al., 1974). Five derivatives of homolysergol (cpd 87a) and six of dihydrohomolysergol (cpd 87b) have been compared in the implantation inhibition test by BERAN et al. (1974) at the dose of 5 mg/kg s.c. All the dihydro compounds were found active, while all homolysergol derivatives did not show any inhibitory effect. Here then are examples of a clear increase of biologic activity by saturation of the double bond Δ9. In the 8α-amino group of compounds, the Δ9 unsaturated lysuride (cpd 96a) is about two times more active than its Δ9 saturated congener (cpd 96c) (AUŠKOVÁ et al., 1974a). From their results in short-term tests with the ergot peptide alkaloid series, CLEMENS et al. (1974) concluded that dihydrogenated derivatives are as active as their parent molecules. When using tests with end points which necessitate a prolonged suppression of prolactin secretion, e.g., the implantation inhibition test (see "Methodological Remarks"), a comparison of the potency of the natural and the dihydrogenated ergot peptides results in a different conclusion: As far as our experimental data presented in Table 3 can be used for comparison it seems that the dihydrogenated compounds are clearly less potent than the natural compounds (FLÜCKIGER et al., 1976). As mentioned before, the discrepancy between our experience and that of CLEMENS et al. (1974) might be due to a difference in the duration of action between the two series of compounds, which would not show up in short-term experiments.

Stereoisomers at position 10. Hydrogenation of the double bond of 9-ergolene compounds produces a new asymmetric carbon atom at position 10. It is possible in principle to have 5, 10-cis compounds besides the usual 5,10-trans compounds, but this, where tested, does not seem to give compounds with biologic activity. CASSADY et al. (1974) have published negative results with three such compounds, one of which is the 10β-stereomer of the active isolysergol (cpd 79e). ZIKAN et al. (1974) have published another example: 1,1-diethyl-4(6-methyl-8α-ergolinyl)-semicarbazide inhibits implantation at 5 mg/kg orally, but its 10β-stereomer showed no activity at this dose.

β) Sites of Action

In 1954 SHELESNYAK pointed out that two possible sites should be considered where ergot alkaloids exert their prolactin secretion inhibitory effect, i.e., the hypothalamus and the pituitary. Only very few ergot alkaloids have been analyzed as to their site of action.

The first experimental proof that ergot alkaloids inhibit prolactin secretion by acting directly at the pituitary level was brought forth in two experiments by ZEILMAKER and CARLSEN (1962): In female rats with functioning corpora lutea, which are hypophysectomized, and the autologous pituitary transplanted under

Table 3. Implantation inhibitory activity of ergot peptide alkaloids and the 9,10-dihydroderivatives

		ED_{50} mg/kg s.c.[a]		
			9,10 dihydro-	
(Cpd 20)	ergotamine	14	>20	(cpd 102b)
(Cpd 21)	ergosine	5.7	20	(cpd 102a)
(Cpd 22)	ergostine	>20	> 3	(cpd 102g)
(Cpd 23)	ergocristine	4.2	> 3	(cpd 102c)
(Cpd 24)	ergocornine	2.7	> 3	(cpd 102d)
(Cpd 25)	α-ergokryptine	1.1	4.8	(cpd 102e)
(Cpd 26)	β-ergokryptine	2.8	—	
(Cpd 108a)	ergovaline	9.0	>20	(cpd 108b)
(Cpd 110a)	ergocornine	4.6	> 3	(cpd 110b)
(Cpd 111a)	ergostine	4.0	> 3	(cpd 111b)

> Denotes highest dose tested, with no or marginal effect.

[a] Drug injected s.c. on day 5 after insemination. Autopsy for the search of implantation sites on day 12.

the kidney capsule, ergocornine (1 mg s.c.), prevented the deciduoma reaction in the traumatised uterus; in intact females the transplantation of two isologous pituitaries under the kidney capsule leads to activation of corpora lutea as evidenced by continuous leukocyte dominance of the vaginal smear. Ergocornine (1 mg s.c.) induced in such animals a cyclic vaginal smear pattern and ovulation. It was concluded from these observations that ergocornine interrupts the luteotropic function of an ectopic pituitary by a direct action at the (ectopic) pituitary level. Later, direct proof using in vitro methods was provided by several laboratories using different alkaloids within a very short time; NICOLL et al. (1970) demonstrated an inhibitory effect of ergotamine on prolactin secretion from rat pituitaries. PASTEELS et al. (1971), using a bioassay method, found less prolactin-like activity in the incubation media of rat and human (fetal) anterior pituitaries when about 10^{-5} M ergocornine or 2-Br-α-ergokryptine (bromocriptine) was present in the incubation media than in the absence of an alkaloid. LU et al. (1971), using a RIA system to measure prolactin, incubated rat pituitaries over 12 h and found ergocronine at about 10^{-7} M to inhibit secretion and synthesis of prolactin. Incubation of the pituitaries in the presence of estradiol stimulated synthesis and secretion, and this was prevented by the addition of ergocornine. ECTORS et al. (1972), using electron microscopic methods, observed that rat pituitaries incubated in vitro contained more secretory material in the presence of ergocornine (at 10^{-6} M) than in its absence. MACLEOD and LEHMEYER (1972) observed that ergocornine, ergokryptine, and ergotamine inhibit the release of freshly labeled prolactin into the medium from incubated rat pituitaries. Using clonal cell cultures of a rat pituitary tumor (GH_3), TASHJIAN and HOYT (1972) found a dose-dependent inhibition of prolactin release into the culture medium in the presence of bromocriptine. Finally, the antagonism by bromocriptine (SCHAMS, 1972) of the prolactin-releasing effect of the directly acting TRH (TASHJIAN et al., 1971) also suggests a direct inhibitory action of this alkaloid. Not only peptide alkaloids but also low-molecular-weight ergoline derivatives act directly at the pituitary to inhibit prolactin secretion, as demonstrated by CLEMENS et al. (1975), incubating rat pituitaries with lergotrile (Lilly 83636).

Some observations suggest that prolactin inhibition is obtained by an action at the hypothalamic level. FUXE and HÖKFELT (1970) first reported that after ergocornine or bromocriptine treatment of lactating rats an inactivation of the tubero-infundibular dopaminergic (TIDA) neurons of the N. arcuatus hypothalami occurred. WUTTKE et al. (1971) found an increase in the hypothalamus of rats of PIF activity after ergocornine. These observations were interpreted as showing a hypothalamic site of action (HÖKFELT and FUXE, 1972). HÖKFELT and FUXE (1972) also observed that hypophysectomy decreases the DA turnover in female and male rats in the TIDA neurons as well, and that treatment of hypophysectomized rats with prolactin increases DA turnover of the same neurons. Obviously, the TIDA neurons respond to alterations in circulating prolactin levels as elements in a short-loop, feed-back system. It is known from other studies that prolactin may inhibit its own secretion (MEITES, 1973; NEILL, 1974). CLEMENS et al. (1971), using an electrophysiologic approach, have actually demonstrated in rabbits the presence of prolactin responsive neurons. The effect of drugs like the aforementioned ergot alkaloids on the transmitter turnover of the TIDA neurons could then be explained as secondary to the suppression of serum prolactin levels by a direct pituitary action. It does not seem necessary to assume a primary hypothalamic site of action of the ergot alkaloids for the suppression of prolactin secretion. On the other hand, all this does not exclude that in addition to acting directly on the pituitary, the ergot alkaloids also influence an hypothalamic neuronal system to release PIF—we are not certain as long as we cannot specifically measure circulating PIF. For practical purposes, the problem seems of secondary importance, but the question will have to be discussed again in the context with changes of secretion of other pituitary hormones, especially FSH and LH.

In summary, there is clear proof that some ergot alkaloids act directly at the pituitary level to inhibit prolactin secretion, but we have no concrete evidence that these drugs also inhibit prolactin secretion by acting at the hypothalamic level (to release PIF). The assumption that they also act by hypothalamic neurons to inhibit prolactin secretion derives support from their well-known effects on dopaminergic neuronal systems in extra-hypophyseotropic areas of the CNS (see Chapter VI) (CORRODI et al., 1973).

γ) Mechanism of Prolactin-Secretion Inhibition

Only very few ergot alkaloids have been subjected to detailed studies as to how they act to reduce serum prolactin levels, α-ergokryptine and bromocriptine being the best investigated compounds.

When bromocriptine (10^{-7} to 10^{-10} M) is incubated together with cultured cells derived of a rat pituitary tumor (GH_3) (TASHJIAN and HOYT, 1972), or when α-ergokryptine is incubated with rat anterior pituitary fragments (MACLEOD and LEHMEYER, 1974; HILL-SAMLI and MACLEOD, 1975) the concentration of prolactin in the medium is reduced dose-dependently, and the intracellular prolactin concentration is increased over control values. During a 5 h incubation period, there was observed only a marginal inhibition of prolactin synthesis. This indicates that the secretory process is primarily inhibited, apomorphine or dopamine acting similarly. YANAI and NAGASAWA (1974), treating proestrus rats with bromocriptine 1–8 h before incubating their pituitaries in vitro in the presence of ^{14}C-leucine found prolactin secretion greatly depressed but prolactin synthesis unaltered. Inhibition of secretion is the primary event, and this is in agreement with morphologic observation using ergocornine (ECTORS et al., 1972) and bromocriptine (FLÜCKIGER et al., 1976). HILL-SAMLI and MACLEOD (1975), using ^{3}H-leucine incorporation into prolactin as a marker for freshly synthetized peptide, found evidence that newly formed prolactin is more sensitive to secretion inhibition by α-ergokryptine than preformed prolactin.

The consequences of prolonged secretion inhibition upon prolactin cell metabolism has been studied in vivo by DAVIES et al. (1974) and LLOYD et al. (1975) with male rats under continuous estrogen stimulation. They found that such rats, when treated with bromocriptine (3 mg/kg·d), have lower serum prolactin levels and show less DNA synthesis in the pituitaries. Also, such pituitaries show less mitotic activity than the controls treated with estrogen alone, the difference being in good quantitative correlation to the differences in serum prolactin levels between bromocriptine-treated and control rats. Assuming that the observed effects are specific of change in prolactin cells, these observations seem to signify that when prolactin accumulates within the cell due to inhibition of hormone release, then a negative feed-back occurs on the overall metabolism of the prolactin cell, including mitotic processes. In a study using rats implanted with the pituitary tumor MtT.W15, QUADRI and MEITES (1973) demonstrated that ergocornine, besides inhibiting prolactin secretion, also induced a time-dependent shrinking of the tumor size over the 3-week treatment period.

Whether this means that spontaneous prolactin-secreting pituitary tumors (e.g., in man) may be arrested or reversed in their development by a continuous inhibition of prolactin secretion remains unanswered.

Bromocriptine inhibits the acute stimulatory effect on prolactin secretion of TRF (SCHAMS, 1972) in vivo which is known to act directly at the pituitary level (TASHJIAN et al., 1971). We have described (FLÜCKIGER et al., 1976) that bromocriptine in rats quantitatively antagonizes the prolactin-releasing action of TRF, suggestive of a competitive antagonism. In vitro, the inhibitory action of α-ergokryptine (4×10^{-10} M) on prolactin secretion by incubated rat pituitary fragments is reduced by TRF (1.11×10^{-8} M) (HILL-SAMLI and MACLEOD, 1975), which also antagonizes the release-inhibitory action of apomorphine (7.5×10^{-8} M) (HILL-SAMLI and MACLEOD, 1974). The fundamental in vitro studies of MACLEOD and his group (for a review of earlier studies, see MACLEOD and LEHMEYER, 1972) has further shown that the inhibitory action of α-ergokryptine, dopamine, or apomorphine is fully antagonized by neuroleptics like haloperidol or perphenazine (MACLEOD and LEHMEYER, 1974a) (Fig. 3). Another neuroleptic, pimozide, was also found to antagonize the effects of dopamine and apomorphine on prolactin release (MACLEOD and LEHMEYER, 1974b; SMALSTIG et al., 1974). Thus, the isolated pituitary displays a prolactin secretion control system by which some ergot alkaloids as well as apomorphine and dopamine act to inhibit secretion, while TRF and the neuroleptics pimozide, haloperidol, and perphenazine act to antagonize these inhibitors. This suggests that these ergot alkaloids inhibit prolactin secretion by directly stimulating dopamine receptors located on the prolactin cells. It is true that MACLEOD's group has found in earlier in vitro studies (MACLEOD and LEHMEYER, 1972) that 1-noradrenaline, 1-adrenaline, and d-adrenaline, but not metanephrine nor 3,4-dihydroxymandelic acid also inhibit prolactin secretion. In these studies, 10^{-5} M amine was used and noradrenaline 2×10^{-7} M was found inactive, while dopamine at 5×10^{-7} M inhibited prolactin secretion by about 90% (MACLEOD and LEHMEYER, 1974a). It thus seems that dopamine is the more specific of the amines studied, which again fits with the assumption that the prolactin release control mechanism is dopaminergic in nature.

There remains the question of how the stimulation of dopamine receptors at the prolactin cell level results in inhibition of prolactin release. Prolactin secretion from pituitaries kept in vitro is stimulated by adding cAMP analogues to the incubation medium (NAGASAWA and YANAI, 1972; PELLETIER et al., 1972) or by adding theophylline (KIMURA et al., 1976), which increased pituitary cAMP content. The stimulatory effect of dibutyryl-cAMP is inhibited by bromocriptine (NAGASAWA et al., 1973), indicating that this drug may interfere with a later step in the process necessary for prolactin release. KIMURA et al. (1976) reported that dopamine blocked the theophylline stimulated rise in cAMP content in incubated rat pitui-

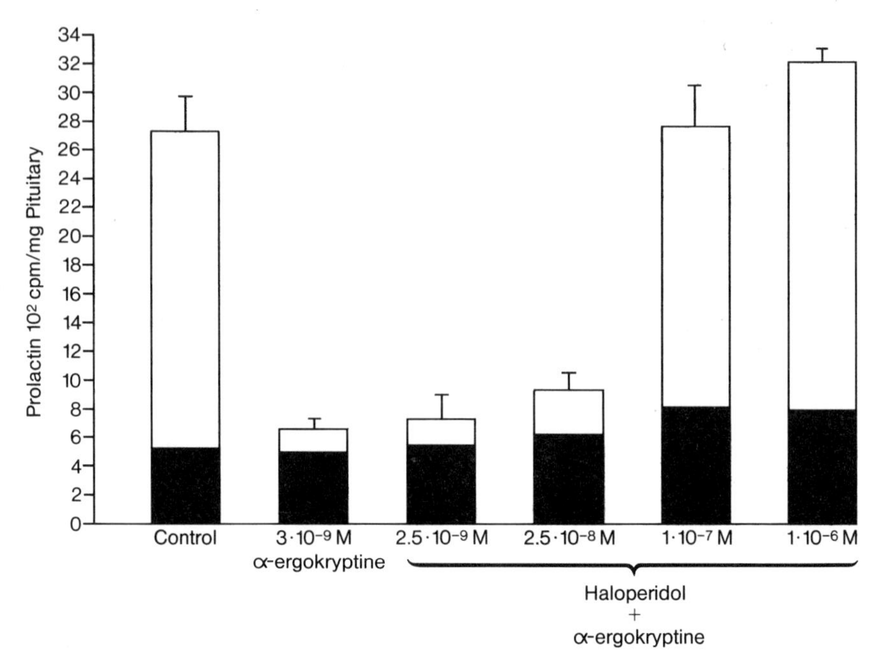

Fig. 3. Blockade of the α-ergokryptine mediated inhibition of prolactin release from rat hemipituitaries by haloperidol. 3×10^{-9} M α-ergokryptine was incubated alone and in the presence of varying concentrations of haloperidol. White columns represent secreted prolactin, black columns retained prolactin. [After MACLEOD and LEHMEYER (1974) with the permission of the Endocrine Society and the J.B. Lippincott Company]

taries as well as the theophylline-induced release of prolactin. GAUTVIK et al. (1973a), using clonal cell cultures derived from a rat pituitary tumor (GH_3), observed that bromocriptine inhibits the increased release of prolactin, which follows an elevation in the potassium concentration of the incubation medium from 5.3 to 30–50 mM. As has been shown earlier, this action on the pituitary of high concentrations of external potassium does not involve an increase in cAMP (ZOR et al., 1970) but depolarizes the pituitary cell membranes (MILLIGAN and KRAICER, 1970) and at the same time increases the Ca^{45} space of rat pituitaries (MILLIGAN and KRAICER, 1969). It is thus possible that bromocriptine and similar drugs act by either polarizing the cell membranes or by reducing free Ca^{++}.

Although we have no information whether dopamine or apomorphine act similarly to bromocriptine, there exists an earlier valuable study on the mechanism of action of PIF extracted from rat hypothalami; PARSONS and NICOLL (1971) observed that PIF activity of rat hypothalamic extracts antagonized prolactin release stimulation by theophylline and attenuated the stimulatory effect of 54 mM potassium but was unable to further suppress the residual prolactin secretion when the calcium concentration in the medium was reduced from 1.8 to ~0.01 mM. These experimental results suggest that PIF acts at the cell membrane and possibly interferes with Ca^{++} influx necessary for the process of secretion (PARSONS, 1969; GAUTVIK and TASHJIAN, 1973b). We have, therefore, certain observational elements to suggest that drugs like bromocriptine and PIF may act in a similar way, but this is not necessarily so.

Not all ergot alkaloids which inhibit prolactin secretion fit into the dopamine concept as applied above. Methysergide (cpd 34a) is such a case: Methysergide (cpd 34a) is characterized as a serotonin receptor blocker (see Chapter III) and was used as such by CALIGARIS and TALEISNIK (1974) in their pharmacologic analysis of the mechanism of the prolactin surge induced in spayed rats by estrogen or estrogen plus progesterone. This prolactin surge was either attenuated by treatment with p-chlorphenylalanine (PCPA) or by the injection of methysergide (10 μg) into the third ventricle. Serotonin injected into the third ventricle stimulates prolactin release. These results form part of a set of observations which led the authors to postulate an inhibitory serotoninergic system impinging on the catecholamine neurons controlling the secretion of PIF. This serotoninergic system would mainly be involved in phasic or episodic release of prolactin, as e.g., in suckling-induced prolactin release (KORDON et al., 1973, 1974; MULLOY and MOBERG, 1975). Thus, GALLO et al. (1975) found that methysergide (25 mg/kg i-p.) fully inhibited in lactating rats the prolactin release induced $3^1/_4$ h later by suckling pups. Further, MARCHLEWSKA-KOJ and KRULICH (1975) observed in male rats complete suppression by 50 mg/kg i.p. methysergide of the prolactin release induced by repeated ether anesthesia and bleeding. No effect of methysergide was reported on prolactin secretion from pituitaries kept in vitro and on basal prolactin secretion of male rats by these authors, but GALLO et al. (1975) described short-lived increases of plasma prolactin levels in anesthetized, ovariectomized rats and in lactating non-suckled rats after injection of methysergide, which effects are unexplained. The two latter groups of authors agree in considering the inhibitory action of methysergide on sensory and stress-evoked prolactin release as being due to central serotonin receptor blockade. Recently, LAWSON and GALA (1976) reported that the pimozide-induced increase of prolactin secretion in ovariectomized, estrogen-stabilized rats could be reduced by methysergide and by the nonergoline serotonin antagonist SQ 10,631 and concluded that "part of the increase in prolactin following dopaminergic blockade may result from the action of a tonically stimulatory serotonin system that is normally masked by the intense tonic inhibition by the dopaminergic system". These findings are complementary to those of CALIGARIS and TALEISNIK (1974) and demonstrate the possibility of interfering at a central level with stimulated prolactin secretion by the use of ergot alkaloids antagonizing serotonin.

It must be assumed that besides methysergide there are further compounds hidden in Table 1 in which serotonin antagonism contributes to their prolactin release inhibitory action.

b) Gonadotropins

Introduction. The gonadotropins [follicle-stimulating hormone (FSH) and luteinizing hormone or interstitial cell-stimulating hormone (LH, ICSH)] have been recognized for many years as the key hormones in reproduction, and their physiologic role in both sexes is well understood and appropriately treated in the text books of physiology or endocrinology. Recently, the subject has been reviewed for the female (GREENWALD, 1974) and for the male (STEINBERGER and STEINBERGER, 1974). The elucidation of the control mechanisms of gonadotropin secretion which attracts most interest today is less advanced (MCCANN, 1974); in males, the secretion of the two gonadotropins is considered to be relatively constant (tonic) and mainly determined by simple negative feed-back mechanisms between steroids and the pituitary-hypothalamic complex. In the female, an additional mechanism is needed to allow for the cyclic events of ovulation, which also necessitates positive feed-back interactions between steroids and the pituitary-hypothalamic complex. The neuronal makeup of the hypothalamic regulatory mechanism is still far from clear. Pharmacologically, the neuronal apparatus in female rodents seems to involve catecholaminergic, serotoninergic, cholinergic, and gabaergic elements. Control of pituitary gonadotropin secretion by the hypothalamus is stimulatory and is effected by the release into the primary plexus of the hypothalamo-pituitary sytem of releasing factors of peptidic nature. There is much experimental evidence that two separate releasing factors for LH and FSH (MCCANN, 1974) exist, but only the structure of LH-RF is known. This LH-RF has been synthetized (MATSUO et al., 1971; MONAHAN et al., 1971) and found to also stimulate the secretion of FSH. Despite this finding, the question of the existence of a separate FSH-RF is not yet settled.

Physiologically and pharmacologically, the regulation of gonadotropin secretion cannot be discussed disconnected from that of prolactin secretion. ROTHCHILD (1960) has pointed out that there seems to exist in the rat a mechanism by which conditions favoring prolactin secretion have an inhibitory effect on gonadotropin secretion. In several species, the anovulatory period during postpartal lactation, the hyperprolactinemia-amenorrhea syndrome in women, as well as the suppression of fertility in the presence of hyperprolactinemia in the human male are well known, just as is the restitution of fertility by drugs that suppress prolactin secretion. It is not clear whether suppression of cyclic gonadotropin secretion in the case of the female is a consequence of the primary event, the increased prolactin secretion, or whether both are due to one and the same cause. It is also not clear how far effects of prolactin at the target systems of the gonadotropins interfere with steroid feed-back control of gonadotropin secretion (MCNATTY et al., 1976).

Methodologic Remarks. Tonic and phasic (cyclic) secretion of the gonadotropins attract pharmacologists differently, probably partly due to methodologic reasons. Whereas it is easy to find the inhibitory action of a drug on phasic LH secretion by simply looking for an ovulation inhibitory effect (with appropriate control experiments to exclude peripheral interference with ovulation), for example, all tonic aspects of gonadotropin secretion either necessitate prolonged administration of the drug and/or prolonged observation periods or necessitate the multiple measurements of circulating LH and FSH radioimmunologically. It seems that nobody has systematically studied the inhibitory or stimulatory action of ergot alkaloids on tonic secretion of FSH or LH in laboratory rodents, and few have looked for effects on phasic gonadotropin secretion. Two main forms of the ovulation-inhibition test in rodents are in use, the pregnant mare serum (PMS)-induced ovulation in prepuberal rats or mice and the spontaneous cyclic event in adult rats or mice. In the past, the two tests were assumed to be equivalent (PIVA et al., 1969), but a recent comparative study in rats (MARKO and FLÜCKIGER,

1974) made clear that important physiologic and pharmacologic differences exist between the two models.

As to the assaying of LH and FSH by bioassay or radioimmunologic methods, the reader will find an introduction to the original literature in McCANN's review (1974).

α) Drug Actions

Inhibition of Gonadotropin Secretion. Ergot alkaloids can inhibit phasic LH secretion, as evidenced by the inhibition of ovulation in rats or mice. This action was first recognized with ergocornine (ZEILMAKER, 1964; KRAICER and STRAUSS, 1970). Table 4 presents the short list of the compounds described to inhibit ovulation. It is interesting to note that the natural peptide alkaloids for which ED_{50} values were obtained show monotonously similar potencies in the adult cycling rat. This potency is greatly reduced in the two compounds where bromine was introduced in position 2 of the indole ring. When comparing the ovulation inhibitory activity and the prolactin secretion inhibitory activity of different ergot alkaloids, no correlation could be found (FLÜCKIGER et al., 1976). Thus, the two actions are probably due to different qualities of these compounds. Another interesting facet is presented by the fact (MARKO and FLÜCKIGER, 1974) that juvenile rats induced to ovulate by pretreatment with pregnant mare serum (PMS) are more sensitive to the inhibitory action of 2-Br-α-ergokryptine than adults, while they seem less sensitive to ergocornine than adults.

KRAICER and STRAUSS (1970) pointed out that adult rats show highest sensitivity towards the ovulation inhibitory action of ergocornine around noon of proestrus, with a sharp decline to zero thereafter. Their animals also responded unexpectedly to ergocornine, if it was injected even a day before the sensitive phase, i.e., in diestrus. It is not known whether this is unique for ergocornine; it is certainly at variance with other types of drugs that inhibit ovulation (EVERETT, 1964). WUTTKE et al. (1971), after injecting ergocornine, 0.05, 0.5, or 2.0 mg/kg i.p. at 1.30 p.m. into proestrus rats, observed a dose-dependent reduction of the increase of LH plasma levels (LH-surge) to be seen at 4 p.m. of the same afternoon. Even with the highest dose used, the attenuation of the LH-surge was not enough to produce ovulation inhibition. Thus, these authors do not confirm the ovulation inhibitory action seen in other studies. Also YOKOYAMA et al. (1972), injecting ~4 mg/kg ergocornine s.c. first in the afternoon of diestrus and again in the morning of proestrus into rats, did not find ovulation inhibited, except in one of six animals. It is not possible to really explain these negative results. Both groups of investigators observed in their experiments the inhibition of the proestrus prolactin surge, and the team of WUTTKE found a dose-dependent reduction of the LH-surge. So it may be permitted to assume that both groups might have observed ovulation inhibition if they had used still higher doses of the drug. In other words, the discrepancy of the findings may be due to different sensitivities of the animal strain used.

Using the spontaneous fall over 6 h in pituitary FSH in 37-days-old female rats immediately before the onset of cyclic ovarian function, BROWN (1971) observed that methysergide (cpd 34a) (~1 mg/kg i.p. or s.c.) blocked this fall. Some very

Table 4. Ovulation inhibiting ergot alkaloids

Compound number	Name	Authors	Remarks
20	Ergotamine	RAJ and GREEP (1973)	Adult rat, fully effective at 10 mg/kg i.p. partially at 4 mg/kg i.p.
		MARKO (unpublished)	Adult rat, $ED_{50} \approx 0.3$ mg/kg s.c.
21	Ergosine	MARKO (unpublished)	Adult rat, $ED_{50} = 0.34$ (0.18–0.63) mg/kg s.c.
22	Ergostine	MARKO (unpublished)	Adult rat, $ED_{50} = 0.63$ mg/kg s.c.
23	Ergocristine	FLÜCKIGER et al. (1976)	Adult rat, $ED_{50} = 1.3$ (0.9–1.8) mg/kg s.c.
24	Ergocornine	ZEILMAKER (1964)	Adult rat, active at 1 mg/rat s.c.
		KRAICER and STRAUSS (1970)	Adult rat, active at 0.5 mg/rat s.c.
		HÖKFELT and FUXE (1972)	Juvenile PMS rat
		MARKO and FLÜCKIGER (1974)	Adult rat, $ED_{50} = 1.7$ (1.2–2.4) mg/kg s.c.
			Juvenile PMS rat, $ED_{50} = 3.2$ (2.2–7.0) mg/kg s.c.
25	α-Ergokryptine	FLÜCKIGER et al. (1976)	Adult rat, $ED_{50} = 1.7$ (1.4–2.1) mg/kg s.c.
26	β-Ergokryptine	FLÜCKIGER et al. (1976)	Adult rat, $ED_{50} = 1.7$ (1.2–2.3) mg/kg s.c.
34a	Methysergide	BROWN (1967)	Adult mouse, 100 μg no effect
			Juvenile PMS mouse, 5–20 μg acting dose-dependently
37c	2-Br-ergocornine	FLÜCKIGER et al. (1976)	Adult rat, $ED_{50} > 20$ mg/kg s.c.
38	Bromocriptine	HÖKFELT and FUXE (1972)	Juvenile PMS rat
		MARKO and FLÜCKIGER (1974)	Adult rat, $ED_{50} = 20$ (13.7–29.0) mg/kg s.c.
			Juvenile PMS rat, $ED_{50} = 1.5$ (0.5–5.9) mg/kg s.c.
73b	LSD-25	BROWN (1967)	Adult mouse, 2 × 100 μg no effect
			Juvenile PMS mouse, 30 μg partially inhibited
108a	Ergovaline	MARKO (unpublished)	Adult rat, $ED_{50} = 0.7$ (0.4–1.2) mg/kg s.c.
110a	Ergonine	MARKO (unpublished)	Adult rat, $ED_{50} = 1.8$ (1.1–2.8) mg/kg s.c.
111a	Ergoptine	MARKO (unpublished)	Adult rat, $ED_{50} = 1.8$ (1.1–2.8) mg/kg s.c.

acute effects on FSH by compound VUFB6683 (cpd 86b) have been reported by CHLEBOUNOVA et al. (1974). Using a simplified STEELMAN and POHLEY test without a standard, they found that pituitaries of rats treated in estrus or metestrus with 0.5 mg/kg of the compound contain statistically significantly more FSH-like activity than control pituitaries. In diestrus and proestrus no effect was found. In a second study pregnant female rats on days 5 and 15 after insemination were used. Compound VUFB6683-treated females on days of pregnancy had less FSH-like activity in their pituitaries than controls, while on day 15 no difference was found. Unfortunately, the bioassay technique used does not permit asessment of the relevance of these results. Ergot alkaloids so far tested have not been reported to inhibit tonic gonadotropin secretion in a functionally relevant measure; long-term treatment of C3H/He mice with ergocornine or bromocriptine did not produce deterioration of vaginal cycles but actually made them more regular than observed in the control animals (YANAI and NAGASAWA, 1970a, b; NAGASAWA and YANAI, 1970). Also, chronic treatment of sheep with bromocriptine in doses necessary to suppress prolactin secretion did not alter serum LH and FSH or progesterone levels nor cycle length (NISWENDER, 1974).

Stimulation of Gonadotropin Secretion. Termination in the rat of early gestation or pseudopregnancy by suppressing prolactin secretion with ergotoxine (SHELESNYAK, 1957; KRAICER and SHELESNYAK, 1965), or any other prolactin secretion inhibiting ergot alkaloid thus far tested is followed by the appearance of estrus vaginal smears and ovulation within 96 h after treatment. This also happens in rats with an ectopic pituitary as a source of hyperprolactinemia, as shown by ZEILMAKER and CARLSEN (1962) with ergocornine and FLÜCKIGER et al. (1976) with bromocriptine. Suppression of prolactin in lactating rats by compound VUFB6638 (cpd 96c) shortened the lactational anestrus period in the rat (AUŠKOVÁ et al., 1974c), and suppression of prolactin secretion in postpartum ewes with bromocriptine also shortened the lactational anestrus (KANN and MARTINET, 1975). AUŠKOVÁ et al. (1974c) reported on four bitches about 2 months out of their last heat, in which daily treatment with compound VUFB6638 (cpd 96d) within 8 days induced enlargement and congestion of the vulva and secretion of mucus, followed by a discharge containing blood, i.e., signs of heat in three of the animals. Two of the bitches were then successfully mated. The authors suggest these observations to indicate that stimulation of gonadotropin secretion is a property of the drug used. Such observations do not in our view necessitate that the drugs used stimulate gonadotropin secretion, a simpler explanation being that suppression of prolactin secretion releases cyclic gonadotropin secretion from its inhibited state, as in the rat model. Prolactin measurements are necessary to clarify the situation.

Another prolactin secretion inhibiting compound VUFB6605 (cpd 83b) (ŘEŽÁBEK et al., 1969), given for 12 days to unilaterally ovariectomized rats, was found to produce a greater weight increase in the remaining ovary (compensatory hypertrophy) than observed in the controls (SEDA et al., 1971). This effect was interpreted as evidence of drug-stimulated FSH secretion. This interpretation seems debatable, as we have learned (WUTTKE and MEITES, 1971; BILLETER and FLÜCKIGER, 1971) that increases of ovarian weight can be obtained through the accumulation of nonregressed corpora lutea if prolactin secretion is inhibited in cycling female rats.

Boyns et al. (1972), treating male rats with 0.1 mg/d of bromocriptine, observed after 10 days of treatment increased plasma LH concentrations, while plasma testosterone levels were at the same time reduced. The authors were uncertain whether to consider these effects as secondary to the suppression of prolactin secretion or to a gonadotropin secretion stimulatory effect of the drug. Bartke (1973, 1974) using male mice and rats, found, after continuous treatment with ergocornine or bromocriptine from 10 days to 3 weeks, reduced plasma testosterone levels, thus confirming Boyns et al., (1972). Bartke (1973, 1974) considers his results as evidence that prolactin is normally involved in the testosterone production by the testis.

There are thus no observations in the literature which provide good evidence for postulating that ergot alkaloids applied systemically stimulate gonadotropin secretion in animals by a direct action.

One abstract of a study, though, provides evidence that with local application different results may be obtained: Borrell et al. (1975) injected bromocriptine bilaterally into the amygdala of adult castrated female rats and measured circulating FSH and LH. Bromocriptine caused LH but not FSH levels to rise above control values. Similarly, apomorphine increased LH and left FSH unaltered. Unfortunately, nothing is said of the prolactin levels of these rats.

β) Sites of Action

Whereas many investigators were interested to know where the prolactin secretion inhibitory action of some of the ergot alkaloids and related compounds takes place, a comparable interest concerning the site of the gonadotropin secretion inhibitory action of these drugs is not evident.

Seki et al. (1974b) published a study aimed at testing whether bromocriptine acted at the pituitary level to suppress LH and FSH secretion. In ovariectomized estrogen-progesterone-stabilized rats 5 mg/kg i.p. of bromocriptine were found to reduce basal secretion of LH by about 30% and to attenuate the LH response to 100 ng i.v. of LH-RF by about 30%. FSH secretion was not altered. Thus, evidence for a direct action at the pituitary level by bromocriptine to suppress basal and LH-RF-stimulated LB but not FSH secretion exists. Nooter and Zeilmaker (1970) reported that in rats ovulation blocked by ergocornine could be induced by electric stimulation in the preoptic area of the hypothalamus, indicating that the pituitary remained capable of releasing LH adequately in response to a hypothalamic stimulus. The two reports are not in conflict, but the study by Nooter and Zeilmaker suggests that the relevant site of action by ergocornine might be at a higher level than the pituitary. Such assumption is supported by the observation by Wuttke et al. (1971) that in ergocornine-treated proestrus rats, LH-RF-like activity in the hypothalalmus is reduced in association with the reduced circulating levels of LH. This suggests (1) that attenuation of LH secretion is the consequence of reduced LH-RF availability and (2) that the hypothalamic level is of relevance to understand the ovulation inhibitory effect of ergot derivatives.

γ) *Mechanisms of Actions*

Inhibition of Gonadotropin Secretion. Concerning the mechanism of the inhibition of phasic gonadotropin secretion and ovulation in female rats or mice, very little experimental evidence exists as a basis of analysis. WUTTKE et al. (1971) have observed in proestrus rats treated with ergocornine a reduction of LH-RF-like activity in the hypothalamus associated with a reduced secretion of LH. This finding is suggestive of an important primary hypothalamic effect of this compound in inhibiting ovulation. It seems, therefore, likely that ovulation inhibitory ergot derivatives interfere with the neuronal events responsible for phasic LH-RF secretion.

Comparing the implantation inhibitory activity and the ovulation inhibitory activity of a number of compounds (Table 5), one can see that the two actions vary independently (FLÜCKIGER et al., 1976), a fact which suggests that they represent two different pharmacologic properties of the drug. As it has been shown that prolactin secretion inhibition is best explained by a DA-receptor stimulatory action, this property cannot be easily used to explain ovulation inhibition, although a certain line of evidence suggests DA to have an inhibitory role in rats in the control of gonadotropin secretion (FUXE and HÖKFELT, 1970).

On the other hand, it has been shown that DA-receptor blocking agents, like the neuroleptics pimozide and fluspirilene, reduced in hypophysectomized female rats serum LH-RF activity (CORBIN and UPTON, 1973). Such drugs are also known to block ovulation in rats (EVERETT, 1964; CHOUDHURY et al., 1974; DICKERMANN et al., 1974). Thus, ovulation inhibition can be brought about by a central DA-receptor blockade. Theoretically, the ergot alkaloids could, besides inhibiting prolactin secretion, also inhibit ovulation if they acted as partial dopamine-receptor agonists being stimulatory in one-dose range and inhibitory in a higher or lower dose range. But DA-receptor blockade also stimulates prolactin secretion, and such an effect is unknown of the ovulation inhibitory ergot alkaloids.

It is well known that in rats α-adrenoceptor blockers also inhibit ovulation (for reviews see EVERETT, 1964; PIVA et al., 1969), and, therefore, the possibility of such a mechanism of action has to be considered with ergot alkaloids. In Table 5 data on α-adrenoceptor antagonistic potency pA_2 of a few ergot alkaloids as assessed on vascular tissue in vitro (Column 4) are included to be compared with the ED_{50} for ovulation inhibition (Column 3). It can be seen that the individual values for the latter range cover more than two orders of magnitude, while the α-receptor blocking activity, with the exception of methysergide is a rather constant quality of the listed drugs. Methysergide, the second most active ovulation inhibitor in our list, is about three orders of magnitude less potent as an α-adrenoceptor blocker than the rest of the series. These data obviously do not lend support to the idea that ovulation inhibition is correlated with the α-receptor blocking activity of these drugs. On the other hand, because the two test systems are fundamentally so different, a lack of correlation does not exclude the possibility that ergot alkaloids inhibit ovulation in rats by inhibiting α-adrenoceptors.

Serotonin is also implicated as a transmitter in the control of phasic gonadotropin secretion (WILSON, 1974; HERY et al., 1975). Because of this, Table 5

Table 5. Comparison of implantation and ovulation inhibitory activity with α- and 5-HT antagonistic activity at vascular receptors

Compound number	Name	ED_{50} mg/kg s.c.		pA_2[a] α-Receptor blockade	pD_2[a] 5-HT-Receptor blockade
		Implantation inhibition	Ovulation inhibition		
20	Ergotamine	14	0.3	8.8	9.6
23	Ergocristine	4.2	1.3	—	—
24	Ergocornine	2.7	1.7	8.8	—
25	α-Ergokryptine	1.1	1.7	8.9	8.6
26	β-Ergokryptine	2.8	1.7	—	—
34a	Methysergide	—	1	5.5	9.1
37c	2-Br-Ergocornine	> 5	> 20	—	—
38	Bromocriptine	0.75	20	8.9	7.6

[a] These values from Chapter III of this Volume.

presents (Column 5) the 5-HT receptor blocking potency (pD_2) as assessed on vascular tissue in vitro for some of the compounds. It can be seen that ergotamine and methysergide are the two most active antagonists to serotonin, while bromocriptine, which is about 60 times less potent as an ovulation inhibitor, is 100 times less potent as a serotonin antagonist than ergotamine. α-ergokryptine was found intermediate in both activities. Here, then, we see two activities varying in parallel between different compounds, suggesting that serotonin-receptor blockade may be involved in ovulation inhibition by these ergot alkaloids. The reader should be aware that the correlation between the two activities may be fortuitous and misleading (MARKO and FLÜCKIGER, 1976), because some ergot alkaloids are known to have at the CNS level receptor actions opposite to what is observed in the periphery (see Chapter VI). Ergocornine, a potent peripheral 5-HT antagonist (CERLETTI and DOEPFNER, 1958), has been characterized by CORRODI et al. (1975) as a central 5-HT receptor agonist.

Induction of Gonadotropin Secretion. Concerning the induction of phasic gonadotropin secretion in rats by certain prolactin secretion inhibitory ergoline derivatives, it would be valuable to know whether the two actions could be attributed to a single mechanism of action, or whether it is necessary to search for two separate mechanisms of action to explain their effects on gonadotropins and on prolactin.

Firstly, no ergot alkaloid has been described to induce sexual cyclicity in rats without at the same time suppressing a state of prolactin dominance (inhibiting early gestation, suppressing physiologically or artificially induced pseudopregnancy, arresting lactation; nobody seems to have searched for an experimental model to test the possibility that ergot alkaloids or related compounds could facilitate cyclicity starting from an acyclic situation not connected with prolactin dominance.

Secondly, in postpartum sheep (KANN and MARTINET, 1975) treatment with bromocriptine shortened the anestrus period while preventing at the same time the high levels of circulating prolactin, but in normal-cycling sheep suppression of serum prolactin levels by the same drug (NISWENDER, 1974; KANN and DENAMUR, 1974) was without effect on gonadotropin secretion and cycle length.

As there is no evidence to the contrary, we shall assume that suppression of prolactin secretion and disinhibition of phasic gonadotropin secretion are due to one and the same property of these compounds, i.e., stimulation of dopamine receptors. The double effect could be brought about by a dopamine-like action at the hypothalamic level to induce gonadotropin secretion as well as at the pituitary level to inhibit prolactin secretion. DA has been implicated as a transmitter in the stimulatory control of gonadotropin secretion (KORDON, 1971; LICHTENSTEIGER and KELLER, 1974; McCann, 1974). But as this concept has been disputed on the ground that the tubero-infundibular dopaminergic (TIDA) neurons have been found to inhibit gonadotropin secretion (HÖKFELT and FUXE, 1972a), a different explanation may be possible. The facilitating effect on gonadotropin secretion may be brought about as a consequence of prolactin secretion inhibition alone. Hypophysectomy, or ergocornine and bromocriptine injected into intact rats, was found by HÖKFELT and FUXE (1972a, b) to decrease the activity of TIDA neurons, which effect could be antagonized by the injection of prolactin. This inhibition of TIDA neurons produces a disinhibition of gonadotropin secretion.

c) Other Pituitary Hormones

There exists only fragmently information from animal studies of actions by ergot alkaloids on the secretion of pituitary hormones other than those treated in the previous two sections. Also, the few observations on altered pituitary hormone secretion after treatment by an ergot alkaloid have rarely stimulated attempts at elucidating the underlying mechanism of action. Therefore, these animal data will be dealt with in a less expansive mode than applied to earlier sections. The pharmacologist interested in endocrinological background reading is invited to consult "The Pituitary Gland and its Neuroendocrine Control," Part 1 and 2 (KNOBIL and SAWYER, eds., 1974) in the *Handbook of Physiology* of the American Physiological Society.

α) Somatotropin (GH)

Ergotamine (cpd 20). MACLEOD and LEHMEYER (1973), using female rat pituitary halves in vitro, observed at 4 and 40 μM ergotamine no effect on GH synthesis and secretion, while prolactin production and release were depressed. In Wistar-Furth rats bearing an ectopic prolactin and GH-secreting tumor (SMtTW5), ergotamine 0.2 mg/day s.c. over 6–7 days reduced tumor size and the GH-dependent spleno-hepatomegaly, while the pituitaries of the treated animals increased to normal size. Typically, pituitaries of ergotamine-treated animals inoculated with a different tumor (MtTW15), when incubated in vitro, were able to synthetize and secrete more GH than pituitaries of untreated tumorbearing rats but still less than pituitaries from normal animals. NICOLL et al. (1970), incubating male rat pituitary fragments for 24 h in the presence of up to 5 μg/ml ergotamine, observed no effect on GH release into the medium.

Ergocornine (cpd 24). YANAI and NAGASAWA (1970) measured prolactin and GH in the pituitaries of C3H/He female mice after prolonged treatment with

0.2 mg·d. GH concentration in the glands was not altered, while prolactin was reduced. SINHA et al. (1974), treating C3H/Bi female mice with 0.2 mg/d for 20 days, found no effect on serum and urine GH, while GH concentration but not GH content in the pituitary was slightly increased.

MACLEOD and LEHMEYER (1973), using female rat pituitary halves incubated for 7 h, observed an inhibitory effect by 10 μM ergocornine on GH synthesis and release. In contrast, when female rats were treated with 0.2 mg ergocornine once daily for 7 days and their pituitaries were then incubated in vitro for 7 hours, the GH synthesis of these pituitaries was increased in comparison to that of control pituitaries. The contrasting effects of ergocornine on GH synthesis and release were not followed up (see also α-ergokryptine, below). Ergocornine, 0.2 mg/d given for 6 days to Wistar-Furth rats with a prolactin and GH-secreting pituitary tumor transplant, inhibited tumor growth and the GH-dependent splenohepatomegaly, while the pituitaries of the treated animals showed somewhat greater weights than those of the untreated animals.

QUADRI and MEITES (1973), using rats inoculated with the MtTW15 pituitary tumor, found during prolonged s.c. treatment with 2 mg/kg·d that ergocornine prevented the growth of the tumor and the rise of serum GH.

α-ergokryptine (cpd 25). MACLEOD and LEHMEYER (1973) reported that the presence of α-ergokryptine (10 μM) in the medium of rat pituitary halves incubated over 7 h reduced the amount of GH synthetized and released. In contrast to this are observations with incubated pituitaries from female rats which had been treated with 0.2 mg of α-ergokryptine daily for 7 days before sacrifice. These pituitaries showed an increased synthesis of GH over 7 h when compared with controls. These contrasting effects are similar to what was observed with ergocornine (see above), but the phenomenon has not been followed up.

Bromocriptine (cpd 38). YANAI and NAGASAWA (1970), treating C3H/He female mice with 0.2 mg/d for 3 weeks, observed no effect by bromocriptine on pituitary GH concentration. SINHA et al. (1974), using C3H/Bi female mice treated with 0.2 mg·d for 20 days, could not observe a change in serum or urine GH, while the pituitary GH content was 10% greater than in the controls. In acute experiments with rats, YANAI and NAGASAWA (1974) injected 0.1 mg bromocriptine per animal between 1 and 8 h before decapitation, after which in vitro incubation of the pituitaries was performed to measure prolactin and GH synthesis and secretion. Bromocriptine did not affect GH in this system. DAVIES et al. (1974), who treated adult male rats with estrogen to stimulate the pituitary to increased DNA prolactin and growth hormone synthesis, observed that bromocriptine reduced pituitary DNA synthesis and prolactin secretion but did not affect the growth hormone response to estrogen.

SMITH et al. (1974) treated lactating Holstein cows with 80 mg s.c. bromocriptine on 2 consecutive days, which depressed prolactin secretion for several days but did not alter GH secretion. In in vitro experiments incubating bovine pituitaries, the same authors found bromocriptine (0.01 to 10 μg/ml) ineffective on GH secretion. Also, in growing sheep 20 mg bromocriptine given 3 times a week over 6 weeks reduced serum prolactin levels to below 1 ng/ml but did not influence GH levels (BROWN et al., 1976).

Similarly, HART (1973), treating lactating goats with 5–20 mg/d of bromocriptine, could not observe an effect on serum GH levels.

Using clonal cell cultures of rat pituitary tumor origin (GH_3), TASHJIAN and HOYT (1972), using concentrations of up to 10 μg/ml bromocriptine and prolonged incubation periods, did not observe an effect by this alkaloid on GH synthesis or secretion. With the same cell system, but in the presence of a depolarizing concentration of potassium, GAUTVIK et al. (1973) also could not observe an effect of bromocriptine on the enhanced GH release by drug concentrations that suppressed prolactin release.

LSD25 (cpd 73b). COLLU et al. (1975) treated growing rats for a month with 0.1 or 0.5 mg/kg i.p. 3 times a week. They observed a reduced gain in body weight and tail length. Plasma GH was found reduced with the high-dose group, while the low-dose group showed only a reduced pituitary GH level.

β) Corticotropin (ACTH)

Ergocornine (cpd 24). SINHA et al. (1974), who treated C3H/Bi mice for 20 days with 0.2 mg/d of ergocornine, observed no difference in adrenal weight when compared to untreated controls. It may be concluded that ergocornine did not influence the pituitary-adrenal axis at the dose used.

Methysergide (cpd 34a). BURDEN et al. (1974), studying the neurotransmitter control of corticotropin-releasing factor (CRF), observed that serotonin, which stimulates CRF release from rat hypothalamic fragments, could be antagonized by methysergide.

Bromocriptine (cpd 38). CAMERON and SCARISBRICK (1973) treated rats for 10, 20, and 30 days with 100 μg/d of bromocriptine and did not observe an effect on adrenal weight nor on plasma corticosterone level. They concluded that prolactin has no effect on adrenal function, but the results also suggest the conclusion that this dose of bromocriptine did not influence the pituitary adrenal axis.

SMITH et al. (1974), treating lactating Holstein cows with 80 mg s.c. of bromocriptine, which effectively suppressed prolactin secretion, did not find an effect on serum cortisol levels at milking.

γ) Melanotropins (MSH)

α-ergokryptine (cpd 25) together with apomorphine, was studied by SMITH (1975), for their effect in frogs (*R. pipiens*) on the state of melanin dispersal in skin melanocytes as indicator for the level of circulating MSH. Both drugs induced pallor of the skin in intact animals but not in hypophysectomized frogs darkened by injected MSH. From this and further experiments, it was concluded that the MSH secreting cells of the frog pituitary have secretion inhibitory dopamine receptors.

Methysergide (cpd 34a) inhibits the depletion of melanocyte-stimulating activity from the pituitary in rats as induced by intra ventricular injection of hypertonic saline or by mechanical stimulation of the vagina at estrus. With this and similar experimental studies in which they used methysergide or other drugs, TALEISNIK et al. (1973/1974) concluded that the hypothalalmic control of MSH secretion in rats comprises, besides a catecholaminergic system, a serotoninergic system also.

Bromocriptine (cpd 38) was reported by HAMILTON et al. (1975) to greatly inhibit in Syrian hamsters chronically treated with diethylstilbestrol the hyperplastics and neoplastic changes in the intermediate pituitary lobe.

Using a RIA for measuring α-MSH in blood and in the pituitary intermediate lobe, PENNY and THODY (1976) found that bromocriptine caused a sharp drop in circulating MSH concentration within half an hour after i.p. application but had no effect on the pituitary MSH level. Haloperidol and other neuroleptics increased blood levels of MSH. These in vivo experiments confirmed earlier in vitro studies which demonstrate that MSH release from the pituitary is under dopaminergic inhibitory control (TILDERS et al., 1975; BAKER 1976).

LSD 25 (cpd 73b) was the first of the ergot compounds for which a pigmentary effect was demonstrated, using the Siamese fighting fish (*Betta splendens*) (ABRAMSON and EVANS, 1954). Other studies using several derivatives other than LSD 25 followed (BERDE and CERLETTI, 1956; EVANS et al., 1956), but it was soon discovered (BERDE and CERLETTI, 1957) that the pigmentary effect could also be elicited in vitro, which means that the central pigmentary control is not necessarily involved. One must be further aware that in the bony fish the pigmentary effectors are doubly innervated, and, therefore, pigmentary changes in such species are not indicative of an endocrine drug effect (PARKER, 1948; FLÜCKIGER, 1962a, b). In amphibians in which pigmentary control is hormonal (FLÜCKIGER, 1963), LSD 25 was also found to induce changes; KAHR and FISCHER (1957) observed in frogs (*R. temporaria*) a short-lasting darkening after injecting 50 µg into intact animals but not when using hypophysectomized frogs. They concluded that LSD 25 acts via the pituitary. In the South African toad *Xenopus laevis*, BURGERS et al. (1958) observed that LSD 25 induced a dose-dependent pallor in intact animals with initially dark skin (expanded melanin) and no effect in pale animals. LSD 25 pretreatment did not influence the melanin dispersing effect of injected ACTH (MSH was not yet available), nor did the presence of LSD 25 influence the melanocyte-stimulation effect of ACTH in vitro. Thus, in amphibians LSD 25 does not act directly on the melanocytes but probably induces inhibition of MSH secretion by the pituitary intermediate lobe. This conclusion later received support by showing an increase in MSH-like activity in the pituitary pars intermedia after treatment of originally dark animals with LSD 25 (BURGERS and IMAI, 1962). Using another toad, *Bufo arenarum*, ITURRIZA and KOCH (1964) observed an increased amount of colloid droplets in the cells of the pituitary pars intermedia, which, based on the aforementioned publication, they considered as indicative of an increase of stored MSH. ITURRIZA (1965) further showed that LSD 25 in vitro did not induce concentration of dispersed melanin granules in skin melanocytes, and more importantly, that in vivo the drug also induced pallor in such toads in which the hypothalamo-pituitary connection had been surgically disrupted. This suggests that LSD 25 acts directly on the hypophyseal intermediate lobe to inhibit MSH secretion.

δ) Ocytocin

Ergotamine (cpd 20) was described by GROSVENOR (1956) to acutely inhibit milk ejection in lactating rats after 3 mg/kg s.c. given on day 9 post partum. When the drug was also injected a second time on day 10, the effect on milk ejection was greatly diminished. Further injections on days 11 and 12 did not bring back the inhibitory effect. In experiments performed to analyze the mechanism of milk ejection inhibition by ergotamine, GROSVENOR and TURNER (1956) observed that a similar effect could also be obtained after 1 mg/kg s.c., and that this effects could be overcome by the injection of ocytocin (0.2–0.4 IU/kg) either before or after ergotamine. Topical application of ergotamine to exposed mammary glands of anesthetized rats resulted in constriction of arterioles but not of venules or of alveolar capillaries. The constrictive effect was transient, and ocytocin applied topically at the height of ergotamine-induced arteriole constriction elicited its usual alveolar contraction. The authors concluded that ergotamine does not inhibit the milk ejection through vasoconstriction, thus preventing the access of ocytocin to elicit the milk ejection. They discussed the possibility of an interference of ergotamine and ocytocin at the myepithelial cell and the possibility that ergotamine centrally inhibits the release of ocytocin.

In a third study, the adrenergic and cholinergic components of the milk ejection reflex in lactating rats was studied, also using various ergot derivatives (GROSVENOR and TURNER, 1957): *Methylergometrine* (cpd 73a), 1–2 mg/kg, *DHE-45*, (cpd 102b), 2–4 mg/kg, and *dihydroergotoxine*, 2–4 mg/kg were injected subcutaneously into lactating rats, and the effect on milk ejection assessed as before. Methylergometrine was more active than the other two drugs in reducing the milk available to the pups. Ocytocin counteracted the inhibitory effect of the ergot drugs. It is unknown how these three drugs produced their inhibitory effect, but it seems impossible that methylergometrine acted in the same way as did DHE-45, for example. These observations, together with those of experiments with nonergot drugs, led to the conclusion that adrenergic and cholinergic links are present in the reflex-arc responsible for ocytocin release.

2. Actions on Peripheral Endocrine Systems

a) Steroidogenic Organs

Ovary. The question of a possible interaction of ergot alkaloids with steroidogenesis has been raised by SHELESNYAK (1975b); the interruption of the progestational state in rats with recurrence of estrus within a few days was attributed to a disturbance of the estrogen/progesterone balance, essential for progestation and implantation, brought about by an interference with progesterone metabolism or action. Based on results from a pilot study in women volunteers (SHELESNYAK et al., 1963) (see Part B of this chapter), it was concluded that ergocornine blocked certain enzyme systems involved in the final steps of progesterone synthesis. Later, LINDNER and SHELESNYAK (1967) studied the ovarian endocrine response to 1 mg ergocornine (cpd 24) in rats on the day 4 of pseudopregnancy. Ergocornine, with a latency of 12 h, induced a fall of ovarian progesterone (P) and a sharp rise of 20-α-hydroxyprogesterone (20αOHP), inversing the ratio P/20αOHP from greater than 1.9 in the controls to less than 0.45. The total P+20βOHP remained constant until 48 h after ergocornine. These changes observed after ergocornine mimic those to be observed in spontaneously cycling rats. They do not support the idea that ergocornine interferes with progesterone synthesis but agree with the assumption that the changes in ovarian steroid metabolism are secondary to the suppression of circulating prolactin by ergocornine (LAMPRECHT et al., 1969).

Bromocriptine (cpd 38) has been similarly studied recently by RODWAY and KUHN (1975). Measuring the 20α-hydroxysteroid-dehydrogenase activity in the ovaries of 5–8-days pregnant rats injected with 1 mg bromocriptine on day 5, the authors found a rise in enzyme activity on two days following treatment, and this drug effect could be fully suppressed by prolactin but not by progesterone plus estrone injections. Bromocriptine given on day 16 of pregnancy in the same dose did not induce an activation of this enzyme. In lactating rats bromocriptine given on days 6 and 7 did not induce a rise in 20α-hydroxysteroid-dehydrogenase activity, but a four-fold rise was obtained when the drug was given on days 13 and 14 of lactation. Prolactin did not inhibit this enzyme. These last findings are certainly not due to a lack of action of bromocriptine on suckling-induced prolactin release in early lactation (FLÜCKIGER, 1976), but they underline the complexity of the control of ovarian steroidogenesis during lactation.

Testis. A reduction of circulating testosterone levels in male rodents under prolonged treatment with either ergocornine (cpd 24) or bromocriptine (cpd 38) has been reported (BOYNS et al., 1972; BARTKE, 1973), but such effects have not been related to a direct action of the ergot alkaloid on steroidogenesis, because it became clear at the same time that prolactin potentiates the effect of LH on testosterone synthesis in rodents (HAFIEZ et al., 1972). Prolactin interacts with steroid metabolism in different ways (BARTKE, 1974; SCHRIEFERS et al., 1975; SCHRIEFERS and WAGNER, 1976) and has also been shown to influence the sensitivity of the testis to the action of LH (BARTKE and DALTERIO, 1976).

Adrenals. Similarly to the findings with the testis, prolactin is also implicated in rat adrenal steroidogenesis (BOYNS et al., 1972; WITORSCH and KITAY, 1972; PIVA et al., 1973; SOLYOM, 1974). This is important to note in view of certain effects of prolactin release inhibitory ergot alkaloids on water and electrolyte metabolism (HORROBIN, 1974, 1975, 1976) and on aldosterone secretion observed in man (see Part B of this chapter). The reader should also be aware of certain ill-understood but probably important interactions between adrenal steroids and prolactin (HORROBIN et al., 1976).

b) The Pancreas (contributed by B.P. RICHARDSON)

α) *Introduction*

The endocrine cells of the mammalian pancreas are arranged in small clusters, the islets of Langerhans, which are dispersed through the exocrine tissue (LANGERHANS, 1869). These islets contain at least three different cell types (LACY, 1957). These are designated α-, β-, and Δ-cells. From immunohistochemical studies it is generally accepted that the α-cells contain glucagon and the β-cells insulin (BAUM et al., 1962; LACY and DAVIES, 1957). The exact function of the Δ-cells remains unknown.

In addition to glucagon- and insulin-containing cells, more recent studies have revealed the presence of gastrin-containing cells within the islet (LOMSKY et al., 1969). It is claimed that the gastrin-containing cells may be a modified form of α- or Δ-cells. The former possibility seems more likely in view of recent claims that the Δ-cell contains somatostatin (LUFT et al., 1974; RUFENER et al., 1975).

The pancreatic nerves originate in the celiac and superior mesenteric plexuses and send rich autonomic innervation to the islets. They enter the gland as a series of mixed nerves containing both a parasympathetic component, which arises from trunks of the vagus, and a sympathetic component arising from the greater and middle splanchnic nerves.

Characteristic cholinergic and adrenergic nerve endings can be found in close association with all islet cell types (WOODS and PORTE, 1974). The parasympathetic component can be selectively activated by electrical stimulation of the vagal nerve, which leads to an increase in the release of insulin which is blocked by atropine (FINDLAY et al., 1969). In contrast to the situation with insulin, the effects of vagal stimulation on glucagon release are less clear. In cats, glucagon secretion is unaffected by vagal stimulation (ESTERHUIZEN and HOWELL, 1970), and atropinization does not affect the glucagon release caused by stimulation of the mixed pancreatic nerve (MARLISS et al., 1973). On the other hand, stimulation of the vagus nerve in calves causes a significant increase in glucagon release (BLOOM et al., 1974).

Selective activation of the sympathetic elements by stimulation of the splanchnic nerve increases the release of both insulin and glucagon (BLOOM et al., 1973). The increased insulin release, but not the increased glucagon release, can be blocked by pretreatment with β-adrenergic blocking agents. Conversely, α-adrenergic blokkade potentiates the insulin release induced by splanchnic nerve stimulation but does not affect glucagon release (KANETO et al., 1975).

Thus, in summary, it is well established that activation of the parasympathetic components of the pancreatic nerves by vagal stimulation leads to insulin release. Activation of the sympathetic components by stimulating the splanchnic nerve also increases insulin release, apparently by a β-adrenergic mechanism. Selective activation of α-adrenergic receptors, by stimulating the splanchnic nerves in the presence of propranolol, conversely inhibits insulin release. The effects of parasympathetic activation on glucagon release are less clear. Sympathetic activation elevates glucagon release, but whether this results from stimulation of α- or β-adrenergic mechanisms is uncertain. Little or nothing is known of the neural control of gastrin or somatostatin release from islets at present.

In agreement with the findings from studies involving vagal nerve stimulation, cholinergic drugs have been shown to stimulate insulin release both in vivo and in vitro, and this effect is blocked by atropine in both cases (MALAISSE, 1972; KANETO et al., 1968). Again, the effects of parasymphatomimetic agents on glucagon release are less clear, although the results obtained thus far seem to indicate that a stimulation probably occurs (IVERSEN, 1973).

As expected from the studies involving stimulation of the splanchnic nerve, isoprenaline stimulates insulin release, and this is antagonized by β-adrenergic blockade (BAUM and PORTE, 1976). In contrast, adrenaline and noradrenaline both inhibit insulin release in vivo and in vitro (CAMPFIELD, 1975; MALAISSE, 1972; WOODS and PORTE, 1974), and this effect is completely antagonized by α-adrenergic blocking agents (MALAISSE et al., 1967; LUNDQUIST, 1972). Thus, the β-cell membrane possesses both α- and β-adrenergic receptors. Activation of the α-receptors inhibits insulin release, while activation of β-receptors enhances release. With glucagon the situation is less clear. Certainly both adrenaline and noradrenaline stimulate release, but whether this effect is mediated through stimulation of α- or β-receptors remains unresolved (WOODS and PORTE, 1974).

In addition to modulation by the secretory products of the pancreatic nerves, the release of insulin is also sensitive to 5-hydroxytryptamine (5-HT). In most species this amine inhibits insulin release by direct effects on the β-cells, although in rats it appears to stimulate (WOODS and PORTE, 1974). As relatively large intracellular pools of 5-HT appear associated with the secretory granules of both α- and β-cells (JAIM-ETCHEVERRY and ZIEHER, 1968; EKHOLM et al., 1971), this substance may act as an endogenous regulator of insulin and glucagon release. The action of 5-HT on glucagon release has not yet been systematically investigated.

β) *Effects on Insulin and Glucagon Release*

Considering the foregoing, it is clear that ergot derivatives with α-adrenergic blokking activity, such as dihydroergotamine (DHE), or those which antagonize the action of 5-HT, such as methysergide, might be expected to influence pancreatic hormone release. In fact, the published works involving the action of ergot derivatives on pancreatic hormones are almost exclusively restricted to studies where one of these two agents has been used.

Methysergide (cpd 34a) has been extensively used as a pharmacologic tool for investigating the physiologic significance of endogenous 5-HT in the control of insulin secretion. It has been reported to potentiate glucose-mediated insulin release from the hamster and rabbit pancreas in vitro (FELDMAN and LEBOVITZ, 1970a; FELDMAN et al., 1972a) and to augment the release of insulin from pieces of rabbit pancreas incubated with tolbutamide (FELDMAN et al., 1972b). The inhibition of glucose-mediated insulin release from either hamster or rabbit pancreas produced by 5-HT in vitro is fully antagonized by methysergide (FELDMAN and LEBOVITZ, 1970a, b; FELDMAN et al., 1972b). On the basis of these findings and similar ones with the 5-HT antagonist cyproheptadine, it has been suggested that endogenous β-cell 5-HT acts as an inhibitory regulator of insulin release. The exact mechanism by which 5-HT produces its effect remains unknown, but it may involve an interference with the action of cAMP on release processes (FELDMAN and LEBOVITZ, 1970b, c). Clinical studies with methysergide have demonstrated a potentiation of glucose-mediated insulin release in maturity-onset diabetics and in acromegalics with impaired glucose tolerance but not in healthy subjects (Fig. 4) (QUICKEL et al., 1971a,b; ARKY, 1972; BIVENS et al., 1972). These findings were later extended to show that tolbutamide-mediated insulin release was also significantly enhanced in maturity-onset diabetics pretreated with methysergide (BALDRIDGE et al., 1974).

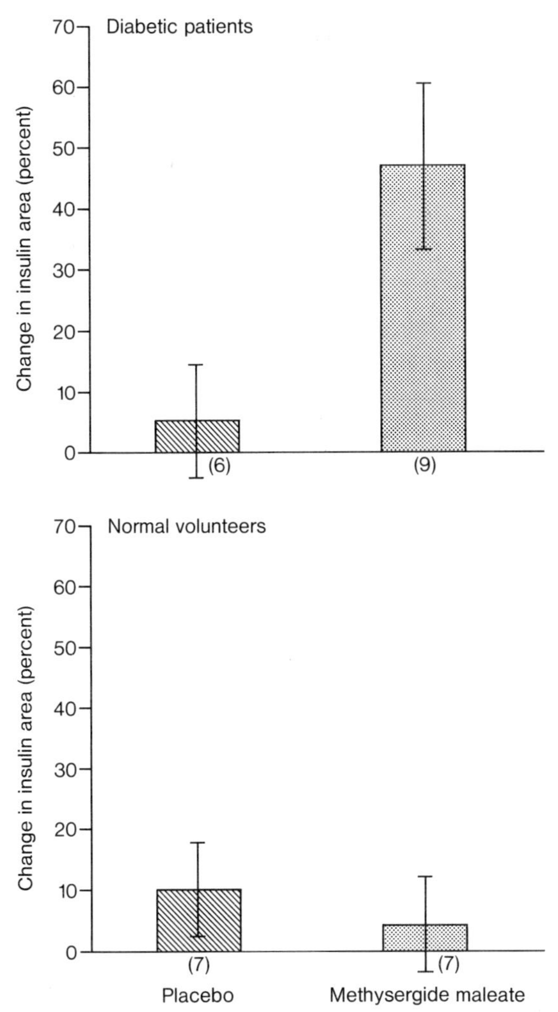

Fig. 4. Effects of pretreatment with 2 mg q.i.d. methysergide on glucose-mediated insulin release in patients with adult onset diabetes mellitus or in normal volunteers. [After QUICKEL et al. (1971b) with the permission of the Journal of Clinical Endocrinology and Metabolism]

These observations have led investigators to suggest a role for endogenous biogenic amines in the pathogenesis of some forms of diabetes mellitus. The recent finding that methysergide slightly enhances glucose-induced insulin biosynthesis by the pancreatic β-cell could give a clue as to its mode of action in increasing the secretory response to a chemical stimulus (LIN and HAIST, 1975).

Recent clinical studies of the effects of methysergide on glucagon secretion have shown that pretreatment with this drug also enhances α-cell function, glucagon release being increased in response to arginine stimulation (MARCO et al., 1976). Since a similar effect is obtained with other 5-HT antagonists or agents which suppress 5-HT synthesis (HEDO et al., 1975), a similar inhibitory role for endogenous α-cell 5-HT in glucagon release has been proposed.

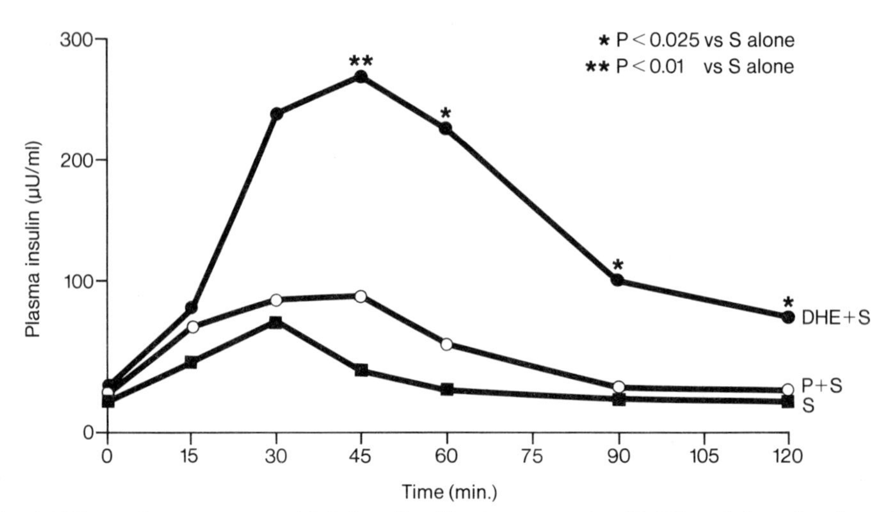

Fig. 5. Effects of pretreatment with 0.2 mg/kg dihydroergotamine (*DHE*) or 0.5 mg/kg phentolamine (*P*) on sulphonylurea-induced (*S*) insulin secretion in dogs. *DHE* or *P* was given 30 min before *S*. All drugs were given intravenously. [After SIREK et al. (1974) with the permission of Diabetologia]

Dihydroergotamine (DHE) (cpd 102b). Studies with DHE on trained conscious dogs have shown it to markedly augment sulphonylurea-mediated insulin release (Fig. 5) (SIREK et al., 1973, 1975a). This potentiation effect appears restricted to sulphonylurea-mediated release, since that produced by glucose or arginine is unaffected by DHE. This amplifying effect seems completely unrelated to the α-adrenergic blocking action of DHE, since neither phentolamine nor ergotamine produce similar effects (SIREK et al., 1975a). As the action of sulphonylureas in stimulating insulin release is believed to involve a primary membrane interaction (HELLMAN et al., 1971; MATTHEWS et al., 1973), it has been suggested that DHE, in binding to a high affinity protein in the β-cell membrane, triggers conformational rearrangements of membrane protein such that more sulphonylurea receptors or binding sites become exposed (SIREK et al., 1974).

As yet there are no reports of the action of DHE on glucagon secretion.

Effects of other Ergot Derivatives. Like DHE (cpd 102b), *2-brom-d-lysergic acid diethylamide* (BOL-148, cpd 37a) can potentiate the insulin release produced by sulphonylureas, but its action is considerably weaker than that of DHE (SIREK et al., 1974). Glucose-mediated release is again unaffected (LERNMARK, 1971). Low concentrations of *ergotamine* (cpd 20) can block the inhibitory action of adrenaline on glucose-mediated insulin release, presumably through its α-adrenergic blocking activity, since phentolamine has an identical effect (ALEYASSINE and LEE, 1972).

Inhibition of prolactin in patients with hyperprolactinemia by the administration of *bromocriptine* (cpd 38) improves both glucose tolerance and glucose-induced insulin release (LANDGRAF et al., 1975). Based on these observations, the investigators suggested a possible role of prolactin in the etiology of diabetes mellitus.

Nicergoline (cpd 104e) reduces glucose-mediated insulin release by an unknown mechanism, which is unrelated to its α-adrenolytic activity (D'ONOFRIO et al., 1975).

Metergoline (cpd 89d), a powerful long-acting 5-HT antagonist, enhances glucose-mediated insulin release in normal subjects but not in chemical diabetics. Conversely, metergoline reduces arginine-induced insulin release significantly in both groups (PONTIROLI et al., 1975).

γ) Interaction With the Peripheral Effects of Insulin and Glucagon

Insulin decreases the phospholipid content of rabbit cerebellum and cerebral cortex in vivo (HINZEN et al., 1970). This effect appears related to a reduction in the blood-sugar levels caused by the insulin and not to a primary action of the hormone per se, since it is abolished when hypoglycemia is prevented by the simultaneous administration of glucose. DHE markedly potentiates the reduction in brain-phospholipid content caused by insulin-induced hypoglycemia (HINZEN et al., 1970). Such an effect of DHE may be explained by its ability to potentiate growth hormone-mediated lipolysis. It is well known that growth hormone is secreted in response to insulin-induced hypoglycemia, and DHE has been shown to potentiate the lipolysis caused by growth hormone both in vivo and in vitro (SIREK et al., 1969, 1972, 1975b; HOTTA et al., 1971). Thus, DHE may potentiate the decrease in brain phospholipid content seen after insulin administration by amplifying the lipolytic action of the growth hormone secreted in response to insulin-induced hypoglycemia. The exact mechanism whereby DHE potentiates the growth hormone-induced lipolysis is not clear. However, its action in this respect appears highly selective, since DHE does not modify the lipolytic actions of ACTH, TSH, or glucagon (SIREK et al., 1969; SIREK et al., 1972; HOTTA et al., 1971). As similar effects are not obtained with phentolamine or BOL-148, this action of DHE, like that on sulphonylurea-mediated insulin release, is not related to either its α-adrenergic blocking or serotonergic-blocking action. Interestingly, the saturation of the double bond at the C9 and C10 positions of the lysergic acid moiety appears to be an essential structural requirement for DHE to function as an amplifier of the stimuli in both systems, suggesting that it may act as a regulatory molecule inducing positive cooperative changes in integral plasma membrane proteins (SIREK et al., 1974; SIREK et al., 1975b). In fact, independent evidence for an action of DHE on adipocyte membranes has already been obtained (VOGEL-CHEVALIER et al., 1971). In vivo studies with male rats have shown DHE to prevent the rise in hepatic cAMP caused by glucagon (PAUK and REDDY, 1970) and thereby to inhibit the normal glucagon-induced uptake of amino acids by the liver (CHAMBERS et al., 1970).

B. Human Data

1. Actions on Pituitary Hormones

Introduction. Although the endocrine effect of ergot derivatives in man had already been investigated in the early 1960's, efforts were mainly concentrated on their action on ovarian function, based on the luteolytic effect of ergocornine found in rats (SHELESNYAK, 1957; SHELESNYAK et al., 1963). In man, the effect of methylergometrine in postpartum lactation has also been the subject of sporadic work at a time in which prolactin had not yet been characterized as a separate entity (SERMENT and RUF, 1955; GUILHEM et al., 1967). It is only recently that selective endocrine actions of ergot compounds have been investigated, based on more precise laboratory techniques. Also, neuroendocrine mechanisms have been the subject of intensive investigations in man, which have led to a better understanding of the control of pituitary hormone release. Thus, dopamine has been found to play an important role within this context, and this was found to be particularly true for prolactin and growth hormone. More recently, serotoninergic and adrenergic pathways have also been implicated in such mechanisms, pointing to the complexity of phenomena involved in single hormone release.

Decisive in the new development of endocrine-active ergot compounds has been the effect of some of these drugs on prolactin and growth hormone. The finding that bromocriptine inhibits prolactin release from the pituitary opened new insights into the pharmacologic control of neurosecretory mechanisms in man. In addition, this drug has been found to effectively suppress growth hormone secretion in acromegalic subjects. The importance of prolactin and growth hormone as indicators of the neuroendocrine action of ergot compounds warrant considerations.

a) Prolactin

α) Characterization of Prolactin in Man

Progress in the field of animal prolactin physiology contrasts with the scarce information concerning the status of this hormone in man. Early work on this hormone was handicapped by the difficulty in segregating it from growth hormone, so that its existence as a separate peptide in man has been seriously doubted. PASTEELS et al. (1963), however, found by culturing human pituitaries that bioassayable prolactin continued to be excreted in the culture medium, whereas immunoassayable growth hormone gradually declined. Further evidence for separate synthesis of prolactin and growth hormone was provided by FRIESEN et al. (1970) by incubating human pituitaries in a medium containing ^{3}H-leucine. They showed that the pituitary from an acromegalic subject would secrete high amounts of growth hormone and very little prolactin, whereas the reverse was found with material obtained from a patient with galactorrhea.

This was followed by the development of a specific radioimmunoassay (RIA) for primate prolactin (HWANG et al., 1971). Later on, and using a fraction derived from acetone-dried human pituitary powder, HWANG et al. (1972) succeeded in purifying prolactin. LEWIS et al. (1971) identified a slow migrating component in extracts of human pituitary glands by gel electrophoresis. This fraction gave a positive response in the pigeon crop assay for prolactin, and it was augmented in the pituitary of a pregnant woman, whereas male subjects had barely detectable amounts. Material obtained by this research group was then utilized to develop a specific RIA for prolactin (SINHA et al., 1973) replacing less sensitive and more tedious bioassay techniques.

Studies in man have shown prolactin to be characterized by episodic secretion with sleep-bound rises. In nocturnal sleep, maximal prolactin elevations are

Table 6. Induction of prolactin release by physiologic stimulation

Estrogen	Thoracic injury	Exercise
Breast feeding	Stress	Sexual intercourse
Breast stimulation	Hypoglycemia	Sleep

recorded between 3 a.m. and 5 a.m. (FRANTZ, 1973; L'HERMITE et al., 1972), and there is a clear dissociation between the prolactin and growth hormone peaks during this period (FRANTZ, 1973). A number of stimuli (Table 6) are effective in inducing prolactin release (FRANTZ, 1973; DEL POZO et al., 1976).

β) Control of Prolactin Secretion

The mechanisms governing the secretion of prolactin are complex, and its release is known to depend on a predominant inhibitory tone from the hypothalamus. Thus, pituitary stalk section in man leads to hyperprolactinemia (TURKINGTON et al., 1971; FRANTZ et al., 1972). This suggests the presence of a prolactin-inhibiting factor (PIF) at suprasellar level. More insight into the mechanisms governing the secretion of prolactin was obtained when the role of dopamine (DA) as a neurotransmitter could be defined in man with the help of centrally acting drugs. Any stimulation of DA synthesis, e.g., the administration of L-DOPA which is endogenously transformed into DA, would in turn increase PIF and subsequently reduce prolactin secretion from the pituitary. A number of neuroleptic drugs, such as the phenothiazines, increase prolactin secretion by blocking DA receptors; others, such as reserpine or α-methyl-DOPA, act by altering the metabolism of catecholamines at different levels. Among these compounds, some are utilized in clinical tests of prolactin reserve (KLEINBERG et al., 1971; ROBYN, 1976; JUDD et al., 1976).

Although thyrotropin-releasing hormone (TRH) does not seem to be involved in the physiologic control of prolactin release, its intravenous administration is followed by a rapid rise in plasma prolactin, presumably through direct action on the pituitary (BOWERS et al., 1971; JACOBS et al., 1971; TASHJIAN et al., 1971; L'HERMITE et al., 1972).

The role of estrogens in the control of prolactin release deserves further comment. Evidence that these steroids promote prolactin secretion and stimulate cell growth of galactotropes has been provided. A close parallelism between plasma estradiol and prolactin concentrations throughout gestation has been reported in humans (DEL POZO et al., 1976). This is in accordance with the increasing pituitary weights and the prolactin cell hyperplasia reported during pregnancy (ERDHEIM and STUMME, 1909; GOLUBOFF and EZRIN, 1969). At the time of delivery, pregnant women exhibit plasma prolactin concentrations approximately 15 times higher than those found in normally menstruating females (HWANG et al., 1971; L'HERMITE et al., 1972; BRUN DEL RE et al., 1973). After birth, these values slowly decline to reach basal nonpregnant levels by postpartum week 3. In human fetuses, the pituitary gland secretes prolactin actively from gestational week 5 to term (SILER-

KHODR et al., 1974), and plasma hormone concentrations have been found to be elevated throughout pregnancy (AUBERT et al., 1975). Since fetal estrogens also increase with growth (SHUTT et al., 1974), it would be reasonable to assume that the prolactin cells undergo the same changes under estrogenic stimulation in the fetus as in the mother, since these steroids freely move across the placental barrier. Studies conducted in animals lend further support to this hormonal interrelationship by showing pituitary adenoma formation following estrogen administration (EL ETREBY and GÜNZEL, 1973) and failure of plasma prolactin concentrations to increase during gestation in monkeys and rats when circulating estrogens remain physiologically low (FRIESEN et al., 1972; YOSHINAGA et al., 1969). The chimpanzee, exhibiting gradual plasma estradiol increases throughout gestation, is the only known species presenting a prolactin secretory pattern similar to man (REYES et al., 1975).

The possible role of serotonin pathways on the release of pituitary prolactin has been the subject of recent clinical investigations. MACINDOE and TURKINGTON (1973) administered intravenously relatively large amounts (5–10 g) of L-tryptophane, a serotonin precursor, to normal individuals. In the organism, this amino acid is first hydroxylated to 5-hydroxy-tryptophane (5-HTP) and then decarboxylated to serotonin or 5-hydroxytryptamine (5-HT). They recorded substantial elevations of plasma prolactin concentrations 20–40 min after initiation of the infusion. Further, KATO et al. (1974) showed that the intravenous administration of 200 mg 5-HTP also enhances prolactin secretion. Recently, LANCRANJAN et al. (1977) were successful in elevating plasma prolactin subsequently to an i.v. infusion of a new soluble ester of L-5-HTP (Ro-35940). This effect, however, reached only statistical significance in females. Indeed, differences in prolactin response between the sexes have already been noticed for other stimuli (JACOBS et al., 1971). In contrast, SMYTHE et al. (1976), giving L-tryptophane or 5-HTP orally, were unable to modify basal plasma prolactin. It can be assumed that the route of administration had some bearing on the absence of response observed after oral administration.

γ) Effect of Ergot Compounds on Prolactin Secretion

Ergometrine (Ergonovine, cpd 19) is a compound with uterotonic properties of current use in obstetric practice. SHANE and NAFTOLIN (1974) recorded a slight but significant decrease in plasma prolactin after single intravenous administration of 0.2 mg ergonovine maleate to postpartum women. The authors concluded that repetitive doses may have an inhibitory effect on lactation, but no pertinent studies have yet been reported. It should be mentioned, however, that LAWRENCE and HAGEN (1972) have reported reestablishment of menses in four women with galactorrhea-amenorrhea after long-term treatment with ergonovine maleate 0.2 mg three times daily. Ovulatory cycles could be confirmed in three by the occurrence of pregnancy.

Methysergide (cpd 34a) is a serotonin receptor antagonist, its clinical indication being the interval treatment of migraine headaches. The attention of endocrinologists, however, was focused on methysergide after a possible participation of serotoninergic pathways in the control of pituitary hormones became apparent from animal experiments. MENDELSON et al. (1975) reported a significant suppression of sleep-related hyperprolactinemia after oral administration of methysergide, 2 mg every 6 h to normal individuals. The authors concluded that serotonin is important in modulating prolactin secretion. More recently, LANCRANJAN and DEL POZO (unpublished) have tested the effect of methysergide on resting prolactin levels as compared with a nonergot serotonin antagonist, a benzocycloheptathiophene (Sandoz BC 105, pizotifen). The oral administration of 1 mg methysergide to normal individuals (Fig. 6) induced a significant fall in plasma prolactin, whereas doses up to 2 mg pizotifen failed to induce any changes. The fact that a serotonin antagonist chemically unrelated to ergot did not modify basal prolactin secretion suggests the presence in methysergide of an active moiety, presumably of dopaminergic nature.

Bromocriptine. First clinical trials with bromocriptine (cpd 38) in man have amply confirmed the antigalactic properties of this compound emanating from animal experimentation (VARGA et al., 1972; LUTTERBECK et al., 1971). Subsequently, its effect on prolactin secretion was investigated. In the first trial, a single dose of 4 mg induced a dramatic fall in plasma hormone concentrations in normal female volunteers (Fig. 7). Prolonged treatment with 3 mg daily will abolish the nyctohemeral rhythm of prolactin secretion, as depicted in Figure 8. Serial prolactin and growth hormone measurements performed during this period clearly demonstrate the specificity of action of this drug on prolactin. Sleep related growth hormone changes are preserved, whereas nocturnal prolactin oscillations are suppressed. As mentioned previously, phenothiazines (chlorpromazine) can cause acute secretion of prolactin in normal individuals. Also, TRH produces a rapid increase in circulating prolactin levels. Bromocriptine, 2.5 mg, administered prior to the test injection, effectively suppressed this effect of both compounds. Knowing that phenothiazines on repeated administration can also cause a sustained release of prolactin, a study with bromocriptine was undertaken in a group of 22 psychiatric patients, receiving chronically 100 mg chlorpromazine or more daily. Average basal prolactin levels were significantly ($p<0.001$) elevated (28 ± 2.6 ng/ml; Normal = 11.1 ± 1.3 ng/ml). Bromocriptine, 3 mg daily, which effectively inhibits prolactin in normal untreated subjects, failed to modify basal prolactin levels or the response to a standard dose of TRH (200 μg). A gradual dosage increase to 2.5 mg three times daily was necessary before basal plasma prolactin was normalized and the peak response to TRH effectively suppressed from 198 ± 9.8 (SE) ng/ml down to 24.4 ± 3.3 (SE) ng/ml. Results were interpreted as reflecting competitive drug antagonism in agreement with observations recorded in rats (FLÜCKIGER, 1977).

The administration of the compound to postpartum women has been successful in suppressing milk letdown (VARGA et al., 1972; BRUN DEL RE et al., 1973). The effect of this therapy on a group of seven women who did not wish to breastfeed their infants is presented in Figure 9. Six normally lactating mothers on no treatment served as controls. The compound was administered three times daily for 7 days. Plasma prolactin was depressed to the low normal range, and no milk was collected from the treated group. The compound also inhibited the prolactin peak that normally occurs in response to suckling. The studies were then extended to established lactation, at a time when basal prolactin had already reached the normal range (BRUN DEL RE et al., 1973; DEL POZO et al., 1975a). Also in this situation, a rapid fall in plasma prolactin was observed and lactation ceased

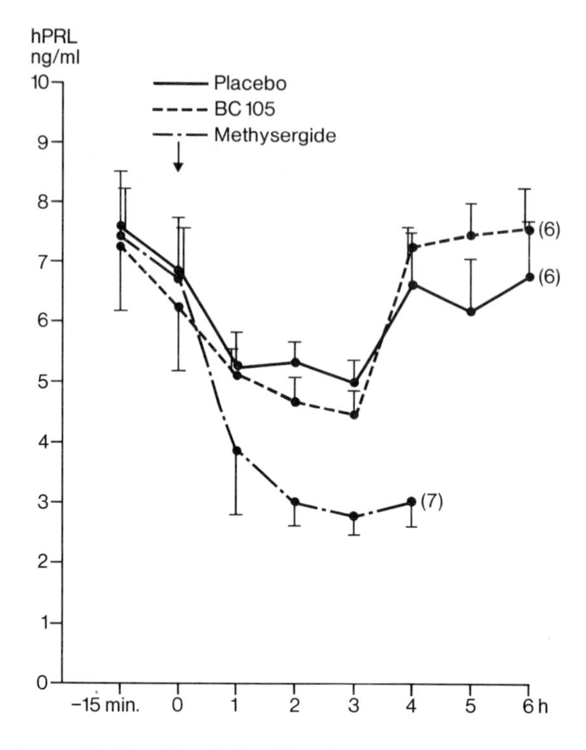

Fig. 6. Effect of methysergide (1 mg) and pizotifen (2 mg) on basal plasma prolactin in normal male subjects as compared with a placebo. There is a significant inhibition ($p < 0.01$) after methysergide administration, but pizotifen shows no action

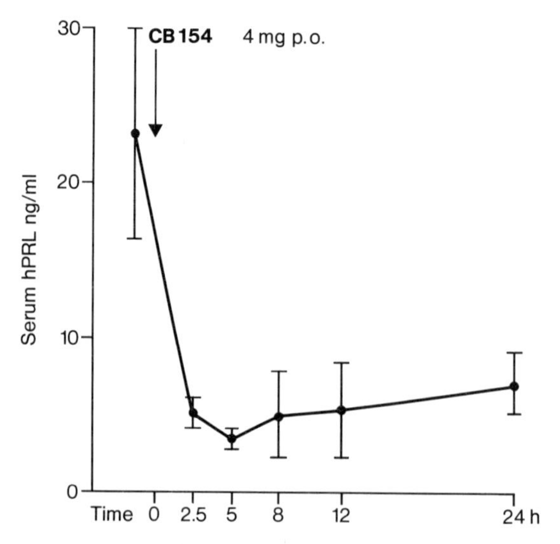

Fig. 7. Single oral administration of 4 mg bromocriptine (CB154) induced a significant fall in plasma prolactin in normal female volunteers ($p < 0.01$)

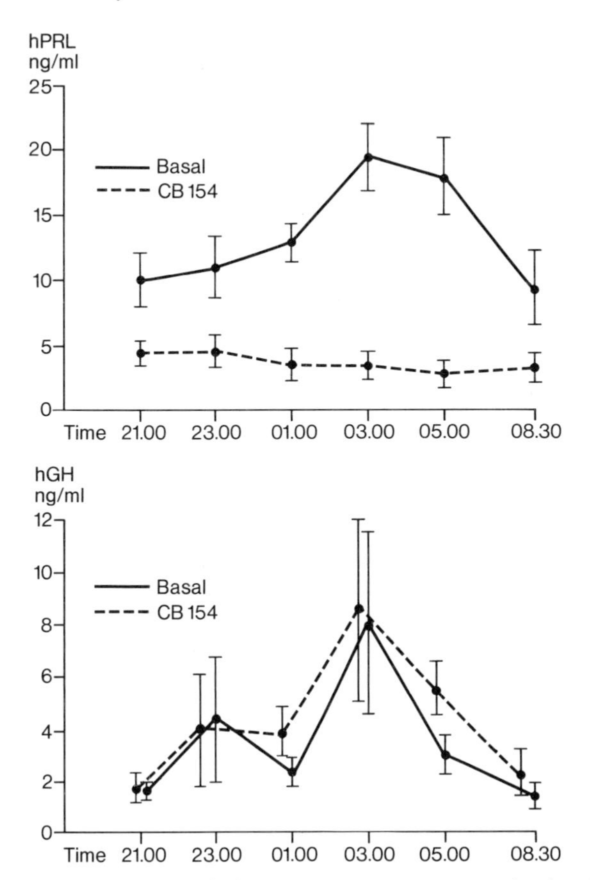

Fig. 8. Overnight prolactin and growth hormone measurements under basal conditions and during treatment with bromocriptine showing inhibition of the nocturnal prolactin surge during the late-sleep phase. Treatment did not alter the sleep-related growth hormone changes (M ± SE), demonstrating selective specific action for prolactin. [After DEL POZO et al. (1975a) with the permission of the American Journal of Obstetrics and Gynecology]

(Fig. 10), demonstrating the importance of prolactin in the maintenance of milk secretion in humans.

Soon after the first trials with bromocriptine were initiated in nonpuerperal galactorrhea, it was reported that, in addition to lactation suppression, menses and fertility were rapidly restored in women with a previous history of amenorrhea or infertility (LUTTERBECK et al., 1971; BESSER et al., 1972; DEL POZO et al., 1974). The fact that hyperprolactinemia had been found to abolish episodic LH secretion required for normal cycling activity (BOYAR et al., 1974) led BOHNET et al. (1975) to investigate the effect of bromocriptine on LH-pulsatile rhythm. They found that this drug restored LH-pulsatility in previously hyperprolactinemic women. By reducing local prolactin concentrations with bromocriptine, the cycling center would resume periodic activity.

Restoration of fertility by bromocriptine in a number of women and occurrence of pregnancy has led us to consider the possible effect of this drug on the endocrine

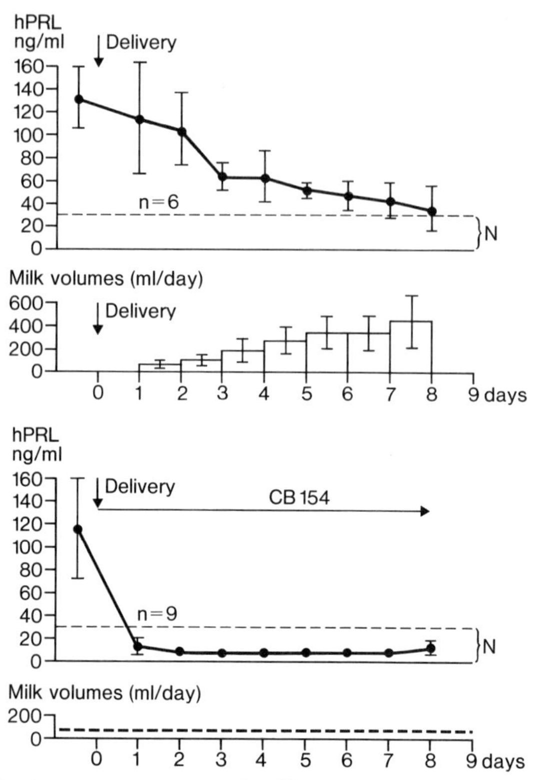

Fig. 9. Human prolactin measurements and milk volumes obtained in six normally breast-feeding women (upper panel) as compared with a prolactin suppressed group (lower panel). Prolactin was readily depressed by 2.5 mg t.i.d. bromocriptine (CB154) to the low normal range. No milk secretion was obtained (M ± SE)

system of the fetus. Data are available from two women receiving daily doses of 5 and 10 mg, respectively, throughout pregnancy. Prolactin and growth hormone were measured in the serum of mothers and newborns and also in amniotic fluid. Bromocriptine suppressed plasma prolactin in both mothers and newborns but did not modify it in the amniotic fluid, nor were growth hormone contents of the physiologic fluids modified by treatment. After delivery, both infants exhibited gradual increases in plasma prolactin to subsequently decline in a similar pattern as observed in untreated newborns (HIBA et al., 1977). The secretory pattern of growth hormone in the neonates was not modified by bromocriptine, and inhibition of prolactin throughout gestation seemed not to influence other possible biologic effects of this hormone, such as fetal growth.

The mechanism by which bromocriptine modifies the release of prolactin by the pituitary in man is not completely clarified. Experience to date suggests two different mechanisms of action. At the level of the CNS a dopamine-receptor stimulating effect can be assumed on the basis of human pharmacologic trials. Thus, prolactin stimulation by chlorpromazine can be readily counteracted by bromocriptine (FRIESEN et al., 1973). The effect of this neuroleptic drug takes

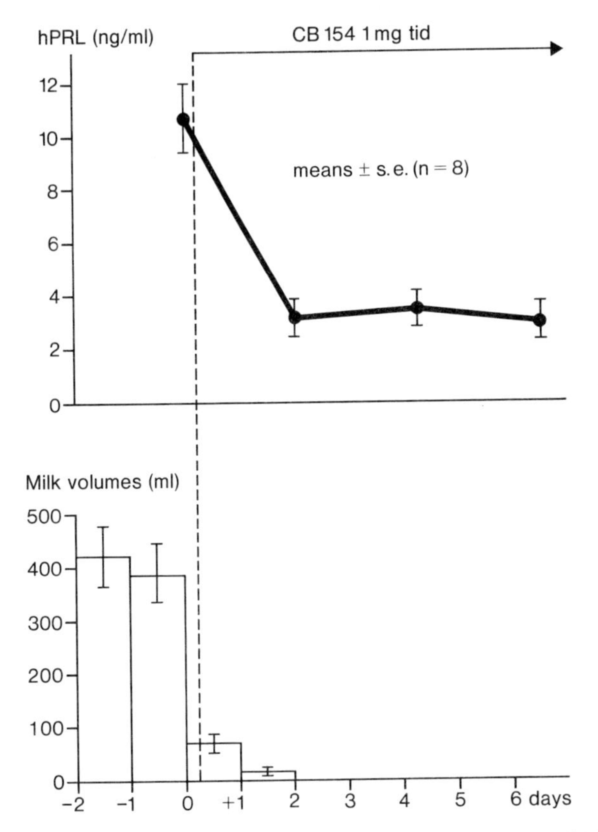

Fig. 10. Response to bromocriptine (CB 154) in eight lactating women exhibiting normal basal plasma prolactin concentrations. There was a significant prolactin fall ($p < 0.002$) accompanied by cessation of lactation within 24 to 48 h ($M \pm SE$). [After DEL POZO et al. (1975a) with the permission of the American Journal of Obstetrics and Gynecology]

place presumably via the TIDA (tubero-infundibular-dopamine) system, since results of experimental work can be reproduced in man through the administration of other compounds interfering with brain turnover of catecholamines, so that dopamine synthesis and/or dopamine-receptor sensitivity is reduced. The reserpines and α-methyl-DOPA belong among these compounds. On the other hand, the stimulatory effect of TRH on prolactin secretion (BOWERS et al., 1971), demonstrated to be a direct one (TASHJIAN et al., 1971), is also abolished by bromocriptine (DEL POZO et al., 1973), supporting experimental and in vitro work showing a direct action of this compound on the prolactin cells (TASHJIAN and HOYT, 1972; PASTEELS et al., 1971). This may suggest the existence of dopamine-receptors on the pituitary cell membrane. Indeed, MACLEOD et al. (1976) have presented in vitro data indicating specific H^3-dopamine binding to pituitary receptors. Thus, bromocriptine would act not only at the level of the hypothalamus but also directly on the pituitary as a dopamine-receptor agonist.

Lergotrile (cpd 39) is an ergoline of the clavine type. After its prolactin-inhibitory properties were demonstrated in the experimental animal, studies in man have

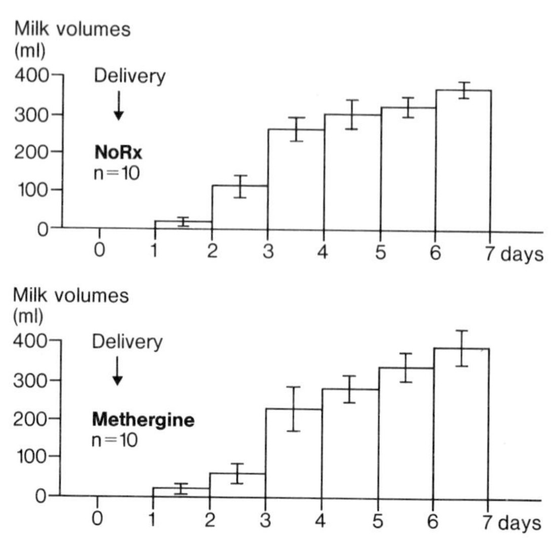

Fig. 11. Milk volumes produced by methergine-treated women (0.25 mg t.i.d.) were not different from volumes recorded in a control group (M ± SE). [After DEL POZO et al. (1975a) with the permission of the American Journal of Obstetrics and Gynecology]

shown doses of 2–6 mg to effectively inhibit serum prolactin levels and also to delay the onset of perphenazine-induced hyperprolactinemia (LEMBERGER et al., 1974). Lergotrile has also been found effective in suppressing nonpuerperal galactorrhea (CLEARY et al., 1975).

Methylergometrine (cpd 73a). Attempts to suppress lactation in humans with methylergometrine (methylergonovine) have shown contradictory results (SERMENT and RUF, 1955; GUILHEM et al., 1968). WEISS et al. (1975) administered 0.2 mg of this compound intramuscularly to a group of postpartum women. They used as a parameter a short-lived prolactin increase observed in the immediate postpartum. The injection of methylergonovine significantly ($p < 0.002$) reduced the magnitude of this elevation when compared with women receiving only saline. Also, studies reported by PEREZ-LOPEZ et al. (1975) have demonstrated a prolactin-inhibitory effect of methylergonovine after intravenous administration of 0.2 mg to women on postpartum day 3. The same treatment was also effective in acutely reducing basal plasma prolactin in normal individuals. This suppressive action was also found by DEL POZO et al. (1976) in normal volunteers. CANALES et al. (1976) extended their investigations with the same compound to postpartum week 1. Ten women received 0.2 mg orally three times daily, which is the routinely recommended dose to favor uterine involution in the postpartum. The authors recorded a significant fall in basal plasma prolactin in comparison with another group on no treatment, but milk letdown occurred in 7 cases. It is noteworthy that in these studies conducted in the postpartum, no mention of the effect of the drug on milk volume was made. DEL POZO et al. (1975b) were unable to find changes in plasma prolactin or milk volume in a group of puerperae treated with oral methylergometrine 0.2 mg three times a day for seven days. Milk volume collected increased in a linear pattern, which was not different from values recorded in a control group (Fig. 11).

Methergoline (cpd 89d). As a specific serotonin receptor blocking agent, methergoline has been found to lower unstimulated basal prolactin in acromegalic subjects, in addition to growth hormone (CHIODINI et al., 1976). The comparison of this drug with other serotonin antagonists and adrenergic drugs led to the conclusion that the inhibitory effect of methergoline on both hormones was probably due to a dopaminergic mechanism of action rather than to serotonin blockade.

b) Somatotropin

α) Control of Growth Hormone Secretion

Growth hormone is a peptide biochemically and biologically related to prolactin and placental lactogen. Experience acquired with the use of radioimmunoassay has shown this hormone to be remarkably sensitive to a variety of stimuli. Thus, hypoglycemia, physical and emotional stress, and exercise will elevate plasma growth hormone levels. A series of amino-acids have also been found to stimulate the release of this hormone, and the intravenous administration of arginine has become a standard clinical test for the capacity of response of the pituitary gland. Another physiologic variable is sleep, which induces nocturnal rises and can also be used as an indicator of somatotrope cell function.

Attention has been recently devoted to the hypothalamus as an important organ in monitoring somatotropin secretion. Releasing (GHRF) and inhibiting (GHIF) factors seem to regulate the function of pituitary somatotropes through the portal system. This seems to be regulated by dopaminergic, serotoninergic, and adrenergic mechanisms (MÜLLER, 1973). Serum growth hormone is acutely increased in normal subjects following ingestion of L-DOPA, the metabolic precursor of dopamine (BOYD et al., 1970; EDDY et al., 1971), or after apomorphine (BROWN et al., 1973), a selective stimulator of dopamine receptors (ANDÉN et al., 1967; LAL et al., 1973). Data collected in normal individuals are in contrast with what has been observed in acromegalic subjects. In this particular situation, administration of L-DOPA can induce a paradoxical fall in basal growth hormone, the effect being only transitory (CHIODINI et al., 1974). Adrenergic stimuli have been found to enhance growth hormone secretion (LAL et al., 1973), and their blockade with phentolamine has been effective in reducing it in acromegalic subjects (CRYER and DAUGHADAY, 1974).

To date, the effect of serotonin precursors on growth hormone secretion is controversial. Direct evidence of the stimulatory role of the serotoninergic system on this hormone in humans was provided by IMURA et al. (1973) through the administration of oral 5-HTP. The authors recorded substantial elevations of plasma growth hormone 2 h after ingestion of 150 mg 5-HTP. Moreover, BIVENS et al. (1973) and NAKAI et al. (1974) demonstrated the suppressive effect of serotonin antagonists on growth hormone. Unlike IMURA et al. (1973), MÜLLER et al. (1974) and HANDWERGER et al. (1975) were unable to induce growth hormone hypersecretion with oral 5-HTP, 70 mg/kg and 200 mg, respectively: There is no explanation for this discrepancy. More recently, LANCRANJAN et al. (1977) observed significant increments after intravenous injection of 200 mg L-5 HTP (Ro-35940) to normal volunteers.

It should be mentioned that decreased brain serotonin turnover has been found in humans by measuring indolamine metabolites in the spinal fluid of subjects treated with L-DOPA (GOODWIN et al., 1971). Also, dopamine receptor antagonists, such as chlorpromazine, are able to induce profound changes in brain serotonin activity in the experimental animal (BRADLEY, 1963). Thus, links between the dopaminergic and serotoninergic systems can be established on the basis of drug profiles. Indeed, SMYTHE et al. (1976) have proposed common serotoninergic pathways for drugs such as L-DOPA and bromocriptine with the nature of response depending on variable receptor occupancy. Subsequently, the authors presented structural similarities between dopamine, serotonin, and ergoline ring systems in order to explain common mechanisms of action.

β) Action of Ergot Compounds on Growth Hormone Secretion

Methysergide (cpd 34a). Based on animal data showing that the hypothalamic content of serotonin increases during insulin-induced hypoglycemia, BIVENS et al. (1973) investigated the effect of the serotonin antagonist methysergide in man on the growth hormone response to this insulin-induced hypoglycemia, as compared with cyproheptadine, a nonergot receptor antagonist. The administration of 4 mg cyproheptadine resulted in a 59% ($p<0.01$) reduction in the overall secretion of growth hormone, whereas 2 mg methysergide induced a moderate fall (35%: $p<0.05$). The authors concluded that serotonin was one of the factors regulating the secretion of growth hormone. It should be mentioned, however, that the clinical relevance of the recorded effect was not investigated until FELDMAN et al. (1976) administered 4 mg methysergide to six acromegalic subjects during a period of 48 h. Treatment lowered basal plasma growth hormone concentrations in only one case, rendering questionable the importance of serotoninergic mechanisms in this particular situation.

MENDELSON et al. (1975) studied the effect of methysergide on physiologic growth hormone fluctuations during sleep. They administered 2 mg every 6 h for 48 h to normal volunteers. In addition to a fall in plasma prolactin concentrations, the authors reported a significant elevation of growth hormone during the sleep period. Paradoxically, methysergide reduced insulin-stimulated (0.1 U/kg) growth hormone secretion by 36%. They suggested different mechanisms for sleep-related and insulin-induced growth hormone secretion and concluded that serotonin may be an important neurotransmitter for the control of this peptide. It is interesting to note that CHIHARA et al. (1976) were able to suppress nocturnal growth hormone secretion in normal volunteers with intravenous cyproheptadine, a nonergot serotonin antagonist.

Bromocriptine (cpd 38). Augmentation in the secretory activity of pituitary somatotropes has been linked to hypothalamic dopaminergic activity. Thus, the administration of L-DOPA and apomorphine (see above) has been followed by elevation of plasma growth hormone concentrations in normal subjects. After a paradoxical decrease was recorded in acromegaly, attention was directed to bromocriptine. Thus, this drug was found to elevate plasma growth hormone in normal individuals in doses of 1–3 mg (CAMANNI et al., 1975b; TOLIS et al., 1975), but this effect was not sustained when the compound was administered chronically (DEL POZO et al., 1977). Of note, the acute effect of bromocriptine on growth hormone can be blocked by previous treatment with pimozide, 1–4 mg administered twice orally (DAMMACCO et al., 1976; CHIODINI et al., 1976). This drug blocks dopamine receptors, and the results are interpreted as demonstrating a dopaminergic control of growth hormone secretion.

First testing of bromocriptine in acromegaly was reported by LIUZZI et al. (1974). A single oral dose of 2.5 mg lowered basal plasma growth hormone in seven patients, and this effect lasted 4 h. This action has also been amply demonstrated in chronic trials (CHIODINI et al., 1975; THORNER et al., 1975; SACHDEV et al., 1975). Doses used in different studies have varied between 10 and 50 mg daily. With this regime a fall in growth hormone significant enough to produce a biologic effect can be expected in about 40% of patients and complete normalization in 20%. The effect on growth hormone is accompanied by prolactin suppression in all instances (UEDA et al., 1975; CHIODINI et al., 1976). It should be mentioned that L-DOPA, which is transformed into dopamine in the organism, induces a sharp but short-lived growth hormone fall when administered orally to acromegalic individuals, whereas a time-lag of several hours has been observed for bromocriptine until maximal suppression is reached (LIUZZI et al., 1976).

This effect of bromocriptine has been compared with three other drugs known to exhibit dopaminergic activity, namely L-DOPA, amantadine (1,3-dimethyl-5-amino-adamantan), and piribedil (1-2-pyrimidil-4-piperonyl-perazine), in a group of acromegalic subjects (CAMANNI et al., 1975a). L-DOPA and bromocriptine at oral doses of 500 mg and 2.5 mg, respectively, were effective in lowering plasma growth hormone, exhibiting maximal suppression 2–3 h after drug administration. In contrast, 100 mg piribedil produced only a moderate suppression and 200 mg amantadine were ineffective. It could be postulated that the difference in activity between the above-mentioned drugs may be due to their different affinity for the dopamine receptors involved.

The role of dopamine has been further articulated by MASSARA et al. (1976a, 1976b). They found that the infusion of 280 μg/min dopamine would not modify basal growth hormone in normal subjects but would induce a substantial fall in acromegalic patients known to be sensitive to bromocriptine. It seemed that the favorable effect observed was due to the presence of pituitary dopaminergic receptors, since dopamine does not cross the blood-brain barrier and, consequently, cannot exert its suppressive action via the hypothalamus. VERDE et al. (1976) were able to confirm these data by administering L-DOPA and dopamine to normal persons and to acromegalics. Both drugs were effective in reducing plasma growth hormone in the patients, but only L-DOPA caused an elevation in the control subjects.

Finally, CHIODINI et al. (1976) compared the effect of 2.5 mg bromocriptine with 4 mg methergoline, both drugs administered orally to acromegalic patients. Treatment was followed by a significant decrease in plasma growth hormone, although the suppressive effect of bromocriptine was more sustained. The authors suggested a dopaminergic mechanism of action for methergoline similar to bromocriptine, in spite of its previous characterization as a serotonin blocking agent.

The mechanism of action of bromocriptine in acromegaly is poorly understood. Considering the effect of this drug on prolactin secretion, considerable differences are found when it is used in acromegaly. Thus, the clinical response rate in this condition (20–40%) is lower than in hyperprolactinemia (>90%), and higher doses are required to lower abnormally elevated growth hormone. The anomalous response to TRH (SAMAAN et al., 1974) recorded in about 80% of acromegalies is preserved after bromocriptine, whereas its effect on prolactin is abolished. The latter would suggest that the site of action of the drug may be located at the level of the hypothalamus. However, data discussed above concerning the effect of dopamine raise the possibility of growth hormone receptors being present in the pituitary gland and probably subjected to changing sensitivity or specificity. This may explain the paradoxical results of dopaminergic therapy in the acromegalic patient.

c) Effect of Ergot Compounds on the Control of Gonadal Function

α) Introduction

The effect of ergot derivatives on the reproductive system of the rat was already the subject of intense research in the early 1950's. Later on, SHELESNYAK (1957) proposed the existence of pharmacologic relationships between ergocornine and progesterone metabolism after showing that it prevented the development of the decidual reaction associated with nidation of the blastocyst. A preliminary report of women treated with ergocornine gave evidence of disturbed progesterone metabolism based on reduced pregnandiol excretion (SHELESNYAK et al., 1963). Further clinical studies, however, were not conclusive enough to justify the use of ergot compounds as luteolytic agents in humans. The availability of more sensitive methods for hormonal determinations and the characterization of prolactin as a separate peptide from growth hormone led to a better understanding of the pituitary dependency of ovarian function and of the effect of ergot derivatives on reproduction.

β) Action of Bromocriptine (cpd 38) on Gonadotropins, and Ovarian Function

The restoration of ovarian cyclicity by this drug in prolactin-dependent infertility has already been commented on (see above), but this action on the restoration of menstrual cycles deserves further attention. Pretreatment with bromocriptine failed to modify the gonadotropin response to a standard dose of 100 μg LHRH in the galactorrhea-amenorrhea syndrome (DEL POZO et al., 1974). This indicates that the inhibitory effect of prolactin on gonadotropins is exerted at suprasellar level. Therapy with bromocriptine is believed to restore normal cycling activity through prolactin suppression, but in some instances this therapy may present interesting features concerning restoration of cycles. We have observed resumption of menses to occur in some women after dosage increase, despite previous adequate prolactin suppression (DEL POZO et al., 1974). It could be speculated that while prolactin suppression may be a sensitive parameter, it may be only one of at least two mechanisms by which this drug normalized cyclic activity. The restoration of clomiphene sensitivity by bromocriptine in nonprolactin-dependent amenorrhea may add some weight to this hypothesis.

It is well established that nursing prolongs the physiologic amenorrhea that follows delivery. Also, decreased pituitary and ovarian responsiveness to releasing stimuli has been documented in the puerperium. Hence, a prolactin-induced block of the pituitary-gonadal axis seems likely, since milk secretion and amenorrhea are outstanding features in pathologic hyperprolactinemia. First evidence of an early normalization of gonadotropin secretion under bromocriptine therapy in the postpartum was provided by SEKI et al. (1974a). In three women treated with bromocriptine, they observed a significant increase in unstimulated plasma FSH from day 7 of puerperium on. NADER et al. (1975) also reported a significant elevation in basal FSH in postpartum women treated with bromocriptine, but there was no discernible response to LHRH. More recently, ROLLAND et al. (1975) have shown that bromocriptine may shorten the period of physiologic amenorrhea following delivery.

More than a decade has elapsed since SHELESNYAK's (1963) work concerning ergocornine and human luteal function was published. Recently, and on the basis of in vitro investigations by MCNATTY et al. (1974) showing prolactin-dependency of human granulosa cells, SCHULZ et al. (1976) administered bromocriptine in increasing doses to normal menstruating women. They found that a dosage increase to 7.5 mg daily would significantly depress plasma progesterone, in contrast to a previous report by DEL POZO et al. (1975a) showing that 1 mg three times daily would not modify the hormonal secretory pattern of the menstrual cycle. These data by SCHULZ et al. (1976) are in agreement with findings by ESPINOSA-CAMPOS et al. (1975), demonstrating prolactin-dependency of luteal function in monkeys. The evolution of the luteal plasma progesterone pattern was severely blunted by bromocriptine treatment, and the authors put forward the hypothesis that prolactin may play a role in the maintenance of granulose cell function in these animals. Their fertility status, however, was not assessed. It is interesting to note that, in our laboratory, BRÜGGEMANN (unpublished data) recorded pregnancies in five rhesus monkeys treated with 0.3 mg/kg bromocriptine for several days.

d) Other Endocrine Actions of Ergot Compounds

α) Effect of Bromocriptine on TSH

The inhibitory effect of bromocriptine in TSH in hypothyroidism reported by KIYOSHI et al. (1974) is an interesting finding restricted to this particular situation.

Evaluation of thyroid function in normal volunteers receiving bromocriptine and also in long-term clinical trials has disclosed normal thyroid function (DEL POZO et al., 1977).

β) Effect of Bromocriptine on ACTH

LAMBERTS and BIRKENHÄGER (1976) investigated the influence of bromocriptine on pituitary-dependent Cushing's disease, after this drug has failed to modify plasma ACTH under basal conditions and after stimulation with lysine-vasopressin. Four out of seven subjects responded to a single oral dose of 2.5 mg bromocriptine with a significant fall in basal plasma ACTH various times after administration of the drug. The authors concluded that dopaminergic mechanisms may have a bearing in the pathogenesis of Cushing's disease. BENKER et al. (1976) have also reported a significant fall in plasma ACTH in Nelson's and Cushing's syndromes after administration of 2.5 mg bromocriptine in an acute trial.

A 4-day treatment with 10 mg daily of methergoline blunted the ACTH response to insulin hypoglycemia in normal subjects (Cavagnini et al., 1976). This was accompanied by a moderate but significant fall in plasma cortisol. In contrast, methergoline failed to affect the ACTH response to lysine-vasopressin. Based on these data and on experience collected in patients, a physiologic stimulating effect of serotonin on ACTH secretion was proposed.

γ) Effect of Bromocriptine on Aldosterone

Edwards et al. (1975) showed that the administration of bromocriptine in increasing doses up to 7.5 mg daily to healthy volunteers inhibited the rise in plasma aldosterone that normally follows the administration of frusemide. The authors suggested that prolactin may modulate the secretion of aldosterone, although a direct action of bromocriptine on the adrenals was also considered. More recently, however, Del Pozo et al. (1977) reported normal aldosterone response to a postural challenge in three subjects treated chronically with 5 mg bromocriptine daily. It can be assumed that, in the case of a block of steroidogenesis induced by bromocriptine, the absence of an aldosterone rise would not vary with the type of the provocative test. Ølgaard et al. (1976) were unable to alter plasma aldosterone levels in anephric patients treated with 2.5 mg bromocriptine twice daily, despite a substantial reduction in plasma prolactin.

C. References

Abramson, H.A., Evans, L.T.: Lysergic acid diethylamide (LSD 25): II. Psychobiological effects on the Siamese fighting fish. Science **120**, 990–991 (1954)

Aleyassine, H., Lee, S.H.: Inhibition of insulin release by substrates and inhibitors of monoamine oxidase. Amer. J. Physiol. **222**, 565–569 (1972)

Andén, N.E., Rubenson, A., Fuxe, K., Hökfelt, T.: Evidence for dopamine receptor stimulation by apomorphine. J. Pharm. Pharmac. **19**, 627–629 (1967)

Arky, R.A.: Diphenylhydantoin and the beta cell. New Engl. J. Med. **286**, 371–372 (1972)

Astwood, E.B.: The regulation of corpus function by hypophyseal luteotrophin. Endocrinology **28**, 309–312 (1941)

Astwood, E.B.: Tests for luteotrophin. In: Ciba Foundation Colloquia on Endocrinology. Wolstenholme, G.E.W. (ed.), Vol. V, pp. 74–89. London: Churchill Livingstone 1953

Aubert, M.L., Grumbach, M.M., Kaplan, S.L.: The ontogenesis of human fetal hormones. III. Prolactin. J. clin. Invest. **56**, 155–164 (1975)

Audibert, A., Forgue, G., Gage, C.: Influence de la chlorpromazine sur l'activité hypophyso-ovarienne. C.R. Soc. Biol. (Paris) **150**, 173–175 (1956)

Aušková, M., Řežábek, K., Semonský, M.: Laktations-Hemmung bei der Ratte nach D-6-Methyl-8-ergolin-I-yl-essigsäureamidtartrat (VUFB-6683). Arzneimittel-Forsch. **23**, 617–618 (1973)

Aušková, M., Řežábek, K., Zikan, V., Semonský, M.: Suppression of lactation in rats with Lysenyl® SPOFA [N-(D-6-methyl-8-isoergolenyl) N′, N′-diethylcarbamide hydrogen maleate] Endocr. exp. (Bratisl.) **8**, 51–58 (1974a)

Aušková, M., Řežábek, K., Zikan, V., Semonský, M.: Laktationshemmende Wirkung von N-[D-6-Methyl-8-isoergolin-I-yl]-N′,N′-diäthylharnstoff (VUFB-6638). Experientia (Basel) **30**, 393–394 (1974b)

Aušková, M., Řežábek, K., Zikan, V., Semonský, M.: Induction of oestrus and ovulation with an ergoline derivative, substance VUFB-6638, an inhibitor of prolactin secretion. Physiol. bohemoslov. **23**, 417–421 (1974c)

Bach, N.J., Hall, D.A., Kornfeld, E.D.: Descarboxylysergic acid (9,10-didehydro-6-methylergoline). J. med. Chem. **17**, 312–313 (1974)

Baker, B.I.: Ability of various factors to oppose the stimulatory effect of dibutyryl cyclic AMP on the release of melanocyte-stimulating hormone by the rat pituitary in vitro. J. Endocr. **68**, 283–287 (1976)

Baldridge, J.A., Quickel, K.E., Feldman, J.M., Lebovitz, K.E.: Potentiation of tolbutamide-mediated insulin release in adult onset diabetics by methysergide maleate. Diabetes **23**, 21–24 (1974)

Bartke, A.: Plasma testosterone levels in male mice and rats treated with inhibitors of prolactin release. Acta endocr. (Kbh.) (Suppl.) **177**, 22 (1973)

Bartke, A.: Effects of inhibitors of pituitary prolactin release on testicular cholesterol stores, seminal vesicles weight, fertility and lactation in mice. Biol. Reprod. **11**, 319–325 (1974)

Bartke, A., Dalterio, S.: Effects of prolactin on the sensitivity of the testis to LH. Biol. Reprod. **15**, 90–93 (1976)

Baum, D., Porte, D.: Beta adrenergic dysfunction in hypoxic inhibition of insulin release. Endocrinology **98**, 359–366 (1976)

Baum, J., Simmons, B.E., Unger, R.H., Madison, L.L.: Localisation of glucagon in the alpha cells of the pancreatic islet by immunofluorescent technics. Diabetes **11**, 371–374 (1962)

Benker, G., Hackenberg, K., Hamburger, B., Reinwein, D.: Effects of growth hormone release-inhibiting hormone and bromocryptine (CB 154) in states of abnormal pituitary-adrenal function. Clin. Endocr. **5**, 187–190 (1976)

Beran, M., Řežábek, K., Seda, M., Semonský, M.: Some O-acyl derivatives of D-6-methyl-8-(2-hydroxyethyl)=ergolene and D-6-methyl-8-(2-hydroxyethyl ergoline (I). Coll. Czech. chem. Commun. **39**, 1768–1772 (1974)

Beran, M., Krepelka, J., Řežábek, K., Seda, M., Semonský, M.: Biological active 2-halogenated derivatives of D-6-methyl-8-ergolin-I-ylacetic acid. Abstract No. 62, Symposium on Ergot Alkaloids, Marienbad (CSSR), 21–25 April 1975

Berde, B., Cerletti, A.: Über den Melanophoreneffekt von D-Lysergsäure-diäthylamid und verwandten Verbindungen. Helv. physiol. pharmacol. Acta **14**, 325–333 (1956)

Berde, B., Cerletti, A.: Über den Angriffspunkt von D-Lysergsäure-diäthylamid und 5-Hydroxytryptamin im Melanophorentest. Z. Ges. exp. Med. **129**, 149–153 (1957)

Besser, G.M., Parke, L., Edwards, C.R.W., Forsyth, I.A., McNelly, A.S.: Galactorrhea: successful treatment with reduction of plasma prolactin levels by Brom-ergocryptine. Brit. med. J. **3**, 669–672 (1972)

Billeter, L., Flückiger, E.: Evidence for a luteolytic function of prolactin in the intact cycling rat using 2-Br-α-Ergokryptine (CB 154). Experientia (Basel) **27**, 464–465 (1971)

Bivens, C.H., Lebovitz, H.E., Skyler, J.S., Feldman, J.M.: Enhancement of insulin secretion in acromegaly by serotonin antagonists. Diabetes **21** (Suppl. 1), 352 (1972)

Bivens, C.H., Lebovitz, H.E., Feldman, J.M.: Inhibition of hypoglycemia-induced growth hormone secretion by the serotonin antagonists cyproheptadine and methysergide. New Engl. J. Med. **289**, 236–239 (1973)

Bloom, S.R., Edwards, A.V., Vaughan, N.J.A.: The role of sympathetic innervation in the control of plasma glucagon concentration in the calf. J. Physiol. (Lond). **233**, 457–466 (1973)

Bloom, S.R., Edwards, A.V., Vaughan, N.J.A.: The role of the autonomic innervation in the control of glucagon release during hypoglycemia in the calf. J. Physiol. (Lond.) **236**, 611–623 (1974)

Bohnet, H.G., Dahlén, H.G., Wuttke, W., Schneider, H.P.G.: Hyperprolactinemic anovulatory syndrome. J. clin. Endocr. **42**, 132–143 (1975)

Borrell, J., Piva, F., Martini, L.: Amygdala and gonadotropin secretion. Exp. Brain Res. **23** (Suppl.), 27 (Abstr. 49) (1975)

Bowers, C.Y., Friesen, H.G., Hwang, P., Guyda, H.J., Folkers, K.: Prolactin and thyrotropin release in man by synthetic pyroglutamyl-histidyl-prolinamide. Biochem. biophys. Res. Commun. **45**, 1033–1041 (1971)

Boyar, R.M., Kapen, S., Finkelstein, J.W., Perlow, M., Sassin, J.F., Fukushima, D.K., Weitzman, E.D., Hellman, L.: Hypothalamic-pituitary function in diverse hyperprolactinemic states. J. clin. Invest. **53**, 1588–1598 (1974)

Boyd, A.E., Lebovitz, H.E., Pfeiffer, J.B.: Stimulation of human-growth-hormone secretion by L-DOPA. New Engl. J. Med. **283**, 1425–1429 (1970)

Boyns, A.R., Cole, E.N., Golder, M.P., Danutra, V., Harper, M.E.: Brownsey, B., Cowley, T., Jones, G.E., Griffiths, K.: Prolactin studies with the prostate. In: Prolactin and Carcinogenesis. Boyns, A.R., Griffiths, K. (eds.), pp. 207–216. Cardiff: Alpha Omega Alpha Publishing 1972

Bradley, P.B.: Tranquilizers: 1. Phenothiazine derivatives. In: Physiological Pharmacology. Root, W.S., Hofmann, F.G. (eds.). Vol. I, Chap. E, pp. 417–477. New York: Academic Press 1963

Brown, P.S.: The effect of 5-hydroxytryptamine and two of its antagonists on ovulation in the mouse. J. Endocrin. **37**, 327–333 (1967)

Brown, P.S.: Pituitary follicle-stimulating hormone in immature female rats treated with drugs that inhibit the synthesis or antagonise the actions of catecholamines and 5-hydroxytryptamine. Neuroendocrinology **7**, 183–192 (1971)

Brown, W.A., Van Woert, M.H., Ambani, L.M.: Effect of apomorphine on growth hormone release in humans. J. clin. Endocrinol. **37**, 463–465 (1973)

Brown, W.B., Driver, P.M., Jones, R., Forbes, J.M.: Growth, prolactin and growth hormone in lambs treated with CB 154. J. Endocr. **69**, 47P (1976)

Brun del Re, R., Del Pozo, E., De Grandi, P., Friesen, H., Hinselmann, M., Wyss, H.: Prolactin inhibition and suppression of puerperal lactation by a br-ergocryptine (CB 154). Obstet. and Gynec. **41**, 884–890 (1973)

Bryant, G.D., Greenwood, F.C.: Radioimmunoassay for ovine, caprine, and bovine prolactin in plasma and tissue extracts. Biochem. J. **109**, 831–840 (1968)

Burden, J.L., Hillhouse, E.W., Jones, M.T.: A proposed model of the neurotransmitters involved in the control of corticotrophin releasing hormone. J. Endocr. **63**, 20P–21P (1974)

Burgers, A.C.J., Leemreis, W., Dominiczak, T., Van Oordt, G.J.: Inhibition of the secretion of intermedine by D-lysergic acid diethylamide (LSD 25) in the toad, *Xenopus laevis*. Acta Endocr. (Kbh.) **29**, 191–200 (1958)

Burgers, A.C.J., Imai, K.: The melanophore-stimulating potency of single pituitary glands of normal and of D-lysergic acid diethylamide (D-LSD) treated *Xenopus laevis*. Gen. comp. Endocr. **2**, 603–604 (1962)

Butler, W.R., Krey, L.C., Lu, K.H., Espinosa-Campos, J., Weiss, G., Knobil, E.: The secretion and action of prolactin in the rhesus monkey. Acta endocr. (Kbh.) (Suppl.) **193**, 155 (1975)

Caligaris, L., Taleisnik, S.: Involvement of neurones containing 5-hydroxytryptamine in the mechanism of prolactin release induced by oestrogen. J. Endocr. **62**, 25–33 (1974)

Camanni, F., Massara, F., Fassio, V., Molinatti, G.M., Müller, E.E.: Effect of five dopaminergic drugs on plasma growth hormone levels in acromegalic subjects. Neuroendocrinology **19**, 227–240 (1975a)

Camanni, F., Massara, F., Belforte, L., Molinatti, G.M.: Changes in plasma growth hormone levels in normal and acromegalic subjects following administration of 2-bromo-α-ergocryptine. J. clin. Endocr. **40**, 363–366 (1975b)

Cameron, E.H.D., Scarisbrick, J.J.: Determination of corticosterone in rat plasma by competitive protein-binding assay and its use in assessing the effects of CB 154 and perphenazine on adrenal function. J. Endocr. **58**, xxvii–xxviii (1973)

Campfield, L.A.: The effects of physiological concentrations of norepinephrine and epinephrine on the secretion of insulin. Dissertation Abstr. Int. B. **36**, 2086–2087 (1975)

Canales, E., Garrido, J.T., Zárate, A., Mason, M., Soria, J.: Effect of ergonovine on prolactin secretion and milk let-down. Obstet. and Gynec. **48**, 228–229 (1976)

Carlsen, R.A., Zeilmaker, G.H., Shelesnyak, M.C.: Termination of early (pre-nidation) pregnancy in the mouse by single injection of ergocornine methanesulfonate. J. Reprod. Fertil. **2**, 369–373 (1961)
Cassady, J.M., Li, G.S., Spitzner, E.B., Floss, H.G.: Ergot alkaloids, ergolines and related compounds as inhibitors of prolactin release. J. med. Chem. **17**, 300–307 (1974)
Castro-Vásquez, A., Esquivel, J.L., Martín, J.L., Rosner, J.M.: Failure of stressful stimuli to inhibit embryo implantation in the rat. Amer. J. Obstet. Gynec. **121**, 968–970 (1975)
Cavagnini, F., Raggi, U., Micossi, P., Di Landro, A., Invitti, C.: Effect of an antiserotoninergic drug, metergoline, on the ACTH and cortisol response to insulin hypoglycemia and lysine-vasopressin in man. J. clin. Endocr. **43**, 306–312 (1976)
Cerletti, A., Doepfner, W.: Comparative study on the serotonin antagonism of amide derivatives of lysergic acid and of ergot alkaloids. J. Pharmacol. exp. Ther. **122**, 124–136 (1958)
Chambers, J.W., Georg, R.H., Bass, A.D.: Effect of glucagon, cyclic 3′5′ adenosine monophosphate and its dibutyryl derivative of amine acid uptake by the isolated perfused rat liver. Endocrinology **87**, 366–370 (1970)
Cheever, E.V., Seavey, B.K., Lewis, U.J.: Prolactin of normal and dwarf mice. Endocrinology **85**, 698–703 (1969)
Chihara, K., Kato, Y., Maeda, K., Matsukura, S., Imura, H.: Suppression by cyproheptadine of human growth hormone and cortisol secretion during sleep. J. clin. Invest. **57**, 1393–1402 (1976)
Chiodini, P.G., Liuzzi, A., Botalla, L., Cremascoli, G., Silvestrini, F.: Inhibitory effect of dopaminergic stimulation on GH release in acromegaly. J. clin. Endocr. **38**, 200–206 (1974)
Chiodini, P.G., Liuzzi, A., Botalla, L., Oppizzi, G., Müller, E.E., Silvestrini, F.: Stable reduction of plasma growth hormone (hGH) levels during chronic administration of 2-Br-α-ergocryptine (CB 154) in acromegalic patients. J. clin. Endocr. **40**, 705–708 (1975)
Chiodini, P.G., Liuzzi, A., Müller, E.E., Botalla, L., Cremascoli, G., Oppizzi, G., Verde, G., Silvestrini, F.: Inhibitory effect of an ergoline derivative, methergoline, on growth hormone and prolactin levels in acromegalic patients. J. clin. Endocr. **43**, 356–363 (1976)
Chlebounova, J., Řežábek, K., Seda, M., Semonský, M.: Effect of D-6-methyl-8-ergoline-I-ylacetamide (Deprenon) on the FSH content of the rat pituitary during the oestrus cycle and pregnancy. Physiol. bohemoslov. **23**, 113–118 (1974)
Choudhury, S.A.R., Sharpe, R.M., Brown, P.S.: The effect of pimozide, a dopamine antagonist on pituitary gonadotrophic function in the rat. J. Reprod. Fertil. **39**, 275–283 (1974)
Cleary, R.E., Crabtree, R., Lemberger, L.: The effect of lergotrile on galactorrhea and gonadotropin secretion. J. clin. Endocr. **40**, 830–833 (1975)
Clemens, J.A., Shaar, C.J., Tandy, W.A., Roush, M.E.: Effects of hypothalamic stimulation on prolactin secretion in steroid treated rats. Endocrinology **89**, 1317–1320 (1971)
Clemens, J.A., Shaar, C.J., Smalstig, E.B., Bach, N.J., Kornfeld, E.C.: Inhibition of prolactin secretion by ergolines. Endocrinology **94**, 1171–1176 (1974)
Clemens, J.A., Smalstig, E.B., Shaar, C.J.: Inhibition of prolactin secretion by lergotrile mesylate: mechanism of action. Acta endocr. (Kbh.) **79**, 230–237 (1975)
Collu, R., Letarte, J., Leboeuf, G., Ducharme, J.R.: Endocrine effects of chronic administration of psychoactive drugs to prepubertal male rats. II. LSD. Canad. J. Physiol. Pharmacol. **53**, 1023–1026 (1975)
Corbin, A.: Postcoital contraceptive effect of 2-Br-α-ergocryptine (CB 154) in the rat. Experientia (Basel) **30**, 1358 (1974)
Corbin, A., Upton, G.V.: Effect of dopaminergic blocking agents on plasma luteinizing hormone releasing hormone activity in hypophysectomized rats. Experientia (Basel) **29**, 1552–1553 (1973)
Corrodi, H., Fuxe, K., Hökfelt, T., Lidbrink, P., Ungerstedt. U.: Effect of ergot drugs on central catecholamine neurons: evidence for a stimulation of central dopamine neurons. J. Pharm. Pharmacol. **25**, 409–411 (1973)
Corrodi, H., Farnebo, L.O., Fuxe, K., Hamberger, B.: Effect of ergot drugs on central 5-hydr-

oxytryptamine neurons: evidence for 5-hydroxytryptamine release or 5-hydroxytryptamine receptor stimulation. Europ. J. Pharmacol. **30**, 172–181 (1975)

Cowie, A.T., Forsyth, A.J.: Biology of prolactin. Pharmac. Therap. B. **1**, 437–457 (1975)

Cryer, P.E., Daughaday, W.H.: Adrenergic modulation of growth hormone secretion in acromegaly: suppression during phentolamine and phentolamine-isoproterenol administration. J. clin. Endocr. **39**, 658–663 (1974)

Dammacco, F., Rigillo, N., Tafaro, E., Gagliardi, F., Chetri, G., Dammacco, A.: Effects of 2-Bromo-α-ergocryptine and pimozide on growth hormone secretion in man. Horm. Metab. Res. **8**, 247–248 (1976)

Davies, C., Jacobi, J., Lloyd, H.M., Meares, J.D.: DNA synthesis and the secretion of prolactin and growth hormone by the pituitary gland of the male rat: effects of diethylstilboestrol and 2-bromo-α-ergocryptine methanesulphonate. J. Endocr. **61**, 411–417 (1974)

Del Pozo, E., Friesen, H., Burmeister, P.: Endocrine profile of a specific prolactin inhibitor: Br-α-ergokryptine (CB 154). A preliminary report. Schweiz. med. Wschr. **103**, 847–848 (1973)

Del Pozo, E., Varga, L., Wyss, H., Tolis, G., Friesen, H., Wenner, R., Vetter, L., Uettwiler, A.: Clinical and hormonal response to bromocriptin (CB 154) in the galactorrhea syndromes. J. clin. Endocr. **39**, 18–26 (1974)

Del Pozo, E., Goldstein, M., Friesen, H., Brun del Re, R., Eppenberger, U.: Lack of action of prolactin suppression on the regulation of the human menstrual cycle. Amer. J. Obstet. Gynec. **123**, 719–723 (1975a)

Del Pozo, E., Brun del Re, R., Hinselmann, M.: Lack of effect of methyl-ergonovine on postpartum lactation. Amer. J. Obstet. Gynec. **123**, 845–846 (1975b)

Del Pozo, E., Flückiger, E., Lancranjan, I.: Endogenous control of prolactin release and its modification by drugs. In: Basic Applications and Clinical Uses of Hypothalamic Hormones. Charro Salgado, A., Fernández Durango, R., López del Campo, J.G. (eds.), pp. 137–150. Amsterdam: Excerpta Medica 1976

Del Pozo, E., Darragh, A., Lancranjan, I., Ebeling, D., Burmeister, P., Bühler, F., Marbach, P., Braun, P.: Effect of bromocriptine on the endocrine system and fetal development. Clin. Endocr. **6** (Suppl.), 47s–55s (1977)

Dickerman, S., Kledzik, G., Gelato, M., Chen, H.J., Meites, J.: Effects of haloperidol on serum and pituitary prolactin, LH and FSH, and hypothalamic PIF and LRF. Neuroendocrinology **15**, 10–20 (1974)

Döhler, K.D., Wuttke, W.: Total blockade of phasic pituitary prolactin release in rats: effect on serum LH and progesterone during the oestrus cycle and pregnancy. Endocrinology **94**, 1595–1600 (1974)

D'Onofrio, F., Torella, R., Sgambato, S., Ungaro, B.: Nicergoline effect on insulin secretion in man. Farmaco, Ed. prat. **30**, 153–162 (1975)

Ectors, F., Danguy, A., Pasteels, J.L.: Ultrastructure of organ cultures of rat hypophyses exposed to ergocornine. J. Endocr. **52**, 211–212 (1972)

Eddy, R.L., Jones, A.L., Chakamkjian, Z.H., Silverthorne, M.C.: Effect of levodopa (L-DOPA) on human hypophyseal trophic hormone release. J. Clin. Endocrinol. Metab. **33**, 709–712 (1971)

Edwards, C.R.W., Thorner, M.O., Miall, P.A., Al-Dujaili, E.A.S., Hanker, J.P., Besser, G.M.: Inhibition of the plasma-aldosterone response to frusemide bromocriptine. Lancet **1975 II**, 903–904

Edwardson, J.A.: The effects of agroclavine, an ergot alkaloid, on pregnancy and lactation in the rat. Brit. J. Pharmacol. **33**, 215 P (1968)

Ekholm, R., Ericson, L.E., Lundquist, I.: Monoamines in the pancreatic islets of the mouse. Subcellular localisation of serotonin by electron microscopic autoradiography. Diabetologia **7**, 339–349 (1971)

El Etreby, M.F., Günzel, P.: Prolaktinzell-Tumoren im Tierexperiment und beim Menschen. Arzneimittel-Forsch. **23**, 1768–1790 (1973)

Erdheim, J., Stumme, E.: Über Schwangerschaftsveränderungen bei der Hypophyse. Beitr. Path. **46**, 1–132 (1909)

Espinosa-Campos, J., Butler, W.R., Knobil, E.: Inhibition of corpus luteum function in the rhesus monkey by 2-br-α-ergocryptine (CB 154). Abstract. The Endocrine Society Meeting, New York, 1975

Esterhuizen, A.C., Howell, S.L.: Ultrastructure of the A-cells of the cat islets of Langerhans following sympathetic stimulation of glucagon secretion. J. Cell Biol. **46**, 593–631 (1970)
Evans, L.T., Geronimus, L.H., Kornetsky, C., Abramson, H.A.: Effect of ergot drugs on Betta splendens. Science **123**, 26 (1956)
Everett, J.W.: Central neural control of reproductive functions of the adenohypophysis. Physiol. Rev. **44**, 373–431 (1964)
Feldman, J.M., Lebovitz, H.E.: Specificity of serotonin inhibition of insulin release from golden hamster pancreas. Diabetes **19**, 475–479 (1970a)
Feldman, J.M., Lebovitz, H.E.: Mechanism of serotonin inhibitory action on insulin release. Clin. Res. **18**, 52 (1970b)
Feldman, J.M., Lebovitz, H.E.: Mechanism of epinephrine and serotonin inhibition of insulin release. Clin Res. **18**, 359 (1970c)
Feldman, J.M., Quickel, K.E., Lebovitz, H.E.: Potentiation of in vitro insulin secretion by serotonin antagonists. Clin. Res. **20**, 56 (1972a)
Feldman, J.M., Quickel, K.E., Lebovitz, H.E.: Potentiation of insulin secretion in vitro by serotonin antagonists. Diabetes **21**, 779–788 (1972b)
Feldman, J.M., Plonk, J.W., Bivens, C.H.: Inhibitory effect of serotonin antagonists on growth hormone release in acromegalic patients. Clin. Endocr. **5**, 71–78 (1976)
Findlay, J.A., Gill, J.R., Lever, J.D., Randler, P.J., Spriggs, T.L.B.: Increased insulin output following stimulation of the vagal supply to the perfused rabbit pancreas. J. Anat. (Lond.) **104**, 580 (1969)
Floss, H.G., Cassady, J.M., Robbers, J.E.: Influence of ergot alkaloids on pituitary prolactin and prolactin-dependent processes. J. pharm. Sci. **62**, 699–715 (1973)
Flückiger, E.: Zur Biologie der Farbwechselhormone. Verh. naturforsch. Ges. Basel **73**, 194–203 (1962a)
Flückiger, E.: Biologie der Melanophorenhormone. In: Gewebs- und Neurohormone, pp. 187–194. Berlin-Göttingen-Heidelberg: Springer 1962b
Flückiger, E.: Die Melanocyten stimulierenden Hormone der Adenohypophyse. Naunyn-Schmiedebergs Arch. exp. Path. Pharmak. **245**, 168–184 (1963)
Flückiger, E.: Drugs and the control of prolactin secretion. In: Prolactin and Carcinogenesis. Boyns, A.R., Griffiths, K. (eds.), pp. 162–171. Alpha Omega Alpha Publishing 1972
Flückiger, E.: Pharmacological characterization of CB 154. Triangle **14**, 153–157 (1975)
Flückiger, E.: The pharmacology of bromocriptine. In: Pharmacological and Clinical Aspects of Bromocriptine (Parlodel). Symposium, Proceedings M.C.S. Consultants, 12–26 (1977)
Flückiger, E., Kovacs, E.: Inhibition by 2-Br-α-ergokryptine-mesylate (CB 154) of suckling-induced pituitary prolactin depletion in lactating rats. Experientia (Basel) **30**, 1173 (1974)
Flückiger, E., Wagner, H.R.: 2-Br-α-Ergokryptin: Beeinflussung von Fertilität und Laktation bei der Ratte. Experientia (Basel) **24**, 1130 (1968)
Flückiger, E., Markó, M., Doepfner, W., Niederer, W.: Effects of ergot alkaloids on the hypothalamo-pituitary axis. Postgrad. med. J. (Suppl. 1) **52**, 57–61 (1976)
Ford, J.J., Yoshinaga, K.: Ergocryptine and pregnancy maintenance in hamsters. Proc. Soc. exp. Biol. (N.Y.) **150**, 425–427 (1975)
Forsyth, I.A., Parke, L.: The bioassay of human prolactin. In: Human Prolactin. Pasteels, J.L., Robyn, C. (eds.), pp. 71–81. Amsterdam: Excerpta Medica 1973
Frantz, A.G.: The regulation of prolactin secretion in humans. In: Frontiers in Neuroendocrinology. Ganong, W.F., Martini, L. (eds.), pp. 337–374. New York: Oxford Univ. Press 1973
Frantz, A.G., Kleinberg, D.L., Noel, G.L.: Studies on prolactin in man. Recent Progr. Hormone Res. **28**, 527–590 (1972)
Friesen, H.G., Guyda, H., Hardy, J.: The biosynthesis of human growth hormone and prolactin. J. clin. Endocr. **31**, 611–624 (1970)
Friesen, H.G., Shome, B., Belanger, C., Hwang, P., Guyda, H., Myers, R.: The synthesis and secretion of human and monkey placental lactogen (HPL and MPL) and pituitary prolactin (HPr and MPr). In: Growth and Growth Hormone. Pecile, A., Müller, E. (eds.), pp. 224–238. Amsterdam: Excerpta Medica 1972
Friesen, H.G., Tolis, G., Shiu, R., Hwang, P.: Studies on human prolactin: chemistry, radiore-

ceptor assay and clinical significance. In: Human Prolactin. Pasteels, J.L., Robyn, C. (eds.), pp. 11–23. Amsterdam: Excerpta Medica 1973
Fuxe, K., Hökfelt, T.: Central monoaminergic systems and hypothalamic function. In: The Hypothalamus. Martini, L., Motta, M., Fraschini, F. (eds.), pp. 123–138. New York: Academic Press 1970
Gala, R.R., Sanford, J.: The influence of 2-Br-α-ergocryptine (CB 154) and apomorphine on induced prolactin secretion in the crab eating monkey (*Macaca fascicularis*). Endocr. Res. Commun. **2**, 95–108 (1975)
Gallo, R.V., Rabii, J., Moberg, G.P.: Effect of methysergide, a blocker of serotonin receptors, on plasma prolactin levels in lactating and ovariectomized rats. Endocrinology **97**, 1096–1005 (1975)
Gautvik, K.M., Hoyt, R.F., Tashjian, A.H.: Effects of colchicine and 2-Br-α-ergokryptine-methanesulfonate (CB 154) on the release of prolactin and growth hormone by functional tumor cells in culture. J. cell. Physiol. **82**, 401–410 (1973a)
Gautvik, K.M., Tashjian, A.H.: Effects of Ca^{++} and Mg^{++} on secretion and synthesis of growth hormone and prolactin by clonal strains of pituitary cells in culture. Endocrinology **92**, 573–583 (1973b)
Goluboff, L.G., Ezrin, C.: Effect of pregnancy on the somatotroph and the prolactin cell of the human adenohypophysis. J. clin. Endocr. **29**, 1533–1538 (1969)
Goodwin, F.K., Dunner, D.L., Gershon, E.S.: Effect of L-dopa treatment on brain serotonin metabolism in depressed patients. Life Sci. **10** (I), 751–759 (1971)
Gräf, K.-J., Neumann, F., Horowski, R.: Effect of the ergot derivative lisuride hydrogen maleate on serum prolactin concentrations in female rats. Endocrinology **98**, 598–605 (1976)
Greenwald, G.S.: Role of follicle-stimulating hormone and luteinizing hormone in follicular development and ovulation. In: Handbook of Physiology, Section 7: Endocrinology, Vol. IV, Knobil, E., Sawyer, W.H. (eds.), pp. 293–324. The Pituitary Gland and its Neuroendocrine Control, Part 2, Washington D.C.: American Physiological Society 1974
Grosvenor, C.E.: Effect of ergotamine on milk-ejection in lactating rat. Proc. Soc. exp. Biol. (N.Y.) **91**, 294–296 (1956)
Grosvenor, C.E., Mena, F.: Evidence for a time delay between prolactin release and the resulting rise in milk secretion rate in the rat. J. Endocr. **58**, 31–39 (1973)
Grosvenor, C.E., Turner, Ch.W.: Ergotamine, oxytocin and milk let-down in lactating rats. Proc. Soc. exp. Biol. (N.Y.) **93**, 466–468 (1956)
Grosvenor, C.E., Turner, Ch.W.: Evidence for adrenergic and cholinergic components in milk let-down reflex in lactating rat. Proc. Soc. exp. Biol. (N.Y.) **95**, 719–722 (1957)
Guilhem, P., Pontonnier, A., Monrozies, M., Bardenat, M., Merle-Beral, A.: Essai de blocage de la galactogénèse par la méthylergobasine. Bull. Fed. Gynec. Obstet. Fr. **19**, 277–279 (1967)
Hafiez, A.A., Bartke, A., Lloyd, C.W.: The role of prolactin in the regulation of testis function: The synergistic effects of prolactin and luteinizing hormone on the incorporation of $[1-{}^{14}C]$ acetate into testosterone and cholesterol by testes from hypophysectomized rats in vitro. J. Endocr. **53**, 223–230 (1972)
Hamilton, J.M. Flaks, A., Saluja, P.G., Maguire, S.: Hormonally induced renal neoplasia in the male Syrian hamster and the inhibitory effect of 2-Bromo-α-ergocriptine methanesulfonate. J. nat. Cancer Inst. **54**, 1385–1400 (1975)
Handwerger, S., Plonk, J.W., Lebovitz, H.E., Bivens, C.H., Feldman, J.M.: Failure of 5-hydroxytryptophan to stimulate prolactin and growth hormone secretion in man. Horm. Metab. Res. **7**, 214–216 (1975)
Harris, G.W.: Neural Control of the Pituitary Gland. London: Edward Arnold 1955
Hart, I.C.: Effect of 2-Br-α-ergocryptine on milk yield and the level of prolactin and growth hormone in the blood of the goat at milking. J. Endocr. **57**, 179–180 (1973)
Hedo, J.A., Martinell, J., Calle, C., Villanueava, M.L., Marco, J.: Potentiation of glucagon secretion by serotonin antagonists in man. Diabetologia **11**, 348 (1975)
Hellman, B., Sehlin, J., Taljedal, J.B.: The pancreatic β-cell recognition of insulin secretagogues: II. Site of action of tolbutamide. Biochem. biophys. Res. Commun. **45**, 1384–1388 (1971)
Hery, M., Laplante, E., Kordon, C.: Role of pituitary sensitivity and adrenal secretion in the effect of serotonin depletion on luteinizing hormone regulation. J. Endocr. **67**, 463–464 (1975)

Hiba, J., Del Pozo, E., Genazzani, A., Pusterla, E., Lancranjan, I., Sidiropoulos, D., Gunti, J.: Hormonal mechanism of milk secretion in the newborn. J. clin. Endocr., **44**, 973–976 (1977)
Hill-Samli, M., Macleod, R.M.: Interaction of thyrotropin-releasing hormone and dopamine on the release of prolactin from the rat anterior pituitary in vitro. Endocrinology **95**, 1189–1192 (1974)
Hill-Samli, M., Macleod, R.M.: Thyrotropin-releasing hormone blockade of the ergocryptine and apomorphine inhibition of prolactin release in vitro. Proc. Soc. exp. Biol. (N.Y.) **149**, 511–514 (1975)
Hinzen, D.H., Becker, P., Mueller, U.: Einfluß von Insulin auf den regionalen Phospholipidstoffwechsel des Kaninchengehirns in vivo. Pflügers Arch. **321**, 1–14 (1970)
Hökfelt, T., Fuxe, K.: On the morphology and the neuroendocrine role of the hypothalamic catecholamine neurons. In: Brain-Endocrine Interaction. Median Eminence: Structure and Function. Knigge, K.M., Scott, D.E., Weindl, A. (eds.), pp. 181–223. Basel: Karger 1972a
Hökfelt, T., Fuxe, K.: Effects of prolactin and ergot alkaloids on the tubero-infundibular dopamine (DA) neurons. Neuroendocrinology **9**, 100–122 (1972b)
Holt, J.A., Richards, J.S., Midgley, A.R., Reichert, L.E.: Effect of prolactin on LH receptor in rat luteal cells. Endocrinology **98**, 1005–1013 (1976)
Horowski, R., Gräf, K.-J.: Prolactin secretion in rats under the influence of different agents acting on the dopaminergic system. Acta endocr. (Kbh.) (Suppl.) **199**, 203 (1975)
Horowski, R., Neumann, F., Gräf, K.-J.: Influence of apomorphine hydrochloride, dibutyrylapomorphine and lysenyl on plasma prolactin concentrations in the rat. J. Pharm. Pharmacol. **27**, 532–534 (1975)
Horrobin, D.F.: Prolactin: Physiology and Clinical Significance. Lancaster: MTP Medical and Technical Publishing 1973
Horrobin, D.F.: Prolactin 1974. Lancaster: MTP Medical and Technical Publishing 1974
Horrobin, D.F.: Prolactin 1975. Montreal: Eden Press 1975
Horrobin, D.F.: Prolactin 1976. Montreal: Eden Press 1976
Hotta, N., Sirek, O.V., Sirek, A.: Studies on the interaction between growth hormone and dihydroergotamine in adipose cells: II. Augmentation of the lipolytic response. Horm. Metab. Res. **3**, 321–325 (1971)
Hwang, P., Guyda, H., Friesen, H.: A radioimmunoassay for human prolactin. Proc. nat. Acad. Sci. (Wash.) **68**, 1902–1906 (1971)
Hwang, P., Guyda, H., Friesen, H.G.: Purification of human prolactin. J. biol. Chem. **247**, 1955–1958 (1972)
Imura, H., Nakai, Y., Yoshimi, T.: Effect of 5-hydroxytryptophan (5-HTP) on growth hormone and ACTH release in man. J. clin. Endocr. **36**, 204–206 (1973)
Itil, T.M., Hermann, W.M., Akpinar, S.: Prediction of psychotropic properties of lisuride hydrogen maleate by quantitative pharmaco-electroencephalogram. Int. J. clin. Pharmacol. **12**, 221–233 (1975)
Iturriza, F.C.: The effect of D-lysergic acid diethylamide on the melanophores of the toad Bufo arenarum under different experimental conditions. Acta endocr. (Kbh.) **48**, 322–328 (1965)
Iturriza, F.C., Koch, O.R.: Effect of the administration of lysergic acid diethylamide (LSD) on the colloid vesicles of the pars intermedia of the toad pituitary. Endocrinology **75**, 615–616 (1964)
Iversen, J.: Effect of acetyl choline on the secretion of glucagon and insulin from the isolated, perfused, canine pancreas. Diabetes **22**, 381–387 (1973)
Jacobs, L.S., Snyder, P.J., Wilber, J.F., Utiger, R.D., Daughaday, W.H.: Increased serum prolactin after administration of synthetic thyrotropin releasing hormone (TRH) in man. J. clin. Endocr. **33**, 996–998 (1971)
Jaim-Etcheverry, G., Zieher, L.M.: Electron microscopic cytochemistry of 5-hydroxytryptamine in the beta cells of guinea pig endocrine pancreas. Endocrinology **83**, 917–923 (1968)
Jones, G.E., Brownstone, A.D., Boyns, A.R.: Isolation of canine prolactin by polyacrylamide gel electrophoresis. Acta endocr. (Kbh.) **82**, 691–705 (1976)
Judd, S.J., Lazarus, L., Smythe, G.: Prolactin secretion by metoclopramide in man. J. clin. Endocr. **43**, 313–317 (1976)

Kahr, H., Fischer, W.: Die Wirkung des 5-Oxytryptamins auf das Pigmentsystem der Haut. Klin. Wschr. **35**, 41–44 (1957)
Kaneto, A., Kajinuma, H., Kosaka, K., Nakao, K.: Stimulation of insulin secretion by parasympathomimetic agents. Endocrinology **83**, 651–658 (1968)
Kaneto, A., Kajinuma, H., Kosaka, K.: Effects on splanchnic nerve stimulation on glucagon and insulin output in the dog. Endocrinology **96**, 143–150 (1975)
Kann, G., Denamur, R.: Possible role of prolactin during the oestrous cycle and gestation in the ewe. J. Reprod. Fertil. **39**, 473–483 (1974)
Kann, G., Martinet, J.: Prolactin levels and duration of postpartum anoestrus in lactating ewes. Nature (Lond.) **257**, 63–64 (1975)
Karg, H., Schams, D., Reinhardt, V.: Effects of 2-Br-α-ergocryptine on plasma prolactin level and milk yield in cows. Experientia (Basel) **28**, 574–576 (1972)
Kato, Y., Nakai, Y., Imura, H., Chihara, K., Ohgo, S.: Effect of 5-hydroxytryptophan (5-HTP) on plasma prolactin levels in man. J. clin. Endocr. **38**, 695–697 (1974)
Kimura, H., Calbro, M.A., MacLeod, R.M.: Suppression of prolactin secretion and cAMP accumulation by dopamine in the pituitary. Fed. Proc. **35**, 305 (1976)
Kisch, E.S., Shelesnyak, M.C.: Studies on the mechanism of nidation. XXXI. Failure of ergocornine to interrrupt gestation in the rat in the presence of foetal placenta. J. Reprod. Fertil. **15**, 401–407 (1968)
Kiyoshi, M., Toshio, O., Mitsuko, H., Kaichiro, I., Yuichi, K.: Inhibition of thyrotropin and prolactin secretions in primary hypothyroidism by 2-br-α-ergocryptine. J. clin. Endocr. **39**, 391–394 (1974)
Kleinberg, D.L., Noel, G.L., Frantz, A.G.: Chlorpromazine stimulation and L-dopa suppression of plasma prolactin in man. J. clin. Endocr. **33**, 873–876 (1971)
Knobil, E., Sawyer, W.H. (eds.) The Pituitary Gland and Its Neuroendocrine Control, Parts 1 and 2, Endocrinology Vol. IV of Handbook of Physiology, Section 7: Washington D.C.: American Physiological Society 1974
Kordon, C.: Blockade of ovulation in the immature rat by local microinjection of α-methyl-dopa into the arcuate region of the hypothalamus. Neuroendocrinology **7**, 202–209 (1971)
Kordon, C., Blake, C.A., Terkel, J., Sawyer, C.H.: Participation of serotonin containing neurons in the suckling-induced rise in plasma prolactin levels in lactating rats. Neuroendocrinology **13**, 213–223 (1973/74)
Kraicer, P.F., Shelesnyak, M.C.: Studies on the mechanism of nidation. XIII: The relationship between chemical structure and biodynamic activity of certain ergot alkaloids. J. Reprod. Fertil. **10**, 221–226 (1965)
Kraicer, P.F., Strauss, J.F.: Ovulation block produced by an inhibitor of luteotrophin, ergocornine. Acta endocr. (Kbh.) **65**, 698–706 (1970)
Krejči, P., Aušková, M., Řežábek, K., Bílek, J., Semonský, M.: The effect of the ergoline derivative VUFB-6683 on the adenohypophysial prolactin concentration in rats. Experientia (Basel) **29**, 1262–1263 (1973)
Kwa, H.G., Vorhofstad, F.: Radioimmunoassay of rat prolactin. Biochim. biophys. Acta (Amst.) **133**, 186–188 (1967)
Lacy, P.E.: Electron microscopic identification of different cell types in the islets of Langerhans of the guinea-pig, rat, rabbit and dog. Anat. Rec. **128**, 255–267 (1957)
Lacy, P.E., Davies, J.: Preliminary studies on the demonstration of insulin in the islets by the fluorescent antibody technic. Diabetes **6**, 354–357 (1957)
Lal, S., de la Vega, C.E., Sourkes, T.L., Friesen, H.G.: Effect of apomorphine on growth hormone, prolactin, luteinizing hormone and follicle-stimulating hormone levels in human serum. J. clin. Endocr. **37**, 719–724 (1973)
Lamberts, S.W.J., Birkenhäger, J.C.: Effect of bromocriptine in pituitary-dependent Cushing's syndrome. J. Endocr. **70**, 315–316 (1976)
Lamprecht, S.A., Lindner, H.R., Strauss, J.F.: Induction of 20α-hydroxysteroid dehydrogenase in rat corpora lutea by pharmacological blockade of pituitary prolactin secretion. Biochim. biophys. Acta (Amst.) **187**, 133–143 (1969)
Lancranjan, I., Wirz-Justice, A., Pühringer, W., del Pozo, E.: Effect of 1–5 hydroxytryptophan infusion on growth hormone and prolactin secretion in man. J. clin. Endocr. **45**, 588–593 (1977)

Landgraf, R., Weissmann, A., Landgraf-Leurs, M., Werder, K.: Glucose tolerance and glucose-induced insulin release in patients with hyperprolactinemia. Acta endocr. (Kbh.) **78**, 65 (1975)

Langerhans, P.: Contributions to the Microscopic Anatomy of the Pancreas (M.D. Thesis). Berlin 1869 (Translated by H. Morrison, Baltimore: The John Hopkins Hospital Press 1937)

Lawrence, A.M., Hagen, T.C.: Ergonovine therapy of nonpuerperal galactorrhea. New Engl. J. Med. **287**, 150 (1972)

Lawson, D.M., Gala, R.R.: The interaction of dopaminergic and serotoninergic drugs on plasma prolactin in ovariectomized estrogen-treated rats. Endocrinology **98**, 42–47 (1976)

Lemberger, L., Crabtree, R., Clemens, J., Dyke, R.W., Woodburn, R.T.: The inhibitory effect of an ergoline derivative (lergotrile, compound 83636) on prolactin secretion in man. J. clin. Endocr. **39**, 579–584 (1974)

Lernmark, A.: The significance of 5-hydroxytryptamine for insulin secretion in the mouse. Horm. Metab. Res. **3**, 305–309 (1971)

Lewis, U.J., Singh, R.N.P., Sinha, Y.N., van der Laan, W.P.: Electrophoretic evidence for human prolactin. J. clin. Endocr. **33**, 153–156 (1971)

L'Hermite, M., Delvoye, P., Nokin, J., Vekemans, M., Robyn, C.: Human prolactin secretion, as studied by radioimmunoassay: some aspects of its regulation. In: Prolactin and Carcinogenesis. Boyns, A.R., Griffiths, K. (eds.), pp. 81–97. Cardiff: Alpha Omega Alpha Publishing 1972

Li, G.S., Robinson, J.M., Floss, H.G., Cassady, J.M., Clemens, J.A.: Ergot alkaloids. Synthesis of 6-methyl-8-ergolenes as inhibitors of prolactin release. J. med. Chem. **18**, 892–895 (1975)

Lichtensteiger, W., Keller, P.J.: Tubero-infundibular dopamine neurons and the secretion of luteinizing hormone and prolactin: extrahypothalamic influences, interaction with cholinergic systems and the effect of urethane anesthesia. Brain Res. **74**, 279–303 (1974)

Lin, B.J., Haist, R.E.: Insulin biosynthesis: the monoaminergic mechanisms and the specificity of the "glucoreceptor". Endocrinology **96**, 1247–1253 (1975)

Lindner, H.R., Shelesnyak, M.C.: Effect of ergocornine on ovarian synthesis of progesterone and 20-α-hydroxy-pregn-4-en-3-one in the pseudopregnant rat. Acta endocr. (Kbh.) **56**, 27–34 (1967)

Liuzzi, A., Chiodini, P.G., Botalla, L., Cremascoli, G., Müller, E.E., Silvestrini, F.: Decreased plasma growth hormone (GH) levels in acromegalics following CB 154 (2-Br-α-ergocryptine) administration. J. clin. Endocr. **38**, 910–912 (1974)

Liuzzi, A., Panerai, A.E., Chiodini, P.G., Secchi, C., Cocchi, D., Botalla, L., Silvestrini, F., Müller, E.E.: Neuroendocrine control of growth hormone secretion: experimental and clinical studies. In: Growth Hormone and Related Peptides. Pecile, A., Müller, E.E. (eds.), pp. 236–251. Amsterdam: Excerpta Medica 1976

Lloyd, H.M., Meares, J.D., Jacobi, J.: Effects of oestrogen and bromocriptin on in vivo secretion and mitosis in prolactin cells. Nature (Lond.) **255**, 497–498 (1975)

Lomsky, R., Langer, F., Vortel, V.: Immunohistological demonstration of gastrin in mammalian islets of Langerhans. Nature (Lond.) **223**, 618 (1969)

Lu, K.H., Koch, Y., Meites, J.: Direct inhibition by ergocornine of pituitary prolactin release. Endocrinology **89**, 229–233 (1971)

Luft, R., Efendic, S., Hökfelt, T., Johansson, O., Arimura, A.: Immunohistochemical evidence for the localisation of somatostatin-like immunoreactivity in a cell population in the pancreatic islets. Med. Biol. **52**, 428–430 (1974)

Lundquist, I.: Interaction of amines and aminergic blocking agents with blood glucose regulation. I. β-adrenergic blockade. Europ. J. Pharmacol. **18**, 225–235 (1972)

Lutterbeck, P.M., Pryor, S., Varga, L., Wenner, R.: Treatment of non-puerperal galactorrhea with an ergot alkaloid. Brit. med. J. **3**, 228–229 (1971)

McCann, S.M.: Regulation of secretion of follicle-stimulating hormone and luteinizing hormone. In: Handbook of Physiology. Section 7: Endocrinology, Vol. IV, Knobil, E., Sawyer, W.H. (eds.). The Pituitary Gland and Its Neuroendocrine Control, Part 2, pp. 489–518. Washington D.C.: American Physiological Society 1974

MacIndoe, J.H., Turkington, R.W.: Stimulation of human prolactin secretion by intravenous infusion of l-tryptophan. J. clin. Invest. **52**, 1972–1978 (1973)

McKeown, B.A.: Effect of 2-Br-α-Ergocryptine on fresh water survival of the teleosts Xiphophorus hellerii and Poecilia latipinna. Experientia (Basel) **28**, 675–676 (1972)
MacLeod, R.M.: Regulation of prolactin secretion. In: Frontiers in Neuroendocrinology. Martini, L., Ganong, W.F. (eds.). Vol. IV, pp. 169–194. New York: Raven Press 1976
MacLeod, R.M., Krieger, D.T.: Differential effect of ergotamine on ACTH and prolactin secretion. The Endocrine Society 58th Annual Meeting, Abstract No. 317, San Francisco, 1976
MacLeod, R.M., Lehmeyer, J.E.: Regulation of the synthesis and release of prolactin. In: Lactogenic Hormones. Wolstenholme, G.E.W., Knight, J. (eds.). Edinburgh-London: Churchill Livingstone 1972
MacLeod, R.M., Lehmeyer, J.E.: Suppression of pituitary tumor growth and function by ergot alkaloids. Cancer Res. **33**, 849–855 (1973)
MacLeod, R.M., Lehmeyer, J.E.: Studies on the mechanism of the dopamine-mediated inhibition of prolactin secretion. Endocrinology **94**, 1077–1085 (1974a)
MacLeod, R.M., Lehmeyer, J.E.: Restoration of prolactin synthesis and release by the administration of monoaminergic blocking agents to pituitary tumor-bearing rats. Cancer Res. **34**, 345–350 (1974b)
MacLeod, R.M., Kimura, H., Login, I.: Inhibition of prolactin secretion by dopamine and piribedil (ET-495). In: Growth Hormone and Related Peptides. Pecile, A., Müller, E.E. pp. 443–453. Amsterdam: Excerpta Medica 1976
McNatty, K.P., Sawers, R.S., McNeilly, A.S.: A possible role for prolactin in control of steroid secretion by the human graafian follicle. Nature (Lond.) **250**, 653–655 (1974)
McNatty, K.P., Neal, P., Baker, T.G.: Effect of prolactin on the production of progesterone by mouse ovaries in vitro. J. Reprod. Fertil. **47**, 155–156 (1976)
Malaisse, W.J.: Hormonal and environmental modification of islet activity. In: Handbook of Physiology. Endocrine Pancreas. Sec. 7, Vol. I, pp. 237–260. Washington D.C.: Am. Physiol. Soc. 1972
Malaisse, W.J., Malaisse-Legae, F., Wright, P.H., Ashmore, J.: Effects of adrenergic and cholinergic agents upon insulin secretion in vitro. Endocrinology **80**, 975–978 (1967)
Mantle, P.G.: Inhibition of lactation in mice following feeding with ergot sclerotia (*Claviceps fusiformis* (Loveless)) from the bulrush millet (*Pennisetum typhoides* (Staph and Hubbard)) and an alkaloid component. Proc. roy. Soc. B **170**, 423–434 (1968)
Mantle, P.G.: Interruption of early pregnancy in mice by oral administration of agroclavine and sclerotia of *Claviceps fusiformis* (Loveless). J. Reprod. Fertil. **18**, 81–88 (1969)
Mantle, P.G., Finn, C.A.: Investigations on the mode of action of D-6-methyl-8-cyanomethylergoline in suppressing pregnancy in the mouse. J. Reprod. Fertil. **24**, 441–444 (1971)
Marchlewska-Koj, A., Krulich, L.: The role of central monoamines in the stress-induced prolactin releaese in the rat. Fed. Proc. **34**, (Abstr. 191) 252 (1975)
Marco, J., Hedo, J.A., Martinell, J., Calle, C., Villanueva, M.L.: Potentiation of glucagon secretion by serotonin antagonists in man. J. clin. Endocr. **42**, 215–221 (1976)
Markó, M.: Unpublished studies.
Markó, M., Flückiger, E.: Inhibition of spontaneous and induced ovulation in rats by nonsteroidal agents. Experientia (Basel) **30**, 1174–1176 (1974)
Markó, M., Flückiger, E.: Inhibition of ovulation in rats by antagonists to serotonin and by a new tricyclic compound. Experientia (Basel) **32**, 491–492 (1976)
Marliss, E.B., Girardier, L., Seydoux, J., Wollheim, C.B., Kanazawa, Y., Orci, L., Renold, A.E., Porte, D.: Glucagon release induced by pancreatic nerve stimulation in the dog. J. clin. Invest. **52**, 1246–1259 (1973)
Massara, F., Camanni, F., Belforte, L., Molinatti, G.M.: Dopamine-induced inhibition of prolactin and growth hormone secretion in acromegaly. Lancet **1976a I**, 485
Massara, F., Camanni, F., Belforte, L., Molinatti, G.M.: Dopamine and inhibition of prolactin and growth-hormone secretion. Lancet **1976b I**, 913
Matsuo, H., Baba, Y., Nair, R.M.G., Arimura, A., Schally, A.V.: Structure of the porcine LH and FSH-releasing hormone. Biochem. biophys. Res. Commun. **43**, 1334–1339 (1971)
Matthews, E.K., Dean, P.M., Sakamoto, Y.: Biophysical effects of sulphonylureas on islet cells. Proc. 5th Int. Congr. Pharmacology. Vol. III, pp. 221–229, San Francisco 1973
Mayer, P., Schütze, E.: Effect of 2-Br-α-Ergokryptine (CB 154) on lactation in the bitch. Experientia (Basel) **29**, 484–485 (1973)

Meites, J.: Control of prolactin secretion in animals. In: Human Prolactin. Pasteels, J.L., Robyn, C. (eds.), pp. 105–118. Amsterdam: Excerpta Media 1973
Meites, J., Clemens, J.A.: Hypothalamic control of prolactin secretion. Vitam. and Horm. **30**, 165–221 (1972)
Mendelson, W.B., Jacobs, L.S., Reichman, J.D., Othmer, E., Cryer, P.E., Trivedi, B., Daughaday, W.H.: Methysergide. Suppression of sleep-related prolactin secretion and enhancement of sleep-related growth hormone secretion. J. clin. Invest. **56**, 690–697 (1975)
Milligan, J.V., Kraicer, J.: Calcium-45 uptake and potassium-induced release of ACTH from the adenohypophyses. Physiologist (Wash.) **12**, 303 (1969)
Milligan, J.V., Kraicer, J.: Adenohypophysial transmembrane potentials. Polarity reversal by elevated external potassium ion concentration. Science **167**, 182–183 (1970)
Monahan, M., Rivier, J., Burgus, R., Amoss, M., Blackwell, R., Vale, W., Guillemin, R.: Synthèse totale par phase solide d'un décapeptide qui stimule la sécretion des gonadotropines hypophysaires LH et FSH. C.R. Acad. Sci. (Paris) (D) **273**, 508–510 (1971)
Mulloy, A.L., Moberg, G.P.: Effects of P-Chlorophenylalanine and raphe lesions on diurnal prolactin release in the rat. Fed. Proc. **34** (Abstr. 188) 251 (1975)
Müller, E.E.: Nervous control of growth hormone secretion. Neuroendocrinology **11**, 338–369 (1973)
Müller, E.E., Brambilla, F., Cavagnini, F., Peracchi, M., Panerai, A.: Slight effect of L-tryptophan on growth hormone release in normal human subjects. J. clin. Endocr. **39**, 1–5 (1974)
Nader, S., Kjeld, J.M., Blair, C.M., Tooley, M., Gordon, H., Fraser, T.R.: A study of the effect of bromocriptine on serum oestradiol, prolactin, and follicle stimulating hormone levels in puerperal women. Brit. J. Obstet. Gynaec. **82**, 750–754 (1975)
Nagasawa, H., Yanai, R.: Estrous cycle of the mouse with subcutaneous pellet implant of ergocornine and 2-Br-α-ergokryptin. Endocr. jap. **17**, 233–235 (1970)
Nagasawa, H., Yanai, R.: Promotion of pituitary prolactin release in rats by dibutyryl-adenosine 3′, 5′-monophosphate. J. Endocr. **55**, 215–217 (1972)
Nagasawa, H., Yanai, R., Flückiger, E.: Counteraction by 2-Br-α-ergocryptine of pituitary prolactin release promoted by dibutyryl-adenosine-3′, 5′-monophosphate. In: Human Prolactin. Pastells, J.L., Robyn, C. (eds.), pp. 313–315. Amsterdam: Excerpta Medica 1973
Nakai, Y., Imura, H., Sakurai, H., Kurahachi, H., Yoshimi, T.: Effect of cyproheptadine on human growth hormone secretion. J. clin. Endocr. **38**, 446–449 (1974)
Nasr, H., Pearson, O.H.: Inhibition of prolactin secretion by ergot alkaloids. Acta endocr. (Kbh.) **80**, 429–443 (1975)
Neill, J.D.: Prolactin: Its secretion and control. In: Handbook of Physiology. Section 7: Endocrinology, Vol. IV. Knobil, E., Sawyer, W.H. (eds.). The Pituitary Gland and Its Neuroendocrine Control, Part 2, pp. 469–488. Washington D.C.: American Physiological Society 1974
Nicoll, C.S.: Physiological actions of prolactin. In: Handbook of Physiology. Section 7: Endocrinology, Vol. IV. Knobil, E., Sawyer, W.H. (eds.). The Pituitary Gland and Its Neuroendocrine Control, Part 2, pp. 253–292. Washington D.C.: American Physiological Society 1974
Nicoll, C.S., Parsons, J.A., Fiorindo, R.P., Nichols, C.W.: Estimation of prolactin and growth hormone levels by polyacrylamide disc electrophoresis. J. Endocr. **45**, 183–196 (1969)
Nicoll, C.S., Yaron, Z., Nutt, N., Daniels, E.: Effects of ergotamine tartrate on prólactin and growth hormone secretion by rat adenohypophysis in vitro. Biol. Reprod. **5**, 59–66 (1970)
Niswender, G.D.: Influence of 2-Br-α-ergocryptine on serum levels of prolactin and the oestrus cycle in sheep. Endocrinology **94**, 612–615 (1974)
Nooter, K., Zeilmaker, G.H.: Effects of ergocornine and hypothalamic stimulation on ovulation in the rat. J. Endocr. **48**, 64 (1970)
Ølgaard, K., Hagen, C., Madsen, S., Hummer, L.: Aldosterone and prolactin. Lancet **1976 II**, 959

Olivereau, M., Lemoine, A.M.: Effet de la 2-Br-α-ergocryptine (CB 154) sur la sécretion de prolactine chez l'anguille. C.R. Acad. Sci. (Paris) (D) **276**, 1883–1886 (1973)

Parker, G.H.: Animal Colour Changes and Their Neurohumours. Cambridge: Cambridge University Press 1948

Parsons, J.A.: Calcium ion requirement for prolactin secretion by rat adenohypophyses in vitro. Amer. J. Physiol. **217**, 1599–1603 (1969)

Parsons, J.A., Nicoll, C.S.: Mechanism of action of prolactin-inhibiting factor. Neuroendocrinology **8**, 213–227 (1971)

Pasteels, J.L.: Tissue culture of human hypophyses. In: Lactogenic Hormones. Wolstenholme, G.E.W., Knight, J. (eds.), pp. 269–286. Edinburgh-London: Churchill Livingstone 1972

Pasteels, J.L., Brauman, H., Brauman, J.: Etude comparée de la sécrétion de l'hormone somatotrope par l'hypophyse humaine in vitro, et de son activité lactogénique. C.R. Acad. Sci. (Paris) (D) **256**, 2031–2033 (1963)

Pasteels, J.L., Danguy, A., Frérotte, M., Ectors, F.: Inhibition de la sécrétion de prolactine par l'ergocornine et la 2-Br-α-ergocryptine: action directe sur l'hypophyse en culture. Ann. Endocr. (Paris) **32**, 188–192 (1971)

Pauk, G.L., Reddy, W.J.: Glucagon control of liver adenosine 3′5′ monophosphate. Clin. Res. **18**, 74 (1970)

Pelletier, G., Lemay, A., Béraud, G., Labrie, F.: Ultrastructural changes accompanying the stimulatory effect of N^6-monobutyryl-adenosine-3′,5′-monophosphate on the release of growth hormone (GH), prolactin (PRL) and adrenocorticotropic hormone (ACTH) in rat anterior pituitary gland in vitro. Endocrinology **91**, 1355–1371 (1972)

Penny, R.J., Thody, A.J.: Preliminary studies on the control of α-melanocyte-stimulating hormone secretion in the rat. J. Endocr. **69**, 2P–3P (1976)

Perez-Lopez, F.R., Delvoye, P., Denayer, P., L'Hermite, M., Roncero, M.C., Robyn, C.: Effect of methylergobasine maleate on serum gonadotrophin and prolactin in humans. Acta endocr. (Kbh.) **79**, 644–657 (1975)

Piva, F., Sterescu, N., Zanisi, M., Martini, L.: Non-steroidal antifertility agents affecting brain mechanisms. Bull. Wld. Hlth. Org. **41**, 275–288 (1969)

Piva, F., Gagliano, P., Motta, M., Martini, L.: Adrenal progesterone factors controlling its secretion. Endocrinology **93**, 1178–1184 (1973)

Pontiroli, A.E., Viberti, G.C., Tognetti, A., Pozza, G.: Effect of metergoline, a powerful and long acting antiserotininergic agent on insulin secretion in normal subjects and in patients with chemical diabetes. Diabetologia **11**, 165–167 (1975)

Quadri, S.K., Meites, J.: LSD-induced decrease in serum prolactin in rats. Proc. Soc. exp. Biol. (N.Y.) **137**, 1242–1243 (1971)

Quadri, S.K., Meites, J.: Effects of ergocornine and CG 603 on blood prolactin and GH in rats bearing a pituitary tumor. Proc. Soc. exp. Biol. (N.Y.) **142**, 837–841 (1973)

Quadri, S.K., Lu, K.H., Meites, J.: Ergot-induced inhibition of pituitary tumor growth in rats. Science **176**, 417–418 (1972)

Quadri, S.K., Clark, J.L., Meites, J.: Effects of LSD, pargyline, and haloperidol on mammary tumor growth in rats. Proc. Soc. exp. Biol. (N.Y.) **142**, 22–26 (1973)

Quickel, K.E., Feldman, J.M., Lebovitz, H.E.: Enhancement of insulin secretion in adult onset diabetes by methysergide maleate. Diabetes **20** (Suppl. 1), 312 (1971a)

Quickel, K.E., Feldman, J.M., Lebovitz, H.E.: Enhancement of insulin secretion in adult onset diabetes by methysergide maleate. Evidence for an endogenous biogenic monamine mechanism as a factor in the impaired insulin secretion in Diabetes Mellitus. J. clin. Endocr. **33**, 877–881 (1971b)

Rabii, J., Gallo, R.V.: Effect of methysergide, a blocker of serotonin receptors, on plasma prolactin levels in lactating and ovariectomized rats. Fed. Proc. **34**, (Abstr. 190) 252 (1975)

Raj, G.H.M., Greep, R.O.: Inhibition of ovulation and luteinizing hormone secretion in the cyclic rat by ergotamine tartrate. Proc. Soc. exp. Biol. (N.Y.) **144**, 960–962 (1973)

Reyes, F.I., Winter, J.S.D., Faiman, C., Hobson, W.C.: Serial serum levels of gonadotropins, prolactin and sex steroids in the nonpregnant and pregnant chimpanzee. Endocrinology **96**, 1447–1455 (1975)

Řežábek, K., Semonský, M., Kucharczyk, N.: Suppression of conception with D-6-methyl-8-cyanomethylergoline (I) in rats. Nature (Lond.) **221**, 666–667 (1969)

Řežábek, K., Cassady, J.M., Floss, H.G.: Nidation inhibition by simple ergoline derivatives. J. pharm. Sci. **64**, 1045–1046 (1975)

Robyn, C., Vekemans, M., Delvoye, P., Joostens-Defleur, V., Caufriez, A., L'Hermite, M.: Prolactin and fertility control in women. In: Growth Hormone and Related Peptides. Pecile, A., Müller, E.E. (eds.), pp. 396–406. Amsterdam: Excerpta Medica 1976

Rodway, R.G., Kuhn, N.J.: Luteal 20-α-hydroxy steroid dehydrogenase and the formation of Δ^4-3-oxo steroids in the rat after weaning or treatment with 2-Br-α-ergocryptine during lactation. Biochem. J. **152**, 445–448 (1975)

Rolland, R., De Jong, F.H., Schellekens, L.A., Lequin, R.M.: The role of prolactin in the restoration of ovarian function during the early post-partum period in the human female. II. A study during inhibition of lactation by bromergocryptine. Clin. endocr. **4**, 27–38 (1975)

Rothchild, I.: The corpus luteum-pituitary relationship: the association between the cause of luteotrophin secretion and the cause of follicular quiescence during lactation; the basis for a tentative theory of the corpus luteum-pituitary relationship in the rat. Endocrinology **67**, 9–41 (1960)

Rufener, C., Amherdt, M., Dubois, M.P., Orci, L.: Ultrastructure immunocytochemical localisation of somatostatin in D-cells of rat pancreatic monolayer culture. J. Histochem. Cytochem. **23**, 866–869 (1975)

Sachdev, Y., Gomez-Pan, A., Tunbridge, W.M.G., Duns, A., Weightman, D.R., Hall, R., Goolamali, S.K.: Bromocriptine therapy in acromegaly. Lancet **1975II**, 1164

Salzmann, R.C.: Beiträge zur Fortpflanzungsbiologie von Meriones shawi. Rev. suisse Zool. **70**, 346–452 (1963)

Samaan, N.A., Leavens, M.E., Jesse, R.H.: Serum growth hormone and prolactin response to thyrotropin-releasing hormone in patients with acromegaly before and after surgery. J. clin. Endocr. **38**, 957–963 (1974)

Schams, D.: Prolactin release effects of TRH in the bovine and their depression by a prolactin inhibitor. Horm. Metab. Res. **4**, 405 (1972)

Schams, D., Karg, H.: Untersuchungen über Prolaktin im Rinderblut mit einer radioimmunologischen Bestimmungsmethode. Zbl. Vet.-Med. (A) **17**, 193–212 (1970)

Schriefers, H., Wagner, W.: Cholesterol 7α-hydroxylase activity of the rat liver after hypophysectomy and administration of hypophyseal hormones. Experientia (Basel) **32**, 18–19 (1976)

Schriefers, H., Keck, E., Klein, S., Schröder, E.: Die Funktion der Hypophyse und des Hypophysenhormons Prolaktin für die Aufrechterhaltung der Sexualspezifität des Stoffwechsels von Testosteron und 5-α-Dihydrotestosteron in Rattenleberschnitten. Hoppe-Seilers Z. physiol. Chem. **356**, 1535–1543 (1975)

Schulz, K.-D., Geiger, W., Del Pozo, E., Lose, K.H., Künzig, H.J., Lancranjan, I.: The influence of the prolactin-inhibitor bromocriptine (CB 154) on human luteal function in vivo. Arch. Gynäk. **221**, 93–96 (1976)

Šeda, M., Řežábek, K., Marhan, O., Semonský, M.: Stimulation of gonadotrophin secretion with the pregnancy inhibitor D-6-methyl-8-cyanomethylergoline (I). J. Reprod. Fertil. **24**, 263–265 (1971)

Seki, K., Seki, M., Okumura, R.: Serum FSH rise induced by CB 154 (2-br-α-ergocryptine) in postpartum women. J. clin. Endocr. **39**, 184–186 (1974a)

Seki, M., Seki, K., Yoshihara, T., Watanabe, N., Okumura, T., Tajima, C., Huang, S.-Y., Kuo, C.-C.: Direct inhibition of pituitary LH secretion in rats by CB 154 (2-Br-α-ergocryptine). Endocrinology **94**, 911–914 (1974b)

Semonský, M., Kucharczyk, N., Beran, M., Řežábek, K., Šeda, M.: Ergot alakloids XXXVIII: some amides of D-6-methyl-ergolin(I)yl acetic acid. Coll. Czech. chem. Commun. **36**, 2200–2204 (1971)

Serment, H., Ruf, H.: Note á propos de l'utilisation thérapeutique de la méthyl-ergobasine "per os". Sem. Hôp. Paris **31**, 2675–2676 (1955)

Shaar, C.J., Clemens, J.A.: Inhibition of lactation and prolactin secretion in rats by ergot alkaloids. Endocrinology **90**, 285–288 (1972)

Shane, J.M., Naftolin, F.: Effect of ergonovine maleate on puerperal prolactin. Amer. J. Obstet. Gynec. **120**, 129–131 (1974)

Shelesnyak, M.C.: Ergotoxine inhibition of deciduoma formation, and its reversal by progesterone. Amer. J. Physiol. **179**, 301–304 (1954a)
Shelesnyak, M.C.: The action of selected drugs on deciduoma formation. Endocrinology **55**, 85–89 (1954b)
Shelesnyak, M.C.: Some experimental studies on the mechanism of ova-implantation in the rat. Recent Progr. Hormone Res. **13**, 269–317 (1957)
Shelesnyak, M.C.: Action de differents alcaloides de l'ergot sur la formation du déciduome chez les rats en pseudogestation. C.R. Acad. Sci. (Paris) (D) **247**, 2525 (1958)
Shelesnyak, M.C., Lunenfeld, B., Honig, B.: Studies on the mechanism of ergocornine interference with decidualization and nidation. III: Urinary steroids after administration of ergocornine to women. Life Sci. **1**, 73–79 (1963)
Shutt, D.A., Smith, I.D., Shearman, R.P.: Oestrone, oestradiol-17β and oestriol levels in human foetal plasma during gestation and at term. J. Endocr. **60**, 333–341 (1974)
Siler-Khodr, T.M., Morgenstern, L.L., Greenwood, F.C.: Hormone synthesis and release from human fetal adenohypophyses in vitro. J. clin. Endocr. **39**, 891–905 (1974)
Sinha, Y.N., Selby, F.W., Lewis, U.J., van der Laan, W.P.: A homologous radioimmunoassay for human prolactin. J. clin. Endocr. **36**, 509–516 (1973)
Sinha, Y.N., Selby, F.W., Vanderlaan, W.P.: Effects of ergot drugs on prolactin and growth hormone secretion, and on mammary nucleic acid content in C3H/Bi mice. J. nat. Cancer Inst. **52**, 189–191 (1974)
Sirek, A., Sirek, O.V., Niki, A., Niki, H., Przybylska, K.: The effect of dihydroergotamine on growth hormone-induced lipolysis in dogs. Horm. Metab. Res. **1**, 276–281 (1969)
Sirek, A.M., Sirek, O.V., Sirek, A.: The effect of dihydroergotamine on lipolysis stimulated by human chorionic somatomammotropin in hypophysectomized dogs. Horm. Res. **3**, 221–227 (1972)
Sirek, A., Sirek, O.V., Policova, Z.: Dihydroergotamine: A potent amplifier of the insulinogenic effect of sulphonylureas. Diabetes **22**, 328 (1973)
Sirek, A., Sirek, O.V., Policova, Z.: Dihydroergotamine: A potent biological amplifier of sulphonylureas. Diabetologia **10**, 267–270 (1974)
Sirek, O.V., Sirek, A., Policova, Z.: Effects of propranolol and of ergot alkaloids on sulphonylurea-stimulated insulin secretion. Diabetes **24**, 444 (1975a)
Sirek, A.M.T., Sirek, A., Sirek, O.V.: Effects of dihydroergotamine and ergotamine on plasma free fatty acid concentration following a single injection of growth hormone in dogs. The Endocrine Society Bethesda 1975b, Md. Abstract 572, p. 337
Smalstig, E.B., Sawyer, B.D., Clemens, J.A.: Inhibition of rat prolactin release by apomorphine in vivo and in vitro. Endocrinology **95**, 123–129 (1974)
Smith, A.F.: The effect of apomorphine and ergocryptine on the release of MSH by the Pars intermedia of *Rana pipiens*. Neuroendocrinology **19**, 363–376 (1975)
Smith, M.S., Freeman, M.E., Neill, J.D.: The control of progesterone secretion during the estrous cycle and early pseudopregnancy in the rat: Prolactin, gonadotrophin and steroid levels associated with rescue of the corpus luteum of pseudopregnancy. Endocrinology **96**, 219–226 (1975)
Smith, V.G., Beck, T.W., Convey, E.M., Tucker, H.A.: Bovine serum prolactin, growth hormone, cortisol and milk yield after ergocryptine. Neuroendocrinology **15**, 172–181 (1974)
Smythe, G.A., Compton, P.J., Lazarus, L.: Serotoninergic control of human growth hormone secretion: the actions of L-dopa and 2-bromo-α-ergocryptine. In: Growth Hormone and Related Peptides. Pecile, A., Müller, E.E. (eds.), pp. 222–235. Amsterdam: Excerpta Medica 1976
Sólyom, J.: Anterior pituitary and aldosterone secretion. Lancet **1974 I**, 507
Sommer, A.F., Buchanan, A.R.: Effects of ergot alkaloids on pregnancy and lactation in the albino rat. Amer. J. Physiol. **180**, 296–300 (1955)
Stähelin, H., Burckardt-Vischer, B., Flückiger, E.: Rat mammary cancer inhibition by a prolactin suppressor, 2-Bromo-α-ergocryptine (CB 154). Experientia (Basel) **27**, 915–916 (1971)
Steinberger, E., Steinberger, A.: Hormonal control of testicular function in mammals. In: Handbook of Physiology. Section 7: Endocrinology, Vol. IV. Knobil, E., Sawyer W.H. (eds.). The Pituitary Gland and Its Neuroendocrine Control, Part 2, pp. 325–346. Washington D.C.: American Physiological Society 1974

Stricker, P., Grüter, F.: Action du lobe antérieur de l'hypophyse sur la montée laiteuse. C.R. Soc. Biol (Paris) (D) **99**, 1978–1980 (1928)
Sulman, F.G.: Hypothalamic Conrol of Lactation. Berlin-Heidelberg-New York: Springer 1970
Sweeney, M.J., Poore, G.A., Kornfeld, E.C., Bach, N.J., Owen, N.V., Clemens, J.A.: Activity of 6-methyl-8-substituted ergolines against the 7,12-dimethyl-benz[a]anthracene-induced mammary carcinoma. Cancer Res. **36**, 106–109 (1975)
Taleisnik, S., Celis, M.E., Tomatis, M.E.: Release of melanocyte-stimulating hormone by several stimuli through the activation of a 5-hydroxytryptamine-mediated inhibitory neuronal mechanism. Neuroendocrinology **13**, 327–388 (1973/74)
Tashjian, A.H., Barowsky, N.J., Jensen, D.K.: Thyrotropin releasing hormone: direct evidence for stimulation of prolactin production by pituitary cells in culture. Biochem. biophys. Res. Commun. **43**, 516–523 (1971)
Tashjian, A.H., Hoyt, R.F.: Transient control of organ specific functions in pituitary cells in culture. In: Molecular Genetics and Developmental Biology. Sussman, M. (ed.), pp. 353–387. New Jersey: Cliffs 1972
Taylor, J.C., Peaker, M.: Effects of bromocriptine on milk secretion in the rabbit. J. Endocr. **67**, 313–314 (1975)
Thorner, M.O., Chait, A., Aitken, M., Benker, G., Bloom, S.R., Mortimer, C.H., Sanders, P., Stuart Mason, A., Besser, G.M.: Bromocriptine treatment of acromegaly. Brit. med. J. **1**, 299–303 (1975)
Tilders, F.J.H., Mulder, A.H., Smelik, P.G.: On the presence of a MSH-release inhibiting system in the rat neurointermediate lobe. Neuroendocrinology **18**, 125–130 (1975)
Tindal, J.S.: Hypothalamic control of secretion and release of prolactin. J. Reprod. Fertil. **39**, 437–461 (1974)
Tolis, G., Pinter, E.J., Friesen, H.: The acute effect of of 2-bromo-α-ergocryptine (CB-154) on anterior pituitary hormones and free fatty acids in man. Int. J. clin. Pharmacol. **12**, 281–283 (1975)
Turkington, R.W., Underwood, L.E., Van Wyk, J.J.: Elevated serum prolactin levels after pituitary-stalk section in man. New Engl. J. Med. **285**, 707–710 (1971)
Ueda, G., Sato, Y., Yamasaki, T., Shioji, T., Aono, T., Kupachi, K.: Effects of CB 154 (2-Br-α-Ergocryptine) on prolactin and growth hormone release in an acromegalic subject with galactorrhea. Endocr. jap. **22**, 265–268 (1975)
Varga, L., Lutterbeck, P.M., Pryor, J.S., Wenner, R., Erb, H.: Suppression of puerperal lactation with an ergot alkaloid: a double-blind study. Brit. med. J. **2**, 743–744 (1972)
Verde, G., Oppizzi, G., Colussi, G., Cremascoli, G., Botalla, L., Müller, E.E., Silvestrini, F., Chiodini, P.G., Liuzzi, A.: Effect of dopamine infusion on plasma levels of growth hormone in normal subjects and in acromegalic patients. Clin. Endocr. **5**, 419–423 (1976)
Vogel-Chevalier, L., Hammer, W., Flückiger, E.: Influence of dihydroergotamine on the lipolytic system of isolated dog fat cells. Experientia (Basel) **27**, 674–676 (1971)
Weiss, G., Klein, S., Shenkman, L., Kataoka, K., Hollander, C.S.: Effect of methylergonovine on puerperal prolactin secretion. Obstet. Gynecol. **46**, 209–210 (1975)
Welsch, C.W., Gribler, C., Clemens, A.: 6-methyl-8β-ergoline-acetonitrile (MEA)-induced suppression of mammary tumorigenesis in C3H/HeJ female mice. Europ. J. Cancer **10**, 595–600 (1974)
Wilson, C.A.: Hypothalamic amines and the release of gonadotropins and other anterior pituitary hormones. In: Advances in Drug Research. Harper, N.J., Simmonds, A.B. (eds.), Vol. VIII, pp. 120–204. London-New York: Academic Press 1974
Witorsch, R.J., Kitay, J.I.: Pituitary hormones affecting adrenal 5α-reductase activity: ACTH, growth hormone and prolactin. Endocrinology **91**, 764–769 (1972)
Woods, S.C., Porte, D.: Neural control of the endocrine pancreas. Physiol. Rev. **54**, 596–619 (1974)
Wuttke, W., Döhler, K.D.: Partial and total blockade of ergocornine on serum prolactin release in rats. Effects on pregnancy and serum progesterone. In: Human Prolactin. Pasteels, J.L., Robyn, C. (eds.), pp. 156–159. Amsterdam: Excerpta Medica 1973
Wuttke, W., Meites, J.: Luteolytic role of prolactin during the estrous cycle of the rat. Proc. Soc. exp. Biol. (N.Y.) **137**, 988–991 (1971)

Wuttke, W., Cassell, E., Meites, J.: Effects of ergocornine on serum prolactin and LH, and on hypothalamic content of PIF and LRF. Endocrinology **88**, 737–741 (1971)
Yanai, R., Nagasawa, H.: Quantitative analysis of prolactin by disc electrophoresis and its relation to biological activity. Proc. Soc. exp. Biol. (N.Y.) **131**, 167–171 (1969)
Yanai, R., Nagasawa, H.: Suppression of mammary hyperplastic nodule formation and pituitary prolactin secretion in mice induced by ergocornine and 2-Br-α-ergocryptine. J. nat. Cancer Inst. **45**, 1105–1112 (1970a)
Yanai, R., Nagasawa, H.: Effects of ergocornine and 2-Br-α-ergocryptine (CB 154) on the formation of mammary hyperplastic alveolar nodules and the pituitary prolactin levels in mice. Experientia (Basel) **26**, 649–650 (1970b)
Yanai, R., Nagasawa, H.: Effect of 2-Br-α-ergocryptine on pituitary synthesis and release of prolactin and growth hormone in rats. Horm. Res. **5**, 1–5 (1974)
Yokoyama, A., Tomogane, H., Ôta, K.: Ergocornine blockade of the surge of prolactin at proestrus failed to block ovulation in cycling rats. Proc. Soc. exp. Biol. (N.Y.) **140**, 169–171 (1972)
Yoshinaga, K., Hawkins, R.A., Stocker, J.F.: Estrogen secretion by the rat ovary in vivo during the estrous cycle and pregnancy. Endocrinology **85**, 103–112 (1969)
Zeilmaker, G.H.: Experimentele Onderzoekingen Over Het Eerste Stadium van de Zwangerschap bij de Rat. Amsterdam: Academisch Proefschrift 1964
Zeilmaker, G.H.: Effect of ergocornine methanesulfonate on the luteotrophic activity of the ectopic mouse trophoblast. Acta endocr. (Kbh.) **59**, 442–446 (1968)
Zeilmaker, G.H., Carlsen, R.A.: Experimental studies on the effect of ergocornine methanesulfonate on the luteotrophic function of the rat pituitary gland. Acta endocr. (Kbh.) **41**, 321 (1962)
Zikan, V., Semonský, M., Řežábek, K., Aušková, M., Šeda, M.: Ergot alkaloids. XL. Some N-(D-6-methyl-8-isoergolin-I-yl) and N-(D-6-methyl-8-isoergolin-II-yl)-N′-substituted ureas. Coll. Czech. chem. Commun. **37**, 2600–2605 (1972)
Zikan, V., Řežábek, J., Semonský, M.: Synthesis of 1,1-diethyl-4-(D-6-methyl-8-ergolin-I-yl) semicarbazide and its isoergolin-I-yl and isoergolin-II-yl isomers. Coll. Czech. chem. Commun. **39**, 3144–3146 (1974)
Zor, U., Kaneko, T., Schneider, H.P.G., McCann, S.M., Field, J.B.: Further studies of stimulation of anterior pituitary cyclic adenosine-3′, 5′-monophosphate formation by hypothalamic extracts and prostaglandins. J. biol. Chem. **245**, 2883–2888 (1970)

CHAPTER X

Metabolic Effects

H. WAGNER

A. Introduction

A chapter about metabolic effects is difficult to write because of the comprehensive textbook definitions of the term metabolism, such as "the numerous chemical processes which occur within the living organisms are encompassed in the term metabolism" (WHITE et al., 1959) or intermediary metabolism: "it includes all chemical processes within cells and tissues that are concerned with either building

Table 1. Concentration of ergot alkaloids used in vitro tests to influence metabolic parameters

Author	Concentr. range molar	Drug	Organ/enzyme	Species
VOGEL-CHEVALIER et al. (1971)	10^{-8}–10^{-7}	DHE	Adipocytes	Dog
MARKSTEIN and WAGNER (1975)	10^{-8}–10^{-6}	Dihydro-ergotoxine	Cerebral cortex slices	Rat
IWANGOFF et al. (1973b)	10^{-7}–10^{-4}	Dihydroergot-derivatives	Brain, ATPase	Cat
HOTTA et al. (1970)	8×10^{-6}	DHE	Adipocytes	Rat
HOTTA et al. (1971a, c)	8.6×10^{-6}	DHE	Adipocytes	Rat
KOWADLO-SILBERGELD et al. (1972)	1.2×10^{-5}	DHE	Adipocytes	Rat
KOWADLO-SILBERGELD et al. (1973)	1.35×10^{-5}	DHE	Adipocytes	Rat
NAKANO et al. (1969)	10^{-5}–10^{-4}	DHE	Adipocytes	Rat
IWANGOFF and ENZ (1972)	10^{-5}–10^{-4}	Dihydro-ergocristine	Brain, PDE	Cat
WARD and FAIN (1971)	2×10^{-5}–10^{-4}	DHE	Adipocytes	Rat
FAIN (1970)	1–2.3×10^{-4}	DHE	Adipocytes	Rat, rabbit
IWANGOFF and ENZ (1973a)	10^{-5}–10^{-3}	Dihydro-ergotoxine	Brain, heart	Cat
		DHE	PDE	
MOSKOWITZ and FAIN (1970)	10^{-4}	DHE	Adipocytes	Rat
WEINRYB et al. (1972)	10^{-4}	Methysergide	Heart, brain PDE	Cat, rat
BERTHET et al. (1957)	1.72×10^{-4}	Ergotamine	Liver homogenate phosphorylase	Dog
CARLSÖÖ et al. (1975)	2×10^{-4}	BOL 148	Submandibular gland secretion of peroxydase and amylase	Guinea-pig

up and breaking down and their functional operation" (WEST et al., 1966), or: "intermediary metabolism which is concerned with specific chemical reactions occurring in the body" (BEST and TAYLOR, 1966). The application of these definitions to this review would also cover the biochemical mechanisms underlying the pharmacologic actions of ergot alkaloids. For this reason, more importance will be given to classical biochemical items like carbohydrate, lipid-, and protein-metabolism. Metabolic actions on the heart and the nervous system are discussed in detail in Chapters V and VI. For review articles, the reader should refer to BARGER (1938), NICKERSON (1949, 1959), SUTHERLAND and ROBISON (1966), HIMMS-HAGEN (1967, 1972), LUNDHOLM et al. (1968), HORNBROOK (1970), FAIN (1973), and BRADLEY and BRIGGS (1974).

The effect of ergot alkaloids on adrenoceptors concerned with metabolic reactions, the closely related adenyl cyclase and cAMP, in connection with the actions of catecholamines will be discussed in relation to the second-messenger concept of SUTHERLAND et al. (1965). In addition to the action of ergot alkaloids on the sympathetic-controlled mobilization of glucose and lipids, these drugs have direct actions on other enzymes.

There is controversy in the literature concerning some of the metabolic effects of ergot alkaloids. One of the reasons for this could be the dose ranges used by the different investigators in in vitro experiments. Some effects were observed with low (10^{-8}–10^{-6}M) and some with much higher (10^{-5}–10^{-3}M) concentrations (Table 1). One could argue that effects obtained with lower concentrations may possibly be of more relevance for the therapeutic applications. Peptide ergot alkaloids are given to man in a dose range of 0.5–5 mg per day. An equal distribution assumed, one can calculate a concentration in the tissues of 10^{-8}–10^{-7}M. However, the effective concentrations at the different receptor sites are not known.

B. In vitro Systems

1. Liver

There are many studies concerning the action of catecholamines and antagonists—mainly glycogenolysis—on liver metabolism. Most studies have been performed in intact animals; only little has been done in vitro using the perfused liver preparation, liver slices, or homogenates. For drug receptor-interaction experiments, the intact animal does not give clear results, because many factors, including insulin, glucagon, glucocorticoids, and oxygen supply, influence liver carbohydrate and fat metabolism measured as plasma glucose or free fatty acid concentration. The secretion of insulin and glucagon is partially controlled sympathetic, as discussed by PORTE and ROBERTSON (1973), ROBERTSON and PORTE (1973), and IVERSEN (1973). But changes in plasma glucose or free fatty acid concentration can also occur by glucose uptake into muscle and fat tissue or by release of fatty acids from adipose tissue under control of hormones like insulin and adrenaline.

a) Isolated Perfused Liver

SHERLINE et al. (1972) investigated the action of different catecholamines, phentolamine, and propranolol on activity of liver phosphorylase, cAMP concentration, and glucose output in the isolated perfused rat liver. Adrenaline (10^{-7}M) increased the glucose output from control values of −3 to over 40 mg/liver during 15 min. This could be blocked completely by phentolamine (10^{-4} M) but not by propranolol (10^{-4} M). Isoproterenol stimulated only liver phosphorylase at 10^{-3} M, an effect which could also be explained by an impurity of 0.1% noradrenaline in the isoproterenol used. The effects of noradrenaline on phosphorylase could be blocked by phentolamine and propranolol. cAMP levels rose in the liver and the perfusate following adrenaline. Phentolamine potentiated while propranolol inhibited this effect. Isoproterenol caused a greater maximal elevation of cAMP than phenylephrine. The authors suggested the occurrence of α- and β-receptors in the rat liver.

NORTHROP (1968), using the perfused guinea-pig liver, found a stimulation of glucose output by adrenaline or cAMP. Dihydroergotamine (DHE) inhibited both responses, but dichloroisoproterenol only blocked the adrenaline effect. The dose of 0.8 mg/liver is rather high, giving a calculated concentration of DHE (assuming a 100% uptake and an equal distribution) of approximately 10^{-4} M. The authors claim an effect of DHE following the stage of cAMP formation. It could well be that DHE blocks one or several of the enzymes concerned with glycogenolysis. Pretreatment of donor rats with adrenaline (1 mg/kg) resulted in an uptake of glucose and α-aminoisobutyric acid (AIB) from the liver perfusate, which was diminished by 1 mg/kg DHE. DHE also reduced the effect on glucagon-stimulated AIB uptake in vitro, which when added in a dose of 300 μg also gives a rather high concentration, $\sim 4 \times 10^{-5}$ M in the liver, calculated as above. This dose did not influence glucagon-stimulated glucose release. But a dose of 900 μg inhibited glycogenolysis induced by (2 mg) cAMP, which is in agreement with the assumption that the interaction of DHE with the liver glycogenolytic system occurs after the stage of adenyl cyclase formation. The action on the AIB uptake could be explained by direct interaction of DHE with the liver cell membrane (CHAMBERS et al., 1968, 1970).

b) Liver Slices

HAYLETT and JENKINSON (1972) demonstrated the existence of α- and β-receptors concerned with glucose release, stimulated respectively by amidephrine (5×10^{-6} M) and isoproterenol (10^{-8} M) in guinea-pig liver slices. The isoproterenol effect was inhibited by propranolol (10^{-6} M) but not by phentolamine (10^{-5} M), whereas the converse held for amidephrine. CHAN and ELLIS (1969) found a shift of the adrenaline dose-response curve for glucose release in rabbit liver slices by 3×10^{-5} M DHE and a corresponding pA_2 value of 6.05. At a concentration 3×10^{-5} M DHE, the response was noncompetitive, suggesting nonspecific interaction of DHE with this system. In rabbit liver slices, DHE blocked the glucose release induced by adrenaline and $CaCl_2$ but did not inhibit the effect of glucagon (ELLIS et al., 1952, 1953).

c) Isolated Liver Cells

EXTON and HARPER (1975) showed that in the perfused rat liver and also in isolated rat liver parenchymal cells, there exist α-adrenoceptors mediating glycogenolysis and gluconeogenesis without influencing cAMP levels. The glycogenolytic actions of adrenaline, noradrenaline, and phenylephrine were inhibited by α-blockers such as phentolamine and dihydroergotamine. There are also β-receptors in rat livers, stimulated by isoproterenol and inhibited by propranolol, effecting increase in cAMP with little influence on carbohydrate metabolism. In the rat, contrary to other species, carbohydrate metabolism in the liver is governed by an α-adrenergic mechanism.

d) Liver Homogenate

BERTHET et al. (1957) used the supernatant of 900 g centrifugation of dog liver homogenate for detecting the effects of adrenaline and glucagon on liver phosphorylase. Cat liver homogenate could also be used but not homogenates from livers of rabbits and rats which did not respond to glucagon and adrenaline. Ergotamine (1.5×10^{-4} M) inhibited the increase of phosphorylase formation due to adrenaline in dog liver but had no effect on the similar action of glucagon (0.04–1 μg/ml). Inhibition of phosphodiesterase by caffeine (10^{-3} M) resulted in a potentiation of the glucagon effect.

MURAD et al. (1962) showed inhibition of adrenaline-stimulated adenyl cyclase in particles of dog liver and heart by ergotamine ($IC_{50} = 3 \times 10^{-5}$ M), but for the dichloroisoproterenol effect in heart particles IC_{50} was 6×10^{-7} M. In a particulate cat liver preparation, MAKMAN and SUTHERLAND (1964), found that neither ergotamine (1.8×10^{-4} M) nor dichloroisoproterenol influenced the response of adenyl cyclase due to glucagon.

2. Adipose Tissue

Ever since WINEGARD and RENOLD (1958) reported that pieces of epididymal rat adipose tissue can be used for studying the influence of insulin on carbohydrate and fat metabolism, and RODBELL (1964) employed isolated fat cells obtained by collagenase treatment for investigating the effects of hormones on glucose metabolism and lipolysis, a wonderful tool for research in this field has been created. The fat tissue has the advantage of consuming only 1/100 of oxygen compared to the liver (ALTMAN and DITTMER, 1968). This means that fat cells can be handled without danger of damage due to oxygen deficiency. A great number of biologically active substances have been tested in this system, ergot alkaloids among them. Lipolysis in adipose tissue is stimulated by a variety of hormones, including catecholamines, ACTH, MSH, TSH, glucagon, GH, and glucocorticoids (RUDMAN, 1963; FAIN et al., 1965; STEINBERG et al., 1959; WHITE and ENGEL, 1958). The lipolytic action of these hormones can be antagonized by a variety of agents, including insulin, the prostaglandins, nicotinic acid, and adrenoceptor blocking agents (TCHERKES and ROSENFELD, 1941; CUATRECASAS, 1971; STEINBERG et al., 1963; MOSINGER, 1965). Most of the activating hormones stimulate adenyl cyclase according to the second-messenger concept of SUTHERLAND and ROBISON (1969). Catecholamine binds to the β-receptor on the surface of the cell, which leads to activation of adenyl cyclase bound to the cytoplasmic membrane part. Adenyl cyclase catalyzes the conversion of ATP to cAMP. The latter activates protein kinase, which promotes the phosphorylation of inactive lipase to the active triglyceride hydrolysing

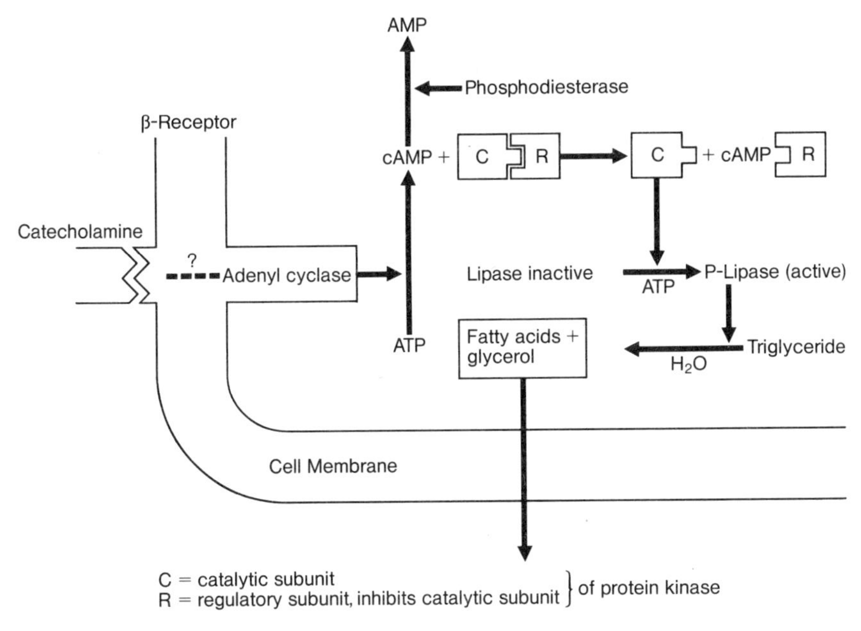

Fig. 1

enzyme (HUTTUNEN et al., 1970) (Fig. 1). Protein kinase is a key regulatory enzyme, which through phosphorylation activates many enzymes, including phosphorylase kinase (WALSH et al., 1968), glycogen synthetase (SODERLING et al., 1970), and influences membrane permeability (JOHNSON et al., 1972) and leads to membrane hyperpolarization (MCAFEE and GREENGARD, 1972).

Much less is known about α-receptors. They occur in human but not in rat fat cells; they have an inhibitory effect on lipolysis and are blocked by phentolamine (BURNS and LANGLEY, 1970; ROBISON et al., 1972).

a) Intact Adipose Tissue

Isolated tissue or perfused isolated tissue has been used to investigate sympathetic neuronal control of lipolysis. WEISS and MAICKEL (1968) electrically stimulated rat epididymal fat pads with intact innervation and showed a lipolytic response, which could be inhibited by the β-blocking agent DCB[1] and enhanced by atropine and theophylline. Pretreatment of the rats with dibenamine, ergotamine, and bretylium antagonized the lipolytic response elicited by nervous stimulation. Nerve stimulation of perfused segments of dog mesenteric adipose tissue leads to a release of glycerol and free fatty acids, which is not influenced by dihydroergotamine (BALLARD and ROSELL, 1968). FREDHOLM and ROSELL (1968, 1970) showed that electrical stimulation of the nerve supply of perfused canine subcutaneous adipose tissue leads to an increased vascular resistance and retention of glycerol, free fatty

[1] [1-(2′,4′-dichlorophenyl)-1-hydroxy-2-(t-butylamino) ethane HCl]

acids and also of noradrenaline and its metabolites. Stopping stimulation normalized resistance and led to an overshoot of the metabolites. Dihydroergotamine inhibited the vascular response and the inhibiting effect on glycerol, free fatty acid, and metabolite release during nerve stimulation. Working with perfused omental adipose tissue, BALLARD and ROSELL (1971) found inhibition of nerve-stimulated glycerol release by propranolol (100 μg i.a.) but not by dihydroergotamine. ROSELL and BELFRAGE (1975) postulate that dihydroergotoxine-mesylate[2] (120–150 μg i.a.) inhibits only the vascular α-receptors in canine subcutaneous adipose tissue but has no influence on lipolysis.

b) Adipose Tissue Slices and Isolated Fat Cells

The influence of α- and β-blockers on lipolysis of rat adipose tissue is known from the publications of SCHOTZ and PAGE (1960), WENKE et al. (1962), LOVE et al. (1963), and SALVADOR et al. (1964). BROOKER and CALVERT (1967) first reported the inhibitory effect of dihydroergotamine on noradrenaline, adrenaline, or isoproterenol-stimulated epididymal fat pads of the rat. In this system DHE is a more active blocker than phentolamine, but rather high concentrations (10^{-4}–10^{-5} M) are needed for a definite blocking activity compared with the pA_2 values of modern β-blockers, such as propranolol of 7.2 and pindolol of 7.4 (own unpublished observations). Using isolated rat fat cells, NAKANO et al. (1969) and ISHII (1969) found that the inhibition of the noradrenaline-induced lipolysis by dihydroergotamine is a non competitive one. This means that DHE probably does not react with the β-adrenergic receptor site. They also showed a competitive inhibition of DHE of the dibutyryl-cAMP stimulated lipolysis with a K_i value of 4.7×10^{-5} M, which is also a rather high concentration. Using even higher concentrations of DHE, FAIN (1970) obtained a potentiation of the dibutyryl-cAMP effect in rat fat cells, which he explained by phosphodiesterase inhibition, because the lipolytic effect of theophylline was also potentiated. But NAKANO and OLIVER (1970a, b) again demonstrated the inhibiting action of 10^{-4}M DHE on noradrenaline-stimulated lipolysis of rat fat cells. WARD and FAIN (1971) investigated the inhibitory effect of DHE on rat white and brown adipose tissue phosphodiesterase in more detail and found a mixed competitive–noncompetitive type. From this, an apparent K_i of ~10^{-4}M can be calculated. They could also show an inhibition of fat cell ghost adenyl cyclase by DHE with an IC_{50} value of 2.7×10^{-5}M. VOGEL-CHEVALIER et al. (1971) stimulated dog adipocytes with noradrenaline ($pD_2 = 7.3$) and DHE ($pD_2 = 7.5$) with the same efficacy. The lipolytic effect of noradrenaline could be inhibited by low concentrations of propranolol, but the lipolytic effect of DHE required 100 times higher concentrations. In the dog fat cell DHE seems to react with a receptor which is not the β-adrenoceptor. Even with 10^{-5}M DHE, adipose tissue phosphodiesterase was not blocked. BURNS and LANGLEY (1970) found that human fat cells contained both β- and α-adrenoceptors, but the maximal lipolysis obtainable in human fat cells was only a fraction of that in rat fat cells. The maximal lipolysis with isoproterenol (μmol glycerol/ml/h) found by these authors was 0.3 in human tissue and 1.4 in rat tissue. They found

[2] Containing equal parts of dihydrogenated ergocristine, ergocornine and ergokryptine = Hydergine.

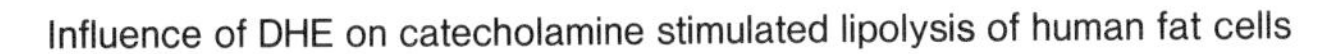

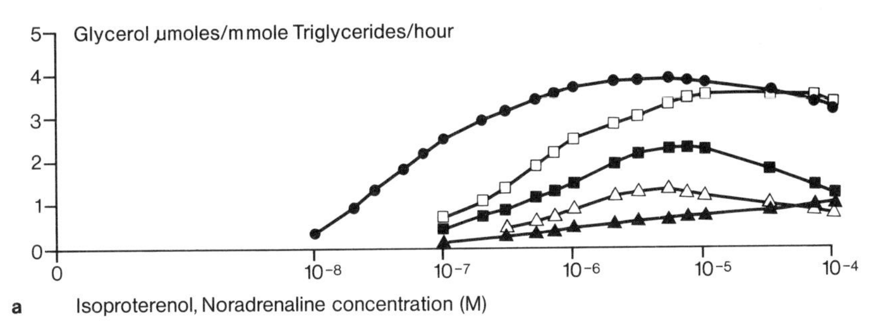

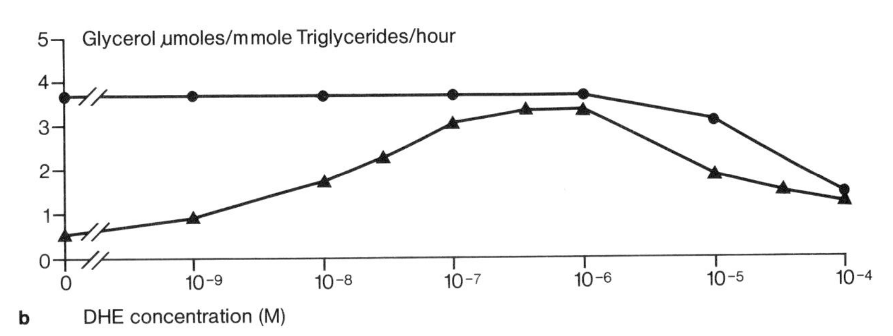

Fig. 2. (a) Typical dose-response curves for catecholamine stimulated lipolysis of human fat cells. Influence of DHE on the noradrenaline effect. Isoproterenol ●, noradrenaline ▲, noradrenaline+DHE 3×10^{-8} M ■, noradrenaline+DHE 10^{-7} M □, noradrenaline+DHE 10^{-4} M △. Basal lipolysis 0.5 µmoles/mmole triglycerides/h was subtracted. Fat cells were isolated by the method of RODBELL (1964), modified so that the medium used for the digestion of the tissue did not contain glucose. The isolated fat cells were incubated for 2 h in a Krebs-Ringer phosphate buffer pH 7.4 with 4% albumin. Glycerol production was measured according to LAURELL and TIBBLING (1966), triglycerides with the method of EGGSTEIN and KREUTZ (1966), modified by Biochemica Test Combination from Boehringer. (b) The effect of DHE on lipolysis induced by 3×10^{-6} M noradrenaline ▲ and 10^{-6} M isoproternol ● (MILAVEC and WAGNER, in preparation)

that isoproterenol produced a higher ceiling effect (higher efficacy) in stimulating lipolysis in human fat cells than adrenaline or noradrenaline. Addition of the α-blocker phentolamine (10^{-5}M) raised the lipolytic response to adrenaline, bringing it to the level of the response to isoproterenol. MILAVEC and WAGNER (in preparation) also found a lower ceiling effect in human fat cells with noradrenaline than with isoproterenol. Addition of dihydroergotamine in concentrations of 10^{-9}–10^{-6}M raised the maximum response to noradrenaline, progressively bringing it to the level of isoproterenol. If even higher concentrations of dihydroergotamine were used, lipolytic responses to both isoproterenol and noradrenaline were depressed noncompetitively (Fig. 2a). DHE alone had no effect on lipolysis.

These results suggest that in human fat cells, stimulation of α-adrenoceptors depresses lipolysis, while α-blockers (phentolamine, dihydroergotamine) stimulate it. The effect of dihydroergotamine on lipolysis of human fat cells is unlikely to be due to phosphodiesterase inhibition, which is maximal at 10^{-5}–10^{-4}M DHE, while the potentiating effect on lipolysis by noradrenaline is reduced at these concentrations (Fig. 2b).

Growth hormone (0.75 μg/ml)+dexamethasone (0.016 μg/ml) stimulated lipolysis in rat white fat cells (MOSKOWITZ and FAIN, 1970), which could be potentiated by DHE (8.6×10^{-6}M) (HOTTA et al., 1970, 1971c). Lipolysis was inhibited by β-hydroxybutyrate (HOTTA et al., 1971a). In the same test system, HOTTA et al. (1971b) investigated the lipolytic effect of DHE and found the maximal lipolysis was five times lower than that of adrenaline. The lipolytic effect of DHE (8.6×10^{-6}M) was increased by theophylline (10^{-5}M) and suppressed by propranolol (6×10^{-6}M), Kö 592 (9×10^{-6}M), phentolamine (2×10^{-5}M), and insulin 25 μU/ml. Adrenaline-induced lipolysis was blocked by DHE (4×10^{-5}M) but not the lipolytic effect caused by ACTH, TSH, and glucagon. KOWADLO-SILBERGELD et al. (1972) confirmed the potentiation of the lipolytic action of growth hormone+dexamethasone by DHE (~ 10^{-5} M) and showed that DHE was even more potent using a pepsin-digested growth hormone fraction. DHE (10^{-5} M) also shifted the dose-response curve of ACTH in rat adipocyte lipolysis to the left (KOWADLO-SILBERGELD et al., 1973). The lipolytic activity in rat adipocytes of β-lipotropin, a pituitary hormone related chemically to ACTH and MSH (LI et al., 1965), was clearly potentiated by dexamethasone (0.02 μg/ml)+DHE (~10^{-5} M) (KOWADLO-SILBERGELD and LARON, 1974). The stimulation of peptide hormone action on lipolysis by DHE is difficult to interprete, because only one dose was used, precluding any assessment of efficacy, affinity, and competitive—noncompetitive antagonism.

3. Various Tissues

Ergotamine and ergotoxine stimulated the transfer of hydrogen to methylene blue in minced frog skeletal muscle in low concentrations ~10^{-9}–10^{-10} M but inhibited the same effect of adrenaline (VON EULER, 1929). HEGNAUER and CORI (1934), using matched frog muscle, showed that adrenaline 5×10^{-8} M–5×10^{-5} M caused an increase in lactate and hexosemonophosphate under aerobic and anaerobic conditions. Ergotamine (1.5–3×10^{-5} M) had no influence on this action of adrenaline. CHAN and ELLENBOGEN in 1974 clearly demonstrated the existence of β-adrenergic receptors on particulate frog erythrocyte adenyl cyclase preparations. Stimulation with isoproterenol was competitively inhibited by propranolol (5×10^{-6} M), noncompetitively by DHE (5×10^{-5}–5×10^{-4} M), and not at all by phentolamine. The noncompetitive action of DHE may indicate that this substance is not a β-adrenoceptor blocking agent but has some influence in higher concentrations on post receptor events. Very high concentrations of LSD (10^{-3} M) inhibited the uptake of phenylalanine by slices of guinea-pig intestine (SEPULVEDA and ROBINSON, 1975). VACCARI et al. (1971) studied the uptake of ^{45}Ca in isolated rat fundal strips. Ca transport and contractions produced by dopamine and serotonin were inhibited by LSD (1.5×10^{-5} M). Using the isolated guinea-pig ileum, BANERJEE (1972) did not find any effect of LSD (10^{-5} M) on ^{45}Ca uptake.

C. Intact Animals and Men

There are many reports about the action of ergot alkaloids on metabolism in intact organisms. MICULICICH (1912) first showed the antagonistic effect of "ergotoxine" on adrenaline-stimulated glycosuria in rabbits, which he explained in terms of the theory of DALE (1906), who first described the action of ergot alkaloids as sympathetic antagonists. The explanation of these and other results, even with the help of modern biochemical and pharmacologic knowledge, is difficult because of the numerous metabolic effects elicited by catecholamines, which comprise direct actions on α- or β-receptors and indirect ones like control of hormone release or vascular changes. Experimental conditions, such as species, the ergot substances used, dose, way of application, and main effects are summarized in Table 2. The lowest metabolically effective i.v. doses in man are of the order of 0.01 mg/kg, but in animals parenteral doses up to 50 mg/kg have been used.

1. Influence on Catecholamine-Stimulated Carbohydrate Mobilization

The first hint of a connection between adrenaline-stimulated metabolism and ergot alkaloids came from MICULICICH (1912) and MORITA (1915), using a mixture of different ergot alkaloids which they called ergotoxine but which were chemically not identical with todays ergotoxine[3]. They used the rabbit as an experimental animal and showed that ergotoxine inhibited the glucosuria provoked by adrenaline (MICULICICH) and adrenaline analogues (MORITA). More than 10 years after STOLL (1920) described the isolation and characterization of ergotamine as a pure chemical entity, NITZESCU and MUNTEANU (1932) in the rabbit and GOLDBLATT (1933a, b) in the rabbit and the cat, demonstrated the inhibitory action of ergotamine on adrenaline-stimulated hyperglycemia but not on lactacidemia. Later MAYER et al. (1961) confirmed this also for the dog. In the rabbit, insulin hypoglycemia was potentiated by ergotamine. In the light of present knowledge, these effects can now be explained by an α-blocking action of the high doses (1–6 mg/kg i.v.) of ergotamine used in causing hypoglycemia. The adrenaline-induced hyperglycemia could arise through β-adrenergic stimulation of muscle glycogenolysis (ARNOLD and SELBERIS, 1968) via hyperprolactacidemia, gluconeogenesis, and α-receptor stimulated inhibition of insulin secretion (PORTE, 1967). Alpha-receptor blockade would then stimulate insulin release and lower blood glucose levels but not influence β-receptor-controlled lactacidemia. The inhibition of adrenaline hyperglycemia in the rabbit applies to ergocristine, ergocornine, ergokryptine, dihydroergotamine, dihydroergocornine, dihydroergokryptine, and dihydroergocristine, as ROTHLIN (1947) showed. But this could not be confirmed by SPITZER (1968) after infusing ergotamine. After giving s.c. dose 0.15 mg/kg of different ergot alkaloids to rabbits, the inhibition of the adrenaline hyperglycemic effect was between 32 and 92%. This was confirmed for DHE in the rabbit by WRIGHT et al. (1958), in the rat by ELLIS and ANDERSON (1950), KENNEDY and ELLIS (1963), NORTHROP and PARKS (1964), KENNEDY and ELLIS (1969a), ADNITT (1969), and for ergotamine, dihydroergocornine, and ergocornine by HARVEY et al. (1952) and also for dopamine and

[3] Ergotoxine contains equal parts of ergocristine, ergocornine and, ergokryptine.

Table 2. Synopsis of in vivo effects of ergot alkaloids on metabolic parameters

Author	Year	Species	Substance	Doses[a] mg/kg	Way	Effect of ergot substance
Miculicich	1912	Rabbit	"Ergotoxine"	0.3–3	s.c.	Inhibition of adrenaline (1 mg/kg s.c.) glucosuria
Morita	1915	Rabbit	"Ergotoxine"	1–3	s.c.	Inhibition of glucosuria evoqued by side chain analogues of adrenaline
Lesser and Zipf	1923	Rabbit	Ergotamine	3–19	s.c.	Short hypoglycemia (–14%)
Hetenyi and Pogany	1926	Man	Ergotamine	0.004–0.007	s.c.	Inhibition of postprandial glucose hyperglycemia
Grunke	1926	Man	Ergotamine	0.005–0.007	i.v.	Inhibition of postprandial glucose hyperglycemia
Nitzescu and Munteanu	1932	Rabbit	Ergotamine	2–2.5	i.v.	Inhibition of adrenaline (0.2 mg/kg s.c.) induced glycemia. No influence on lactacidemia
Orestano	1933a, b	Rat	Ergotamine	3	s.c.	Lowered basal metabolic rate
				0.1–1	s.c.	Inhibited adrenaline and pilocarpine induced metabolism
Goldblatt	1933a	Cat	Ergotamine	1.1–2.8	i.v.	Adrenaline (1 mg/kg s.c. induced hyperglycemia partially, lactacidemia not inhibited
Goldblatt	1933b	Rabbit	Ergotamine	4.2–6.3	i.v.	Insulin hypoglycemia potentiated, adrenaline hypoglycemia inhibited
Issekutz and Harangozo-Oroszy	1942	Rat	Ergotamine	1.5–3	s.c.	No influence on oxygen consumption induced by adrenaline
Spühler	1947	Man	DHE	0.007–0.028	i.v.	Lowers fasting blood glucose, inhibits adrenaline hyperglycemia and glucose absorption (only p.o. glucose is inhibited
Rothlin	1947	Rabbit	Ergotamine	0.15	s.c.	These substances inhibited adrenaline (0.15 mg/kg) stimulated hyperglycemia in the range of 32–92%
Rothlin	1947	Rabbit	Ergocristine	0.15	s.c.	
Rothlin	1947	Rabbit	Ergocornine	0.15	s.c.	
Rothlin	1947	Rabbit	Ergokryptine	0.15	s.c.	
Rothlin	1947	Rabbit	DHE	0.15	s.c.	
Rothlin	1947	Rabbit	Dihydro-ergocornine	0.15	s.c.	
Rothlin	1947	Rabbit	Dihydro-ergokryptine	0.15	s.c.	
Rothlin	1947	Rabbit	Dihydro-ergocristine	0.15	s.c.	
Freis et al.	1948	Man	Dihydro-ergokryptine	0.014	i.v.	Suppressed the hyperglycemic effect of 0.0036 mg/kg adrenaline i.m.

ISSEKUTZ and GYERMEK	1949	Rat	Dihydro-ergotamine	4–6	s.c.	Inhibition of amphetamine induced O_2-consumption
			Dihydro-ergocornine	1–6	s.c.	Inhibition of amphetamine induced O_2-consumption
LINDNER and BRAUNER	1950	Rat	DHE	2	s.c.	Partially inhibited the adrenaline (2 mg/kg s.c.) induced metabolic rate. DHE alone slightly increases, dihydroergocornine slightly decreases metabolic rate
			Dihydro-ergocornine	2	s.c.	
			Ergotamine	2	s.c.	
			Methergine	2	s.c.	
ELLIS and ANDERSON	1950	Rat	DHE	3	i.p.	Inhibited adrenaline (0.1 mg/kg i.p.) hyperglycemia
PETRIDES and SCHÄFER	1950	Man	Dihydro-ergotoxine	0.004	i.v.	Improved p.o. glucose balance in patients with high sympathetic tone
HARVEY et al.	1952	Cat	Ergotamine	0.3 (ED_{50})	i.v.	Inhibition of hyperglycemia produced by 0.1 mg/kg adrenaline s.c.
HARVEY et al.	1952	Cat	DHE	0.6 (ED_{50})	i.v.	
HARVEY et al.	1952	Cat	Dihydro-ergocornine	1.0 (ED_{50})	i.v.	
HARVEY et al.	1952	Cat	Ergonovine	3.5 (ED_{50})	i.v.	
HARVEY et al.	1952	Rabbit	Ergotamine	0.06 (ED_{50})	s.c.	
HARVEY et al.	1952	Rabbit	DHE	0.03 (ED_{50})	s.c.	
HARVEY et al.	1952	Rabbit	Dihydro-ergocornine	0.15 (ED_{50})	s.c.	
HARVEY et al.	1952	Rabbit	Ergonovine	2.5 (ED_{50})	s.c.	
WOOL et al.	1954	Rat	Ergotamine	2.5	s.c.	Inhibited like adrenalectomy the fatty liver inducing effect of ethionine (counteracts cortisone)
FENN and ASANO	1956	Cat	DHE	10.7	i.v.	Inhibited increase in blood K^+ after inhalation of 30% CO_2 but not hyperglycemia and hyperphosphatemia
KONZETT	1956	Rabbit	LSD	0.15	s.c.	Hyperglycemia, inhibited by hexamethonium
			Dihydro-ergotoxine	0.1–0.2	s.c.	Inhibited LSD effect and also adrenaline hyperglycemia
SIREK O.V. et al.	1957	Dog	DHE	0.11	i.v.	Inhibition of hyperglycemia induced by injection of HG-stimulated hyperglycemic factor in pancreatoduodenal vein. Glucagon is not antagonized
LEVY and RAMEY	1958	Rat	Ergotamine	5	s.c.	Inhibition of depot fat mobilization after adrenalectomy. Dibenamine (2 mg/kg) was inactive
WRIGHT et al.	1958	Rabbit	DHE	0.2–0.4	i.v.	Inhibited adrenaline induced hyperglycemia
GOODMAN and KNOBIL	1959	Rat	Ergotamine	2.5–7.5	s.c.	Inhibited adrenaline-induced increase in plasma FFA but no fasting induced

Table 2 (continuation)

Author	Year	Species	Substance	Doses[a] mg/kg	Way	Effect of ergot substance
Mansour	1959	Liver fluke	LSD	10^{-6} M	Bath	Serotonin and LSD increased lactate
			BOL 148	10^{-5} M	Bath	Antagonizes serotonin effect
Galansino et al.	1960	Dog	DHE	0.4	Intra-portal	Inhibited hyperkalemia but not hyperglycemia due to serotonin (intra-portal or intra-femoral, 10 mg/kg)
Mayer et al.	1961	Dog	Ergotamine	0.5–8	i.v.	Inhibited adrenaline (1 µg/kg infusion 15′) hyperglycemia but not hyperlactacidemia
Sawyer and Lipner	1961	Rat	DHE	0.4	s.c.	No influence on thyroxine induced oxygen consumption and blood glucose levels
Tobe et al.	1961	Rat	DHE	3.5–7.5	s.c.	Inhibition of glucose tolerance (also dibenamine or tolazoline). Dibenamine does not inhibit adrenaline (0.2 mg/kg i.v.) hyperglycemia, DHE does
McElroy and Spitzer	1961	Dog	Ergotamine	0.4–0.5/15′	i.v.	Inhibited adrenaline hyperglycemia (0.01 mg/kg) one dog, three other dogs no effect
Kennedy and Ellis	1963	Rat	DHE	0.1–1	i.p.	Inhibited-like phentolamine adrenaline (0.1–1 mg/kg i.p.) induced glycogenolysis, DCI does not
Northrop and Parks	1964	Rat	DHE	5.6	i.p.	Inhibited adrenaline (0.1 mg/kg i.p.) and cAMP (100 mg/kg i.p.) induced hyperglycemia. DCI only decreased adrenaline effect
Elder	1964	Cat	LSD	0.3	i.v.	Phenoxybenzamine (PBA) or pentolinium inhibited LSD hyperglycemia, DBA adrenaline hyperglycemia not inhibited
Ellis and Kennedy	1965	Rat	DHE	10	i.p.	Inhibited like phentolamine adrenaline (0.1–1 mg/kg i.p.) induced glycogenolysis, DCI did not
Sirek A. et al.	1966	Dog	BOL 148	0.1	i.v.	Inhibited serotonin (12.5 µg/kg) hyperglycemia or GH treated donor blood hyperglycemia
Levassort	1967	Rabbit	DHE	10	i.v.	Gave higher oxygen consumption, lowered CO_2 excretion, and lowered fat oxidation
Sanders and Riggs	1967a	Rat	DHE	0.3	i.p.	Inhibition of adrenaline (1 mg/kg s.c. stimulated liver and heart uptake of model aminoacids (ACPC[b], AIB[b])
Sanders and Riggs	1967b	Rat	DHE	0.3	i.p.	Inhibition of insulin (0.2–2 U/kg) induced uptake of model amino acids (ACPC[b], AIB[b]) by liver but not by diaphragm

CHARBONNIER and CACHIN	1967a, b	Man	DHE	0.03	i.v.	Inhibited galactosuria after 0.6 g/kg galactose i.v. and had retardation effect on galactose hyperglycemia
FOY	1967	Rat	DHE	5	i.p.	Inhibited hyperglycemic action of ethacrynic acid (100 mg/kg i.p.)
VIGAS and NEMETH	1967	Rabbit	DHE	0.5	s.c.	No influence on endotoxine-induced hyperglycemia
HAUDE	1967	Rat	DHE	50	i.p.?	Lowered plasma free fatty acids in newborn rats
PINTER and PATTEE	1968	Man	DHE	0.03/30′	i.v.	Increase in plasma free fatty acids but no hyperglycemia. Phenoxybenzamine caused the same effect
SPITZER	1968	Rabbit	Ergotamine	0.25 0.75/20′	i.v. i.v.	Inhibited adrenaline (4 μg/kg 140′) induced rise in plasma free fatty acids. No effect on plasma glucose and glycerol
SCHIRMEISTER et al.	1968	Man	Dihydroergotoxine	4 × 0.004/day	sublingual	Inhibited furosemide (0.1 mg/kg p.o.) induced lactacidemia. Stress reaction due to plasma volume reduction
SIREK, A. et al.	1968	Dog hypophysect.	DHE	0.2	i.v.	Inverted the decrease of plasma free fatty acid after GH (2.5 mg/kg i.v.) to an increase
SCRIABINE et al.	1968	Dog	DHE	0.125–0.5	i.v.	Dose dependent increase of plasma free fatty acids not inhibited by propranolol but by nicotinic acid
SIREK, A. et al.	1969	Dog	DHE	0.2	i.v.	DHE + GH no effect in Houssay dogs
IWATA	1969	Rat	DHE	3.5	s.c.	Inhibited clonidine hyperglycemia. Propranolol inactive
MALYGINA	1969	Rabbit	DHE	0.1		Inhibited ethymizol (10 mg/kg) hyperglycemia as did adrenalectomy or adrenal denervation
SIREK, O. et al.	1969	Dog pancreatect.	DHE BOL 148	0.2	i.v.	Inhibited the GH (2.5–5 mg/kg i.v.) induced reduction of plasma amino nitrogen
KENNEDY and ELLIS	1969a	Rat	DHE	10	i.p.	Inhibited adrenaline (1 mg/kg i.p.) induced glycogenolysis like phentolamine (10 mg/kg i.p.) but not in heart and muscle
ADNITT	1969	Rat	DHE	1	s.c.	Inhibited adrenaline (0.1–1 mg/kg s.c.) hyperglycemia in fed rats. Propranolol only inhibited in fasted rats
KENNEDY and ELLIS	1969b	Rat	DHE	10	i.p.	Inhibited adrenaline (0.5 mg/kg i.p.) induced increase of plasma free fatty acids
CHARBONNIER et al.	1969	Man	DHE	0.03	i.v.	Increased like phentolamine (0.15 mg/kg i.v.) plasma free fatty acids. Propranolol (0.15 mg/kg) decreased

Table 2 (continuation)

Author	Year	Species	Substance	Doses[a] mg/kg	Way	Effect of ergot substance
ARNOLD and MCAULIFF	1970	Mouse	DHE	3.16	s.c.	Inhibited adrenaline hyperglycemia but not lactacidemia in fed mice
MANSOUR and STONE	1970	Liver fluke	LSD	10^{-5} M	Bath	Increased like serotonin phosphofructokinase activity in the liver
KULINSKY	1970	Mouse	DHE	1	s.c.	Inhibited the adrenaline (1 mg/kg) induced reduction of oxygen tension in muscle, liver and spleen
NEUVONEN et al.	1971	Rat	DHE	10	i.m.	Phentolamine (10–15 mg/kg i.m.), but not Kö 592, inhibited dopamine (2.3 mg/kg i.m.) and noradrenaline (0.1 mg/kg i.m.) induced hyperglycemia. α-blockers had no effect on free fatty acids, but Kö 592 increased
QUICKEL et al.	1971 a, b	Man	Methysergide	8 × 2 mg/ 2 dogs	p.o.	After i.v. glucose tolerance in adult onset diabetic patients increase in insulin output, but not in normal volunteers
PAUK and REDDY	1971	Rat	DHE	5.6	i.p.	Inhibited glucagon stimulated increase in liver cAMP but not glucagon hyperglycemia in fasted rats
SIREK, O. and SIREK, A.	1971	Hypophysect. pancreatect.	BOL 148	0.1	i.v	BOL 148 did not show the DHE effect
SIREK, A.M. et al.	1972	Dog	DHE	0.2	i.v.	Potentiated the lipolytic effect of human chorionic somatomammotropin (25 mg/kg i.v.)
MORETTI and ARCARI	1972	Rat	Nicergoline	1.5–20	s.c.	Phenoxybenzamine (7 mg/kg s.c.) restored adrenaline (s.c.) and noradrenaline (s.c.) impaired oxidative phosphorylation of heart mitochondria
VILLA and PANCERI	1973	Mouse	Nicergoline	10	i.p.	Increased fatigue resistance like dipyridamole and caffeine
MASTEN	1973	Rabbit	Ergonovine	4	i.v.	Hexamethonium (10 mg/kg i.v.) inhibited ethanol acetaldehyde induced hyperglycemia
MORETTI et al.	1973	Rat	Nicergoline	5	s.c. in sesame oil	Inhibited ISO-, NA-, and A-induced glycogenolysis but only A and NA, Ca uptake in rat heart

WEBLING	1973	Rabbit	DHE	0.1–1	i.v.	Decreased glucose tolerance after i.v. and increased tolerance after p.o. glucose load. Vascular effects?
SIREK, A. et al.	1974	Dog	DHE	0.2	i.v.	Potentiated action of sulfonylurea on insulin secretion. Phentolamine (0.5 mg/kg i.v.) and BOL 148 (0.1 mg/kg) had no effect
CHARBONNIER et al.	1974	Man	DHE	0.14	i.v.	No influence on galactosemia after an i.v. galactose load
DONOWITZ and BINDER	1974	Man	Methysergide	?	p.o.	Inhibited diarrhea in carcinoid syndrome
DYNAROWICZ	1974	Rat	DHE	4	i.v.	Inhibited glycogenolysis and activity of phosphorylase a and b in skeletal muscle and phosphorylase in heart muscle
LANG et al.	1974	Man	Methysergide	8×0.03	p.o.	No influence on glucose stimulated insulin secretion
BOGDANOWICZ et al.	1974	Rabbit	DHE	1	i.v.	Inhibited angiotensin II hyperglycemia (2 μg/kg i.v.)
BOGDANOWICZ and MIROSZ	1968					
TOLIS et al.	1974	Man	CB 154	0.03	p.o.	Increased plasma free fatty acids and GH, suppressed prolactin and prevented diurnal fall of cortisol
EXTON and HARPER	1975	Rat liver	Dihydro-ergotoxine phentolamine	10^{-5} M 10^{-4}–10^{-5} M		Inhibited adrenaline, noradrenaline and phenylephrine stimulated glycogenolysis, but no increase in cAMP
D'ONOFRIO et al.	1975	Man	Nicergoline	0.14–0.28	i.v.	Impaired i.v. glucose tolerance and insuline secretion
MELTZER	1975	Rat	LSD	0.6	i.p.	No influence on rat plasma creatine phosphokinase
PONTIROLI et al.	1975	Man diabetes	Methergoline	12×0.03/ 2 days	p.o.?	No influence on i.v. glucose tolerance hyperglycemia Slight increase in insulin secretion in non diabetics
MAHAJAN et al.	1975	Rat	CB 154	6.7	i.p.	Increased plasma Ca, lowers urinary Ca, Na and K

[a] Partially calculated from data of original papers. If body weights are not given there, estimated values have been used

[b] ACPC = 1-aminopentanecarboxylic acid, AIB = α-aminoisobutyric acid

noradrenaline-stimulated hyperglycemia by NEUVONEN et al. (1971) for DHE. MORETTI et al. (1973) reported inhibition of isoproterenol-, adrenaline-, and noradrenaline-stimulated rat heart glycogenolysis by s.c. doses of nicergoline. HARVEY et al. (1952) inhibited adrenaline-induced hyperglycemia in the cat by ergotamine, dihydroergotamine, dihydroergocornine, and ergometrine. The infusion of ergotamine into dogs, inhibited the adrenaline-stimulated hyperglycemia but not the lactacidemia. With lower doses of ergotamine, MCELROY and SPITZER (1961) only saw this effect in one of three dogs. ARNOLD and MCAULIFF (1970) reported that dihydroergotamine-inhibited adrenaline stimulated hyperglycemia also in mice but had no influence on blood lactate levels. In man, SPÜHLER (1947) and FREIS et al. (1948) found that low intravenous doses of dihydroergotamine inhibited the hyperglycemia due to adrenaline. FOY (1967) explained the hyperglycemic action of the diuretics hydroflumethazide, ethacrynic acid, and disulphamide as adrenergic, because adrenalectomy or dihydroergotamine abolished this effect. Using perfused rat liver or isolated liver cells, EXTON and HARPER (1975) showed that adrenaline, noradrenaline, and phenylephrine stimulated glycogenolysis and gluconeogenesis mediated by α-adrenergic receptors without involvement of cAMP, because the effect was inhibited by phentolamine and dihydroergotamine. They also found a β-adrenergic system influencing cAMP levels but of little importance for carbohydrate metabolism in rat liver.

Investigating the clonidine-induced hyperglycemia in the rat, IWATA (1969) found that this effect depended on a stimulation of α-receptors in the liver, because it could not be inhibited by pretreatment with hexamethonium, reserpine, and propranolol or adrenalectomy. However, dihydroergotamine depresses this clonidine hyperglycemia.

2. Influence on Catecholamine-Stimulated Lipolysis

The influence of ergot alkaloids on catecholamine-stimulated lipolysis has also been studied. GOODMAN and KNOBIL (1959) found that ergotamine in rats inhibited the increase of plasma free fatty acids due to adrenaline injection but had no influence on the high free fatty acid level during fasting. In the same species, ELLIS and KENNEDY (1965) and KENNEDY and ELLIS (1969b) showed that dihydroergotamine also inhibited the adrenaline-dependent increase of plasma free fatty acids (SPITZER, 1968).

3. Influence on Other Catecholamine-Stimulated Metabolic Processes

SANDERS and RIGGS (1967a) studied the uptake of the model amino acids l-aminopentanecarboxylic and α-aminoisobutyric acid in liver and heart. They found that dihydroergotamine inhibited the stimulation of uptake provoked by adrenaline. The action of ergot alkaloids on adrenaline-stimulated basal metabolic rate has also been investigated. Ergotamine applied s.c. in doses from 3 mg/kg to rats lowered basal metabolic rate and in a lower dose of 1–3 mg/kg inhibited adrenaline-stimulated metabolism (ORESTANO, 1933a). This author could also show that the stimulating effect of pilocarpine on basal metabolic rate was completely inhibited by ergotamine (from 0.3 mg/kg) (ORESTANO, 1933b). ISSEKUTZ and HARANGOZO-

OROSZY (1942) did not detect any influence of ergotamine and sensibamine[4] on adrenaline enhanced metabolism. Dihydroergotamine and dihydroergocornine also had no effect but inhibited amphetamine-induced increase in metabolism (ISSEKUTZ and GYERMEK, 1949). In the rat, ergotamine, dihydroergotamine, dihydroergocornine, and methergine (all 2 mg/kg s.c.) partially inhibited the adrenaline-stimulated oxygen consumptions (LINDNER and BRAUNER, 1950). KULINSKY (1970) showed in mice that dihydroergotamine counteracted the adrenaline-induced reduction of oxygen tension measured by oxygen electrode in muscle, liver, and spleen, but MORETTI and ARCARI (1972) found that the ergot derivative nicergoline reversed impairment of oxydative phosphorylation of rat heart mitochondria by adrenaline or noradrenaline.

4. Influence on Stress-Stimulated Metabolic Parameters

In cats breathing air containing 30% CO_2, in which the level of K^+, glucose, and PO_4^{3-} was raised in plasma, dihydroergotamine inhibited the hyperkalemia but had no influence on glucose and phosphate plasma levels (FENN and ASANO, 1956). SCHIRMEISTER et al. (1968) showed in man that dihydroergotoxine inhibited furosemide-induced lactacidemia and explained this effect by the assumption of a counteraction of the stress reaction due to plasma volume reduction. VILLA and PANCERI (1973) showed in mice increased resistance against fatigue with nicergoline and also with dipyridamole and caffeine.

5. Influence on the Effects of Adrenalectomy or Sympathectomy

In the rat, the fatty liver-producing effect of ethionine was inhibited by adrenalectomy or s.c. administration of ergotamine (WOOL et al., 1954). During a 12-h fast, adrenalectomized rats mobilize relatively more fat from the epididymal depot than normal animals. Administration of ergotamine produced marked inhibition of fat movement out of this depot. Dibenzyline or hexamethonium had no effect on this process (LEVY and RAMEY, 1958). In the rabbit, administration of dihydroergotamine or adrenalectomy inhibited ethymizol hyperglycemia (MALYGINA, 1969).

6. Influence on Glucose or Galactose Tolerance

In man, HETENYI and POGANY (1926) und GRUNKE (1926) showed that ergotamine inhibits postprandial glucose hyperglycemia. SPÜHLER (1947) found that dihydroergotamine inhibited hyperglycemia only in oral glucose tolerance tests but had no influence on the i.v. test. Dihydroergotoxine also improves oral glucose tolerance (PETRIDES and SCHÄFER, 1950) in patients with high sympathetic tone. In the rat, the α-blockers dibenamine, tolazoline, dihydroergotamine, and dihydroergotoxine inhibited the response to i.v. glucose administration (TOBE et al., 1961).

QUICKEL et al. (1971a and 1971b) showed in methysergide-treated patients during i.v. glucose tolerance an increase in insulin secretion not seen in normal volunteers (also LANG et al., 1974). Methysergide produced no change in the plasma

---

[4] Sensibamine: an equimolecular mixture of ergotamine and ergotaminine.

glucose disappearance rate. WEBLING (1973) treated rabbits with dihydroergotamine and found that i.v. glucose tolerance was impaired and oral tolerance ameliorated, but urinary excretion of glucose was diminished independently of the route of administration. This decrease in urinary excretion was also shown for galactose i.v. or p.o. and is in agreement with the results of CHARBONNIER and CACHIN (1967a, b) and CHARBONNIER et al. (1974) in man. WEBLING explains this by a decrease in renal and enteral blood flow rates provoked by dihydroergotamine. In man, nicergoline treatment (D'ONOFRIO et al., 1975) inhibited insulin secretion and free fatty acid release due to an i.v. glucose load which is not in agreement with its α-blocking properties (ARCARI et al., 1968), because phentolamine enhances insulin release (CERASI et al., 1969). For methergoline, PONTIROLI et al. (1975) showed that this substance had no influence on i.v. glucose tolerance hyperglycemia, although it caused some increase in insulin secretion in nondiabetic subjects.

7. Influence on Serotonin Effects

In the dog, intraportal injection of serotonin gives a hyperglycemia which is abolished by dihydroergotamine administered by the same route (GALANSINO et al., 1960), an effect also produced by 2-bromo-lysergic-acid-diethylamide (BOL 148) (SIREK, A. et al., 1966). In the liver fluke *(Fasciola hepatica)*, serotonin and lysergic-acid-diethylamide (LSD) cause an increase in lactate which is inhibited by BOL 148 (MANSOUR, 1959). Serotonin and LSD increased cAMP formation, but the effect of LSD was not dose dependent (MANSOUR et al., 1960). MANSOUR and STONE (1970), further investigating this effect, showed that a 10^{-5} M concentration of LSD increased the activity of the liver phosphofructokinase in these animals.

8. Interaction With Pancreas, Hypophysis, and Thyroidea

In hypophysectomized dogs, growth hormone (GH), phentolamine, or both decreased plasma free fatty acid (FFA) levels; GH+dihydroergotamine increased FFA levels; additional pancreatectomy, pancreatectomy alone, or puromycin abolished the dihydroergotamine effect; BOL 148 had no influence (SIREK, A. et al., 1969; SIREK, O. and SIREK, A., 1971). Dihydroergotamine also failed to influence the increase in plasma FFA in hypophysectomized dogs after administration of ACTH, TSH, and prolactin but stimulated and accelerated the lipolytic effect of chorionic somatomammotropin, also called placental lactogen (SIREK, A. et al., 1968; SIREK, A. et al., 1969; SIREK, O. and SIREK, A., 1971; SIREK, A.M. et al., 1972). In the dog, the action of the GH-stimulated hyperglycemic factor, injected into the pancreatoduodenal vein, was inhibited by i.v. dihydroergotamine, but dihydroergotamine had no influence on glucagon injection. Infusion of the hyperglycemic factor into pancreatectomized dogs also resulted in a rise in blood sugar levels. This effect was inhibited by BOL 148, inducing the authors to speculate whether the hyperglycemic factor is identical with serotonin (SIREK, O.V. et al., 1957; SIREK, A. et al., 1968). In man, another ergot alkaloid, 2-bromo-α-ergokryptine (CB 154), besides its well known inhibition of prolactin secretion, also increases plasma free fatty acids (TOLIS et al., 1974). SIREK, O. et al. (1969) and SIREK,

O. and SIREK, A. (1971) also studied the influence of dihydroergotamine and BOL 148 on plasma aminonitrogen in pancreatectomized dogs after GH injection. Both substances inhibited the fall in amino nitrogen induced by GH partially; only addition of puromycin resulted in complete suppression.

SANDERS and RIGGS (1967b) showed that dihydroergotamine also seems to inhibit the insulin-induced uptake of amino acids in rat diaphragm. A further influence of DHE on the pancreas was seen in experiments of SIREK, A. et al. (1974) in the dog, showing a potentiating effect of this ergot alkaloid on sulfonylurea-stimulated insulin secretion. The α-blocker phentolamine and the serotonin antagonist BOL 148 were inactive. In man, nicergoline impaired i.v. glucose tolerance and insulin secretion, but methergoline showed no effect (D'ONOFRIO et al., 1975; PONTIROLI et al., 1975); the serotonin antagonist methergoline also did not influence these parameters (LANG et al., 1974).

In dog, dihydroergotamine applied intraportally inhibited the hyperkalemia but not the hyperglycemia induced by glucagon given by the same route (GALANSINO et al., 1960). PAUK and REDDY (1970, 1971) found a similar effect of dihydroergotamine in the rat. Again, the hyperglycemia was not suppressed, but the increase of cAMP in the liver due to glucagon was inhibited.

In thyroidectomized rats, dihydroergotamine had no influence on thyroxine-induced hyperglycemia and oxygen consumption. The adrenaline-induced hyperglycemia was inhibited; the increased respiration was not influenced by dihydroergotamine (SAWYER and LIPNER, 1961). In rabbits, dihydroergotamine inhibited angiotensin II-induced hyperglycemia (BOGDANOWICZ and MIROSZ, 1968; BOGDANOWICZ et al., 1974).

9. Actions of Ergot Alkaloids Alone on Metabolic Parameters

After giving high subcutaneous doses of ergotamine to rabbits, a short hypoglycemia occurred (LESSER and ZIPF, 1923), an effect also shown for therapeutic doses of dihydroergotamine in man by SPÜHLER (1947). Perhaps this can be explained by the work of DYNAROWICZ (1974), who showed an inhibitory action of dihydroergotamine on phosphorylase a and b in skeletal muscle and on heart muscle phosphorylase.

KONZETT (1956) reported that LSD produced hyperglycemia in rabbits, which he could inhibit by hexamethonium. In cats (ELDER, 1964), LSD produced the same effect, which was inhibited by pentolinium and phenoxybenzamine. Because the latter could not antagonize adrenaline-induced hyperglycemia, this metabolic effect of LSD was assumed to have its origin in the central nervous system.

Using very high doses (50 mg/kg i.p.) in newborn rats, HAUDE (1967) could see a decrease in plasma FFA. PINTER and PATTEE (1968) infused dihydroergotamine and phenoxybenzamine into man. Both drugs induced a rise in plasma free fatty acids. This was confirmed by CHARBONNIER et al. (1969), who also found an inhibitory effect of propranolol on free fatty acids. TOLIS et al. (1974) found an increase in plasma FFA after administration of CB 154. The hyperlipidacidemia produced by dihydroergotamine in dog could not be inhibited by propranolol (SCRIABINE et al., 1968). The effect of these ergot alkaloids is probably due to their α-adrenergic blocking properties. BURNS and LANGLEY (1970), using isolated human fat cells, found that phentolamine increased the lipolytic activity of adrenaline to the value of isoproterenol, proving the existence of inhibitory α-receptors on the cell membrane.

High intravenous doses of dihydroergotamine (10 mg/kg) in rabbit accelerated oxygen consumption, lowered carbon dioxyde excretion, and resulted in a lower respiratory quotient, pointing to a greater use of fat as an energy source (LEVASSORT, 1967).

D. Various Actions of Ergot Alkaloids

In rabbits, VIGAS and NEMETH (1967) found no influence of dihydroergotamine on endotoxin-induced hyperglycemia. Ethanol-induced hyperglycemia in rabbits is due to the production of acetaldehyde. The effect may be of central origin, because it can be inhibited by hexamethonium and high doses of ergonovine (MASTEN, 1973). For LSD, MELTZER (1975) could not find any influence on rat plasma creatine phosphokinase. High doses (6.7 mg/kg i.p.) of CB 154 increased plasma Ca and lowered urinary Ca, Na, and K (MAHAJAN et al., 1975). In some patients with carcinoid syndrome, increased electrolyte secretion was reversed by glucose and methysergide (DONOWITZ and BINDER, 1974).

E. References

Adnitt, P.I.: Hepatic glycogen and blood glucose control. Biochem. Pharmacol. **18**, 2599–2604 (1969)
Altman, Ph.L., Dittmer, D.S.: Metabolism, pp. 387/389. Bethesda (Maryland): Federation of American Societies for Experimental Biology 1968
Arcari, G., Dorigotti, L., Fregnan, G.B., Glässer, A.H.: Vasodilating and alpha-receptor blocking activity of a new ergoline derivative. Brit. J. Pharmacol. **34**, 700P (1968)
Arnold, A., Selberis,, W.H.: Activities of catecholamines on the rat muscle glycogenolytic (β-2) receptor. Experientia (Basel) **24**, 1010–1011 (1968)
Arnold, A., McAuliff, J.P.: α-adrenergic receptor mediated hyperglycemia in the laboratory rodent. Pharmacol. **12** (Abstr. No. 582), 306 (1970)
Ballard, K., Rosell, S.: Nervous and pharmacological influences on fat metabolism in mesenteric adipose tissue. Acta physiol. scand. **74**, 18A–19A (1968)
Ballard, K., Rosell, S.: Adrenergic neurohumoral influences on circulation and lipolysis in canine omental adipose tissue. Circulat. Res. **28**, 389–396 (1971)
Banerjee, A.K.: The influence of drugs upon the movements of calcium ions in smooth muscle. Comp. gen. Pharmacol. **3**, 41–51 (1972)
Barger, G.: The alkaloids of ergot. Effect of ergotamine on metabolism. In: Handbuch der experimentellen Pharmakologie (Ergänzungswerk). Heubner, W., Schüller, J. (eds.), Vol. VI, pp. 150–169. Berlin-Heidelberg-New York: Springer 1938
Berthet, J., Sutherland, E.W., Rall, T.W.: The assay of glucagon and epinephrine with use of liver homogenates. J. biol. Chem. **229**, 351–361 (1957)
Best, Ch.H., Taylor, N.B.: The physiological basis of medical practice, 9th ed., p. 1270. Baltimore: Williams and Wilkins 1966
Bogdanowicz, S., Mirosz, J.: Wpływ angiotensyny na poziom glukozy krwi królików. Acta physiol. pol. **19**, 651–655 (1968)
Bogdanowicz, S., Mirosz, J., Wyszynska-Koko, M.: The effect of drugs influencing the level of cyclic AMP on angiotensin hyperglycaemia in rabbits. Acta physiol. pol. **25**, 251–256 (1974)

Bradley, P.B., Briggs, I.: Ergot alkaloids and related substances. In: Neuropoisons. Their Pathophysiological Actions. Simpson, L.L., Curtis, D.R. (eds.), pp. 249–296. New York-London: Plenum Press 1974
Brooker, W.D., Calvert, D.N.: Blockade of catecholamine mediated release of free fatty acids from adipose tissue in vitro. Arch. int. Pharmacodyn. **169**, 117–130 (1967)
Burns, T.W., Langley, P.E.: Lipolysis by human adipose tissue: the role of cyclic 3′,5′-adenosine monophosphate and adrenergic receptor sites. J. Lab. clin. Med. **75**, 983–997 (1970).
Carlsöö, B., Danielsson, A., Marklund, S., Stigbrand, T.: Inhibition of catecholamine and 5-hydroxytryptamine induced enzyme secretion from the guinea-pig submandibular gland by 2-bromo-d-lysergic acid diethylamide. Experientia (Basel) **31**, 395–397 (1975)
Cerasi, E., Effendic, S., Luft, R.: Role of adrenergic receptors in glucose-induced insulin secretion in man. Lancet **1969**, 301–302/II
Chambers, J.W., Georg, R.H., Bass, A.D.: Effects of catecholamines and glucagon on amino acid transport in the liver. Endocrinology **83**, 1185–1192 (1968)
Chambers, J.W., Georg, R.H., Bass, A.D.: Effect of glucagon, cyclic 3′,5′-adenosine monophosphate and its dibutyryl derivative on amino acid uptake by the isolated perfused rat liver. Endocrinology **87**, 366–370 (1970)
Chan, P.S., Ellis, S.: Dihydroergotamine antagonism of glucose release by rabbit liver slices induced by catecholamines, glucagon and 3′,5′-AMP. Fed. Proc. **28**, Abstr. No. 2706, 742 (1969)
Chan, P.S., Ellenbogen, L.: New evidence for the β-adrenergic receptor blocking activity of dihydroergotamine. Arch. int. Pharmacodyn. **209**, 204-213 (1974)
Charbonnier, A., Cachin, M.: Influence de la dihydroergotamine sur certaines fonctions hépatiques de l'homme. Sem. Hôp. (Paris) **43**, 1673–1684 (1967a)
Charbonnier, A., Cachin, M.: Influence de la dihydroergotamine sur certaines fonctions hépatiques de l'homme. Symp. de St.-Germain-en-Laye, 15.–16. Oct. 1966, Paris: Sandoz 1967b, pp. 117–141
Charbonnier, A., Cachin, M., Bernard, G.: Influence d'une administration unique de dihydroergotamine sur les acides gras non estérifiées plasmatiques chez l'homme. Therapie **24**, 399–417 (1969)
Charbonnier, A., Nepveux, P., Fluteau, G., Fluteau, D.: Etude de l'influence de la dihydroergotamine sur les résultats de l'épreuve de perfusion intraveineuse de galactose. Ann. Gastroent. Hépatol. **10**, 197–208 (1974)
Cuatrecasas, P.: Unmasking of insulin receptors in fat cells and fat cell membranes. J. biol. Chem. **246**, 6532–6542 (1971)
Dale, H.H.: On Some physiological actions of ergot. J. Physiol. (Lond.) **34**, 163–206 (1906)
D'Onofrio, F., Torella, R., Sgambato, S., Ungaro, B.: Nicergoline effect on insulin secretion in man. Farmaco **30**, 153–162 (1975)
Donowitz, M., Binder, H.J.: Jejunal electrolyte secretion in carcinoid syndrome. Clin. Res. **22**, 356A (1974)
Dynarowicz, I.: Adrenergic regulation of glycogen breadkdown in the heart and skeletal muscle. Acta pysiol. pol. **25**, 145–150 (1974)
Eggstein, M., Kreutz, G.H.: Eine neue Bestimmung der Neutralfette im Blutserum und Gewebe. Klin. Wschr. **44**, 262–267 (1966)
Elder, J.T.: Antagonism of lysergic acid diethylamide (LSD)-induced hyperglycemia. Int. J. Neuropharmacol. **3**, 295–300 (1964)
Ellis, S., Anderson, H.L.: Effect of sympathomimetic amines and sympatholytics on blood sugar and lactate of the rat. Fed. Proc. **9**, 269–270 (1950)
Ellis, S., Kennedy, B.L.: Interactions of sympathomimetic amines and adrenergic blocking agents at receptor sites mediating lipolysis in the intact rat. Pharmacol. **7** Abstr., 137 (1965)
Ellis, S., Anderson, H.L., Turtle, M.A.: A study of the mechanism of action of epinephrine on liver slices. J. Pharmacol. exp. Ther. **106**, 383 (1952)
Ellis, S., Anderson, H.L., Collins, M.C.: Pharmacologic differentiation between epinephrine- and HGF-hyperglycemia: Application in analysis of cobalt-hyperglycemia. Proc. Soc. exp. Biol. (N.Y.) **84**, 383–386 (1953)
Exton, J.H., Harper, S.C.: Role of c-AMP in the actions of catecholamines on hepatic carbohydrate metabolism. Adv. Cyclic Nucleotide Res. **5**, 519–532 (1975)

Fain, J.N., Kovacev, V.P., Scow, R.O.: Effect of growth hormone and dexamethasone on lipolysis and metabolism in isolated fat cells of the rat. J. biol. Chem. **240**, 3522–3529 (1965)
Fain, J.N.: Dihydroergotamine, propranolol and the beta adrenergic receptors of fat cells. Fed. Proc. **29**, 1402–1407 (1970)
Fain, J.N.: Biochemical aspects of drug and hormone action on adipose tissue. Pharmacol. Rev. **25**, 67–118 (1973)
Fenn, W.O., Asano, T.: Effects of carbon dioxide inhalation on potassium liberation from the liver. Amer. J. Physiol. **185**, 567–576 (1956)
Foy, J.M.: Acute diuretic induced hyperglycaemia in rats. Life Sci. **6**, 897–902 (1967)
Fredholm, B., Rosell, S.: Effects of adrenergic blocking agents on lipid mobilization from canine subcutaneous adipose tissue after sympathetic nerve stimulation. J. Pharmacol. exp. Ther. **159**, 1–7 (1968)
Fredholm, B.B., Rosell, S.: Fate of ^{3}H-noradrenaline in canine subcutaneous adipose tissue. Acta physiol. scand. **80**, 404–411 (1970)
Freis, E.D., Stanton, J.R., Wilkins, R.W.: The effects of certain dihydrogenated alkaloids of ergot in hypertensive patients. Amer. J. med. Sci. **216**, 163–171 (1948)
Galansino, G., D'Amigo, G., Kanameishi, D., Berlinger, F.G., Foa, P.P.: Hyperglycemic substances originating in the pancreatoduodenal area. Amer. J. Physiol. **198**, 1059–1062 (1960)
Gill, G.N., Garren, L.D.: A cyclic-3′,5′-adenosine monophosphate dependent protein kinase from the adrenal cortex: Comparison with a cyclic AMP binding protein. Biochem. biophys. Res. Commun. **39**, 335–343 (1970)
Goldblatt, M.W.: Ergotamine and the effect of adrenaline on blood lactate. J. Physiol. (Lond.) **78**, 96–105 (1933a)
Goldblatt, M.W.: Insulin and adrenaline. J. Physiol. (Lond.) **79**, 286–300 (1933b)
Goodman, H.M., Knobil, E.: Effect of adrenergic blocking agents on fatty acid mobilization during fasting. Proc. Soc. exp. Biol. (N.Y.) **102**, 493–495 (1959)
Grunke, W.: Über den Mechanismus der alimentären Hyperglykämie. Z. exp. Med. **52**, 488–498 (1926)
Harvey, S.C., Wang, C.Y., Nickerson, M.: Blockade of epinephrine-induced hyperglycemia. J. Pharmacol. exp. Ther. **104**, 363–376 (1952)
Haude, W.: Wlijanie gormonow nadpotschniko, golod anija i aloksanowo diabeta na soderschanie swobodnich schirnich kislot w plasme krisinich embrionow i noworoschdennich. Pat. Fiziol. éksp. Ter. **11**, 48–51 (1967)
Haylett, D.G., Jenkinson, D.H.: The receptors concerned in the actions of catecholamines on glucose release, membrane potential and ion movements in guinea-pig liver. J. Physiol. (Lond.) **225**, 751–772 (1972)
Hegnauer, H., Cori, G.T.: The influence of epinephrine on chemical changes in isolated frog muscle. J. biol. Chem. **105**, 691–703 (1934)
Hetenyi, S., Pogany, J.: Ergotaminversuche zur Frage des Kohlehydratstoffwechsels. Verhandlungen des Kongress für Innere Medizin 1926, pp. 306–308
Himms-Hagen, J.: Sympathetic regulation of metabolism. Pharmacol. Rev. **19**, 367–461 (1967)
Himms-Hagen, J.: Effects of catecholamines on metabolism. In: Handbook of Experimental Pharmacology. Blaschko, H., Muscholl, E. (eds.), Vol. XXXIII, pp. 363–462. Berlin-Heidelberg-New York: Springer 1972
Hornbrook, K.R.: Adrenergic receptors for metabolic responses in the liver. Fed. Proc. **29**, 1381–1385 (1970)
Hotta, N., Sirek, O.V., Sirek, A.: Effect of dihydroergotamine and growth hormone on lipolysis in isolated fat cells of the rat. Canad. J. Physiol. Pharmacol. **48**, 324–326 (1970)
Hotta, N., Sirek, O.V., Sirek, A.: Studies on the interaction between growth hormone and dihydroergotamine in adipose cells. Horm. Metab. Res. **3**, 161–166 (1971a)
Hotta, N., Sirek, O.V., Sirek, A.: Studies on the Interaction between growth hormone and dihydroergotamine in adipose cells. Horm. Metab. Res. **3**, 321–325 (1971b)
Hotta, N., Sirek, A., Sirek, O.V.: Inhibitory effect of beta-hydroxybutyrate on lipolysis stimulated by dihydroergotamine and growth hormone in vitro. Canad. J. Physiol. Pharmacol. **49**, 87–91 (1971c)

Huttunen, J.K., Steinberg, D., Mayer, S.E.: Protein kinase activation and phosphorylation of a purified hormone-sensitive lipase. Biochem. biophys. Res. Commun. **41**, 1350–1356 (1970)
Ishii, T.: Effect of dihydroergotamine (DHE) and nicotinic acid (NIA) on dibutyryl cyclic AMP-induced lipolysis in isolated rat fat cells. Tex. Rep. Biol. Med. **27**, 921 (1969)
Issekutz, B., Gyermek, L.: Die Wirkung von Dihydroergotamin und Dihydroergocornin auf den Gaswechsel. Arch. int. Pharmacodyn. **78**, 174–195 (1949)
Issekutz, B. von, Harangozo-Oroszy, M. von: Über Beeinflussung der Wirkung von Adrenalin auf den Gasstoffwechsel durch die Schilddrüse und Sympathicolytica. Naunyn-Schmiedergs Arch. exp. Path. Pharmak. **199**, 292–305 (1942).
Iversen, J.: Adrenergic receptors and the secretion of glucagon and insulin from the isolated, perfused canine pancreas. J. clin. Invest. **52**, 2101–2116 (1973)
Iwangoff, P., Enz, A.: The influence of various dihydroergotamine analogues on cyclic adenosine-3′,5′-monophosphate phosphodiesterase in the grey matter of cat brain in vitro. Agents Actions **5**, 223–230 (1972)
Iwangoff, P., Enz, A.: Inhibition of phosphodiesterase by dihydroergotamine and hydergine in various organs of the cat in vitro. Experientia (Basel) **29**, 1067–1069 (1973a)
Iwangoff, P., Chappuis, A., Enz, A.: The effect of different dihydroergot alkaloids on the noradrenaline-activated ATP-ase of the cat brain. IRCS (73-8) 3-10-20 (1973b)
Iwata, Y.: Hyperglycemic action of 2-(2,6-Dichlorphenyl-amino)-2-imidazoline hydrochloride in relation to its hypertensive effect. Jap. J. Pharmacol. **19**, 249–259 (1969)
Johnson, E.M., Ueda, T., Maeno, H., Greengard, P.: Adenosine 3′,5′-monophosphate-dependent phosporylation of a specific protein in synaptic membrane fractions from rat cerebrum. J. biol. Chem. **247**, 5650–5662 (1972)
Kennedy, B.L., Ellis, S.: Interactions of sympathomimetic amines and adrenergic blocking agents at receptor sites mediating glycogenolysis. Fed. Proc. **22** (Abstr.), 1725 (1963)
Kennedy, B.L., Ellis, S.: Interactions of sympathomimetic amines and adrenergic blocking agents at receptor sites mediating glycogenolysis. Arch. int. Pharmacodyn. **177**, 390–406 (1969a)
Kennedy, B.L., Ellis, S.: Interactions of catecholamines and adrenergic blocking agents at receptor sites mediating glycogenolysis in the rat. Proc. Soc. exp. Biol. (N.Y.) **130**, 1223–1229 (1969b)
Konzett, H.: Zur Wirkung von LSD (und LSD-Derivaten) auf den Blutzucker. XXe Congrès International de Physiologie, Brussels, July 30–August 4, 1956. Résumés des communications, p. 518
Kowadlo-Silbergeld, A., Laron, A.: Lipolytic effects of sheep β-lipotropin in rat adipose tissue: Interaction with theophylline and dihydroergotamine. Horm. Metab. Res. **6**, 303–306 (1974)
Kowadlo-Silbergeld, A., Klipper, I., Assa, S., Laron, Z.: Augmentation by Dihydroergotamine of lipolysis stimulated by whole and pepsin-digested human growth hormone. Horm. Metab. Res. **4**, 187–190 (1972)
Kowadlo-Silbergeld, A., Klipper, I., Laron, Z.: The effect of dihydroergotamine on ACTH-stimulated lipolysis in rat adipocytes. Acta endocr. (Kbh.) **73**, 250–258 (1973)
Kulinsky, V.I.: Concerning the mechanism of catecholamine action on oxygen tension in tissues. Probl. Endocrinol. (Mosk.) **16**, 67–72 (1970)
Lang, I., Littmann, L., Stützel, M., Balazsi, I.: Insulin response of healthy and diabetic subjects to oral glucose tolerance test before and after the administration of methysergide maleate. Diabetologia **10**, 375 (1974)
Laurell, S., Tibbling, G.: An enzymatic fluorometric micro-method for the determination of glycerol. Clin. chim. Acta **13**, 317–322 (1966)
Lesser, E.J., Zipf, K.: Über Herabsetzung des Blutzuckers beim normalen Kaninchen durch Ergotamin. Biochem. Z. **140**, 612–615 (1923)
Levassort, C.: Action de quelques agents pharmacodynamiques hyperthermisants et hypothermisants sur le métabolism de base du lapin. Modifications apportés par différents hypothermisants. Ann. Pharm. Fr. **25**, 43–57 (1967)
Levy, A.C., Ramey, E.R.: Effect of autonomic blocking agents on depot fat mobilization in normal and adrenalectomized animals. Proc. Soc. exp. Biol. (N.Y.) **99**, 637–639 (1958)

Li, C.H., Barnafi, L., Chretien, M., Chung, D.: Isolation and amino acid sequence of β-LPH from sheep pituitary glands. Nature (Lond.) **208**, 1093–1094 (1965)
Lindner, A., Brauner, F.: Der hemmende Einfluß von Mutterkornalkaloiden und ihrer Dihydroderivate auf die Stoffwechselsteigerung durch Adrenalin. Z. Vitamin-, Hormon- u. Fermentforsch. **3**, 278–287 (1950)
Love, W.C., Carr, L., Ashmore, J.: Lipolysis in adipose tissue: Effects of dl-3,4-dichloroisoproterenol and related compounds. J. Pharmacol. exp. Ther. **140**, 287–294 (1963)
Lundholm, L., Mohme-Lundholm, E., Svedmyr, N.: Metabolic effects of catecholamines. In: the Biological Basis of Medicine. Bittar, E.E., Bittar, N. (eds.), Vol. II, pp. 101–130. New York: Academic Press 1968
McAfee, D.A., Greengard, P.: Adenosine 3′,5′-monophosphate: electrophysiological evidence for a role in synaptic transmission. Science **178**, 310–312 (1972)
McElroy, W.T., Spitzer, J.J.: Effects of adrenergic blocking agents on plasma free fatty acid concentrations. Amer. J. Physiol. **200**, 318–322 (1961)
Mahajan, K.K., Horrobin, D.F., Robinson, C.J.: Metabolic effects of 2-bromo-ergocryptine-methane-sulphonate (CB 154) in the rat. J. Endocr. **64**, 587–588 (1975)
Makman, M.H., Sutherland, E.W.: Use of liver adenyl cyclase for assay of glucagon in human gastro-intestinal tract and pancreas. Endrocrinology **75**, 127–134 (1964)
Malygina, E.I.: Drug equivalence: Ethymizol—a derivative of imidazoldicarboxylic acid. Farmakol. i Toksikol. **32**, 586–588 (1969)
Mansour, T.E.: The effect of serotonin and related compounds on the carbohydrate metabolism of the liver fluke, *Fasciola hepatica*. J. Pharm. exp. Ther. **126**, 212–216 (1959)
Mansour, T.E., Stone, D.B.: Biochemical effects of lysergic acid diethylamide on the liver fluke *Fasciola hepatica*. Biochem. Pharmacol. **19**, 1137–1146 (1970)
Mansour, T.E., Sutherland, E.W., Rall, T.W., Bueding, E.: The effect of serotonin (5-hydroxytryptamine) on the formation of adenosine 3′,5′-phosphate by tissue particles from the liver fluke, *Fasciola hepatica*. J. biol. Chem. **235**, 466–470 (1960)
Markstein, R., Wagner, H.: The effect of dihydroergotoxine, phentolamine and pindolol on catecholamine-stimulated adenyl-cyclase in rat cerebral cortex. FEBS lett. **55**, 275–277 (1975)
Masten, L.W.: The role of acetaldehyde in selected acute toxic responses to ethanol in the rabbit. Diss. Abstr. **34**, 16-67-68 (1973)
Mayer, S., Moran, N.C., Fain, J.: The effect of adrenergic blocking agents on some metabolic actions of catecholamines. J. Pharmacol. exp. Ther. **134**, 18–27 (1961)
Meltzer, H.Y.: Plasma creatine phosphokinase levels in rats following lysergic acid diethylamide. Psychopharmacologia **44**, 91–93 (1975)
Miculicich, M.: Über den Einfluß von Ergotoxin auf die Adrenalin- und Diuretinglykosurie. Naunyn-Schmiedebergs Arch. exp. Path. Pharmak. **69**, 133–148 (1912)
Milavec, M., Wagner, H.: (1978) (in preparation)
Moretti, A., Arcari, G.: Protection by nicergoline from the catecholamine-induced impairment of the oxidative phosphorylation in the rat heart. Farmaco **27**, 800–807 (1972)
Moretti, A., Arcari, G., Laterza, L., Suchowsky, G.K.: The effect of catecholamines and adrenergic blocking agents on the calcium and glycogen content in the rat heart. Farmaco **28**, 3–7 (1973)
Morita, S.: Untersuchungen über die zuckertreibende Wirkung adrenalinähnlicher (sympathomimetischer) Substanzen. Naunyn Schmiedeberg's Arch. exp. Path. Pharmak. **78**, 245–276 (1915)
Mosinger, B.: Action of lipomobilizing hormones on adipose tissue. In: Handbook of Physiology, Sect. 5, Adipose Tissue. Renold A.E., Cahill G.F. (eds.). Washington, D.C.: American Physiological Society 1965
Moskowitz, J., Fain, J.N.: Stimulation by growth hormone and dexamethasone of labeled cyclic adenosine 3′,5′-monophosphate accumulation by white fat cells. J. biol. Chem. **245**, 1101–1107 (1970)
Murad, F., Chi, Y.M., Rall, T.W., Sutherland, E.W.: Adenyl cyclase. III. The effect of catecholamines and choline esters on the formation of adenosine 3′,5′-phosphate by preparations from cardiac muscle and liver. J. biol. Chem. **237**, 1233–1238 (1962)
Nakano, J., Oliver, R.D.: Effect of histamine, betazole and histidine on the lipolysis in isolated rat fat cells. Clin. Res. **18**, 53 (1970a)

Nakano, J., Oliver, R.D.: Effect of histamine and its derivatives on lipolysis in isolated rat fat cells. Arch. int. Pharmacodyn. **186**, 339 (1970b)
Nakano, J., Ishii, T., Oliver, R.D., Gin, A.C.: Effect of dihydroergotamine and propranolol on dibutyryl cyclic 3′,5′-AMP-induced lipolysis in isolated rat fat cells. Proc. Soc. exp. Biol. (N.Y.) **132**, 150–153 (1969)
Neuvonen, P.J., Vapaatalo, H.I., Westerman, E.: Some metabolic effects of dopa and dopamine in rats. Acta pharmacol. (Kbh.) **29** (Suppl. 4), 40 (1971)
Nickerson, M.: The pharmacology of adrenergic blockade. Pharmacol. Rev. **1**, 27–101 (1949)
Nickerson, M.: Blockade of the actions of adrenaline and noradrenaline. Pharmacol. Rev. **11**, 443–461 (1959)
Nitzescu, I.I., Munteanu, N.: L'ergotamine et l'hyperlactacidémie adrénalique. C.R. Soc. Biol. (Paris) **109**, 311–313 (1932)
Northrop, G.: Effects of adrenergic blocking agents on epinephrine- and 3′,5′-AMP- induced responses in the perfused rat liver. J. Pharmacol. exp. Ther. **159**, 22–28 (1968)
Northrop, G., Parks, R.E.: The effects of adrenergic blocking agents and theophylline on 3′,5′-AMP-induced hyperglycemia. J. Pharmacol. exp. Ther. **145**, 87–91 (1964)
Orestano, G.: Azione dei farmaci simpatico e parasimpatico-mimetici sugli scambi gassosi. V.—Influence della ergotamina sull'azione eccitometabolica della adrenalina. Boll. Soc. ital. Biol. sper. **8**, 1148–1150 (1933a)
Orestano, G.: Azione dei farmaci simpatico e parasimpatico-mimetici sugli scambi gassosi. VI.—Influenza della ergotamina sull'azione eccitometabolica della pilocarpina. Boll. Soc. ital. Biol. sper. **8**, 1150–1151 (1933b)
Pauk, G.L., Reddy, W.J.: Glucagon control of liver adenosine 3′,5′-monophosphate. Clin. Res. **18**, 74 (1970)
Pauk, G.L., Reddy, W.J.: Evaluation of the liver adenosine 3′,5′-monophosphate response to glucagon. Diabetes **20**, 129–133 (1971)
Petrides, P., Schäfer, E.: Zur Frage der Wirkung der hydrierten Mutterkornalkaloide auf den Kohlenhydratstoffwechsel. Schweiz. med. Wschr. **80**, 844–853 (1950)
Pinter, E.J., Pattee, C.J.: Fat-mobilizing action of amphetamine. J. clin. Invest. **47**, 394–402 (1968)
Pontiroli, A.E., Viberti, G.C., Tognetti, A., Pozza, G.: Effect of metergoline, a powerful and long-acting antiserotoninergic agent, on insulin secretion in normal subjects and in patients with chemical diabetes. Diabetol. **11**, 165–167 (1975)
Porte, D.: Beta adrenergic stimulation of insulin release in man. Diabetes **16**, 150–155 (1967)
Porte, D., Robertson, R.P.: Control of insulin secretion by catecholamines, stress, and the sympathetic nervous system. Fed. Proc. **32**, 1792–96 (1973)
Quickel, K.E., Feldman, J.M., Lebovitz, H.E.: Enhancement of insulin secretion in adult onset diabetics by methysergide maleate. Diabetes **20** (Suppl. 1) Abstr., p. 321 (1971a)
Quickel, K.E., Feldman, J.M., Lebovitz, H.E.: Enhancement of insulin secretion in adult onset diabetics by methysergide maleate: evidence for an endogenous biogenic monoamine mechanism as a factor in the impaired insulin secretion in diabetes mellitus. J. clin. Endocr. **33**, 877–881 (1971b)
Robertson, R., Porte, D.: Adrenergic modulation of basal insulin secretion in man. Diabetes 22, 1–8 (1973)
Robison, G.A., Langley, P.E., Burns, T.W.: Adrenergic receptors in human adipocytes—divergent effects on adenosine 3′,5′-monophosphate and lipolysis. Biochem. Pharmacol. **21**, 589–592 (1972)
Rodbell, M.: Metabolism of isolated fat cells. I. Effects of hormones on glucose metabolism and lipolysis. J. biol. chem. **239**, 375–380 (1964)
Rosell, S., Belfrage, E.: Adrenergic receptors in adipose tissue and their relation to adrenergic innervation. Nature (Lond.) **253**, 738–739 (1975)
Rothlin, E.: The pharmacology of the natural and dihydrogenated alkaloids of ergot. Bull. schweiz. Akad. med. Wiss. **2**, 249–273 (1947)
Rudman, D.: The adipokinetic action of polypeptide and amine hormones upon the adipose tissue of various animal species. J. Lipid Res. **4**, 119–129 (1963)
Salvador, R.A., Colville, K.I., April, S.A., Burns, J.J.: Inhibition of lipid mobilization by N-isopropyl methoxamine (B.W. 61–43). J. Pharmacol. exp. Ther. **144**, 172–180 (1964)

Sanders, R.B., Riggs, T.R.: Effects of epinephrine on the distribution of two model amino acides in the rat. Molec. Pharmacol. **3**, 352–358 (1967a)
Sanders, R.B., Riggs, T.R.: Modification by insulin of the distribution of two model amino acids in the rat. Endocrinology **80**, 29–37 (1967b)
Sawyer, H.K., Lipner, H.J.: Effects of dihydroergotamine in athyroid and thyroxinized rats. Amer. J. Physiol. **201**, 264–266 (1961)
Schirmeister, J., Man, N.K., Hallauer, W.: Zum Mechanismus des Blutlactatanstiegs nach Diuretikagaben. Klin. Wschr. **46**, 1062–1064 (1968)
Schotz, M.C., Page, I.H.: Effect of adrenergic blocking agents on the release of free fatty acids from rat adipose tissue. J. Lipid Res. **1**, 466–468 (1960)
Scriabine, A., Bellet, S., Kershbaum, A., Feinberg, L.J.: Effect of dihydroergotamine on plasma free fatty acids (FFA) in dogs. Life Sci. **7**, 453–463 (1968)
Sepulveda, F.V., Robinson, J.W.L.: New characteristics of harmaline inhibition of intestinal transport systems. Naunyn Schmiedeberg's Arch. Pharmacol. **291**, 201–212 (1975)
Sherline, P., Lynch, A., Glinsmann, W.H.: Cyclic AMP and adrenergic receptor control of rat liver glycogen metabolism. Endocrinology **91**, 680–690 (1972)
Sirek, A., Geerling, E., Sirek, O.V.: Serotonin as the hyperglycemic substance released by growth hormone. Amer. J. Physiol. **211**, 1018–1020 (1966)
Sirek, A., Niki, A., Niki, H., Sirek, O.V.: The effect of dihydroergotamine on plasma free fatty acid concentrations in hypophysectomized dogs following a single injection of growth hormone. Acta Diabetol. Lat. **5**, 167–172 (1968)
Sirek, A., Sirek, O.V., Niki, A., Niki, H., Przybylska, K.: The effect of dihydroergotamine on growth hormone-induced lipolysis in dogs. Horm. Metab. Res. **1**, 276–281 (1969)
Sirek, A., Sirek, O.V., Policova, Z.: Dihydroergotamine: A potent biological amplifier of Sulphonylureas. Diabetologia **10**, 267–270 (1974)
Sirek, A.M., Sirek, O.V., Sirek, A.: The effect of dihydroergotamine on lipolysis stimulated by human chorionic somatomammotropin in hypophysectomized dogs. Horm. **3**, 221–227 (1972)
Sirek, O.V., Sirek, A., Best, C.H.: Pituitary growth hormone and the question of pancreatic secretion of glucagon. Amer. J. Physiol. **188**, 17–20 (1957)
Sirek, O.V., Niki, A., Niki, H., Sirek, A.: Serotonin and the plasma amino acid reduction caused by a single injection of growth hormone. Canad. J. Physiol. Pharmacol. **47**, 611–617 (1969)
Sirek, O.V., Sirek, A.: Acute effects of growth hormone on plasma free amino acids and free fatty acids in dogs. In: Actions of Hormones, Genes to population Foa, C., Foa, R. (eds.), pp. 433–450. Whitty, Springfield, Ill.: Thomas 1971
Soderling, T.R., Hickenbottom, J.P., Reimann, E.M., Hunkeler, F.L., Walsh, D.A., Krebs, E.G.: Inactivation of glycogen synthetase and activation of phosphorylase kinase by muscle adenosine 3′,5′-monophosphate-dependent protein kinases. J. biol. Chem. **245**, 6317–6328 (1970)
Spitzer, J.A.: Dissociation of epinephrine-induced free fatty acid and glycerol release by adrenergic blocking drugs. Biochem. Pharmacol. **17**, 2205–2213 (1968)
Spühler, O.: Die experimentelle Untersuchung eines neuen Sympathiocolyticums, des Dihydroergotamins (DHE 45). Schweiz. med. Wschr. **77**, 28–32 (1947)
Steinberg, D., Shafrir, E., Vaughan, M.: Direct effect of glucagon on release of unesterified fatty acids (UFA) from adipose tissue. Clin. Res. **7**, 250 (1959)
Steinberg, D., Vaughan, M., Nestel, P.J., Bergström, S.: Effects of prostaglandin E opposing those of catecholamines on blood pressure and on triglyceride breakdown in adipose tissue. Biochem. Pharmacol. **12**, 764–766 (1963)
Stoll, A.: Zur Kenntnis der Mutterkornalkaloide. Verh. schweiz. naturforsch. Ges. **1920**, 190–191
Sutherland, E.W., Robison, G.A.: Metabolic effects of catecholamines. A. The role of cyclic-3′,5′-AMP in responses to catecholamines and other hormones. Pharmacol. Rev. **18**, 145–161 (1966)
Sutherland, E.W., Robison, G.A.: The role of cyclic AMP in the control of carbohydrate metabolism. Diabetes **18**, 797–819 (1969)
Sutherland, E.W., Øye, I., Butcher, R.W.: Action of epinephrine and the role of the adenyl cyclase system in hormone action. Recent Progr. Hormone Res. **21**, 623–642 (1965)

Tcherkes, L.A., Rosenfeld, E.L.: The influence of nicotinic acid on the blood sugar level and its relation to adrenaline hyperglycemia. Biokhimiya **6**, 58–66 (1941)
Tobe, M., Kurihara, N., Takeuchi, S.: Studies on intravenous glucose tolerance curve. 6. Effect of adrenergic blocking agents. Endocr. jap. **8**, 77–85 (1961)
Tolis, G., Pinter, E.J., Friesen, H.: Metabolic and endocrine actions of 2-bromo-α-ergocryptine (CB 154). Int. J. clin. Pharmacol. **10**, 151 (1974)
Vaccari, A., Vertua, R., Furlani, A.: Decreased calcium uptake by rat fundal strips after pretreatment with neuraminidase or LSD in vitro. Biochem. Pharmacol. **20**, 2603–2612 (1971)
Vigas, M., Nemeth, S.: Participation of catecholamines and glucocorticoids in metabolic changes during endotoxin fever in rabbits. Med. Pharmacol. Exp. **16**, 337–342 (1967)
Villa, R.F., Panceri, P.: Action of some drugs on performance time in mice. Farmaco **28**, 43–48 (1973)
Vogel-Chevalier, L., Hammer, W., Flückiger, E.: Influence of dihydroergotamine on the lipolytic system of isolated dog fat cells. Experientia (Basel) **27**, 674–676 (1971)
Von Euler, U.: Zur Kenntnis des Antagonismus zwischen Adrenalin und Ergotamin. Naunyn-Schmiedebergs Arch. exp. Path. Pharmak. **139**, 373–377 (1929)
Walsh, D.A., Perkins, J.P., Krebs, E.G.: An adenosine 3′,5′-monophosphate-dependent protein kinase from rabbit skeletal muscle. J. biol. Chem. **243**, 3763–3765 (1968)
Ward, W.F., Fain, J.N.: The effects of DHE upon adenyl cyclase and phosphodiesterase of rat fat cells. Biochim. biophys. Acta (Amst.) **237**, 387–390 (1971)
Webling, D.D'A.: Effects of dihydroergotamine on glucose and galactose tolerance in the rabbit. J. Pharm. Pharmacol. **25**, 500–501 (1973)
Weinryb, I., Chasin, M., Free, C.A., Harris, D.N., Goldenberg, H., Michel, I.M., Paik, V.S., Phillips, M., Samaniego, S., Hess, S.M.: Effects of therapeutic agents on cyclic AMP metabolism in vitro. J. pharm. Sci. **61**, 1556–1567 (1972)
Weiss, B., Maickel, R.P.: Sympathetic nervous control of adipose tissue lipolysis. Int. J. Neuropharmacol. **7**, 393–403 (1968)
Wenke, M., Mühlbachova, E. Hynie, S.: Effects of some sympathicotropic agents on the lipid metabolism. Arch. int. Pharmacodyn. **136**, 104–112 (1962)
West, E.St., Todd, W.R., Mason, H.S., van Bruggen, J.T.: Textbook of Biochemistry, 4th ed., p. 849. New York-London: Macmillan 1966
White, J.E., Engel, F.L.: Lipolytic action of corticotropin on rat adipose tissue in vitro. J. clin. invest. **37**, 1556–1563 (1958).
White, A., Handler, Ph., Smith E.L., Stetten, D.: Principles of Biochemistry, 2nd ed., p. 297. New York-Toronto-London: McGraw-Hill 1959
Winegrad, A.I., Renold, A.E.: Studies on rat adipose tissue in vitro. J. biol. Chem. **233**, 267–272 (1958)
Wool, I.R., Goldstein, M.S., Ramey, E.R., Levine, R.: Role of epinephrine in the physiology of fat mobilization. Amer. J. Physiol. **178**, 427–432 (1954)
Wright, P.A., Jordan, E.J., Haight, A.S.: Effectiveness of DHE in blocking epinephrine-induced hyperglycemia in rabbits and bullfrogs. Endocrinology **62**, 696–698 (1958)

CHAPTER XI

Biopharmaceutical Aspects

Analytical Methods, Pharmacokinetics, Metabolism and Bioavailability

H. ECKERT, J.R. KIECHEL, J. ROSENTHALER, R. SCHMIDT and E. SCHREIER

A. Introduction

The aim of every rational pharmacotherapy is to supply to the organism the necessary amount of drug for a certain time in order to govern the extent and duration of the biologic effect. Biopharmaceutics provides the necessary data on the fate of the pharmaceutical preparation and the drug in the organism with regard to bioavailability, absorption, distribution, metabolism and excretion. This knowledge not only makes it possible to work out the dosage regimen, but contains in addition the elements necessary for construction of the drug-release pattern of the pharmaceutical preparation, e.g., immediate release of initial dose or sustained release kinetics.

The majority of drugs are given orally, and we should take into account that the orally administered drug must pass several membranes and compartment-like barriers before it reaches the receptor sites (Fig. 1).

In general, the pharmaceutical preparation disintegrates when it comes into contact with the gastrointestinal (GI) juices. If the drug is soluble in polar solvents, it diffuses out of the particles formed and becomes available to the membranes of the GI tract for absorption. Even insoluble substances can be absorbed if the particle size is small enough. In the GI tract the drug may be altered by chemical or metabolic processes.

An absorbed substance reaches the liver via the portal vein, and from the liver it can reach quantitatively the systemic circulation. From the liver it can be secreted with the bile into the intestine where it either is excreted with the feces or reabsorbed.

The substance can be metabolized partially or completely. This reduction of the amount of absorbed drug by hepatic extraction is called the "first pass effect." The percentage of the drug that reaches the systemic circulation unchanged is, in general terms, its "bioavailability." The general circulation distributes the drug throughout the whole organism, and if the substance can permeate through the various membranes, it reaches the target organ and ultimately its receptor site.

From a biopharmaceutical standpoint, ergot compounds form a very special class in many respects. The great majority of ergot alkaloids are pharmacologically very potent, which means that they are administered in low doses. The low dose and consequently the minute drug concentration in the organism pose an analytic problem. In blood and urine, drug concentrations are in the nanogram or picogram per milliliter range. Therefore, none but the most sensitive analytic methods can be used to measure ergot concentrations in biologic material. There are, however,

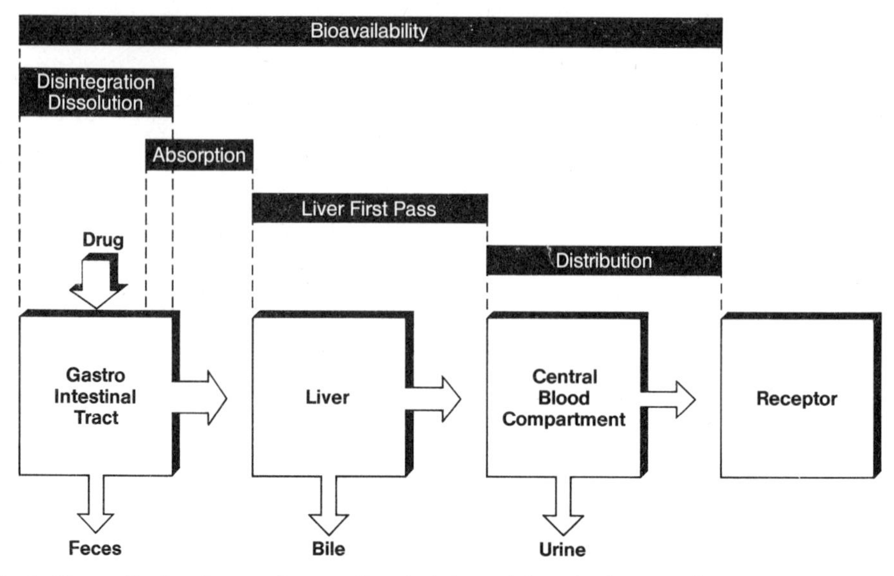

Fig. 1. Generalized pathway of an orally administered drug in the organism

still other reasons for the difficulty in analysing ergot compounds. Their low volatility and thermal instability, especially in the case of peptide alkaloids, preclude the use of gas chromatography and gas chromatography with mass-spectrometry. This limitation in analytic possibilities is reflected in the almost complete lack of bioavailability data on ergot compounds. It is hoped that the recent progress in radioimmunoassay technique will, in the near future, provide the missing information.

The only tool so far available for biopharmaceutical studies of ergot compounds is the use of radioactively labeled compounds. This procedure introduces many problems, such as radiochemical purity, label stability and the relationship between measured radioactivity and drug concentration. In view of these special analytical difficulties, we have devoted considerable space to the analytical chapter, with special emphasis on radioactivity.

With regard to absorption, bioavailability and excretion, the ergot compounds have been classified in three groups: the ergolenes with a high bioavailability and a fairly high urinary excretion; the lysergic acid and derivatives, whose absorption is between that of the ergolenes and that of the third group, the peptide alkaloids, which have a minor bioavailability and are excreted mainly with the bile. The dihydro ergot peptide alkaloids in general show the lowest bioavailability. The term bioavailability is used here in its wider sense: because of the lack of specific detection methods, most studies have been carried out measuring total radioactivity instead of unchanged drug.

In the chapter on metabolism, the same classification has been used as in the preceding chapters. Here also the methodologic problem plays a predominant role because of the minute quantities of substances to be isolated and identified. These problems are mirrored in the heterogeneity and paucity of valid information on this large and important class of chemical compounds. Recent developments in isolation and separation techniques, e.g., reversed phase high-pressure liquid chromatography, should throw more light on this.

Surveying the biopharmaceutical scene on ergot compounds in the last few decades, we must state that the relevant questions about bioavailability, placental transfer and passage through the blood-brain barrier were asked long ago, and have been answered according to the technology available at the time. The bioavailability of hydrogenated ergot alkaloids was investigated by ROTHLIN et al. (1951) using a pharmacologic test for the detection of drug concentration. Today we are in a period of high technologic development where we are able, and will be to a greater degree in the future, to detect minute amounts of drugs and their metabolites.

The pharmacologist will be increasingly called upon to quantify the biologic activity of a drug and possibly of some of its metabolites as a basis for correlating drug and metabolite concentration with pharmacologic effect.

Further developments in biopharmaceutical research will make for better characterization of the properties of existing and future drugs and will enable us to establish rational dosage regimens, controled drug release geared to therapeutic needs, and hence, improved efficacy. All these facets of biopharmaceutical research contribute to more effective and safer drug therapy.

B. Assay of Ergot Alkaloids

1. Introduction

The criteria for the acceptance of new drugs for therapeutic use in man have become very stringent. Before any drug can be accepted and used clinically some knowledge of its disposition, quantitative behavior and metabolic fate in vivo is commonly required. The investigation of these basic requirements necessitates highly sensitive analytic methods capable of detecting amounts in the nanogram to picogram range. This also applies to most of the new as well as to the oldestablished drugs belonging to the class of ergot alkaloids. Owing to their high biologic activity, the ergot alkaloids, especially their peptide analogs, are administered in very low dosage, a few milligrams a day; thus they attain very low concentrations in the body fluids. It is essential to be able to assay reproducibly the concentration of the drug in the blood, for this is the central compartment from which the compound is further distributed throughout the organism. A knowledge of blood or plasma levels, moreover, permits the calculation of pharmacokinetic values such as the apparent volume of distribution, the elimination rate constant and the plasma clearance.

To illustrate the situation in the field of ergot alkaloids, the approximate maximum therapeutic plasma concentrations in man produced by some ergot alkaloid drugs (Table 1) are contrasted with the detection limits of the analytic methods in current use (Table 2).

Owing to the analytic method used, the peak plasma concentrations in Table 1 represent the sum of the parent drug and its labeled metabolites. Because of

Table 1. Maximum plasma concentrations of some ergot compounds in man

Substance	(No.)	Dose regimen	ng/ml[a]	Ref.
Nicergoline (MNE)	(104e)	4–5 mg[b]	approx. 100–200	1
LSD	(73b)	0.16 mg[b]	approx. 3–5[e]	2
Methysergide	(34a)	1 mg[b]	16	3
		3 × 1 mg daily[c]	20 (8.5–30)	3
		3 × 2 mg daily[c]	40 (17–60)	3
Ergotamine	(20)	1 mg[b] (solution)	1.5	5
		2 mg[b] (capsule)	1	4
1-Methylergotamine	(34c)	2 mg[b]	4.5	5
Bromocriptine	(38)	3 mg[b]	6–7	5
Dihydroergotamine	(102b)	1 mg[b]	0.6	3,5
		2.5 mg[b]	1.5	3
		3 × 1 mg daily[c]	2–3	3
		3 × 2.5 mg daily[c]	5–7.5	3
Dihydroergocristine	(102c)	1 mg[b]	approx. 0.6	6
Dihydroergotoxine[d]		1 mg[b]	0.5	5

[a] Based on total radioactivity, therefore considerably lower concentration of parent drug due to extensive biotransformation.
[b] Single oral dose.
[c] Steady state.
[d] Active ingredient of the pharmaceutic speciality Hydergine.
[e] Fluorometric determination.

References: 1. ARCAMONE et al. (1972); 2. UPSHALL and WAILLING (1972); 3. MEIER and SCHREIER (1976); 4. SCHMIDT and FANCHAMPS (1974); 5. AELLIG and NÜESCH (1977); 6. BERDE et al. (1970).

Table 2. Approximate sensitivities of the most commonly used analytic methods

Analytic method	Limits of detection in plasma and urine (ng/ml)
Photometry (colorimetry)	1000–750
Fluorometry	10– 5
Phosphorimetry	10– 5
Thin-layer chromatography	10
High-pressure liquid chromatography	5
Gas chromatography	10– 0.5
Combined gas chromatography and mass spectrometry	1– 0.1
Radioimmunoassay	1– 0.1
Measurement of total radioactivity[a]:	
tritium	0.02
carbon-14	0.5

[a] Maximum single radioactive dose in man limited to 1 mCi (^3H) and 0.3 mCi (^{14}C).

the known rapid rate of biotransformation, the true plasma concentrations of the unchanged drugs are much lower, the maxima seldom exceeding 1 ng/ml in the steady state, thus rendering assay and pharmacokinetic evaluation even more difficult. For a satisfactory pharmacokinetic study it is necessary to follow the plasma concentration/time course down to at least one-tenth of the maximum concentration.

Therefore, only the methods (Table 2) which allow the determination of picogram quantities are potential analytic tools for the ergot alkaloid drugs. The method used for analysis of biologic samples obtained from a drug experiment is important. The choice of method, which should be governed by the objectives of the experiment, largely depends upon the feasibility, efficiency and sensitivity of the analytic techniques.

Even though great progress has been made during the last decade in the development of very sensitive nonradioisotopic bioanalytic techniques, the methods in current use have not proved adequate for the assay of ergot alkaloids in biologic samples at concentrations of 1 ng/ml and below. The highly sensitive gas chromatography–mass spectrometry method is of limited applicability since few ergot alkaloids are sufficiently volatile and stable to withstand gas chromatographic treatment. Therefore, the only currently available methods which satisfy the analytic requirements of human biopharmaceutical research are radioimmunoassay and the use of drugs labeled with radioisotopes.

2. Radiotracer Methods

This article gives a brief account of the most important current methods for the assay of radioactive samples obtained from labeled drug experiments. Furthermore, it touches upon problems of methodology and the disadvantages sometimes associated with the use of radioisotopic tracers.

In studies carried out with labeled drugs the measurement of total radioactivity may satisfactorily account for the total quantity of the active substance and its labeled metabolites.

Attempts at determining either the bioavailability of the active substance from an oral drug delivery system, or the bioequivalence of different dosage forms, or attempts at correlating drug concentration with degree and duration of a pharmacologic effect are more likely to be fruitful if methods more specific for the unchanged drug or for a well-established principal metabolite are used. If a reasonably complete picture of the metabolism of a drug in both the chemical and physiologic sense is desired, several analytic techniques are usually needed. Particularly useful are combinations with chromatographic separation methods, such as thin-layer, partition, liquid, or gas chromatography.

The usefulness of radioactive tracers ultimately depends upon the availability of suitably labeled drugs, reliable, rapid and accurate methods for measuring the radioactivity of the tracer isotope, and techniques for the analysis and identification of its labeled compounds.

a) Radiolabeling of Ergot Compounds

The labeling process employed must ensure that the labeled product is suitable for the use to which it will be put, i.e., the compound must possess high radiochemical purity, label stability, and adequate specific activity. Depending on the species used and the dose to be administered, specific activity may range from 0.1 to 1 mCi/mg for ^{3}H compounds and from 5 to 100 µCi/mg for ^{14}C compounds. Labeled compounds for radioimmunoassay techniques and studies on drug-binding sites should have molar specific activities exceeding 10 Ci/mmol.

A full description of what has been achieved in radioisotopic labeling of ergot alkaloids is beyond the scope of this handbook. More than a hundred papers dealing with the preparation of labeled ergot alkaloids had appeared in the literature to the end of 1976.

The application of tracers to research problems in the biosynthesis of ergot alkaloids has produced a great variety of labeled ergot alkaloids. However, only rarely are these products labeled compounds useful as intermediates for the synthesis of labeled ergot alkaloid drugs or for direct application in studies on drug disposition, pharmacokinetics and metabolism; the yield is usually too small, the specific activity too low, or the isotope may not be incorporated in the desired position in the molecule.

Only a few papers report the radiolabeling of proper ergot compounds suitable for biopharmaceutical tracer studies. Presently lysergic acid diethylamide (LSD) and dihydroergokryptine are the only labeled ergot alkaloids commercially available. Table 3 is an almost complete list of the published radiolabeled ergot alkaloids. A large number of additional ergot compounds has been labeled by SCHREIER and VOGES at the Synthetic Isotope Laboratories of Sandoz Ltd., work which hitherto has not been published.

Another unwelcome property of radiochemicals is that they are liable to decompose as a result of autoirradiation, this adversely affecting their shelf-life. All compounds labeled with radioisotopes are subject to this phenomenon, although the extent to which it occurs varies greatly depending upon the circumstances. Decomposition increases with increasing specific activity. The decomposition phenomena involved are highly complex and not yet fully understood.

The instability of tritium-labeled ergot alkaloids due to autoradiolysis is a problem of growing concern, as increasing use is being made of these compounds for radioimmunoassay (RIA) methods needing very high specific activities. Dispersion of the radioactive compounds by dissolution, in order to control the autodecomposition, is only practicable for those ergot alkaloids which are chemically stable in the appropriate solvents. As discussed by EVANS (1974), the autodecomposition rate of radioactive compounds in solution is a function both of specific activity and of radioactive concentration. In general, for high specific activities the rate of decomposition is proportional to the radioactive concentration and independent of specific activity, while for low specific activities it is proportional to specific activity and less dependent on radioactive concentration. The point at which the rate of decomposition in solution becomes independent of specific activity occurs in the range of specific activities from 1–10 Ci/mmol at radioactive concentrations of about 1 mCi/ml and less.

In practice tritiated ergot alkaloids with a high specific activity, including most ergolines, clavines and dihydrolysergic acid derivatives, are dissolved in ethanol, ethanol/benzene or ethanol/water mixtures at a radioactive concentration not exceeding 1 mCi/ml and stored under nitrogen in glass ampules, preferably in the dark below $-20°$ C. Most ergot alkaloids derived from lysergic acid cannot be stored in solution as they are unstable in the solvents commonly employed. With these compounds radiolytic autodecomposition may be minimized by storage in the dry solid state under vacuum at a temperature of $-20°$ C in sealed borosilicate-glass ampules.

Table 3. Ergot compounds labeled with radioisotopes

Compound (No.)	Labeling	Reference
Ergolines		
Methergoline MCE (89d)	9,10-^{3}H	MINGHETTI et al. (1969)
Nicergoline MNE (104e)	G-^{3}H 17-^{3}H 17-^{3}H, *nicotinic* [^{14}C]*acid*	ARCAMONE et al. (1972)
Lysergic acid derivatives		
Ergometrine (19)	4,5-^{3}H	VICARIO et al. (1967)
LSD (73b)	G-^{3}H	BRADLEY and CANDY (1970)
	2-^{3}H	Commercial product
	di[1-^{14}C]*ethyl-amine*	STOLL et al. (1954a), BARNES (1974). Commercial product
Methysergide (34a)	6-*methyl*-^{14}C	MEIER and SCHREIER (1976)
Ergot peptide alkaloids		
Ergotamine (20)	13-^{3}H 4-^{14}C	SCHREIER (1976)
1-Methylergotamine MY 25 (34c)	13-^{3}H	SCHREIER (1976)
Ergostine (22)	2-^{3}H 12-^{3}H 13-^{3}H	SCHREIER (1976)
Bromocriptine CB 154 (38)	12-^{3}H 4-^{14}C	SCHREIER (1976)
	2-^{82}Br	MARKEY et al. (1976)
5′β-Methylergoalanine MD 121 (119a)	12-^{3}H	SCHREIER (1976)
Dihydrogenated ergot peptide alkaloids		
Dihydroergotamine DHE 45 (102b)	9,10-^{3}H	MEIER and SCHREIER (1976)
Dihydroergokryptine[a]	9,10-^{3}H	WILLIAMS and LEFKOWITZ (1976) Commercial product
Dihydroergotoxine[b]	9,10-^{3}H	PLEISS and ZERJATKE (1975)

[a] Not specified if α- or β-, or mixture of both.
[b] Mixture of dihydroergocornine and dihydroergokryptine.

b) Radiochemical Purity

Radiochemical purity is one of the well-known problems associated with the use of radiolabeled compounds. It is important to use compounds which have a high radiochemical purity, or at least compounds which do not contain impurities that affect the interpretation of the experimental data. The usual criteria for chemical purity, such as melting point, ultraviolet (UV), infrared (IR), nuclear magnetic resonance (NMR) spectra and elemental analysis, are helpful, but not sufficient on their own. Chromatographic separations used in conjunction with sensitive radioactivity detection techniques are generally the most effective method of establishing radiochemical purity. In order to obtain reliable information a variety of chromatography systems should be used.

As a pure radioactive substance may undergo radiation-induced chemical decomposition on storage, it is important to know the radiochemical purity at the time the experiment is begun. Depending on the objectives of the experiment it may be necessary to repurify the labeled compound. In metabolism studies the same chromatography systems used to detect metabolites should also be used to characterize the administered drug in order to avoid the discovery of metabolites which are in reality degradation products originally present in the labeled substance.

The procedure generally used in our laboratories (SCHREIER, 1976) to assess the radiochemical purity of ergot alkaloids labeled with ^{3}H and ^{14}C is as follows: samples equivalent to 0.05–0.1 μCi (^{14}C compounds) and 1–2 μCi (^{3}H compounds), dissolved in methanol or chloroform, are chromatographed on commercial plates ($5 \times 20 \times 0.025$ cm) precoated with silica gel 60 F254 or aluminium oxide F254. At least two different solvent systems are used for each support. After development the thin-layer chromatograms are assayed for radioactivity with a commercial thin-layer scanner. Quantitative values are obtained by electronic peak integration of the ratemeter curve or by scraping 5 mm wide zones from the plates for analysis by liquid scintillation techniques.

The method is readily capable of detecting and estimating 0.2–0.5% of radiochemical impurities. Up to 5% of radiochemical impurities is generally of little consequence in biologic tracer work. However, it is advantageous to be aware of any impurities present since they affect the reliability of data on excretion, tissue localization, etc., of small amounts of radioactivity and trace metabolites.

The chemical purity of labeled ergot alkaloids and their identity with unlabeled reference compounds is usually checked by UV and IR spectroscopy and by thin-layer chromatography of 50-μg samples. The spots are best visualized by UV (254 nm), followed by spraying with Van Urk or Dragendorff reagent.

Further proof of radiochemical purity may occasionally be obtained by "inverse isotope dilution analysis" (Review: e.g. Radiochemical Centre Amersham, 1964). In addition to radio thin-layer chromatography, this technique has been applied in our laboratories to check the purity of "superactive" dihydrogenated ergot alkaloids labeled with ^{3}H (30–50 mCi/mg) for use as radioactive antigens in RIA procedures. The compounds are prepared from the 13-bromo precursors by catalytic halogen-tritium replacement and stored in ethanol at a concentration of 10 μg/ml (radioactive concentration approximately 300–500 μCi/ml).

Analytical checks have shown that, if properly stored, "superactive" dihydro[13-^{3}H]ergot alkaloids of the peptide type, such as dihydroergotamine, dihydroergonine, dihydroergocristine, dihydroergocornine, and dihydroergokryptine, remain suitable for RIA purposes for a period of about one year from the date of preparation.

c) Label Stability

Another very important factor in appraising the usefulness of ^{3}H and ^{14}C compounds as radioactive tracers is the stability of the label under the experimental conditions. The use of radioisotopes as tracers presupposes that the radioactive atoms remain attached to the molecules being traced.

One aspect of this problem concerns the stability of tritium attached to carbon atoms. If tritium does not "leak" from the compound in a hydroxylic solvent over a wide range of pH values, this is taken as sufficient evidence of chemical stability.

A simple procedure in which aqueous test solutions were maintained under acidic, neutral and alkaline conditions at 50° for 24 h was used to check the tritium label of tritiated ergot alkaloids for resistance to chemical exchange (SCHREIER, 1976). The currently available information on the chemical stability of ^{3}H-labeled positions in ergot alkaloids is summarised in Table 4. Tritium atoms located at positions 4, 5 and 13 of the tetracyclic ergolene system and at positions 9, 10 and 13 of the ergoline derivatives proved stable in both acidic and alkaline medium. For the ergot alkaloids labeled at position 12, the tritium-hydrogen exchange rate occasionally reached 12% under alkaline conditions, whereas the label at this position is stable in neutral and acidic medium. A tritium atom in position 2 was found to be by far the most unstable under acidic conditions. The tritium label at position 8 of 9-ergolene derivatives with an 8-carboxyl group is partially lost by change of configuration at this chiral centre, as was observed by AGURELL (1966b). The tritium label in a variety of side-chains linked to carbon 8 was found to be stable over the entire pH range. The $-CT_2CN$ group of homolysergic acid nitrile (83a)[1] was an exception; tritium was almost completely lost on alkaline hydrolysis to homolysergic acid (84a).

Although the stability of the label to chemical exchange was not very satisfactory in some cases, most of the [^{3}H]ergot alkaloids bearing an acid-labile tracer proved adequate for biological experiments. It should, however, be noted that even tritium atoms which have proved stable in chemical tests may prove labile under biological conditions.

The loss of a radioactive atom may ensue in a biotransformation process resulting in a chemical change of the molecule. Examples of this are the oxidation of a ^{14}C-labeled N-methyl group to [^{14}C]carbon dioxide or the replacement of an aromatic tritium atom by a hydroxyl group. Furthermore, even if tritium is biologically stable in the parent compound, it may come to occupy an unstable position in its metabolites.

Clearly when isotope loss occurs, measurement of radioactivity may no longer serve for quantitative characterization of the fate of the parent compound and its metabolites since part of the radioactivity detected may be due simply to the presence of tritiated body water, hydrogen[^{14}C]carbonate or compounds in which ^{3}H or ^{14}C from tritiated water or [^{14}C]carbonate have been incorporated by biosynthesis. On the other hand, if the purpose of the experiment is to detect major metabolites rather than to measure their actual concentrations, fairly marked label instability may be of no consequence.

Biolability of ^{14}C labels can generally be recognized by assaying the expired air for [^{14}C]carbon dioxide or the urinary excreted urea for ^{14}C-content.

In the present incomplete state of our knowledge of metabolism of ergot alkaloids, definite evidence of the biologic stability of labels can only be obtained by the actual experiment. In the case of ergot alkaloids, metabolic attack at a

[1] Numbers in parentheses following the name of a compound refer to structural formula given in Chapter II.

Table 4. Stability of the tritium label to chemical exchange of generally and specifically labeled ergot alkaloids in acidic, alkaline, and neutral aqueous media determined after treatment at 50° for 24 h

Label position[d]	Alkaloid types tested	Stability[a] of ^{3}H-label		
		pH ~1	pH ~13	pH ~7–8
Generally (labeling pattern not determined)	Lysergic acid[b]	Moderate to unstable	Stable	
	6-Methyl-8-amino-ergoline[c]	Stable	Stable	
	Bromocriptine (CB154)[c]	Stable	Stable	
2	Lysergic acid amides, ergot peptide alkaloids, dihydroergot peptide alkaloids	Unstable	Stable	Stable to moderate
4,5	Paspalic acid, lysergic acid	Stable	Stable	
8	Lysergic acid	^{3}H-loss by change of the configuration at C-8 (AGURELL, 1966b)		
9,10	Ergolines, dihydrolysergic acid and derivatives: amides, esters; dihydroergot peptide alkaloids	Stable	Stable	
12	Paspalic acid, lysergic acid, ergot peptide alkaloids, 1-methyl and 2-bromo-lysergic acid derived alkaloids	Stable	Moderate to unstable	Stable
13	Paspalic acid, lysergic acid, ergot peptide alkaloids, dihydrolysergic acid and derivatives, dihydroergot peptide alkaloids	Stable to moderate	Stable	Stable
17	Lysergol, lysergylamines: PTR 17–402 (88e), 18–658 (88f); CF 25–397 (90d)	Stable	Stable	
	Homolysergic acid nitrile (83a)	Stable	Unstable	
8′	Aminocyclol (ergotamine series)	Stable	Stable	

[a] Stable: tritium loss <5%; moderate: tritium loss >5 and <10%; unstable: tritium loss >10%.
[b] Platinum catalyzed exchange labeling with tritiated water.
[c] Exchange labeling with platinum oxide and tritium gas in dimethylformamide.
[d] Numbering according to the nomenclature of Chapter II. Chemical Background.

labeled position followed by the loss of the tracer atom has so far been observed only in compounds with a labeled methyl group in position 1 of the indole ring, e.g., [1-*methyl*-^{14}C]methysergide (34a) and [1-*methyl*-^{14}C]1-methylergotamine (34c).

The biostability of the [6-*methyl*-^{14}C] label of bromocriptine (38) was verified by comparing the excretion in urine and feces of intact rats and the excretion in bile and urine of rats with bile duct fistulas following oral administration of [4-^{14}C]bromocriptine and [6-*methyl*-^{14}C]bromocriptine (KIECHEL, 1976). For the [4-^{14}C]-labeled compound, the loss of the label by a biotransformation process is improbable.

The biologic stability of tritium labels can be tested in various ways:

1. Retention of specific activity: In this test the specific activity of the material recovered from the biologic system is compared with that of the administered compound. The test is only valid for compounds which are exogenous to the particular biologic system, so that there is no isotopic dilution by endogenous synthesis.

2. Urinary tritium water: The absence of tritium as tritiated water in the distillate of urine samples collected after administration of the ^{3}H-compound is another general test for the biostability of the tritium label. The test is valid even when the compound is metabolized and is the method of choice in our laboratories for determining total tritiated water formed in pharmacokinetic studies of [^{3}H]ergot alkaloids (NIMMERFALL and ROSENTHALER, 1976; SCHMIDT and FANCHAMPS, 1974; MEIER and SCHREIER, 1976). However, it must be borne in mind that tritium and hydrogen may transfer intra- and intermolecularly without actual exchange with body water.

3. Double isotope technique: In this method pharmacokinetic rate constants, for example the biologic half-life of the tritiated compound, are compared with the corresponding constants for the same compound labeled with carbon-14. If the values are identical for both labeled compounds it may be inferred that no tritium is lost by exchange in vivo. An extension of this method consists in administering the compound doubly labeled with tritium and carbon-14 and comparing the ratio of ^{3}H:^{14}C before administration with that in the body fluids and excretion products. Identical isotope ratios demonstrate the integrity of both ^{3}H and ^{14}C labeling.

Double isotope techniques have been applied to verify the biostability of the label of [13-^{3}H]ergotamine (20) and of [12-^{3}H]bromocriptine (38) by comparing the elimination characteristics with those of the corresponding ^{14}C-labeled compounds [4-^{14}C]ergotamine and [4-^{14}C]bromocriptine, respectively.

d) Measurement of Radioactivity

Liquid scintillation counting has become the method of choice for the measurement of radioactivity in pharmacokinetic and metabolic studies of all kinds of organic compounds, including biochemicals and drugs usually labeled with pure low energy β-particle emitters such as tritium and carbon-14.

Besides scintillation measurement, gas ionization counting is used in radio paper and thin-layer chromatography and in radio gas chromatography. The distribution pattern of radioactivity on paper and thin-layer chromatograms and in animal whole body or tissue sections can be visualized by autoradiography.

Scintillation counting has proved highly versatile and convenient for the determination of both tritium and carbon-14, hence it is not surprising that numerous publications, including many reviews, have appeared on the subject. For more detailed information on general or particular aspects of liquid scintillation counting, the reader is referred to recently published textbooks. DYER (1974), NEAME and HOMEWOOD (1974), provide a useful introduction to the subject. HORROCKS (1974), KOBAYASHI and MAUDSLEY (1974), SIMON (1974), deal with the application of the techniques. STANLEY and SCOGGINS (1974) and CROOK and JOHNSON (1974), contain reports of papers read at symposia, etc. BIRKS (Koch-Light, 1975), NICOLL and EWER (Nuclear Enterprises, 1971), RAPKIN (Intertechnique), RAPKIN (New England Nuclear), TURNER (Radiochemical Centre Amersham, 1971), and Laboratorium Prof. Dr. Berthold (1973), are publications by manufacturers of radioisotopes and measuring equipment.

Apart from radioimmunoassay (RIA) there are no radioanalytic methods specific to ergot alkaloids, hence a brief account will now be given of the general procedure employed in our laboratories for measuring the radioactivity of samples collected from tracer experiments with radiolabeled ergot alkaloids (MESZAROS et al., 1975; NIMMERFALL and ROSENTHALER, 1976; MEIER and SCHREIER, 1976; SCHREIER, 1976).

Samples of plasma, bile and urine containing ^{14}C, urine samples containing ^{3}H, as well as pure ^{3}H- and ^{14}C-ergot alkaloids in organic solvents (chloroform, methanol or mixtures of both) are directly assayed for radioactivity by mixing duplicate 0.1- or 0.5 ml aliquots of each sample with 5 ml or 15 ml of a liquid scintillation cocktail in counting vials. Instagel (Packard) or a solution of 0.6% of butyl-PBD in ethanol-toluene 6:4 is generally used.

Radioactivity due to tritium water in urine samples is determined in the distillates of freeze-dried urine aliquots by the same procedure and subtracted from total radioactivity. Since tritium water radioactivity may account for a considerable proportion of the total radioactivity of plasma samples containing ^{3}H, 0.4 ml aliquots of each sample are dried at 80° for 45 min and combusted in a sample oxidizer. The tritiated water formed is trapped in either Instagel or Monophase.

Blood, tissue and feces are combusted for determination of radioactivity. Prior to combustion, feces are first homogenized with water to a fine slurry, and aliquots of the homogenized material are then processed like blood and tissue. Duplicate samples of known wet weight, dispensed on special filter papers, are vacuum dried at 40° overnight and combusted either by the oxygen flask technique of KALBERER and RUTSCHMANN (1961) or by means of a commercially available sample oxidizer. The labeled oxidation products are absorbed in liquid scintillant mixtures to yield homogenous counting solutions.

In work on the biotransformation of ergot alkaloids and the structure of their metabolites, the radioactive constituents of body fluids after administration of the labeled compounds may be efficiently separated by column chromatography. The detection of the radioactive fractions in the column effluent may be performed either discontinuously by taking an aliquot of every collected fraction for radioactivity measurement or continuously by splitting (9:1) the effluent of the column and mixing the one-tenth split continuously with scintillant for counting in a commercially available liquid scintillation flow counter which registers the counts on a suitable recorder (SCHRAM, 1970; WENZEL, 1974). FIGGE et al. (1975) describe a measuring system which permits the use of detectors for counting homogenous mixtures of effluent and scintillant as well as a detector equipped with a solid scintillator. Solid scintillators are less suitable for ^3H compounds since the counting efficiency is less than 0.1%.

e) Autoradiography

Autoradiographic techniques may be used to locate radioactivity in radiochromatograms as well as in whole body and tissue sections of animals (FISCHER and WERNER, 1971). In autoradiography the specimen containing the radioactive material is placed in contact with a photographic emulsion. The β particles from the disintegration of the radioactive isotope affect the grains of silver halide in the emulsion in the same manner as light. Developing and fixing the emulsion produces a photographic image which locates the radioactivity.

α) Autoradiography of Radiochromatograms

Autoradiographic detection of pure low energy β-particle emitters on paper and thin-layer chromatograms is routinely used in many laboratories for checking the radiochemical purity of labeled compounds and for elucidating the metabolic pattern in biotransformation studies.

A typical TLC autoradiogram of [^{14}C]paspalic acid (7) biosynthesised from DL-[^{14}C]tryptophan in submerged cultures of *Claviceps paspali* has been published by AGURELL (1966a).

β) Macroautoradiography

Macroautoradiography is the method of choice for determining the distribution of a labeled substance throughout the whole body. The alternative method of obtaining the same information is to carry out a normal dissection and examine the tissue samples as described in the previous chapter.

The limitations of macroautoradiography are that it can be employed only for small animals such as mice, rats, cats, guinea pigs and rabbits (KALBERER, 1969a) and that the information obtained is mainly qualitative. Its great advantage is that the whole distribution pattern can be seen as a picture, and that concentrations of labeled substances can be detected in areas in the body which are not usually included in dissection.

Several techniques habe been described (ULLBERG, 1963; KALBERER, 1966). The first step is common to all methods. The test animal is frozen in a mixture of dry-ice/acetone, dry-ice/heptane or other freezing medium. Freezing prevents the test substance from diffusing and gives the animal the right consistency for sectioning.

Sectioning can be performed on a microtome in a freezing cabinet at about −15° C (ULLBERG, 1963) or with a circular hard-metal saw (KALBERER, 1966).

The microtome sections are mounted on adhesive tape for stability and freeze-dried. The dried sections are then placed on film for exposure.

The sawed sections are kept in the frozen state and placed on a precooled X-ray film for exposure at −25° to −30° C. The exposure time depends on the isotope used, the dose of radioactivity administered and the characteristics of the film. KALBERER (1966) recommends 30 days exposure for a dose of 10 mCi ^{3}H per kg body wt. and 10 days exposure for a dose of 50 μCi ^{14}C per kg body wt.

Although macroautoradiography is mainly used to obtain qualitative information, quantitative evaluation is possible by measuring the blackening of the film (ECKERT and HOPF, 1969; CROSS et al., 1974).

γ) High-Resolution Microautoradiography

Ergot alkaloids are diffusible substances and cannot therefore be investigated by conventional autoradiography. They are soluble in the fixation and dehydration media which are used in the histologic preparation.

Various techniques used for autoradiography of diffusible substances have been reviewed by ROTH and STUMPF (1969). The essential points are the following: Tissues must be removed from the experimental animal without delay and frozen quickly to prevent diffusion of the substances to be detected; freeze-sectioning of the tissues is performed in a cryostat, and the sections are brought in contact with a nuclear emulsion; exposure is performed at a temperature below −15° C.

An alternative method to freeze-sectioning is freeze-drying, followed by embedding and conventional autoradiographic techniques. This alternative is limited in its applications by the difficulty of finding an embedding medium in which the test substance is not soluble.

ARNOLD et al. (1958) published a study on the distribution of [^{14}C]LSD (73b) in the brain, liver and kidney of mice killed 20 or 60 min after intraperitoneal administration of a dose of about 10 mg [^{14}C]LSD per kg body wt., equivalent to about 70 μCi ^{14}C per kg body wt. The ^{14}C was located in the ethyl groups of the side-chain. After the animals had been sacrificed, the blood vessels of the brain were flushed with Compensan. The various specimens were frozen in propane, cooled with liquid nitrogen, and freeze-dried. They were then embedded in paraffin wax and processed by conventional histologic methods.

DIAB et al. (1971) studied the cellular localization of [^{3}H]LSD in the rat brain. One half of the brain was processed by the freeze-sectioning technique, the other half was processed by conventional histologic methods for investigation of binding. In this way it was possible to differentiate between free and bound LSD in the brain tissue. In this experiment a dose of 1.7 mg d-lysergic acid diethylamide tartrate, randomly labeled with ^{3}H in the side-chain (520 μCi/mg), was administered intravenously.

Techniques are available for electron-microscopic autoradiography of diffusible substances (ROTH and STUMPF, 1969), but they have not yet been applied to the ultrastructural localization of ergot alkaloids.

3. Nonradioisotopic Physicochemical Methods

The most important analytic methods in current use for the separation and assay of ergot alkaloids have been briefly presented in Chapter II of this monograph.

The present section deals in greater depth with analytic procedures which have been applied or are thought to be suitable for the assay of ergot alkaloids either in body fluids and tissues after administration of unlabeled ergot alkaloid drugs or in biologic in vitro systems.

a) Spectrophotometry and Colorimetry

The distinct UV-absorption maximum and the high extinction of LSD (73b) at 311 nm in ethanol solution were used by NEKRASOV and DAVYDOVA (1970) to determine microgram amounts of the drug in cat blood following administration of 0.5–0.8 mg/kg body wt. The procedure consists in the thin-layer chromatographic separation of a 50 µl blood sample on silica gel with 9:1 dichloromethane/methanol as the mobile phase, location of the LSD spot by UV light, double elution of the marked zone with 5 ml 95% ethanol, measurement of the optical density of the eluate, and comparison of the data with a standard concentration curve for LSD. Linearity was observed over a concentration range of 5–25 µg/ml.

KOPET and DILLE (1942) employed a colorimetric method to evaluate the rate of elimination of ergotoxine, ergotamine (20) and ergometrine (19) from the blood and muscle of guinea pigs after intracardial administration of sublethal doses of ergotoxine ethanesulphonate (16 mg/kg), ergotamine tartrate (25 mg/kg) and ergometrine tartrate (25 mg/kg). This analytic method is based on the color reaction of ergot alkaloids with p-dimethylaminobenzaldehyde as described by VAN URK (1929) and later developed to a standard procedure by SMITH (1930) and ALLPORT and COCKING (1932).

The procedure involves the extraction of the alkaloid from blood (10–15 ml) or tissues (about 50 g) with ether, reextraction of the alkaloid from the ether phase into aqueous tartaric acid solution, treatment of this solution with the Van Urk reagent, and estimation of the intensity of the blue color in a photoelectric colorimeter. The concentration of the alkaloid is then determined from a standard concentration curve. The limit of detection was about 5 µg. The method proved sufficiently sensitive for estimating drug concentrations for about 5–7 h after administration. The method entailed sacrificing an animal at given intervals of time, this giving rise to additional variations due to individual differences.

The colorimetric assay is not specific unless the constituents of an alkaloid mixture are separated prior to analysis.

b) Fluorescence Spectrometry

The versatile and very sensitive fluorometric method of BOWMAN et al. (1955) for the assay of 9-ergolene derivatives has been widely used for estimation of LSD (73b) in biologic materials such as body fluids and tissue homogenates. The accuracy and specificity of the LSD assay largely depends on the extraction and purification procedures used for preparation of the samples.

α) LSD and Related Lysergic Acid Amides

In the method of AXELROD et al. (1957) LSD is extracted from biologic material (up to 5 ml plasma, cerebrospinal fluid, bile, or tissue homogenates of experimental animals) with n-heptane containing 2% isoamylalcohol (25 ml), saturated with sodium chloride (3 g) and rendered alkaline with 1 *N* sodium hydroxide (0.5 ml). The drug is subsequently extracted from the heptane phase (20 ml) with 0.004 *N* hydrochloric acid (3 ml). The drug content is determined by measuring fluorescence of an aliquot of the acid extract at 445 nm after activation at 325 nm. This method permits the determination of LSD in concentrations as low as 1 ng/5 ml. The drug added to biologic material was recovered quantitatively ($95 \pm 6\%$).

This fluorometric assay method has been widely employed for the determination of submicrogram quantities of LSD in biologic fluids and tissue preparations for a wide range of biologic and biochemical experiments in vivo and in vitro, e.g., to study drug distribution in rats (DOEPFNER, 1962), distribution in macroscopic areas and subcellular fractions of monkey brain (SNYDER and REIVICH, 1966) and of rat brain (FARAGALLA, 1972); elimination from rat brain after various intraperitoneal doses of LSD (ROSECRANS et al., 1967); binding to rat brain preparations (MARCHBANKS, 1966). It has also been employed for in vitro studies of binding to calf thymus deoxyribonucleic acid (YIELDING and STERGLANZ, 1968), etc.

A modified fluorometric procedure developed by NIWAGUCHI and INOUE (1971) has been used to determine the unchanged substrate and the products of enzymatic transformation obtained by incubating LSD and closely related compounds with rat liver microsomes in vitro (NIWAGUCHI et al., 1974b). The unchanged substrate and metabolites were extracted and separated by thin-layer chromatography and were assayed by fluorometric scanning, either directly or with the aid of internal standards such as quinine. The excitation and emission wavelengths were 330 and 410 nm, respectively.

This fluorometric assay was later developed to a standard procedure for the assay of ergot alkaloids, permitting accurate estimation of 15–200 ng (EICH and SCHUNACK, 1975).

The more sensitive method of AXELROD was adopted by AGHAJANIAN and BING (1964) to determine the plasma levels of LSD over an 8-hour period following intravenous administration to human subjects of 2 µg LSD tartrate/kg body wt. The study confirmed that the fluorometric method permitted the assay of LSD in concentrations down to 1 ng/5 ml in plasma samples. The assay proved reliable provided fluorescent contaminants were eliminated. With plasma samples, excellent linearity was obtained with internal standards, the deviation ranging from 0 to 6.5%.

When the Axelrod method was used to determine LSD in human plasma after administration of a single oral dose of 0.16 mg, it was noted that a fluorescent blank of variable intensity was present, and that it was of sufficient magnitude to interfere seriously with the assay (UPSHALL and WAILLING, 1972). The interference was eliminated by exploiting an observation of STOLL and SCHLIENTZ (1955). They noted that UV irradiation of LSD in aqueous solution catalyzed the addition of water to the 9,10 double bond, producing a nonfluorescent lumiderivative. The difference in fluorescence of plasma extracts before and after intense UV irradiation was taken as a measure of LSD concentration.

The improved method for assaying LSD in human plasma is carried out as follows:

1. Plasma is immediately separated from the blood samples by centrifugation and stored at −20° C.

2. Extraction with n-heptane: plasma (2 ml), sodium chloride (1 g), 1 *N* sodium hydroxide (0.1 ml), n-heptane (10 ml) are shaken for 30 min. The heptane extract is separated off by centrifugation at 1500 *g* for 5 min.

3. Extraction with acid: the heptane extract (8 ml) is added to 0.004 *N* hydrochloric acid (3 ml) and shaken for 10 min. The two phases are separated by centrifugation, the heptane layer is removed by suction and an aliquot (1 ml) of the acid extract is transferred to a quartz cuvette.

4. Spectrofluorometry: a wavelength of 318 nm is used for activation and the emission wavelength is 413 nm.

5. UV irradiation: after measurement of the fluorescence the acid extract is transferred to a glass tube and exposed to UV light (254 nm) for 3 h. The fluorescence is then read again. The difference of the readings corresponds to the fluorescence of the drug, and the residual fluorescence is the blank reading.

A method for screening the urine of persons taking LSD is described by FAED and MCLOED (1973). The Axelrod extraction procedure had to be modified for the assay in urine since it was necessary to carry out enzymatic hydrolysis before extraction in order to detect the drug. The extraction from heptane with dilute acid was also found to be unsuitable for urine samples, and to avoid high background fluorescence it was necessary to use a chromatographic step to separate LSD from some of the interfering urinary constituents. LSD and its metabolites were still detectable in human urine for as long as 4 days after ingestion of 0.2 mg of the drug.

Difficulties experienced in an attempt to screen human gastric fluid for LSD are reported by MUELLER and LANG (1973).

It has been reported that LSD and related lysergic and isolysergic acid amides can be conveniently assayed in biologic material by fluorometric techniques: isoergine (=isolysergic acid amide) (VOGEL et al., 1972), BOL 148 (37a) (=2-bromolysergic acid diethylamide) (NIWAGUCHI et al., 1974b), methergine (73a) (BIANCHINE et al., 1967), methysergide (34a) (DOEPFNER, 1962; BIANCHINE et al., 1967).

β) Ergot Peptide Alkaloids

Ergot alkaloids derived from lysergic acid and containing a cycloltype peptide moiety fluoresce strongly at 400–425 nm in absolute or aqueous ethanolic solution when activated at about 340 nm. Based on these properties, a fluorometric method for assaying ergotamine (20) and related peptide alkaloids in plasma has been developed by PACHA (1969a) and EADIE (1972).

EADIE does not give the detailed procedure, but reports a lower limit of detection of about 2 ng/ml for ergotamine in 5-ml samples of human plasma.

In PACHA's method the drug is extracted with diethyl ether from plasma rendered alkaline (pH 8–10) with 1 *N* sodium carbonate. The drug is extracted from the ether phase with 0.2 *N* aqueous tartaric acid. For the fluorometric measurement ethanol is added to the tartaric acid extract to give a final ethanol content of 60%. This procedure permitted the determination of approximately 10 ng peptide alkaloid in 2–5 ml of rat plasma. Since it is the lysergic acid moiety of the ergot alkaloid molecule which fluoresces, any metabolites extracted by the solvent systems used would be included in the assay.

Neither procedure was sensitive enough for measurement of plasma levels in human subjects receiving therapeutic doses.

Peptide alkaloids derived from dihydrolysergic acid do not have the 9,10 double bond and their fluorescense maxima are both less intense and shifted to shorter wavelengths (290/360 nm). Exploiting the fact that suitably fluorescent derivatives may be obtained by reacting indoles, for example serotonin (MAICKEL and MILLER, 1966) or pindolol (PACHA, 1969b), with o-phthalaldehyde in the presence of sulphuric acid, PACHA (1971) developed a sensitive fluorometric assay for dihydrogenated peptide alkaloids of ergot. The procedure was found to be sufficiently accurate for quantities down to 10 ng using 1- to 5-ml plasma samples, but was not suitable for the assay of dihydrogenated ergot alkaloids in urine, as interference gave rise to variable, high blank values.

c) Gas Chromatography

Relatively few reports have appeared on the analysis of ergot alkaloids by gas chromatography (RADECKA and NIGAM, 1966; LERNER, 1967; LERNER and KATSIAFICAS, 1969; AGURELL and OHLSSON, 1971; JANE and WHEALS, 1973; BARROW and QUIGLEY, 1975). None of the methods described has so far been used to assay ergot alkaloids in biologic material. They have been used primarily to test the suitability of gas chromatography for the separation, characterization and identification of ergot alkaloids, particularly in conjunction with spectroscopic techniques such as UV spectroscopy, IR spectroscopy, spectrofluorometry or mass spectrometry.

In the light of our present knowledge it may be stated that all clavine alkaloids of low molecular weight (240–300) can be gas chromatographed satisfactorily. The peaks are generally acceptable, but clavine alkaloids containing hydroxyl groups show tailing. Attempts to overcome this by the formation of suitable derivatives has so far proved unsuccessful.

Of the lysergic acid derivatives, only the simpler amides such as lysergic acid amide (18), LSD (73b) and lysergic acid methylcarbinolamide (12) (the latter after pyrolysis in the injector to lysergic acid amide) could be chromatographed at relatively high column temperatures (240°–270°). The more complex amides of higher molecular weight and the ergot peptide alkaloids may be expected to decompose in the injection port or on the column to give a pattern of several fragments.

A general gas-liquid chromatographic screening system designed to detect common poisons, drugs, and human metabolites encountered in forensic toxicology has been proposed for demonstrating the presence or absence of ergot alkaloids (e.g., methysergide, ergotamine, ergocristine and ergokryptine) in human blood, urine and tissue specimens after appropriate extraction (FINKLE et al., 1971). The lower limit of detection is 2 μg/ml.

Mass spectrometric analysis of the gas chromatographic effluent is the best technique at present available for measurement of nanogram to picogram quantities. Several small, mobile mass spectrometers equipped with combined electron impact/chemical ionization sources designed specifically for the direct coupling of a gas chromatograph with a mass spectrometer are now commercially available. However, the recent phenomenal growth of the literature on combined gas chromatography and mass spectrometry is in marked contrast to the meager use of this analytic tool in the field of ergot alkaloids. Although useful mass spectra of quite a number of individual, pure ergot alkaloids have been recorded (BARBER et al., 1965; CHAN LIN et al., 1967; RAMSTAD et al., 1967; SHOUGH and TAYLOR, 1969; NIWAGUCHI et al., 1974a, b; VOIGT et al., 1974), all attempts to use the gas chromatography/mass spectrometry technique to assay ergot alkaloids which are known to chromatograph satisfactorily have failed to give reproducible results.

The principal difficulties encountered in the detection of ergot alkaloids in trace amounts may arise from several causes, such as uncontrollable fragmentation, column adsorption, memory effects, interfering background due to the stationary phase, and unsuitable trapping of the substance in the effluent from the gas chromatograph. Attempts to overcome these problems have not yet met with success.

Plasma chromatography, another recently developed method for the detection and assay of ultratraces of organic compounds is reported to be especially well suited for the analysis of gas chromatographic effluents (KARASEK et al., 1975). In this technique use is made of the characteristic positive and negative ion mobility spectra which are produced by an ion-molecule reaction between the trace amount of organic compound and the reactant ions or electrons generated. Ions for the reaction are generated by the action of 60-KeV electrons emitted from a nickel-63 foil into purified nitrogen or air carrier gas containing a trace of water vapor. The procedure operates at atmospheric pressure and the lower limit of detection is in the microgram to picogram range.

The value of this method for the analysis of ergot alkaloids cannot yet be assessed since so far LSD is the only ergot compound for which a reference mobility spectrum has been published.

d) High-Pressure Liquid Chromatography

Of the various chromatographic methods for separation and assay of ergot alkaloids, pressure-assisted liquid chromatography appears to be superior to gas chromatographic methods. Because of the low vapor pressure and the thermal instability of lysergic acid amides and ergot peptide alkaloids, liquid chromatographic systems (paper chromatography, thin-layer chromatography, and high-pressure liquid chromatography) are the only suitable methods for chromatographic separations.

In a preliminary study HEACOCK et al. (1973) confirmed the value of high-pressure liquid chromatography (HPLC) for the separation and determination of ergot alkaloids. The procedure was subsequently adopted for the assay and identification of LSD in a wide variety of illicit preparations (WITTWER and KLUCKHOHN, 1973; JANE and WHEALS, 1973). The best results were obtained by using a reversed-phase system (e.g., stationary phase: Corasil C_{18}, mobile phase: 6:4 methanol–0.1% aqueous ammonium carbonate).

Recently a combination of HPLC and thin-layer chromatography has been found to be satisfactory for the isolation and identification of LSD in biologic liquids, especially in the urine of suspected illicit users (CHRISTIE et al., 1976). Mass spectrometry has been employed for additional confirmation of identity.

Occasionally, the extracts of some preparations screened with the UV detector gave large signals on the chromatogram due to coextractives derived from tablet excipients. This problem was solved by using a fluorometric detector which yielded chromatograms displaying a linear relationship between signal and quantity of LSD injected over the range 0–750 ng. The lower limit of detection for LSD was about 2–10 ng.

For high-pressure liquid chromatography, another reversed-phase system with solvent gradient has been reported to be an efficient method for testing the purity of ergotamine and assaying the ergotamine content of pharmaceutical preparations (BETHKE et al., 1976). Because of its good resolution, this system can be used not only for the selective assay of ergotamine, but also for the identification and assay of isomerization and degradation products.

An additional advantage of the liquid chromatographic method over other chromatographic methods is that it permits collection of the compound for further examination, notably for identification by mass spectrometry. The major limitation of the use of high-pressure liquid chromatography for the analysis of body fluids and tissue preparations is the lack of sensitivity of the available UV detectors.

4. Radioimmunoassay

Another technique is the competitive inhibition between labeled and unlabeled ligand by using antibodies to detect compounds in biologic fluids. Suitable antibodies are produced by immunizing animals with an ergot alkaloid bound to some carrier molecule, e.g., protein. The compound to be measured competes with the labeled species for the available binding sites on the antibody. This method allows the detection of an amount of ergot alkaloid in the picogram range.

a) Lysergic Acid and Derivatives

VAN VUNAKIS et al. (1971) obtained an antiserum by immunizing rabbits with a conjugate of polylysine and lysergic acid amide (ergine) (18) bound to succinylated hemocyanin. The antibody was tested for specificity against psychomimetic compounds, neurotransmitter substances and a number of compounds with various chemical structures. The method was not very specific: 50% inhibition of the antigen-antibody reaction using ergine as the antigen was attained with a quantity of 3–5 pmol of various lysergic acid derivatives [ergonovine (19), methylergonovine (73a) and LSD (73b) as well as with ergot peptide alkaloids ergotamine (20) and ergosine (109a)]. *d*-Lysergic acid (8) produced the same level of inhibition only in 8–10 times higher concentration. The discrepant low inhibitory effect of the free lysergic acid is attributed to the nature of the conjugate binding: amide linkages are formed when the lysergic acid molecules combine with free amino groups of the homopolymer. An antiserum produced in this way reacts particularly with ergine and also with N-substituted lysergic acid amides. In the presence of a lysergic acid conjugate labeled with iodine-125 the antiserum has been used to detect LSD. To separate the bound fraction from the free fraction the LSD protein complex was precipitated with goat anti-rabbit γ-globulin. This test would detect quantities of LSD down to 1 pmol (approximately 300 pg).

As a modification of the method discussed TAUNTON-RIGBY et al. (1973) coupled LSD with serum albumin with the aid of the Mannich reaction (BLICKE, 1942) between phenols (here the tyrosine residues of the albumin) and secondary amines (LSD) in the presence of formaldehyde. The LSD is presumably linked to the albumin at the indole-nitrogen. Immunization of New Zealand rabbits with the conjugate yielded an antiserum with exclusive specificity against LSD. A number of possible competitive inhibitors were tested and an inhibitory effect in the antigen-antibody reaction of 50% was taken as the reference value. This degree of cross reaction was observed with 0.16 nmol (50 ng) *l*-LSD (61). Ergine exerted an inhibitory effect of this magnitude only in quantities in excess of 40 nmol (10 μg). In a test procedure similar to that of VAN VUNAKIS et al. (1971) as little as 0.06 pmol (20 pg) were detectable in 0.1 ml sample.

The Mannich reaction for coupling serum albumin to the indole-nitrogen of LSD was also employed by CASTRO et al. (1973). An estimated 40 molecules of LSD were bound to each molecule of protein. New Zealand rabbits were immunized with the conjugate thus obtained. As in the method of TAUNTON-RIGBY et al. (1973) binding to the nitrogen in position 1 yielded antiserum which was specific for LSD. The antiserum was incubated in the reaction mixture with tritium-labeled LSD. Free hapten was separated from the soluble complex by means of dextran-coated charcoal. The lower limit of detection was 30 pmol (10 ng) LSD per ml buffer solution. Serotonin, tryptophan and lysergic acid had no inhibitory effect in concentrations of up to 6, 5 and 4 nmol, respectively (~1 μg compound).

Another radioimmunoassay for LSD was published by LOEFFLER and PIERCE (1973). Lysergic acid was bound by covalent linkage to human serum albumin by the carbodiimide method (SHEEHAN and HESS, 1955). Sheep were immunized with this conjugate, and the antiserum obtained was employed in dilutions ranging from 1:100 to 1:400. The free hapten was separated from the soluble complex by adsorption of the low molecular weight fraction with dextran-coated charcoal. The lower limit of detection was 3 pmol (1 ng) LSD per 0.2 ml sample (plasma, serum, urine). The antiserum obtained was not very specific, showing similar cross-reactions to those described by VAN VUNAKIS et al. (1971).

b) Dihydrogenated Ergot Peptide Alkaloids

ROSENTHALER and MUNZER (1976) have described a radioimmunoassay for detection of intact ergot peptide alkaloids. 6-Nor-6-carboxymethyl-9,10-dihydroergotamine was coupled to bovine serum albumin, and silver fawn rabbits were immunized with the conjugate. The antiserum obtained was employed in a dilution of 1:640. Experiments with Dihydergot (2.5 mg dihydroergotamine (102b) mesylate per tablet) in rhesus monkeys showed that the active compound could still be assayed in the blood up to 4 h after oral administration of two tablets. The lower limit of detection in 0.5-ml sample volumes of plasma or serum was 0.1 pmol (60 pg) dihydroergotamine. The peptide moiety of the ergot peptide alkaloids is especially susceptible to metabolic degradation (see D. Metabolism). It is well known that dihydrolysergic acid amide (74a) is formed in small quantities in the metabolism of dihydro-β-ergokryptine (102f) and some other alkaloids. In the range of concentrations investigated which extended up to 2 pmol dihydroergotamine no cross reaction was observed either with dihydrolysergic acid amide or with the cyclic tripeptide moiety. However, starting at 6 pmol cyclolcarbonic acid (see II. Chemical Background, general formula (32), R^1=methyl, R^2=benzyl, free acid) in the reaction mixture a measurable degree of competitive inhibition (approximately 20%) was observed, whereas even as much as 50 pmol dihydrolysergic acid amide had no effect. This different contribution of the two halves of the ergot peptide alkaloids can be explained by assuming that the antiserum formed combines preferentially with the structures of the intact peptide moiety which would be the immunodeterminant site and has less affinity for the tetracyclic structural elements of the dihydrolysergic acid molecule.

c) Antisera Against Ergot Alkaloids and Their Specificity

When assaying compounds of the indole type in biologic fluids it should be borne in mind that there is frequently some interference by endogenous indoles. MCMENAMY et al. (1961) estimated that this "background" was equivalent to a molar concentration of approximately 10^{-6}. Tryptamine and various N-substituted tryptamine and phenylethylamine derivatives exert, under assay conditions, an inhibitory effect of 50% in nanomol quantities, as VAN VUNAKIS et al. (1971) have shown. With the small sample volumes employed in radioimmunoassay biogenic amines are not likely to be present in the reaction mixture in these concentrations.

INMAN et al. (1973) and GOPALAKRISHNAN et al. (1973) pointed out that the affinity of antibodies for large ligand molecules (molecular weight 800–1000) is characterized by a high binding constant. The information content of the low molecular hapten is considerably less than that of a more complex molecule, i.e., the small ligand group supplies some, but possibly not the complete, decisive part of the immunodeterminant structure. This fact offers a plausible explanation for the fact that an antiserum produced with the aid of an immunogen having haptenic groups has low avidity for the hapten itself. An example of this is the antiserum against LSD described by VAN VUNAKIS et al. (1971); here, probably because the amide linkage is missing in lysergic acid, LSD was several times more effective in inhibiting the reaction between copolymer ergine and antiserum (see Fig. 2). LOPATIN and VOSS (1974) discussed the immunodeterminant structure of LSD and concluded that rings C and D made the greatest contribution to immunologic specificity. This was confirmed experimentally inasmuch as the diethylamide substituent at ring D was immunodeterminant in haptenic LSD coupled at the indole nitrogen (see Fig. 2). TAUNTON-RIGBY et al. (1973) compared the competitive inhibition by *d*-LSD and *l*-LSD of the reaction between *d*-LSD copolymer and its antiserum, and found that a 1000 times higher concentration of the *l*-LSD enantiomer was needed to bring about 50% inhibition. It may therefore be stated that the linkage of the haptenic indole nitrogen to the macromolecule yields a monovalent antiserum highly specific for *d*-LSD, while coupling the carboxyl group of lysergic acid to the macromolecule yields a multivalent antiserum which displays greater or lesser avidity for the basic tetracyclic structure of lysergic acid and its amide derivatives.

The cyclol structure (32) of the ergot peptide alkaloid was the immunodeterminant component of an antiserum against dihydroergotamine as has been published by ROSENTHALER and MUNZER (1976) (see Fig. 2). The tetracyclic ergoline structure had only a small effect since no crossreaction occurred even with 25 times greater concentrations of dihydrolysergic acid amide. On the other hand, the cyclic peptide

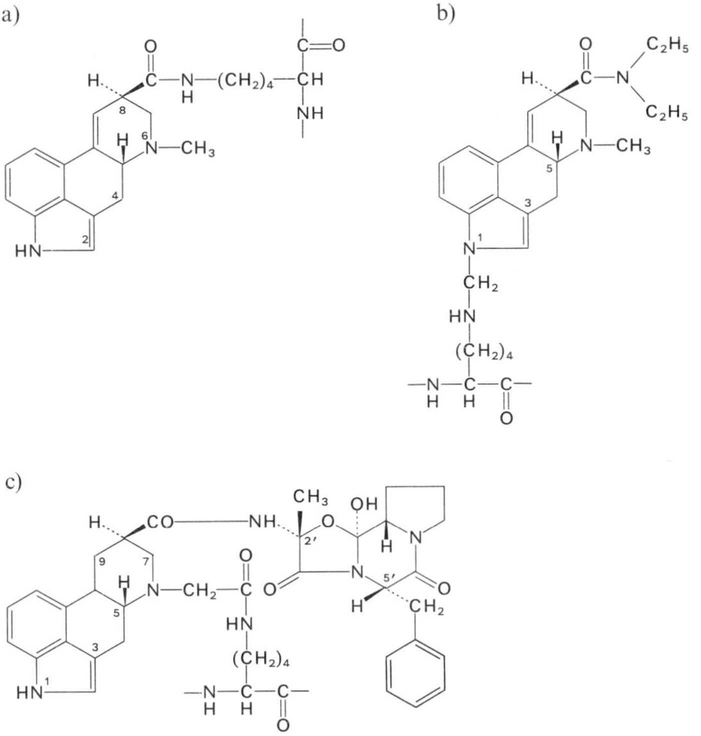

Fig. 2. *d*-Lysergic acid (a) and *d*-lysergic acid diethylamide (b) bound to a lysine side chain of a protein. *d*-Lysergic acid was coupled by means of the carbodiimide-activated carboxyl group at position 8, and *d*-lysergic acid diethylamide by means of the Mannich type reaction at the indole nitrogen (position 1). In both cases, specificity is preferably directed toward *d*-LSD, but binding at the indole nitrogen produces an antiserum with several times a higher avidity for *d*-LSD. 9,10-Dihydrogenated ergot peptide alkaloids are bound to a protein carrier at either the indole nitrogen as for b) or, c) their carboxymethyl derivative (position 6) is coupled to protein by means of the carbodiimide-activated compound. Antisera produced by conjugates bound at positions 1 and 6 are very specific to the tricyclic peptide moiety of the alkaloid

moiety of the alkaloid was a competitive inhibitor in concentrations only three times greater than the concentration of dihydroergotamine. These findings indicate that, provided the stereochemical configuration remains unchanged, substitution in position 2′ has little effect on specificity, and the immunodeterminant site is probably located in other parts of the cyclic peptide moiety.

C. Pharmacokinetics

1. Introduction

Pharmacokinetics is the branch of biopharmaceutics which treats the mathematical relationship of drug and metabolite concentrations in different parts of the body and develops models to interpret such data. Primarily pharmacokinetics is the study of the time course with respect to the concentrations of active compounds and their metabolites, mainly in the plasma and the excreta, but also in the tissue and organs.

The emphasis here will be on the characteristic pharmacokinetic properties of ergot alkaloids. The findings for the individual compounds will also be discussed with regard to the physicochemical and physiologic behavior by determining whether the compounds or any metabolites are excreted in the bile or remain in the plasma and ultimately are eliminated in the urine.

2. Experiments in Animals

a) Absorption, Hepatic Distribution and Excretion in the Rat, Dog and Monkey

α) *Absorption and Bioavailability: Definitions and Methodologic Problems*

Enteral absorption is the overall process whereby an active compound crosses the intestinal barrier, finding its way into the mesenteric venous blood or into the lymph-channels either as unchanged compound or as one or more metabolites. The physicochemical properties of a drug, e.g., its solubility, degree of ionization and its distribution ratio between lipid and water are decisive factors in its absorption. Passive transport through the epithelial membrane is the most important transport mechanism for drugs, although, as has been reported by SCHANKER (1962) and RUMMEL and FORTH (1964), special systems also appear to play a minor role. Passage through the epithelial cells into the subepithelial fluid cannot be measured with accuracy. Once it has passed into the capillaries or lymph-channels, the active compound and any metabolites which may already have been formed by gut-wall metabolism are accessible to exact assay. Drug and metabolites find their way into the systemic circulation via the portal vein or thoracic duct.

To measure intestinal absorption it is common practice to label the compound with a radioactive tracer.

The labeled compound must be biologically stable, for example, tritium should not be interchanged with the protons of body water. Measurement of total radioactivity in the products of excretion provides an estimate of the quantity (A) of compound absorbed. Special problems arise with compounds which are excreted with the bile and only appear in small amounts in the urine, e.g., ergot peptide alkaloids. In the liver the absorbed compound or its metabolites are distributed between the plasma and bile. NIMMERFALL and ROSENTHALER (1976) used such data to calculate the hepatic distribution ratio Q. Experiments on rats using biliary cannulae have shown that this ratio differs widely depending on whether the active compound is administered intravenously (i.v.) or orally (p.o.). For dihydro-[9,10-^{3}H]ergocristine (102c) mesylate, for example

$$Q_{\text{i.v.}} = \frac{A^{\infty}_{\text{b,i.v.}}\,\%}{A^{\infty}_{\text{u,i.v.}}\,\%} = 24.9 \quad \text{and} \quad Q_{\text{p.o.}} = \frac{A^{\infty}_{\text{b,p.o.}}\,\%}{A^{\infty}_{\text{u,p.o.}}\,\%} = 11.8$$

A^{∞}_{b}, A^{∞}_{u} = cumulative amounts of radioactivity excreted in bile (A^{∞}_{b}) and urine (A^{∞}_{u}) after oral and intravenous administration.

Assay of the amount eliminated by one route of excretion, as suggested by DOST (1968), yields a false estimate of intestinal absorption if the hepatic distribution ratios differ for intravenous and oral administration ($Q_{i.v.} \neq Q_{p.o.}$). Both ratios must therefore be determined separately. A simpler way of determining enteral absorption as applied to ergot alkaloids was described by NIMMERFALL and ROSENTHALER (1976): The cumulative quantities of radioactivity excreted in the bile and in the urine are summed, A (as a percentage of the dose) = $A^{\infty}_{b,p.o.}\% + A^{\infty}_{u,p.o.}\%$. This method presupposes that practically all the radioactivity absorbed is excreted by these routes, and this can be tested by means of a balance study on bile fistula animals.

In one method described by DOST and GLADTKE (1967) the absorption after various routes of administration is calculated by comparing the areas under the blood level curves ($t = \infty$) with that for intravenous administration, these areas being obtained by integration. There is a problem associated with this method due to the first-pass effect after oral administration of a drug. The problem does not stem directly from metabolic degradation of the active compound but, as a result of degradation, from the unequal distribution of the metabolites and drug respectively between plasma and bile by the liver.

For substances which are mainly absorbed into the lymph-channels, the above precondition does not apply since the lymph flows directly into the subclavian vein.

The bioavailability of a drug differs from its enteral absorption in that it concerns only the fraction of the compound which reaches the systemic circulation unchanged. Bioavailability has acquired major importance for the assessment of the bioequivalence of two or more experimental pharmaceutical dosage forms. In keeping with the relation between dose and effect it may be assumed that similar concentrations of identical drugs in the plasma should produce comparable effects. Bioavailability has been shown by LEVY (1963) to be determined by integrating the area under the plasma concentration curve from time of administration to infinite time. If the dosage forms are administered in widely differing doses, it should be borne in mind that this may bring about a change in the volume of distribution and elimination rate constant. In this case, the integrated area from time zero to infinity for the fraction of unchanged drug in the systemic circulation, divided by the volume of distribution and elimination rate constant, is then compared with the value obtained for the same dose of the standard preparation.

β) Hepatic Distribution and Estimation of the Biliary and Urinary Excretion in Bile Fistula Animals

The biliary route of excretion is the most important of the various ways in which metabolites may be secreted into the intestinal tract. HANZON (1952) investigated the mechanism of elimination with the bile in the rat using fluorescein. It was found that the metabolites formed in the liver penetrate the parenchymal cells from the plasma and are actively transported from there into the bile canaliculi. Using sliced liver tissue WILLIAMS et al. (1965) have shown that compounds with different lipid solubilities penetrate the parenchymal cells very readily. The subsequent transfer to the canaliculi is not very dependent on the chemical structure of the molecules transported by means of the above-mentioned active mechanism.

The conditions for excretion by the liver in the bile are outlined briefly herein. Metabolites appearing in the bile are highly polar and have a molecular weight of a least 300. SMITH (1966) has found certain structural elements to be necessary, but their effect has not been clearly defined.

When STOLL et al. (1955) administered [^{14}C]LSD (73b) to bile fistula rats, 70% of the radioactivity was excreted via the liver with the bile. Only 30 min after intravenous administration of LSD and [^{14}C]LSD to rats, ROTHLIN (1956) found the highest concentration in the liver and this was approximately six times greater than the amount measured in the plasma. These results were confirmed by BOYD (1959) in subsequent studies in which it was shown that after intravenous or intraperitoneal administration of [^{14}C]LSD to intact rats in a dose of 0.01–1 mg/kg body wt., 60%–80% of the dose administered was found in the intestinal tract. Under these conditions only 8% of the radioactive dose was excreted in the urine. Essentially similar results were obtained by SIDDIK et al. (1975) in bile fistula rats. The hepatic distribution and excretion of parenterally administered LSD are thus well established, and as other experiments with ergot alkaloids will show, the pattern is very characteristic for this class of compounds.

MESZAROS et al. (1975) and NIMMERFALL and ROSENTHALER (1976) demonstrated in bile fistula rat and rhesus monkey that most of the absorbed quantity of ergotamine (20) and dihydroergotamine (102b) is likewise excreted with the bile when these compounds are administered intravenously, orally or intraduodenally. A striking difference was found between ergotamine which contains lysergic acid and dihydroergotamine with its dihydrolysergic acid moiety. Absorption of the two compounds in bile fistula monkeys differed by a factor of approximately 3; it was about 30% for ergotamine and about 10% for the dihydro derivative. The reasons for the difference, which is due to the double bond in the 9,10 position, are not known.

Unlike the peptide alkaloids, such as ergotamine and dihydroergotamine, the ergolines, e.g., methergoline (89d), nicergoline (104e) and the lysergic acid derivative methysergide (34a), differ considerably among themselves in pattern of excretion when given orally to monkeys (*Macaca mulatta* and *patas*). The percentage excretion in monkeys by various routes is shown in Table 5. In rhesus monkeys the ratio of radioactivity excreted in the bile to that excreted in the urine is approximately 3:1 for the peptide alkaloids ergotamine and dihydroergotamine. In monkeys the greater part of an oral dose of the ergolines and lysergic acid and its derivatives is eliminated via the kidneys with the urine. In the dog, excretion of nicergoline and methysergide in the urine after oral administration is similar to that observed in rhesus monkeys. However, under the same conditions a considerably smaller amount of an oral dose of methergoline appears in the urine (see Table 6). Excretion was not investigated in bile fistula animals; hence it is not possible to estimate intestinal absorption or hepatic distribution, and the lower level of excretion via the kidneys cannot necessarily be ascribed to reduced enteral absorption.

In the rat a different pattern of distribution is found. Table 7 illustrates the differences in biliary and urinary excretion after oral administration of the two ergolines, the lysergic acid derivative methysergide and various ergot peptide alka-

Table 5. Biliary, urinary, and fecal excretion of orally administered [^{3}H] and [^{14}C] labeled ergot alkaloids in monkeys (mean ±S.D.)

Compound	Dose (mg/kg)	Number of animals	Radioactivity as a percentage of total dose in		
			Bile (A_b^∞)	Urine (A_u^∞)	Feces (A_f^∞)
Ergolines					
[9,10-^{3}H]Methergoline maleate or ascorbate (89d)	1 [a]	— [b]	—	32.0	15.0
[8β-*hydroxymethyl*-^{3}H]Nicergoline tartrate (104e)	1 [a]	— [c]	—	64.1	10.7
Lysergic acid and derivatives					
[6-*methyl*-^{14}C]Methysergide hydrogen maleate (34a)	0.5 [a]	— [c]	—	30.6 ± 6.5	42.6 ± 16.7
Ergot peptide alkaloids					
[4-^{14}C]Ergotamine tartrate (20)	0.25	6 [c]	24.1 ± 5.7	7.4 ± 1.6	68.2 ± 6.4
Dihydro-[9,10-^{3}H]ergotamine mesylate (102b)	0.25	6 [c]	7.6 ± 1.3	2.8 ± 0.7	91.9 ± 5.0

[a] Intact animals. [b] Patas. [c] Macaca mulatta.
A_b^∞, A_u^∞, A_f^∞ = cumulative amounts of radioactivity excreted in bile, urine, and feces, respectively.

loids. The hepatic distribution of the radioactivity observed in the monkey and dog in which different amounts of the orally administered doses of an ergoline or lysergic acid derivative are excreted with the urine is also observed in the rat. Nicergoline is mainly excreted via the kidneys in the rat, dog and monkey; methysergide follows this urinary pattern of excretion, characteristic of the ergolines and lysergic acid and its derivatives, in the dog and monkey; and methergoline conforms to this pattern only in the monkey.

ARCAMONE et al. (1971) demonstrated that methergoline is metabolized in a very similar fashion in all three species, the 8β-(carbobenzoxyamino)-methyl group resisting metabolic degradation. According to HIROM et al. (1976) this compound with its molecular weight of approximately 400 lends itself equally well to excretion either in the urine or in the bile. It was shown experimentally in the rat that when one of the routes of excretion was blocked by ligation, compounds with a molecular weight of approximately 350–450 were excreted by the other route. This flexibility in the route of excretion was not observed with compounds having a lower or higher molecular weight. In the metabolic degradation of nicergoline the methyl 8β-5′-bromonicotinate of the side chain is split off by hydrolysis, thus reducing the molecular weight to approximately 300, and the metabolite is then excreted in the urine. On the other hand LSD is largely excreted in the bile, although its molecular weight is approximately 320, thus very similar to that of the metabolite formed from nicergoline (1,6-dimethyl-8β-hydroxymethyl-10α-

Table 6. Urinary and fecal excretion of orally administered [^{3}H] and [^{14}C] labeled ergot alkaloids in dogs (mean ± S.D.)

Compound	Dose (mg/kg)	Number of animals	Radioactivity as a percentage of total dose in	
			Urine (A_u^∞)	Feces (A_f^∞)
Ergolines				
[9,10-^{3}H]Methergoline maleate or ascorbate (89d)	1	–	15.0	67.4
[8β-*hydroxymethyl*-^{3}H]Nicergoline tartrate (104e)	0.2	–	74.4	18.6
Lysergic acid and derivatives				
[6-*methyl*-^{14}C]Methysergide hydrogen maleate (34a)	5	3[a]	37.7 ± 1.6	43.1 ± 8.0

[a] Beagle.

A_u^∞, A_f^∞ = cumulative amounts of radioactivity excreted in urine and feces, respectively.

Table 7. Biliary, urinary, and fecal excretion of orally administered [^{3}H] and [^{14}C] labeled ergot alkaloids in rats (mean ± S.D.)

Compound	Dose (mg/kg)	Number of animals	Radioactivity as a percentage of total dose in		
			Bile (A_b^∞)	Urine (A_u^∞)	Feces (A_f^∞)
Ergolines					
[9,10-^{3}H]Methergoline maleate or ascorbate (89d)	1	–[a]	–	16.6	77.6
[8β-*hydroxymethyl*-^{3}H]Nicergoline tartrate (104e)	20	–[a]	–	63.6	18.6
Lysergic acid and derivatives					
[6-*methyl*-^{14}C]Methysergide hydrogen maleate (34a)	5	7	72.7 ± 6.0	11.7 ± 3.4	8.3 ± 2.0
	5	5[a]	–	12.6 ± 1.8	79.1 ± 10.9
Ergot peptide alkaloids					
[^{3}H]Ergotamine tartrate (20)	1	7	32.8 ± 9.3	–	–
	1	6[a]	–	8.6 ± 2.1	63.9 ± 6.7
Dihydro-[9,10-^{3}H]ergotamine mesylate (102b)	1	6	10.4 ± 3.3	–	–
	1	6[a]	–	1.9 ± 0.2	93.2 ± 1.6
Dihydro-[9,10-^{3}H]ergocristine mesylate (102c)	1	7	13.8 ± 2.4	1.2 ± 0.3	88.6 ± 6.4

[a] Intact animals.

A_b^∞, A_u^∞, A_f^∞ = cumulative amounts of radioactivity excreted in bile, urine, and feces, respectively.

methoxyergoline) by hydrolysis of the ester linkage. LSD and the nicergoline metabolite differ considerably in chemical structure (see D. Metabolism).

Molecular weight is one of the properties of a compound which determines its route of excretion. Another factor can be the structural features of the molecule, although this has not been thoroughly investigated. For compounds within the above-indicated range of molecular weights in particular, structural differences may well explain why the route of excretion varies from species to species.

The hepatobiliary route of excretion of ergot alkaloids permits the enterohepatic circulation of the metabolites eliminated with the bile. BOYD (1959) and NIMMERFALL and ROSENTHALER (1976) have studied this problem by examining intestinal absorption of the metabolites from the diverted bile. Dihydro-[9,10-^{3}H]ergocristine was administered orally to a bile fistula rat, and the bile from this animal was infused into the duodenum of a second animal which had not received the drug. The bile from this second animal was then infused into the duodenum of a third untreated animal. Reabsorption as a fraction of the dose administered to the first animal, namely 1 mg/kg body wt. was approximately 1.5%. A similar result was obtained by BOYD (1959) in earlier studies with LSD. After oral administration of 1 mg [^{14}C] LSD/kg body wt. to rats, the bile from the first animal was infused into the duodenum of a second. If complete absorption had taken place the bile from this rat ought to have contained approximately 70% of the radioactivity administered to the first animal. However, only 0.05%–1.3% of the dose administered to the first animal was recovered. It may therefore be assumed that for the ergot alkaloids the enterohepatic circulation does not play a very significant role in the intact rat. NIMMERFALL and ROSENTHALER (1976) employed a similar method to study the effect of bile on intestinal absorption in the rat. Bile was not found to have any effect.

γ) Estimation of Enteral Absorption Using Intact and Bile Fistula Animals

As was discussed above, the enteral absorption of compounds which are excreted mainly with the bile and to only a small extent with the urine cannot be directly estimated from the ratio of urinary excretion after oral and after intravenous administration. Experiments with dihydro-[9,10-^{3}H]ergocristine by NIMMERFALL and ROSENTHALER (1976) and with [6-*methyl*-^{14}C]methysergide by ZEHNDER (1976) in bile fistula rats have shown that the enteral absorption values determined by different methods may vary. On the other hand KALBERER (1969b, 1970) did show that there is no statistically significant difference between the values obtained for the absorption either of [^{3}H]ergotamine or of dihydro-[9,10-^{3}H]ergotamine in the rat, whether determined from the ratio of urinary excretion after oral and after intravenous administration or from the sum of the fractions of radioactivity excreted in the bile and urine (see Table 9). It should, however, be pointed out that if there is a great disparity between the dose administered orally and that administered intravenously, this may possibly affect the pattern of hepatic distribution. In bile fistula animals absorption is calculated from the sum of the fractions excreted with the bile and with the urine. Data for peptide alkaloids from studies

Table 8. Intestinal absorption of [^{3}H] and [^{14}C] labeled ergot alkaloids in rhesus monkeys (for dose, see Table 5)

Compound	A(% dose)[a] $=A^{\infty}_{b,po}\% + A^{\infty}_{u,po}\%$	Q_{po}[a] $= \frac{A^{\infty}_{b,po}\%}{A^{\infty}_{u,po}\%}$
Ergot peptide alkaloids		
[4-^{14}C]Ergotamine tartrate (20)	31.5 ± 5.2	3.4 ± 1.2
Dihydro-[9,10-^{3}H]ergotamine mesylate (102b)	10.3 ± 1.5	2.9 ± 1.0

[a] Mean ± S.D.

A^{∞}_{b}, A^{∞}_{u} = cumulative amounts of radioactivity excreted in bile and urine, respectively.

in the rat and rhesus monkeys have been published by MESZAROS et al. (1975) and NIMMERFALL and ROSENTHALER (1976) (see Tables 8, 9).

The enteral absorption of ergot peptide alkaloids is very much lower than that of the alkaloids containing only the lysergic acid moiety. This difference in absorption is possibly attributable in part to low aqueous solubility, but more likely it is due to the fact that the peptide alkaloids have both hydrophilic and lipophilic (amphipathic) properties because of their chemical structure. Passage through the stomach appears to have some effect on enteral absorption, as has been shown in the case of ergotamine by MESZAROS et al. (1975). When this compound is administered intraduodenally to rhesus monkeys the radioactivity excreted in the bile and urine as a percentage of dose is about one-third greater (44.8 ± 8.0) than after oral administration (31.5 ± 5.2). With regard to their enteral absorption the ergot peptide alkaloids fall into two categories, the 9,10-unsaturated and the corresponding saturated compounds. In the rat and rhesus monkey the enteral absorption of ergotamine is approximately three times greater than that of the analogous 9,10-dihydro derivative. It may be that a conformational change by conferring enhanced lipophilic properties on the molecule facilitates passage through the intestinal barrier.

b) Distribution in Tissue and Organs

α) *Ergolines*

Two representatives of the ergoline class of compounds, the semisynthetic active compounds methergoline (89d) and nicergoline (104e) were the subject of pharmacokinetic studies described by ARCAMONE et al. (1971) and ARCAMONE et al. (1972). Methergoline labeled with tritium was administered intravenously to rats in a dose of 1 mg/kg body wt. and found its way rapidly from the blood to various tissues, but not the brain. The level of radioactivity in the plasma measured after 1 hour yielded a value equivalent to 0.55 μg active compound/ml. The half-life in the plasma was estimated at 60–70 min. A similar distribution pattern was obtained after oral administration.

Table 9. Intestinal absorption of [^{3}H] and [^{14}C] labeled ergot alkaloids in rats (for dose, see Table 7)

Compound	Intestinal absorption[a]			Hepatic distribution ratio[a]	
	A (% dose) = $A^{\infty}_{b,po}\% + A^{\infty}_{u,po}\%$	$A_U\% = \frac{100 \cdot A^{\infty}_{u,po}\%}{A^{\infty}_{u,iv}\%}$	$A_B\% = \frac{100 \cdot A^{\infty}_{b,po}\%}{A^{\infty}_{b,iv}\%}$	$Q_{iv} = \frac{A^{\infty}_{b,iv}\%}{A^{\infty}_{u,iv}\%}$	$Q_{po} = \frac{A^{\infty}_{b,po}\%}{A^{\infty}_{u,po}\%}$
Lysergic acid and derivatives					
[6-*methyl*-^{14}C]Methysergide hydrogen maleate (34a)	84.4 ± 6.9	92.0 ± 23.5	85.7 ± 7.9	13.9 ± 3.3	5.5 ± 0.8
				$p < 0.005$	
Ergot peptide alkaloids					
[^{3}H]Ergotamine tartrate (20)	41.4 ± 9.5	44.3 ± 13.7	47.3 ± 14.8	3.6 ± 0.8	3.8 ± 1.4
Dihydro-[9,10-^{3}H]ergotamine mesylate (102b)	12.3 ± 3.3	13.9 ± 1.9	14.0 ± 4.7	5.4 ± 0.8	5.5 ± 1.8
Dihydro-[9,10-^{3}H]ergocristine mesylate (102c)	15.0 ± 2.5	30.8 ± 11.0	15.2 ± 2.7	24.9 ± 6.5	11.8 ± 2.2
				$p < 0.001$	

[a] Mean ± S.D.

A^{∞}_b, A^{∞}_u = cumulative amounts of radioactivity excreted in bile and urine, respectively.

Table 10. Distribution of nicergoline (104e) and LSD (73b) in tissue and organs at various time intervals after administration. a) Oral administration of [^{3}H]nicergoline (20 mg/kg) to *rats*. Values are calculated as microgram-equivalents nicergoline either per gram of tissue or per milliliter of plasma (ARCAMONE et al., 1972). b) Intravenous administration of LSD (1 mg/kg body wt.) to *cats*. Values obtained by the fluorimetric method are calculated as microgram of LSD per gram of tissue (AXELROD et al., 1957)

Tissue	30 min	90 min	6 h	12 h
a) *Ergolines:* [^{3}H]nicergoline				
Plasma	4.3	1.9	1.1	0.2
Liver	67.3	34.7	17.6	6.1
Lung	22.3	11.8	8.8	4.4
Kidney	20.8	16.8	5.8	3.0
Heart	10.1	7.2	3.5	0.3
Fat	1.3	–	1.0	0.6
Brain	0.7	0.5	0.3	0.1
Stomach	223.2	195.0	20.6	2.0
Intestines:				
small	36.8	39.3	21.7	3.5
large	11.2	5.5	8.9	12.6
b) *Lysergic acid and derivatives*: LSD				
Plasma		1.75		
Liver		0.67		
Lung		0.87		
Kidney		0.53		
Heart		0.30		
Fat		0.20		
Brain		0.52		
Intestines		0.39		

The mode of distribution of the radioactivity of labeled nicergoline (see Table 10) in the tissues was similar to that of methergoline. In the rat maximum radioactivity in the blood after an oral dose of 2 mg/kg body wt. was attained after only 30 min. This concentration was equivalent to 0.52 μg active compound/ml. The half-life calculated from the time course of the plasma concentration was approximately 1 hour and thus comparable with that of methergoline, LSD (73b) and methysergide (34a). The level of radioactivity measured in various organs was highest in the liver and kidneys. Contrary to expectations, however, the greater part of the radioactivity was excreted in the urine in all the animal species investigated, namely the rat, dog and rhesus monkey. This has already been discussed in connection with hepatic distribution.

β) Lysergic Acid and Its Derivatives

Very much more is known about the distribution of LSD. On administration of 1 mg LSD/kg body wt. to rats by the intraperitoneal route, BOYD et al. (1955a) found that the major part of the dose appeared in the intestinal tract due to biliary excretion. Further studies in rats by BOYD et al. (1955b) with [^{14}C]LSD showed that it was distributed uniformly in very low concentrations in all tissues.

When 1 mg/kg was administered intravenously to bile fistula rats 64% of the administered dose of radioactivity was excreted with the bile within a time interval of only 3 hours. Probably as little as 10%–20% of an intraperitoneal dose reaches the systemic circulation, the greater part being excreted in the bile by the liver.

Since no specific and sensitive method was available for the detection of LSD, LANZ et al. (1955) employed a biologic test, the antagonistic effect of LSD on contractions of isolated uterus in response to serotonin, to study the distribution in mice. One to two micrograms of LSD per liter sufficed as the threshold dose for this method of detection. Studies in the intact mouse revealed that after an intravenous dose of 35 mg/kg body wt. the concentration measured in the liver was roughly three times greater than in the blood and skeletal muscle. The concentration in the brain was lower than in the blood and declined very rapidly, independently of the blood concentration. The half-life in the blood was 37 min.

AXELROD et al. (1957) assayed LSD in biologic material using a fluorimetric method and published quantitative data on its distribution (see Table 10). Various tissues and organs of the cat were investigated 90 min after an intravenous injection of 1 mg/kg body wt. Unlike the ergot peptide alkaloids, LSD was found in appreciable amounts in the plasma (1.75 mg/kg), the levels being very similar to those determined in the bile (1.85 mg/kg). The half-life calculated from the first-order rate constant in plasma was 130 min. The somewhat different half-life should not be ascribed to species-dependent elimination but seem to reflect lower specificity of the assay method as compared to the earlier biologic test of LANZ et al. (1955).

Brain tissue distribution of LSD has been the subject of much interest from an early date. Several workers became interested in where pharmacodynamic interaction of LSD in brain tissue would occur, and therefore tissue levels of the various brain sections were studied. AXELROD et al. (1957), using the fluorimetric assay, attempted to detect LSD in various regions of the brain. Considerable quantities were found in the cat brain after intravenous administration of 1 mg/kg body wt. To investigate the relationship between plasma concentrations and levels attained in the cerebrospinal fluid, LSD was administered intravenously to rhesus monkeys in a dose of 0.2 mg/kg body wt. The maximum concentration in the cerebrospinal fluid (0.04 μg/ml) was attained after only 10 min and was comparable at this time with the level of free compound (0.03 μg/ml) in the plasma (half-life 100 min).

HALEY and RUTSCHMANN (1957) injected [^{14}C]LSD (25 μg) either intravenously or intracerebrally into mice. Changes in behavior of the animals were similar after either administration, confirming that the drug penetrated the blood-brain barrier. ARNOLD et al. (1958) employed autoradiography after injection of [^{14}C]LSD (~1 μCi) into mice. Distribution in tissue and organs confirmed work already done, but unequal distribution of the radioactivity in different regions of brain was found. BOYD (1959) administered [^{14}C]LSD by the intraperitoneal and intravenous route in a dose of 1 mg/kg body wt. to rats and demonstrated that the amount present in the brain was never more than approximately 0.01% of the dose (~100 ng). WINTER (1971), who employed the fluorimetric method, found LSD in the brain in a concentration of 30–35 ng/g tissue 10–20 min after intraperitoneal administration of 96 μg/kg body wt. to rats. SNYDER and REIVICH (1966) studied the regional localization of LSD in the brain of squirrel monkey (*Saimiri sciureus*) using the fluorimetric method. The animals were infused with 0.5, 1 and 2 mg/kg body wt. i.v. Specific distribution in different regions of brain was confirmed.

IDÄNPÄÄN-HEIKKILÄ and SCHOOLAR (1969) employed an autoradiographic method to study the tissue distribution of [^{14}C]LSD in mice. Autoradiograms were taken from the sagittal sections through the frozen body using ULLBERG'S technique (1963). The radioactivity in the brain was higher than in the blood and was distributed over the whole brain. The greatest amount of radioactivity was found in the hippocampus and thalamus, followed by the cerebellum and medulla. These levels were approximately the same as those in the spinal cord. High uptake was also found in the salivary and lacrimal glands, indicating some excretory function of these organs for LSD. Besides the adrenals the pituitary contained the greatest quantity of radioactivity. It was not possible to pinpoint the distribution in the pituitary more accurately by macroautoradiography. This prompted DIAB et al. (1971) to investigate this aspect of the distribution of [^{3}H]LSD in the rat brain in greater depth. The results obtained in rats showed that [^{3}H]LSD (1.7 μg/g ∼1 μCi/g) penetrated the brain within 5 min after administration, attained its maximum concentration 15 min later and was no longer detectable 1 hour after injection. Earlier work by ROSECRANS et al. (1967) showed that plasma levels after intraperitoneal administration of 260–2600 μg LSD/kg body wt. to rats reached a peak after approximately 10 min and after 45 min dropped to less than 100 ng/g brain tissue. Lastly, DIAB et al. (1971) investigated the distribution of [^{3}H]LSD in individual cerebral structures using microautoradiography. In freeze-dried sections of the pituitary and pineal glands and of the hippocampus a generalized nonspecific pattern of radioactively labeled compound was found. When the same sections were prepared by the conventional method they were devoid of any radioactivity indicating that [^{3}H]LSD has been lost in the several extractions involved in tissue processing. The granular layer and the Purkinje cells in the cerebellum contained radioactivity when processed by freeze-drying. The conventional method, however, revealed [^{3}H]LSD to be present only in the Purkinje cells where it was firmly bound. Binding seems to occur also on the membranes of the multipolar cells in the midbrain and the medulla, especially in the periphery of specific neurons.

FARAGALLA (1972) studied the subcellular distribution of LSD in rat brain homogenates. The results obtained were at variance with earlier work of FREEDMAN and COQUET (1965), who showed that after an intravenous dose (500 μg/kg) of LSD to rats the larger amount was taken up in the particulate fraction. However, the data of FARAGALLA (1972) did generally agree with those of SNYDER and REIVICH (1966).

Other studies on the distribution of LSD in the rat were carried out by BOYD (1959) using [^{14}C]LSD as described by STOLL et al. (1954a). However, earlier work of AXELROD et al. (1957) in the cat using the fluorimetric method revealed a distribution pattern which differed considerably from that obtained in the rat with the radioactively labeled compound. The differences are probably due to metabolic degradation since the radioactive label is not completely resistant to metabolic breakdown (see D. Metabolism).

Transplacental passage of LSD was examined by INDÄNPÄÄN-HEIKKILÄ and SCHOOLAR (1969). They injected [^{14}C]LSD (9.9 μg/g) intravenously into mice during the last week of pregnancy. Five minutes after administration approximately 0.5% of the label was found in the fetus. The amount of radioactivity transferred through the placental barrier was higher during the first trimester of pregnancy (2.3% of the dose), the distribution pattern in the fetus being very similar to that in the mother.

BIANCHINE (1968) investigated another lysergic acid derivative, methysergide, in the rabbit using a modified version of the well-known fluorimetric procedure of AXELROD et al. (1957). The highest concentration was found in the kidneys and the lowest in the brain and adipose tissues. The half-life estimated from the plasma concentration time curve was 40 min. The concentration in the cerebrospinal fluid remained throughout approximately one-seventh of the plasma concentration.

γ) Ergot Peptide Alkaloids

Little is known about the distribution of the ergot peptide alkaloids in the tissues and organs. ROTHLIN (1946) made an attempt to detect the presence of unchanged active compound in the blood and urine of rats which had received a dose of 2.7 mg and rabbits which had received a dose of 45 mg ergotamine (20) tartrate by measuring the adrenolytic effect on isolated organs. In accordance with the dose-effect relation this method should be capable of detecting active compound in a concentration of 1.7–3 ng/ml sample. These studies showed that the concentration in the blood rapidly falls and that only very small quantities are excreted in the urine, findings which were confirmed in the main by MESZAROS et al. (1975), ROSENTHALER and MUNZER (1976), and NIMMERFALL and ROSENTHALER (1976). Earlier work has centered on measurable biologic effects. Such techniques were employed to investigate the distribution of dihydroergokryptine (102e) in rabbits. Active compound was localized in the liver, kidneys, spleen and muscle tissue in quantities which were fairly large compared with the low concentration in the blood. ROTHLIN (1946/1947) also found active compound in the aqueous humor and in the cerebrospinal fluid, but not in the brain. Further experiments in the rabbit with dihydroergotamine (102b) and dihydroergocornine (102d) showed that a dose of 20 mg/kg body wt. was rapidly distributed, and ergot alkaloid was found in decreasing order of concentration in the liver, kidneys, lungs, spleen and skeletal muscle. No active compound was detectable after 16 hours. A rise in concentration after 60 min was noted by ROTHLIN (1947), especially in the excretory organs, namely in the liver and, to a much less extent, in the kidneys, whereas after the same period the concentration in the lungs had fallen to half and that in the heart had fallen to one-tenth of the maximum concentration attained shortly after injection.

Administration of dihydroergotoxine mesylate to anesthetized cats (ROTHLIN et al., 1951) by intraduodenal infusion of 56 μg/kg body wt. and intraportal injection of 14 μg/kg body wt. had the same adrenaline-inhibiting effect on the renal vessels as an intravenous dose of 7 μg/kg body wt. This result pointed to an enteral absorption rate of approximately 25%, but half of the active compound was removed in the passage through the liver. When 14 μg/kg was injected into the

Table 11. Distribution of ergotamine (20) and dihydroergotamine (102b) in tissue and organs at various time intervals after administration. a) Either oral or intravenous administration of [^{3}H]ergotamie tartrate (1 mg/kg body wt.) to *rats*. Values are calculated as microgram-equivalents ergotamine tartrate per gram of fresh tissue (KALBERER, 1970). b) Intravenous administration of dihydro-[9,10-^{3}H]ergotamine (0.5 mg/kg body wt.) to *rats*. Values are calculated as microgram-equivalents dihydroergotamine per gram of fresh tissue (KALBERER, 1969b)

Tissue	30 min	2 h		8 h	
	i.v.	i.v.	p.o.	i.v.	p.o.
a) *Ergot peptide alkaloids*: [^{3}H]ergotamine					
Blood		0.09	0.02	0.02	0.02
Liver		1.36	0.37	0.52	0.26
Lung		1.09	0.04	0.44	0.02
Kidney		0.74	0.09	0.17	0.07
Heart		0.26	0.03	0.03	0.02
Brain		0.05	0.02	0.01	0
b) *Dihydrogenated ergot peptide alkaloids*: dihydro-[9,10-^{3}H]ergotamine					
Blood	0.04	0.03		0.005	
Liver	0.87	0.61		0.15	
Lung	0.74	0.72		0.17	
Kidney	0.86	0.50		0.06	
Heart	0.29	0.10		0.02	
Brain	0.005	0.01		0.005	
Stomach	0.32	0.19		0.04	
Intestines:					
small	0.57	0.24		0.04	
large	0.14	0.17		0.19	

brachial artery the effect was equivalent to the intravenous dose of 7 μg/kg body wt. In relation to the weight of tissue supplied by the brachial artery the liver retained more active compound than the extremity per unit weight. This shows that the liver, as the central compartment, plays a major role in the distribution of dihydroergotoxine. The distribution of radioactively labeled ergotamine and dihydroergotamine in tissue and organs of the rat was studied by KALBERER (1969b, 1970). A fairly high amount of radioactivity after intravenous injection (1 and 0.5 mg/kg) was found in the liver, lung and kidney (see Table 11). Unlike the ergolines and lysergic acid and its derivatives the ergot peptide alkaloids yield very low plasma levels 2 hours after administration, namely 90 ng-equiv ergotamine and 30 ng-equiv dihydroergotamine/g blood.

In experiments with the anesthetized bile fistula dog, MARZO et al. (1975) showed that after intravenous injection of dihydro-[^{3}H]ergocristine (102c) (80 μg/kg) and dihydro-[9,10-^{3}H]ergotamine (102b) (20 μg/kg) the level of radioactivity in the blood decreased quite rapidly. Levels of radioactivity equivalent to 40 ng dihydroergocristine and 10 ng dihydroergotamine/ml plasma were found after one hour.

LEIST and GRAUWILER (1973) investigated the transplacental passage of an ergot peptide alkaloid by using ergotamine as a typical representative of this class of compounds. After intravenous administration of [^{3}H]ergotamine (2.5 μg/kg) to pregnant rats 14 days after mating, approximately three times more radioactivity was found in the uterus, placenta and yolk-sac than in the blood. Radioactivity was detectable in the amniotic fluid and fetal tissues only in a small quantity, findings which likewise have been obtained by IDÄNPÄÄN-HEIKKILÄ and SCHOOLAR (1969) in their investigations on the transplacental passage of LSD. This limited transplacental passage was attributed to the pharmacodynamic effects of the peptide alkaloid, partly to its vasoconstrictive effect and partly also to its known uterotonic effect, which may have reduced placental blood flow.

The distribution of dihydro-[9,10-^{3}H]ergotoxine in the cat brain was investigated (MEIER-RUGE et al., 1973) by infusion of 2 mg/kg body wt. into the left common carotid artery during a period of 60 min. The highest concentration was found in the pituitary (4730 ng-equiv/g tissue). The hypothalamus and sacral cord contained approximately 100 ng-equiv/g tissue. The levels found in the cerebellum, the cerebral cortex and the hippocampus (78 ng-equiv/g tissue) were lower than those found in the hypothalamus, and the difference was statistically significant ($p < 0.05$). The distribution pattern seemed to be similar to that of LSD. Further work on brain uptake of dihydro-[9,10-^{3}H]ergotoxine was done by IWANGOFF et al. (1976) who injected 2 mg/kg body wt. into the left common carotid artery of cats. Distribution of the radioactivity in the brain and subcellular fractions was investigated by using autoradiography and zone centrifugation. The radioactivity was not uniformely distributed, but was localized in certain cells, especially in synaptic structures. Per unit weight of fresh tissue the cerebellum contained some 15% more radioactivity than the cerebrum. An average concentration of 10^{-7} M dihydroergotoxine equivalent was calculated for the brain tissue, except the pituitary gland which showed higher levels of radioactivity.

3. Experiments in Man

Therapeutic doses of ergot alkaloids amount to only a few milligrams, and consequently the concentrations in blood and urine are correspondingly low. The main requirement for kinetic studies is therefore a very sensitive analytic method. Since the capabilities of chemical methods of estimation are limited due to technical problems (see B. Assay of Ergot Alkaloids) most studies have been conducted using radioactively labeled substances. ROSENTHALER and MUNZER (1976) have recently developed a radioimmunoassay for unchanged dihydroergotamine (102b) which ought to make it possible to study the steady-state kinetics of this substance in man without multiple administrations of radioactivity. Due to methodologic difficulties it is only in recent years that pharmacokinetic studies other than with LSD (73b) have been carried out in man.

The pharmacokinetic data of all ergot alkaloids investigated up to now show some common characteristics. Absorption is rapid and elimination takes place in two phases with a shorter α- and a longer β-half-life. Differences exist concerning the extent of absorption, the maximal plasma concentration (cp max) and the amount of substance excreted in urine and feces. The following is the description of pharmacokinetic data in man classified as follows: ergolines, lysergic acid and derivatives, and nonhydrogenated and hydrogenated ergot peptide alkaloids.

In Tables 12 and 13 all relevant pharmacokinetic data are presented. The values for cp max have been extrapolated for the administration of 1 mg, but as the linearity of the pharmacokinetics of the ergot alkaloids in man has not yet been demonstrated these standardized cp max values may vary within certain limits. Plasma concentration is given as nanogram equivalents per milliliter, i.e., nanograms of the substance calculated from the radioactivity measured and therefore also including labeled metabolites.

a) Ergolines (see Table 12)

ARCAMONE et al. (1972) have shown that the oral administration of [^{3}H]nicergoline (104e) tartrate (4.16 and 5.0 mg) leads within about $1^1/_2$ hours to a cp max of radioactivity equivalent to 100–200 ng/ml. By extrapolation, plasma concentrations up to 50 ng-equiv/ml may be assumed after a 1 mg oral dose. After i.v. administration, about two thirds of the radioactivity is excreted in the urine, whereby only 6%–7% represent unchanged substance. The spectrum of metabolites excreted in the urine after i.v. and oral administration was similar. After the oral dose cumulative urinary excretion amounted to about 80% and approximately 10% were eliminated in the feces within 3 or 4 days. From these data it is assumed that the substance is completely absorbed. ARCAMONE et al. (1971) also investigated the excretion of [^{3}H]methergoline (89d) after an oral dose of 0.15 mg/kg body wt., and found that 44% and 39% of the administered amount of radioactivity were excreted within 5 days in urine and feces, respectively. In the urine 2.2% of the administered dose was excreted as unchanged substance, 16% as nonconjugated and 9% as glucuronized metabolites while the rest (17%) was not identifiable. The high excretion of the ergolines in the urine and the high plasma levels are comparable to the LSD and derivatives and differs distinctly from the hydrogenated and nonhydrogenated ergot peptide alkaloids.

b) Lysergic Acid and Derivatives (see Table 12)

Plasma concentrations of LSD (73b) were estimated fluorimetrically by UPSHALL and WAILLING (1972). A maximum concentration of 2–8 ng/ml was reached 1.0–1.25 h after an oral dose of 160 μg. Extrapolated to a 1–mg dose this would represent 12–50 ng/ml. By measuring for up to 8 hours, AGHAJANIAN and BING (1964) gave a value of 2.9 h for the elimination half-life of LSD from plasma. This value probably relates only to the α-phase since FAED and MCLEOD (1973) were able to demonstrate the excretion of LSD-like substances in the urine for up to 4 days. AGHAJANIAN and BING (1964) found plasma levels after an intravenous injection of LSD (2 μg/kg body wt.) which were very similar to those reported by UPSHALL and WAILLING (1972) following a comparable oral dose. This would suggest that LSD is very well absorbed.

BIANCHINE (1968) studied methysergide (34a), another lysergic acid derivative, in man after oral administration of 2 mg. Roughly 20% of the administered dose of a fluorescent substance was found in urine after 5 hours. The same author demonstrated, with a thin-layer chromatographic method, that 90% of that which is excreted in urine is demethylated in the 1-position and consequently dealkylated to form methylergonovine (73a). The half-life of elimination from the plasma was about 1.0 hour. After oral administration of [^{14}C]methysergide, MEIER and

Table 12. Kinetic parameters of ergolines, lysergic acid and derivatives, and nonhydrogenated ergot alkaloids in man

Ergot alkaloids	t max (h) p.o. time to maximal plasma level	cp max/1 mg p.o. (ng-equiv/ml) maximal plasma concentration	Plasma half-lives (h)					Cumulative urinary excretion (Cu(∞)) in %		Absorption in % ratio of p.o. to i.v. urinary excretion	Half-lives from urinary excretion (h)			
			Absorption p.o.	α-phase		β-phase					α-phase		β-phase	
				p.o.	i.v.	p.o.	i.v.	p.o.	i.v.		p.o.	i.v.	p.o.	i.v.
[^{3}H]Nicergoline (104e) (ARCAMONE et al., 1972)	~1.5	20–50		1.2				>80	>66	90–100				
[^{3}H]Methergoline (89d) (ARCAMONE et al., 1971)								>44						
LSD (73b) (UPSHALL and WAILLING, 1972)	~1.0	12–50												
[^{14}C]Methysergide (34a) (MEIER and SCHREIER, 1976)			0.38	2.7		10.0		56.4						
[^{3}H]Bromocriptine (38) (AELLIG and NÜESCH, 1977)	1.4	2.15	0.12	6.2	3.3	50	44	6.4	6.7	95	4.2	5.3	48	35
[^{3}H]Ergotamine (20) (AELLIG and NÜESCH, 1977)	2.1	1.52	0.38	2.7	1.9	21	21	4.3	6.7	62	2.8	1.4	31	18
[^{3}H]l-Methylergotamine (34c) (AELLIG and NÜESCH, 1977)	2.0	2.29	1.12	1.9	1.5	24	21	13.3	18.8	71	1.7	2.1	16	18

SCHREIER (1976) found an absorption half-life of 0.38 hour and elimination half-lives of 2.7 and 10.0 hours. The amount of radioactivity excreted in the urine was 56%, which allows the conclusion that the substance is well absorbed. The authors have also simulated steady-state plasma levels and found them to be 8.5–30 ng/ml with a dosage of 1 mg t.i.d.

c) Nonhydrogenated Ergot Peptide Alkaloids (see Table 12)

AELLIG and NÜESCH (1977) have investigated [^{3}H]bromocriptine (38), [^{3}H]ergotamine (20) and [^{3}H]methylergotamine (34c). They administered the labeled substances (SCHREIER, 1976) orally and intravenously in a cross-over design to groups of six patients in each case. The solution injected intravenously corresponded to that in marketed ampules and in the case of investigational substances was similar in composition to ampules used in clinical trials. Oral doses were given to fasting patients along with 200 ml of a xanthine-free beverage. Radioactivity was measured up to 48 and 72 or 96 hours in plasma and urine, respectively. A calculation of kinetic parameters was done using phenomenologic nonlinear regression methods using a sum of exponentials. The nonhydrogenated ergot peptide alkaloids have a short absorption half-life of 0.1–1.1 hour and produce the maximal plasma concentration at 1.4–2.1 hours after oral administration similarly to the hydrogenated ergot peptide alkaloids. The nonhydrogenated ergot peptide alkaloids lead, however, to a higher plasma maximum (1.5–2.3 ng-equiv/ml) than the hydrogenated ergot peptide alkaloids.

Elimination of the nonhydrogenated ergot peptide alkaloids occurs typically in two phases. The α-phase in plasma varies between 1.5 and 6.2 hours. Values found from plasma and urine data for the β-phase of ergotamine and methylergotamine were 16–31 hours after i.v. and oral administration and corresponded to those found for the hydrogenated substances. [^{3}H]Bromocriptine is an exception with a long β-phase of elimination from plasma of 50 and 44 hours after oral and i.v. administration, respectively. A correspondingly long therapeutic effect was found by DEL POZO et al. (1972) who registered a drop in serum prolactin concentration for over 24 hours. Cumulative urinary excretion of the nonhydrogenated ergot peptide alkaloids after oral administration is, with values of 6%–13%, somewhat greater than that of the hydrogenated peptide ergot alkaloids but much smaller than that of the ergolines as well as lysergic acid and derivatives.

Assuming that the metabolism is the same after oral and i.v. administration one can postulate that the ratio of the urinary excretion after oral and i.v. administration is a measure of the absorption (NÜESCH, 1973). The 62%–95% absorption of the nonhydrogenated ergot peptide alkaloids is in the same range as that of the ergolines and LSD and derivatives. SCHMIDT (1977) found in six patients that the relative bioavailability of the marketed bromocriptine tablet was equal to that of a solution or a capsule (solution = 95% absolute bioavailability).

d) Hydrogenated Ergot Peptide Alkaloids (see Table 13)

Using a method similar to that used for studying the nonhydrogenated ergot peptide alkaloids, AELLIG and NÜESCH (1977) have also investigated [^{3}H]dihydroergotamine (102b), [^{3}H]dihydroergovaline (108b), [^{3}H]dihydroergostine, [^{3}H]dihydroergonine (110b), tritiated Hydergine and [^{3}H]dihydroergocornine (102d). The

Table 13. Kinetic parameters of hydrogenated ergot alkaloids in man. (After AELLIG and NÜESCH, 1977)

Ergot alkaloids	t max (h) p.o. time to maximal plasma level	cp max/1 mg p.o. (ng-equiv/ml) maximal plasma concentration	Plasma half-lives (h)					Cumulative urinary excretion (Cu(∞)) in %		Absorption in % ratio of p.o. to i.v. urinary excretion	Half-lives from urinary excretion (h)			
			Absorption p.o.	α-phase		β-phase					α-phase		β-phase	
				p.o.	i.v.	p.o.	i.v.	p.o.	i.v.		p.o.	i.v.	p.o.	i.v.
[^{3}H]Dihydroergotamine (102b)	2.7	0.63	0.32	2.0	1.4	21	20	3.0	10.6	30	2.0	1.7	21	21
[^{3}H]Dihydroergovaline (108b)	1.3	0.49	0.35	1.9	1.5	23	27	2.1	19.1	11	2.3	1.4	22	19
[^{3}H]Dihydroergostine	2.3	0.42	—	—	1.5	—	16	2.9	10.7	26	2.7	1.8	23	24
[^{3}H]Dihydroergonine (110b)	1.0	0.77	0.84	1.8	1.5	14	14	2.9	18.7	17	1.9	2.0	15	13
[^{3}H]Hydergine	2.3	0.50	0.52	4.1	1.5	—	13	2.0	8.4	25	—	—	12	13
[^{3}H]Dihydroergocornine (102d)	1.4	0.57	0.32	3.0	2.5	13	17	2.5	10.6	25	3.0	1.8	17	12

cp max found were 0.4–0.8 ng-equiv/ml. The absorption half-lives were short, generally 0.3 hour. Longer values of 0.5 and 0.8 hour were found only for tritiated Hydergine and [^{3}H]dihydroergonine, respectively. Peak plasma concentrations were found at 1.0–2.7 hours.

The shorter elimination plasma half-life (α-phase) was, in general, the same after i.v. and oral administration (i.v.: 1.4–2.5 hours; oral: 1.9–4.1 hours). The longer elimination plasma half-life (β-phase) was also practically identical after oral and i.v. administration and varied between 13 and 20 hours. Only in the case of [^{3}H]dihydroergovaline (27 hours) was it somewhat higher, although here the urine data gave a value of 19–22 hours. Cumulative urinary excretion is small and, even when extrapolated to infinity, amounts to only 8.4%–19.1% and 2.5%–3.0% of the administered dose of radioactivity after intravenous and oral administration, respectively. Absorption varies between 11% and 30% for the different hydrogenated ergot peptide alkaloids. For tritiated Hydergine, LODDO et al. (1976) confirmed these results in healthy volunteers who received the stubstance orally as solution and tablets (marketed formulation) and intravenously in the form of an infusion. They found a urinary excretion of 8.45% 72 hours after the infusion. The values for the oral administration of solution and tablets were 1.8% and 2.1%, respectively, which would correspond to an absorption of 21% and 24%. The bioavailability of the marketed Hydergine tablets is therefore equal to that of the solution. From urinary data AELLIG and NÜESCH (1977) calculated the elimination half-lives of some hydrogenated ergot peptide alkaloids and found them to be the same for oral and i.v. administration. In general they are in the same range for all substances and confirm the values from plasma data. Table 13 contains the most important kinetic parameters. What is striking is the small difference in the kinetic parameters for the various substances. That this is not due to the method of estimation or calculation is revealed by comparing the differences to those found for the nonhydrogenated ergot peptide alkaloids. Moreover for both nonhydrogenated and hydrogenated substances the procedure in performing the clinical studies and evaluation were the same.

MEIER and SCHREIER (1976) calculated, on the basis of data from AELLIG and NÜESCH (1977), several kinetic parameters for [^{3}H]dihydroergotamine based on a multicompartment model. They obtained the same invasion half-life but a somewhat longer elimination half-life in plasma (α-phase 5.3 hours, β-phase 30.3 hours). A steady-state plasma level of 2–3 ng/ml was calculated on the basis of a dose of 1 mg t.i.d.

Until now it has been possible to demonstrate a correlation beween pharmacokinetic data and therapeutic activity in two experimental studies in man. On the human hand vein, AELLIG (1974) noted a very rapid onset of action of dihydroergotamine after oral administration, which is in keeping with the short absorption half-life. In accordance with the moderately long β-elimination half-life ROUBICEK (1975) found the duration of the activity of Hydergine after intravenous administration to be at least 8 hours as judged from the EEG.

4. Interactions in Man

The absorption of orally administered LSD seems to be decreased and retarded by the simultaneous intake of food. The size of the meal taken also seems to have a slight influence on absorption, maximal plasma concentration and the time needed to attain maximal plasma level (t max) (UPSHALL and WAILLING, 1972).

It was assumed by ZOGLIO et al. (1969) that the better antimigraine effect of ergotamine when given orally together with caffeine instead of alone (FRIEDMAN and VON STORCH, 1951) might be due to the formation of a complex which improved the absorption. BERDE et al. (1970) showed, in a cross-over study in patients, that the absorption of 1 mg [^{3}H]dihydroergocristine (102c) was improved by the simultaneous administration of 100 mg hydroxypropyltheophylline. Both plasma levels and urinary excretion were higher after the combination than after dihydroergocristine alone. An effect on the urinary excretion due to theophylline could be excluded. Therefore, higher plasma levels and the greater amount of radioactivity excreted in the urine must be due to a better absorption. While SUTHERLAND et al. (1974) were unable to demonstrate any improvement in ergotamine absorption when ergotamine and caffeine were given sublingually, SCHMIDT and FANCHAMPS (1974) showed a significantly greater urinary excretion of radioactivity following oral administration of 2 mg [^{3}H]ergotamine along with 200 mg caffeine. In this case it was also possible to exclude the possibility of a diuretic effect due to caffeine. The cumulative urinary excretion of radioactivity up to 24 hours following administration of the combination was 73% greater than the amount excreted after ergotamine alone ($p<0.01$). Plasma levels after the combination were not only higher but also appeared sooner ($p<0.05$). This is an indication that the onset of action is more rapid with the combination, which is certainly of importance in the treatment of migraine.

The kinetics and metabolism of [^{14}C]methysergide (34a) were investigated by BIANCHINE and FRIEDMAN (1970). They studied migraine patients, who had developed retroperitoneal fibrosis as a result of chronic treatment with methysergide, and normal volunteers. Neither the amount of radioactivity excreted in the urine nor the quantity of $^{14}CO_2$ in expired air were different in the two groups. In addition, the time course of elimination of radioactivity in urine and in expired air were the same. Hence there is no alteration in the kinetics due to the disease, and there is no indication that the latter is caused by any error of metabolism.

5. Physicochemical Properties of Ergot Alkaloids Which May Affect Enteral Absorption

The ergot alkaloids are weak bases which are presumably absorbed like most drugs by passive diffusion of the nonionized form of the molecule. The pH at the site of absorption determines the degree of ionization. The section of the gastrointestinal tract in which compounds of this class are absorbed is not known. However, it may be assumed that no absorption occurs in the stomach where the ergot molecule is presumably in the form of a salt.

Of the physicochemical influences exerted by the internal environment, particular importance attaches to the pH value, i.e., the hydrogen ion concentration. Properties of a compound which are decisive for the absorption process are its solubility and the distribution ratio between lipid and water. The effect of membrane potential and permeability, which must be taken into account when considering the penetration of the active compound through the various membrane barriers, is not readily accessible to experimental investigation. The known physicochemical properties of ergot alkaloids which permit assessment of their enteral absorption will be discussed briefly below.

a) Solubility

The ergot alkaloids in the form of the free bases are poorly soluble in water. BERCEL (1950) and FRIEDMAN (1954) established that the pharmacologic effect of ergotamine (20) is enhanced when it is administered together with caffeine, and from this finding ZOGLIO et al. (1969) assumed that this combination might improve the enteral absorption of ergotamine. It was, in fact, shown in in vitro experiments that caffeine increases the aqueous solubility of ergotamine tartrate. Maximum solubility was attained in distilled water at 30° C with a molar ratio of caffeine to ergotamine tartrate of 30:1. ZOGLIO et al. (1969) and ZOGLIO and MAULDING (1970a) also found that the solubility was dependent on the pH inasmuch as the tartrate was best soluble in strongly acid medium (0.1 *N* HCl), the solubility declining with increasing formation of free base. As ZOGLIO and MAULDING (1970a) and MAULDING and ZOGLIO (1970a, 1970b) demonstrated, a parallel effect is observed with various xanthines, in that their effect on solubility decreases with increasing pH (see Table 14). It was suggested by ZOGLIO et al. (1969) that ergotamine tartrate might form a complex with caffeine, but no experimental evidence was adduced to support this hypothesis. From the available data it is not possible to say definitely whether the enhancement of solubility is due, as postulated, to formation of a complex or to solubilization. MAULDING and ZOGLIO (1970a) interpreted the influence of 7-β-hydroxypropyltheophylline on the solubility of dihydroergocristine mesylate as a solubilization effect. Increasing the concentration of xanthine above 50 mg/ml does not lead to any further increase in the solubility of the ergot alkaloid. Further investigations by MAULDING and ZOGLIO (1970b) and ZOGLIO and MAULDING (1970b) yielded similar findings. Neither the stoichiometry of the hypothetic complex nor the constants governing its formation have been demonstrated, so that the manner in which xanthines interact with the ergot alkaloids must remain an open question.

b) The Ionization Constants

K_a is the dissociation constant of an acid and K_b that of a base in dilute aqueous solution[2]. The following reversible reaction (conjugate base $\rightleftharpoons$ acid) is an important one for ergot alkaloids:

$$[\rhd \underline{N}^6\text{—}CH_3]+[H^+] \rightleftharpoons \left[>\overset{+}{\underset{\substack{| \\ H}}{\underline{N}^6}}\text{—}CH_3 \right].$$

[2] K_a and K_b can only be accurately determined by taking into account the activity coefficient, i.e., the factor by which the ionic concentration must be multiplied in order to obtain the concentration of the free ions which are not subject to electrostatic constraints. The data employed are based on concentrations, not on activities, and strictly speaking should be designated K'_a, K'_b and pK'_a and pK'_b. However, for the sake of simplicity, these symbols will be employed here without the prime.

Table 14. Effect of the molar proportions of caffeine to ergotamine on the solubility of ergotamine at various pH values

pH	Molar ratio of caffeine to ergotamine affording maximum solubility	Solubility of ergotamine tartrate (mg/ml)
1	20:1	20
5.5	30:1	9
6.65	800:1	0.3

Single bonds and free electron pair (underline) are indicated. Superscript to the right of the nitrogen refers to the nitrogen at position 6 in the tetracyclic structure of ergot alkaloids.

To simplify the terminology the negative logarithm of the dissociation constants pK_a are employed in accordance with the HENDERSON-HASSELBALCH equation:

$$pH = pK_a + \log \frac{[\text{conjugate base}]}{[\text{acid}]},$$

and $pH = pK_a$ when half the conjugate base is in the ionized form. pK_b may then be calculated from the relation $pK_a + pK_b = 14$. With increasing pK_a the basicity of basic compounds increases, and conversely with increasing acidity, pK_a decreases for an acidic compound.

Since lysergic acid forms the basis of the tetracyclic structure of ergot alkaloids, the pK_{a_1} values[3] of lysergic acid and its isocompound will be dealt with first and compared. CRAIG et al. (1938) determined the dissociation constants of lysergic acid and derivatives in aqueous solution. They found pK_{a_1} values of 3.19 and 3.44 for lysergic acid and pK_{a_1} values of 3.21 and 3.44 for isolysergic acid. HOFMANN (1964) measured the dissociation constants in 80% aqueous methylcellosolve and found values deviating from those of CRAIG et al. (1938) and, furthermore, different values for lysergic acid ($pK_{a_1} = 4.4$) and isolysergic acid ($pK_{a_1} = 4.0$). By definition dissociation constants apply to dilute aqueous solutions, hence comparisons between values obtained in mixed solvents must be interpreted with caution, even on extrapolating to zero concentrations of solvent. In the same paper by CRAIG et al. (1938) other pK_a values were published for lysergic acid and isolysergic acid derivatives. With the limited analytic methods available at the time there were only restricted means of verifying the purity of the compounds investigated. Despite this shortcoming the data published will serve as rough estimates. Surprisingly enough, the pK_a values measured by CRAIG et al. (1938) for ergonovine (19) (6.73 ± 0.16 at 24° C) approximates very closely the pK_a value for methylergonovine (73a) (6.65 ± 0.03 at 24° C) determined by MAULDING and ZOGLIO (1970c).

In their studies of the stereochemistry of lysergic acids and dihydrolysergic acids STOLL et al. (1954b) also determined pK_a values in 80% cellosolve. As already

[3] For compounds with more than one pK_a value, e.g., a dipolar ion, the value is that for the conjugate base when titration is carried out with strong acid (pK_{a_1}) and conversely the value is that for the acid when strong base is employed for the titration (pK_{a_2}).

pointed out pK_a values determined in this way are not to be equated with the thermodynamic constants and should not therefore be employed to assess the behavior of ergot alkaloids in physiologic fluids.

The low solubility of the ergot peptide alkaloid bases render determination of the pK_a values in aqueous solution either difficult or impossible. For this reason HOFMANN (1964) measured these values in 80% methylcellosolve, while MAULDING and ZOGLIO (1970c) carried out their measurements on aqueous solutions containing 10%–20% 7-β-hydroxypropyltheophylline. These pK_a values must also be regarded as approximations and may show appreciable variation in different solvent mixtures. MAULDING and ZOGLIO (1970c) succeeded in determining the thermodynamic dissociation constants of two lysergic acid derivatives, namely methysergide (34a) ($pK_a = 6.62 \pm 0.02$ at 24° C) and methylergonovine (73a) ($pK_a = 6.65 \pm 0.03$ at 24° C).

c) The Distribution Ratio Between Lipid and Water

The pH partition hypothesis was developed by HOGBEN et al. (1959) on the basis of experimental studies. One of the conclusions from the experiments relates to the pK_a values of acids and bases. Acids with a pK_a of less than 3 and bases with a pK_a of more than 7.8 are absorbed to only a limited extent. These experimental data were interpreted as follows: absorption of the nonionized form of an active compound should be favored by its more rapid penetration of the intestinal barrier. The distribution of ergotamine (20) tartrate between 0.1 *N* hydrochloric acid and chloroform was little affected by caffeine, whereas the latter had a considerably greater effect on the distribution of this compound between 0.1 *M* phosphate buffer at pH 6.65 and the organic phase. ZOGLIO et al. (1969) have also established for caffeine itself that the rate of transfer between the phases increases at higher pHs. In further studies of dihydroergotoxine mesylate ZOGLIO and MAULDING (1970a) have shown that the rate of distribution between an aqueous solution (pH 6.65) and chloroform proceeds three times more rapidly in the presence of 100-fold excess of caffeine than in the absence of it. The more rapid attainment of equilibrium between the solvents employed is to be attributed to the probable solubilization effect of caffeine. On the other hand, at strongly acid pHs at which the ergot alkaloid is present in the form of a salt ZOGLIO and MAULDING (1970a) found that caffeine had less effect. Solubility and distribution are inversely proportional to the pH, i.e, the free base with its poor aqueous solubility is taken up more readily in the organic phase than the protonated molecule. The rate of transfer of the base into the lipophilic phase depends on the concentration, and since it is the rate-limiting process, it may possibly be a factor which limits absorption.

6. Synopsis

The treatment of pharmacokinetics in Section C. 2.a) assigned a central position to the role of the liver in its distribution of ergot alkaloids and their metabolites. It will be recalled that the compounds are not readily fitted into a scheme of classification according to the route of elimination. However, the different compounds, e.g., those of the ergoline class such as nicergoline (104e) and methergoline

(89d), are classified as being mainly excreted either in the bile or in the urine by the various animal species investigated (rat, dog and monkey). This differing pattern of excretion is doubtless mainly governed by the way in which the compounds are metabolized, the hepatic distribution varying with the structure of the molecules. To take the case of two compounds of similar molecular weight (m.w.), a metabolite of nicergoline (1,6-dimethyl-8β-hydroxymethyl-10α-methergoline, m.w. 300) and LSD (73b) (m.w. 320), the former is mainly excreted with the urine, whereas LSD is excreted with the bile. Compounds in this intermediate range of molecular weights may either be excreted with the bile or with the urine. It is probably the structural characteristics of the molecule which decide the route of excretion. Precisely since distribution between plasma and bile is dependent on both structure and molecular weight, it is not possible, at the present time at least, to establish any general rules concerning the route of excretion. Basically, however, ergot alkaloids may be classified in a rough and ready fashion according to molecular weight as a means of predicting the route of excretion. Substances with a molecular weight of less than 350 are excreted in the renal tubules with the urine. For compounds in the molecular range 350–450 it is presumably the structure which determines whether excretion occurs by one route or the other. Above m.w. 450, the bile is the preferred route of excretion. The ergot peptide alkaloids and the majority of their metabolites (see D. Metabolism: dihydro-β-ergokryptine) fall into this category. These two possible routes of excretion of the ergot alkaloids are species-dependent inasmuch as metabolic degradation presumably varies qualitatively and quantitatively from species to species, and as a consequence either one route or the other will predominate in a given species.

Enteral absorption in the intact animal and in human subjects after oral and intravenous administration can be estimated from the fraction excreted in the urine if the amount excreted is sufficient. This method of determining enteral absorption is valid if the hepatic distribution ratio is the same for orally administered as for intravenously administered doses of active compound, i.e., provided $Q_{i.v.} = Q_{p.o.}$. Ergot alkaloids sometimes do not fulfil this precondition. Moreover, plasma levels are low and the pattern of absorption, as determined from the area under the plasma level time curve, which frequently shows great variation, would appear to be much affected by the metabolic capacity of the liver (first-pass effect). Nevertheless, studies in the intact organism are feasible and they are practiced.

The enteral absorption of ergot compounds has been investigated in bile fistula animals. Broadly speaking the ergolines and lysergic acid and derivatives are better absorbed than the nonhydrogenated ergot peptide alkaloids which, in turn, are better absorbed than the hydrogenated ergot peptide alkaloids.

Most experiments in man have been carried out with [^{3}H] labeled ergot alkaloids. The findings reflect the absorption pattern in animals, inasmuch as the same decreasing order of intestinal absorption is found: the ergolines and lysergic acid and derivatives are best absorbed, followed by the nonhydrogenated ergot peptide alkaloids and, lastly, the dihydrogenated ergot peptide alkaloids. After oral administration of the dihydrogenated ergot peptide alkaloids the amount of radioactivity in the plasma was low and after a dose of 1 mg attained a maximum of 1 ng-equiv/ml. Urinary excretion under these conditions amounted to approximately 3% of the oral dose (t = ∞). Plasma levels were considerably higher (1.5–2.3 ng-equiv/ml) for nonhydrogenated ergot peptide alkaloids and highest (10–50 ng-equiv/ml) for ergolines and lysergic acid and derivatives. The ratio of the very small amounts of radioactivity excreted in the urine after oral and after intravenous administration of the nonhydrogenated and dihydrogenated ergot peptide alkaloids can be regarded as a rough estimate of intestinal absorption. However, if the hepatic distribution pattern differed for either route of administration, and this has been shown in bile fistula animals to be the case for some ergot alkaloids, the oral/i.v. urinary excretion ratio would not yield a reliable value for intestinal absorption.

D. Metabolism

1. Introduction

Despite considerable interest in ergot alkaloids and derivatives, particularly d-lysergic acid diethylamide LSD (73b), complete information on biotransformation is lacking for most of these compounds. There are two reasons for this – first the chemistry is difficult, and second the compounds are highly potent and are given in small doses, so that the levels attained in biologic materials are very low. As a result the isolation of metabolites from the blood and organs and their identification and assay pose a daunting problem to the chemist.

A review of the metabolic studies of ergot alkaloids during the last decade must give due consideration to the information and techniques available at the time. Mass spectrometry and nuclear magnetic resonance spectrometry, for example, have become routine methods in the study of drug metabolism only in the last 10 years.

Moreover, it was not until 1955 that BRODIE showed microsomal enzyme systems to be responsible for the metabolism of many drugs, and at that time the experimental techniques of microsomal incubation were still in their infancy.

The literature is characterized by its heterogeneity, the metabolic studies being performed either in vitro with liver microsomes or in vivo by analysis of urine or bile from different animal species. The only human data so far published relate to metabolites of methysergide (34a), methergoline (89d) and nicergoline (104e).

From the available data, the different sites of biotransformation mentioned in the literature can be depicted diagrammatically for each of the three structural classes – the 1-methyl-ergolines, lysergic acid derivatives and peptide alkaloids of ergot. The literature references are not given in the diagrams but will be found in the text and tables.

Even a cursory examination of the three diagrams (Fig. 3, 4 and 5) reveals the great difference between the ergolines and the lysergic acid derivatives on one hand and the peptide alkaloids of ergot on the other. The former are biotransformed at the 1-methyl, the 6-methyl, and the 8-substituent and in the aromatic ring structure, while the latter are mainly metabolized in the proline ring of the peptide moiety.

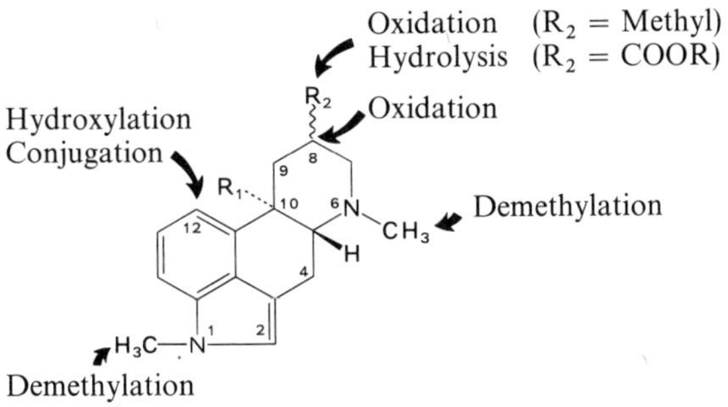

Oxidation (R_2 = Methyl)
Hydrolysis (R_2 = COOR)
Oxidation
Hydroxylation
Conjugation
Demethylation
Demethylation

R_1 = H, OCH_3
C_8—C_9 = Single or double bond

Fig. 3. Sites of biotransformation in compounds with the 1-methylergoline structure

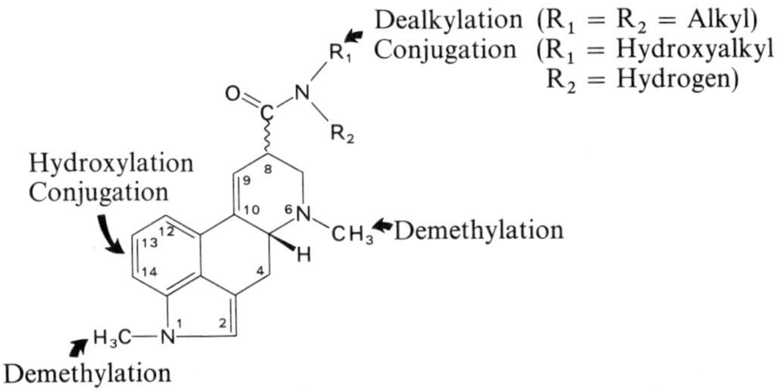

Dealkylation (R_1 = R_2 = Alkyl)
Conjugation (R_1 = Hydroxyalkyl
R_2 = Hydrogen)
Hydroxylation
Conjugation
Demethylation
Demethylation

C-8 Substituent: axial or equatorial position

Fig. 4. Sites of biotransformation in compounds with the 1-methyl-lysergic acid structure

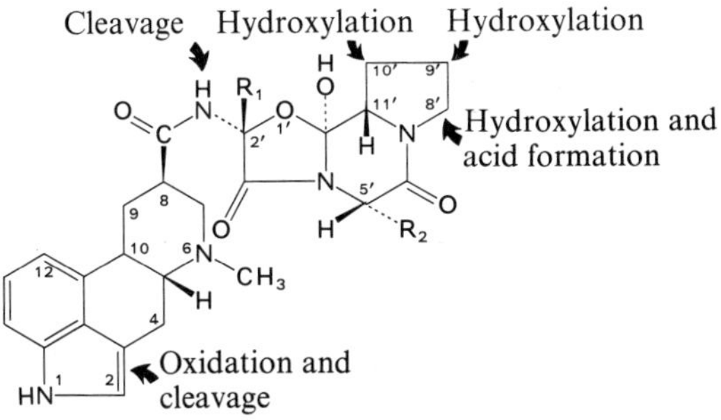

Cleavage Hydroxylation Hydroxylation
Hydroxylation and acid formation
Oxidation and cleavage

R_1 and R_2 = Alkyl
C_9—C_{10} = Single or double bond

Fig. 5. Sites of biotransformation in the hydrogenated and nonhydrogenated peptide alkaloids of ergot

However, the links between the results of incubation experiments and in vivo studies and the blood or tissue metabolites and biliary or urinary excretion products still have to be elucidated. Furthermore, until recently no systematic work had been published on the biotransformation of a given compound in different species or on the metabolism of a series of ergot alkaloids of different structure in the same in vitro or in vivo model.

2. Experiments

In this chapter in vitro and in vivo work will be discussed separately and details will be given of the purpose of the experiment as well as the animals and materials used. The assay methods employed will be described as will the methods employed in elucidating the chemical structure of the metabolites and in their preparation. The conditions of in vitro incubation and the yields obtained, the chromatographic solvent systems and mass spectrometric fragmentation patterns are summarized for convenience in Tables 15 and 16 and Fig. 6.

a) In Vitro Experiments

α) Ergolines

[^{14}C]Agroclavine (5) isolated from cultures of Claviceps grown in the presence of generally labeled [^{14}C]tryptophan was incubated with liver microsomes by WILSON et al. (1971). Table 15 indicates the incubation conditions and the yields of noragroclavine and elymoclavine (6). Formaldehyde formed by demethylation of agroclavine was assayed by the method of NASH (1953). The in vitro metabolism of agroclavine by microsomal fractions from rat livers was further studied by WILSON and ORRENIUS (1972).

The intubation mixture was rendered alkaline and agroclavine and its metabolites were extracted with chloroform. The extract was submitted to thin-layer chromatography in different solvent systems (Table 16) together with appropriate synthetic reference compounds for purposes of identification. The metabolites were characterized by their Rf values, fluorescence and color reactions with Van Urk reagent.

β) Lysergic Acid and Derivatives

When AXELROD et al. (1957) first investigated LSD (73b), many aspects of the cellular processes involved in drug metabolism were still unknown. In preliminary experiments slices of various guinea pig tissues were incubated with LSD in Krebs Ringer buffer and the liver was found to be the site of metabolic breakdown. By separation into nuclear, mitochondrial, microsomal and soluble fractions it was shown that both the microsomal and the soluble fractions were necessary for metabolic activity. An enzyme system generating NADPH, consisting of glucose-6-phosphate dehydrogenase and NADP, was added to the microsomal fraction and found to be as effective as the soluble fraction for biotransformation of LSD (Table 15).

By the time SZARA (1963) was conducting his studies, discrepancies had been noted between the results of the previous in vitro studies with guinea pig liver microsomes and those obtained in vivo in bile fistula rats (SLAYTOR and WRIGHT, 1962). Incubations were therefore carried out with liver microsomes from both species—male guinea pigs and male albino rats (the conditions and yields are given in Table 15). No radioactive material was used in this study and LSD was estimated by AXELROD's fluorimetric method. A "phenolic" metabolite was extracted and the absorption spectrum of the reaction product with diazotized sulphanilic acid was recorded and compared to 6-hydroxy-indole.

In one of the latest in vitro studies of the metabolism of LSD, NIWAGUCHI et al. (1974a) centrifuged liver homogenates from male Wistar rats, male guinea pigs and male albino rabbits at 9000 *g* and employed the supernatant fraction for their experiments. The authors carried out these studies in vitro in order to investigate species differences and inhibition by SKF 525-A, chlorpromazine, nitrazepam, meprobamate and brain monoamines. (For incubation conditions, see Table 15.) The mass spectra of the metabolites were published by NIWAGUCHI et al. (1974a) and the origin of two fragments is indicated in the structural formula of LSD. A discussion of the mass-spectra of lysergic acid derivatives can be found in the publication of INOUE et al. (1972). Figure 6 shows fragments of the lysergamide moiety of relevance to the structural elucidation of compounds of this class. In a later paper, NIWAGUCHI and INOUE (1975) investigated the relation between metabolic degradation by rat liver microsomes and the binding of LSD to cytochrome P450.

A microsomal suspension obtained by ultracentrifugation at 105,000 *g* for 60 min was employed for these studies. The LSD was incubated in the presence of NADPH, nicotinamide and magnesium chloride as cofactors. LSD was assayed as described previously.

In another paper the same authors (1974b) compared the biotransformation of various lysergic acid derivatives in order to gain an insight into the pharmacologic action of LSD.

SIDDIK et al. (1975) perfused isolated rat livers with ^{14}C-ethyl-labeled LSD. The perfusate consisted of resuspended human cells. Bile from the rat liver was chromatographed on paper (for solvents, see Table 16), and the perfusate was extracted with chloroform and chromatographed on thin-layer silica gel plates (Table 16) for identification and assay of the metabolites. Rat liver perfusion was employed to permit the isolation of metabolites in preparative quantities.

b) In Vivo Experiments

α) Ergolines

ARCAMONE et al. (1971) administered [9,10-^{3}H]methergoline (89d) to rats, guinea pigs, dogs, monkeys (Patas), rabbits and humans. The urine was analysed by paper chromatography (Table 16) and was also extracted with organic solvents before and after incubation with glucuronidase, so that the metabolite groups could be classified. Bile from bile fistula rats was chromatographed under identical conditions. The partially purified extracts were incubated with glucuronidase.

Table 15. Summary of relevant information on in vitro experiments with ergot alkaloids

Compound and reference	Species	Conditions	Cofactors	Rate of conversion or quantity converted
Agroclavine (5) Wilson et al. (1971)	Sprague Dawley male rats; Albino male guinea pigs	Microsomal suspension; 4 mg protein in 2 ml total volume; 2.5 µmol substrate; Buffer: succinic acid/Tris pH 7.5	5 mM $MgCl_2$; 0.005 mM $MnCl_2$; 1 mM NADP; 5 mM isocitrate; 0.4 IU pig heart isocitrate dehydrogenase	1.7 nmol formaldehyde min/mg protein; Rat[a]: 5.6% nor-agroclavine, 1.8% elymoclavine; Guinea pig[a]: 5.8% nor-agroclavine, 2.7% elymoclavine
LSD (73b) Niwaguchi et al. (1974a)	Wistar male rats; Hartley male guinea pigs; Albino male rabbits	Homogenate: 9000 *g* fraction from 1.5 g liver; 5 ml total volume; 0.63 µmol substrate; Buffer: phosphate pH 7.4 (0.5 ml of 0.8 M solution)	1 µmol NADP; 100 µmol nicotinamide; 100 µmol $MgCl_2$	0.5 µmol in 2 h (80%); Rat: 27.3 nmol/mg protein/2 h; Guinea pig: 25.4 nmol/mg protein/2 h; Rabbit: 21.7 nmol/mg protein/2 h
Lysergic acid derivatives Niwaguchi et al. (1974b)	Wistar male rats	Homogenate: 9000 *g* fraction from 1.5 g liver; 5 ml total volume; 0.5–3 µmol substrate; Buffer: 0.4 mmol phosphate pH 7.4	1 µmol NADP; 100 µmol nicotinamide; 100 µmol $MgCl_2$	27–83% in 2 h depending on substrate
LSD (73b) Szara (1963)	Male guinea pigs; Male albino rats	Homogenate from 750 mg tissue; 5 ml total volume; 0.58 µmol substrate; Buffer: 400 µmol phosphate pH 7.2	0.3 µmol NADP; 100 µmol $MgCl_2$	Rat: 0.23 µmol in 2 h (40%); Guinea pig: 0.30 µmol in 2 h (52%)
LSD (73b) Axelrod et al. (1957)	Guinea pigs	Homogenate from 200 mg tissue; 5 ml total volume; 0.6 µmol substrate; Buffer: 500 µmol phosphate pH 7.9	0.2 µmol NADP; 50 µmol nicotinamide; 25 µmol $MgCl_2$	0.46 µmol in 2 h (77%)
LSD (73b) Axelrod et al. (1957)	Guinea pigs	Pure microsomal fraction without supernatant	Similar as above + 35 µmol glucose-6-phosphate; 1 mg glucose-6-phosphate dehydrogenase	0.48 µmol in 2 h (80%)

[a] Time of incubation: 30 min

1-Demethyl-methergoline was isolated from rabbit urine, human urine and rat bile and compared chromatographically with reference compounds (Table 16). A phenol glucuronide of methergoline was isolated from rat bile by paper chromatography (Table 16) and hydrolyzed with glucuronidase. The 12-OH derivative for which a synthetic reference compound was available, was assayed in rabbit urine by isotope dilution and in rat bile after treatment with glucuronidase.

Nicergoline (104e) (ARCAMONE et al., 1972) was administered in different radioactive forms: randomly labeled with ^{3}H, labeled in the 17 position with ^{3}H, doubly labeled with ^{14}C and ^{3}H (with ^{14}C in the nicotinic acid residue and in position 17 with ^{3}H). These compounds were administered orally to Sprague-Dawley rats, female Beagle dogs, female rhesus monkeys and to four human subjects, and the metabolites excreted in the urine were analyzed by paper and thin-layer chromatography (Table 16). Paper chromatography, UV spectrometry and mass spectrometry were employed to compare the metabolites with reference compounds for purposes of identification.

β) Lysergic Acid and Derivatives

BOYD et al. (1955a, b) administered LSD (73b) labeled in the ethyl group with ^{14}C intravenously to female rats with cannulated bile ducts. The bile itself or an alkaline extract was chromatographed on paper (Table 16). $^{14}CO_2$ in the expired air was absorbed in potassium hydroxide solution in order to measure the extent of deethylation. STOLL et al. (1955) determined the levels of unchanged LSD in the organs of white mice using isotope dilution, but following a procedure otherwise similar to that employed by BOYD et al.

In a longer paper, BOYD (1959) gave additional details concerning LSD. As before they used LSD labeled with ^{14}C in the ethyl group in order to check the yields of all analytic steps by radioactivity counting. $^{14}CO_2$ was assayed as in their previous paper. Rat bile (sex and breed of rats not indicated) was chromatographed on paper in three solvent systems (Table 16). Three successive chromatographies yielded relatively pure preparations of two main metabolites. Color reactions with Van Urk, ninhydrin or cinnamaldehyde reagents and fluorescence under the UV lamp characterized the different chromatographic zones. With very small quantities of material IR spectra were recorded. UV spectra of the two main metabolites were compared with LSD.

Absorption spectra were recorded after reaction with paradimethylaminobenzaldehyde in 6 *N* sulphuric acid. The UV spectra at different pH values yielded some evidence suggesting the presence of a phenolic group. The compounds were incubated with β-glucuronidase since titration revealed the presence of an acidic group.

The only investigations using nonradioactive compounds are those published by SLAYTOR and WRIGHT (1962) on LSD and ergometrine (19). They collected bile, exhaustively extracted it and used the concentrated methanol extracts for paper chromatography in three solvent systems (Table 16) for analytic work. The metabolites of LSD separated by chromatography were cleaved by β-glucuronidase to a product containing possibly a phenolic hydroxyl group. The same separation method and analytic tests were carried out on ergometrine metabolites excreted in rat bile. But in this case two dose levels (3 and 45 mg/kg body wt.) were used for preparative work since some new metabolites were seen at a high dose level. Chromatography of the phenols obtained after glucuronidase treatment led to a product with the same Rf values as the authentic 12-hydroxyergometrine. The parent compound and its isomer were isolated as glucuronides.

In the latest work on LSD (SIDDIK et al., 1975) ethyl ^{14}C-labeled material was injected intraperitoneally into adult female Wistar rats or intravenously (femoral vein) into bile duct cannulated rats. Urine, bile and fecal homogenates were chromatographed on paper (Table 16). $^{14}CO_2$ was determined in the expired air by an undescribed method. A sample of 12-hydroxy LSD was synthesized for mass-spectrometric and chromatographic analysis and comparison. Mass-spectrometric analysis of some metabolites were performed.

BIANCHINE (1968) administered methysergide (34a) intravenously to male New Zealand rabbits and orally to human subjects. The metabolites were separated by thin-layer chromatography (Table 16). The analysis was probably preceded by an extraction step. Studies of the [6-*methyl*-^{14}C]compound have been carried out by KALBERER et al. (1975) in Wistar rats, Beagle dogs, rhesus monkeys and human subjects. The urine samples were analyzed on thin-layer silica gel plates (Table 16) after extraction of the metabolites with Amberlite XAD-2.

γ) Ergot Peptide Alkaloids

For dihydro-*β*-ergokryptine (102f) the work by MAURER (1977) describes an interesting method of obtaining sufficient quantities of starting material for isolation of metabolites and structural elucidation. Every week for five weeks 18 male Wistar bile fistula rats were operated on and kept in metabolism cages for 5 days. Three times a day a dose of dihydro-*β*-ergokryptine was administered to the rats by intraperitoneal catheters. During 4 days of each week this pattern was followed and the bile produced collected continuously. On one day a dose of radioactive [9,10-^{3}H]dihydro-*β*-ergokryptine was injected to provide a check on excretion, yield, and separation in the subsequent preparative steps. The bile was kept as a freeze-dried powder.

The preliminary purification was carried out in a chromatographic column of Amberlite XAD-2, a polystyrene-divinyl polymer which had been suggested for use as a chromatographic support by GRIESER and PIETRZYK (1973) and by CHI-HONG CHU and PIETRZYK (1974). Elution was performed with a gradient of methanol-water in a manner similar to that employed for reversed phase chromatography; this permitted separation into five peaks. Depending upon the polarity of the peak constituents they were then submitted to column chromatography on the ion-exchanger Sephadex DEAE A25 or chromatographed on silica gel and eluted with chloroform containing a varying amount of methanol. The final purification stage was unusual for preparative work, namely high performance liquid chromatography on 5 μm Lichrosorb in glass columns, followed by elution with chloroform saturated with water and containing varying percentages of methanol. Preparative thin-layer chromatography was employed for the final purification of the polar metabolites (Table 16).

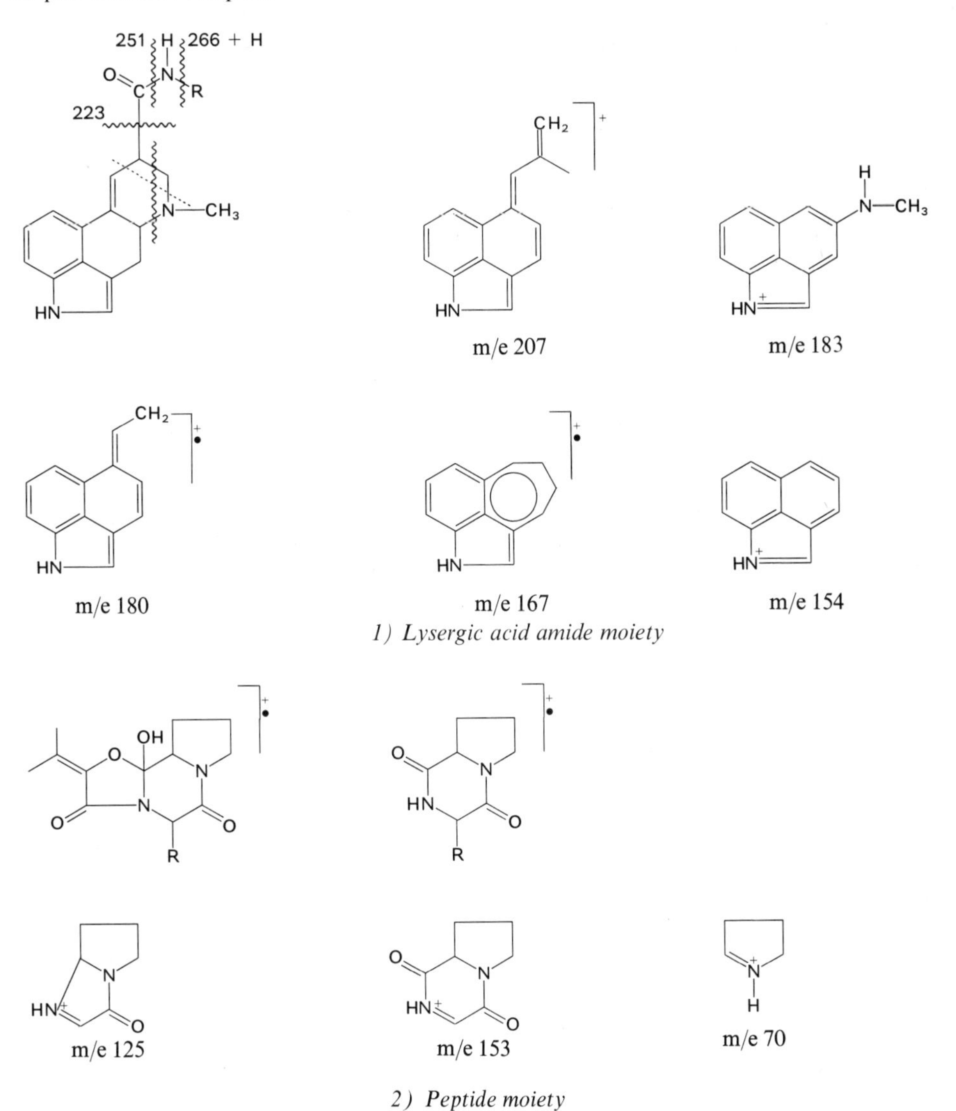

Fig. 6. Fragments in the mass spectra of lysergic acid amide, related compounds and peptide alkaloids of ergot, relevant to biotransformation studies

The metabolites were characterized by their Rf values in appropriate solvent systems (Table 16), by Van Urk, ninhydrin and 1,3-naphthalindiol reactions and in the case of nonpolar derivatives by their elution volumes. Except for dihydrolysergamide (74a) no reference compounds were available for structural elucidation.

It was therefore necessary to employ a combination of ultraviolet, infrared, mass and nuclear magnetic resonance spectroscopy techniques to determine the structures of these highly complex molecules. In addition, an amino acid analysis

Table 16. List of solvents used in thin-layer or paper chromatography of metabolites of the ergot alkal

Compounds and reference	Sample containing metabolites	Carrier	Solvent system	
Agroclavine (5) WILSON et al. (1971)	Chloroform extract of microsomal incubation product	Silica gel G	$CHCl_3$:EtOH $CHCl_3$:MeOH:NH_4OH $CHCl_3$:$(Et)_3N$ $CHCl_3$:$(Et)_2NH$ iPrOH:H_2O:NH_4OH iPrOH:AcOEt:NH_4OH	5:1 50:20:0.2 9:1 9:1 80:18:2 35:45:20
Nicergoline (104e) ARCAMONE et al. (1972)	Urine	Paper (Whatman No. 1) Silica gel G (Merck)	n-BuOH:AcOH:H_2O n-BuOH:Py:H_2O AcOEt:DMF:n-BuOH:H_2O	4:1:5 } uppe 4:1:5 } phas 4:3:3:1
Methergoline (89d) ARCAMONE et al. (1971)	Urine	Paper (Whatman No. 1)	n-BuOH:Py:H_2O	4:1:5
LSD (73b) SZARA (1963)	Extract of microsomal incubation product	Whatman No. 1	n-BuOH:AcOH	10:1 saturate with H_2
LSD (73b) Ergometrine SLAYTOR and WRIGHT (1962)	Bile or methanol extract of bile	Whatman No. 1 or 3	n-BuOH:AcOH:H_2O n-BuOH:H_2O (saturated) n-BuOH:NH_4OH (saturated)	4:1:5
d-Lysergic acid dimethylamide NIWAGUCHI et al. (1974b)	Chloroform extract of microsomal incubation product	Silica gel G (Merck)	MeOH:$CHCl_3$ Acetone:AcOEt:DMF MeOH:$CHCl_3$	1:4 5:5:1 4:1
d-Isolysergic acid dimethyl-amide NIWAGUCHI et al. (1974b)	Chloroform extract of microsomal incubation product	Silica gel G (Merck)	MeOH:$CHCl_3$ MeOH:$(Et)_2NH$:$CHCl_3$ MeOH:$CHCl_3$	1:3 0.2:1:9 1:3
Lysergic acid amide and isoform NIWAGUCHI et al. (1974b)	Chloroform extract of microsomal incubation product	Silica gel G (Merck)	MeOH:$CHCl_3$ Acetone:AcOEt:DMF MeOH:$CHCl_3$	1:4 5:5:1 1:3
Methysergide (34a) Methylergo-metrine (73a) NIWAGUCHI et al. (1974b)	Chloroform extract of microsomal incubation product	Silica gel G (Merck)	MeOH:$CHCl_3$ Acetone:AcOEt:DMF MeOH:$CHCl_3$:n-Hexane	1:4 5:5:1 1:4:2
d-Isolysergic acid-L-2-butanolamide NIWAGUCHI et al. (1974b)	Chloroform extract of microsomal incubation product	Silica gel G (Merck)	MeOH:$CHCl_3$ Acetone:AcOEt:DMF Acetone:$CHCl_3$	1:4 5:5:1 4:1

ıble 16 (continued)

ɔmpounds and ference	Sample containing metabolites	Carrier	Solvent system	
SD (73b) ɔYD (1958)	Bile Urine	Whatman No. 1	n-BuOH:AcOH:H_2O n-BuOH saturated with $1.5 \cdot 10^{-3}$ M NH_4OH Collidine:lutidine	6:1:5 1:1 saturated with H_2O
SD (73b) ɔDIK et al. (1975)	Bile Urine Fecal homogenates	Whatman No. 1 (No. 3 for preparative work)	n-BuOH:AcOH:H_2O	4:1:2
	Chloroform extract of perfusate	Silica gel HF_{254}	$CHCl_3$:MeOH	4:1
SD (73b) WAGUCHI et al. (1974a)	Chloroform extract of microsomal incubation product	Silica gel G (Merck)	MeOH:$CHCl_3$:n-Hexane MeOH:$CHCl_3$ Acetone:$CHCl_3$	1:4:2 1:4 4:1
ɔLSD WAGUCHI et al. (1974b)	Chloroform extract of microsomal incubation product	Silica gel G (Merck)	MeOH:$CHCl_3$ Acetone:AcOEt:DMF $(Et)_2NH$:$CHCl_3$	1:4 5:5:1 1:9
Bromo-d-lysergic acid diethylamide (37a) WAGUCHI et al. (1974b)	Chloroform extract of microsomal incubation product	Silica gel G (Merck)	Acetone:$CHCl_3$ Acetone:$CHCl_3$ Cyclohexane:$CHCl_3$:$(Et)_2NH$	4:1 1:1 5:4:1
ethysergide (34a) ANCHINE (1968) ALBERER et al. (1975)	Urine	Silica gel G	$CHCl_3$:MeOH $CHCl_3$:MeOH:NH_4OH $CHCl_3$:MeOH:iPrOH:H_2O CH_2Cl_2:MeOH Acetone:MeOH	4:1 70:30:2 65:35:10:10 85:15 70:30
hydro-β-ergokryptine (102f) AURER (1977)	Bile extract	Silica gel F_{254} (Merck)	$CHCl_3$:MeOH:AcOH:H_2O $CHCl_3$:MeOH:NH_4OH:H_2O n-BuOH:AcOH:H_2O n-PrOH:NH_4OH:H_2O $CHCl_3$:MeOH $CHCl_3$:MeOH:H_2O n-PrOH:MeOH:NH_4OH	80:18:0.5:1.5 80:23:2:1.5 4:1:1 8:1:1 9:1 80:18:2 70:30:10

eOH: methanol; EtOH: ethanol; iPrOH: isopropanol; n-PrOH: propanol; n-BuOH: butanol; DMF: ıethylformamide: Py: pyridine; AcOH: acetic acid; AcOEt: ethyl acetate; NH_4OH: 25% solution.

of the hydrolyzed metabolites yielded information on the presence of proline and isoleucine residues in the peptide moiety. Valuable information was also forthcoming from analysis of the mass spectra which did not display a molecular peak but which revealed the presence of the dihydrolysergamide fragment and the peptide moiety. The fragments were similar or identical to those described by VOKOUN et al. (1974), VOKOUN and REHACEK (1975), and VOIGT et al. (1974) for peptide alkaloids of ergot and those described by INOUE et al. (1972) for lysergic acid derivatives. The fragments of lysergamide and of the peptide moiety employed for the structural elucidation are shown in Figure 6.

In the examination by nuclear magnetic resonance spectroscopy use was made of deuterated pyridine, dimethylsulphoxide and chloroform to elucidate regions of interest and to investigate the known effect of the solvents on chemical shifts undergone by some of the protons. Double-resonance experiments were performed on the mono- and dihydroxylated metabolites to measure the coupling constants and to determine the angles of vicinal protons with a view to exploring the stereochemistry of the metabolites.

Methyl esters were prepared from acids, and acetates were prepared from alcohols, in order to demonstrate the presence of these functional groups. The introduction of an acetyl group into the alcohol produces a typical shift of the geminal proton to lower fields. This phenomenon helped to assign signals to individual protons. A metabolite conjugated with glutathione was split by reduction with Raney Nickel and the reaction product was identified.

3. Biotransformation Sites in the Molecule

a) Ergolines

Agroclavine (5) (cf. Table 17): The structure of agroclavine, an 8-ergolene, offers a number of possible sites for oxidation by liver microsomes, such as the aromatic rings, the double bond in the 8,9 position, the N-methyl and the C-methyl group.

WILSON et al. (1971) showed that rat liver and guinea pig liver microsomes demethylated agroclavine at N-6 to noragroclavine and oxidized the C-8 methyl to a hydroxymethyl group (elymoclavine) (6).

Demethylation at N-6 was also demonstrated by assaying the formaldehyde formed during incubation. Incubation with rat liver microsomes yielded setoclavine, isosetoclavine and sometimes penniclavine. These compounds have a double bond in the 9,10 position, like the majority of natural ergot alkaloids, indicating that the original double bond in the 8,9 position of agroclavine has undergone rearrangement. Of still greater interest was the formation of the alcohols setoclavine and isosetoclavine by oxidation at the C-8 methyl and the formation of penniclavine by oxidation of C-8 and of the C-8 methyl group. The paper also mentions that phenolic derivatives of agroclavine were formed but does not adduce definite evidence or precise information of these compounds.

Nicergoline (104e) (cf. Table 17): Nicergoline is 8β-(5-bromonicotinoylhydroxymethyl)-1,6-dimethyl-10α-methoxyergoline. It lacks the double bond in position

9,10 characteristic of the natural ergot alkaloids and has a methoxy group in position 10. Typical features of the molecule are the methyl at N-1 and the ester group at C-17. The metabolic degradation of nicergoline has been investigated by ARCAMONE et al. (1971, 1972) who concentrated mainly on the excretion products in the urine which account for 60%–80% of the administered dose.

In vitro, nicergoline was resistant to gastric juice and to phosphate buffer, but it was hydrolyzed by blood. Hydrolysis may also occur in the organs.

Nicergoline appears to be rapidly hydrolyzed in vivo since all human and animal metabolites have lost the 5-bromonicotinic acid residue and moreover, the rate of excretion of the molecule nicergoline closely approximates that of 5-bromonicotinic acid when administered as such.

After administration of low doses to various animal species and to human subjects, little or no parent drug was found in the urine. After administration in a dose of 100 mg/kg body wt. to rats, measurable amounts of unchanged compound were found in the urine. However, when a dose of 1.1 mg was administered intravenously to human subjects, less than 6%–7% of the administered dose appeared in the urine.

Two metabolites, 1,6-dimethyl-8β-hydroxymethyl-10α-methoxyergoline and 8β-hydroxymethyl-10α-methoxy-6-methylergoline, were isolated from rat urine. The glucuronides were incubated with glucuronidase and the aglykons were identified by chromatography.

A comparison of the metabolites in different species showed that nicergoline was biotransformed in a similar manner in the rat, dog, rhesus monkey and man. However, there were some quantitative differences. In particular only a small amount of glucuronides was found in human subjects and 40% of the radioactivity was in the form of conjugates in the rhesus monkey. In all species the nonconjugated metabolites were excreted in greater quantity than the conjugated metabolites, and the quantity of metabolite still retaining the 1-methyl group was greater than the quantity of demethylated metabolite.

One interesting observation was that the metabolic pattern in monkeys was the same after a single dose as after 6 weeks' treatment with 50 mg/kg daily.

Three metabolic pathways were deduced: first, hydrolysis of the ester group with the formation of 5-bromonicotinic acid and the ergoline derivative having a hydroxymethyl group in position C-8; secondly demethylation at position 1 of the ergoline nucleus. (Surprisingly, no nicergoline demethylated at N-1 was detected, perhaps another indication of the rapid rate of hydrolysis.) The third mode of metabolic transformation appeared to be conjugation of the free alcohols with glucuronic acid apparently at the C-17 hydroxyl group.

Methergoline (89d) (cf. Table 17): Methergoline, 1-methyl-N-carbobenzoxy-dihydrolysergylamine, is another semisynthetic ergoline whose metabolism was investigated by ARCAMONE et al. (1971). The characteristic features of its structure are a hydrogenated double bond in position 9,10 and an amine group at C-17 which is coupled to a phenylacetic acid residue by an amide bond. It has a methyl group at N-1. Although in the rat only 60% and in man only 44% of the administered dose of radioactivity appears in the urine after administration of [^{3}H]methergoline, only the urinary metabolites were examined in a comparison of the metabolic pathways in various animal species. However, in the rat the bile was also analyzed and was used for preparative work. The quantity of unchanged drug excreted by rats, guinea pigs, dogs, monkeys (Patas), and human subjects was very low, accounting for 0.1% of the administered dose in rats and 2.2% of the administered dose in human subjects. This indicates that the molecule undergoes extensive biotransformation.

The principal nonconjugated metabolite, 1-demethyl methergoline, was identified in the urine of all species except the dog. This metabolite was also isolated from rabbit and human urine and from rat bile.

Isotope dilution experiments showed that the phenol formed by hydroxylation of C-12 was present in rat bile as the glucuronide and in rabbit urine as the aglykone. This is probably not a major metabolic pathway, as the nonconjugated phenol was not present in measurable amounts in urine samples from the different species studied. Rabbit urine and rat bile contained only small amounts of the nonconjugated phenol.

Metabolic patterns in the various species were compared by analyzing the quantity of unchanged drug, nonconjugated metabolites, glucuronides and residual water-soluble products and by determining the percentage of the dose excreted in the urine and feces. The metabolic pattern in monkeys most closely resembled that in man.

Despite the incomplete data, three metabolic pathways can be deduced: demethylation at N-1, oxidation of the aromatic ring at C-12 and conjugation of the oxidation product with glucuronic acid. The pharmacologic evidence presented in the paper suggests that hydroxylated metabolites other than the 12-hydroxy derivative could be present as glucuronides and as aglykones.

b) Lysergic Acid and Derivatives

Lysergic acid diethylamide (73b) (cf. Table 18): It was already indicated in the first papers (BOYD et al., 1955a, b; STOLL et al., 1955; and ROTHLIN, 1956) that no unchanged LSD was excreted in the bile in rats. Neither lysergic acid nor lysergic acid monoethylamide—two potential metabolites—was found (BOYD et al., 1955a, b). However, it was shown in the same paper by intraperitoneal administration of ^{14}C-labeled LSD to rats the expired air contained 3.5% of $^{14}CO_2$, indicating that the ethyl side-chain underwent oxidation. Paper chromatography of rat bile revealed polar zones which gave positive Ehrlich reactions but were not identified.

AXELROD et al. (1956, 1957) showed that an enzyme system in microsomes from guinea pig liver transformed LSD to 2-oxy-LSD, a metabolite giving a negative Ehrlich reaction. FRETER et al. (1957) and TROXLER and HOFMANN (1959) synthesised 2-oxy-LSD by two different routes, but comparison of the synthetic compound with the metabolite did not provide absolute proof of identity, possibly owing to the instability of the material of biologic origin.

In a later paper BOYD (1959) suggested that two of the four radioactive zones in paper chromatograms of rat bile were glucuronides of phenolic derivatives.

It was shown by hydrolysis of metabolites with glucuronidase that they were conjugated with glucuronic acid, and titration indicated the presence of an acidic group. The presence of a new phenolic function was also indicated by titration of the metabolites.

After administration of LSD to rats, SLAYTOR and WRIGHT (1962) demonstrated the biliary excretion of two metabolites which were most probably glucuronides of hydroxy-LSD and hydroxy-isoLSD, the hydroxylation occurring in the benzene ring. Enzymic hydrolysis of the two compounds with glucuronidase was positive and evidence of isomerization was obtained by incubating the pure compounds in buffer solution. The presence of phenols was also suggested by the fact that the UV spectra differed from that of LSD itself and the metabolites gave a wine color reaction with diazotized sulphanilamide. C-12 was proposed as the site of hydroxylation by analogy with ergometrine which will be discussed later. SZARA (1963) conducted incubation experiments with microsomal fractions and suggested, but without proof, that hydroxylation at C-13 occurred in the rat while 2-oxy-LSD was formed in the guinea pig.

Use has again been made recently of in vitro systems (NIWAGUCHI et al., 1974a) and further information has been forthcoming. The formation of lysergic acid monoethylamide and of 6-demethyl lysergic acid diethylamide has been demonstrated in incubation experiments using microsomes from rat liver, guinea pig liver and rabbit liver. The first-mentioned compound was a major component in all species which showed differences in rate of metabolism. In the same paper it was shown that dealkylations were mediated by an enzyme present in liver microsomes and dependant on NADPH and oxygen, this enzyme being inhibited by SKF 525-A. These authors did not detect any phenols.

The most recent paper has revealed differences between biotransformation by microsomal incubation and biotransformation in the intact animal (SIDDIK et al., 1975). The principal metabolic pathway in the rat was hydroxylation of the benzene ring to phenols which are excreted as glucuronic acid conjugates, mainly in the bile. The position of the hydroxyl group was not determined, but C-12 was excluded by comparison with synthetic reference compounds. The formation of a phenol was demonstrated by mass spectrometry of the phenol itself in one case and of the methylated derivatives which were more stable. Since two hydroxylated derivatives were found, C-13 and C-14 were proposed as the oxidation sites. Possible isomerization at C-8 to the iso form was not discussed in this paper, as it had previously been mentioned by SLAYTOR and WRIGHT (1962).

Demethylation and deethylation were shown to be minor routes, as 6-nor-LSD and the monoethylamide were found in the perfusate in a liver perfusion experiment. Some 2-oxy-LSD was tentatively identified in excretion products. Deethylation was confirmed by the discovery of 3% of $^{14}CO_2$ in the expired air of rats which had received ^{14}C-ethyl LSD. However, this is not a principal metabolic pathway for LSD in the rat.

Ergometrine (19) (cf. Table 18): Ergometrine has an isopropanol side chain instead of the ethyl groups of LSD.

SLAYTOR and WRIGHT (1962) isolated two pairs of polar compounds which, as they were hydrolyzed by glucuronidase, were probably glucuronides.

The hydrolysis of one pair of metabolites yielded the parent compound and its iso form. It was assumed that the glucuronic acid was conjugated with the alcohol group of the amide side chain, this being the most obvious site.

Color reactions given by the second pair after incubation with glucuronidase indicated the possible presence of a phenolic substituent in the molecule. Chromatographic comparison with synthetic reference compound suggested C-12 as the possible position of the OH. As the authors themselves pointed out in the discussion, it may not be possible by this method to distinguish between C-12, C-13 and C-14. The occurrence of the normal and of the iso form (the two stereoisomeric configurations at C-8) was again demonstrated by incubation with buffer solutions.

Methylergometrine (73a) (cf. Table 18): The butanolamide analog of ergometrine was incubated with rat liver microsomes (NIWAGUCHI et al., 1974b). The two metabolites formed indicated demethylation at C-6 and hydroxylation in the aromatic moiety but again the position of the OH was unknown.

Methysergide (34a) (cf. Table 18): Methysergide (Deseril) is identical in structure to methylergometrine except that the indole nitrogen bears an additional methyl substituent.

The demethylated derivative, which is identical with methylergometrine, is the principal metabolite, as has been shown by BIANCHINE (1968) in rabbits and human subjects and by KALBERER et al. (1975) in other animal species and in human subjects.

Microsomal incubations (NIWAGUCHI et al., 1974b) confirmed demethylation at N-1 to methylergometrine and also revealed the presence of an N-1 hydroxymethyl derivative. This metabolite is probably an intermediate in formation of the demethylated compound.

Miscellaneous lysergic acid derivatives (cf. Table 18): The derivatives studied by NIWAGUCHI et al. (1974b) by incubation with rat microsomes fall into two categories. The first has the normal stereochemical configuration at C-8 (2-bromolysergic acid diethylamide, lysergic acid dimethylamide, lysergamide) and the second comprises the epimers (isoLSD, isolysergic acid dimethylamide, isolysergic acid amide and isolysergic acid L-2-butanolamide).

It is interesting to note that for the iso derivatives, demethylation of the basic nitrogen in position 6 was the most important biotransformation since the 6-nor compounds were the only metabolites isolated and identified.

In the series of compounds with the normal stereochemical configuration at C-8 the metabolites not only included the nor derivatives, but also monoethylamide and monomethylamide, indicating that the amide group also underwent dealkylation. In the case of the bromo derivative, biotransformations occurred at both sites simultaneously. Hydroxylation of the aromatic moiety, reported to occur with methylergometrine, was not detected with any of the compounds.

Another interesting point to emerge from the investigations of NIWAGUCHI et al. (1974b) was that isomerization from the normal form to the iso form was a non enzymic process.

c) **Ergot Peptide Alkaloids** (cf. Table 19)

It was shown by pharmacologic tests on urine extracts that for the series of natural and hydrogenated peptide alkaloids of ergot only 1/1000–1/10,000 of the original intravenous dose of the alkaloid was present in the urine as pharmacologically active parent drug or metabolites (ROTHLIN, 1947). This was an early indication of low urinary excretion and probably of extensive biotransformation.

It was later shown (NIMMERFALL and ROSENTHALER, 1976; MESZAROS et al., 1975) that the bile was the main pathway of excretion for this class of compounds, only a small percentage of the administered dose appearing in the urine.

Not surprisingly, therefore, the work of isolating and elucidating the structure of metabolites has been mainly concerned with the biliary excretion products.

The compound for which the most structural information has been amassed is dihydro-β-ergokryptine (102f), a hydrogenated ergot alkaloid (MAURER, 1977). Rat bile (2.5 liters) was employed as the starting material, and 16 metabolites were isolated from it and identified.

Strangely enough, all the metabolites isolated, except the amide of dihydrolysergic acid (a minor metabolite) had undergone oxidation of the proline moiety. Oxidation at C-8′ of the proline was a major route of biotransformation since most of the metabolites had either a hydroxyl or a carboxylic group in this position.

Two types of dihydroxylated compounds were isolated: metabolites with hydroxyls at C-8′ and C-9′ and metabolites with hydroxyls at C-8′ and C-10′, the former series occurring in greater quantities. The stereochemical configuration of the hydroxyl groups differed: β at C-8′ and α at C-9′, α,α at C-8′ and C-9′, α at C-8′ and β at C-9′, α at C-8′ and β at C-10′, β at C-8′ and α at C-10′. Other combinations may have been present, but in amounts too small to be isolated.

Apart from a glutamic acid derivative with the acid group at C-8′, hydroxyglutamic acid derivatives were also isolated with OH groups at C-9′ or C-10′. The glutamic acid derivative and the dihydroxylated derivatives were the metabolites produced in greatest quantity, administration of low doses favoring production of the dihydroxylated metabolites and administration in high doses favoring production of the glutamic acid metabolite.

MAURER (1977) proposed a metabolic pathway which assigned a central role to the stereo-isomeric metabolites hydroxylated at C-8′. These had been isolated, and according to this hypothesis the other compounds were all derived from them. The complete picture was very complex. It can be more readily understood by referring to Fig. 5 which shows the main sites of metabolic attack.

The formation of the glutamic acid derivatives resembles the metabolic opening of the ring in the pyrrolidine fragment of nicotine with the formation of γ-3-pyridyl-γ-methylamino butyric acid (PARKE, 1968). The site of oxidation α to the nitrogen is not the same in the two cases since in nicotine the nitrogen is basic and in dihydro-β-ergokryptine it forms part of an amide group.

Another interesting observation is that proline itself is biotransformed to glutamic acid via Δ^1-pyrroline-5-carboxylic acid (STETTEN, 1955) in a manner similar to the biotransformation of the proline fragment of the ergot alkaloid (Fig. 7). In proline the nitrogen is also basic. The biotransformation step corresponding to Δ^1-pyrroline-5-carboxylic acid is the monohydroxy derivative (Fig. 7). This metabolite is probably stable since water cannot be eliminated from it as it is in the case of proline.

Of the minor metabolites, four types are of interest: first the glucuronides of the monohydroxy (C-8′) and dihydroxy (C-8′ and C-9′) derivatives. Contrary to expectations, for glucuronidation is one of the most common detoxification

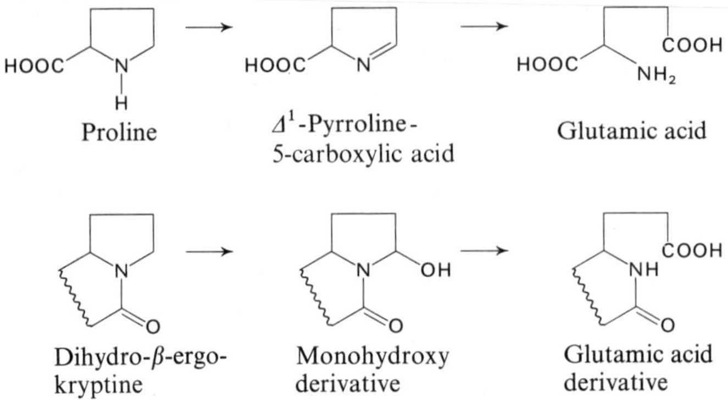

HOOC N H → HOOC N → HOOC COOH NH₂

Proline — Δ^1-Pyrroline-5-carboxylic acid — Glutamic acid

N O → N OH O → NH COOH O

Dihydro-β-ergokryptine — Monohydroxy derivative — Glutamic acid derivative

Fig. 7. Comparison of the biotransformation sequence of the amino acid proline and the proline fragment of dihydro-β-ergokryptine

mechanisms (WILLIAMS, 1959), these metabolites were found in only small amounts in rat bile.

The occurrence of dihydrolysergic acid amide (18) formed by cleavage of the molecule also calls for an explanation. This compound may possibly stem from the glutamic acid derivative which is more readily hydrolyzed than the parent drug. The amide may therefore be only indirectly of enzymic origin.

A metabolite containing glutamic acid instead of proline was oxidized simultaneously in the indole structure to an anilinoacetone. This oxidation corresponds to the formation of anthranilic acid in the metabolic degradation of indole (KING et al. 1966). It was the only example of indole oxidation cited.

The last minor metabolite of the series is hydroxylated at C-9′ and conjugated with glutathione. The exact position of the substituent is unknown but there is some evidence to report position C-8′. Reductive cleavage with Raney nickel showed that the hydroxyl group was at C-9′. The discovery of this metabolite together with the occurrence of derivatives dihydroxylated at C-8′ and C-9′ suggests that an epoxide may be formed as an intermediate, as occurs with aromatic compounds (JERINA and DALY, 1974).

On surveying all the structures elucidated, it is curious to note that these do not include any demethylated derivatives or N-oxides. The basic nitrogen of xenobiotics is generally a favored site of metabolic transformation. These results are in keeping with the small extent of demethylation observed with the previously mentioned compounds having a normal stereochemical configuration at C-8 of the lysergic acid moiety.

Another surprising feature is that the aromatic structure of the molecule does not undergo substitution. From a knowledge of the biotransformation of drugs in general and from the results of biotransformation studies of LSD and ergometrine, it might have been expected that phenols would have been formed.

4. Interaction of Ergot Derivatives With Cytochrome P450

The interactions of compounds with cytochrome P450 as evidenced by characteristic spectral changes may be of three types: type I, type II and modified type II

(MANNERING, 1971). It has been suggested that the spectral changes of type I reflect the formation of a complex between enzyme and substrate since compounds giving rise to such a spectrum are metabolized by cytochrome P450.

Some authors hold the view that the type II change results from the interaction of the cytochrome with compounds containing a basic nitrogen and that it is associated with ferrihemochrome formation. In the introduction to their paper WILSON and ORRENIUS (1972) add that compounds giving rise to the type II spectral change are not, as a rule, oxidized by cytochrome P450, aniline being an exception.

It was an obvious step, therefore for investigators who have worked on microsomal fractions, such as NIWAGUCHI et al. (1974a) who investigated lysergic acid diethylamide and WILSON et al. (1971) who worked on agroclavine, to examine the spectral changes produced by interaction of the substrate with cytochrome P450 (NIWAGUCHI and INOUE, 1975; WILSON and ORRENIUS, 1972). In both cases a type II spectral change was observed at higher concentrations, shifting gradually to type I with decreasing concentration. Both groups of workers suggested that the type II spectra were in reality type I superimposed on type II components.

Both were able to derive type I component of the ergot derivative by subtracting the spectra recorded in the presence of both type I compound and the ergot derivative from the spectrum recorded for the ergot derivative alone. The spectral dissociation constant calculated from the type I interaction with LSD was almost exactly equal to the Km value obtained for the disappearance of LSD as a result of enzymatic transformation. The same applied to the rate of N-demethylation for agroclavine.

In spite of the satisfactory results obtained in these instances, it must be stated that the relation between binding spectra and metabolization as well as the relation between the dissociation constant and the metabolization constant are still a matter for controversy.

5. Conclusions and Prospects

By way of conclusion the various metabolic pathways which have been delineated for the ergot alkaloids will now be summarized and an attempt will be made to indicate their importance. Possible ways in which future work could help to fill the gaps in our knowledge will also be mentioned.

Demethylation is the principal metabolic pathway for all compounds with a methyl group at N-1, the indole nitrogen. The assay of the demethylated metabolites and of the parent compound in the blood and organs would, if combined with carefully designed kinetic studies, cast light on the true significance of this route of degradation and its relevance to pharmacologic activity. It is possible that the nor metabolite is the only form of the compound excreted.

Although 6-nor derivatives are produced in vitro in the incubation mixture, demethylation at that site is only a minor pathway. Isolation in the studies cited, including work on dihydro-β-ergokryptine which has been extensively investigated, has shown that the nor metabolites never figure very prominently. This contrasts with the many examples of biotransformation of xenobiotics. The metabolic "inertness" of this nitrogen is borne out by the absence of N-oxides or products of oxidation α to this basic nitrogen.

Table 17. Summary of data on metabolites of ergot alkaloids and related compounds: Ergolines

Compound	In vitro system, species, administration	Characterized or identified metabolites	Proof of structure	Reference
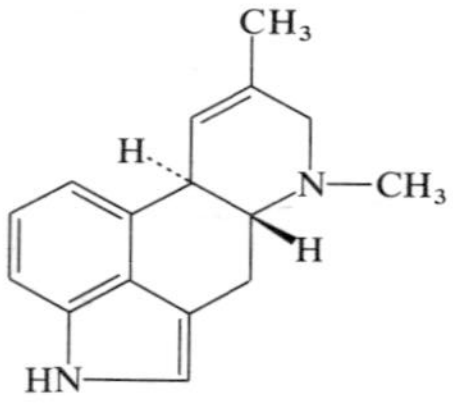 Agroclavine (5)	Rat and guinea pig liver microsomes	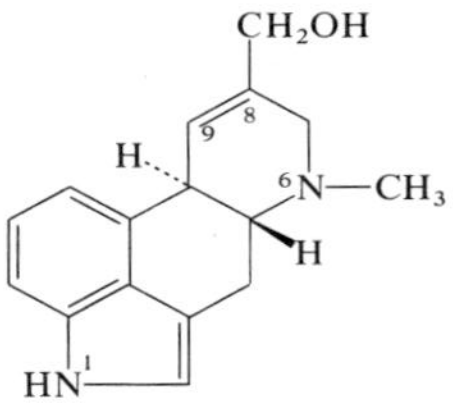 Elymoclavine (6)	Thin-layer chromatography in different solvent systems and comparison with reference	WILSON et al. (1971)
		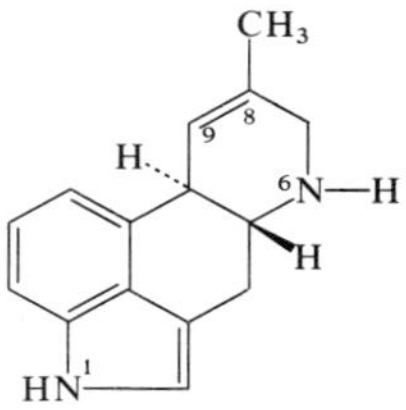 Nor-agroclavine	Thin-layer chromatography in different solvent systems and comparison with reference Demethylation also measured by assay of formaldehyde	
		A number of other, nonidentified zones		
	Rat liver microsomes only	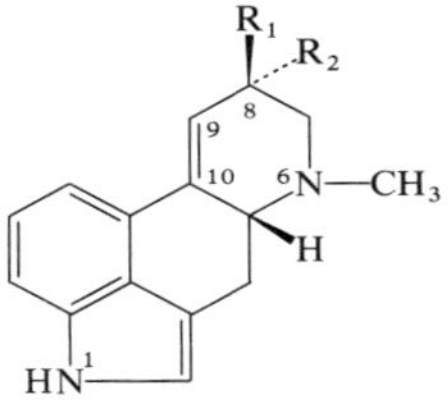 R_1 R_2 CH_3 OH Setoclavine OH CH_3 Isosetoclavine	Comparison with reference compound by two-dimensional thin-layer chromatography	

Drug	Species, material, dose	Metabolite	Identification	Reference
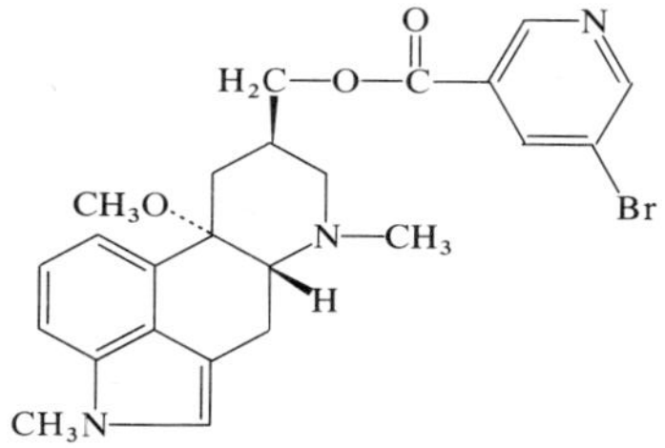	Isolation from rat urine 100 mg/kg p.o. Dog, monkey urine 0.2 mg/kg p.o. Man urine 1.1 mg i.v.	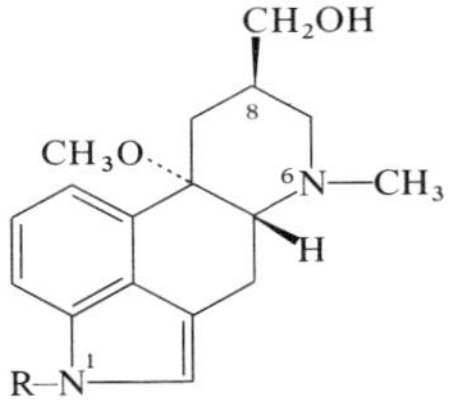 a) $R = CH_3$; b) $R = H$	Chromatographic comparison with reference compound UV and mass-spectral comparison with reference compound	ARCAMONE et al. (1971) ARCAMONE et al. (1972)
Nicergoline (104e)		Glucuronides of a and b	Hydrolysis with glucuronidase	
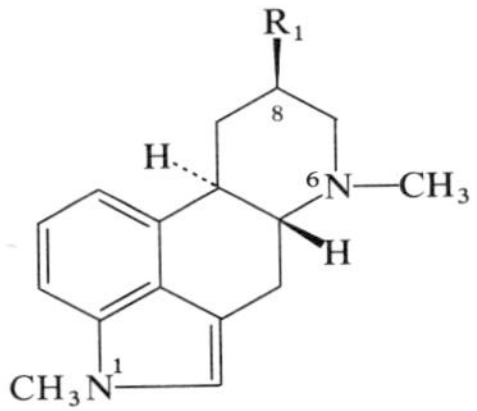	Rat, guinea pig, monkey urine 1 mg/kg p.o. Man urine 0.15 mg/kg p.o.	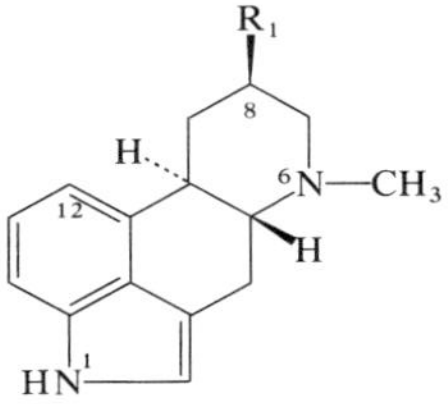	Chromatographic comparison with reference compound	ARCAMONE et al. (1971)
Methergoline $R_1 = CH_2NH\text{-}COO\text{-}CH_2\text{-}C_6H_5$	Isolation from rat bile (R_2 = Gluc) 12 mg/kg p.o. or rabbit urine (R_2 = H)	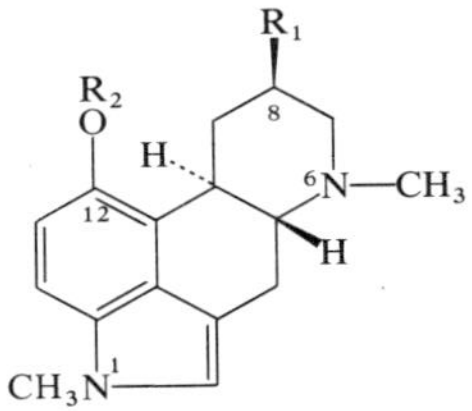 R_2 = H, or glucuronic acid (Gluc)	Direct isotope dilution (rabbit urine) or after treatment with glucuronidase (rat bile)	

Table 18. Summary of data on metabolites of ergot alkaloids and related compounds: Lysergic acid and derivatives

Compound	In vitro system, species, administration	Characterized or identified metabolites	Proof of structure	Reference
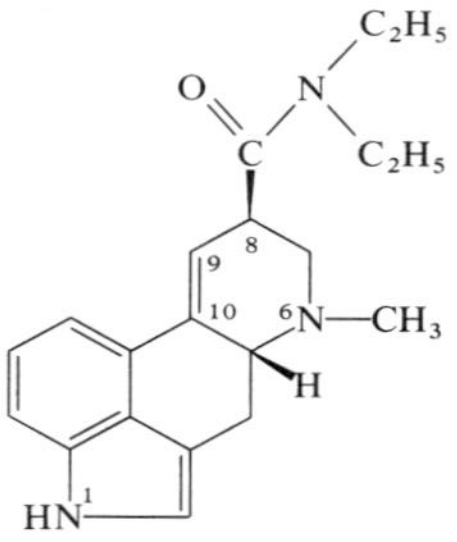 Lysergic acid diethylamide (73b)	Bile fistula rats 1 mg/kg i.v.	Two principal, polar chromatographic zones with positive Ehrlich reaction	IR of metabolites and reference compound	BOYD et al. (1955)
		No lysergic acid or lysergic acid monoethylamide		
	Bile fistula rats Dose unknown i.v.	Three polar chromatographic zones, Van Urk positive; traces of LSD	Rf-value	STOLL et al. (1955), ROTHLIN (1956)
	Guinea pig liver microsomes	No lysergic acid or nor-lysergic acid diethylamide	Chromatography with reference compound	AXELROD et al. (1956)
		2-Oxy-lysergic acid diethylamide	Color reactions	
			Degradation to aniline derivative	
	Guinea pig liver microsomes	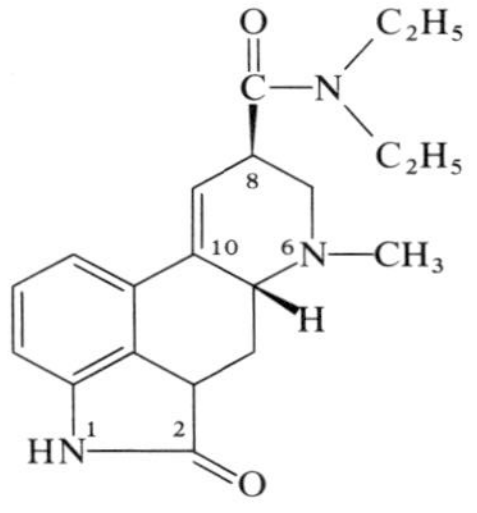	Color reactions, UV spectra	AXELROD et al. (1957)
			Analogy to synthetic reference compound in UV, Rf, partition coefficient	FRETER et al. (1957), TROXLER and HOFMANN (1959)
		No 6-nor-derivative	Negative formaldehyde test	AXELROD et al. (1957)

1 mg/kg i.p.	graphic zones No 2-oxy-lysergic acid amide derivative		BOYD (1959)
	Two glucuronides of phenols	Color reactions, UV, pK, glucuronidase	
Bile fistula rats 3 mg/kg i.v.	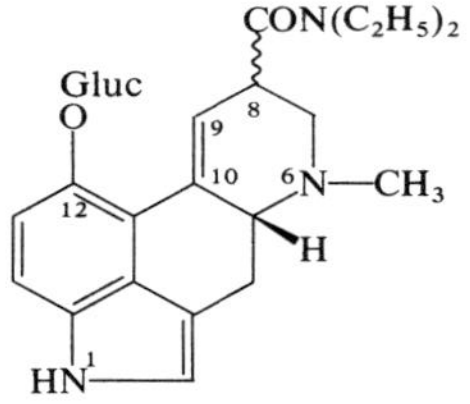 12-OH glucuronides of lysergic and isolysergic acid derivatives	Isomerization, color reactions, glucuronidase, UV-spectrum, analogy to ergometrine	SLAYTOR and WRIGHT (1962)
Guinea pig liver microsomes	None; disappearance of LSD measured		SZARA (1963)
	Hydroxyl in position 13	Color reactions No proof; analogy with indole metabolism	
Rat, guinea pig and rabbit liver microsomes	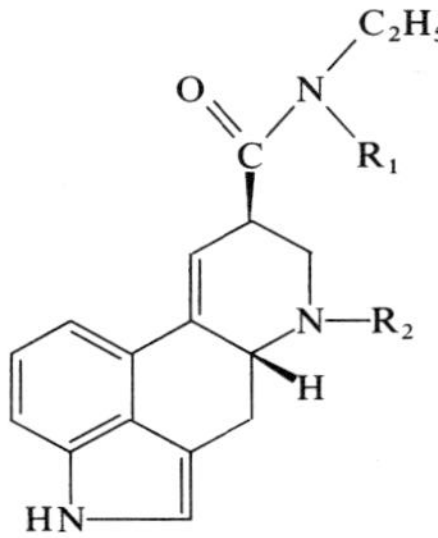 a) $R_1 = H$, $R_2 = CH_3$ b) $R_1 = C_2H_5$, $R_2 = H$	Chromatographic comparison with reference compound UV and fluorescence spectra, mass spectra, determination of molecular peak	NIWAGUCHI et al. (1974a)

Table 18 (continued)

Compound	In vitro system, species, administration	Characterized or identified metabolites	Proof of structure	Reference
Lysergic acid diethylamide (continued)	Bile fistula rats, intact rats 1 mg/kg i.v. or i.p.	Eight radioactive chromatographic zones:		
		a) Two glucuronides and their aglycone	Glucuronidase, color reactions, mass spectrometry of methylated aglycones	SIDDIK et al. (1975)
		RO– not in position 12 $R = H$, or Gluc	Chromatographic comparison with reference compound	
		b) 2-Oxy derivative	No proof	
		c) Deethylated derivative	Comparative TLC	
	Isolated perfused rat liver	a) In bile: Two glucuronides and aglycones + unchanged LSD	See above	SIDDIK et al. (1975)
		b) In perfusate:	Chromatography with reference compound	

Compound	System	Metabolite	Identification	Reference
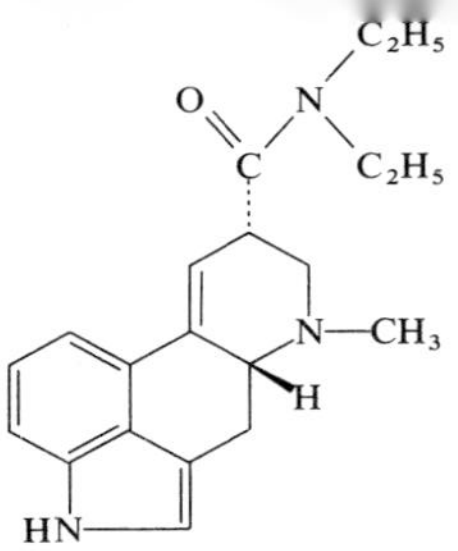 Isolysergic acid diethylamide	Rat liver microsomes	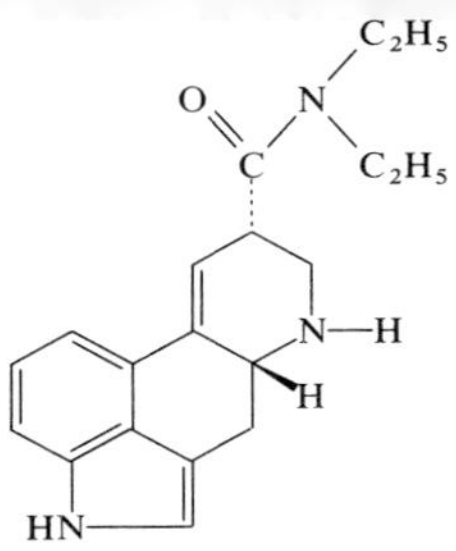	UV, mass spectra, determination of molecular peak, shift technique analysis of ion fragments	NIWAGUCHI et al. (1974b)
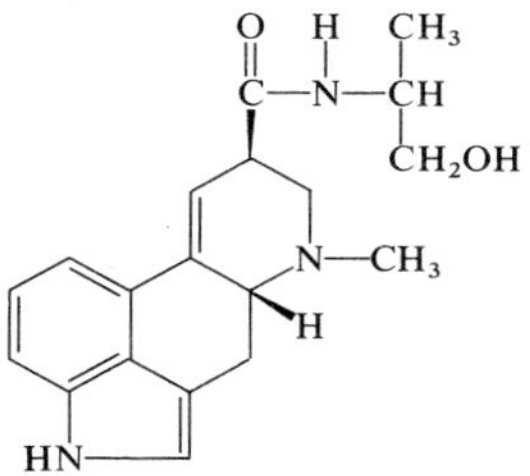 Ergometrine (19)	Bile fistula rats 3 mg/kg i.v.	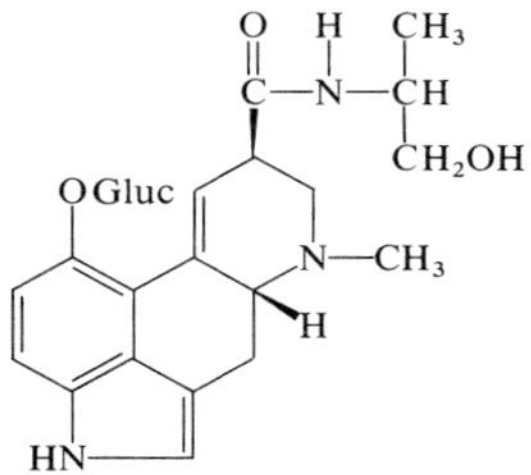 Isoform is also present	Chromatographic comparison with synthetic compound after treatment with glucuronidase	SLAYTOR and WRIGHT (1962)
			Isomerization from normal form to isoform	
		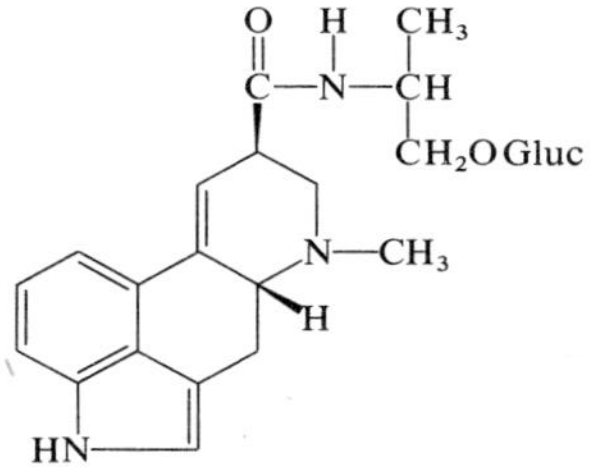 Isoform is also present	Hydrolysis product identical with reference compound after chromatography	

Table 18 (continued)

Compound	In vitro system, species, administration	Characterized or identified metabolites	Proof of structure	Reference
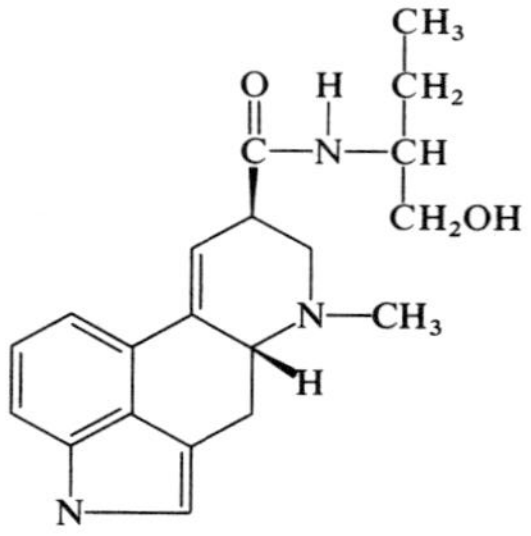 Methysergide (34a)	Rabbit no dosage indicated, i.v. Man 2 mg/kg p.o.	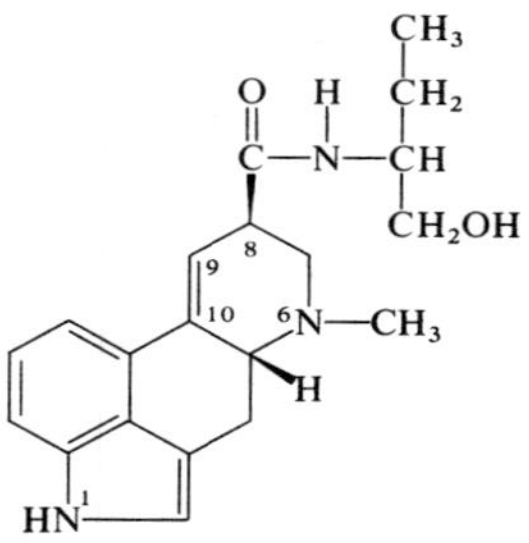 [structure]	Thin-layer chromatographic comparison with reference compound	BIANCHINE (1968)
	Rat 1 mg/kg p.o. Dog 1 mg/kg p.o. Rhesus monkey 0.1 mg/kg i.v. Man 1 mg p.o.	Many radioactive zones; methylergometrine main metabolite except in dog	Thin-layer chromatographic comparison with reference compound	KALBERER et al. (1975)
	Rat liver microsomes	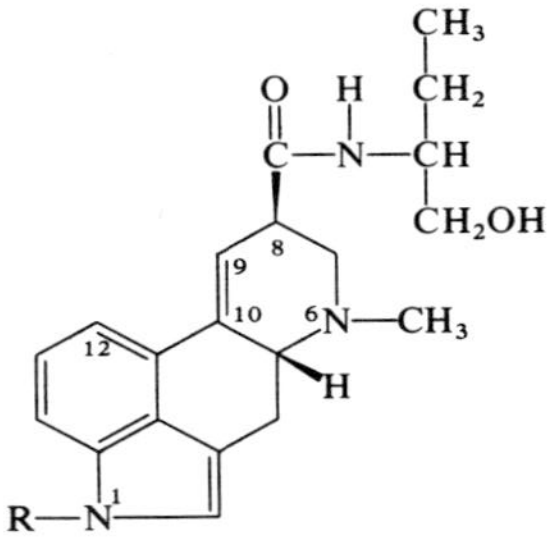 [structure] a) R = H, b) R = CH_2OH	UV and high resolution mass spectra, determination of molecular peak, shift technique analysis of ion fragments	NIWAGUCHI et al. (1974b)

Compound	System	Metabolites	Identification	Reference
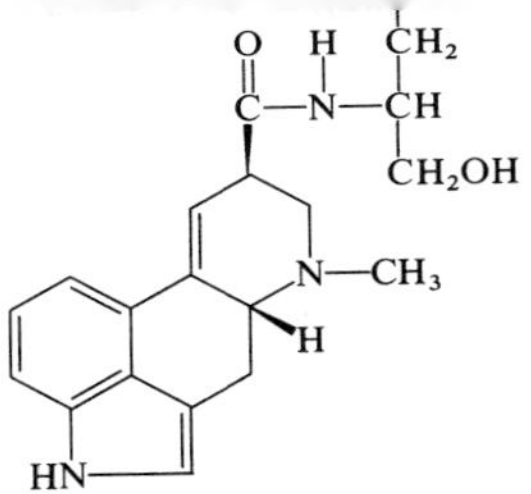 Methylergometrine (73a)		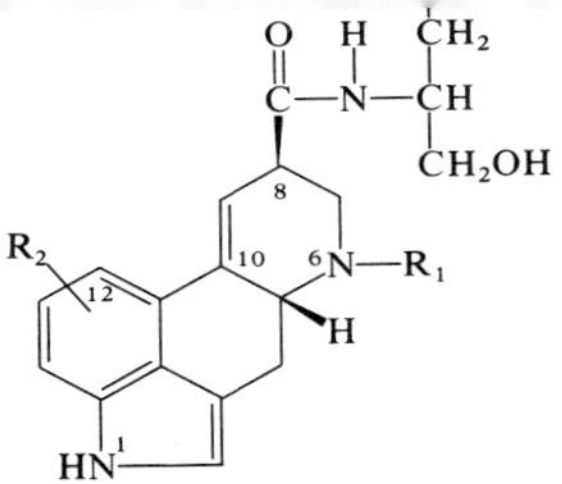 a) $R_1 = R_2 = H$ b) $R_1 = CH_3$, $R_2 = OH$	spectra, molecular peak determination, shift technique analysis of ion fragments	(1974b)
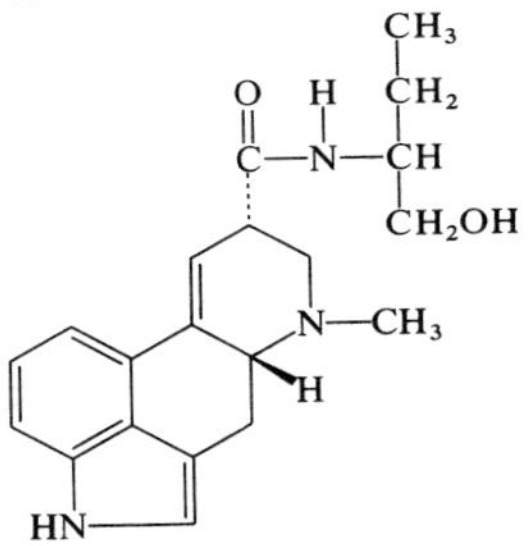 d-Isolysergic acid L-2-butanolamide	Rat liver microsomes	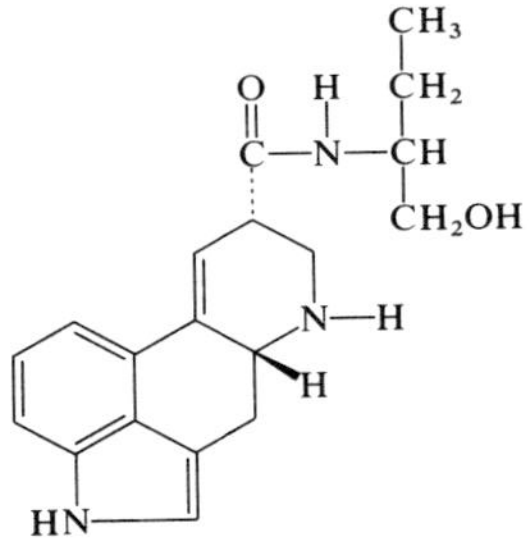	UV, high resolution mass spectra, determination of molecular peak, shift technique analysis of ion fragments	NIWAGUCHI et al. (1974b)
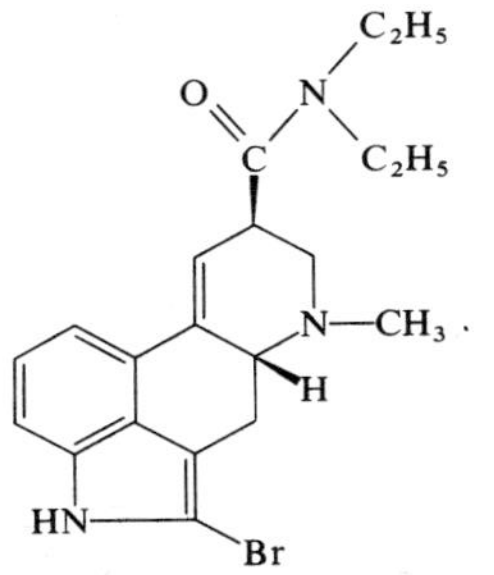 2-Bromo-d-lysergic acid diethylamide (37a)	Rat liver microsomes	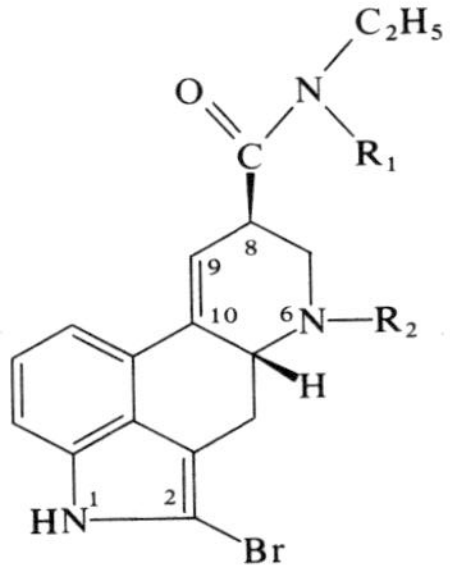 a) $R_1 = H$, $R_2 = CH_3$ b) $R_1 = C_2H_5$, $R_2 = H$ c) $R_1 = R_2 = H$	UV and mass spectra, molecular peak determination, shift technique analysis of ion fragments	NIWAGUCHI et al. (1974b)

Table 18 (continued)

Compound	In vitro system, species, administration	Characterized or identified metabolites	Proof of structure	Reference
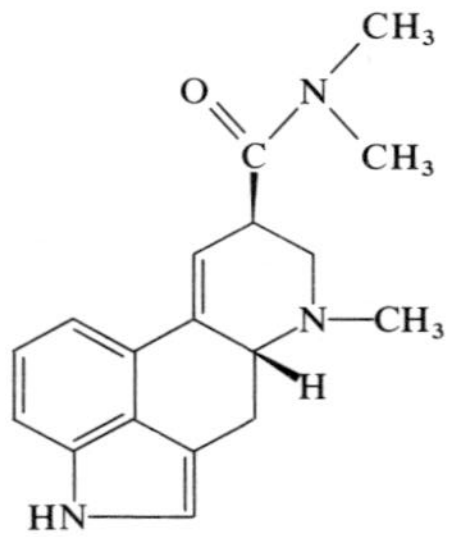 Lysergic acid dimethylamide	Rat liver microsomes	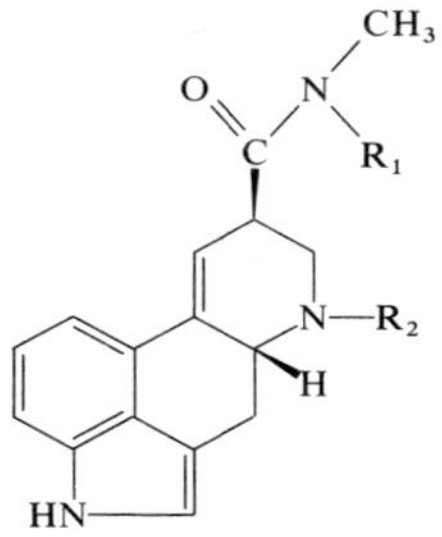 a) $R_1 = H$, $R_2 = CH_3$ b) $R_1 = CH_3$, $R_2 = H$	UV and mass spectra, molecular peak determination, shift technique analysis of ion fragments	NIWAGUCHI et al. (1974b)
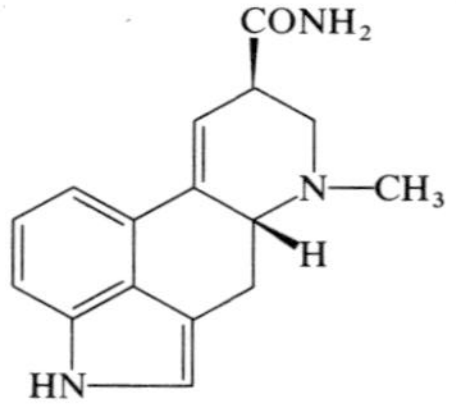 Lysergic acid amide (18)	Rat liver microsomes	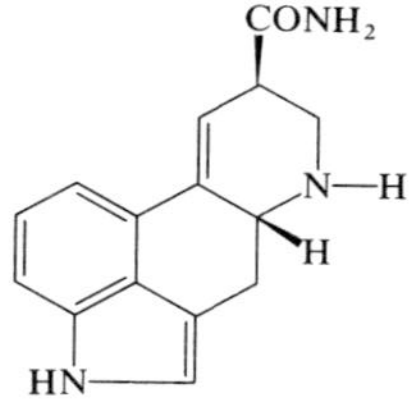	UV and mass spectra, molecular peak determination, shift technique analysis of ion fragments	NIWAGUCHI et al. (1974b)
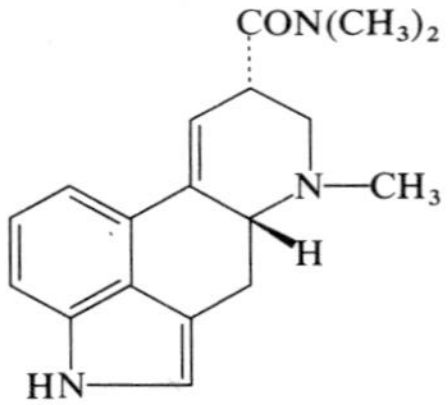 Isolysergic acid dimethylamide	Rat liver microsomes	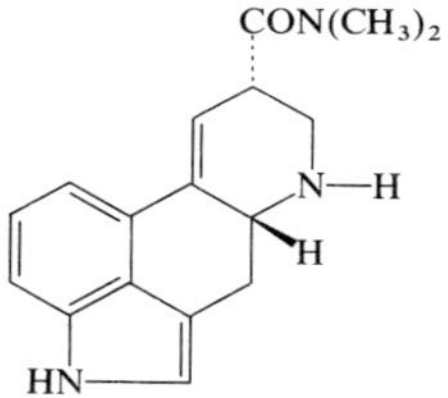	UV and mass spectra, molecular peak determination, shift technique analysis of ion fragments	NIWAGUCHI et al. (1974b)

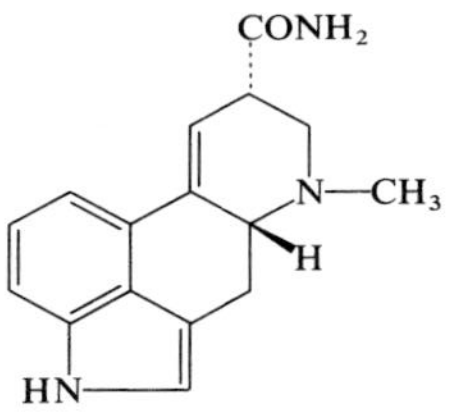 Isolysergic acid amide	Rat liver microsomes	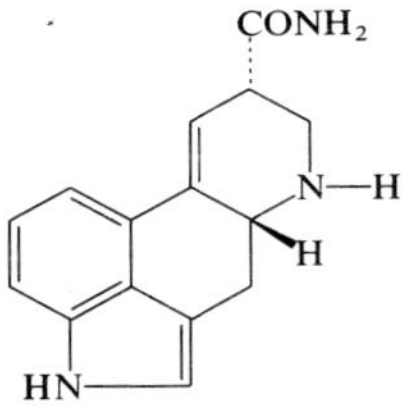	UV and mass spectra, molecular peak determination, shift technique analysis of ion fragments	NIWAGUCHI et al. (1974b)

Table 19. Summary of data on metabolites of ergot alkaloids and related compounds: Ergot peptide alkaloids

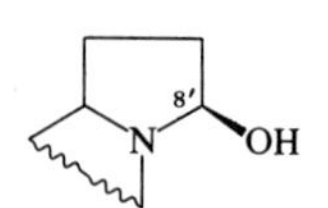

Compound: Dihydro-β-ergokryptine (102f)
Reference: MAURER (1977)

Species and administration: Rat 30 mg/kg 3 times daily

Characterized or identified metabolites: Rat bile

a) Monohydroxy- derivatives

b) Dihydroxy- derivatives

c) Derivatives with a carboxylic acid group

d) Conjugates

Gluc = $C_6H_9O_6$

$R_1 = -CH_2CH(CONHCH_2COOH)(NHCOCH_2CH_2CH(COOH)NH_2)$

e) Miscellaneous

It would appear from the results of in vitro experiments that this type of degradation is more important for the iso series with its different stereochemical configuration at C-8 than it is for the normal series. It would be of interest to examine how demethylation kinetics vary with structure.

The biotransformation of the substituent at C-8 of the ergoline unit follows different pathways depending upon the nature of the substituent. There is nothing unusual in the fact that nicergoline undergoes ester hydrolysis, but the rate and extent to which this occurs is worthy of note. For nicergoline also it would be interesting to have data on the compound or compounds circulating in the blood and present in the organs. Moreover, the oxidation of the methyl substituent at C-8 of agroclavine to the alcohol was observed in vitro, and information is needed on the situation in vivo.

The deethylation of LSD seems to occur to a greater extent in incubation studies than in animal experiments. Further investigations are needed in order to throw light on this problem, especially as differing results were obtained in recent work (in vitro studies by NIWAGUCHI et al., 1974a, and in vivo studies by SIDDIK et al., 1975).

Many papers describe the formation of one or two phenols. Chromatographic and isotope dilution studies suggested that the OH is in position 12 of the lysergic acid moiety of methergoline and ergometrine. The results published in the most recent paper on LSD (SIDDIK et al., 1975) are again at variance with previous findings. It has now been established that phenols are produced, but the structure of these metabolites has yet to be fully elucidated.

Another question still to be resolved for LSD and lysergic acid is the significance of metabolites found in excretion products such as bile and urine. The metabolites of LSD found in the bile differ from those found in liver perfusates. It is noteworthy that the metabolites found in the perfusate were the deethylated or the demethylated derivatives of LSD. It was precisely these metabolites which were found by NIWAGUCHI et al. (1974a, b) in the incubation medium in his microsomal experiments. It may be that these two metabolites are those which occur in the organs. The phenols and phenol conjugates may only be excretion forms which have no great relevance for pharmacology and toxicology.

A curious feature which has emerged from work on peptide alkaloids of ergot is that the proline fragment is the almost exclusive site of biotransformation. The site of metabolic attack in this class of compounds, therefore, differs greatly from that in the other compounds discussed which possess the same ergoline fragment. It should be stressed that these findings relate to metabolites excreted in rat bile. No information is as yet available on urinary metabolites and biotransformation in other animal species and in man. The effect of structural variations on biotransformation would also be of interest, since many other derivatives of this same chemical family have now been synthesized. Another worthwhile approach would be to investigate whether the double bond in the 9,10 position of the natural ergot alkaloids affects the way in which they are metabolized.

Regarding the avenues still to be explored in future work, a few general remarks are called for.

In many instances (LSD, methergoline, methysergide, and methylergometrine, for example) the structure of the metabolites has still to be fully elucidated.

Species differences have still to be investigated for the same compounds and for the peptide alkaloids of ergot. Good data for a variety of species is available in the literature only for nicergoline.

The data obtained in in vitro studies of some compounds have still to be correlated with the in vivo findings, especially with regard to the kinetics of metabolism.

For all the compounds information is still needed on the identity of metabolites in body tissues.

Finally, the relation between structure and metabolic degradation has still to be investigated for the various classes of compounds.

The conclusion is, therefore, that the metabolism of the ergot alkaloids must still be pieced together for most compounds, commencing with the elucidation of the chemical structures of the metabolites.

E. References

Aellig, W.H.: Venoconstrictor effect of dihydroergotamine in superficial hand veins. Europ. J. clin. Pharmacol. **7**, 137–139 (1974)

Aellig, W.H., Nüesch, E.: Comparative pharmacokinetic investigations with tritium labelled ergot alkaloids after oral and after intravenous administration in man. Int. J. clin. Pharmacol. **15**, 106–112 (1977)

Aghajanian, G.K., Bing, O.H.L.: Persistence of lysergic acid diethylamide in the plasma of human subjects. Clin. Pharmacol. Ther. **5**, 611–614 (1964)

Agurell, S.: Biosynthesis of ergot alkaloids in *Claviceps paspali*. Part II. Incorporation of labelled agroclavine, elymoclavine, lysergic acid and lysergic acid methylester. Acta pharm. Suec. **3**, 23–32 (1966a)

Agurell, S.: Biosynthesis of ergot alkaloids in *Claviceps paspali*: Incorporation of 6-methyl-$\Delta^{8,9}$-ergolene-8-carboxylic acid-^{14}C and lysergic acid-8-^{3}H. Acta pharm. Suec. **3**, 65–70 (1966b)

Agurell, S., Ohlsson, A.: Gas chromatography of ergot alkaloids. J. Chromatogr. **61**, 339–342 (1971)

Allport, N.L., Cocking, T.T.: The colorimetric assay of ergot. Quart. J. Pharm. Pharmacol. **5**, 341–346 (1932)

Arcamone, F., Glässer, A.H., Minghetti, A., Nicolella, V.: Studi sul metabolismo di derivati ergolinici. Boll. chim. farm. **110**, 704–711 (1971)

Arcamone, F., Glässer, A.G., Grafnetterova, J., Minghetti, A., Nicolella, V.: Studies on the metabolism of ergoline derivatives. Metabolism of nicergoline in man and in animals. Biochem. Pharmacol. **21**, 2205–2213 (1972)

Arnold, O.H., Hofmann, G., Leupold-Löwenthal, H.: Untersuchungen zum Schizophrenieproblem. Wien. Nervenheilk. **15**, 15–27 (1958)

Axelrod, J., Brady, R.O., Witkop, B., Evarts, E.V.: Metabolism of lysergic acid diethylamide. Nature (Lond.) **178**, 143–144 (1956)

Axelrod, J., Brady, R.O., Witkop, B., Evarts, E.V.: The distribution and metabolism of lysergic acid diethylamide. Ann. N.Y. Acad. Sci. **66**, 435–444 (1957)

Barber, M., Weisbach, J.A., Douglas, B., Dudek, G.O.: High resolution mass spectroscopy of the clavine and ergot peptide alkaloids. Chem. Ind. **1965**, 1072–1073

Barnes, R.D.: Synthesis of ^{14}C-labelled diethylamine and lysergic acid diethylamide. J. Labelled Compds. **10**, 207–212 (1974)

Barrow, K.D., Quigley, F.R.: Ergot alkaloids. II. Determination of agroclavine by gas-liquid chromatography. J. Chromatogr. **105**, 393–395 (1975)

Bercel, N.A.: Treatment of migraine. Results with dihydroergocornine methanesulfonate (DHO-180) and other ergot derivatives. Calif. Med. (San Francisco) **72**, 234–238 (1950)

Berde, B., Cerletti, A., Dengler, H.J., Zoglio, M.A.: Studies of the interaction between ergot alkaloids and xanthine derivatives. In: Background to Migraine. 3rd Migraine Symposium, London, 1969. Cochrane, A.L. (ed.), pp. 80–102. London: William Heinemann Medical Books 1970

Bethke, H., Delz, B., Stich, K.: Determination of the content and purity of ergotamine preparations by means of high-pressure liquid chromatography. J. Chromatogr. **123**, 193–203 (1976)

Bianchine, J.R.: Metabolism of methysergide (MS) in the rabbit and man. Fed. Proc. **27**, 238 (1968)

Bianchine, J.R., Friedman, A.P.: Metabolism of methysergide and retroperitoneal fibrosis. Arch. intern. Med. **126**, 252–254 (1970)

Bianchine, J.R., Niec, A., Macaraeg, P.V.J.: Thin-layer chromatographic separation and detection of methysergide and methergine. J. Chromatogr. **31**, 255–257 (1967)

Birks, J.B.: An Introduction to Liquid Scintillation Counting and Solutes and Solvents for Liquid Scintillation Counting. Colnbrook: Koch-Light Laboratories 1975

Blicke, F.F.: The Mannich reaction. In: Organic Reactions. Adams, R., Bachmann, W.E., Fieser, L.F., Johnson, J.R., Snyder, H.R. (eds.), Vol I. New York: Wiley 1942

Bowman, R.L., Caulfield, P.A., Udenfriend, S.: Spectrophotofluorometric assay in the visible and ultraviolet. Science **122**, 32–33 (1955)

Boyd, E.S.: Metabolism of lysergic acid diethylamide. Fed. Proc. **17**, 352 (1958)

Boyd, E.S.: The metabolism of lysergic acid diethylamide. Arch. int. Pharmacodyn. **120**, 292–311 (1959)

Boyd, E.S., Rothlin, E., Bonner, J.F., Slater, I.H., Hodge, H.C.: Preliminary studies on the metabolism of lysergic acid diethylamide. J. Pharmacol. exp. Ther. **113**, 6–7 (1955a)

Boyd, E.S., Rothlin, E., Bonner, J.F., Slater, I.H., Hodge, H.C.: Preliminary studies of the metabolism of lysergic acid diethylamide using radioactive carbon-marked molecules. J. nerv. ment. Dis. **122**, 470–471 (1955b)

Bradley, P.B., Candy, J.M.: Iontophoretic release of acetylcholine, noradrenaline, 5-hydroxytryptamine and LSD 25 from micropipettes. Brit. J. Pharmacol. **40**, 194–201 (1970)

Castro, A., Grettie, D.P., Bartos, F., Bartos, D.: LSD radioimmunoassay. Res. Commun. Chem. Pathol. Pharmacol. **6**, 879–886 (1973)

Chan Lin, W.N., Ramstad, E., Taylor, E.H.: Enzymology of ergot alkaloid biosynthesis. III. 10-Hydroxyelymoclavine, an intermediate in the peroxidase conversion of elymoclavine to penniclavine and isopenniclavine. Lloydia **30**, 202–208 (1967)

Chi-Hong Chu, Pietrzyk, D.J.: High pressure chromatography on XAD-2, a porous polystyrene-divinylbenzene support. Separation of organic bases. Anal. Chem. **46**, 330–336 (1974)

Craig, L.C., Shedlovsky, TH., Gould, R.G., Jacobs, W.A.: The ergot alkaloids. XIV. The positions of the double bond and the carboxyl group in lysergic acid and its isomer. The structure of the alkaloids. J. biol. Chem. **125**, 289–298 (1938)

Christie, J., White, M.W., Wiles, J.M.: A chromatographic method for the detection of LSD in biological liquids. J. Chromatogr. **120**, 496–501 (1976)

Crook, M.A., Johnson, P. (eds.): Liquid Scintillation Counting, Vol III. London: Heyden 1974

Cross, S.A.M., Groves, A.D., Hesselbo, T.: A quantitative method for measuring radioactivity in tissues sectioned for whole-body autoradiography. Int. J. appl. Radiat. Isot. **25**, 381–386 (1974)

Del Pozo, E., Brun Del Re, R., Varga, L., Friesen, H.: The inhibition of prolactin secretion in man by CB 154 (2-Br-α-ergocryptine). J. clin. Endocr. **35**, 768–771 (1972)

Diab, I.M., Freedman, D.X., Roth, L.J.: [^{3}H]Lysergic acid diethylamide. Cellular autoradiographic localization in rat brain. Science **173**, 1022–1024 (1971)

Doepfner, W.: Biochemical observations on LSD 25 and Deseril. Experientia (Basel) **18**, 256–257 (1962)

Dost, F.H.: Grundlagen der Pharmakokinetik, 2nd. ed., pp. 267–268. Stuttgart: Georg Thieme 1968

Dost, F.H., Gladtke, E.: Die enterale Absorption schwer löslicher Sulfanilamide beim Kind. Arzneimittel-Forsch. **17**, 772–774 (1967)

Dyer, A.: An Introduction to Liquid Scintillation Counting. London: Heyden 1974
Eadie, M.J.: The use of ergotamine in migraine. Med. J. Aust. (Suppl.) **2**, 26–29 (1972).
Eckert, H., Hopf, A.: Autoradiographic studies on the distribution of psychoactive drugs in the rat brain. Int. Pharmacopsychiatry **2**, 12–26 (1969)
Eich, E., Schunack, W.: Direct quantitative evaluation of thin-layer chromatograms by remission and fluorescence measurements. Part 4. Determination of ergot alkaloids from medicaments and ergot by fluorescence measurements. Planta Med. **27**, 58–64 (1975)
Evans, E.A.: Tritium and Its Compounds, 2nd ed. London: Butterworths 1974
Faed, E.M., McLeod, W.R.: A urine screening test of lysergide (LSD 25). J. Chromatogr. Sci. **11**, 4–6 (1973)
Faragalla, F.F.: The subcellular distribution of lysergic acid diethylamide in the rat brain. Experientia (Basel) **28**, 1426–1427 (1972)
Figge, K., Piater, H., Kolbe, W.: Radio-Flüssigkeitssäulen-Chromatographie. GIT-Fachzeitschr. für das Laborat. **19**, 192–202 (1975)
Finkle, B.S., Cherry, E.J., Taylor, D.M.: A GLC based system for the detection of poisons, drugs and human metabolites encountered in forensic toxicology. J. Chromatogr. Sci. **9**, 393–419 (1971)
Fischer, H.A., Werner, G.: Autoradiographie. Berlin: De Gruyter 1971
Freedman, D.X., Coquet, C.A.: Regional and subcellular distribution of LSD and effects of 5-HT levels. Pharmacologist **7**, 183 (1965)
Freter, K., Axelrod, J., Witkop, B.: Studies on the chemical and enzymatic oxidation of lysergic acid diethylamide. J. Amer. chem. Soc. **79**, 3191–3193 (1957)
Friedman, A.P.: Treatment of migraine. New Engl. J. Med. **250**, 600–602 (1954)
Friedman, A.P., von Storch, T.J.C.: Recent advances in treatment of migraine. J. Amer. med. Ass. **145**, 1325–1329 (1951)
Gopalakrishnan, P.V., Hughes, W.S., Kim, Y., Karush, F.: Antibody affinity-IV. The synthesis and immunogenicity of a large β-lactoside hapten. Immunochemistry **10**, 191–196 (1973)
Grieser, M.D., Pietrzyk, D.J.: Liquid chromatography on a porous polystyrene-divinylbenzene support. Separation of nitro- and chlorophenols. Anal. Chem. **45**, 1348–1353 (1973)
Haley, T.J., Rutschmann, J.: Brain concentrations of LSD 25 (Delysid) after intracerebral or intravenous administration in conscious animals. Experientia (Basel) **13**, 199–200 (1957)
Hanzon, V.: Liver cell secretion under normal and pathologic conditions studied by fluorescence microscopy on living rats. Acta physiol. scand. (Suppl. 101) **28**, 1–268 (1952)
Heacock, R.A., Langille, K.R., McNeil, J.D., Frei, R.W.: A preliminary investigation of the high-speed liquid chromatography of some ergot alkaloids. J. Chromatogr. **77**, 425–430 (1973)
Hirom, P.C., Millburn, P., Smith, R.L.: Bile and urine as complementary pathways for the excretion of foreign organic compounds. Xenobiotica **6**, 55–64 (1976)
Hofmann, A.: Die Mutterkornalkaloide. Stuttgart: F. Enke 1964
Hogben, C.A.M., Tocco, D.J., Brodie, B.B., Schanker, L.S.: On the mechanism of intestinal absorption of drugs. J. Pharmacol. exp. Ther. **125**, 275–282 (1959)
Horrocks, D.L.: Application of Liquid Scintillation Counting. New York: Academic Press 1974
Idänpään-Heikkilä, J.E., Schoolar, J.C.: LSD: autoradiographic study of the placental transfer and tissue distribution in mice. Science **164**, 1295–1297 (1969)
Inman, J.K., Merchant, B., Claflin, L., Tacey, S.E.: Coupling of large haptens to proteins and cell surfaces: preparation of stable, optimally sensitized erythrocytes for hapten-specific, hemolytic plaque assays. Immunochemistry **10**, 165–174 (1973)
Inoue, T., Nakahara, Y., Niwaguchi, T.: Studies on lysergic acid diethylamide and related compounds. II. Mass spectra of lysergic acid derivatives. Chem. Pharm. Bull. (Tokyo) **20**, 409–411 (1972)
Iwangoff, P., Meier-Ruge, W., Schieweck, C., Enz, A.: The uptake of DH-ergotoxine by different parts of the cat brain. Pharmacology **14**, 27–38 (1976)
Jane, I., Wheals, B.B.: The characterization of LSD in illicit preparations by pressure-assisted liquid chromatography and gas chromatography. J. Chromatogr. **84**, 181–186 (1973)

Jerina, D.M., Daly, J.N.: Arene oxides: a new aspect of drug metabolism. Science **185**, 573–582 (1974)
Kalberer, F.: A new method of macroautoradiography. In: Adv. Tracer Methodology. Rothchild, S. (ed.), Vol. III. New York: Plenum Press 1966
Kalberer, F.: Macroautoradiography of larger laboratory animals. Proc. 9th Jpn. Conf. Radioisotopes, Tokyo, 1969a
Kalberer, F.: Absorption and excretion of dihydro-[9,10-^{3}H]ergotamine in the rat. Internal report SANDOZ Ltd., Basel (1969b)
Kalberer, F.: Absorption, distribution and excretion of [^{3}H]ergotamine in the rat. Internal report SANDOZ Ltd., Basel (1970)
Kalberer, F., Rutschmann, J.: Eine Schnellmethode zur Bestimmung von Tritium, Radiokohlenstoff und Radioschwefel in beliebigem organischem Probenmaterial mittels des Flüssigkeits-Scintillations-Zählers. Helv. chim. Acta **44**, 1956–1966 (1961)
Kalberer, F., Baldeck, J.P., Renella, M.C.: Métabolisme du Deseril chez le rat, le chien, le singe et l'homme. Internal report SANDOZ Ltd., Basel (1975)
Karasek, F.W., Karasek, D.E., Kim, S.H.: Detection of lysergic acid diethylamide, Δ^9-tetrahydrocannabinol and related compounds by plasma chromatography. J. Chromatogr. **105**, 345–352 (1975)
Kiechel, J.R.: Stability of the label in [6-*methyl*-^{14}C]CB 154 in rats. Internal report SANDOZ Ltd., Basel (1976)
King, L.J., Parke, D.V., Williams, R.T.: The metabolism of [2-^{14}C]indol in the rat. Biochem. J. **98**, 266–277 (1966)
Kobayashi, Y., Maudsley, D.V.: Biological Application of Liquid Scintillation Counting. New York: Academic Press 1974
Kopet, J.C., Dille, J.M.: The elimination of ergotoxine, ergotamine and ergonovine. J. Amer. pharm. Ass. **31**, 109–113 (1942)
Laboratorium Prof. Dr. Berthold: Probenpräparation und Messung. Eine Arbeitsanleitung zur Radioaktivitätsbestimmung mit der Flüssigkeitsscintillationsspektrometrie. Wildbach: Laboratorium Prof. Dr. Berthold 1973
Lanz, U., Cerletti, A., Rothlin, E.: Über die Verteilung des Lysergsäurediäthylamids im Organismus. Helv. physiol. pharmacol. Acta **13**, 207–216 (1955)
Leist, K.H., Grauwiler, J.: Transplacental passage of ^{3}H-ergotamine in the rat, and the determination of the intra-amniotic embryotoxicity of ergotamine. Experientia (Basel) **29**, 764 (1973)
Lerner, S.: LSD analysis in seizures. Bull. Narc. **19**, 39–45 (1967)
Lerner, M., Katsiaficas, M.D.: Analytical separations of mixtures of hallucinogenic drugs. Bull. Narc. **21**, 47–51 (1969)
Levy, G.: Biopharmaceutical considerations in dosage form design and evaluation. In: Prescription Pharmacy. Sprowls, J.B. (ed), pp. 31–94. Philadelphia: Lippincott 1963
Loddo, P., Spano, P.F., Trabucchi, M.: Urinary elimination of dihydro-ergotoxine after oral administration and intravenous infusion. Boll. Chim. Farm. **115**, 570–574 (1976)
Loeffler, L.J., Pierce, J.V.: Radioimmunoassay for lysergide (LSD) in illicit drugs and biological fluids. J. pharm. Sci. **62**, 1817–1820 (1973)
Lopatin, D.E., Voss, E.W.: Antilysergyl antibody: measurement of binding parameters in IgG fractions. Immunochemistry **11**, 285–293 (1974)
McMenamy, R.H., Lund, C.C., van Marcke, J., Oncley, J.L.: The binding of L-tryptophan in human plasma at 37° C. Arch. Biochem. Biophys. **93**, 135–139 (1961)
Maickel, R.P., Miller, F.P.: Fluorescent products formed by reaction of indole dervatives and o-phthalaldehyde. Anal. Chem. **38**, 1937–1938 (1966)
Mannering, G.J.: Microsomal enzyme systems which catalyze drug metabolism. In: Fundamentals of Drug Metabolism and Drug Disposition. La Du, B.N., et al. (eds.). Baltimore: Williams and Wilkins 1971
Marchbanks, R.M.: Serotonin binding to nerve ending particles and other preparations from rat brain. J. Neurochem. **13**, 1481–1493 (1966)
Markey, S.P., Colburn, R.W., Kopin, I.J.: Synthesis and purification of 2-bromo-α-ergokryptine-^{82}Br. J. Labelled Compds. Radiopharmac. **12**, 627–630 (1976)
Marzo, A., Ghirardi, P., Parenti, M.A., Merlo, L., Marchetti, G.: Livelli plasmatici ed eliminazione biliare e urinaria della raubasina, della diidroergocristina e della diidroergotamina

somministrate per vena nel cane anestetizzato. Boll. Soc. ital. Biol. sper. **51**, 684–686 (1975)

Maulding, H.V., Zoglio, M.A.: Complexes of ergot alkaloids and derivatives III: interaction of dihydroergocristine with xanthine analogs in aqueous media. J. pharm. Sci. **59**, 384–386 (1970a)

Maulding, H.V., Zoglio, M.A.: Complexes of ergot alkaloids and derivatives IV: investigations into the nature of ergot alkaloid-xanthine complexes. J. pharm. Sci. **59**, 1673–1675 (1970b)

Maulding, H.V., Zoglio, M.A.: Physical chemistry of ergot alkaloids and derivatives I: ionization constants of several medicinally active bases. J. pharm. Sci. **59**, 700–701 (1970c)

Maurer, G.: Isolement et Structure de Métabolites Biliaires de la Dihydro-β-ergokryptine Chez le Rat. Thèse du docteur d'état es-sciences présentée devant l'Institut National des Sciences Appliquées de Lyon et l'Université Claude Bernard Lyon I. No. d'ordre IDE 77014 (1977)

Meier, J., Schreier, E.: Human plasma levels of some antimigraine drugs. Headache **16**, 96–104 (1976)

Meier-Ruge, W., Schieweck, C., Iwangoff, P.: The distribution of [^{3}H]Hydergine in the cat brain. Int. Res. Commun. Syst. Pharmacol. II (73-4) 7–10–3 (1973)

Meszaros, J., Nimmerfall, F., Rosenthaler, J., Weber, H.: Permanent bile duct cannulation in the monkey. A model for studying intestinal absorption. Europ. J. Pharmacol. **32**, 233–242 (1975)

Minghetti, A., Arcamone, F., Nicollela, V., Dubini, M., Vicario, G.P.: Synthesis of 1,6-dimethyl-8β-carbobenzyloxyaminomethyl-10α-ergoline-9,10-^{3}H and method for the analysis of its metabolites in the excreta of rat, dog and man. In: Int. Conference on Radioactive Isotopes in Pharmacology. Waser, P.G., Glasson, B. (eds.), p. 61 London: Wiley-Interscience 1969

Mueller, R.G., Lang, G.E.: Fluorescent spectra of lysergic acid diethylamide. Observations on a gastric extract. Amer. J. clin. Path. **60**, 487–492 (1973)

Nash, T.: The colorimetric estimation of formaldehyde by means of the Hantzsch reaction. Biochem. J. **55**, 416–421 (1953)

Neame, K.D., Homewood, C.A.: Introduction to Liquid Scintillation Counting. London: Butterworths 1974

Nekrasov, V.I., Davydova, O.N.: Spectrophotometric determination of lysergic acid diethylamide and salts in blood of animals. Farmatsiya (Mosk.) **19**, 39–40 (1970). Chem. Abstr. **73**, 69907 (1970)

Nicoll, D.R., Ewer, M.J.C.: Liquid Scintillation Sample Preparation Techniques for Organic Materials. Beenham: Nuclear Enterprises 1971

Nimmerfall, F., Rosenthaler, J.: Ergot alkaloids: hepatic distribution and estimation of absorption by measurement of total radioactivity in bile and urine. J. Pharmacokinet. Biopharm. **4**, 57–66 (1976)

Niwaguchi, T., Inoue, T.: Studies on the quantitative *in situ* fluorometry of lysergic acid diethylamide on thin-layer chromatograms. J. Chromatogr. **59**, 127–133 (1971)

Niwaguchi, T., Inoue, T.: Studies on the P-450 difference spectra induced by lysergic acid diethylamide in rat liver microsomes. Chem. Pharm. Bull. (Tokyo) **23**, 1300–1303 (1975)

Niwaguchi, T., Inoue, T., Nakahara, Y.: Studies on enzymatic dealkylation of d-lysergic acid diethylamide (LSD). Biochem. Pharmacol. **23**, 1073–1078 (1974a)

Niwaguchi, T., Inoue, T., Sakai, T.: Studies on the *in vitro* metabolism of compounds related to lysergic acid diethylamide (LSD). Biochem. Pharmacol. **23**, 3063–3066 (1974b)

Nüesch, E.: Proof of the general validity of Dost's law of corresponding areas. Europ. J. clin. Pharmacol. **6**, 33–43 (1973)

Pacha, W.L.: Fluorometric determination of ergotamine and other nonhydrogenated ergot derivatives. Internal report SANDOZ Ltd., Basel (1969a)

Pacha, W.L.: A method for the fluorimetric determination of 4-(2-hydroxy-3-isopropylamino-propoxy)-indole (LB46), a β-blocking agent, in plasma and urine. Experientia (Basel) **25**, 802–803 (1969b)

Pacha, W.L.: Fluorimetrische Bestimmungsmethode für Dihydroergotamin und analoge Verbindungen. Internal report SANDOZ Ltd., Basel (1971)

Parke, D.V.: The Biochemistry of Foreign Compounds. London: Pergamon Press 1968
Pleiss, U., Zerjatke, W.: Markierung von 9,10-Dihydroergotoxinen mit Tritium. Isotopenpraxis (Berl.) **11**, 427–429 (1975)
Radecka, C., Nigam, I.C.: Detection of trace amounts of lysergic acid diethylamide in sugar cubes. J. pharm. Sci. **55**, 861–862 (1966)
Radiochemical Centre Amersham: Radioactive isotope dilution analysis. Review **2** (1964)
Ramstad, E., Chan Lin, W.N., Shough, H.R., Goldner, K.J., Parikh, R.P., Taylor, E.H.: Norsetoclavine, a new clavine-type alkaloid from *Pennisetum* ergot. Lloydia **30**, 441–444 (1967)
Rapkin, E.: Sample Preparation for Liquid Scintillation Counting. Part I: Solubilization techniques. Digitechniques No. 2. Part II: Solvents and scintillators. Digitechniques No. 3. Gel and emulsion counting of aqueous solutions. Digitechniques No. 5. Preparation of samples for liquid scintillation counting by combustion. Digitechniques No. 6. Plaisir (France): Intertechnique
Rapkin E.: Guide to Preparation of Samples for Liquid Scintillation Counting. Dreieichenhain (Germany): New England Nuclear Chemicals
Rosecrans, J.A., Lovell, R.A., Freedman, D.X.: Effects of lysergic acid diethylamide on the metabolism of brain 5-hydroxytryptamine. Biochem. Pharmacol. **16**, 2011–2021 (1967)
Rosenthaler, J., Munzer, H.: 9,10-Dihydroergotamine: production of antibodies and radioimmunoassay. Experientia (Basel) **32**, 234–236 (1976)
Roth, L.J., Stumpf, W.E.: Autoradiography of Diffusable Substances. New York-London: Academic Press 1969
Rothlin, E.: Recherches expérimentales sur le sort dans l'organisme des alcaloïdes natifs et dihydrogénés de l'ergot de seigle. Helv. chim. Acta **29**, 1290 (1946)
Rothlin, E.: The pharmacology of the natural and dihydrogenated alkaloids of ergot. Bull. schweiz. Akad. med. Wiss. **2**, 249–273 (1946/47)
Rothlin, E.: Über das Schicksal der natürlichen und dihydrierten Mutterkornalkaloide im Organismus. Schweiz. med. Wschr. **77**, 1161–1163 (1947)
Rothlin, E.: Metabolism of lysergic acid diethylamide. Nature (Lond.) **178**, 1400–1401 (1956)
Rothlin, E., Berde, B., Fernandez, E.: Über die enterale Resorption hydrierter Mutterkornalkaloide. Helv. physiol. pharmacol. Acta **9**, C76–C77 (1951)
Roubicek, J.: Hydergina en la terapia geriátrica. Invest. Méd. Internac. **2**, 61–71 (1975)
Rummel, W., Forth, W.: Aktiver Transport und enterale Resorption. Pharm. Ztg. **109**, 1053–1054 (1964)
Schanker, L.S.: Passage of drugs across body membranes. Pharm. Rev. **14**, 501–530 (1962)
Schmidt, R.: Pharmacocinétique de la Bromocriptine chez l'Homme. In: La Bromocriptine, Colloque de Paris 1976. Sandoz Paris (ed.) 1977
Schmidt, R., Fanchamps, A.: Effect of caffeine on intestinal absorption of ergotamine in man. Europ. J. clin. Pharmacol. **7**, 213–216 (1974)
Schram, E.: Flow-monitoring of aqueous solutions containing weak beta-emitters. In: The Current Status of Liquid Scintillation Counting. Bransome, E.D. (ed.). New York: Grune and Stratton 1970
Schreier, E.: Radiolabelled peptide ergot alkaloids. Helv. chim. Acta **59**, 585–606 (1976)
Sheehan, J.C., Hess, G.P.: A new method of forming peptide bonds. J. Amer. chem. Soc. **77**, 1067–1068 (1955)
Shough, H.R., Taylor, E.H.: Enzymology of ergot alkaloid biosynthesis. IV. Additional studies on the oxidation of agroclavine by horseradish peroxidase. Lloydia **32**, 315–326 (1969)
Siddik, Z.H., Barnes, R.D., Dring, L.G., Smith, R.L., Williams, R.T.: The fate of lysergic acid di[^{14}C]ethylamide ([^{14}C]LSD) in the rat. Biochem. Soc. Trans. **3**, 290–292 (1975)
Simon, H.: Messung von radioaktiven und stabilen Isotopen. Berlin-Heidelberg-New York: Springer 1974
Slaytor, M.B., Wright, S.E.: The metabolites of ergometrine and lysergic acid diethylamide in rat bile. J. Med. Pharm. Chemistry **5**, 483–491 (1962)
Smith, M.I.: A quantitative colorimetric reaction for the ergot alkaloids and its application in the chemical standardization of ergot preparations. U.S. Public Health Reports **1930**, 1466–1481

Smith, R.L.: The biliary excretion and enterohepatic circulation of drugs and other organic compounds. In: Progress in Drug Research. Jucker, E. (ed.), Vol. IX, pp. 299–360. Basel-Stuttgart: Birkhäuser 1966
Snyder, S.H., Reivich, M.: Regional localization of lysergic acid diethylamide in monkey brain. Nature (Lond.) **209**, 1093–1095 (1966)
Stanley, P.E., Scoggins, B.A.: Liquid Scintillation Counting, Recent Developments. New York: Academic Press 1974
Stetten, M.R.: Metabolic relationship between glutamic acid, proline, hydroxyproline and ornithine. In: A Symposium on Amino Acid Metabolism. McElroy, W.D. and Glass, H.B. (eds.). Baltimore: The Johns Hopkins Press 1955
Stoll, A., Schlientz, W.: Über Belichtungsprodukte von Mutterkornalkaloiden. Helv. chim. Acta **38**, 585–594 (1955)
Stoll, A., Rutschmann, J., Hofmann, A.: Über die Synthese von ^{14}C-Diäthylamin und ^{14}C-Lysergsäure-diäthylamid. Helv. chim. Acta **37**, 820–824 (1954a)
Stoll, A., Petrzilka, T., Rutschmann, J., Hofmann, A., Günthard, H.H.: Über die Stereochemie der Lysergsäuren und der Dihydrolysergsäuren. Helv. chim. Acta **37**, 2039–2057 (1954b)
Stoll, A., Rothlin, E., Rutschmann, J., Schalch, W.R.: Distribution and fate of ^{14}C-labeled lysergic acid diethylamide (LSD25) in the animal body. Experientia (Basel) **11**, 396–397 (1955)
Sutherland, J.M., Hooper, W.D., Eadie, M.J., Tyrer, J.H.: Buccal absorption of ergotamine. J. Neurol. Neurosurg. Psychiat. **37**, 1116–1120 (1974)
Szara, S.: Enzymatic formation of a phenolic metabolite from lysergic acid diethylamide by rat liver microsomes. Life Sci. **9**, 662–670 (1963)
Taunton-Rigby, A., Sher, S.E., Kelley, P.R.: Lysergic acid diethylamide: radioimmunoassay. Science **181**, 165–166 (1973)
Troxler, F., Hofmann, A.: Oxydation von Lysergsäure-Derivaten in 2,3-Stellung. Helv. chim. Acta **42**, 739–802 (1959)
Turner, J.C.: Sample preparation for liquid scintillation counting. Review No. 6. Amersham: The Radiochemical Centre 1971
Ullberg, S.: Autoradiographic localization in the tissues of drugs and metabolites. In: Proceedings of the First International Pharmacological Meeting, Uvnäs, B. (ed.), Vol. V, pp. 29–37. Oxford: Pergamon Press 1963
Upshall, D.G., Wailling, D.G.: The determination of LSD in human plasma following oral administration. Clin. chim. Acta **36**, 67–73 (1972)
Van Urk, H.W.: Een nieuwe gevoelige reactie op de moederkoornalkaloiden ergotamine, ergotoxine en ergotinine en de toepassing voor het onderzoek en de colorimetrische bepaling in moederkoornpreparaten. Pharm. Weekbl. **66**, 473–481 (1929)
Van Vunakis, H., Farrow, J.T., Gjika, H.B., Levine, L.: Specificity of the antibody receptor site to d-lysergamide: model of a physiological receptor for lysergic acid diethylamide. Proc. nat. Acad. Sci. (Wash.) **68**, 1483–1487 (1971)
Vicario, G.P., Dubini, M., Minghetti, A., Arcamone, F.: Synthesis of ^{3}H-ergometrine and its use for biosynthetic studies in *Claviceps paspali* and *Claviceps purpurea*. J. Labelled Compds. **3** (Suppl. 2), 492–493 (1967)
Vogel, W.H., Carapellotti, R.A., Evans, B.D., Der Marderosian, A.: Physiological disposition of isoergine and its effect on the conditioned avoidance response in rats. Psychopharmacologica (Berl.) **24**, 238–242 (1972)
Voigt, D., Johne, S., Gröger, D.: Untersuchungen zur Massenspektrometrie von Mutterkornalkaloiden. Pharmazie **29**, 697–700 (1974)
Vokoun, J., Rehacek, Z.: Mass spectra of ergot peptide alkaloids. Coll. Czechoslov. Chem. Commun. **40**, 1731–1737 (1975)
Vokoun, J., Sajdl, P., Rehacek, Z.: Mass spectrometry determination of some natural clavines and lysergic acid derivatives. Zbl. Bakt., II. Abt. **129**, 499–519 (1974)
Wenzel, M.: Radiochromatographie. In: Messung von radioaktiven und stabilen Isotopen. Simon, H. (ed.). Berlin-Heidelberg-New York: Springer 1974
Williams, L.T., Lefkowitz, R.J.: Alpha-adrenergic receptor identification by [^{3}H]dihydroergokryptine binding. Science **192**, 791–793 (1976)
Williams, R.T.: Detoxication Mechanisms, 2nd ed. London: Chapman and Hall 1959

Williams, R.T., Millburn, P., Smith, R.L.: The influence of enterohepatic circulation on toxicity of drugs. Ann. N.Y. Acad. Sci. **123**, 110–124 (1965)

Wilson, B.J., Orrenius, S.: A study of the modified type II spectral change produced by the interaction of agroclavine with cytochrome P-450. Biochim. biophys. Acta (Amst.) **261**, 94–101 (1972)

Wilson, B.J., Ramstad, E., Jansson, J., Orrenius, S.: Conversion of agroclavine by mammalian cytochrome P 450. Biochim. biophys. Acta (Amst.) **252**, 348–356 (1971)

Winter, J.C.: Tolerance to a behavioral effect of lysergic acid diethylamide and cross-tolerance to mescaline in the rat: absence of a metabolic component. J. Pharmacol. exp. Ther. **178**, 625–630 (1971)

Wittwer, J.D., Kluckhohn, J.H.: Liquid chromatographic analysis of LSD. J. Chromatogr. Sci. **11**, 1–3 (1973)

Yielding, K.L., Sterglanz, H.: Lysergic acid diethylamide binding to deoxyribonucleic acid (DNA). Proc. Soc. exp. Biol. (N.Y.) **128**, 1096–1098 (1968)

Zehnder, K.: Unpublished results on the excretion of radioactivity after oral administration of [6-*methyl*-^{14}C]methysergide to bile fistula rats and intact dogs. SANDOZ Ltd., Basel (1976)

Zoglio, M.A., Maulding, H.V.: Complexes of ergot alkaloids and derivatives II: interaction of dihydroergotoxine with certain xanthines. J. pharm. Sci. **59**, 215–219 (1970a)

Zoglio, M.A., Maulding, H.V.: Complexes of ergot alkaloids and derivatives V: interaction of methysergide maleate and caffeine in aqueous solution. J. pharm. Sci. **59**, 1836–1837 (1970b)

Zoglio, M.A., Maulding, H.V., Windheuser, J.J.: Complexes of ergot alkaloids and derivatives I: the interaction of caffeine with ergotamine tartrate in aqueous solution. J. pharm. Sci. **59**, 222–225 (1969)

CHAPTER XII

Toxicologic Considerations

R.W. GRIFFITH, J. GRAUWILER, CH. HODEL, K.H. LEIST, and B. MATTER

A. Introduction

Toxic effects of ergot compounds have been recognized since the discovery that consumption of infected cereals could cause severe illnesses; this is reflected in some of the names given to the early compounds extracted, e.g., chrysotoxin, secalintoxin (BARGER and DALE, 1907). One such name persists even today: ergotoxine. The purpose of this chapter is to review the information available on the toxicity of chemically defined ergot derivatives, both in animals and in man. The topics chosen are: Systemic Toxicity, Effects on Reproductive Processes, Potential Genetic Effects, and Interactions. The nomenclature for ergot derivatives used is that given in Chapter II.

Inevitably, available data on human toxicity are anecdotal or consist of a series of case reports. Good experimental animal work is also limited, as these compounds have been known for many years, and most animal studies were done at a time before toxicology techniques had reached a sufficient degree of sophistication to yield reproducible results. In the recently researched areas of reproduction and mutagenicity testing, more data are available for review. The borderlines between exaggerated pharmacodynamic effects, undesired side-effects, and clear-cut toxicity are often ill-defined, so that a degree of overlap in this book is unavoidable. Indeed, some of the effects on reproduction could equally well belong in other chapters. Good historical descriptions of epidemic ergotism in animals and man are available (BARGER, 1931; CHAUMARTIN, 1946; GUILHON, 1955; BOVÉ, 1970) and are not treated here.

B. Systemic Toxicity

1. Animals

a) Acute Toxicity

The purpose of acute toxicity tests in animals is to determine the mean lethal single dose and the clinical signs and effects of acute overdosage. Normally, groups of animals are given various dose levels, and the LD_{50} is calculated by probit analysis, using such statistical procedures as the methods of MILLER and TAINTER (1944) or LITCHFIELD and WILCOXON (1949).

As the ergot derivatives were chemically identified, their acute toxicity was studied, but the results were only occasionally published (BROWN and DALE, 1935;

KAPPERT, 1949; ROTHLIN, 1957). Moreover, these results were obtained before standardized methods of LD_{50} determination were developed, so that they are not readily reproducible. Since considerable data on acute toxicity experiments with ergot derivatives under standard conditions are available in the Sandoz laboratories, we have included them in this section:

The method used for LD_{50} determination in the Sandoz laboratories is as follows: mice (albino, MF2), rats (albino, OFA Sandoz SPF), and rabbits (mixed breeds or hare-type or Silver-Fawn) of both sexes were used. For intravenous or subcutaneous injection, compounds were dissolved, usually in equimolar concentrations, with the appropriate acid (i.e. tartaric, methane-sulfonic or hydrochloric) at concentrations of 1 or 2% to provide a stock solution. A few compounds (e.g., bromocriptine) had to be dissolved in 5% glucose with the addition of dimethylsulfoxide (DMSO). Stock solutions were diluted with 0.9% sodium chloride or 5% glucose, or preferably with distilled water, prior to injection. For oral administration compounds were suspended in 2% gelatin. Appropriate dilutions were made with gelatin solution. Injected or ingested concentrations were chosen to give administration volumes of up to 25 ml/kg for mice and 10 ml/kg for rats, for both routes respectively, and for rabbits 1 or 2 ml/kg intravenously and 5 ml/kg orally. Records were kept of the signs before death, those elicited by the maximum tolerated dose (or the maximum dose given) and the overall mortality for a period of 7 days. LD_{50} values were determined according to the method of MILLER and TAINTER (1944) or calculated using a statistical-mathematical probit analysis according to the theory of FINNEY (1971). Pigeons used were wild-caught animals of both sexes with a body weight between 280 and 380 g. The substances were administered orally by gavage, intravenously into the alar vein, or intramuscularly into the pectoralis muscle. The total volumes were 10 ml/kg for oral administration and 5 ml/kg both for intravenous and intramuscular injection.

LD_{50} values are given in Table 1. It can be seen that the range of toxicity is considerable. Of the animal species used most frequently (mice, rats, and rabbits), the rabbit is almost invariably the most susceptible. Table 2 demonstrates this phenomenon using the example of ergotamine and its dihydrogenated derivative. This example also confirms the general trend that dihydrogenated derivatives are less toxic than their original alkaloids.

A comparison between the different ergot alkaloids can be made taking the rabbit as being the most sensitive species. Table 3 lists the intravenous LD_{50} values in rabbits for 29 derivatives. LSD (d-lysergic acid diethylamide) and ergokryptine are the most toxic compounds (LD_{50} $\sim$0.3 mg/kg), and lysergic acid is the least toxic (LD_{50} 100 mg/kg). All the dihydrogenated alkaloids have values above 10 mg/kg. The methylated derivatives l-methylergotamine and methysergide have a low acute toxicity, whereas methylergometrine (methergine) is slightly more toxic than its nonmethylated derivative ergometrine.

It is not possible to administer lethal doses of the peptide alkaloids by mouth in many instances, suggesting that their absorption may be poor or rather slow, with the result that high lethal peak levels are not readily achieved.

Subtoxic or toxic doses in mammals usually produce restlessness and mydriasis. Piloerection and tachypnoea were described in *mice, rats, rabbits,* and *guinea-pigs* after treatment with ergotamine and ergobasine (ROTHLIN, 1923; ROTHLIN, 1935) and, with higher doses, convulsions were seen in all three species after ergotamine, ergotoxine, and ergometrine (DAVIS et al., 1935). Tail gangrene occurred in 20% of rats 5–7 days after intraperitoneal administration of 25 mg/kg of ergotoxine (GÖRÖG and KOVÁCS, 1971). Bromocriptine in subtoxic doses evoked motor excita-

Table 1. LD_{50} values (in mg/kg) for some ergot derivatives (unpublished results from Sandoz Toxicology Laboratories – methods described in text). MILLER and TAINTER (1944) determination used except where otherwise indicated

Compound	Species	Route	LD_{50} Result
Clavine alkaloids			
Agroclavine (5)[a]	Rabbit	i.v.	< 1.0
Elymoclavine (6)	Mouse	i.v.	36
	Rabbit	i.v.	1.2
d-Lysergic acid (8)	Mouse	i.v.	240
	Rabbit	i.v.	100
Ergometrine (19)	Mouse	i.v.	160
	Mouse	s.c.	370
	Mouse	p.o.	460
	Rat	i.v.	120
	Rat	p.o.	671
	Rabbit	i.v.	3.2
	Rabbit	p.o.	27.8
	Pigeon	i.v.	38
Peptide alkaloids			
Ergotamine (20)	Mouse	i.v.	265
	Mouse	s.c.	> 1000
	Mouse	p.o.	3200
	Rat	i.v.	38
	Rat	s.c.	200
	Rat	p.o.	1300
	Rabbit	i.v.	3.0
	Rabbit	s.c.	6.6
	Rabbit	p.o.	550
	Pigeon	i.v.	0.88
	Pigeon	p.o.	340
Ergosine (21)	Mouse	i.v.	33.5
	Rat	i.v.	30
	Rat	s.c.	> 200
	Rabbit	i.v.	1.23
	Rabbit	s.c.	0.7
Ergostine (22)	Mouse	i.v.	125
	Mouse	p.o.	1700
	Rat	i.v.	47
	Rat	s.c.	> 500
	Rat	p.o.	> 1000
	Rabbit	i.v.	1.2
	Rabbit	s.c.	22
	Rabbit	p.o.	~ 1000
	Pigeon	p.o.	> 10,000
Ergonine (110a)	Rabbit	i.v.	1.1
	Rabbit	s.c.	1.4
	Rabbit	p.o.	150
Ergostinine	Mouse	i.v.	180
	Rat	i.v.	180
	Rabbit	i.v.	5.3
Ergocristine (23)	Mouse	i.v.	110

Table 1 (continued)

Compound	Species	Route	LD_{50} result
	Rat—male	i.v.	64
	Rat—female	i.v.	150
	Rabbit	i.v.	1.9
	Cat	s.c.	30
Ergocornine (24)	Mouse	i.v.	275
	Mouse	p.o.	2000
	Rat	i.v.	95
	Rat	s.c.	>500
	Rat	p.o.	>500
	Cat	s.c.	30
α-Ergokryptine (25)	Mouse	i.v.	275
	Rat	i.v.	140
	Rabbit	i.v.	0.95
β-Ergokryptine (26)	Mouse	i.v.	210
	Rat	i.v.	49
	Rabbit	i.v.	0.78
Ergokryptine (both isomers)	Mouse	i.v.	300
	Mouse	p.o.	870
	Rat	i.v.	58
	Rat	s.c.	10
	Rabbit	i.v.	0.34
	Rabbit	s.c.	1.0
	Cat	s.c.	19.5
Ergotoxine	Mouse	i.v.	90
	Mouse	s.c.	450
	Rat	i.v.	76
Ergovaline (29)	Mouse	i.v.	175
	Rabbit	i.v.	1.7
Hydrogenated alkaloids			
DH-Ergometrine (74c)	Mouse	i.v.	74
DH-Ergotamine (102b)	Mouse	i.v.	160
	Mouse	s.c.	1170
	Mouse	p.o.	>8000
	Rat	i.v.	130
	Rat	s.c.	>500
	Rat	p.o.	>2000
	Rabbit	i.v.	37
	Rabbit	s.c.	>60
	Rabbit	p.o.	>1000
	Pigeon	i.v.	31.5
	Pigeon	p.o.	>3000
	Cat	s.c.	70
DH-Ergonine (110b)	Mouse	i.v.	178
	Mouse	p.o.	>2000
	Rat	i.v.	80
	Rat	p.o.	>2000
	Rabbit	i.v.	19
	Rabbit	p.o.	1300
DH-Ergosine (102a)	Mouse	i.v.	190
	Rabbit	i.v.	21

Table 1 (continued)

Compound	Species	Route	LD_{50} result
DH-Ergostine (102g)	Mouse	i.v.	150
	Mouse	p.o.	> 8000
	Rat	i.v.	36
	Rat	p.o.	> 4000
	Rabbit	i.v.	12.5
	Rabbit	p.o.	> 2000
DH-Ergocristine (102c)	Mouse	i.v.	150
	Mouse	s.c.	900
	Mouse	p.o.	5000
	Rat	i.v.	66
	Rat	p.o.	> 2000
	Rabbit	i.v.	33.2
	Rabbit	p.o.	> 1400
	Cat	s.c.	54
DH-Ergocornine (102d)	Mouse	i.v.	193
	Mouse	s.c.	1050
	Mouse	p.o.	> 8000
	Rat	i.v.	125
	Rabbit	i.v.	34.5
	Cat	s.c.	66
DH-α-Ergokryptine (102c)	Rat	i.v.	88
	Rabbit	i.v.	14.2
DH-β-Ergokryptine (102f)	Rat	i.v.	87
	Rabbit	i.v.	19.5
DH-Ergokryptine (both isomers)	Mouse	i.v.	164
	Mouse	s.c.	750
	Rat	i.v.	66
	Rabbit	i.v.	20
	Cat	s.c.	45
DH-Ergotoxine mesylate (Hydergin)	Mouse	i.v.	180
	Mouse	s.c.	> 4000
	Mouse	p.o.	> 1000
	Rat	i.v.	86
	Rat	s.c.	> 2000
	Rat	p.o.	> 1000
	Rabbit	i.v.	18.5
	Rabbit	s.c.	~ 105
	Rabbit	p.o.	> 1000
DH-Ergovaline (108b)	Mouse	i.v.	152
	Mouse	p.o.	> 2000
	Rat	i.v.	250
	Rat	p.o.	> 2000
	Rabbit	i.v.	19
	Rabbit	p.o.	325
Synthetic lysergic acid amides			
d-Lysergic acid-diethylamide (LSD 25) (73b)	Mouse	i.v.	41
	Mouse	s.c.	240
	Mouse	p.o.	120
	Rat	i.v.	16.5

Table 1 (continued)

Compound	Species	Route	LD_{50} result
	Rat	s.c.	21
	Rabbit	i.v.	0.305
	Rabbit	s.c.	0.25
	Rabbit	p.o.	4.5
d-Lysergic acid-L-2-butanolamide (73a) (methylergometrine)	Mouse	i.v.	85
	Mouse	s.c.	64
	Mouse	p.o.	140
	Rat	i.v.	23
	Rat	s.c.	17.5
	Rat	p.o.	93
	Rabbit	i.v.	2.0
	Rabbit	s.c.	3.0
	G-Pig	i.v.	45
Alkylated derivatives			
Methysergide (34a)	Mouse	i.v.	185
	Mouse	p.o.	440
	Rat	i.v.	125
	Rat	p.o.	2450
	Rabbit	i.v.	28
	Rabbit	s.c.	25
	Pigeon	i.v.	100
	Pigeon	p.o.	>2000
I-Methyl-dihydrolysergic acid-L-2-butanolamide (35b)	Mouse	i.v.	43
	Rat	i.v.	56
	Rabbit	i.v.	27
	Pigeon	i.v.	55
I-Methylergotamine (34c)	Mouse	i.v.	185
	Mouse	p.o.	>8000
	Rat	i.v.	169
	Rat	p.o.	>4000
	Rabbit	i.v.	21
	Rabbit	p.o.	~2500
	Pigeon	i.v.	138
	Pigeon	p.o.	>2000
Halogenated derivatives			
2-Bromo-α-ergokryptine (bromocriptine) (38)	Mouse	i.v.	230[b]
	Mouse	p.o.	2620[b]
	Rat	i.v.	120[b]
	Rat	p.o.	>2000[b]
	Rabbit	i.v.	12[b]
	Rabbit	p.o.	>1000[b]

[a] Chemical reference number in Chapter II.
[b] Calculated after FINNEY (1971).

Table 2. LD_{50} values (in mg/kg) for ergotamine and dihydroergotamine in three species (data from Table 1)

	Mouse	Rat	Rabbit
Ergotamine			
i.v.	265	38	3.0
s.c.	> 1000	~ 200	6.6
p.o.	3200	1300	550
Dihydroergotamine			
i.v.	160	130	37
s.c.	1170	> 500	> 60
p.o.	> 8000	> 2000	> 1000

Table 3. Intravenous LD_{50} values (in mg/kg) for the rabbit, arranged in order of toxicity (data from Table 1)

d-Lysergic acid diethylamide	0.305	DH-Ergostine	12.5
Ergokryptine	0.34	DH-α-Ergokryptine	14.2
β-Ergokryptine	0.78	DH-Ergotoxine mesylate	18.5
Ergocornine	0.9	DH-Ergonine	19
α-Ergokryptine	0.95	DH-Ergovaline	19
Ergonine	1.1	DH-β-Ergokryptine	19.5
Elymoclavine	1.2	DH-Ergokryptine	20
Ergostine	1.2	1-Methylergotamine	21
Ergosine	1.23	DH-Ergosine	21
Ergovaline	1.7	DH-Methysergide	27
Ergocristine	1.9	Methysergide	28
Methylergometrine	2.0	DH-Ergocristine	33.2
Ergotamine	3.0	DH-Ergocornine	34.5
Ergometrine	3.2	DH-Ergotamine	37
Ergostinine	5.3	Lysergic acid	100
2-Bromo-α-ergokryptine	12		

tion, leading to rhythmic cramps, dyspnea, bradypnea, and finally coma in all three species (GRAUWILER and GRIFFITH, 1974).

The predominant signs in *cats* and *dogs* given toxic doses of ergotamine or ergotoxine were excitement, restlessness, excess salivation, vomiting, piloerection, miosis, mydriasis, and tachypnea (ROTHLIN, 1923 and unpublished results). Muscular weakness occurred in cats several hours after subcutaneous administration of ergotamine, and tremor and rigidity of extensor muscles was seen in dogs after ergotamine and ergotoxine (BARGER, 1938). Both species exhibited profuse salivation and vomiting after being given either alkaloid. With dihydrogenated derivatives this effect was 6–8 times weaker than with the nonhydrogenated compounds (ROTHLIN, 1946).

Ergotamine tartrate administration to *Rhesus monkeys* in single intravenous doses of up to 1 mg/kg did not cause any marked adverse effects. On the other hand, 3 mg/kg i.v. or 100 mg/kg p.o. of 5′β-methyl-ergoalanine resulted in tachypnea, mydriasis, headwagging, and tonic cramps. No vomiting was seen. (Unpublished results from our laboratories.)

The *cock* has been used for many years to demonstrate gangrenous ergotism. Cyanosis of the comb and wattles, followed within 1–1½ h by gangrene, occurred after subcutaneous, oral, or intramuscular administration of 2–3 mg/kg of ergotamine, ergometrine, and ergotoxine (ROTHLIN, 1923; BARGER, 1938; DAVIS et al., 1935). This sign was consistent enough to allow the model to be used for a bioassay of ergot toxicity. In addition, signs of overdosage in the cock included tachypnea, ataxia, salivation, defecation, and drowsiness. Vomiting in the *pigeon* can also be used for bioassay purposes. The ED_{50} for ergotamine has been estimated as 5 mg/kg p.o., 0.14 mg/kg i.m., and 0.068 mg/kg i.v. (unpublished experimental results; see above for method). These findings are also referred to in Chapter VI of this book.

The acute toxic effects of LSD have been investigated in numerous species. In rats, LSD given intraperitoneally at doses of 0.18–0.5 mg/kg produced marked hyperactivity with violent headshaking and delay in performance time in a conditioned avoidance test (WINTER and FLATAKER, 1956). Within 15 min profuse salivation and abnormal behavior was noted. Similar signs were seen after intravenous administration of 1 mg/kg, while 3 and 10 mg/kg produced generalized body tremors and convulsive movements (DOEPFNER, 1962). LSD given in doses of 0.25 mg/kg s.c. to guinea-pigs caused frequent scratching, coughing, and restlessness, and the animals bit the cage bars (SIVADJIAN, 1969). The effects of intraperitoneal administration in rats could be antagonized completely by administration of serotonin 0.9–2 mg/kg i.p., whereas reserpine (0.5–5 mg/kg) intensified and prolonged these signs (WINTER and FLATAKER, 1956).

LSD has also been studied in nonhuman primates. Doses up to 1 mg/kg i.v. given to *Macaca mulatta* produced within 20 min a prone extended posture with increased muscle tone, followed by ataxia and lack of response to visual or noxious stimuli (EVARTS, 1956). COLE and GLEES (1967) described similar signs following lower doses (0.1–0.5 mg/kg) given intravenously to *M. mulatta*, *M. nemestrina*, and *Papio*. Here too, the lack of response to visual stimuli was striking, as well as mydriasis, cold extremities, and palor of the anogenital region. Vomiting, nausea, or vocalization were not induced. The signs produced by LSD in an Asian elephant are described by WEST et al. (1962). Within a few minutes of receiving 0.1 mg/kg i.m. (a massive dose, totally ~300 mg), the animal became restless and began trumpeting; this was followed by ataxia and collapse. A prolonged epileptiform fit was associated with hyperextension of the limbs, spasm of the orbital muscles, and mydriasis. Death supervened after 1 h and 40 min, following dyspnea due to laryngeal spasm.

b) Chronic Toxicity

Prolonged administration of ergot derivatives to animals was undertaken by some early research workers, in an attempt to find out more about classical ergotism. Up to the early 1930's, such studies involved the use of impure or only partially purified extracts, usually in excessive doses, and the changes produced corresponded to those seen in ergotism in man, i.e., involving chiefly the circulatory and nervous system. In more recent studies, using purified materials and carefully monitored doses, the central nervous effects have been less pronounced. It is, therefore, uncertain whether convulsive effects are due to contaminants, as suggested by MELLANBY (1931) and STOCKMAN (1934), or are the results of excessive dosage. In recent years, the endocrine actions of ergots have received more attention (FLÜCKIGER and WAGNER, 1968).

The first studies with pure alkaloids were done with ergotamine, but later experiments employed other peptide alkaloids. Extremely few studies have been done using the clavine alkaloids, the lysergic acids, or the lysergic acid amides. Prolonged toxicity studies reported with ergot alkaloids are listed in Table 4. In general, the dihydrogenated derivatives were less toxic than the original alkaloids. In nearly all cases, the principal effect produced was ischemia of some part of the body – the comb and wattles in the case of cocks, the tails of rats, the margins of the external ear in dogs and rabbits, and the tongue-tip in sheep. The pathogenesis of this effect has been studied quite extensively, using chiefly the cock's comb or rat tail model. A literature review as well as extensive experimental work on the rat model has been published by LUND (1951). LEWIS (1935) described the histology of gangrene of the hen's comb produced by 10 mg ergotoxine given i.m. daily. Unrelieved vasoconstriction led to marked degenerative changes in the endothelium within a few days, which was followed by stasis in the capillaries and clot formation in the central vessels, leading to necrosis. LEWIS pointed out that vascular spasm in ergot poisoning did not arrest the circulation and so did not cause gangrene directly but rather by the chain of events he described. ANDERSON and WELLS (1948), however, threw some doubt on the role of thrombosis as a contributory factor; they were unable to impede ergotamine-induced gangrene in the rat tail using heparin or dicoumarin. They concluded that thrombosis was incidental to the vascular occlusion, and that the degree of vasoconstriction produced by the ergot alkaloid was critical. BRAUN (1942) was able to show that the vasodilator benzylimidazoline could exert a protective effect. Dihydroergotamine and dihydroergocornine also have a protective action, as does dihydroergotoxine mesylate (STUCKI, 1952); in these cases a receptor-blocking mechanism should be considered.

Since obliterative vascular disease is more common in men than in women, the possible protective role of female sex hormones was of interest; ergotamine-induced necrosis of the rat tail was used as a test model (MCGRATH, 1935; SUZMAN et al., 1938; SIMON, 1946; MESSINA, 1964). The results were not conclusive and are probably without significance for human therapeutics. BIGGIO et al. (1964) reported a protective action of griseofulvin on ergotamine-induced rat tail necrosis, which cannot be explained by the mycotoxic action of the compound.

A relatively large number of the published studies (Table 4) concern methysergide. These were stimulated by the attempts to find an animal model for the fibrosing condition which occurs occasionally in man (see Section 2f). In addition to the standard toxicity studies listed, extra experiments employing various possible cofactors have been done (HODEL and GRIFFITH, 1973); in none of their standard or supplemental animal studies was there any evidence for the occurrence of lesions corresponding to retroperitoneal fibrosis. Seven different species, periods of drug administration up to $2\frac{1}{2}$ years, and manipulations such as provocation of fibrosis

Table 4. Prolonged animal toxicity studies with ergot derivatives

Derivative	Species	Route	Duration (wks)	Dose (mg/kg/day)	Reference
Ergometrine	Cock	i.m.	1	65 mg/day	BROWN and DALE (1935)
	Cock	i.m.	4	0.06–0.48	CUSTER (1938)
	Cock	i.m.	3	1.0 mg/day	DAVIS et al. (1935)
	Dog	i.v.	3	0.5, 1.0	DAVIS et al. (1935)
Ergotamine	Frog	lymph sac	6	0.5	LANGECKER (1932)
	Mouse	feed	8	0.25 mg/day	LANGECKER (1932)
	Rat	feed	8	1.0 mg/day	LANGECKER (1932)
	Rat	s.c.	1	1.0	BARNARD (1961)
	Rat	s.c.	8	0.25, 0.5	BARNARD (1961)
	Rat	s.c.	15	0.6, 1.2	SMITH and ZALMAN (1949)
	Rat	i.v.	1	1.0, 1.25, 2.5	ORTH and RITCHIE (1947)
	G-pig	s.c.	6	1.0	BARNARD (1961)
	Rabbit	i.v.	4	2, 3, 4 mg/day	PENTSCHEW (1929)
	Rabbit	i.v.	4	1.0	BARNARD (1961)
	Dog	s.c.	14	0.25, 0.5	ORTH and RITCHIE (1947)
	Dog	s.c.	22	0.025→0.4	STAHNKE (1928)
	Sheep	p.o.	2	1.0	GREATOREX and MANTLE (1973)
Ergotoxine	Rat	feed	52+	5% in feed	FITZHUGH et al. (1944)
	Cock	i.m.	1	10 mg/day	LEWIS (1935)
DH-Ergotamine	Rat	s.c.	15	1.3, 2.5, 5.0	SMITH and ZAHLMAN (1949)
	Rat	i.v.	4	5, 10	ORTH (1946)
	Rat	i.v.	6	5, 10, 20	ORTH and RITCHIE (1947)
	Rabbit	i.v.	4	1.0	BARNARD (1961)
	G-pig	s.c.	4	1.0	BARNARD (1961)
	Dog	s.c.	14	0.5, 1.0	ORTH and RITCHIE (1947)
DH-Ergocristine	Rat	s.c.	15	0.3–2.3	SMITH and ZALMAN (1949)
DH-Ergocornine	Rat	s.c.	17	0.8–3.4	SMITH and ZALMAN (1949)
DH-Ergotoxine mesylate	Rat	s.c.	14	0.2–1.5	SMITH and ZALMAN (1949)
	Rabbit	i.v.	4	1.0	BARNARD (1961)
d-Lysergic acid diethylamide	Rat	p.o.	4	0.04	MATVEEV (1970)
Methysergide	Mouse	i.p.	2	20	LANGGARD and ULRICH (1973)
	Rat	p.o.	52	5, 20, 50	HODEL and GRIFFITH (1973)
	Rat	feed	52	0.9, 9.0	HODEL and GRIFFITH (1973)
	Rat	s.c.	26	0.1, 1.0	HODEL and GRIFFITH (1973)
	Rat	s.c.	10	5–15 μg/day	ALBERTI et al. (1968)
	Rat	i.p.	26	0.1, 1.0	HODEL and GRIFFITH (1973)
	Rat	i.p.	10	5–15 μg/day	ALBERTI et al. (1968)
	Rabbit	i.v.	8	20	HODEL and GRIFFITH (1973)
	Rabbit	s.c.	3	12	HODEL and GRIFFITH (1973)
	Rabbit	s.c.	10	25–50 μg/day	ALBERTI et al. (1968)
	G-pig	feed	52	0.5, 5.0	HODEL and GRIFFITH (1973)
	Cat	p.o.	104	1.0→6.0	HODEL and GRIFFITH (1973)
	Dog	p.o.	52	0.3, 3.0	HODEL and GRIFFITH (1973)
	Dog	p.o.	30	5.0	HODEL and GRIFFITH (1973)
	Minipig	p.o.	104	0.3, 1.0	HODEL and GRIFFITH (1973)
	Rhesus	p.o.	156	1.3, 2.6	HODEL and GRIFFITH (1973)
Bromocriptine	Rat	feed	53	5, 20, 82	GRIFFITH (1974)
	Dog	p.o.	62	1.0, 3.0, 10	GRIFFITH and RICHARDSON (1975)
	Rhesus	p.o.	13	2, 8, 32	GRIFFITH (1976)

and hormone imbalance were used. ALBERTI et al. (1968) reported fibrotic changes in rats and rabbits after intraperitoneal and subcutaneous administration of methysergide, but HODEL and GRIFFITH (1973) could not reproduce these results, in spite of using higher doses given for longer periods. LANGGARD and ULRICH (1973) were also unable to detect any connective tissue lesions in mice given methysergide parenterally.

Although it is our intention to confine ourselves to experiments employing pure ergot derivatives, a study by FITZHUGH et al. (1944) should be mentioned. These workers fed crude ergot to rats for periods of up to 2 years. A high percentage of rats given 5% of ergot in the diet developed tumors on the ears, which were diagnosed histologically as neurofibromas. The frequency of occurrence was dose-dependent, rarely being seen with 1% dietary admixture. Removal of ergot from the feed led to regression of the tumors. No cutaneous gangrene or vascular lesions attributable to ergot were seen (possibly because the dosage was relatively low). In a parallel study done with ergotoxine, tumors also occurred but with a far lower frequency. The authors concluded that an impurity in the crude ergot was either directly responsible or an enhancing factor.

Endocrine effects of ergots were hinted at by FITZHUGH et al. (1944) when they described "corpus luteum hyperplasia" after more than 1 year of crude ergot administration. Bromocriptine, which has marked dopamine receptor agonist activities, produced persistent corpora lutea and endometritis in rats (GRIFFITH, 1974) and cystic corpora lutea in dogs (GRIFFITH and RICHARDSON, 1975). It is possible that other ergot derivatives can have such actions, but experience is lacking from long-term studies. (The endocrine actions of ergot derivatives are reviewed in Chapter IX.)

The emetic action of ergot derivatives in dogs is well known. It is especially pronounced with bromocriptine, being observed after oral doses of only 0.1 mg/kg (GRIFFITH and RICHARDSON, 1975). This effect is discussed more fully in Chapter VI.

Long-term toxicity studies may also give a clue as to possible beneficial drug effects. In rats given bromocriptine for 52 weeks, the frequency and degree of degenerative renal lesions were markedly reduced compared to those in controls, due to the compound's action on circulating prolactin levels (RICHARDSON, 1973).

This brief survey has been limited to experiments in laboratory animals. Earlier reports, based on acute poisoning in many different species, have indicated that some species have considerable resistance to ergot overdosage—for instance, herbivores are far more resistant than carnivores (CUSHNY, 1924).

2. Man

The effects of overdosage of ergot derivatives in man cannot be treated conventionally as acute (one dose) or chronic, as with animals. In some cases, brief exposure to ergot compounds is followed by the onset of side effects, but the time interval is often variable, depending on the dosage and the condition of the patient. The adverse effects are considered here under various organ-system headings. Unfortunately, systematic analyses of reported side effects are rare, most publications being concerned with individual case reports.

a) Effects on the Heart

The pharmacologic actions of ergot derivatives on the heart are well known in animals, and changes in cardiac function in man have also been reported in therapeutic doses (Chapter V).

The first report of myocardial ischemia precipitated by ergotamine tartrate used therapeutically is attributed to LABBÉ et al. (1929); 0.5 mg i.m. given to a 49-year-old woman to treat thyrotoxicosis produced typical signs of angina pectoris. ZIMMERMANN (1935) and GOULD et al. (1936) had similar cases. GOLDFISCHER (1960) described a case of myocardial infarction in a 35-year-old migrainous woman who was given a total dose of only 2.5 mg of ergotamine—2 mg orally followed by 0.5 mg intramuscularly.

In the late 1940's, several clinical investigators tried using intravenous ergot derivatives as a diagnostic aid in differentiating functional from organic ECG changes. SCHERF and SCHLACHMAN (1948) gave ergotamine or dihydroergotamine at doses of 0.5 mg i.v. STEIN (1949) used doses of 0.2 to 0.4 mg of ergometrine maleate. MCNERNEY and LEEDHAM (1950) used 0.5 mg ergotamine, and MASTER et al. (1950) combined intravenous ergotamine with a "two-step" exercise test. All these workers reported one or more incidents of precipitation of angina or acute coronary insufficiency and have recommended abandoning this use of ergots.

Oral administration should theoretically have a lower risk of causing cardiac complications, based on considerations of hypothetical circulating drug concentrations. However, BERNREITER (1965) described a case of acute cardiac ischemia in a 45-year-old woman who took only four tablets of a combination compound containing ergotamine and caffeine (a total dose of 4 mg ergotamine tartrate).

Ergometrine does not usually cause increased blood pressure in the low i.m. doses used in obstetrics. However, it can exert undesired effects. BAILLIE (1969a) studied 100 patients anesthetized for obstetric or minor gynecologic procedures, who received ergometrine maleate 0.5 mg intravenously; ECG monitoring revealed depression of sinoatrial node activity, associated with nodal rhythm in 12 cases, within a few seconds of injection. Normal sinus rhythm could be restored with atropine or gallamine triethiodide. He concluded that ergometrine shares a common tendency with suxamethonium and halothane to increase vagal tone. Hypotension was not detected in any case, but a slight elevation of blood pressure (10 mm Hg on average) occurred. The same author reported a further case in which ergometrine given during anesthesia for manual removal of the placenta caused ventricular ectopic beats (BAILLIE, 1969b). BROWNING (1974) described a patient in whom cardiac arrest under general anesthesia for delivery occurred 2–3 min after intravenous administration of 0.5 mg of ergometrine; the patient responded to external cardiac massage, and no residual effects were detected. The diagnosis was not, however, supported by ECG monitoring, and it seems more likely that this was a case of severe arrhythmia, similar to those reported by BAILLIE (1969b) and STEIN and WEINSTEIN (1950).

Angina pectoris has occasionally been reported in susceptible patients taking methysergide; GRAHAM (1960) first drew attention to this possibility. In 1967, HUDGSON et al. reported three cases of myocardial infarction in connection with methysergide medication; coronary insufficiency is, therefore, clearly a contraindication to the use of this drug.

b) Vascular Effects

The vascular effects of ergot poisoning have been known for centuries. Vivid descriptions of "St. Anthony's fire" are numerous. However, therapeutic doses of ergot compounds in sensitive individuals, as well as overdosage, can lead to equally dramatic effects. The offending derivative is usually ergotamine, often in combination with caffeine, taken orally or rectally for the treatment of migraine. Less commonly methysergide is responsible. The clinical picture is that of vascular ergotism, i.e., numb, cold or blue limbs, paresthesia, intermittent claudication, absent peripheral arterial pulses, and, on arteriography, abrupt narrowing at various sites. Good descriptions have been given by YATER and CAHILL (1936), CAMERON and FRENCH (1960), DALESSIO et al. (1961), URELES and ROB (1963), EDGERLY and STEWART (1963), CRANLEY et al. (1963), BYRNE-QUINN (1964), GRAHAM (1964), DANIELL (1964), IUEL and MUNE (1967), HIRSCH and EGER (1972), DIAMANT-BERGER et al. (1972).

The standard treatment is usually intraarterial administration of vasodilators, such as tolazoline, isoproterenol, or papaverine. CRANLEY et al. (1963) used heparin with some success in one case; ELOFF et al. (1963) recommended hyperbaric oxygen therapy; and HANSTEEN (1966) used hydrocortisone effectively. Low-molecular-weight dextran combined with epidural anaesthesia is a more recent approach (LONDON et al., 1970).

In most cases, the vessels of the limbs are chiefly affected, but this is not invariable. Effects on the coronary circulation have been considered in the previous section. Necrosis of the tongue has been attributed to oral ergotamine tartrate administration in a patient with temporal arteritis (WOLPAW et al., 1973). In this disease, pathologic occlusive changes in the lingual arteries occur (MISSEN, 1961); gangrene was probably precipitated by the additional insult of ergotamine administration. Spasm of the internal carotid artery, with associated ptosis, nystagmus, hypalgesia, and facial dropping, occurred in a patient with migraine taking oral ergotamine and methysergide concurrently (RICHTER and BANKER, 1973). Unilateral occlusion of the carotid artery has also been reported in a 20-year-old woman following oral ingestion of LSD (LIEBERMAN et al., 1974); angiography indicated that the underlying mechanism was probably vasoconstriction, followed by stenosis and secondary thrombosis. A similar case was reported earlier by SOBEL et al. (1971). DE MARGERIE et al. (1972) described obliteration of the central retinal artery in a patient who misused LSD and amphetamine simultaneously. Spasm of the retinal artery has also been reported after dihydroergotamine overdosage (HANSELMAYER and WERNER, 1973).

Involvement of the renal arteries has been described. FEDOTIN and HARTMAN (1970) reported ergotism in a woman given 10 mg of ergotamine tartrate rectally over a period of 3 days, in whom aortography revealed constriction of the aorta and its major branches, together with bilateral renal arterial stenosis. Creatinine clearance was reduced during the acute phase but rose again after ergotamine had been discontinued, and plasma renin activity fell from high levels back to normal. In the patient described by Luke et al. (1970), renal failure developed 2 weeks after delivery, at which time she had received 0.2 mg methylergometrine intramuscularly, followed by 0.6 mg daily by mouth for 3 days; a causal relationship here, however, is by no means certain. Methysergide has also been implicated in several cases of renal artery spasm (Graham and Parnes, 1965). Buenger and Hunter (1966) have reported a case of reversible stenosis of the superior mesenteric artery related to methysergide therapy. Arteriography showed multiple vascular narrowings, which disappeared after cessation of medication.

Some authors (von Storch, 1938; Glazer et al., 1966) postulate that migrainous subjects may be inherently less prone to the vascular side effects of ergot derivatives. Thus, Appenzeller et al. (1963) showed that migraine sufferers have a diminished reflex vasodilator response in the hand to warming the thorax. The relative infrequency of reports of vascular ergotism in patients with migraine seems at first sight to support this concept. More likely, however, this is due to the intermittent nature of treatment (Young and Humphries, 1961). Horton and Peters (1963) failed to detect toxic reactions from ergotamine tartrate in any case of classical migraine (where ergotamine use was intermittent), whereas migraine-tension headaches were associated with more intensive or even continuous use of ergotamine, and vasospastic disturbances occurred in almost half the patients.

Less dramatic vascular actions of ergot derivatives include hypertension and venous effects. There is no doubt that a rise in blood pressure can occur in a proportion of patients receiving therapeutic doses of ergometrine in obstetric practice (Forman and Sullivan, 1952), and it is recommended that the drug should not be used in patients who are already hypertensive, especially those with preeclampsia. Baillie (1963) surveyed 266 patients who received ergometrine intravenously in connection with general anesthesia for Caesarian section or instrumental delivery. A rise in both systolic and diastolic blood pressure, often exceeding 20 mm Hg, was noted in patients suffering from preeclamptic toxemia, whereas no response occurred in normotensive patients. Similarly, patients with chronic hypertension showed little or no change in blood pressure. These results confirmed those of McGinty (1956), who also examined methylergometrine, and Casady et al. (1960).

Intravenous administration of ergometrine (0.5 mg) in a normotensive postpartum patient was shown by Hendricks and Brenner (1970) to be associated with increased uterine activity and arterial pressure increases of 20 mm Hg in both the systolic and diastolic values; they concluded that ergot derivatives should be given only by the intramuscular route in normal obstetric practice. Certainly, they should never be used in conjunction with vasopressor therapy in spinal anesthesia in obstetrics (Gottschalk, 1972).

The veins are responsive to ergot alkaloids. Occasionally, toxic effects have been reported. Von Storch (1938) mentioned pains in varicose veins as a rare side effect of ergotamine therapy. Clarke (1957) has seen a patient with migraine who had spasm of the saphenous vein lasting several hours after ergotamine tartrate administration. Thrombophlebitis after single doses of ergotamine tartrate has been reported by Carter (1958) in three patients—two of these also suffered from varicose veins. Graham (1964) mentioned thrombophlebitis as a rare complication of methysergide therapy. It is clear that side effects involving the veins are less frequent than those affecting the arteries; in general, such effects are also less serious.

c) Central Nervous System Effects

Traditional descriptions of ergot poisoning divide the effects into two main groups: gangrenous ergotism and convulsive ergotism. The latter form is rarely encountered nowadays; this possibly reflects a change from the accidental ingestion of large amounts of crude ergots in earlier times to the therapeutic misadventures of today. Convulsions occurred in a newborn infant accidently given 0.5 mg of ergometrine (KENNA, 1972), but respiratory depression was predominant in this case, as in another reported by BRERETON-STILES et al. (1972). FISHER and UNGERLEIDER (1967) reported *grand mal* seizures following LSD; however, this compound also can produce respiratory arrest (KLOCK et al., 1974).

It is clearly beyond the scope of this chapter to consider the effects of ergot derivatives, and especially LSD, on psychic functions. These aspects are treated more fully in Chapter VIII. The results of overdosage, such as schizoid reactions, paranoid behavior, severe depression, or acute panic states will not be reviewed here. They have been adequately described, for LSD, by ROSENTHAL (1964), COHEN (1966), and SARWER-FONER (1972). The evidence suggests that hallucinogens like LSD, apart from acute effects, may unmask but cannot directly cause a variety of psychiatric disorders (HOLLISTER, 1975). In 1972, PERSYKO warned of possible psychotic effects of methysergide in certain individuals. This risk, however, has not been confirmed by any other reports. Bromocriptine, like other dopamine receptor agonists, may cause hallucinations in patients with Parkinson's disease (CALNE et al., 1976).

Nausea and vomiting are the most commonly observed symptoms of overdosage of ergot derivatives (VON STORCH, 1938; LAUERSEN and CONRAD, 1974). In some patients they occur at therapeutic doses, occasionally constituting a disabling side effect (FRIEDMAN et al., 1959). Higher doses of ergots, in addition to vascular effects, may lead to fatigue, insomnia, restlessness, excitement, delirium, and dementia (VON STORCH, 1938). LSD overdosage has been reported to cause extreme hyperthermia (FRIEDMAN and HIRSCH, 1971), as may also occur after amphetamine abuse (LISKOW, 1971). VOLTOLINA (1970) reported that creatine phosphokinase levels in the cerebrospinal fluid of LSD abusers were clearly elevated for a period after use. This parameter is regarded as evidence of brain damage. Organic brain dysfunction persisting for a long period after recovery from LSD overdosage in a 5-year-old child has been described by MILMAN (1967). It seems evident that LSD poisoning in children runs a different course from that in adults, possibly due to increased susceptibility of the immature brain. This is supported by the findings of SCHIEFER et al. (1972), who found that the EEG changes in nine children with LSD intoxication were the reverse of those normally encountered in adults given therapeutic doses. The children had evidence of synchronization with increased slow (delta and theta) waves, whereas adults have been shown to exhibit desynchronization, with acceleration of alpha rhythm and increased beta activity (BENTE et al., 1958).

PETERS and HORTON (1951), ROWSELL et al. (1973), and PEARCE (1976) have drawn attention to the problem of headaches following overdosage of ergotamine for the treatment of tension headache. These occur with increasing frequency when ergotamine is being taken regularly. They are not usually accompanied by nausea and vomiting, and paradoxically they are only relieved by further doses of ergotamine. They can be cured by discontinuing ergotamine, but withdrawal headaches occur in many cases. ANDERSSON (1975), in describing the problems met in diagnosing and treating this interesting syndrome, concluded that ergotamine should be used intermittently and for only a few days each month. Headache patients who are unduly anxious or subjected to prolonged stress run a real risk of abusing ergot derivatives; LUCAS and FALKOWSKI (1973) reported six such cases – five misused ergotamine and one methysergide.

KRAVITZ (1935) described optic neuritis in a woman who took ~1 mg daily of crude ergot to procure an abortion – bilateral papillitis led to subsequent optic atrophy. GUPTA and STROBOS (1972) reported a similar case with signs first appearing after 40 mg ergotamine taken orally over a 6-day period. Neuritis was probably due to ischemia secondary to arteriolar constriction, with subsequent damage to intraneural capillaries. A typical ring-type scotoma developed due to selective involvement of the paraxial optic fibers. Transitory cortical blindness was described in a patient given methylergometrine (0.2 mg i.v.) at delivery (CREZE et al., 1976). This was accompanied by severe headache and hallucinations, all of which resolved within half an hour. The mechanism here is uncertain.

d) Autonomic and Peripheral Nervous System Effects

Mydriasis and hyperreflexia have been reported in several cases of intoxication with different ergot derivatives (IANZITO et al., 1972; LARCAN and LAMBERT, 1972; BÄHR et al., 1972; NICAISE, 1972). Formication, another common symptom of severe intoxication, is probably related to ischemia. While peripheral symmetrical sensory loss and paresthesia are often described as part of the vascular ergotism symptomatology, selective ischemic neuritis is less common. PERKIN (1974) described a case of lateral popliteal nerve palsy due to ergotamine overdosage.

Nasal stuffiness is reported with high doses of dihydrogenated peptide derivatives, especially after parenteral administration (KAPPERT, 1949); this is clearly an exaggerated α-adrenoceptor blocking effect.

e) Endocrine Effects

In 1950, NASSAR et al. described a patient with postpartum necrosis of the anterior pituitary, which developed in association with hemorrhagic shock and ergometrine therapy. The authors postulated a possible etiologic relationship to ergot administration and described a rat experiment supporting this hypothesis. Since then, however, no reports of a similar nature have been published.

Recently, the endocrinologic actions of ergot derivatives have received attention due to the therapeutic use of 2-bromo-α-ergokryptine (bromocriptine) in treating disorders and conditions associated with high serum levels of prolactin (BESSER et al., 1972). SHANE and NAFTOLIN (1974) showed that ergometrine lowers prolactin levels in postpartum patients 3 days after delivery; they reported a modest but significant fall with 0.2 mg per os. This raised the question as to whether an ergot alkaloid used as an oxytocic could interfere with lactation. DEL POZO et al. (1975) have shown that methylergometrine, a commonly used oxytocic, has no lactation-suppressing effect of clinical relevance in mothers wishing to breastfeed. Certainly the possible endocrinologic side effects of most ergot derivatives are overshadowed by their more obvious actions on the cardiovascular and central nervous systems.

f) Effects on Fibrous Tissue

The first indication that an ergot alkaloid derivative could be responsible for an inflammatory fibrosing process was when GRAHAM (1964) described two cases of retroperitoneal fibrosis occurring during methysergide treatment. Further cases were discovered, and in 1967 GRAHAM et al. published a review of 27 patients where a causal relationship had been established. Retroperitoneal fibrosis is a rare condition in which the ureters and other retroperitoneal structures become encased in a mass of dense fibrous tissue. Symptoms are usually related to mechanical ureteric obstruction, although nonspecific signs are encountered (e.g., raised sedimentation rate, anemia). The retroperitoneal mass can be removed relatively easily at operation, but in cases associated with methysergide therapy this is not usually necessary. Withdrawal of the drug is followed by partial or complete regression of the symptoms, signs, and X-ray changes (GRAHAM et al., 1966). SCHWARTZ and DUNEA (1966), however, reported two cases in which spontaneous regression did not follow methysergide withdrawal. No dose- or time-dependence is evident for this uncommon effect. However, since regression usually follows drug withdrawal, it was recommended in 1967 that prolonged methysergide treatment should be interrupted occasionally by 1-month drug-free intervals. Since then, reports of retroperitoneal fibrosis have been less frequent (information from Sandoz—Adverse Drug Reaction Department).

The fibrotic process is not always confined to the retroperitoneal tissues. In 1967, GRAHAM drew attention to the occurrence of cardiac murmurs in patients taking methysergide and suggested that valvular changes might be responsible. MISCH (1974) described the postmortem appearance of the mitral valve in such a patient; there was mild stenosis with uniform fibrous thickening of the valve cusps and chordae tendinae; the tricuspid valve was also involved. BANA et al. (1974) have reviewed this complication of methysergide therapy. GRAHAM et al. (1967) described pleural pulmonary fibrosis in several patients taking methysergide, and pleural effusion associated with such fibrosis has been reported in some instances (HINDLE et al., 1970; DUNN and SLOAN, 1973). Fibrosis of the adventitia of the mesenteric vessels, leading to luminal narrowing with subsequent infarction, was reported in a patient given methysergide who had no other signs of fibrosis (REGAN and POLETTI, 1968). This case is to be differentiated from those rare cases of mesenteric artery spasm due to the vasoconstrictor action of ergot derivatives in sensitive individuals (BUENGER and HUNTER, 1966).

Although a causal relationship between methysergide ingestion and the occurrence of retroperitoneal fibrosis in some sensitive individuals has been established, the mechanism of this effect is still uncertain (HODEL and GRIFFITH, 1973). Of the different hypotheses put forward, that of an autoimmune mechanism remains the most likely. Other compounds have been implicated as possible etiologic factors in this condition. GRAHAM et al. (1967) described two patients who developed retroperitoneal fibrosis while taking in one case dihydroergotamine and in the other ergotamine tartrate. SEILER et al. (1973) implicated ergotamine as a possible cause of mitral insufficiency in a patient who had symptoms of chronic ergotism, and TOURNIGAND et al. (1974) described a case of retroperitoneal fibrosis after prolonged use of ergotamine. Dihydroergotamine taken orally for 8 years for ophthalmic migraine was considered to be the etiologic factor in a patient reported by VERIN et al. (1974), but details of concomitant medication (analgesics) were not given. STECKER et al. (1974) described a patient with retroperitoneal fibrosis who gave no history of medication other than intermittent use of LSD over a 6-month period; a causal relationship here seems somewhat questionable. LEWIS et al. (1975) drew attention to two patients with retroperitoneal fibrosis who had taken a combination preparation containing phenacetin, aspirin, and codeine for many years. In a retrospective search, the authors found seven patients with retroperitoneal fibrosis labeled "idiopathic" who had, on analysis, histories of analgesic abuse. They concluded that some cases at least might be related to generalized analgesic abuse. This may explain the very rare instances reported after ergotamine or dihydroergotamine, where analgesic comedication was likely to have been employed.

g) Miscellaneous Side Effects

Respiratory depression has been reported in severe cases of acute poisoning (NICAISE, 1972; KENNA, 1972; BRERETON-STILES et al., 1972). Because of their uterotonic action, some ergot derivatives have been used for many years in obstetrics and gynecology. The risk of uterine rupture is well known (WINKLER, 1965).

Hematologic effects of ergot derivatives are uncommon. Hemolytic anemia, with a positive direct Coombs test, was reported in a patient receiving methysergide who also had retroperitoneal fibrosis and mitral regurgitation (SLUGG and KUNKEL, 1970). Drug-induced lupus erythematosus, histologically confirmed, has been described in relation to methysergide administration by RACOUCHOT et al. (1968).

Pigmentation of the skin is a side effect of methysergide which is occasionally seen (GRAHAM, 1964). LEYTON (1964) reported hair loss in 1% of his 850 patients on methysergide therapy. SADJADPOUR (1974) described reversible alopecia in connection with methysergide medication in a 30-year-old woman.

Allergic conditions have been reported only rarely following ergot medication. NAVA (1972) described a case of Quincke's edema with urticaria after LSD consumption; the causal relationship was confirmed by patch testing.

A tumor-promoting effect of ergot derivatives in man has not been described. STEVENS and CALLAWAY (1940) reported the development of a mixed-type epithelial tumor in a patient who had, for more than 20 years, self-administered a skin paint containing phenol and an unspecified ergot derivative. It seems likely that this represents the well-recognized response to chronic irritation rather than a carcinogenic effect of phenol or ergot per se.

C. Effects on Reproductive Processes

Poisoning with ergot alkaloids has long been known to be a possible cause of reproductive failure in herbivorous mammals and man; thus, ergots can induce abortion, stillbirth, agalactia, malnutrition, or clinical disorders in the progeny (see reviews by Bové, 1970; Floss et al., 1973; Moir, 1974). Few pertinent experimental investigations in laboratory animals were done, however, before 1945. The effects of ergot alkaloids on the reproduction process are considered here under three headings:

1. Effects on implantation and early pregnancy.
2. Effects on embryonic and fetal development.
3. Effects on lactation and the offspring.

Potential mutagenic effects are discussed in the next section of this chapter.

1. Implantation and Early Pregnancy

Pioneer experimental work was done by Shelesnyak, working with a number of collaborators, who studied the site and mechanism of action of ergotoxine, the natural ergot alkaloid having three components: ergocornine, ergokryptine, and ergocristine. A single subcutaneous injection of ergotoxine ethanesulfonate given to rats in early gestation (up to day 7 post coitum) terminated pregnancy within 1–3 days; threshold doses ranged between 0.1 and 1.0 mg/rat. Rats given ergotoxine after implantation was established (day 8 p.c.) delivered normal litters (Shelesnyak, 1955, 1956). A mixture of the three components (1:1:1) as their mesylates was as active as the natural alkaloid (Shelesnyak, 1957a). Of the three components, ergocristine was only weakly active, the other two being equally potent (Bovet-Nitti and Bovet, 1959; Shelesnyak, 1957a, 1961; Kraicer and Shelesnyak, 1964, 1965). Termination of pregnancy was associated with suppressed deciduoma formation (Shelesnyak, 1954a, 1954b, 1955) and with the occurrence of proestrus and estrus within 48–98 h after drug administration (Shelesnyak, 1955, 1961; Kraicer and Shelesnyak, 1964, 1968; Lobel et al., 1966). The action of these alkaloids of the ergotoxine group could be blocked or reversed by administration of progesterone (Shelesnyak, 1954a, 1956); this suggested that the effect was not a direct toxic action or an end-organ competitive reaction between the alkaloids and the hormone but rather an interference with the endocrine balance necessary for normal implantation. Further investigations showed that: (1) ergotoxine had no inherent estrogenic or gonadotrophic activity (Shelesnyak, 1957a); (2) ergotoxine in doses effective in terminating pregnancy did not modify the gonadotrophin content of the pituitary (Shelesnyak, 1957b); (3) the presence of the adrenals was not essential for this action of ergotoxine (Shelesnyak, 1956); (4) exogenous prolactin was effective in stimulating the ovary to produce enough additional progesterone to reverse the ergotoxine action (Shelesnyak, 1958); (5) reserpine was effective in overcoming the action of ergotoxine (Shelesnyak, 1961). This evidence suggested that after ergotoxine treatment the uterus could still respond to progesterone, the ovary to prolactin, and the pituitary to reserpine, i.e., a direct toxic action on these target organs may be excluded; Shelesnyak and BARNEA (1963) reported in confirmation that ergocornine placed directly on the uterus, ovaries, or the pituitary gland had no effect.

However, ZEILMAKER and CARLSEN (1962) reemphasized the importance of the pituitary for nidation in the rat. They showed that ergocornine inhibited the secretion of prolactin necessary for corpora lutea function and, hence, the maintenance of pregnancy; after implantation (about day 8 of gestation), the placenta becomes the major source of luteotrophic hormone (MEITES and SHELESNYAK, 1957; MATTHIES, 1967; KISCH and SHELESNYAK, 1968). Later, additional evidence (TUROLLA et al., 1969; CARPENT and DESCLIN, 1969) supported the current view that certain ergot alkaloids inhibit the release of prolactin from the pituitary but not from the placenta, and that the resulting inhibition of nidation is mediated through this interference with pituitary secretion. (The site of ergot activity on pituitary secretion is discussed in Chapter IX.)

The phenomenon of nidation inhibition in rats has been confirmed in other rodent species and with other ergot compounds. MANTLE (1969) found that agroclavine given in the diet during the preimplantation period prevented establishment of pregnancy in mice, although not when given subcutaneously. Agroclavine was also found to be active orally in rats (FINN and MANTLE, 1969; EDWARDSON and MACGREGOR, 1969) but not intraperitoneally (EDWARDSON, 1968). This raises the question as to whether metabolic activation is necessary for agroclavine to exert its effect. MANTLE (1969) found that ergotoxine, ergosine, and lysergic acid-α-hydroxyethylamide could also interrupt pregnancy in mice when given mixed in the diet. CARLSEN et al. (1961) showed that in mice the implantation-inhibiting effect of ergocornine was confined to the prenidation period; with treatment from day 5 onwards the animals delivered normal litters. FORD and YOSHINAGA (1975) observed that ergokryptine terminated pregnancy in hamsters only when given up to or on day 5. The relative potency of the representatives of the ergopeptine series for inhibiting nidation and prolactin secretion are given in Table 5. It can be seen that ergokryptine was the most potent, whereas ergotamine and ergometrine were not nearly as effective. The 9,10 dihydrogenated derivatives generally showed less activity, with a similar ranking to their parent compounds (SHELESNYAK, 1957a; FLÜCKIGER et al., 1976a). Substitution of a bromine atom in position 2 of ergokryptine resulted in a compound with an increased potency for inhibition of implantation but with less general toxic effects – bromocriptine (FLÜCKIGER and WAGNER, 1968). The implantation-inhibitory activities of the nonpeptide series are also discussed in Chapter IX.

In addition to inhibition of implantation, the possibility of a direct embryotoxic effect must also be considered. When ergot alkaloids were given during the post-implantation period, normal litters resulted (EDWARDSON, 1968; EDWARDSON and MACGREGOR, 1969; MANTLE, 1969). However, if treatment in the preimplantation period did not inhibit nidation completely, or when this action was suppressed by administration of progesterone or prolactin, a dose-dependent increase of resorptions was reported (SHELESNYAK, 1956 and 1958; EDWARDSON and MACGREGOR, 1969). Ergocornine in doses which are effective in inhibiting implantation was found to have no direct toxic effect on the blastocysts in rats (VARAVUDHI and LOBEL, 1965). However, another study with ergocornine yielded pronounced effects on rat fetus morphology (CARPENT and DESCLIN, 1969). Doses up to 1 mg given

Table 5. Comparison of serum prolactin-reducing and implantation-inhibiting activities in rats

	Percentage reduction of serum prolactin[a]	Relative potency for implantation inhibition (ergokryptine = 100)[b]	ED_{50} for implantation inhibition[c] (mg/kg daily)
Ergometrine	59%	< 5.5	209
Ergotamine	45%	5.5	133
Ergocornine	84%	50.7	1.4
Ergokryptine	73%	100.0	—
Ergonine	—	23.9	5.0
DH-Ergotamine	—	< 5.5	> 30
DH-Ergocornine	70%	27.5	14.2
DH-Ergokryptine	78%	22.9	> 30
DH-Ergonine	—	< 5.5	59

[a] Data from MEITES and CLEMENS (1972) and FLÜCKIGER et al. (1976a)—s.c. or i.p. administration.

[b] Data from FLÜCKIGER et al. (1976a)—single s.c. administration.

[c] Unpublished data from Sandoz laboratories—maternal dose levels in mg/kg/day p.o. on days 6–15 p.c. needed to produce a 50% reduction in pregnancy rate in a standardized teratology experiment (GRAUWILER and SCHÖN, 1973).

on day 4 p.c. did not in all cases inhibit implantation but had a very deleterious effect on the maintenance of pregnancy. This treatment did not increase the incidence of embryopathies. However, 1 mg ergocornine given on day 7, while no longer effective in terminating pregnancy, resulted in a high incidence or resorptions and visceral malformations. Treatment at a later stage of gestation had no detrimental effect on pregnancy. Both embryonic mortality and fetal malformations were diminished by supplemental progesterone injections. The authors concluded, therefore, that the embryotoxic and, in this case, teratogenic effect was not caused directly by ergocornine but indirectly by induced progesterone deficiency.

It is important to consider whether the effects observed in mice and rats have relevance for other animals, including man. This is dependent on whether prolactin plays a similarly essential role in the process of early gestation in species other than rats and mice. Feeding ergot-contaminated rye and barley to guinea-pigs (NORDSKOG and CLARK, 1945) and pigs (BAILEY et al., 1973) did not inhibit implantation. Ergocornine and its more potent analogue bromocriptine, although lowering prolactin levels, did not disturb luteal function in ferrets, sheep, and cows (BLATCHLEY and DONOVAN, 1974; NISWEDER, 1974; HOFFMANN et al., 1974). FLOSS et al. (1973) postulated that only in rats and mice does prolactin have an important role to play in maintaining corpora lutea during early pregnancy, so that the implantation-inhibiting effects of ergot alkaloids are strictly species-specific. The irrelevance of these particular animal results for man is emphasized by the clinical use of bromocriptine in treating hyperprolactinemic conditions in women, in whom pregnancy and normal delivery frequently results (THORNER et al., 1975; BESSER and THORNER, 1976). These endocrinologic aspects are discussed further in Chapter IX.

2. Embryonic and Fetal Development

Early experimental investigations into possible embryotoxic actions of ergot alkaloids provided conflicting results. Both ORTH et al. (1947), who gave pregnant rats ergotamine tartrate 2.5 mg/kg i.v. twice weekly, and GIROUD and TUCHMANN-DUPLESSIS (1962), who gave ergotamine in unspecified dosages, reported no adverse effects on rat fetuses, although the dams occasionally had evidence of ergotism. On the other hand, SOMMER and BUCHANAN (1955) and TINDAL (1956), using i.p. and s.c. administration, respectively, showed that ergotamine tartrate caused increased fetal death and postnatal mortality. Opacities of the lens in newborn rabbits were seen by VASSILEV et al. (1959) after ergotamine tartrate i.v. on day 10 of pregnancy. This finding could not be confirmed in rats, however (PITEL and LERMAN, 1964). Abortions and fetal deaths in sheep and cows (associated with signs of ergotism in the dams) have been reported following ergotamine administration in midpregnancy (MANTLE and GUNNER, 1965; GREATOREX and MANTLE, 1974).

A systematic study of the effects of ergotamine in pregnant mice, rats, and rabbits was done by GRAUWILER and SCHÖN (1973). They found that oral doses given during the organogenetic phase—days 6–15 post coitum (p.c.) in mice and rats, days 6–18 p.c. in rabbits—which affected maternal weight gain, caused an increase in prenatal mortality in rats and evidence of fetal retardation with delayed skeletal ossification in the surviving offspring in all three species. No specific teratogenic activity was seen. They concluded that the effects on the offspring were largely due to an indirect disturbance of fetal development, secondary to impairment of normal gestation produced by doses subtoxic to the dams. This was postulated to be via a pharmacodynamic action on the cardiovascular system. In investigating this effect further, SCHÖN et al. (1975) gave pregnant rats 10 mg/kg ergotamine tartrate p.o. on single days between days 4 and 19 of gestation. A clear phase-specificity of embryotoxicity was seen; from days 4 to 10 no adverse effects were observed, but from day 11 onwards prenatal mortality increased, reaching a maximum on day 14 of gestation. In addition, during this critical phase (days 13–16) characteristic anomalies occurred—cleft palates and bilateral limb defects (shortening or absence of nails, phalanges, and digits). The phase-specific fetal mortality and the type of anomalies closely resembled those seen following temporary clamping of the main uterine vessels in the rat (LEIST and GRAUWILER, 1973a, b, 1974a; SCHÖN et al., 1975). In contrast to single-day ergotamine treatment, uterine vessel clamping caused additional anomalies of the heart and the axial skeleton before day 12 of gestation (LEIST and GRAUWILER, 1973b; SCHÖN et al., 1975). Interruption of uterine blood flow as well as placental hypoxia with subsequent impairment of embryonic nutrition can lead to embryonic death if a certain threshold is exceeded (FRANKLIN and BRENT, 1964; SENGER et al., 1967); this depends less on the degree of impaired blood flow than on its duration (LEIST and GRAUWILER, 1973a, b). It is probably irrelevant whether this effect is achieved mechanically or pharmacologically. Hypoxia has been shown to be a teratogenic factor in several mammalian species (INGALLS et al., 1950; WERTHEMANN and REINIGER, 1950; DEGENHARDT, 1954; TEDESCHI and INGALLS, 1956; MURAKAMI and KAMEYAMA, 1963; NOGUCHI et al., 1967). Furthermore, it may be assumed that the increasing susceptibility of rat fetuses to ergotamine from day 10 onwards is related to the change from dependence on the yolk sac placenta to the chorioallantoic placenta at this time (WITSCHI, 1956; KREYBIG, 1968).

The hypothesis that embryotoxicity in rats given ergotamine is caused by α-adrenoceptor stimulation producing hypoxia is strengthened by studies showing that the ergotamine effect can be totally antagonized by α-adrenoceptor blockade (phenoxybenzamine 10 mg/kg s.c.) (GRAUWILER and LEIST, 1973; LEIST and GRAUWILER, 1973c; SCHÖN et al., 1975).

LEIST and GRAUWILER (1973c) found that the intra-amniotic dose of ergotamine needed to produce a similar embryolethal effect at day 14 of gestation was 50 times higher than the amount of radioactive-labeled substance reaching the fetus via the placenta following administration to the dam of an embryolethal dose (2.5 mg/kg i.v.). Using intra-amniotic injection, 50% fetal mortality was obtained with a dose of 0.55 μg per implantation site. This result confirmed the findings of PITEL and LERMAN (1964) that intrauterine injection of ergotamine on days 17–19 p.c. at a comparable dosage resulted in a high percentage of fetal deaths (67%). Therefore, a direct toxic action of ergotamine on the fetus could hardly be responsible for the embryotoxic effects obtained. The low transplacental passage of ergotamine (~2.8%) can be explained partly by its pharmacodynamic action; GRAUWILER and LEIST (1973) showed that ergotamine (2.5 mg/kg i.v.) reduced the transplacental passage of ^{3}H-1-leucine, as a marker for uteroplacental blood supply, for at least 3 h, and that this effect could be antagonized by phenoxybenzamine.

Theoretically, impaired uteroplacental blood supply could also be due in part to the uterotonic potential of ergotamine (ROTHLIN, 1946). However, LEIST and GRAUWILER (1974b) showed that ergometrine (10 mg/kg i.v. on day 14 of gestation) produced no inhibition of uteroplacental blood circulation and had no adverse effect on the fetuses; this derivative has a uterotonic activity comparable to ergotamine's but only very slight vasoconstrictor potential.

Obviously, different ergot alkaloids have varying potentials for causing embryotoxicity. SOMMER and BUCHANAN (1955) found that whereas ergotoxine given i.p. to rats during the second half of pregnancy caused fetal mortality, similar doses of dihydroergotoxine mesylate and methylergometrine failed to have any adverse effects on fetal development. ORTH and RITCHIE (1947) and ORTH et al. (1947) found no adverse effects with dihydroergotamine or dihydroergocornine in pregnant rats. Considerable experience has been gained at the Sandoz laboratories, using a standardized rat teratology experiment design, as described for ergotamine by GRAUWILER and SCHÖN (1973). Table 6 gives the maternal dose level (in mg/kg p.o. daily from day 6–15 p.c.) needed to produce 50% embryonic mortality for various ergot alkaloids. In general, the 9,10 dihydro-derivatives had diminished potential for interfering with embryonic and fetal development. This relationship, as well as the order ascribed to the peptide derivatives, correlates with the compounds' potential for vasoconstriction, which supports the concept of the mechanism of action outlined above.

What relevance do the animal results have for man? The abortifacient action of uterotonic ergots has been known for many years and has led to their misuse, often with disastrous consequences to the mother, due to precipitation of acute

Table 6. Doses of ergot derivatives required in pregnant rats to cause 50% embryonic deaths (mg/kg daily p.o. from day 6–15 p.c.)—partially unpublished data from Sandoz laboratories using a standardized teratology experiment (GRAUWILER and SCHÖN, 1973)

	Unsaturated form	9, 10 dihydrogenated
Ergometrine	86.9	—
Ergotamine	27.3	617
Ergostine	11.8	1095
Ergovaline	9.7	21.4
Ergonine	4.5	104
Ergotoxine	—	100[a]
Ergoalanine	5.1	—
1-Methylergotamine	6889	—
5-Methylergoalanine	10.9	—
2-Bromo-α-ergokryptine	300[b]	—

[a] Dihydroergotoxine mesylate.

[b] Administration on days 8–15 p.c.

vascular ergotism. There have been no substantiated reports, however, of a teratogenic action of ergot derivatives except in the case of LSD, which is discussed below. DAVID (1972, 1973) reported a collection of 24 patients with the Poland anomaly (congenital unilateral hypoplasia or absence of the sternocostal part of the pectoralis major muscle with ipsilateral cutaneous syndactyly and shortening of the fingers to a variable degree). Attempted (but failed) abortion by ingestion of ergotamine, ergometrine, or crude ergot infusion had been undertaken by the mothers of four of these patients. DAVID postulated a connection between ergot alkaloid ingestion in the first trimester and the occurrence of the Poland anomaly in the child, but the evidence is extremely weak. Attempted abortion by different means may play a part in the etiology of certain congenital defects (GARDNER et al., 1971; KUČERA, 1972). However, SUGIURA (1976), in describing 45 cases of Poland's syndrome in Japan, was unable to find a history of attempted abortion or threatened miscarriage in the mothers of his patients. The Poland anomaly is considered to be genetic rather than environmentally-induced (DEGENHARDT and KLEINEBRECHT, 1972). It seems highly improbable that in fact ergot alkaloids are responsible. Their widespread therapeutic use could hardly be associated with the occurrence of such a rare but specific anomaly without this being noted prior to 1972. WAINSCOTT et al. (1978) reported on the occurrence of congenital abnormalities in babies born to mothers attending a migraine clinic, where it may be assumed that at least 50% would have taken ergot compounds at some stage during the first trimester. The frequency and type of abnormalities were strictly comparable with those in a normal population.

Controversy still exists as to whether LSD is teratogenic in animals or man. The first suggestion that maternal intake of LSD during pregnancy could cause an abnormality in the child was raised by ZELLWEGER et al. (1967). This led to extensive animal experiments in various species. In *rats*, ALEXANDER et al. (1967) showed that 5 μg/kg of LSD given subcutaneously in early pregnancy (up to day 7) caused resorptions, retardations, and even embryonic and fetal death. No effects occurred however when the drug was given late in pregnancy (after day 7), and no specific deformities were encountered. Indeed teratogenicity during a particular organogenetic phase was not demonstrated. These investigators confirmed their results with a larger collective but using a similar experimental design (ALEXANDER et al., 1970). In contrast to these results, numerous other workers have failed to show any adverse effects of large doses of LSD in pregnant rats, using both the same experimental design as ALEXANDER and his colleagues and also other routes and periods of administration (WARKANY and TAKACS, 1968; GAGNON, 1969; NOSAL, 1969; ROUX et al., 1970; UYENO, 1970; SATO et al., 1969; NAIR et al., 1970; BEALL, 1972). WEST (1962), investigating three lysergic acid derivatives – LSD, 2-bromo-LSD, and methysergide – could not detect any toxic effects on the rat fetus. On the other hand, SAM and JOSEPH (1973) were able to show that while an oral dose of 200 µg/kg LSD in early pregnancy had no adverse effects, subcutaneous administration produced decreased litter size, fetal retardation, and increased perinatal mortality. These workers also failed to find any specific deformities. Increased prenatal mortality and retardation of the offspring were noted by NAIR (1974) after high s.c. doses (100 µg/kg) on days 1–3, 9–12, or 13–15. A conspicuous finding was lowered brain 5-HT levels in the offspring, which persisted until maturity and was associated with hyperactivity in behavior tests. No gross organ anomalies were seen.

Various types of malformation have been described in *mice*, apparently depending on the strain used. AUERBACH and RUGOWSKI (1967) reported that large doses of LSD – 0.2 to 35 µg/kg – given intraperitoneally on days 6–7 resulted in a high rate of malformations of the central nervous system with modifications of the facial contours. No effects occurred with exposure later than day 7. However, a retardation of development by 1 or 2 days can also result in fetuses of similar appearance to those described by AUERBACH and RUGOWSKI. DIPAOLO et al. (1968) reported facial anomalies (hare lip, cleft palate, or micrognathia) in A/Cum mice, but there was no evidence of teratogenic effects in NIH general-purpose mice. HANAWAY (1969) gave large doses to Swiss Webster mice and found apparent abnormalities of the lens but no malformations of the brain or other organs. ARASZKIEWICZ and BARTEL (1972), using a mixed strain, observed a high rate of malformed fetuses exhibiting circulatory disorders, hernias, and deformities of the CNS. On the other hand, ROUX et al. (1970) and BRO-RASMUSSEN et al. (1972) were unable to induce malformations, although the latter found increased resorptions and fetal deaths. In an attempt to explain the marked strain differences yielding these conflicting results, AUERBACH (1970) pointed out that the drug may act against a background of genetically influenced susceptibility; thus, LSD administration leads to an increased incidence of those spontaneous defects specific for the strains used.

In *hamsters,* GEBER (1967) reported malformations of the brain, spinal cord, liver, and other organs after giving LSD and 2-bromo-LSD in very high s.c. doses on day 8 (0.8–240 µg/kg LSD, 2–410 µg/kg 2-bromo-LSD); a dose-dependent increase in resorptions, fetal deaths, and retardations was also noted. On the other hand, DIPAOLO et al. (1968) and ROUX et al. (1970) failed to confirm these results, using even higher doses of LSD (up to 3000 and 500 µg/kg, respectively). In *rabbits,* FABRO and SIEBER (1968) found no adverse effects of LSD on the course or outcome of pregnancy in a study using thalidomide as a positive control.

The results in rodents and rabbits reveal a wide variation of individual, strain, and species susceptibility. However, positive effects, except for those of NAIR (1974), were invariably obtained when LSD was given early in gestation. These results are not unlike those found with other ergot alkaloids—ergotoxine, ergocornine, ergokryptine (see above); embryotoxicity with LSD in rodents may well be an indirect effect of progesterone deficiency due to drug-related prolactin inhibition, as with the other alkaloids. In fact, LSD has been reported to be a potent prolactin inhibitor (QUADRI and MEITES, 1971).

A preliminary study in *Rhesus monkeys,* described by KATO et al. (1970), yielded one normal and two still-born infants, one of which had a facial deformity. A fourth baby died at 1 month of age. The doses used in the study were extremely high—the lowest (0.125 mg/kg subcutaneously) exceeded by 100 times the average human dose. WILSON (1972) treated eight pregnant Rhesus monkeys orally three times per week for 4 weeks between days 20 and 45 of gestation, and six further females on single days with doses of 200 μg (~20 times the human "trip" dose on a mg/kg basis). One female aborted; one had a retarded fetus; and 12 produced normal 100-day fetuses at hysterotomy. Chromosomal abnormalities were not significantly increased in mother or fetus (WILSON, 1973).

Other animal models have been used: the *Xenopus laevis* embryo (BAKER, 1971) and chick embryo (HART and GREENE, 1971; MESSIER, 1973; HART, 1975; LEE et al., 1975). LSD has a possible retarding effect on cellular movement during the segmentation of paraxial mesoderm, resulting in fewer somite pairs in explanted chick embryos and biochemical changes involving 5-HT metabolism in the *Xenopus* model.

In *humans,* it is even more difficult to get a precise answer to the question of whether LSD is a teratogenic agent. Therapeutic use of LSD is extremely limited today and would never be considered in a pregnant woman. Retrospective (or even prospective) surveys are hampered by the vagueness and uncooperative attitude of the patients, as well as uncertainty as to drug abuse by the father or mother prior to conception (i.e., the risk of a potential mutagenic effect cannot be readily differentiated). In addition, drug abusers frequently take more than one drug and often suffer from severe ill-health (malnutrition, hepatitis, multiple infections), so that nonspecific factors may contribute to the results evaluated. Small prospective surveys made by AASE et al. (1970), ROBINSON et al. (1974), and a retrospective study by DUMARS (1971) indicate that parental use of illicit LSD does not in itself constitute a valid reason for a higher incidence of chromosomal or congenital abnormalities in the progeny. More extensive retrospective surveys by MCGLOTHLIN et al. (1970) and JACOBSON and BERLIN (1972) did not permit the establishment of clear causal relationships, although the incidences of abortion and malformations were increased with illicit LSD exposure in both surveys. DISHOTSKY et al. (1971), in a comprehensive review, concluded that cases of congenital malformations occurred almost exclusively among illicit drug users and could be related to drug abuse generally; there was no reported instance of a woman delivered of a malformed child after taking pure LSD during pregnancy, and they inferred that LSD is not a teratogen in humans. LONG (1972) reviewed 161 cases reported in the literature. After excluding known genetic and familial defects, only seven children (4.3%) remained where a causal relationship between maternal ingestion of LSD and an abnormal child existed. More recently, NISHIMURA and TANIMURA (1976), after differentiating between mutagenicity and teratogenicity in the cases reported in the literature, recalculated the prevalence of congenital malformations as 16.7% (seven of 42 established pregnancies "at risk"). SMITHELLS (1976) explained that a difficulty in interpreting these figures stems from what he called the "me-too" phenomenon. For example, after a publication in which an association between LSD and congenital "amputations" was reported (ZELLWEGER et al., 1967), the presentation of infants with such lesions automatically prompted a search for a history of LSD abuse. SMITHELLS postulated that the risk of terminal defects in the offspring of mothers taking LSD is, therefore, likely to be much lower than the 12% suggested by published cases (LONG, 1972).

To summarize, available clinical and experimental data at present are not sufficient to establish chemically-pure LSD as a teratogen in man. Expert opinions (LONG, 1972; WILSON, 1973) have estimated the hazard, if any, to be extremely small.

3. Lactation and the Offspring

Feeding cereal infected with ergot causes hypogalactia in sheep (GREATOREX and MANTLE, 1974), cows, pigs, and rats but not in guinea-pigs (NORDSKOG and CLARK, 1945). Further experimental evidence for such an effect in rats has been reported by NORDSKOG (1946) for ergotoxine, SOMMER and BUCHANAN (1955) for ergotamine and ergotoxine, and by EDWARDSON (1968) for agroclavine; MANTLE (1968) also showed this effect of agroclavine in mice. In positive cases, there is impaired mammary gland development, with diminished total milk yield and reduced fat content (SOMMER and BUCHANAN, 1955). Dihydroergotoxine and methylergometrine do not produce such an effect (SOMMER and BUCHANAN, 1955), nor does dihydroergotamine (ORTH and RITCHIE, 1947; TINDAL, 1956) or dihydroergocornine (ORTH et al., 1947).

The reasons for failure of lactation after administration of ergots have been ascribed to impaired maternal instinct (ORTH and RITCHIE, 1947), impaired mammary development (NORDSKOG and CLARK, 1945; SHONE et al., 1959), reduced maternal food intake (TINDAL, 1956), and inhibition of the milk ejection reflex (GROSVENOR, 1956). SOMMER and BUCHANAN (1955) suggested that suckling might overcome the adverse effect of ergot alkaloids on lactation.

ZEILMAKER and CARLSEN (1962) provided the first experimental proof of inhibition of prolactin release from the pituitary by ergot alkaloids. They showed that in rats lactation inhibition could be prevented by simultaneous administration of prolactin. The effect of agroclavine in mice could also be partially inhibited by administration of prolactin, ACTH, or oxytocin (MANTLE, 1968). SHAAR and CLEMENS (1972) correlated serum prolactin levels in rats with the potency in inhibiting lactation of ergocornine, ergokryptine, ergometrine, ergotamine, and dihydroergocornine, and concluded that reduced lactation was at least partly due to the suppression of prolactin release. The correlation was not perfect in all cases, however, suggesting that some alkaloids may have additional pharmacodynamic effects, both on the mother and the pups, contributing to their overall action on lactation – e.g., vasoconstriction in the mammary gland due to α-adrenoceptor stimulation.

Comparisons of the ability of various ergot alkaloids to suppress lactation with their potential to inhibit nidation (SHELESNYAK, 1957a; ZEILMAKER and CARLSEN, 1962; KRAICER and SHELESNYAK, 1965; SHAAR and CLEMENS, 1972; CLEMENS et al., 1974) showed a good correlation in some cases: while ergotoxine, ergocornine, ergokryptine and dihydroergocornine were effective in both directions, ergometrine and dihydroergotamine were ineffective. On the other hand, ergotamine showed adverse effects on lactation but little activity in inhibiting implantation. This raises doubt as to whether both responses depend entirely on the same primary effect, or whether additional pharmacodynamic effects are involved.

FLÜCKIGER and WAGNER (1968) studied this in some depth for ergokryptine and bromocriptine in the rat and came to the conclusion that the nidation- and lactation-inhibition effects are unlikely to be governed by a single mechanism of action. It is possible, as NICHOLL et al. (1971) have suggested, that the compounds have different additional actions – e.g., an oxytocic effect. Thus, various ergot derivatives may interfere with regulatory mechanisms in different ways, depending on the end-organ in each case. For instance, a typical oxytocic agent, such as ergometrine (PAUERSTEIN, 1973), will react differently from a typical vasoconstrictor with minor oxytocic activity, such as ergotamine (CHU et al., 1976). It must be assumed that ergot derivatives can pass into the milk, so that a direct toxic effect may be produced in the pups. This possibility was examined for the rabbit with bromocriptine by FLÜCKIGER et al. (1976b). A dosage of 1 mg s.c. of bromocriptine given to suckling pups had no adverse effect on milk intake or growth rate. On the other hand, FOMINA (1934) reported the presence of ergot derivatives in human milk from mothers given liquid or dry extract of ergot; of babies nursed with milk containing active substance, 90% were reported to show some signs of ergotism, but they were not further described. It seems probable that in most species ergot derivatives can pass into the milk and exert an effect on postnatal development due to their pharmacodynamic actions.

COWIE and TINDAL (1971) suggested that the principal functions of prolactin are promotion of growth of the mammary glands and the initiation and maintenance of lactation. Administration of bromocriptine to lactating cows, while markedly lowering serum prolactin levels, had little effect on the mild yield (KARG et al., 1972). On the other hand, treatment just before parturition effectively inhibited the onset of lactation (SCHAMS et al., 1972). These results have been confirmed in goats (HART, 1973). In contrast, the rabbit (FLÜCKIGER et al., 1976b) and the dog (MAYER and SCHÜTZE, 1973) respond to bromocriptine with a dose-dependent reduction of milk yield. In mice, prolactin and adrenal cortical steroids play only minor roles in initiating lactation, whereas they are indispensable for the maintenance of lactation (NAGASAWA and YANAI, 1973). The inhibitory actions of ergot derivatives on lactation have recently been used therapeutically with success in the treatment and prevention of puerperal mastitis, as well as for the suppression of lactation in women when breast feeding is contraindicated or undesired. The compounds used have been bromocriptine and 2-chloro-6-methyl-ergoline-8β-acetonitrile, as cited by LUTTERBECK et al. (1971), DEL POZO et al. (1974), LEMBERGER et al. (1974), and CLEARY et al. (1975).

D. Potential Genetic Effects

In recent years the possibility that drugs may produce mutagenic effects has been studied on an ever-increasing scale, and LSD has been a prominent candidate for such investigations. Less attention has been paid to other ergot alkaloids.

1. LSD

Several hundred articles, including numerous surveys and individual case reports, have been published on possible genetic effects of LSD in humans; these have been reviewed by SMART and BATEMAN (1968), HOUSTON (1969), MOORHEAD et al. (1971), DISHOTSKY et al. (1971), NICHOLS (1972), LONG (1972) and SANKAR (1975). This section will consider results and viewpoints of these reviewers as well as some results from more recent work, particularly on laboratory animals. For detailed literature survey, the reader is referred to the above-mentioned reviews, and, if necessary, to the Environmental Mutagen Information Center, Oak Ridge, National Laboratory, Tennessee, USA.

a) Studies on Human Material

The most extensive information available is from examination of chromosomes from leukocyte cultures derived from persons exposed to LSD and from unexposed controls. DISHOTSKY et al. (1971) have reviewed 21 different studies involving a total of 310 subjects; 126 subjects were exposed to pure and 184 to impure (i.e., illicit) LSD. Only 14% of those exposed to pure LSD had slightly increased frequencies of chromosomal aberrations; in contrast, 49% of those taking illicit LSD had an increased frequency of chromosome aberrations. Similarly, HOUSTON (1969), MOORHEAD et al. (1971), NICHOLS (1972), LONG (1972), TITUS (1972), and SANKAR (1975), all reviewing human investigations, came to the conclusion that LSD treatment had either no effect or caused only a slight transitory increase in chromosome aberrations in leukocytes of peripheral blood of exposed subjects. More recently, well-controlled studies on leukocytes from a large number of exposed individuals have failed to show any chromosome-damaging effect of LSD (OBE and HERHA, 1973; FERNANDEZ et al., 1973, 1974; JARVIK et al., 1974; SIMMONS et al., 1974; ROBINSON et al., 1974).

Some of the reviews cited contain results from individual case reports and planned studies where fresh bone-marrow aspirates, testis biopsies, or peripheral blood lymphocytes from children whose parents took LSD before or during pregnancy were examined. Several isolated case reports deal with birth defects in infancy, where fathers and/or mothers had ingested LSD prior to conception. From these limited data, no clear, consistent evidence of a chromosome-damaging effect of LSD emerges. A number of reports deal with the question as to whether chromosomal aberrations produced by LSD are associated with leukemia or other forms of neoplasia; there is to date no evidence that a causal relationship exists between LSD, genetic damage, and cancer (DISHOTSKY et al., 1971).

When human leukocyte cultures are treated with LSD in vitro, chromosome damage is frequently observed, although clearcut dose-response relationships are not always obtained (COHEN et al., 1967a, 1967b; KATO and JARVIK, 1969; COREY et al., 1970). However, negative results with this test system have also been reported (STURELID and KIHLMAN, 1969).

b) Studies on Laboratory Mammals and Nonmammalian Systems

Several in vivo cytogenetic studies have been performed in laboratory mammals. In those involving LSD-treated Rhesus monkeys, a slight transient increase in chromosome aberrations was obtained in peripheral leukocytes, but no such effects were seen in testicular biopsy material from the same animals (EGOZCUE and IRWIN, 1969; KATO et al., 1970). In the baboon, LSD induced a questionable increase in frequency of aneuploid metaphases in peripheral blood leukocytes (RUFFIÉ et al., 1972).

In the mouse, an increased frequency of chromosomal aberrations was found in spermatocytes after LSD treatment (COHEN and MUKHERJEE, 1968; SKAKKEBAEK et al., 1968; SKAKKEBAEK and BEATTY, 1970). JAGIELLO and POLANI (1969) and EGOZCUE and IRWIN (1969), on the other hand, could not confirm these results. The most extensive cytogenetic work on mouse and rat spermatocytes has been done by GOETZ et al. (1974). They found no evidence of chromosomal damage except for a questionable increase in the yield of spermatocytes with autosomal univalents; the significance of this finding is, at present, still obscure. SRAM et al. (1974) have reported a slight, but dose-dependent increase of dominant lethal mutations in male and female mice after parenteral administration of high doses of LSD. These effects, however, pertain mainly to preimplantation loss of embryos, which may be of nongenetic origin; it is debatable, therefore, whether the effect observed was caused by dominant lethal mutations. NICHOLSON et al. (1973) and AMAROSE et al. (1973) found no chromosome damage in peripheral blood leukocytes of LSD-treated Syrian hamsters or rabbits. After treating pregnant rats with LSD, SATO et al. (1971) and EMERIT et al. (1972) studied chromosomes from embryos and maternal bone marrow; neither source revealed a significant increase of chromosome aberrations above control values. On the other hand, LSD has been shown to produce antimitotic effects and chromosome aberrations in embryos of the amphibian *Pleurodeles waltlii Michah* (CHIBON and BÉLANGER-BARBEAU, 1972; BÉLANGER et al., 1975).

In vitro studies using LSD and animal cells in culture have, as with human cells in in vitro tests, led to contradictory results. When leukocyte cultures of the marsupial *Potorus tridactylus* were treated with LSD, a dose-dependent increase of chromosome breaks was found (BICK, 1970). On the other hand, LSD did not produce chromosomal aberrations in treated fibroblast cultures of the Chinese hamster (STURELID and KIHLMAN, 1969).

Mutagenicity experiments have also been done in submammalian models. Early experiments using *Drosophila melanogaster* failed to reveal any effects of LSD on recessive lethal mutations or translocations (GRACE et al., 1968; TOBIN and TOBIN, 1969). However, significant increases in recessive lethal mutations have been reported by BROWNING (1968), MARKOWITZ et al. (1969), VANN (1969), ŠRÁM (1970), and BARNETT and MUÑOZ (1971) after exposing *Drosophila* males to LSD.

Chromosome losses and/or mosaic mutations have also been reported in *Drosophila* after LSD exposure (BROWNING, 1968).

Similar contradictory results have been obtained using plants and microorganisms. Cytogenetic effects of LSD were reported in germinated barley seeds (SINGH et al., 1970), whereas no such changes were seen in onion or *Vicia faba* root tips (STURELID and KIHLMAN, 1969; RILEY and NEUROTH, 1970). LSD has been shown to produce auxotrophic mutations in *Escherichia coli*, depending on dose (VANN et al., 1970). On the other hand, negative results were obtained with the fungus *Ophiostoma multiannuatum* (ZETTERBERG, 1969), as well as in *Salmonella typhimurium G46*, both in vitro and in an in vivo mouse host-mediated assay (LEGATOR, 1970).

c) Interactions With DNA

Several studies examining the mechanism of interaction between LSD and DNA have been reviewed by DORRANCE et al. (1974). Earlier observations on the ability of LSD to bind to or to intercalate with DNA of mammalian cells in culture could not be confirmed in more recent studies. LSD does not affect DNA synthesis (TROSKO, 1971) nor the repair-synthesis of UV-induced DNA damage in human cell material in vitro (DORRANCE et al., 1974). The question of specificity of LSD/DNA interactions at present remains unsolved.

2. Other Ergot Alkaloids

Only very few reports exist on the possible mutagenic potential of ergot derivatives other than LSD. In an in vivo cytogenetic study, nine children received therapeutic doses of methysergide and eight a combination of LSD and methysergide (SANKAR et al., 1969); examination of peripheral blood lymphocytes revealed no increase in the frequency of chromosome aberrations in either group. Dihydroergotoxine mesylate has been studied in vivo in laboratory mammals, using the bone marrow micronucleus test in mice and Chinese hamsters, and metaphase analysis of bone marrow cells from Chinese hamsters; it did not produce any cytogenetic damage in these studies (MATTER and GRAUWILER, 1975). In addition, ergotamine and methysergide failed to show any cytogenetic effect in these test systems (MATTER, 1976). Negative results with dihydroergotoxine mesylate have also been obtained in a study involving peripheral blood lymphocyte examination in normal human volunteers taking the compound in therapeutic doses over a period of 3 months (TSUCHIMOTO and STALDER, 1976). Ergometrine has been tested in vitro in cultured human lymphocytes, in comparison with LSD; both compounds were similarly effective in inducing chromosome aberrations (KATO and JARVIK, 1969).

3. Conclusions

Whereas the data for LSD effects in microorganisms, plants, or mammalian cells in vitro are both limited and contradictory and, therefore, inconclusive, there seems to be no doubt that LSD at high dose levels produces mutations in *Drosophila*. On the other hand, the majority of in vivo studies in laboratory mammals and man indicate that chemically pure LSD at moderate doses does not produce genetic damage at the chromosome level.

There are reasons to believe that the sporadically observed chromosomal damage in various organisms and test systems, both in vivo and in vitro, is the result of a nonspecific, indirect action of LSD. For instance, very high doses are needed (in terms of human exposure, dose levels far exceeding those used therapeutically even with prolonged treatment), little evidence of dose-dependence is apparent, and there is no clear association between the action of LSD at the molecular level (e.g., DNA) and sporadically observed effects on the genetic material. Studies on human chromosomes prior to 1970 were not always carried out in an optimal fashion, mainly due to insufficient material or lack of standardization of experimental design and technical methodology (e.g., scoring of chromosome aberrations); they are, therefore, unlikely to contribute much to our knowledge. More recently, techniques have improved, and well-designed and well-controlled human studies done since 1970 have failed to show any chromosome-damaging effects of LSD (OBE and HERHA, 1973; FERNANDEZ et al., 1973, 1974; JARVIK et al., 1974; SIMMONS et al., 1974; ROBINSON et al., 1974). Furthermore, the clearcut difference between results with pure and illicit LSD (DISHOTSKY et al., 1971) have shown that chromosome aberrations, if present, were mainly found under conditions of drug abuse. The high incidence of hepatitis and other viral infections as well as the concomitant use of numerous other hallucinogens or powerful drugs, in addition to the general ill-health and malnutrition associated with drug abuse, could contribute to chromosome damage (NICHOLS, 1972; SADASIVAN and RAGHURAM, 1973).

On the basis of available evidence from well-designed and well-controlled studies, it is concluded that pure LSD does not produce chromosomal defects in humans under therapeutic conditions.

The total body of positive and negative data, conflicting results, and unresolved work should encourage a cautious view concerning the condemnation or support of LSD usage on the basis of genetic considerations alone. Some workers assume that LSD, especially under conditions of drug abuse, could constitute a potential genetic risk for man; EBERLE (1973) even claims that this risk may be of the same order of magnitude as that of permissible levels of ionizing radiation, in terms of occupational exposure. ŠRÁM and GOETZ (1974) believe that LSD usage should be limited to therapeutic indications in carefully controlled medical practice and not permitted during pregnancy. Nevertheless, the potential genetic risk seems to be low and, therefore, far less important than the problems associated with drug abuse (i.e., psychologic and physical disorders) and the possibility of embryotoxicity (see Section C).

Formal studies with other ergot derivatives are scanty; however, results available so far from in vivo studies on mammalian systems are negative.

E. Interactions Leading to Enhanced Toxicity

In this section, we shall consider types of conditions in which ergot toxicity in man may be enhanced:

1. Disease processes affecting the response to ergot derivatives.
2. Concomitant medication affecting the response to ergot derivatives.

Possible drug interactions in laboratory animals, such as the effects of hormone pretreatment on ergotamine-induced rat tail necrosis (McGRATH, 1935), are discussed in Section B.

1. Disease Processes

It has long been known that certain conditions may aggravate toxic effects of ergot drugs: febrile states, sepsis, malnutrition, thyrotoxicosis, pregnancy, hepatic disease, renal disease, hypertension, coronary artery disease, and peripheral vascular disease (VON STORCH, 1938; FUCHS and BLUMENTHAL, 1950; FELIX and CARROLL, 1970). In 1929, SAENGER reported the significance of bacterial toxin-induced changes as a cofactor in the occurrence of puerperal gangrene following ergotamine administration. Later, ergotamine came into use for the treatment of pruritus associated with jaundice, and peripheral gangrene was seen more frequently than might have been expected (YATER and CAHILL, 1936; GOULD et al., 1936). The rationale for the use of this drug in pruritus was that the mild decrease in skin temperature produced symptomatic relief (COMFORT and ERICKSON, 1939). The increased susceptibility to side effects in patients with liver disease might be related to impaired drug metabolism, which would lead to higher circulating blood levels for longer periods. ABRAMSON and LICHTMAN (1937) were unable to show any differences in blood flow response after ergotamine between normal subjects and patients with liver disease. This suggests that ergotamine metabolism is not changed markedly in such patients. However, the effects of repeated administration were not studied. More recently, KATZ and MASSRY (1966) described how viral hepatitis facilitated the appearance of prolonged arterial spasm after ergotamine tartrate was given orally at a normally safe dosage. WHELTON et al. (1968) described a patient who took ergot derivatives for many years, but on developing acute hepatic failure exhibited severe peripheral gangrene.

2. Concomitant Medication

The possibility that two ergot derivatives can have a synergistic effect on vasoconstriction was raised by JOHNSON (1966), who described a case of peripheral arterial constriction in a patient with migraine who was taking methysergide and ergotamine together. RICHTER and BANKER (1973) reported internal carotid artery spasm under similar circumstances. On the other hand, it is known that LSD can antagonize the uterotonic action of ergotamine (RICHARD and RAPPOLT, 1970).

In 1969, HAYTON drew attention to the emergence of ergotism in a patient who had been treated with ergotamine for several years, and then received triacetyloleandomycin. This antibiotic is known to have a potential for hepatotoxicity, so it is possible that the effect observed was related to impaired metabolism of ergotamine secondary to hepatic insufficiency. BIGORIE et al. (1975) have described another instance of this potentially dangerous interaction. BAUMRUCKER (1973) reported the occurrence of ergotism in a man who was given propranolol added to continuous use of ergotamine-containing suppositories for the prevention of headache. In another example, a man taking ergotamine for migraine and subsequently given propranolol for angina pectoris found that his migraine was exacerbated and became refractory to ergot preparations (BLANK and RIEDER, 1973). Currently, there is no satisfactory explanation for the discrepancy between these two case-reports – the ergot response was apparently increased by propranolol in one case and diminished in the other.

In comparison with the majority of widely used medicines, interaction reports for ergot alkaloids are relatively infrequent.

F. Summary

The data reviewed in this chapter show that the ergot derivatives possess fairly specific toxic effects. These are, in the main, related to their pharmacodynamic actions. For instance, the occurrence of gangrene in various species correlates closely with the vasoconstrictor potential of the compounds. Embryotoxicity when the drug is given to rats during midpregnancy correlates also with vasoconstrictor activity. On the other hand, impairment of implantation following administration in early pregnancy in rats is related to the endocrinologic profile of the compounds. However, administration of high toxic doses will lead to a more uniform picture, where gangrene, embryotoxicity, and implantation inhibition may be produced by the same compound, provided high enough doses can be given.

The spectrum of toxicity of ergot compounds, both in animals and in man, has changed in recent times. Whereas convulsive ergotism was an important type earlier, it is nowadays encountered infrequently; this is possibly related to increased purity of the preparations administered (both therapeutically and in the laboratory). Another reason for this is that acute poisoning in man (either iatrogenic or accidental) is at present relatively rare, compared with prolonged overdosage due to therapeutic error. Convulsions are still encountered in acute toxicity experiments in animals with very high doses.

Most side effects of ergot derivatives are predictable from animal experiments, although different species vary in their responses. An important exception is the fibrosing process induced in sensitive patients by methysergide, for which as yet there is no adequate explanation of the mechanism and no suitable animal model.

Certain effects found in animals have not been reported in man – chiefly those involving the reproductive processes. There is no evidence that ergot derivatives have an undesirable effect in human pregnancy if taken therapeutically in doses unlikely to stimulate uterine contractions.

Only scanty information is available concerning potential mutagenic effects of ergot alkaloids, except for LSD. Most investigations demonstrate that this compound has no adverse effects on the chromosome complement of man and laboratory animals. Some unequivocal effects of LSD on the genetic material have been observed in vitro and in nonmammalian systems; it is improbable that these have any practical relevance for man.

G. References

Aase, J.M., Laestadius, N., Smith, D.W.: Children of mothers who took LSD in pregnancy. Lancet **1970/II**, 100–101

Abramson, D.I., Lichtman, S.S.: Influence of ergotamine tartrate upon peripheral blood-flow in subjects with liver disease. Proc. Soc. exp. Biol. (N.Y.) **37**, 262–267 (1937)

Alberti, C., Macaluso, G., Bocchi, R., Potenzoni, D.: Contributo sperimentale allo studio delle periureteriti da farmaci. Nota preliminare. Ateneo parmense, Acta bio-med. **39**, 1–19 (1968)
Alexander, G.J., Miles, B.E., Gold, G.M., Alexander, R.B.: LSD: Injection early in pregnancy produces abnormalities in offspring of rats. Science **157**, 459–460 (1967)
Alexander, G.J., Gold, G.M., Miles, B.E., Alexander, R.B.: Lysergic acid diethylamide intake in pregnancy: fetal damage in rats. J. Pharmacol. exp. Ther. **173**, 48–59 (1970)
Amarose, A.P., Schuster, C.R., Muller, T.P.: An animal model for the evaluation of drug-induced chromosome damage (Rabbit). Oncology (Basel) **27**, 550–562 (1973)
Anderson, L.H., Wells, J.A.: Attempts to prevent ergot gangrene with heparin and dicumarol. Vascular effects of ergot by fluorescein technic. Proc. Soc. exp. Biol. (N.Y.) **67**, 53–56 (1948)
Andersson, P.G.: Ergotamine headache. Headache **15**, No. 2 (1975)
Appenzeller, O., Davison, K., Marshall, J.: Reflex vasomotor abnormalities in the hands of migrainous subjects. J. Neurol. Neurosurg. Psychiat. **26**, 447–450 (1963)
Araszkiewicz, H., Bartel, H.: Teratogenic action of LSD-25 on the central nervous system in mouse fetuses. Folia morph. (Warszawa) **31**, 502–509 (1972)
Auerbach, R.: LSD: Teratogenicity in mice. Science **170**, 558 (1970)
Auerbach, R., Rugowski, J.A.: Lysergic acid diethylamide: effect on embryos. Science **157**, 1325–1326 (1967)
Bähr, G., Borselle, I., Kuefer, B.: Kurzer Bericht über eine LSD-Vergiftung bei neun Kindern. Mschr. Kinderheilk. **120**, 287–288 (1972)
Bailey, J., Wrathall, A.E., Mantle, P.G.: The effect of feeding ergot to gilts during early pregnancy. Brit. vet. J. **129**, 127–133 (1973)
Baillie, T.W.: Vasopressor activity of ergometrine maleate in anaesthetized parturient women. Brit. med. J. **1963/I**, 585–588
Baillie, T.W.: The influence of ergometrine on the initiation of cardiac impulse. J. Obstet. Gynaec. Brit. Cwlth **76**, 34–40 (1969a)
Baillie, T.W.: Ventricular ectopic activity following intravenous ergometrine. Anaesthesia **24**, 253–255 (1969b)
Baker, P.C.: LSD: Its effects upon 5-hydroxytryptamine in embryonic development of *Xenopus laevis*. Experientia (Basel) **27**, 536–537 (1971)
Bana, D.S., MacNeal, P.S., Le Compte, P.M., Shah, Y., Graham, J.R.: Cardiac murmurs and endocardial fibrosis associated with methysergide therapy. Amer. Heart J. **88**, 640–655 (1974)
Barger, G.: Ergot and Ergotism. London-Edinburgh: Gurney and Jackson 1931
Barger, G.: The alkaloids of ergot. In: Handbuch der experimentellen Pharmakologie **6**, 84–226 (1938)
Barger, G., Dale, H.H.: Ergotoxine and some other constituents of ergot. Biochem. J. **2**, 240–299 (1907)
Barnard, P.J.: The role of vasospasm in the pathogenesis of experimental embolic endarteritis obliterans. Cent. Afr. J. Med. **7**, 355–360 (1961)
Barnett, B.M., Muñoz, E.R.: Genetic effects of LSD in *Drosophila melanogaster* sperm. Mutation Res. **11**, 441–444 (1971)
Baumrucker, J.F.: Drug interaction—propranolol and cafergot. New Engl. J. Med. **288**, 916–917 (1973)
Beall, J.R.: A teratogenic study of chlorpromazine, orphenadrine, perphenazine, and LSD-25 in rats. Toxicol. appl. Pharmacol. **21**, 230–236 (1972)
Bélanger, M., Brugal, G., Chibon, P.: Embryologie expérimentale: Effets du LSD-25 sur le cycle cellulaire d'embryons de *Pleurodeles waltlii Michah.* traités en fin de gastrulation. C.R. Acad. Sci. (Paris) **281**, 1987–1990 (1975)
Bente, D., Itil, T., Schmid, E.E.: Elektroenzephalographische Studien zur Wirkungsweise des LSD 25. Psychiatr. Neurol. **135**, 273 (1958)
Bernreiter, M.: Drug reaction. Severe angina pectoris and electrocardiographic changes after Cafergot medication. J. Kans. med. Soc. **66**, 464–466 (1965)
Besser, G.M., Thorner, M.O.: Bromocriptine in the treatment of the hyperprolactinaemia-hypogonadism syndromes. Postgrad. med. J. **52** (Suppl. 1), 64–70 (1976)
Besser, G.M., Parkes, L., Edwards, C.R.W., Forsyth, I.A., McNeilly, A.S.: Galactorrhea:

successful treatment with reduction of plasma prolactin levels by brom-ergocryptine. Brit. med. J. **1972/III**, 669–672
Bick, Y.A.E.: Comparison of the effects of LSD, Heliotrine and X-irradiation on chromosome breakage, and the effects of LSD on the rate of cell division. Nature (Lond.) **226**, 1165–1167 (1970)
Biggio, P., Gessa, G.L., Pinetti, P.: Azione protetiva della griseofulvina sulla necrosi ischemica da ergotamina della coda del ratto. Boll. Soc. ital. Biol. sper. **40**, 785–787 (1964)
Bigorie, B., Aimez, P., Soria, R.J., Samama, F., di Maria, G., Guy-Grand, B., Baur, H.: L'association triacétyl oléandomycine-tartrate d'ergotamine est-elle dangereuse? Nouv. Presse méd. **4**, 2723–2725 (1975)
Blank, N.K., Rieder, M.J.: Paradoxical response to propranolol in migraine. Lancet **1973/II**, 1336
Blatchley, F.R., Donovan, B.T.: Effect of ergot alkaloids upon luteal function in the ferret. J. Endocr. **60**, 91–99 (1974)
Bové, F.J.: The Story of Ergot. Basel-New York: Karger 1970
Bovet-Nitti, F., Bovet, D.: Action of some sympatholytic agents on pregnancy in the rat. Proc. Soc. exp. Biol. (N.Y.) **100**, 555–557 (1959)
Braun, H.: Tierexperimentelle Gefäßstudien. Derm. Wschr. **115**, 1008–1012 (1942)
Brereton-Stiles, G.G., Winship, W.S., Goodwin, N.M., Roos, R.F.: Accidental administration of Syntometrine to a neonate. S. Afr. med. J. **46**, 2052 (1972)
Bro-Rasmussen, F., Jensen, B., Sorensen, A.H.: "Spontaneous" amputations. Lancet **1972/I**, 907–908
Brown, G.L., Dale, H.: The pharmacology of ergometrine. Proc. roy. Soc. B. **118**, 446–447 (1935)
Browning, D.J.: Serious side effects of ergometrine and its use in routine obstetric practice. Med. J. Aust. **1**, 957–958 (1974)
Browning, L.S.: Lysergic acid diethylamide: mutagenic effects in Drosophila. Science **161**, 1022–1023 (1968)
Buenger, R.E., Hunter, J.A.: Reversible mesenteric artery stenoses due to methysergide maleate. J. Amer. med. Ass. **198**, 558–560 (1966)
Byrne-Quinn, E.: Prolonged arteriospasm after overdose of oral ergotamine tartrate in migraine. Brit. med. J. **1964/II**, 552–553
Calne, D.B., Kartzinel, R., Shoulson, I.: An ergot derivative in the treatment of Parkinson's disease. Postgrad. med. J. **52** (Suppl. 1), 81–82 (1976)
Cameron, E.A., French, E.B.: St. Anthony's fire rekindled: gangrene due to therapeutic dose of ergotamine. Brit. med. J. **1960/II**, 28–30
Carlsen, R.A., Zeilmaker, G.H., Shelesnyak, M.C.: Termination of early (pre-nidation) pregnancy in the mouse by single injection of ergocornine methanesulphonate. J. Reprod. Fertil. **2**, 369–373 (1961)
Carpent, G., Desclin, L.: Effects of ergocornine on the mechanism of gestation and on fetal morphology in the rat. Endocrinology **84**, 315–324 (1969)
Carter, E.R.: Bilateral thrombophlebitis after a single dose of ergotamine tartrate for migraine. Brit. med. J. **1958/II**, 1452–1453
Casady, G.N., Moore, D.C., Bridenbaugh, L.D.: Postpartum hypertension after use of vasoconstrictor and oxytocic drugs. Etiology, incidence, complications, and treatment. J. Amer. med. Ass. **172**, 1011–1015 (1960)
Chaumartin, H.: Le Mal des Ardents et le Feu Saint-Antoine. Paris: Chaumartin 1946
Chibon, P., Bélanger-Barbeau, M.: Embryologie expérimentale: Effets du LSD sur le développement embryonnaire et les chromosomes de l'Amphibie Urodèle *Pleurodeles waltlii Michah.* C.R. Acad. Sci. (Paris) **274**, 280–283 (1972)
Chu, D., Owen, D.A.A., Stürmer, E.: Effects of ergotamine and dihydroergotamine on the resistance and capacitance vessels of skin and skeletal muscle in the cat. Postgrad. med. J. **52** (Suppl. 1), 32–36 (1976)
Clarke, C.A.: Analgesics. Practitioner **178**, 33–42 (1957)
Clearly, R.E., Grabtree, R., Lemberger, L.: The effect of Lergotrile on galactorrhea and gonadotropin secretion. J. clin. Endocr. **40**, 830–833 (1975)
Clemens, J.A., Shaar, C.J., Smalstig, E.B., Bach, N.J., Kornfeld, E.C.: Inhibition of prolactin secretion by ergolines. Endocrinology **94**, 1171–1175 (1974)

Cohen, M.M., Hirschhorn, K., Frosch, W.A.: In vivo and in vitro chromosomal damage induced by LSD-25. New Engl. J. Med. **277**, 1043–1049 (1967a)
Cohen, M.M., Marinello, M.J., Back, N.: Chromosomal damage in human leukocytes induced by lysergic acid diethlyamide. Science **155**, 1417–1419 (1967b)
Cohen, M.M., Mukherjee, A.B.: Meiotic chromosome damage induced by LSD-25. Nature (Lond.) **219**, 1072–1074 (1968)
Cohen, S.: A classification of LSD complications. Psychosomatics **7**, 182–186 (1966)
Cole, J., Glees, P.: Behavioural effects of lysergic acid diethlyamide in monkeys. Arzneimittel-Forsch. **17**, 401–404 (1967)
Comfort, M.W., Erickson, C.W.: Untoward effects from the use of ergot and ergotamine tartrate. Ann. intern. Med. **13**, 46–60 (1939)
Corey, M.J., Andrews, J.C., McLeod, M.J., McLean, J.R., Wilby, W.E.: Chromosome studies on patients (in vivo) and cells (in vitro) treated with lysergic acid diethylamide. New Engl. J. Med. **282**, 939–943 (1970)
Cowie, A.T., Tindal, J.S.: The physiology of lactation. In: Monographs of the Physiological Society. Davson, H., Whittorn, R., (eds.), No. 22. London: E. Arnold 1971
Cranley, J.J., Krause, R.J., Strasser, E.S., Hafner, C.D.: Impending gangrene of four extremities secondary to ergotism. New Engl. J. Med. **269**, 727–729 (1963)
Creze, B., Truelle, J.L., Denis, A., Boutin, P., Grosieux, P.: Cécité corticale transitoire après délivrance dirigée au méthergin. Rev. franç. Gynéc. **71**, 353–356 (1976)
Cushny, A.R.: Mutterkorn. In: Handbuch der Exper. Pharmakologie. Heffter, A. (ed.). Vol. II, Sect. 2, pp. 1297–1354. Berlin: J. Springer 1924
Custer, R.P., The experimental pathology of ergotism. With reference to some newer ergot derivatives. Amer. J. med. Sci. **195**, 452–457 (1938)
Dalessio, D.J., Camp, W.A., Goodell, H., Wolff, H.G.: Studies on headache. The mode of action of UML-491 and its relevance to the nature of vascular headache of the migraine type. Arch. Neurol. Psychiat. (Chic.) **4**, 235–240 (1961)
Daniell, H.W.: Vasospastic reaction to methysergide maleate simulating Leriche syndrome. Ineffective treatment with adrenergic blockade. Ann. intern. Med. **60**, 881–885 (1964)
David, T.J.: Nature and etiology of the Poland anomaly. New Engl. J. Med. **287**, 487–489 (1972)
David, T.J.: The Poland anomaly in the South West of England. Excerpta Medica, Int. Congress Series No. 297, 4th Int. Conf. on Birth Defects, Vienna, Sept. 2–8, 1973
Davis, M.E., Adair, F.L., Rogers, G., Kharasch, M.S., Legault, R.R.: A new active principle in ergot and its effects on uterine motility. Amer. J. Obstet. Gynec. **29**, 155–167 (1935)
Degenhardt, K.-H.: Durch O_2-Mangel induzierte Fehlbildungen der Axialgradienten bei Kaninchen. Z. Naturforsch. **9**, 530–536 (1954)
Degenhardt, K.-H., Kleinebrecht, J.: Poland-Syndrom durch secale Alkaloide? Dtsch. Ärztebl. **52**, 3413–3415 (1972)
Del Pozo, E., Varga, L., Wyss, H., Tolis, G., Friesen, H., Wenner, R., Vetter, L., Uettwiler, A.: Clinical and hormonal response to bromocryptine (CB 154) in the galactorrhea syndromes. J. clin. Endocr. **39**, 18–26 (1974)
Del Pozo, E., Brun del Re, R., Hinselmann, M.: Lack of effect of methyl-ergonovine on postpartum lactation. Amer. J. Obstet. Gynec. **123**, 845–846 (1975)
De Margerie, J., Mondon, H., Magis, C.-C.: Oblitération de l'artère centrale de la rétine et intoxication par absorption conjointe de LSD et amphétamine. Bull. Soc. Ophtal. Fr. **72**, 853–858 (1972)
Diamant-Berger, F., Pasticier, A., Haas, Cl., Soyer, R., Ricordeau, G., Dubost, Ch.: Intolérance vasculaire périphérique nécrosante à l'ergotamine thérapeutique. Toxicologie clinique. Europ. J. Toxikol. **5**, 366–370 (1972)
DiPaolo, J.A., Givelber, H.M., Erwin, H.: Evaluation of teratogenicity of lysergic acid diethylamide. Nature (Lond.) **220**, 490–491 (1968)
Dishotsky, N.I., Loughman, W.D., Mogar, R.E., Lipscomb, W.R.: LSD and genetic damage. Is LSD chromosome damaging, carcinogenic, mutagenic, or teratogenic? Science **172**, 431–440 (1971)
Doepfner, W.: Biochemical observations on LSD-25 and deseril. Experientia (Basel) **18**, 256–257 (1962)
Dorrance, D.L., Beighlie, D.J., Yoshii, V., Janiger, O., Brodetsky, A.M., Teplitz, R.L.: Studies

on the mechanism of interaction between lysergic acid and chromosomes. J. Lab. clin. Med. **84**, 36–41 (1974)
Dumars, Jr., K.W.: Parental drugs usage: effect upon chromosomes of progeny. Pediatrics **47**, 1037–1041 (1971)
Dunn, J.M., Sloan, H.: Pleural effusion and fibrosis secondary to Sansert administration. Ann. thorac. Surg. **15**, 295–298 (1973)
Eberle, P.: Verursachen Halluzinogene Chromosomendefekte und Mißbildungen? Nervenarzt **44**, 281–284 (1973)
Edgerly, W.S., Stewart, C.F.: Ergotism. New Engl. J. Med. **269**, 1385–1386 (1963)
Edwardson, J.A.: The effect of agroclavine, an ergot alkaloid, on pregnancy and lactation in the rat. Brit. J. Pharmacol. **33**, 215P–216P (1968)
Edwardson, J.A., MacGregor, L.A.: The effect of progesterone and some other agents on the failure of pregnancy produced by feeding agroclavine, an ergot alkaloid, in the rat. Brit. J. Pharmacol. **35**, 367P–369P (1969)
Egozcue, J., Irwin, S.: Effect of LSD-25 on mitotic and meiotic chromosomes of mice and monkeys. Humangenetik **8**, 86–93 (1969)
Eloff, S.J., Brummelkamp, W.H., Boerema, I.: A case of "ergot-foot" treated with hyperbaric oxygen drenching. Case report. J. cardiovasc. Surg. (Torino) **4**, 747–751 (1963)
Emerit, I., Roux, C., Feingold, J.: LSD: No chromosomal breakage in mother and embryos during rat pregnancy. Teratology **6**, 71–74 (1972)
Evarts, E.V.: Some effects of bufotenine and lysergic acid diethlylamide on the monkey. Arch. Neurol. Psychiat. (Chic.) **75**, 49–53 (1956)
Fabro, S., Sieber, S.M.: Is lysergide a teratogen? Lancet **1968/I**, 639
Fedotin, M.S., Hartman, C.: Ergotamine poisoning producing renal arterial spasm. Case report. New Engl. J. Med. **283**, 518–520 (1970)
Felix, R.H., Carroll, J.D.: Upper limb ischaemia due to ergotamine tartrate. Practitioner **205**, 71–72 (1970)
Fernandez, J., Browne, I.W., Cullen, J., Brennan, T., Matheu, H., Fischer, I.: LSD—an in vivo retrospective chromosome study. Ann. hum. Genet. **37**, 81–91 (1973)
Fernandez, J., Brennan, T., Masterson, J., Power, M.: Cytogenetic studies in the offspring of LSD users. Brit. J. Psychiat. **124**, 296–298 (1974)
Finn, C.A., Mantle, P.G.: The influence of agroclavine on the preparation of the uterus for implantation in the mouse. J. Reprod. Fertil. **20**, 527–529 (1969)
Finney, P.J.: Probit analysis, 3rd ed. London: Cambridge Univ. Press 1971
Fisher, D., Ungerleider, T.: Grand mal seizures following ingestion of LSD-25. Calif. Med. **106**, 210–211 (1967)
Fitzhugh, O.G., Nelson, A.A., Calvery, H.O.: The chronic toxicity of ergot. J. Pharmacol. exp. Ther. **82**, 364–376 (1944)
Floss, H.G., Cassady, J.M., Robbers, J.E.: Influence of ergot alkaloids on pituitary prolactin and prolactin-dependent processes. J. pharm. Sci. **62**, 699–715 (1973)
Flückiger, E., Wagner, H.R.: 2-Br-α-Ergokryptine: Beeinflussung von Fertilität und Laktation bei der Ratte. Experientia (Basel) **24**, 1130–1131 (1968)
Flückiger, E., Markó, M., Doepfner, W., Niederer, W.: Effects of ergot alkaloids on the hypothalamic pituitary axis. Postgrad. med. J. **52** (Suppl. 1), 57–61 (1976a)
Flückiger, E., Billeter, E., Wagner, H.R.: Inhibition of lactation in rabbits by 2-Br-α-Ergokryptine-mesilate (CB 154). Arzneimittel-Forsch. **26**, 51–53 (1976b)
Fomina, P.I.: Untersuchungen über den Übergang des aktiven Agens des Mutterkorns in die Milch stillender Mütter. Arch. Gynäk. **157**, 275–285 (1934)
Ford, J.J., Yoshinaga, K.: Ergokryptine and pregnancy maintenance in hamsters. Proc. Soc. exp. Biol. (N.Y.) **150**, 425–427 (1975)
Forman, J.B., Sullivan, R.L.: The effects of intravenous injections of ergonovine and methysergide on the postpartum patient. Amer. J. Obstet. Gynec. **63**, 640–644 (1952)
Franklin, J.B., Brent, R.L.: The effect of uterine vascular clamping on the development of rat embryos three to fourteen days old. J. Morph. **115**, 273–290 (1964)
Friedman, A.P., von Storch, J.C., Araki, S.: Ergotamine tartrate: its history, action, and proper use in the treatment of migraine. N.Y. St. J. Med. **6** (10.12), 2359–2366 (1959)

Friedman, S.A., Hirsch, S.E.: Extreme hyperthermia after LSD ingestion. J. Amer. med. Ass. **217**, 1549–1550 (1971)
Fuchs, M., Blumenthal, L.S.: Use of ergot preparations in migraine. J. Amer. med. Ass. **143**, 1462–1464 (1950)
Gagnon, R.: Le LSD est-il tératogène? Un. méd. Can. **98**, 123 (1969)
Gardner, L.I., Assemany, S.R., Neu, R.L.: Syndrome of multiple osseous defects with pretibial dimples. Lancet **1971/II**, 98
Geber, W.F.: Congenital malformations induced by mescaline, lysergic acid diethlyamide, and bromolysergic acid in the hamster. Science **158**, 265–267 (1967)
Giroud, A., Tuchmann-Duplessis, H.: Malformations congénitales: rôle des facteurs exogènes. Pathol. Biol. **10**, 119–151 (1962)
Glazer, G., Myers, K.A., Davies, E.R.: Ergot poisoning. Postgrad. med. J. **42**, 562–568 (1966)
Görög, P., Kovács, I.B.: Ergotamine gangrene in various inflammatory conditions. Angiologica **8**, 57–64 (1971)
Goetz, P., Šrám, R.J., Zudová, Z.: The mutagenic effect of lysergic acid diethylamide. I. Cytogenetic analysis. Mutation Res. **26**, 513–516 (1974)
Goldfischer, J.D.: Acute myocardial infarction secondary to ergot therapy. Report of a case and review of the literature. New Engl. J. Med. **262**, 860–863 (1960)
Gottschalk, W.: Principles of obstetric anesthesia. In: Obstet. Gynecol. Annual **1**, 199 (1972)
Gould, S.E., Price, A.E., Ginsberg, H.I.: Gangrene and death following ergotamine tartrate (Gynergen) therapy. J. Amer. med. Ass. **106**, 1631–1635 (1936)
Grace, D., Carlson, E.A., Goodman, P.: *Drosophila melanogaster* treated with LSD: absence of mutation and chromosome breakage. Science **161**, 694–696 (1968)
Graham, J.R.: Use of a new compound, UML-491 (1-methyl-d-lysergic acid butanolamine) in the prevention of various types of headache. New Engl. J. Med. **263**, 1273–1277 (1960)
Graham, J.R.: Methysergide for prevention of headache. Experience in five hundred patients over three years. New Engl. J. Med. **270**, 67–72 (1964)
Graham, J.R.: Cardiac and pulmonary fibrosis during methysergide therapy for headache. Amer. J. med. Sci. **254**, 1–12 (1967)
Graham, J.R., Parnes, L.R.: Possible cardiac and reno-vascular complications of Sansert therapy. Headache **5**, 14–18 (1965)
Graham, J.R., Suby, H.I., LeCompte, P.R., Sadowsky, N.L.: Fibrotic disorders associated with methysergide therapy for headache. New Engl. J. Med. **274**, 359–368 (1966)
Graham, J.R., Suby, H.I., LeCompte, P.M.: Inflammatory fibrosis associated with methysergide therapy. Res. clin. studies Headache **1**, 123–164 (1967)
Grauwiler, J., Griffith, R.W.: Acute toxicity studies with 2-bromo-α-ergocryptine mesylate (CB 154). IRCS Med. Sci. **2**, 1516 (1974)
Grauwiler, J., Leist, K.-H.: Impairment of uteroplacental blood supply by ergotamine as a cause of embrytoxicity in rats. Teratology **7**, A-16 (1973)
Grauwiler, J., Schön, H.: Teratological experiments with ergotamine in mice, rats and rabbits. Teratology **7**, 227–235 (1973)
Greatorex, J.C., Mantle, P.G.: Experimental ergotism in sheep. Res. Vet. Sci. **15**, 337–346 (1973)
Greatorex, J.C., Mantle, P.G.: Effect of rye ergot on the pregnant sheep. J. Reprod. Fertil. **37**, 33–41 (1974)
Griffith, R.W.: Toxicity studies with 2-bromo-α-ergocryptine mesylate (CB 154). Prolonged administration in rats. IRCS Med. Sci. **2**, 1661 (1974)
Griffith, R.W.: Toxicity studies with 2-bromo-α-ergocryptine (CB 154): effect of prolonged oral administration in monkeys. IRCS Med. Sci. **4**, 386 (1976)
Griffith, R.W., Richardson, B.P.: Toxicity studies with 2-bromo-α-ergocryptine (CB 154): Effects of prolonged oral administration in dogs. IRCS Med. Sci. **3**, 298–299 (1975)
Grosvenor, C.E.: Effect of ergotamine on milk-ejection in lactating rat. Proc. Soc. exp. Biol. (N.Y.) **91**, 294–296 (1956)
Guilhon, J.: L'ergotisme des animaux domestiques. Rev. Path. gén. comp. **55**, 1467–1478 (1955)
Gupta, D.R., Strobos, R.J.: Bilateral papillitis associated with cafergot therapy. Neurology (Minneap.) **22/8**, 793–797 (1972)

Hanaway, J.K.: Lysergic acid diethylamide: effects on the developing mouse lens. Science **164**, 574–575 (1969)
Hanselmayer, H., Werner, W.: Netzhautarterienspasmus nach oraler überdosierter DHE-Medikation. Klin. Mbl. Augenheilk. **162**, 807–811 (1973)
Hansteen, V.: Ergotisme. Nord. Med. **75**, 447–449 (1966)
Hart, I.C.: Effect of 2-bromo-α-ergocryptine on milk yield and the level of prolactin and growth hormone in the blood of the goat at milking. J. Endocr. **57**, 179–180 (1973)
Hart, N.H.: The effect of LSD on somite number in explanted chick embryos. Experientia (Basel) **31**, 97–98 (1975)
Hart, N.H., Greene, M.: LSD: Teratogenic action in chick blastoderms. Proc. Soc. exp. Biol. (N.Y.) **137**, 371–373 (1971)
Hayton, A.C.: Precipitation of acute ergotism by triacetyloleandomycin. N.Z. med. J. **69**, 42–43 (1969)
Hendricks, C.H., Brenner, W.E.: Cardiovascular effects of oxytocic drugs used post partum. Amer. J. Obstet. Gynec. **108**, 751–760 (1970)
Hindle, W., Posner, E., Sweetnam, M.T., Tan, R.S.H.: Pleural effusion and fibrosis during treatment with methysergide. Brit. med. J. **1970/I**, 605–606
Hirsch, M., Eger, M.: Angiography in diagnosis of ergotism. Radiology **103/1,** 89–90 (1972)
Hodel, Ch., Griffith, R.W.: Inability to reproduce retroperitoneal fibrosis in animal toxicity studies with methysergide. Excerpta medica, Int. Congress Series No. 311, Proc. Eur. Soc. Study Drug Tox. **15**, 317–322 (1973)
Hoffmann, B., Schams, D., Bopp, R., Ender, M.L., Giménez, T., Karg, H.: Luteotrophic factors in the cow; evidence for LH rather than prolactin. J. Reprod. Fertil. **40**, 77–85 (1974)
Hollister, L.E.:: Social drugs. Chap. 3. In: Meyler's Side Effects of Drugs. Dukes, M.N.G. (ed.), Vol. VIII, pp. 47–63. Amsterdam-Oxford: Excerpta Medica; New York: Elsevier 1975
Horton, B.T., Peters, G.A.: Clinical manifestations of excessive use of ergotamine preparations and management of withdrawal effect. Headache **20**, 214–227 (1963)
Houston, B.K.: Review of the evidence and qualifications regarding the effects of hallucinogenic drugs on chromosomes and embryos. Amer. J. Psychiat. **126**, 251–254 (1969)
Hudgson, P., Foster, J.B., Walton, J.N.: Methysergide and coronary-artery disease. Lancet **1967/I**, 444–445.
Ianzito, B., Liskow, B., Stewart, M.A.: Reaction to LSD in a two-year-old child. J. Pediat. **80**, 643–647 (1972)
Ingalls, T.H., Curley, F.J., Prindle, R.A.: Anoxia as a cause of fetal death and congenital defect in the mouse. Amer. J. Dis. Child. **80**, 34–45 (1950)
Iuel, J., Mune, O.: Peripheral arterial insufficiency in ergotism. Review of the literature and foot plethysmographic studies in ergotamine poisoning. Vasc. Dis. **4**, 159–166 (1967)
Jacobson, C.B., Berlin, C.M.: Possible reproductive detriment in LSD users. J. Amer. med. Ass. **222**, 1367–1373 (1972)
Jagiello, G., Polani, P.E.: Mouse germ cells and LSD-25. Cytogenetics **8**, 136–147 (1969)
Jarvik, L.Y., Fu-Sun Yen, Dahlberg, C.C., Fleiss, J.L., Jaffe, J., Kato, T., Moralishvili, E.: Chromosome examinations after medically administered lysergic acid diethylamide and dextroamphetamine. Dis. nerv. Syst. **74**, 399–407 (1974)
Johnson, T.D.: Severe peripheral arterial constriction. Acute ischemia of lower extremity with use of methysergide and ergotamine. Arch. intern. Med. **117**, 237–241 (1966)
Kappert, A.: Untersuchungen über die Wirkungen neuer dihydrierter Mutterkornalkaloide bei peripheren Durchblutungsstörungen und Hypertonie. Helv. med. Acta, Ser. A **16** (Suppl. 22), pp. 66–67 (1949)
Karg, H., Schams, D., Reinhardt, V.: Effects of 2-Br-α-ergocryptine on plasma prolactin level and milk yield in cows. Experientia (Basel) **28**, 574–576 (1972)
Kato, T., Jarvik, L.F.: LSD-25 and genetic damage. Dis. nerv. Syst. **30**, 42–46 (1969)
Kato, T., Jarvik, L.F., Roizin, L., Moralishvili, E.: Chromosome studies in pregnant rhesus macaque given LSD-25. Dis. nerv. Syst. **31**, 245–250 (1970)
Katz, A.I., Massry, S.G.: Arteriospasm after ergotamine tartrate in infectious hepatitis. Arch. intern. Med. **118**, 62–64 (1966)

Kenna, A.P.: Accidental administration of syntometrine to a newborn infant. J. Obstet. Gynaec. Brit. Cwlth. **79**, 764–766 (1972)
Kisch, E.S., Shelesnyak, M.C.: Studies on the mechanism of nidation. XXXI. Failure of ergocornine to interrupt gestation in the rat in the presence of foetal placenta. J. Reprod. Fertil. **15**, 401–407 (1968)
Klock, J.C., Boerner, U., Becker, C.E.: Coma, hyperthermia and bleeding associated with massive LSD overdose. West. med. J. **120**, 183–188 (1974)
Kraicer, P.F., Shelesnyak, M.C.: Studies on the mechanism of nidation. IX. Analysis of the responses to ergocornine—an inhibitor of nidation. J. Reprod. Fertil. **8**, 225–233 (1964)
Kraicer, P.F., Shelesnyak, M.C.: Studies on the mechanism of nidation. XIII. The relationship between chemical structure and biodynamic activity of certain ergot alkaloids. J. Reprod. Fertil. **10**, 221–226 (1965)
Kraicer, P.F., Shelesnyak, M.C.: Interruption of pregnancy, induction of ovulation and delayed pseudopregnancy following suppression of luteal function. Acta endocr. (Kbh.) **58**, 251–260 (1968)
Kravitz, D.: Neuroretinitis associated with symptoms of ergot poisoning. Report of a case. Albrecht v. Graefes Arch. Klin. Ophthal. **13**, 201–206 (1935)
Kučera, J.: Syndrome of multiple osseous defects. Lancet **1972/I**, 260
Labbé, M., Justin-Besançon, Gouyen, J.: Accidents consécutifs au traitement de la maladie de Basedow par le tartrate d'ergotamine. Ann. Méd. Interne (Paris) **53**, 429–432 (1929)
Langecker, H.: Zur experimentellen Mutterkornvergiftung. Naunyn-Schmiedebergs Arch. exp. Path. Pharmak. **165**, 291–298 (1932)
Langgard, H., Ulrich, J.: Absence of effects of methysergide on connective tissue in mice. Acta pharmacol. toxicol. (Kbh.) **33/1**, 53–56 (1973)
Larcan, A., Lambert, H.: Aspects cliniques des intoxications par dérivés de l'ergot de seigle. Ann. Méd. (Nancy) **11/2**, 289–292 (1972)
Lauersen, N.H., Conrad, P.: Effect of oxytocic agents on blood loss during first trimester suction curettage. Obstet. and Gynec. **44**, 428–433 (1974)
Lee, H.Y., Hart, N.H., Kalmus, G.W.: Teratologic effects of LSD in explanted early chick embryos. Teratology **11**, 187–192 (1975)
Legator, M.S.: The host mediated assay, a practical procedure for evaluating potential mutagenic agents. In: Chemical Mutagenesis in Mammals and Man. Vogel, F., Röhrborn, G. (eds.), pp. 260–270. Berlin-Heidelberg-New York: Springer 1970
Leist, K.H., Grauwiler, J.: Influence of the developmental stage on embryotoxicity following uterine vessel clamping in the rat. Teratology **8**, 227–228 (1973a)
Leist, K.H., Grauwiler, J.: Influence of the developmental stage on embryotoxicity following uterine vessel clamping in the rat. Acta Univ. Carol. [Med.] (Praha) Monographia **56–57**, 173–176 (1973b)
Leist, K.H., Grauwiler, J.: Transplacental passage of ^{3}H ergotamine in the rat, and determination of the intraamniotic embryotoxicity of ergotamine. Experientia (Basel) **29**, 764 (1973c)
Leist, K.H., Grauwiler, J.: Fetal pathology in rats following uterine-vessel clamping on day 14 of gestation. Teratology **10**, 55–68 (1974a)
Leist, K.H., Grauwiler, J.: Ergometrine and uteroplacental blood supply in pregnant rats. Teratology **10**, 316 (1974b)
Lemberger, L., Crabtree, R., Clemens, J., Dyke, R.W., Woodburn, R.T.: The inhibitory effect of an ergoline derivative (Lergotrile, Compound 83636) on prolactin secretion in man. J. clin. Endocr. **39**, 579–584 (1974)
Lewis, T.: The manner in which necrosis arises in the fowl's comb under ergot poisoning. Clin. Sci. **2**, 43–55 (1935)
Lewis, C.T., Molland, E.A., Marshall, V.R., Tresidder, G.C., Blandy, J.P.: Analgesic abuse, ureteric obstruction and retroperitoneal fibrosis. Brit. med. J. **1975/II**, 76–78
Leyton, N.: Methysergide in the prophylaxis of migraine. Lancet **1964/I**, 830
Lieberman, A.N., Bloom, W., Kishore, P.S., Lin, J.P.: Carotid artery occlusion following ingestion of LSD. Stroke **5**, 213–215 (1974)
Liskow, B.: Extreme hyperthermia from LSD. J. Amer. med. Ass. **218**, 1049 (1971)

Litchfield, J.T., Wilcoxon, F.: A simplified method of evaluating dose-effect experiments. J. Pharmacol. exp. Ther. **96**, 99–113 (1949)
Lobel, B.L., Shelesnyak, M.C., Tic, L.: Studies on the mechanism of nidation. XIX. Histochemical changes in the ovaries of pregnant rats following ergocornine. J. Reprod. Fertil. **11**, 339–348 (1966)
London, M., Magora, F., Rogel, S., Romanoff, H.: Acute ergot poisoning. Angiology **21**, 565–567 (1970)
Long, S.Y.: Does LSD induce chromosomal damage and malformations? A review of the literature. Teratology **6**, 75–90 (1972)
Lucas, R.N., Falkowski, W.: Ergotamine and methysergide abuse in patients with migraine. Brit. J. Psychiat. **122**, 199–203 (1973)
Luke, R.G., Talbert, W., Siegel, R.R., Holland, N.: Heparin treatment for postpartum renal failure with microangiopathic haemolytic anaemia. Lancet **1970/II**, 750–753
Lund, F.: Vasodilator drugs against experimental peripheral gangrene. A method of testing the effect of vasodilator drugs on constricted peripheral vessels. Acta physiol. scand. **23** (Suppl. 82), 1–141 (1951)
Lutterbeck, P.M., Pryor, J.S., Varga, L., Wenner, R.: Treatment of non-puerperal galactorrhoea with an ergot alkaloid. Brit. med. J. **1971/III**, 228–229
McGinty, L.B.: A study of the vasopressor effects of oxytocics when used intravenously in the third stage of labor. West. J. Surg. **64**, 22–28 (1956)
McGlothlin, W.H., Sparkes, R.S., Arnold, D.O.: Effect of LSD on human pregnancy. J. Amer. med. Ass. **212**, 1483–1487 (1970)
McGrath, E.J.G.: Experimental peripheral gangrene. Arch. intern. Med. **55**, 942 (1935)
McNerney, J.J., Leedham, C.L.: Acute coronary insufficiency pattern following intravenous ergotamine studies. Report of a case. Amer. Heart J. **39**, 629–632 (1950)
Mantle, P.G.: Inhibition of lactation in mice following feeding with ergot sclerotia [*Claviceps fusiformis*, (Loveless)] from the bulrush millet [*Pennisetum typhoides,* (Staph and Hubbard)] and an alkaloid component. Proc. roy. Soc. B **170**, 423–434 (1968)
Mantle, P.G.: Interruption of early pregnancy in mice by oral administration of agroclavine and sclerotia of *Claviceps fusiformis* (loveless). J. Reprod. Fertil. **18**, 81–88 (1969)
Mantle, P.G., Gunner, D.E.: Abortions associated with ergotised pastures. Vet. Rec. **77**, 885–886 (1965)
Markowitz, E.H., Brosseau, G.E., Markowitz, E.: Genetic effects of LSD treatment on the post-meiotic stages of spermatogenesis in *Drosophila melanogaster*. Mutation. Res. **8**, 337–342 (1969)
Master, A.M., Pordy, L., Kolker, J., Blumenthal, M.J.: The 'two-step' exercise electrocardiogram in functional heart disturbances and in organic heart disease: the use of ergotamine tartrate. Circulation **1**, 629–699 (1950)
Matter, B.E.: Failure to detect chromosome damage in bone-marrow cells of mice and Chinese hamsters exposed in vivo to some ergot derivatives. J. int. med. Res. 4, 382–392 (1976)
Matter, B.E., Grauwiler, J.: The micronucleus test as a simple model, in vivo, for evaluation of drug-induced chromosome aberrations. Comparative studies with 13 compounds. Mutation. Res. **29**, 198–199 (1975)
Matthies, D.L.: Studies of the luteotropic and mammotropic factor found in trophoblast and maternal peripheral blood of the rat at mid-pregnancy. Anat. Rec. **159**, 55–68 (1967)
Matveev, V.F.: Pathomorphological brain changes in experimental animals during chronic intoxication with lysergic acid amide. Zh. Nevropat. Psikhiat. **70**, 1856–62 (1970)
Mayer, P., Schütze, E.: Effect of 2-Br-α-ergokryptine (CB 154) on lactation in the bitch. Experientia (Basel) **29**, 484–485 (1973)
Meites, J., Clemens, J.A.: Hypothalamic control of prolactin secretion. VII. Effect of ergot derivatives on prolactin secretion. Vitam. and Horm. **30**, 198–203 (1972)
Meites, J., Shelesnyak, M.C.: Effect of prolactin on duration of pregnancy, viability of young and lactation in rats. Proc. Soc. exp. Biol. (N.Y.) **94**, 746–749 (1957)
Mellanby, E.: The experimental production and prevention of degeneration in the spinal cord. Brain **54**, 247–290 (1931)
Messier, P.-E.: Effects of LSD on the development, histology and fine structure of the chick embryo. Toxicol. appl. Pharmacol. **25**, 54–59 (1973)

Messina, C.: Effetti del trattamento con H.C.G. e con ergotamina in ratti integri ed ipofisectomizzati. Boll. Soc. ital. Biol. sper. **40**, 439–443 (1964)
Miller, L.C., Tainter, M.L.: Estimation of the ED_{50} and its error by means of a logarithmic probit graph paper. Proc. Soc. exp. Biol. (N.Y.) **57**, 261–264 (1944)
Milman, D.H.: An untoward reaction to accidental ingestion of LSD in a 5-year-old girl. J. Amer. med. Ass. **201**, 821–824 (1967)
Misch, K.A.: Development of heart valve lesions during methysergide therapy. Brit. med. J. **1974/II**, 365–366
Missen, G.A.K.: Gangrene of the tongue. Brit. med. J. **1961/I**, 1393–1394
Moir, J.C.: Ergot: From 'St. Anthony's Fire' to the isolation of its active principle, ergometrine (ergonovine). Amer. J. Obstet. Gynec. **2**, 291–296 (1974)
Moorhead, P.S., Jarvik, L.F., Cohen, M.M.: 11. Cytogenetic methods for mutagenicity testing. In Drugs of Abuse. Epstein, S.S. (ed.), pp. 140–170. Cambridge-London: The MIT Pr. 1971
Murakami, U., Kameyama, Y.: Vertebral malformation in the mouse foetus caused by maternal hypoxia during early stages of pregnancy. J. Embryol. exp. Morph. **11**, 107–118 (1963)
Nagasawa, H., Yanai, R.: Effects of adrenalectomy and/or deficiency of pituitary prolactin secretion on initiation and maintenance of lactation in mice. J. Endocr. **58**, 67–73 (1973)
Nair, V.: Prenatal exposure to drugs: effect on the development of brain monoamine systems. Advanc. behav. Biol. **8**, 171–197 (1974)
Nair, V., Bau, D., Siegel, S.: Effect of LSD in pregnancy on the biochemical development of brain and liver in the offspring. Pharmacologist **12**, 296 (1970)
Nassar, G., Greenwood, Ms., Djanian, A., Shanklin, W.: The etiological significance of ergot in the incidence of postpartum necrosis of the anterior pituitary. Amer. J. Obstet. Gynec. **60**, 140–145 (1950)
Nava, C.: Descrizione di un caso di allergia a lisergidi (Derivati dell'amide dell'acido lisergico). Med. d. Lavoro **63**, 57–61 (1972)
Nicaise, B.: L'ergot de seigle. Intoxications aiguës par ses dérivés médicamenteux. Univ. Nancy U.E.R. Sciences méd. A + B No. 144, 1972
Nicholl, G.S., Yaron, Z., Nutt, N., Daniels, E.: Effects of ergotamine tartrate on prolactin and growth hormone secretion by rat adenohypophysis in vitro. Biol. Reprod. **5**, 59–66 (1971)
Nichols, W.W.: The relationship of chromosome aberrations to drugs. In: Drug-Induced Diseases. Meyler, L., Peck, H.M. (eds.), Vol. IV, pp. 60–80. Amsterdam: Excerpta Medica 1972
Nicholson, M.T., Pace, H.B., Davis, W.M.: Effects of marihuana and lysergic acid diethylamide on leukocyte chromosomes of the golden hamster. Chem. Pathol. Pharmacol. **6**, 427–434 (1973)
Nishimura, H., Tanimura, T.: Clinical Aspects of the Teratogenicity of Drugs: Psychotomimetic Drugs. New York: Elsevier 1976
Nisweder, G.D.: Influence of 2-Br-α-ergokryptine on serum levels of prolactin and the oestrus cycle in sheep. Endocrinology **94**, 612–615 (1974)
Noguchi, Y., Nakayama, Y., Kowa, Y.: Teratogenic action of hypoxia under normal atmospheric pressure. Jap. J. vet. Sci. **29**, 11–19 (1967)
Nordskog, A.W.: Reproductive failure and agalactia in ergotized female rats. Amer. J. vet. Res. **7**, 490–497 (1946)
Nordskog, A.W., Clark, R.T.: Ergotism in pregnant sows, female rats and guinea pigs. Amer. J. vet. Res. **6**, 107–116 (1945)
Nosal, G.: Complications et dangers des hallucinogènes. Aspects cytopharmacologiques. Laval méd. **40**, 48–55 (1969)
Obe, G., Herha, J.: Genetische Schäden durch LSD? In vivo-Untersuchungen an 11 LSD-Konsumenten. Fortschr. Med. **91**, 533–536 (1973)
Orth, O.S.: Studies of the sympathicolytic drug dihydroxyergotamine (DHE 45). Fed. Proc. **5**, 196 (1946)
Orth, O.S., Ritchie, G.: A pharmacological evaluation of dihydroergotamine methanesulfonate (DHE 45). J. Pharmacol. exp. Therap. **90**, 166–173 (1947)
Orth, O.S., Capps, R.A., Suckle, H.M.: Some pharmacological properties of dihydroergocornine (DHO 180). Fed. Proc. **6**, 361 (1947)

Pauerstein, C.J.: Use and abuse of oxytocic agents. Clin. Obstet. Gynecol. **16**, 262–277 (1973)
Pearce, J.: Hazards of ergotamine tartrate. Brit. med. J. **1976/I**, 834–835
Pentschew, A.: Experimentelle Untersuchungen über Pellagra, Ergotismus und Bleivergiftung. Krankheitsforschung **7**, 399–414 (1929)
Perkin, G.D.: Ischaemic lateral popliteal nerve palsy due to ergot intoxication. J. Neurol. Neurosurg. Psychiat. **37**, 1389–1391 (1974)
Persyko, I.: Psychiatric adverse reactions to methysergide. J. nerv. ment. Dis. **154**, 299–301 (1972)
Peters, G.A., Horton, B.T.: Headache: with special reference to the excessive use of ergotamine preparations and withdrawal effects. Proc. Mayo Clin. **26**, 153–161 (1951)
Pitel, M., Lerman, S.: Further studies on the effects of intrauterine vasoconstrictors on the foetal rat lens. Amer. J. Ophthal. **58**, 464–470 (1964)
Quadri, S.K., Meites, J.: LSD-induced decrease in serum prolactin in rats. Proc. Soc. exp. Biol. (N.Y.) **137**, 1242–1243 (1971)
Racouchot, M.J., Gaillard, L., Guilaine, J.: Lupus erythémateux subaigu et méthysergide. Bull. Soc. franç. Derm. Syph. **75**, 513–515 (1968)
Regan, J.F., Poletti, B.J.: Vascular adventitial fibrosis in a patient taking methysergide maleate. J. Amer. med. Ass. **203**, 1069–1071 (1968)
Richard, T., Rappolt, S.: Clinical observation: Apparent antagonism of ergotamine on the gravid uterus by LSD-25. Europ. J. Toxicol. **3**, 138–139 (1970)
Richardson, B.P.: Evidence for a physiological role of prolactin in osmoregulation in the rat after its inhibition by 2-bromo-alpha-ergokryptine. Brit. J. Pharmacol. **47**, 623–624 (1973)
Richter, A.M., Banker, V.P.: Carotid ergotism. Radiology **106**, 339–340 (1973)
Riley, H.P., Neuroth, J.V.: LSD and plant chromosomes. J. Hered. **61**, 283–284 (1970)
Robinson, J.T., Chitham, R.G., Greenwood, R.M., Taylor, J.W.: Chromosome aberrations and LSD. A controlled study in 50 psychiatric patients. Brit. J. Psychiatry **125**, 238–244 (1974)
Rosenthal, S.H.: Persistent hallucinosis following repeated administration of hallucinogenic drugs. Amer. J. Psychiatry **121**, 238–244 (1964)
Rothlin, E.: Recherches expérimentales sur l'ergotamine, alcaloïde spécifique de l'ergot de seigle. Arch. int. Pharmacodyn. **27**, 459–479 (1923)
Rothlin, E.: Sur les propriétés pharmacologiques d'un nouvel alcaloïde de l'ergot de seigle, l'ergobasine. C.R.Soc. Biol. (Paris) **119**, 1302–1304 (1935)
Rothlin, E.: The pharmacology of the natural and dihydrogenated alkaloids of ergot. Bull. schweiz. Akad. med. Wiss. **2**, 249–273 (1946)
Rothlin, E.: Lysergic acid diethylamide and related substances. Ann. N.Y. Acad. Sci. **66**, 668–676 (1957)
Roux, C., Dupuis, R., Aubry, M.: LSD: No teratogenic action in rats, mice, and hamsters. Science **169**, 588–589 (1970)
Rowsell, A.R., Neylan, C., Wilkinson, M.: Ergotamine induced headaches in migrainous patients. Headache **13**, 65–67 (1973)
Ruffié, M.M.J., Colombiès, P., Grozdea, J.: Nouvelle étude de l'action expérimentale de fortes doses de diéthylamide de l'acide lysergique (LSD 25) sur la réactivité lymphocytaire à la phytohémagglutinine et sur le caryotype du babouin (Papio papio). Bull. Acad. nat. Méd. (Paris) **156**, 345–351 (1972)
Sadasivan, G., Raghuram, T.C.: Chromosomal aberrations in malnutrition. Lancet **1973/II**, 574
Sadjadpour, K.: Methysergide alopecia. J. Amer. med. Ass. **229**, 639 (1974)
Saenger, H.: Über Puerperalgangrän bei septischen Zuständen und Gynergenmedikation. Zbl. Gynäk. **53**, 586–594 (1929)
Sam, V., Joseph, T.: Effect of lysergic acid diethylamide on oestrus cycle and offspring in rats. Indian J. Physiol. Pharmacol. **17**, 277–282 (1973)
Sankar, D.V.S.: Genetic aspects. In: LSD: A Total Study. Sankar, D.V.S. (ed.), pp. 470–500. Westbury: PJD Publications 1975
Sankar, D.V.S., Rozsa, P.W., Geisler, A.: Chromosome breakage in children treated with LSD-25 and UML-491. Compr. Psychiatry **10**, 406–410 (1969)
Sarwer-Foner, G.J.: Some clinical and social aspects of lysergic acid diethylamide. Psychosomatics **13**, 309–316 (1972)

Sato, H., Pergament, E., Nair, V.: Lysergic acid diethylamide in pregnancy. Fed. Proc. **28**, 549 (1969)
Sato, H., Pergament, E., Nair, V.: LSD in pregnancy: chromosomal effects. Life Sci. **10**, 773–779 (1971)
Schams, D., Reinhardt, V., Karg, H.: Effects of 2-Br-α-ergokryptine on plasma prolactin level during parturition and onset of lactation in cows. Experientia (Basel) **28**, 697–699 (1972)
Scherf, D., Schlachman, M.: Electrocardiographic and clinical studies on the action of ergotamine tartrate and dihydro-ergotamine 45. Amer. J. med. Sci. **216**, 673–679 (1948)
Schiefer, I., Bähr, G., Boiselle, I., Kiefer, B.: EEG-Veränderungen von 9 Kindern mit einer LSD-Vergiftung. Klin. Pädiatrie **184**, 307–311 (1972)
Schön, H., Leist, K.H., Grauwiler, J.: Single day treatment of pregnant rats with ergotamine. Teratology **11**, 32A (1975)
Schwartz, F.D., Dunea, G.: Progression of retroperitoneal fibrosis despite cessation of treatment with methysergide. Lancet **1966/I**, 956–957
Seiler, K., Jenzer, H.R., Kácl, J.: Verlauf eines Falles von Ergotismus mit Femoralarterienverschlüssen und Mitralinsuffizienz. Cor Vasa **2**, 366–371 (1973)
Senger, P.L., Lose, E.D., Ulberg, L.C.: Reduced blood supply to the uterus as a cause for early embryonic death in the mouse. J. exp. Zool. **165**, 335–343 (1967)
Shaar, C.J., Clemens, J.A.: Inhibition of lactation and prolactin secretion in rats by ergot alkaloids. Endocrinology **90**, 285–288 (1972)
Shane, J.M., Naftolin, F.: Effect of ergonovine maleate on puerperal prolactin. Amer. J. Obstet. Gynec. **120**, 129–131 (1974)
Shelesnyak, M.C.: Ergotoxine inhibition of deciduoma formation and its reversal by progesterone. Amer. J. Physiol. **179**, 301–304 (1954a)
Shelesnyak, M.C.: Reversal of ergotoxine inhibition of deciduoma by M.E.D. of progesterone in spayed pseudopregnant rats. Proc. Soc. exp. Biol. (N.Y.) **87**, 377–378 (1954b)
Shelesnyak, M.C.: Disturbance of hormone balance in the female rat by a single injection of ergotoxine ethanesulphonate. Amer. J. Physiol. **180**, 47–49 (1955)
Shelesnyak, M.C.: Progesterone reversal of ergotoxine induced suppression of early—preimplantation—pregnancy. Acta endocr. (Kbh.) **23**, 151–157 (1956)
Shelesnyak, M.C.: III. Aspects of reproduction. Some experimental studies on the mechanism of ova-implantation in the rat. In: Recent Progress in Hormone Research. Proc. of the Laurentian Hormone Conference 1956. Pincus, G. (ed.), Vol. XIII, pp. 269–322. New York: Academic Press 1957a
Shelesnyak, M.C.: Gonadotrophin content of pituitary of pregnant and pseudopregnant rats following single injection of ergotoxine. Endocrinology **60**, 802–803 (1957b)
Shelesnyak, M.C.: Maintenance of gestation in ergotoxine-treated pregnant rats by exogenous prolactin. Acta endocr. (Kbh.) **27**, 99–109 (1958)
Shelesnyak, M.C.: Further studies on the mechanism of ergocornine (ergotoxine) interference with hormonal requirements for decidualization and nidation. Bull. Soc. roy. belge Gynéc. Obstét. **31**, 375–379 (1961)
Shelesnyak, M.C., Barnea, A.: Studies on the mechanism of ergocornine (ergotoxine) interference with decidualization and nidation: II. Failure of topical application of ergocornine to reveal the site of action of the alkaloid. Acta endocr. (Kbh.) **43**, 469–476 (1963)
Shone, D.K., Philip, J.R., Christie, G.J.: Agalactia of sows caused by feeding the ergot of the bullrush millet, Pennisetum typhoides. Vet. Rec. **71**, 129–132 (1959)
Simmons, J.Q., Sparkes, R.S., Blake, P.R.: Lack of chromosomal damaging effects by moderate dosis of LSD in vivo. Clin. Genet. **5**, 59–61 (1974)
Simon, G.: Gangrènes et hormones stéroïdes. Etude expérimentale sur l'antagonisme des hormones sexuelles et de quelques stéroïdes vis-à-vis de l'action vaso-constrictive de l'ergotamine. Sem. Hôp. Paris **22**, 1420–1424 (1946)
Singh, M.P., Kalia, C.S., Jain, H.K.: Chromosomal aberrations induced in barley by LSD. Science **169**, 491–492 (1970)
Sivadjian, J.M.: Psychopharmacologie. L'action de la mescaline et du diéthylamide de l'acide lysergique (LSD-25) sur le comportement du Cobaye. C.R. Acad. Sci. (Paris) **268**, 984–985 (1969)
Skakkebaek, N.E., Beatty, R.A.: Studies on meiotic chromosomes and spermatozoan heads in mice treated with LSD. J. Reprod. Fertil. **22**, 141–144 (1970)

Skakkebaek, N.E., Philip, J., Rafaelsen, O.J.: LSD in mice: abnormalities in meiotic chromosomes. Science **160**, 1246–1248 (1968)
Slugg, P.H., Kunkel, R.S.: Complications of methysergide therapy. J. Amer. med. Ass. **213**, 297–298 (1970)
Smart, R.G., Bateman, K.: The chromosomal and teratogenic effects of lysergic acid diethylamide: a review of the current literature. Canad. med. Ass. J. **99**, 805–810 (1968)
Smith, J.A., Zalman, S.: Some effects of large doses of ergot products on rats. Proc. Soc. exp. Biol. (N.Y.) **72**, 13–15 (1949)
Smithells, R.W.: Environmental teratogens in man. In: Human Malformations. Berry, C.L. (ed.). Brit. med. Bull. **32**, 27–33 (1976)
Sobel, J., Espinas, O.E., Friedman, S.A.: Carotid artery obstruction following LSD capsule ingestion. Arch. intern. Med. **127**, 290–291 (1971)
Sommer, A.F., Buchanan, A.R.: Effects of ergot alkaloids on pregnancy and lactation in the albino rat. Amer. J. Physiol. **180**, 296–300 (1955)
Šrám, R.J.: Mutagenic effects of LSD in *Drosophila melanogaster*. Acta nerv. super. (Praha) **12**, 265–266 (1970)
Šrám, R.J., Goetz, P.: The mutagenic effect of lysergic acid diethylamide. III. Evaluation of the genetic risk of LSD in man. Mutation Res. **26**, 523–528 (1974)
Šrám, R.J., Zudovà, Z., Goetz, P.: The mutagenic effect of lysergic acid diethylamide. II. Dominant lethal test in mice. Mutation Res. **26**, 517–522 (1974)
Stahnke, E.: Studien zur Wirkung des Ergotamins. Klin. Wschr. **7**, 23–25 (1928)
Stecker, J.F., Rawls, H.P., Devine, C.J., Devine, P.C.: Retroperitoneal fibrosis and ergot derivatives. J. Urol. (Baltimore) **112**, 30–32 (1974)
Stein, I.: Observations on the action of ergonovine on the coronary circulation and its use in the diagnosis of coronary artery insufficiency. Amer. Heart J. **37**, 36–45 (1949)
Stein, I., Weinstein, J.: Further studies of the effect of ergonovine on the coronary circulation. J. Lab. clin. Med. **36**, 66–81 (1950)
Stevens, J.B., Callaway, J.L.: Mixed epithelioma of the back arising from daily application of a phenol and ergot ointment. Amer. J. Cancer **38**, 364–366 (1940)
Stockman, R.: The cause of convulsive ergotism. J. Hyg. (Lond.) **34**, 235–241 (1934)
Stucki, P.: Der Einfluß des Hydergin auf die experimentelle Ergotamingangrän des Rattenschwanzes. Beitrag zur Frage der Wirkungsbeziehungen zwischen genuinen und hydrierten Mutterkornalkaloiden. Arch. int. Pharmacodyn. Thér. **90**, 159–168 (1952)
Sturelid, S., Kihlman, B.A.: Lysergic acid diethylamide and chromosome breakage. Hereditas (Lund) **62**, 259–262 (1969)
Sugiura, Y.: Poland's syndrome. Clinico-roentgenographic study on 45 cases. Congen. Anom. **16**, 17–28 (1976)
Suzman, M.M., Freed, C.C., Prag, J.J.: Studies on experimental peripheral vascular disease with special reference to thrombo-angeitis obliterans. S. Afr. J. med. Sci. **3**, 29–39 (1938)
Tedeschi, C.G., Ingalls, T.H.: Vascular anomalies of mouse fetuses exposed to anoxia during pregnancy. Amer. J. Obstet. Gynec. **71**, 16–28 (1956)
Thorner, M.O., Besser, G.M., Jones, A., Dacie, J., Jones, A.E.: Bromocriptine treatment of female infertility: report of 13 pregnancies. Brit. med. J. **1975/IV**, 694–697
Tindal, J.S.: The effect of ergotamine and dihydroergotamine on lactation in the rat. J. Endocr. **14**, 268–274 (1956)
Titus, R.J.: Lysergic acid diethylamide: Its effects on human chromosomes and the human organism in utero. Int. J. Addict. **7**, 701–714 (1972)
Tobin, J.M., Tobin, J.M.: Mutagenic effects of LSD-25 in Drosophila melanogaster. Dis. nerv. Syst. **30** (Suppl.), 47–52 (1969)
Tournigand, P., Marino Di, V., Mercier, C.: Une cause rare de compression veineuse intra-abdominale. La fibrose rétropéritonéale (à propos d'un cas). Phlébologie **27**, 161–165 (1974)
Trosko, J.E.: Studies on deoxyribonucleic acid metabolism in human cells treated with lysergic acid diethylamide. Biochem. Pharmacol. **20**, 3213–3218 (1971)
Tsuchimoto, T., Stalder, G.: Effect of an Ergot derivative on human lymphocyte chromosomes in vivo. Arzneimittel-Forsch. **26**, 2101–2103 (1976)
Turolla, E., Baldratti, G., Scrascia, E., Ricevuti, G.: Effect of ergocornine on the luteal

20-α-hydroxysteroid dehydrogenase in pseudopregnant and pregnant rats. Experientia (Basel) **25**, 415–416 (1969)
Ureles, A.L., Rob, C.: Acute ischemia of a limb complicating methysergide maleate therapy. J. Amer. med. Ass. **183**, 1041–1042 (1963)
Uyeno, E.T.: Lysergic acid diethylamide in gravid rats. Proc. West. Pharmacol. Soc. **13**, 200–203 (1970)
Vann, E.: Lethal mutation rate in Drosophila exposed to LSD-25 by injection and ingestion. Nature (Lond.) **223**, 95–96 (1969)
Vann, E., Matlen, C., Rossmoore, H.: Genetic effects of LSD-25 on E. Coli. Mutation Res. **10**, 269–275 (1970)
Varavudhi, P., Lobel, B.L.: Studies on the mechanism of nidation. XXI. Viability of blastocysts in ergocornine-treated pregnant rats. J. Reprod. Fertil. **10**, 451–453 (1965)
Vassilev, I., Dabov, S., Rankov, B.: Contribution à l'étude de l'action de l'ergotine sur les yeux. Les cataractes acquises et congénitales provoquées expérimentalement par l'ergotamine. Arch. Ophtal. (Paris) **19**, 524–528 (1959)
Vérin, P., Bresque, E., Vizdy, A., Lagoutte, F.: Fibrose rétro-péritonéale et dérivés de l'ergot. Bull. Soc. Ophtal. Fr. **74**, 281–286 (1974)
Voltolina, E.J.: Spinal fluid creatine phosphokinase. Abnormalities following LSD usage. Clin. Toxicol. **3**, 85–87 (1970)
Von Kreybig, T.: Experimentelle Praenatal-Toxikologie. Arzneimittel-Forsch. **17** (Suppl.), 11–40 (1968)
Von Storch, T.J.C.: Complications following the use of ergotamine tartrate. Their relation to the treatment of migraine headache. J. Amer. med. Ass. **111**, 293–300 (1938)
Wainscott, G., Sullivan, F., Volans, G.N., Wilkinson, M.: The outcome of pregnancy in women suffering from migraine. Postgrad. med. J. (1978, in press)
Warkany, J., Takacs, E.: Lysergic acid diethylamide (LSD): No teratogenicity in rats. Science **159**, 731–732 (1968)
Werthemann, A., Reiniger, M.: Über Augenentwicklungsstörungen bei Rattenembryonen durch Sauerstoff-Mangel in der Frühschwangerschaft. Acta anat. (Basel) **11**, 329–347 (1950)
West, G.B.: Drugs and rat pregnancy. J. Pharm. Pharmacol. **14**, 828–830 (1962)
West, L.J., Pierce, C.M., Thomas, W.D.: Lysergic acid diethylamide: its effects on a male asiatic elephant. Science **138**, 1100–1103 (1962)
Whelton, M.J., Allaway, A., Stewart, A., Kreel, L.: Ergot poisoning in acute hepatic necrosis. Gut **9**, 287–289 (1968)
Wilson, J.G.: Use of primates in teratological investigations. In: Medical Primatology 1972. Part III: Infectious Diseases, Oncology, Pharmacology and Toxicology, Cardiovascular studies. Proc. 3rd Conf. Exp. Med. Surg. Primates, Lyon, 1972. Goldsmith, E.I., Moor-Jankowski, J. (eds.), pp. 286–295. Basel: Karger 1972
Wilson, J.G.: Present status of drugs as teratogens in man. Teratology **7**, 3–15 (1973)
Winkler, E.: Rzadki przypadek bezobjawowego zupelnego pekniecia macicy z urodzonym zywym plodem. Ginek. pol. **36/12**, 1423–1425 (1965)
Winter, C.A., Flataker, L.: Effects of lysergic acid diethylamide upon performance of trained rats. Proc. Soc. exp. Biol. (N.Y.) **92**, 285–289 (1956)
Witschi, E.: Development of Vertebrates. Philadelphia: W.B. Saunders 1956
Wolpaw, J.R., Brottem, J.L., Martin, H.L.: Tongue necrosis attributed to ergotamine in temporal arteritis. J. Amer. med. Ass. **225**, 514–515 (1973)
Yater, W.M., Cahill, J.A.: Bilateral gangrene of feet due to ergotamine tartrate used for pruritus of jaundice. J. Amer. med. Ass. **106**, 1625–1631 (1936)
Young, J.R., Humphries, A.W.: Severe arteriospasm after use of ergotamine tartrate suppositories. Report of a case. J. Amer. med. Ass. **175**, 1141–1145 (1961)
Zeilmaker, G.H., Carlsen, R.A.: Experimental studies on the effect of ergocornine methanesulphonate on the luteotrophic function of the rat pituitary gland. Acta endocr. (Kbh.) **41**, 321–335 (1962)
Zellweger, H., McDonald, J.S., Abbo, G.: Is lysergic-acid diethylamide a teratogen? Lancet **1967/II**, 1066–1068
Zetterberg, G.: Lysergic acid diethylamide and mutation. Hereditas (Lund) **62**, 263–265 (1969)
Zimmermann, O.: Störung der Coronardurchblutung durch Ergotamin. Klin. Wschr. **14**, 500–503 (1935)

Author Index

Page numbers in *italics* refer to bibliography

Subject Index

Handbuch der experimentellen Pharmakologie/ Handbook of Experimental Pharmacology

Heffter-Heubner, New Series

Volume 4:
General Pharmacology

Volume 10:
Die Pharmakologie anorganischer Anionen

Volume 11:
Lobelin und Lobeliaalkaloide

Volume 12:
Morphin und morphinähnlich wirkende Verbindungen

Volume 14: Part 1
The Adrenocortical Hormones I
Part 2
The Adrenocortical Hormones II
Part 3
The Adrenocortical Hormones III

Volume 16:
Erzeugung von Krankheitszuständen durch das Experiment/ Experimental Production of Diseases
Part 1
Blut (In Vorbereitung)
Part 2
Atemwege
Part 3
Heart and Circulation
Part 4
Niere, Nierenbecken, Blase
Part 5
Liver
Part 6
Schilddrüse
(In Vorbereitung)
Part 7
Zentralnervensystem
Part 8
Stütz- und Hartgewebe
Part 9
Infektionen I
Part 10
Infektionen II
Part 11A
Infektionen III
Part 11B
Infektionen IV
Part 12
Tumoren I
Part 13
Tumoren II
Part 14
Tumoren III
(In preparation)
Part 15
Kohlenhydratstoffwechsel, Fieber/ Carbohydrate Metabolism, Fever

Volume 17: Part 1
Ions alcalino-terreux I
Part 2
Ions alcalino-terreux II

Volume 18: Part 1
Histamine
Part 2
Anti-Histaminics

Volume 19:
5-Hydroxytryptamine and Related Indolealkylamines

Volume 20: Part 1
Pharmacology of Fluorides I
Part 2
Pharmacology of Fluorides II

Volume 21:
Beryllium

Volume 22: Part 1
Die Gestagene I
Part 2
Die Gestagene II

Volume 23:
Neurohypophysial Hormones and Similar Polipeptides

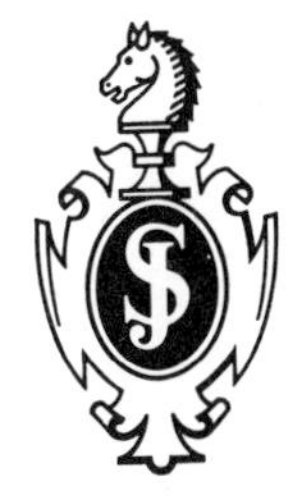

Springer-Verlag
Berlin
Heidelberg
New York

Handbuch der experimentellen Pharmakologie/ Handbook of Experimental Pharmacology

Heffter-Heubner, New Series

Volume 24:
Diuretica

Volume 25:
Bradykinin, Kallidin and Kallikrein

Volume 26:
Vergleichende Pharmakologie von Überträgersubstanzen in tiersystematischer Darstellung

Volume 27:
Anticoagulantien

Volume 28: Part 1
Concepts in Biochemical Pharmacology I
Part 3
Concepts in Biochemical Pharmacology III

Volume 29:
Oral wirksame Antidiabetika

Volume 30:
Modern Inhalation Anesthetics

Volume 32: Part 1
Insulin I
Part 2
Insulin II

Volume 34:
Secretin, Cholecystokinin, Pancreozymin and Gastrin

Volume 35: Part 1
Androgene I
Part 2
Androgens II and Antiandrogens/ Androgene II und Antiandrogene

Volume 36:
Uranium – Plutonium – Transplutonic Elements

Volume 37:
Angiotensin

Volume 38: Part 1
Antieoplastic and and Immunosuppressive Agents I
Part 2
Antineoplastic and Immunosuppressive Agents II

Volume 39:
Antihypertensive Agents

Volume 40:
Organic Nitrates

Volume 41:
Hypolipidemic Agents

Volume 42:
Neuromuscular Junction

Volume 43:
Anabolic-Androgenic Steroids

Volume 44:
Haem and Haemoproteins

Volume 45: Part 1
Drug Addiction I
Part 2
Drug Addiction II

Volume 46:
Fibrinolytics and Antifibrinolytics
(In Preparation)

Volume 47:
Kinetics of Drug Action

Volume 48:
Arthropod Venoms

Volume 49:
Gangliomic Transmission (In preparation)

Volume 50:
Inflammation and Antiinflammatory Drugs
(In preparation)

Volume 51:
Ergot Alkaloids and Related Compounds
(In preparation)

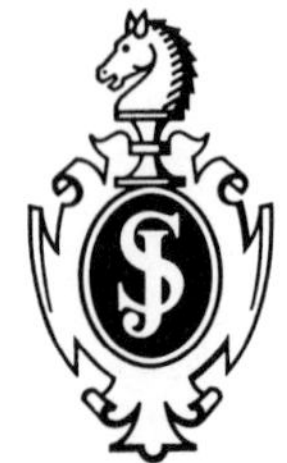

Springer-Verlag
Berlin
Heidelberg
New York